Fundamentals
of Aquatic Toxicology

Fundamentals of Aquatic Toxicology

Methods and Applications

Edited by

Gary M. Rand, Ph.D.
FMC Corporation
Princeton, New Jersey

Sam R. Petrocelli, Ph.D.
Battelle New England Marine Research Laboratory
Duxbury, Massachusetts

⬤HEMISPHERE PUBLISHING CORPORATION, Washington

A subsidiary of Harper & Row, Publishers, Inc.

Cambridge   New York   Philadelphia   San Francisco
London   Mexico City   São Paulo   Singapore   Sydney

This book was set in Press Roman by Hemisphere Publishing Corporation. The editors were Bettie Loux Donley and Mary Dorfman; the production supervisor was Miriam Gonzalez; and the typesetter was Peggy M. Rote.
Edwards Brothers, Inc. was printer and binder.

FUNDAMENTALS OF AQUATIC TOXICOLOGY:
Methods and Applications

4 5 6 7 8 9 0   E B E B   8 9 8 7

Library of Congress Cataloging in Publication Data

Main entry under title:

Fundamentals of aquatic toxicology.

    Includes bibliographies and index.
    1. Water quality bioassay. 2. Toxicity testing.
3. Water—Pollution—Toxicology. 4. Aquatic organisms—
Effect of water pollution on. I. Rand, Gary M.,
date. II. Petrocelli, Sam R.
QH90.57.B5F86 1984   574.5′263   84-4529
ISBN 0-89116-302-6 (hard cover)
ISBN 0-89116-382-4 (soft cover)

Contents

TOXICITY TESTING

SUBLETHAL EFFECTS

SPECIFIC CHEMICAL EFFECTS

CHEMICAL DISTRIBUTION/FATE

HAZARD EVALUATION

Contributors

G. L. BAUGHMAN
S.E. Environmental Research Laboratory
U.S. Environmental Protection Agency
Athens, Georgia

W. E. BISHOP, Ph.D.
Environmental Safety Department
The Procter and Gamble Company
Cincinnati, Ohio

A. W. BOURQUIN, Ph.D.
Environmental Research Laboratory
U.S. Environmental Protection Agency
Gulf Breeze, Florida

L. A. BURNS, Ph.D.
S.E. Environmental Research Laboratory
U.S. Environmental Protection Agency
Athens, Georgia

R. B. FOSTER
Aquatic Toxicology Laboratory
Springborn Bionomics, Inc.
Wareham, Massachusetts

R. D. GELBER, Ph.D.
Dana Farber Cancer Institute
Harvard University School of Public
    Health
Boston, Massachusetts

T. R. GILBERT, Ph.D.
Department of Chemistry
Northeastern University
Boston, Massachusetts

J. L. HAMELINK, Ph.D.
Toxicology Division
Lilly Research Laboratories
Eli Lilly & Co.
Greenfield, Indiana

J. D. HENDRICKS, Ph.D.
Department of Food Science and
  Technology
Food Toxicology Laboratory
Oregon State University
Corvallis, Oregon

J. P. KAKAREKA
Department of Chemistry
Tufts University
Medford, Massachusetts

J. S. KUWABARA, Ph.D.
U.S. Department of the Interior
Geological Survey
Menlo Park, California

P. T. LAVIN, Ph.D.
Dana Farber Cancer Institute
Harvard University School of Public
  Health
Boston, Massachusetts

J. J. LECH, Ph.D.
Department of Pharmacology and
  Toxicology
The Medical College of Wisconsin
Milwaukee, Wisconsin

H. V. LELAND, Ph.D.
U.S. Department of the Interior
Geological Survey
Menlo Park, California

K. J. MACEK, Ph.D.
EG&G Environmental Group
Wellesley, Massachusetts

A. W. MAKI, Ph.D.
Research and Environmental Health
  Division
Medical Department
Exxon Corporation
East Millstone, New Jersey

L. L. MARKING
U.S. Department of the Interior
Fish and Wildlife Service
National Fishery Research Laboratory
LaCrosse, Wisconsin

F. L. MAYER, Ph.D.
U.S. Department of the Interior
Fish and Wildlife Service
Columbia National Fisheries Research
  Laboratory
Columbia, Missouri

J. M. McKIM, Ph.D.
Environmental Research Laboratory
U.S. Environmental Protection Agency
Duluth, Minnesota

P. M. MEHRLE, Ph.D.
U.S. Department of the Interior
Fish and Wildlife Service
Columbia National Fisheries Research
  Laboratory
Columbia, Missouri

C. R. MEHTA, Ph.D.
Dana Farber Cancer Institute
Harvard University School of Public
  Health
Boston, Massachusetts

T. R. MEYERS, Ph.D.
School of Fisheries and Science
University of Alaska
Juneau, Alaska

J. M. NEFF, Ph.D.
New England Marine Research
   Laboratory
Battelle
William F. Clapp Labs., Inc.
Duxbury, Massachusetts

D. R. NIMMO, Ph.D.
Department of Fishery and Wildlife
   Biology
Colorado State University
Ft. Collins, Colorado

P. R. PARRISH
8330 Wilde Lake Road
Pensacola, Florida

S. R. PETROCELLI, Ph.D.
Battelle New England Marine
   Research Laboratory
Duxbury, Massachusetts

P. H. PRITCHARD, Ph.D.
Environmental Research Laboratory
U.S. Environmental Protection Agency
Gulf Breeze, Florida

G. M. RAND, Ph.D.
Corporate Toxicology
FMC Corporation
Princeton, New Jersey

R. C. RUSSO, Ph.D.
Fisheries Bioassay Laboratory
Montana State University
Bozeman, Montana

W. M. SANDERS III, Ph.D.
S.E. Environmental Research Laboratory
U.S. Environmental Protection Agency
Athens, Georgia

D. A. SCHOENFELD, Ph.D.
Dana Farber Cancer Institute
Harvard University School of Public
   Health
Boston, Massachusetts

A. SPACIE, Ph.D.
Department of Forestry and Natural
   Resources
Purdue University
West Lafayette, Indiana

J. B. SPRAGUE, Ph.D.
College of Biological Science
Department of Zoology
University of Guelph
Guelph, Ontario

M. J. VODICNIK, Ph.D.
Department of Pharmacology and
   Toxicology
The Medical College of Wisconsin
Milwaukee, Wisconsin

Preface

Fundamentals of Aquatic Toxicology is designed to fill the need for a single, comprehensive source of information concerning aquatic toxicology. It presents a definitive description of basic concepts and test methods employed in aquatic toxicology studies as well as examples of typical data and their interpretation.

This volume is designed to be used as a textbook for courses in aquatic and environmental toxicology. In addition, it should be a useful reference for those whose responsibilities include managing industrial plant operations and interacting with agencies charged with regulating chemical impacts on aquatic ecosystems.

The contributors are scientists and managers from academic, government, and industrial institutions. In addition to their extensive knowledge of the theoretical aspects of the individual topics, each contributor is experienced in the practical application of these theories to actual environmental situations.

The 23 chapters are divided into five parts. The first part—Toxicity Testing—describes the basic concepts and methodologies used in aquatic toxicity testing. Sublethal Effects, the second part, presents information on sublethal effects testing and its utility in evaluating the less obvious effects of chemical exposure on aquatic organisms. The third part—Specific Chemical Effects—summarizes the available literature on the toxicity of generic types of chemicals (such as pesticides and metals) to aquatic organisms. Chemical Distribution/Fate, the fourth part, discusses the various factors that affect the distribution and fate of chemicals in the aquatic environment and thus influence the chemical concentrations to which aquatic organisms may be exposed. The concluding fifth part—Hazard Evaluation—discusses the manner in which environmental fate and biological effects data are integrated to provide an assessment of the potential hazard posed by the use or discharge of chemicals in the aquatic environment. It also identifies the specific laws that provide regulatory agencies with enforcement powers to control discharges into the aquatic environment.

Since aquatic toxicology is a specialized discipline, with its own terminology, a glossary of the most commonly used terms is included.

This book represents an attempt to provide a broad perspective on the subject of aquatic toxicology. We are grateful to the contributors, whose combined theoretical knowledge and practical experience make a volume of this scope possible. We will consider that our objective has been met if this book proves pertinent to the needs of its readers and if it provides a stimulus for further advancement in this evolving science.

Gary M. Rand, Ph.D.
Sam R. Petrocelli, Ph.D.

Fundamentals
of Aquatic Toxicology

Chapter 1

Introduction

G. M. Rand and S. R. Petrocelli

AQUATIC TOXICOLOGY

Aquatic toxicology is the qualitative and quantitative study of the adverse or toxic effects of chemicals and other anthropogenic materials or xenobiotics on aquatic organisms. Toxic effects may include both lethality (mortality) and sublethal effects such as changes in growth, development, reproduction, pharmacokinetic responses, pathology, biochemistry, physiology, and behavior. Effects may be expressed by quantifiable criteria such as number of organisms killed, percent egg hatchability, changes in length and weight, percent enzyme inhibition, number of skeletal abnormalities, and tumor incidence. Aquatic toxicology is also concerned with the concentrations or quantities of chemicals that can be expected to occur in the aquatic environment in water, sediment, or food. Therefore, it includes the study of the transport, distribution, transformation, and ultimate fate of chemicals in the aquatic environment.

As a result of these concerns, aquatic toxicology has evolved as a multidisciplinary field of study, which borrows freely from several other basic sciences (Fig. 1). It is necessary to understand the chemical (e.g., hydrolysis, oxidation, and photolysis), physical (e.g., molecular structure, solubility, volatility, and sorption), and biological (e.g., biotransformation) factors that affect environmental concentrations of chemicals in order to determine how potentially toxic agents act in the environment and how the environment acts on these agents and to estimate the potential exposure of aquatic organisms. A knowledge of aquatic ecology, physiology, biochemistry, histology, and behavior is needed in order to understand the effects of toxic agents on aquatic organisms.

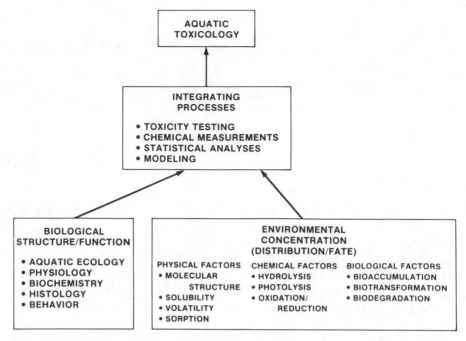

Figure 1 Aquatic toxicology—a multidisciplinary science.

Statistical analysis and mathematical modeling are used to quantitate and predict biological effects and determine the probability of their occurrence. Finally, it is essential to comprehend sophisticated analytical chemistry methodologies and instrumentation in order to accurately identify and quantify extremely low concentrations of chemicals in various aquatic environmental compartments (e.g., sediment, water, and tissues).

THE AQUATIC ENVIRONMENT

The aquatic environment is complex and diverse. It includes several distinct ecosystem types—freshwater streams, lakes, ponds and rivers; estuaries; and marine coastal and deep ocean waters—within which exist many different biotic and abiotic components. The biotic or living components consist of many combinations of plants, animals, and microorganisms that inhabit specific ecological niches in each ecosystem. The abiotic or nonliving components include the physical environment

(e.g., water, substrate, and suspended material) within the boundaries of the ecosystem. Each aquatic ecosystem is thus a product of complex interactions of living and nonliving components.

The physical and chemical properties of aquatic ecosystems can have a profound effect on the biological activity and impact of chemicals and other xenobiotics. The vulnerability of the aquatic environment to chemical insult depends on several factors, including the (1) physical and chemical properties of the chemical and its transformation products; (2) concentrations of the chemical entering the ecosystem; (3) duration and type of inputs (acute or chronic, intermittent spill or continuous discharge); (4) properties of the ecosystem that enable it to resist changes which could result from the presence of the chemical (e.g., pH buffering capacity of seawater) or return it to its original state after the chemical is removed from the system (e.g., flushing of water from estuaries by tidal action); and (5) location of the ecosystem in relation to the release site of the chemical.

Since ecosystems involve complex interactions of physical, chemical, and biological factors, it is difficult to understand the response of a system to a chemical unless the relationships among components of the system are well defined. Assessment is further complicated by the ability of the biotic components to adapt, the diversity of species present in the ecosystem (which normally changes over time), and the differences in structural and functional responses among the biological components. Furthermore, similar ecosystems are not necessarily affected similarly by addition of the same chemical. Minor differences in the chemical and physical environment and in species composition can result in differences in the fate of a chemical and to different effects on the systems. Therefore, site-specific conditions must be considered in evaluating potential chemical hazards.

All aquatic ecosystems have in common the fact that the indigenous species of animals, plants, and microorganisms are generally inescapably immersed in the water medium throughout their lives. This is significant since aquatic ecosystems may serve as reservoirs or sinks for various chemicals.

TOXICANTS AND TOXICITY

A *toxicant* is an agent that can produce an adverse response (effect) in a biological system, seriously damaging its structure or function or producing death. The adverse response may be defined in terms of a measurement that is outside the "normal" range for healthy organisms. A toxicant or foreign substance may be introduced deliberately or accidentally into the aquatic ecosystem, impairing the quality of the water and making it unfavorable for aquatic life. Toxicants enter aquatic ecosystems from (1) nonpoint sources such as agricultural runoff from land, contaminated ground water and bottom sediments, urban runoff, dredged sediment disposal, and atmospheric fallout, and (2) point sources such as discharges (effluents) from manufacturing plants, hazardous

waste disposal sites, and municipal waste water treatment plants.

This book focuses on anthropogenic materials, especially those known to cause significant problems in the aquatic environment. These include synthetic organic pesticides, other industrial chemicals from chemical manufacturing, petroleum hydrocarbons, metal salts, and other inorganic compounds and liquid industrial waste discharges (effluents). The biological and toxicological effects of some of these chemicals are discussed in Chapters 12 through 15. Although some of these chemicals (e.g., certain metal salts or other inorganics) may normally be found in minimal nutritive background concentrations, most of those discussed here are foreign, nonnutritive, and not normally present in significant background concentrations in the aquatic environment.

The most innocuous chemical substances can have undesirable or distinctly harmful effects when taken up by an organism in sufficient amounts. In contrast, the uptake of minute quantities of toxic chemicals may result in no apparent adverse effects. Therefore, it is an important concept in toxicology that in general no chemical is completely safe and no chemical is completely harmful. The factor that determines whether a chemical agent is potentially harmful or safe is the relationship between the concentration (quantity) of the chemical to which an organism is exposed and the duration of the exposure. A measure of the severity of the response resulting from the exposure is the concentration-response relationship. For any chemical, contact with a biological membrane or system may not produce an adverse effect if the concentration of the chemical is below some minimal effective (threshold) level. This also implies that all chemicals are capable of producing a deleterious effect if a high enough concentration of the chemical comes into contact with a biological membrane or system.

Toxicity is a relative property of a chemical which refers to its potential to have a harmful effect on a living organism. It is a function of the concentration of the chemical and the duration of exposure. Toxicity data are commonly used in comparing chemical substances. Information about the biological mechanisms affected and the conditions under which the toxicant is harmful is also important for this comparison. *Toxicity tests* are used to evaluate the adverse effects of a chemical on living organisms under standardized, reproducible conditions which permit a comparison with other chemicals tested.

FACTORS THAT AFFECT THE ENVIRONMENTAL CONCENTRATION OF TOXICANTS

In the aquatic environment the concentration, transport, transformation, and disposition (fate) of a chemical are primarily controlled by (1) the physical and chemical properties of the compound, (2) the physical, chemical, and biological properties of the ecosystem, and (3) the sources and rate of input of the chemical into the environment.

The physical and chemical properties of the compound that are important include molecular structure, solubility in water, and vapor pressure. Rate constants for hydrolysis, photolysis, biological degradation, evaporation, sorption, uptake, and depuration by organisms and partition coefficients (air:water, sediment:water, octanol:water) also provide significant information.

Some of the properties of aquatic environments that may affect the fate of a chemical are surface area to volume relationships, temperature, salinity, pH, flow, depth, amount of suspended material, sediment particle size, and carbon content in sediment.

Knowledge of the average rates of input and the occurrence of single large "slugs" of chemicals entering the aquatic environment is important for predicting environmental concentrations. However, the average rates of entry and the short-term higher inputs associated with manufacture, use, and disposal are variable and are difficult to estimate; hence they can only be crudely approximated. Information on background concentrations

of chemicals and on transformation products is also important for predicting concentrations in the aquatic environment.

The types of data outlined above are used not only to predict environmental concentrations but also to determine (1) the mobility of a chemical and the parts of the aquatic environment in which it would most likely be distributed, (2) the kinds of chemical and biological reactions that take place during transport and after deposition, (3) the eventual chemical form, and (4) the persistence of the chemical.

Knowledge of the physical and chemical properties of a compound permits an estimate of the part of the aquatic environment likely to receive the greatest exposure and the ability of the compound to move within and through the environment. For example, chemicals with high vapor pressure and low water solubility tend to dissipate from the water into the atmosphere (volatilize). Chemicals with low vapor pressure and low water solubility tend to become associated with sediment and particulate matter, and chemicals with high water solubility tend to remain in water. Water-soluble chemicals also tend to be more widely and homogeneously distributed than insoluble chemicals in the aquatic environment.

In water, a chemical can exist in three different forms which affect its availability to organisms (bioavailability): (1) dissolved, (2) adsorbed to a biotic or abiotic component and suspended in the water column or deposited on the bottom, and (3) incorporated (accumulated) in organisms. Dissolved chemicals are readily available to organisms in the water column. Hydrophobic chemicals may be adsorbed on sediments, suspended colloids, or microparticulates and may be irreversibly bound and generally unavailable. However, some of the bound chemicals may be available to benthic organisms through ingestion or direct uptake from interstitial water. Sediment-bound chemicals may also be covered and unavailable until the sediment is disturbed. Chemicals can be accumulated by organisms in various tissues, biotransformed (metabolized), and excreted back into the water.

Bioaccumulation and bioavailability are discussed in Chapter 17.

Water-soluble chemicals may persist and retain their physical and chemical characteristics while being transported and distributed in the aquatic environment. Chemicals that are persistent (not significantly degraded) can accumulate in the environment to toxic levels. The persistence of a chemical may be expressed in terms of its *half-life*, which is defined as the time required to reduce the initial concentration of the chemical by one-half. Chemicals may also be converted to other forms as a result of biotic and abiotic transformations. The predominant abiotic transformation reactions in water are hydrolysis, oxidation, and photolysis. These reactions may render a chemical more or less available for biotic transformation (biotransformation). Fish, invertebrates, microorganisms, and plants transform chemicals to various metabolites after their uptake and absorption. These biotransformations are enzymatically mediated, unlike the purely nonmetabolic chemical and photochemical reactions that occur in the aquatic environment. Biotransformations mediated by plants and animals affect the environmental concentrations of chemicals. However, for most organic compounds in the aquatic environment, these effects are insignificant in comparison to those of microbial transformations. Generally, biotransformation tends to degrade a chemical to a more polar and water-soluble form of lower toxicity. However, this is not always the case, and the transformation products may also be toxic. Biotic transformations are discussed in Chapter 8 (microbial) and Chapter 18 (fish and invertebrates), and abiotic transformations are discussed in Chapter 19.

Mathematical modeling can be used to integrate data on complex mechanisms such as transport, degradation and transformation processes, transfers between environmental media (e.g., air, water, and sediment), and biological uptake into a mathematical picture of the behavior of a chemical. The model may be used to predict the concentrations of the chemical in the aquatic environment, the potential exposure areas, and the fate of the chemical. The use of mathematical modeling is described in Chapter 19.

FACTORS THAT INFLUENCE TOXICITY

Factors Related to Exposure

For a chemical, its metabolites, or its conversion products to elicit an adverse response or have a toxic effect on aquatic organisms, the compound must come into contact and react with an appropriate receptor site on the organism at a high enough concentration and for a sufficient length of time. The concentration and time required to produce an adverse effect vary with the chemical, species of organism, and severity of the effect. This contact-reaction between the organism and the chemical is called *exposure*. In the assessment of toxicity the most significant factors related to exposure are the kind, duration, and frequency of exposure and the concentration of the chemical.

Aquatic organisms may be exposed to chemicals present in water, sediment, or food items. Water-soluble (hydrophilic) chemicals are more readily available to organisms than water-insoluble (hydrophobic) chemicals that are tightly adsorbed or otherwise bound to suspended particles, organic matter, or biological systems. Water-soluble chemicals may enter an organism through the general body surface, gills, or mouth. Chemicals in food may be ingested and absorbed through the gastrointestinal tract. Adsorbed chemicals may also enter the body through the body surface and gills as they gradually dissociate from particles to the water in immediate contact with these areas. The route of exposure may affect kinetic factors such as absorption, distribution, biotransformation, and excretion and may ultimately determine the toxicity of a chemical. Kinetic factors are discussed in Chapters 8, 17, and 18.

Adverse or toxic effects can be produced in the laboratory or in the natural environment by acute (short-term) or chronic (long-term) exposure to chemicals or other potentially toxic agents. In *acute exposure,* organisms come in contact with the chemical delivered either in a single event or in multiple events that occur within a short period of time, generally hours to days. Acute exposures to chemicals that are rapidly absorbed generally produce immediate effects, but they may also produce delayed effects similar to those resulting from chronic exposure. During *chronic exposure,* organisms are exposed to low concentrations of a chemical delivered either continuously or at some other periodic frequency over a long period of time (weeks, months, or years). Chronic exposure to chemicals may induce rapid, immediate effects similar to acute effects, in addition to effects that develop slowly. Acute and chronic exposure and toxicity are discussed in Chapters 2 and 4, respectively.

In general, an acute exposure involves a short period of time compared to the life cycle of an organism, whereas a chronic exposure may involve the entire reproductive life cycle. Exposures that are intermediate in duration (a month to several months) are less than a complete reproductive life cycle and include exposure during sensitive early stages of development. These are referred to as subchronic exposures. In aquatic toxicology, studies involving subchronic exposure are generally called early life stage, critical life stage, embryo-larval, or egg-fry tests. These tests are discussed in Chapter 3.

The frequency of exposure may also affect toxicity. For example, one acute exposure to a single concentration of a chemical may have an immediate adverse effect on an organism, while two successive exposures cumulatively equal to the single acute exposure may have little or no effect. This may occur as a result of metabolism (detoxification) of the chemical between exposures or acclimation of the organism to the chemical. However, if there is minimal metabolism the chemical may not be easily transformed and excreted and may remain in the organism, eventually producing a chronic effect.

The importance of the threshold concentration of a chemical in toxicity has been discussed. Chemicals elicit an adverse effect only if the or-

ganism is exposed to a high enough concentration. At a low concentration, a minimal effect or no effect may result from exposure.

Factors Related to the Organism

Species differ in susceptibility to chemicals. This may be due to differences in accessibility, with certain species effectively excluding a toxic medium for short periods of time (e.g., clams can close and maintain anaerobic metabolism). In addition, rates and patterns of metabolism and excretion can substantially affect susceptibility. Differences in susceptibility to chemical agents among fish of different strains also result from genetic factors. Evidence for genetic selection in the natural environment has been observed in mosquito fish after exposure to high levels of insecticides.

Dietary factors also influence toxicity, by producing changes in body composition, physiological and biochemical functions, and nutritional status of the organism.

Immature or young neonatal organisms in general appear to be more susceptible to chemical agents than are adult organisms. This may be due to differences in degree of development of detoxification mechanisms between young and adult organisms. Differences in rates of excretion of toxic chemicals may also be involved in age-dependent toxicity effects.

The toxicity of a particular chemical agent is traditionally evaluated on the basis of tests carried out with healthy organisms. However, test organisms that are in poor health or are stressed in some other manner, such as by previous or concurrent exposure to other toxicants, are likely to be more susceptible to a toxic chemical.

External Environmental Factors

External environmental factors that may influence the toxicity of a chemical include factors associated with the bioavailability of the chemical in the water medium, such as dissolved oxygen, pH, temperature, and dissolved solids. These factors are discussed in Chapter 6.

Factors Related to the Chemical

The toxicity of a chemical agent can be influenced by its composition. Impurities or contaminants that are considerably more toxic than the chemical itself may be present. Impurities may vary from one batch of the chemical to another, so that the results obtained with a particular batch may not be reproducible. Therefore, the identity and purity of chemicals are important in toxicity testing. However, toxicity tests conducted with highly purified samples of a chemical agent may not accurately predict the aquatic hazard associated with exposure to the chemical when it is discharged into the environment. Other factors that are directly related to the chemical are its physical and chemical properties such as solubility, vapor pressure, and pH. These factors affect the bioavailability, persistence, transformation, and ultimate fate of the chemical in the aquatic environment.

Certain chemicals are *nonselective* in their mode of activity in that they may have an undesirable effect on numerous cells and tissues of aquatic organisms. These chemicals may also be effective in small concentrations. In contrast, a chemical may be so *selective* that it adversely affects only one type of cell or tissue without harming others that are in close contact. The affected and nonaffected cells or tissues may be in the same or different organisms. If they are in different organisms, the chemical is *species-specific* in its selective activity. If they are in the same organism, the chemical may or may not be species-specific, but it will be selectively active on certain types of cells or tissues within a species. *Selective activity* or *toxicity* results from biological diversity and variability in the response of cells and tissues to chemicals. This diversity may prevent the toxicologist from predicting the effects of a chemical in one species from results of experiments performed in another species. There appear to be two significant mechanisms for the selective action of a chemical. The first mechanism involves the presence or absence of specific *target* or receptor sites in the exposed cell system, since selectivity indicates that the chemical reacts only with specific normal components (or targets) of the cell. The target may be vital to the cell and may be altered by the chemical so that it can no longer carry on its function; as a result, its viability is altered. Or the target may be a protein or lipid that is not vital to the function of the cell, so that the reaction between the chemical and the target does not produce a direct alteration in cell function. The second mechanism involves factors that are responsible for the distribution and alteration of the concentration of the chemical at specific cells or tissue sites. This is usually the result of such processes as selective absorption, translocation, biotransformation, and excretion.

Small changes in the structure of a chemical agent may alter its biological activity. This is because chemical-biological effects are the result of a physical-chemical reaction or interaction between the chemical and some target in the living aquatic system. The study of the type of chemical structure that will react with a specific target is referred to as the study of *structure-activity relationships*. Such studies are used to define as precisely as possible the limits of variation in chemical structure that are consistent with the production of a specific biological effect. If enough of these studies are performed, a hypothesis may be developed concerning the most likely targets or receptors in a reaction with the chemical. These studies also enable the investigator to synthesize analogs of the chemical that may be more active in producing the same biological effect or that may be inactive in the biological system under investigation. Such information is also important for the development of a hypothesis concerning the structure of the target.

EFFECTS

Just as a distinction is made between acute and chronic exposures, so should one be made between acute and chronic effects. *Acute effects* are those that occur rapidly as a result of short-term exposure to a chemical. In fish and other aquatic organisms, effects that occur within a few hours, days, or weeks are considered acute. Generally, acute effects are relatively severe. The most common one measured in aquatic organisms is lethality or mortality. A chemical is considered acutely toxic if by its direct action it kills 50% or more of the exposed population of test organisms in a relatively short period of time, such as 96 h to 14 d. *Chronic* or *subchronic toxic effects* may occur when the chemical produces deleterious effects as a result of a single exposure, but more often they are a consequence of repeated or long-term exposures. There may be a relatively long latency (time to occurrence) period for the expression of these effects, particularly if the exposure concentration is very low. *Chronic effects* may be lethal or sublethal. A typical lethal effect is failure of the chronically exposed organisms to produce viable offspring. The most common *sublethal effects* are behavioral changes (e.g., swimming, attraction-avoidance, and prey-predator relationships), physiological changes (e.g., growth, reproduction, and development), biochemical changes (e.g., blood enzyme and ion levels), and histological changes. Some sublethal effects may indirectly result in lethalities. For example, certain behavioral changes (e.g., swimming or olfactory) may diminish the ability of aquatic organisms to find food or to escape from predators and may ultimately lead to death. Some sublethal effects may have little or no effect on the organism because they are rapidly reversible or diminish or cease with time (e.g., growth may be reduced at high concentrations early in a toxicity study but not be significantly different from that in controls by the end of the study). In laboratory studies, sublethal effects may be unnoticed in acute tests. The only way to study sublethal toxicity in the laboratory is by using longer term exposures. Subchronic and chronic exposure studies and the sublethal effects that may result from these exposures are discussed throughout this book.

In general, effects may be manifested *immediately* during exposure or after termination of exposure to a chemical, or they may be *delayed* until some time after exposure. This is determined by the properties of the chemical and the ability of the organism to metabolize (or biotransform) the chemical. For example, chemicals that are susceptible to biotransformation will have a short half-life in the organisms and therefore be excreted rapidly. Chemicals with a short half-life should not produce delayed effects. In the natural aquatic environment, chemicals may have a short half-life in the water and sediment because they are transformed by chemical and physical processes as well as biological processes.

Some toxic effects are *reversible* and others are *irreversible.* They may be reversible by normal repair mechanisms, such as by regeneration of damaged tissue. In many cases effects are reversible only if the organism can escape the toxic medium and find a toxicant-free environment. Serious damage or injury to an organism may be irreversible and may eventually result in death. In the laboratory, the reversibility or irreversibility of chemical effects may be studied by transferring organisms from a medium containing the toxicant to a medium that is free of the toxicant (e.g., a recovery study).

A distinction can be made on the basis of the general site of action of a toxicant. *Local effects* occur at the primary site of contact. An example of a local effect is a skin or gill reaction (e.g., discoloration, inflammation, or erosion) in fish exposed to various organic and inorganic compounds. For a chemical to have an effect at a site other than the primary site of contact, it must gain access to the internal environment of the organism, generally by transport through the circulatory system. *Systemic effects* are those that require absorption and distribution of the chemical to a site distant from the original contact or entry site. Effects on the nervous system or various organs are classified as systemic effects.

In assessing chemically induced effects (responses), it is important to consider that in the natural aquatic environment organisms are exposed not to a single chemical but rather to a myriad of different substances that form mixtures. Exposure to mixtures may result in toxicological interactions. A *toxicological interaction* is one in which exposure to two or more chemicals results in a biological response quantitatively or qualitatively different from that expected from the action of each of the chemicals alone. The multiple chemical exposures may be *sequential* or *simultaneous* in time, and the altered response may be greater or smaller in magnitude. See Chapter 7 for a complete discussion of interactions.

CONCENTRATION–RESPONSE RELATIONSHIPS

Substantial differences may exist among individual organisms in a supposedly homogeneous population. These differences become evident when the organisms are challenged by exposure to a chemical or potentially toxic stress. For example, not all of the organisms would respond in a quantitatively identical manner to the same concentration of a toxicant. The effects of such an exposure might vary from very intense in some organisms to minimal or none in other organisms. That is, some organisms may die and others survive with apparently minimal adverse effects. These differences in response are due to biological variation. The variation is normally small for organisms of the same species and similar age and health, and generally greater between species.

In measuring the toxicity of a chemical, the objective is to estimate as precisely as possible the range of chemical concentrations that produce some selected, readily observable, quantifiable response in groups of the same test species under controlled laboratory conditions. The results of the exposure are plotted on a graph that relates the concentration of the test chemical to the percentage of organisms in test groups exhibiting the defined response. Such a correlation is commonly referred to as a *concentration-response relationship*. It is analogous to the dose-response relationship employed in mammalian toxicological testing. In the case of mammalian testing, the exposure takes place by direct introduction of a measured amount (dose) of the test chemical onto (dermal or ocular exposure) or into (feeding or injection)

the test animals. Therefore, the *dose* is known and the response can be correlated with it. In aquatic toxicity testing, the test organism is exposed to the chemical indirectly by mixing the chemical into the water in which the animal lives, thus producing a test *concentration*. There is generally no measure of the amount of the chemical that actually enters the organisms, even if the concentration of the chemical in the exposure medium is measured. Therefore, the response observed is more correctly correlated with the exposure concentration, hence the term concentration-response relationship.

The concentration of a test chemical in water is usually expressed in parts per million (ppm), or units of test chemical (usually expressed as mass) per 10^6 units of untreated dilution water (diluent). The commonly used ratio is milligrams of test chemical per liter of water (1 ppm = 1 mg/l). The concentration may also be expressed in parts per billion (ppb), or units of test chemical per 10^9 units of diluent water. Here the commonly used ratio is micrograms of test chemical per liter of water (1 ppb = 1 μg/l). If the organisms are exposed to test solutions of liquid industrial wastes of an effluent, the concentration of effluent in water is usually expressed as a volume percent [100 × (volume of effluent)/(volume of effluent plus volume of dilution water)]. For example, a 10% dilution equals 1 volume of effluent in 9 volumes of dilution water. Corresponding expressions of chemical concentrations in solid media such as tissues and sediments are in parts per million or milligrams of test chemical per kilogram of tissue or sediment (1 ppm = 1 mg/kg), which is equivalent to micrograms of test chemical per gram of tissue or sediment. Likewise, parts per billion correspond to micrograms of test chemical per kilogram of tissue or sediment or nanograms per gram. Weight-specific concentrations are generally expressed on the basis of tissue wet weight and sediment wet or dry weight.

The concentration-response relationship is the most fundamental concept in aquatic toxicology. It extends to all kinds of adverse responses and implies that for each chemical agent there exists a threshold concentration below which, under defined conditions, no harmful effect is produced.

There are several assumptions underlying the concentration-response relationship. The first is an implicit assumption of causality. To derive a quantitative statement of the relationship between a toxic chemical and an observed effect or response, it must be known with reasonable certainty that the relationship is indeed a causal one. However, there may be some doubt about the identity of the chemical, which may have changed during the exposure, about the concentration to which the organism is actually exposed in water, or even about the specificity of the response, since aquatic organisms may respond similarly to a variety of stresses. It is thus only a reasonable presumption that in the concentration-response relationship the effect observed is a result of exposure to the known chemical. The second assumption is that the production and severity of a response are functions of the concentration of the chemical.

The concentration-response relationship is a graded relationship between the concentration of the test chemical to which the organisms are exposed and the severity of the response elicited. Generally, within certain limits, the greater the concentration of the test chemical, the more severe the response. The curve drawn to represent this relationship will generally be asymptotic, since at all concentrations below some minimum (threshold) value no measurable adverse response will be elicited, while at all concentrations above some maximum value most or all of the test group will be adversely affected. The steeper the slope of the central portion of the curve, the sharper the threshold of effect— that is, the more intense the response over a narrow range of concentrations. Figure 2 shows the typical sigmoid form of the concentration-response curve. For a statement about the concentration-response relationship to have a precise meaning, the duration of exposure must also be defined.

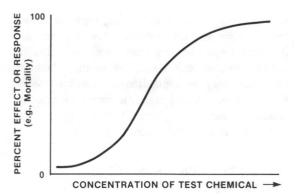

Figure 2 Typical form of the concentration-response curve.

Criteria for Effects and LC50

In evaluating the safety of chemical substances, it is necessary to have a precise means of expressing the toxicity and a quantitative method of measuring it. There are a variety of *criteria for effects* or end points of toxicity that could be used to compare chemically exposed organisms with unexposed organisms. The ideal criteria are those closely associated with the molecular events that result from exposure to the chemical. However, in aquatic toxicology this is difficult to achieve because the molecular events are usually unknown. Alternatively, one may select a measure of toxicity that is unequivocal, clearly relevant, readily observable, describable, measurable, biologically significant, and reproducible. For the initial test measurement in toxicological evaluation, it is customary to use lethality (or mortality) as an index.

Measurement of lethality is precise, important, unequivocal, and therefore useful for estimating the concentration and potency of a chemical. It provides a means of comparing substances whose actions may be quite different and indicates whether further toxicity studies should be conducted. Mortality and survival over a specific period of time are typical effect criteria in short-term (acute) exposure tests. Data from lethality tests are quantal; that is, the animals live or die (all-or-none response). However, it is important to have sublethal effect criteria that indicate toxic stress at a stage before death, so that early observation will permit rapid action to prevent mortalities. Growth (length and weight), number of normal embryos, morphological anomalies (e.g., double-headedness and deformed spines), and number of offspring produced are typical sublethal effect criteria in long-term (chronic) exposure tests. All these responses are quantitative (or graded); they are measured not in terms of incidence but in some unit of response (milligrams, centimeters) that can be used to compare test organisms with unexposed controls and determine whether the differences between them are statistically significant. Since there are usually many test organisms, a series of several graded measurements is generated for each concentration. Whereas in a quantal test it is sufficient merely to determine for every organism whether or not the selected response (effect) has occurred, a quantitative test requires measuring the extent of the response shown by each organism.

Whatever the effect or response selected for measurement, the relationship between the degree of response of the organisms and the quantity (or concentration) of the chemical almost always assumes a classic concentration-response form. In Fig. 3 the ordinates represent percent mortality and the abscissas represent concentration of the chemical; both measures increase with increasing distance from the origin. The graphs represent the results of tests in which groups of test organisms of the same species were exposed to various concentrations of a chemical for a specific length of time. In Fig. 3a the mean percent mortality for each test group has been plotted on ordinary graph paper (arithmetic scale) against the concentration producing that mortality. The responses of test organisms to the different chemical concentrations yield a characteristic S-shaped curve. Each point on the curve represents the mean response to the concentration corresponding to that point, and each mean has an associated variation due to different responses of individual organisms. The least variability in the curve is at the 50% level of response. The concentration at

which 50% of the individuals react (the median) after a specified length of exposure (e.g., 24 or 48 h) is therefore used as a measure of the activity or toxicity of the chemical agent.

In determining the relative toxicity of a new chemical to aquatic organisms, an acute toxicity test is first conducted to estimate the median lethal concentration (LC50) of the chemical in the water to which test organisms are exposed. The *LC50* is the concentration estimated to produce mortality in 50% of a test population over a specific time period. The length of exposure is usually 24 to 96 h, depending on the species (see Chapter 2). When effects other than mortality are measured, the expression EC50 is used. The *EC50* (median effective concentration) is the concentration of a chemical estimated to produce a specific effect (e.g., behavioral or physiological) in 50% of a population of test species after a specified length of exposure (e.g., 24 or 48 h). Typical effect criteria include immobility, a developmental abnormality or deformity, loss of equilibrium, failure to respond to an external stimulus, and abnormal behavior.

The LC50 can be interpolated from the curve in Fig. 3a by drawing a horizontal line from the 50% mortality point on the ordinate to the concentration-response curve and then drawing a vertical line from the point of intersection with the curve to the abscissa. The vertical line intersects the abscissa at the LC50 value, which is then read off the graph. The LC50 is an *estimate* of the concentration of a chemical that would produce a specific effect (mortality) in 50% of an infinitely large population of the test species under the stated conditions.

The normally distributed sigmoid curve in Fig. 3a approaches a mortality of 0% as the concentration is decreased and approaches 100% as the concentration is increased, but theoretically never passes through 0 and 100%. The middle portion of the curve, in the region between 16 and 84%, is linear. These values represent the limits of 1 standard deviation (SD) of the mean (and the median) in a normally distributed population of

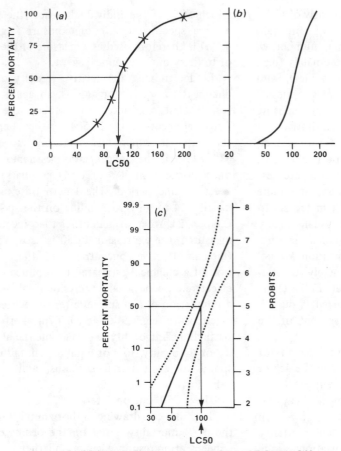

Figure 3 Mortality in a fish population exposed to a range of concentrations of a chemical in water. (a) Percent mortality versus concentration plotted on an arithmetic scale. (b) The same data as in (a), but with mortality on an arithmetic scale and concentration on a logarithmic scale. (c) The same data as in (a), but with mortality expressed as probits versus concentration on a logarithmic scale. The dotted lines on each side of the curve represent the 95% confidence limits.

organisms. In a normally distributed population, the mean ±1 SD represents 68.3% of the test population, the mean ±2 SD 95.5% of the test population, and the mean ±3 SD 99.7% of the test population.

Figure 3b is a plot of the data in Fig. 3a, but with the concentration shown on a logarithmic scale (transformed data). The sigmoid shape is again evident but the curve approaches a straight line. Figure 3c represents another transformation of the same data, with the logarithm of concen-

tration plotted against percent mortality expressed as probits. The probit transformation adjusts mortality data to an assumed normal population distribution, which results in a straight line being the best-fit curve. The LC50 is obtained by drawing horizontal and vertical lines in the same manner described for Fig. 3a.

The logarithmic conversion was introduced by Krogh and Hemmingsen (1928) and later by Gaddum (1933). Since concentration-response data are normally distributed, the percent response was converted to units of deviation from the mean or normal equivalent deviations (NEDs) by Gaddum (1933). The NED for a 50% response is zero and that for an 84.1% response is +1. Bliss (1934a,b) later suggested that 5 be added to the NED to eliminate negative numbers. The converted units of NED plus 5 were called *probits*. The log-probit conversion is valuable for description and statistical analysis (see Chapter 5). The LC50 estimated by graphical interpolation is accurate and usually similar to the LC50 obtained by formal statistical analysis.

Confidence Limits

The degree of scatter of observed values may be evaluated by calculation and expressed as *confidence limits*. Confidence limits are shown by dotted lines on both sides of the solid line in Fig. 3c. The limits indicate the area or range within which the concentration-response line would be expected to fall in replicate tests in 19 of 20 samples (95% confidence limits) taken at random from the same test population under the same conditions. A series of such curves would be well correlated with each other at the 50% mortality level but probably not well correlated as the mortality approaches 0 or 100%. This indicates that the LC50 may be estimated more precisely than greater or lesser effects (e.g., LC99 or LC1).

Slope

Figure 4 shows concentration-response curves (log-probit scale) for two chemicals, X and Z. The LC50 values for the chemicals are the same but the slopes of the concentration-mortality curves are different. The curve corresponding to Z represents a set of data of greater variability, as reflected by the larger confidence limits. The flat slope of line Z indicates that mortality increases by small increments as the concentration of the chemical to which the organisms are exposed increases. Conversely, the steep slope of line X indicates that large increases in mortality are associated with relatively small increases in the concentration to which the test organisms are exposed. The *slope*

is thus an index of the range of sensitivity to the chemical within the test sample of fish.

A flat slope, as for chemical Z, may also be indicative of slow absorption, rapid excretion or detoxification, or delayed toxification. A steep slope, as for chemical X, usually indicates rapid absorption and rapid onset of effects. Although the slope alone is not a reliable indicator of toxicological mechanisms, it is a useful parameter and should always be reported along with the confidence limits.

More information on the statistical procedures used to determine the LC50, the slope, and the confidence limits is given in Chapters 2 and 5. Chapter 5 also discusses statistical procedures used to evaluate quantitative responses in long-term exposure tests.

Toxicity Curves

If a toxicity test such as the 96-h LC50 is conducted, mortality data are generated for various intermediate time periods. The LC50s for these time periods can be used during the test to plot a toxicity curve (Fig. 5), using logarithmic scales for exposure time and concentration. Such a curve

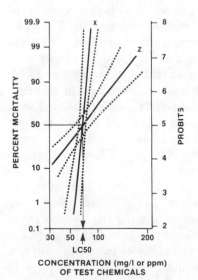

Figure 4 Hypothetical concentration-response curves for two chemicals, X and Z, demonstrating differences in slope.

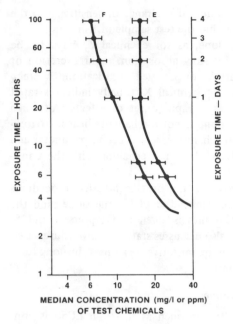

Figure 5 Hypothetical time-toxicity curves for two chemicals, E and F, to evaluate incipient LC50.

(Sprague, 1969). Straight and curved lines are usually fitted to the points by eye. The shape of the curve may provide information about the mode of action of the chemical or may indicate the presence of more than one chemical agent in the water.

TOXICITY TESTING

Aquatic toxicology has been defined as the study of the effects of chemicals and other foreign agents on aquatic organisms with special emphasis on adverse or harmful effects. *Toxicity tests* are used to evaluate the concentrations of the chemical and the duration of exposure required to produce the criterion effect. The effects of a chemical may be of such minor significance that the aquatic organism is able to carry on its functions in a normal manner and that only under conditions of additional stress (e.g., changes in pH, dissolved oxygen, and temperature) can a chemically induced effect be detected. The influence of these factors on chemical toxicity is discussed in Chapter 6. Effects may also result from the interaction of small amounts of some chemicals and larger amounts of other chemicals without these additional stresses.

Aquatic toxicity tests are used to detect and evaluate the potential toxicological effects of chemicals on aquatic organisms. Since these effects are not necessarily harmful, a principal function of the tests is to identify chemicals that can have adverse effects on aquatic organisms. These tests provide a data base that can be used to assess the risk associated with a situation in which the chemical agent, the organism, and the exposure conditions are defined.

The aquatic toxicity test is frequently and erroneously called a *bioassay*. An appropriate definition of a bioassay is "a test to evaluate the relative potency of a chemical by comparing its effect on a living organism with that of a standard preparation." A bioassay is performed to determine the strength of the chemical from the degree of response elicited in the test organisms, not to estimate the concentration of the chemical that is

gives the investigator an idea of how the test is progressing, and it may indicate when acute lethality has ceased. This would be indicated where the curve is asymptotic to the time axis. The LC50 for a specific exposure time that is in the asymptotic part of the curve is called the *threshold* or *incipient LC50* (also called the asymptotic LC50, incipient lethal level, ultimate median tolerance limit, or lethal threshold concentration). This is the concentration at which 50% of the test population can live for an indefinite time or the lethal concentration for 50% of the test organisms in long-term exposure.

For chemical E in Fig. 5 the vertical asymptote after approximately 24 h indicates that acute mortality has ceased and the test may be terminated. For chemical F, the lack of an asymptote at the end of the test indicates that acute mortality was continuing and it may be advantageous to continue the test beyond 96 h to determine whether a threshold exists.

The toxicity curve may be a straight line rather than a curve and may assume a variety of shapes toxic to those organisms. A toxicity test is performed to measure the degree of response produced by a specific level of stimulus (test chemical concentration). Bioassays are frequently used in the pharmaceutical industry to evaluate the potency of vitamins and other pharmacologically active compounds.

Criteria and Approaches to Testing

Before discussing general approaches to toxicity testing, the criteria used to determine the suitability of a test procedure should be established. These criteria may include some of the following:

- The test should be widely accepted by the scientific community.
- It should be able to predict the effects of a wide range of chemicals on different organisms.
- The test procedures should have a sound statistical basis and should be repeatable in different laboratories with similar results.
- The data should include effects of a range of concentrations within realistic durations of exposure. They should also be quantifiable through graphical interpolation, statistical analysis, or other accepted methods of quantitative evaluation.
- The data should be useful for risk assessment.
- The test should be economical and easy to conduct.
- The test should be sensitive and as realistic as possible in design to detect and measure the effect.

Current test methods have been designed predominantly to examine the responses of a few individuals within a species (single-species tests). Considerably less attention has been given to the impact of chemicals on species interactions and on structure and function within different aquatic ecosystems (ecosystem tests). Tests on single species, species interactions (multispecies tests), and ecosystems are all important for evaluating the potential impact of a chemical on an aquatic ecosystem.

Two general approaches may be used to conduct these tests, and each has advantages and limitations.

1 Effects can be studied in controlled laboratory experiments with a limited number of variables.
2 Effects can be studied in a natural ecosystem (*in situ*).

Most single-species tests are conducted in the laboratory. These tests can provide a great deal of information on the concentrations of chemicals and duration of exposure that produce changes in mortality, growth, reproduction, pathology, behavior, physiology, and biochemistry of organisms within species. However, the results cannot be used to assess the chemical impact above this level of biological organization.

Cause-and-effect relationships can easily be established from single-species tests because of the degree of control over laboratory conditions. These tests are also easy to conduct, and many are standardized and can be replicated. Current single-species tests are conducted with individual species that are considered representative of broad classes of organisms (e.g., fish or invertebrates), so that the results provide information on the toxicity of specific chemicals in different types of organisms under given conditions. The utility of single-species laboratory tests is, however, a function of the criteria used to select the test organisms, and these will be discussed below. The main limitation of these studies is that effects observed in the laboratory may not occur in the same way or to the same degree in the natural environment. Single-species laboratory tests cannot account for the adaptive ability of natural populations of organisms. Effects observed in laboratory tests may thus appear more severe than those seen in the field. Furthermore, laboratory studies are unrealistic in that they do not simulate the complex species interactions and environmental influences in natural systems.

Multispecies tests and ecosystem tests may also be conducted in the laboratory. These studies often involve "laboratory microcosms" or "model ecosystems." Laboratory microcosms are small-scale enclosures (plastic or glass) containing samples from the natural ecosystem (water, sediment, fish, invertebrates, and plants). Their advantage is that effects beyond the level of a single species can be identified, providing information more directly related to ecological consequences of the chemical. In principle, if conditions are uniform, these tests should be easy to replicate and standardize for different chemical substances; however, the literature indicates that this is not always the case. Since the environmental influences are controlled, cause-and-effect relationships are more easily analyzed than in natural systems. Microcosms have several limitations, since they are oversimplifications of natural systems. For example, the impact of the physical environment (e.g., temperature and seasonal changes) on natural aquatic ecosystems can be very different from that represented by the microcosm. In addition, significant biotic components of the natural system (e.g., invaders) may be absent. Laboratory microcosm studies are described in Chapter 17.

Single-species, multispecies, and ecosystem tests are most realistically conducted in the field or natural ecosystem. The ecosystem may be a pond or a stream, and it is usually selected because of the possibility of chemical exposure. Some influences and interactions of biotic and abiotic components that are not present in laboratory studies can be identified in field studies. Field studies can also be used to validate laboratory studies and mathematical ecosystem models and to determine environmental concentrations. They may be more useful for predicting the potential fate and effects of chemicals on the aquatic environment. There are, however, limitations of field studies. Environmental variables are not stable, so that field work is difficult to monitor and replicate. Results are often equivocal because they can be attributed to many factors. Cause-and-effect relationships are difficult to establish and interpret because there are too many variables that are not adequately controlled and many are undefined. Field studies are discussed in Chapter 21.

Ideally, data should be obtained from a combination of laboratory and field studies. In designing these studies, consideration should be given to the site-specific factors appropriate to the particular ecosystem. No single test can provide enough information to make adequate predictions of the impact of a chemical on the aquatic environment. Tests should be conducted to detect effects on single species, species interactions, and the ecosystem. However, the development and standardization of tests beyond the single-species level is difficult because of the complexity of species interactions and ecosystems.

Since most aquatic toxicity tests have been laboratory studies of single species, the discussion throughout most of this book concerns these types of test systems. Many single-species tests have yielded results that are well correlated with the observed ecological effects of chemicals. Mathematical models are used to link the data obtained from laboratory toxicity tests with predicted field effects. The combined data can provide more complete information about the potential impact of chemicals on the aquatic environment.

General Test Design

Toxicity testing in the laboratory usually follows a stepwise tier approach, progressing from simple short-term tests to more complex and sophisticated longer-term tests based on the results of the previous tests. Although the specific details of the tests may differ, the general test design is similar; it requires careful control of conditions such as pH, temperature, dissolved oxygen concentration, and photoperiod. Test organisms are exposed in test chambers (e.g., glass tanks) to various concentrations of the test material (e.g., pesticides or industrial effluents) in water solutions. The criteria for effects (e.g., mortality, growth, and reproduction), which are established before testing, are then evaluated by comparing the chemically exposed (treated) organisms with the untreated organisms (controls), which are exposed only to the diluent.

All toxicity tests should include a concurrent control to ensure that the effects observed are associated with or attributable to exposure to the test material. There are three basic types of controls.

1 The untreated (negative) water control consists of a group of organisms with the same dilution water (without test material or solvent added) and the same conditions and procedures. The organisms are from the same source as those used in the remainder of the treatments (exposed to the test material concentrations). This type of control is used to determine the inherent background effects in the test, such as effects related to the health of the organisms and the quality of the dilution water. It provides a baseline for interpreting the test results.

2 In some tests with water-insoluble or poorly soluble test materials, an organic solvent or carrier may be used to prepare stock solutions of the test material. When this occurs, a solvent or vehicle control should be included. A solvent is an organic chemical that is miscible with water and in which the test material is more soluble than it is in the diluent water. The solvent control is essentially an untreated control, except that the maximum volume of solvent used to prepare a test material concentration is added. This control also provides a baseline, taking into account effects of the solvent on the test organisms. The toxicity of the solvent to the test species should be relatively low compared with that of the test material. Typical solvents are acetone, dimethyl formamide (DMF), dimethyl sulfoxide (DMSO), and triethylene glycol (TEG). The toxicities (96-h LC50s) of these solvents to fish are: acetone, 9,100 mg/l; DMF, 10,410 mg/l; DMSO, 33,500 mg/l; and TEG, 92,500 mg/l (C. E. Stephan, personal communication; Willford, 1968).

3 A positive (reference) control which is a material known from previous experience to produce a defined effect on the test organisms. An ideal reference toxicant is toxic at low concentrations, rapidly lethal, stable, nonselective, and detectable by known analytical techniques. It is used to determine the health and sensitivity of the organisms, to compare the relative toxicities of substances by using the control as an internal standard, to perform interlaboratory calibrations, and to evaluate the reproducibility of test data

with time. A positive control is not generally considered necessary if an untreated or solvent control is maintained. Compounds used or evaluated as reference toxicants include sodium pentachlorophenate (Adelman and Smith, 1976; Davis and Hoos, 1975), dehydroabietic acid (Davis and Hoos, 1975), phenol and sodium azide (Klaverkamp et al., 1975), p,p'-DDT (Marking, 1966), the surfactant dodecyl sodium sulfate (DSS) (LaRoche et al., 1970; Pessah et al., 1975), antimycin (Hunn et al., 1968), and sodium chloride (Adelman and Smith, 1976). Based on the characteristics of an ideal reference toxicant, sodium pentachlorophenate has been recommended with phenol as an alternative (Lee, 1980).

Whenever possible, chemical analysis should be performed to measure the concentrations to which test organisms are exposed. In addition, it is valuable to measure chemical residues in tissues of exposed organisms. Methods and instrumentation for the analysis of chemical residues in water and tissues of aquatic organisms are described in Chapter 16.

Test Organisms

Criteria for Selection

In order to extrapolate meaningful, relevant, and ecologically significant results from aquatic toxicity tests, not only appropriate tests but also appropriate organisms should be used. Several criteria should be considered in selecting organisms for toxicity testing.

1 Since sensitivities vary among species, species representing a broad range of sensitivities should be used whenever possible.

2 Widely available and abundant species should be considered.

3 Whenever possible, species should be studied which are indigenous to or representative of the ecosystem that may receive the impact.

4 Species that are recreationally, commercially, or ecologically important should be included.

5 Species should be amenable to routine maintenance in the laboratory and techniques should be available for culturing and rearing them in the laboratory so that chronic toxicity tests can be conducted.

6 If there is adequate background information on a species (i.e., its physiology, genetics, and behavior), the data from a test may be more easily interpreted.

The species selected for testing may differ from ecosystem to ecosystem and the selection will often be based on site-specific considerations. For example, when assessing the potential impact of a chemical on cold water streams, a salmonid such as a trout would be selected, while for warm water streams, a centrarchid such as a sunfish would be chosen. There is no standard test species that can be used for all ecosystems. The kinds and number of species will depend on the complexity of the ecosystem. However, criteria 1, 5, and 6 above are so important at times that several standard aquatic organisms have been used. These include the water flea (*Daphnia* sp.), fathead minnow (*Pimephales promelas*), bluegill (*Lepomis macrochirus*), rainbow trout (*Salmo gairdneri*), mysid shrimp (*Mysidopsis* sp.), and sheepshead minnow (*Cyprinodon variegatus*).

Because of the variation between species in sensitivity to chemicals, a range of different effects and degrees of effect may be expected when different species are exposed to the same concentration of the same chemical. It is therefore important to conduct tests with several species, perhaps from different taxonomic groups, to get some indication of the natural variability. The selection of test species should be based on as many of the criteria listed above as possible.

Species Types

Toxicity tests have traditionally been performed with a variety of freshwater and saltwater test species representing algae, fish, and invertebrates. These are listed in Chapter 2. These species are recommended for use in toxicity tests because there is a substantial amount of toxicity information available for many of them. If one of these

species is not available, organisms from the recommended genus should be considered. Test species can be collected from wild populations in relatively unpolluted areas, purchased from commercial suppliers, or cultured in the laboratory. Species should not be collected by use of electroshock or chemicals because of the physiological stress induced. All species in a particular test should be from the same source.

Exposure Systems

In aquatic toxicity tests the controls and treated organisms can be exposed to the dilution water or the test water solutions containing the chemical toxicant by four different techniques.

1 In a *static test* the organisms are exposed in still water. The test material is added to the dilution water to produce the desired test concentrations. The control and test organisms are then placed in test chambers and there is no change of water for the duration of the test.

2 A *recirculation test* is similar to a static test except that the test solutions and control water are pumped through an apparatus, such as a filter, to maintain water quality but not reduce the concentration of test material. The water is returned to the test chamber. This type of test is not routinely used because it is expensive to set up and maintain and because of uncertainty about the effect of the apparatus (aerator, filter, sterilizer) on the test material.

3 A *renewal test* is similar to a static test because it is conducted in still water, but the test solutions and control water are renewed periodically (usually at 24-h intervals) by transferring the test organisms to chambers with freshly prepared material or by removing and replacing the material in the original containers.

4 In a *flow-through test,* the test solutions and control water flow into and out of the chambers in which the test organisms are maintained. The once-through flow may be intermittent or continuous. A stock solution of test material to be mixed with dilution water to prepare the test material concentrations may be prepared once at the beginning of the test, or fresh stock solutions may be

prepared daily. In either case, metering pumps or diluters control the flow (and thus the volume) of dilution water and test material stock solution so that the proper proportions of each will be mixed. Chapter 2 describes the flow-through technique in detail.

The static and flow-through techniques are the most widely used means of exposure. Although the static technique is uncomplicated and inexpensive, it has disadvantages:

• The test material may be degraded and volatilized, adsorbed onto the test chambers or test organisms, or otherwise changed. The concentrations to which the organisms are exposed thus decrease as the test progresses.
• The test material may have a high biochemical oxygen demand (BOD) so that the toxicity is masked by depletion of dissolved oxygen from the test solution.
• The metabolic products of the test organisms build up and may react with the material being tested, producing a toxic response different from the one that would have been produced had the excretory products been removed.

If any of these conditions exist to a significant extent, the results of the static test may not accurately represent the effects of the chemical being tested. Therefore, the flow-through procedure should be used wherever possible. This results in more uniform and stable test conditions, with the test material concentration, dissolved oxygen concentration, and other water quality characteristics remaining relatively constant while the waste products are removed. Although flow-through tests may involve a more complex delivery system, they yield the best and most accurate estimate of toxicity.

Most of the toxicity tests discussed in this book involve static or flow-through techniques. Both are used for acute tests, but for subchronic and chronic tests the flow-through technique is preferred because there is a greater degree of assurance that the concentrations of test material and conditions to which the organisms are exposed during the test period have remained constant. Cause-and-effect relationships can thus be more easily established.

Standard Procedures

A variety of test methods have been developed by the American Public Health Association (APHA), U.S. Environmental Protection Agency (U.S.EPA), American Society for Testing and Materials (ASTM), and Organization for Economic Cooperation and Development (OECD) to evaluate the hazard and potential toxicity of materials to aquatic organisms. Doudoroff et al. (1951) first recognized the need to develop uniform, standardized test procedures to maximize the comparability of data from tests. The advantages of using standardized test procedures were summarized by Davis (1977) as follows:

• Allows selection of one or more uniform and useful tests by a variety of laboratories.
• Facilitates comparison of data and results and thus increases usefulness of published data.
• Increases accuracy of the data.
• Allows replication of the test.
• Allows the test to be easily initiated and conducted by a variety of personnel (if the procedure is well documented).
• Legal advantage if procedures are accepted by the courts.
• Useful for routine monitoring purposes.

Davis (1977) stated that the initial step to standardization is a thorough knowledge of the various chemical, physical, and biological factors that affect toxicity test results. Standardization can then be achieved by:

• Adoption of detailed test protocols that minimize or standardize disturbing effects.
• Use of a standard test species.
• Selection of specific test types designed to meet specific objectives.
• Use of reference toxicants or "disease-free" certified test animals.

A standardized method (protocol) with reference toxicants and standard test species theoretically maximizes comparability, replicability, and reliability and thus is essential for answering questions of relative toxicity and sensitivity or of replicability of tests (Buikema et al., 1982).

While there is an obvious need for standardized toxicity test protocols, there is also a danger in overstandardization since it "may stifle innovative and creative work," especially if regulatory agencies "do not recognize work that does not coincide with their own priorities" (Davis, 1977). For example, a standardized toxicity test may not be appropriate for answering specific questions about a particular body of water. For assessing the hazard of a particular chemical to an indigenous fish community in a body of water, it may not be useful to employ standard test species that are not normally present in that body of water. Furthermore, it is desirable to conduct the tests under the physical and chemical conditions characteristic of that body of water.

Toxicity test protocols typically specify the exposure of test organisms to fixed concentrations of chemical compounds for a defined time period. However, chemicals rarely, if ever, enter the environment at a constant concentration (Cairns and Thompson, 1980). Most chemicals enter the aquatic environment sporadically in "pulses," intermittently as "slugs," or as a one-time "spill." Therefore, the toxicant is present in high concentration for a relatively short period of time and is usually diluted to lower concentrations with time. In these cases mortality is a function of toxicant concentration and length of exposure. Generally, organisms can tolerate high concentrations for short periods of time and lower concentrations for longer periods of time (Buikema et al., 1982). Since most test methods do not consider the concentration-time relationship, these data cannot be readily applied to predict the effects of the chemical in the field. A typical standard test, in which all test conditions are kept constant or maintained optimally, may be inappropriate for a changing natural system. In that case, site-specific studies should be conducted.

The aim of the toxicity test will determine which test design is most applicable. If the results are to be used to compare the toxicity of one chemical to another, rigid standardization is necessary. However, if the data are to be used to describe or predict the behavior of the chemical in a specific water system, there is a danger in overstandardization.

Some methods that have been widely accepted and are standardized protocols and others that have been proposed are listed in Table 1. They are categorized in Table 1 according to species of fish, invertebrates, and algae and acute, subchronic, and chronic exposures.

Description of Test Methods

Aquatic toxicity test methods may be categorized according to length of exposure, test situation, criteria of effects to be evaluated, and organisms to be tested. The data generated in these tests may enable the researcher to determine the *no observed effect concentration* (NOEC) or *no-effect concentration,* which is the maximum concentration of the test material that produces no statistically significant harmful effect on test organisms compared to controls in a specific test. The *lowest observed effect concentration* (LOEC) or *minimum threshold concentration* (MTC) may also be obtained. This is the lowest concentration that has a statistically significant deleterious effect on test organisms compared to controls in a specific test. The effects evaluated are biological end points selected because they are important to the survival, growth, behavior, and perpetuation of a species. These end points differ depending on the type of toxicity test being conducted and the species used. The statistical approach also changes with the type of toxicity test conducted. Some of the commonly used tests and the end points (effect criteria) that they measure are briefly described below.

Acute Toxicity Tests

These are tests designed to evaluate the relative toxicity of a chemical to selected aquatic organisms on short-term exposure to various concen-

Table 1 Methods for Toxicity Testing and Evaluation

Organization	Fish Acute	Fish Early life stage	Fish Partial chronic	Fish Complete chronic	Macroinvertebrates[b] Acute	Macroinvertebrates[b] Chronic	Phytoplankton	Special
American Public Health Association, American Public Water Works Association, Water Pollution Control Federation (APHA, AWWA, WPCF)[c]	X				X	X	X	Ciliated protozoans, scleractiniar coral, marine polychaete annelids, aquatic insects
American Society for Testing and Materials (ASTM)[d]	X	X	X	X	X	X	X	Bioconcentration, hazard assessment, effluent
Organization for Economic Cooperation and Development (OECD)[e]	X				X	X	X	Bioaccumulation
United States Environmental Protection Agency (U.S. EPA)[f]	X		X		X	X	X	Dredged material, effluent

Type of test[a]

[a] A cross (X) indicates that a type of test has a method that is either standardized or in draft form (proposed) and being reviewed for approval by scientific authorities.

[b] Macroinvertebrates here may include one or more of the following: *Daphnia* sp., *Acartia* sp., *Mysidopsis* sp., crabs, shrimp, or oysters.

[c] APHA, AWWA, WPCF (1981).

[d] ASTM (1980a–k).

[e] OECD (1981).

[f] Committee on Methods for Acute Toxicity Tests with Aquatic Organisms (1975), Brusick et al. (1980), Duke et al. (1977), Miller et al. (1978), Peltier (1978), U.S. EPA (1971, 1972a,b,c, 1974, 1976, 1977, 1978, 1979, no date).

trations of the test chemical. Common effect criteria for fish are mortality; for invertebrates, immobility and loss of equilibrium; and for algae, growth. These tests may be conducted for a predetermined length of time (*time-dependent test*) to estimate the 24- or 96-h LC50 or the 48-h EC50. An acute toxicity test may also have a duration that is not predetermined, in which case it is referred to as a *time-independent* (TI) test. In a TI test, exposure of the test organisms continues until the toxic response manifested has ceased or economic or other practical considerations dictate that the test be terminated. For example, the acute TI test may be allowed to continue until acute toxicity (mortality or a defined sublethal effect) has ceased or nearly ceased and the toxicity curve indicates that a threshold or incipient concentration can be estimated. With most test materials this point is reached in 7–14 d, but it may not be reached within 21 d.

In the early development of acute toxicity tests, data were expressed as the *median tolerance limit* (TLm or TL50)—the test material concentration at which 50% of the test organisms survive for a specified exposure time (usually 24–96 h). This term has been replaced by median lethal concentration (LC50) and median effective concentration (EC50). Acute toxicity tests are discussed in Chapter 2.

Chronic Toxicity Tests

The fact that a chemical does not have adverse effects on aquatic organisms in acute toxicity tests does not necessarily indicate that it is not toxic to these species. Chronic toxicity tests permit evaluation of the possible adverse effects of the chemical under conditions of long-term exposure at sublethal concentrations. In a chronic toxicity test, the test organism is exposed for an entire reproductive life cycle to at least five concentrations of the test material. Partial life cycle (or partial chronic) toxicity tests include only a portion of a life cycle involving several sensitive life stages; these include reproduction and growth during the first year but do not include exposure of very

early juvenile stages. In chronic toxicity tests exposure is generally initiated with an egg or zygote and continues through development and hatching of the embryo, growth and development of the young organism, attainment of sexual maturity, and reproduction to produce a second-generation organism. Tests may also begin with the exposed adult and continue through egg, fry, juvenile, and adult to egg. With fish, for example, exposure begins with fertilized eggs and criteria for effect include growth, reproduction, development of sex products, maturation, spawning success, hatching success, survival of larvae or fry, growth and survival of different life stages, and behavior. The duration of a chronic toxicity test varies with the species tested; it is approximately 21 d for the water flea *Daphnia magna* and can be 275–300 d for the fathead minnow, *Pimephales promelas*.

From the data obtained in partial life cycle and complete life cycle tests the *maximum acceptable toxicant concentration* (MATC) can be estimated. This is the estimated threshold concentration of a chemical within a range defined by the highest concentration tested at which no significant deleterious effect was observed (NOEC) and the lowest concentration tested at which some significant deleterious effect was observed (LOEC) (Mount and Stephan, 1967). Since it is not possible to test an unlimited number of intermediate concentrations, an MATC is generally reported as being greater than the NOEC and less than the LOEC (NOEC < MATC < LOEC; e.g., 0.5 ppm < MATC < 1.0 ppm).

Life cycle tests are also used for the determination of application factors (AFs). Historically (Mount and Stephan, 1967), the AF was the numerical value of the ratio of the MATC to the time-independent or incipient LC50 estimated in a dynamic acute toxicity test, if possible. If the TI LC50 was not available, a time-dependent LC50 (e.g., 96-h LC50) was used; that is, AF = MATC/LC50. The AF was intended to provide an estimate of the relationship between a test material's chronic and acute toxicity, which could then be applied to aquatic organisms for which an MATC could not be derived due to difficulties in conducting a chronic toxicity test. In order to obtain an MATC for these organisms, the assumption was made that the AF for a given toxicant is relatively constant over a range of test species. The AF derived for species 1 and the LC50 for species 2 could then be used to estimate the MATC for species 2; that is, $AF_1 \times LC50_2 = MATC_2$. Although the AF has a value as a crude estimator, there are a number of cases in which this proportion does not hold true (Mount, 1976). Chronic toxicity tests are discussed in Chapter 4.

Early Life Stage Tests

These tests include continuous exposure of the early life stages (e.g., egg, embryo, larva, and fry) of aquatic organisms to various concentrations of a chemical for 1–2 mo, depending on the species. Although these tests do not provide total life cycle exposure and lack a full assessment of reproduction, they do include exposure during the most sensitive life stages. They have been used to accurately predict MATC values estimated in the life cycle tests. Early life stage tests are discussed in Chapter 3.

Bioaccumulation Tests

Chemicals with low solubility in water usually have an affinity for fatty tissues and thus can be stored and concentrated in tissues with a high lipid content. Such hydrophobic chemicals may persist in water and demonstrate cumulative toxicity to organisms. Chemicals with these characteristics are usually considered for bioconcentration tests, which are designed to determine or predict the *bioconcentration factor* (BCF). The BCF is the ratio of the average concentration of test chemical accumulated in the tissues of the test organisms under equilibrium conditions to the average measured concentration in the water to which the organisms are exposed.

Bioconcentration is the process by which chemicals from the water enter organisms, through gills or epithelial tissue, and are accumulated. *Bioaccumulation* is a broader term and includes not only bioconcentration but also accumulation of chemicals through consumption of food. *Biomagnification* refers to the total process, including bioconcentration and bioaccumulation, by which tissue concentrations of accumulated chemicals increase as the chemical passes through several trophic levels. Bioaccumulation tests are discussed in Chapter 17.

Other Sublethal Effects Tests

In the aquatic environment organisms are not usually exposed to high, acutely toxic concentrations of chemicals unless they are restricted to the vicinity of a chemical release site or spill area. Beyond the initial impact site dilution and dispersion occur, decreasing these acute concentrations to lower, sublethal levels. In general, a greater biomass is exposed to sublethal concentrations of chemicals than to acutely toxic lethal concentrations. The lower concentrations may not produce death, but they may have a profound effect on the future survival of the organisms.

Sublethal effects may be studied in the laboratory by a variety of procedures and generally are divided into three classes: biochemical and physiological, behavioral, and histological. Biochemical and physiological tests include studies of enzyme inhibition, clinical chemistry, hematology, and respiration. Since behavior represents an integrated response corresponding to complex biochemical and physiological functions, chemically induced behavioral changes may reflect effects on internal homeostasis. Behavioral end points may thus be sensitive indicators of sublethal effects. Behavioral effects that have received considerable attention in aquatic organisms are locomotion and swimming, attraction-avoidance, prey-predator relationships, aggression and territoriality, and learning. These are all ecologically significant behaviors. Histological studies are also useful because changes in histological structure may often significantly modify the function of tissues and organs. Together, behavioral, biochemical and physiological, and histological tests are useful for evaluating the environmental hazard of a chemical, and they may provide important information on its mode of action. These tests are discussed in Chapters 9, 10, and 11.

Data Usage

Aquatic toxicity test data have a variety of applications, including:

- Corporate industrial decisions on product development, manufacture, and commercialization.
- Registration of products to satisfy regulatory requirements.
- Permitting for the discharge of municipal and industrial wastes.
- Environmental hazard evaluations.
- Prosecution and defense of chemical-related activities in environmental litigation.

In developing a chemical as an intermediate or a final product it is necessary to consider the potential impact of that chemical on human health and on the terrestrial and aquatic environments. Corporate industrial decisions to proceed with the development of a chemical may include consideration of the potential effects on the aquatic environment resulting from its manufacture, transport, use, and disposal. Government authorization for the manufacture of new chemicals is regulated under the Toxic Substances Control Act (TSCA), which requires that a premanufacturing notification (PMN) be submitted for U.S. EPA review prior to full-scale manufacture of the chemical. For chemicals expected to be used, transported, or otherwise released into the aquatic environment, the PMN should include information on their potential toxicity to aquatic organisms. Many industrial chemicals do not survive the initial stages of development because they are toxic to aquatic organisms or are persistent in the aquatic environment.

For biocides such as insecticides, rodenticides, fungicides, and herbicides, the U.S. EPA requires that specific aquatic toxicity tests be conducted to evaluate the potential hazard to nontarget aquatic species and that the resulting data be submitted in support of registration permits for sale and use of these chemicals. In addition, biocide manufacturers frequently conduct aquatic toxicity tests to evaluate the efficacy of chemicals proposed to control pests (piscicides, molluscicides, algicides) in the aquatic environment.

Aquatic toxicity test data are also used to evaluate the potential hazard resulting from the discharge of municipal and industrial wastes (effluents) into the aquatic environment. Industrial discharges are regulated by the U.S. EPA under the National Pollutant Discharge Elimination System (NPDES) permit program. Permits, in fact, may require biomonitoring of industrial discharges. The *biomonitoring* required in the permits is a water quality surveillance program in which aquatic toxicity tests are conducted periodically (e.g., once every month or every 3–4 mo) to ascertain whether aquatic life may be endangered by discharge of the wastes.

Aquatic toxicity tests with indigenous species and site-specific conditions can be used to evaluate the potential environmental hazard of an unanticipated, accidental release of a chemical into the aquatic environment. This evaluation includes the potential human health hazard posed by contamination of commercially important aquatic species with a chemical. For example, bioconcentration studies indicate the extent to which a chemical present at some measurable concentration in the aquatic environment can be accumulated in the tissues of aquatic organisms consumed by humans.

With the relatively recent trend toward use of litigation to resolve concerns about environmental pollutants, aquatic toxicity tests have been used to evaluate the effects of accidental spills as well as long-term chemical releases under controlled conditions which permit the evaluation of causal relationships. That is, toxicity tests can be used to confirm or refute a relationship between observed effects and the concentrations of a chemical shown to exist or to have existed in the aquatic environment.

Some of these applications and uses of aquatic toxicity data are discussed in Chapters 20, 22, and 23.

Good Laboratory Practices

Important in all phases of aquatic toxicity testing, but especially critical with respect to regulatory and litigious matters, is quality assurance (QA) in the laboratory and adherence to good laboratory practices (GLPs) to promote the development of quality test data. Good laboratory practice is concerned with the conditions under which laboratory studies are planned, performed, monitored, recorded, and reported. Aquatic toxicity testing programs are classified as nonclinical laboratory studies, and GLP regulations published by the U.S. Department of Health, Education and Welfare, Food and Drug Administration (1978), and the U.S. Environmental Protection Agency (1980) describe the requirements for an acceptable study. These GLP requirements deal with all related aspects of testing, including *personnel*—their qualifications, responsibilities, management, and QA function; *facilities*—test animal maintenance and handling, chemical handling and storage, laboratory testing areas, specimen storage, and data handling and storage; *equipment*—design, maintenance, and calibration; *laboratory operations*—standard operating procedures, methods of animal care, and standard reagents and solutions; *test chemicals*—handling and storage, characterization, and use of solvents or carriers; *protocols*—test methods, data collection, and data handling; *reports*—data storage, retrieval, verification, use in reports, and retention; and *disqualification of testing facilities*—grounds for disqualification and public notice of such. These comprehensive regulations must be closely adhered to and the adherence must be supported by documentation capable of passing government inspection before a study is considered to meet the minimum test of adequacy. Failure to meet the major provisions of the GLP requirements can result in a ruling by the FDA or U.S. EPA that a study is unacceptable and must be repeated. A testing facility that has failed to comply with the GLP regulations can also be disqualified. Furthermore, these regulations apply to any facilities, including academic and industrial laboratories, that prepare data for submission to the FDA and U.S. EPA in support of regulated products.

CONCLUSION

Aquatic toxicology is a relatively new and still evolving discipline which has resulted from concern for the safety and preservation of the aquatic environment. Scientists from academic, industrial, and government institutions have made and are making significant contributions in this multidisciplinary science. The following chapters were written by scientists with expertise in the respective subdisciplines of aquatic toxicology. They present a comprehensive overview of the general concepts and state of the art in techniques, methodologies, research, and assessment of aquatic toxicology.

LITERATURE CITED

Adelman IR, Smith, LL, Jr: Fathead minnow (*Pimephales promelas*) and goldfish (*Carassius auratus*) as a standard fish in bioassays and their reaction to potential reference toxicants. J Fish Res Bd Can 33:209–214, 1976.

American Society for Testing and Materials: Standard practice for conducting acute toxicity tests with fishes, macroinvertebrates, and amphibians. ASTM E729-80. Philadelphia: ASTM, 1980a.

American Society for Testing and Materials: Standard practice for conducting toxicity tests with larvae of four species of bivalve molluscs. ASTM E724-80. Philadelphia: ASTM, 1980b.

American Society for Testing and Materials: Proposed standard practice for assessing the hazard of a material to aquatic organisms. In subcommittee E47.01, 1980c.

American Society for Testing and Materials: Proposed standard practice for conducting bioconcentration tests with fishes and saltwater bivalve molluscs. In subcommittee E47.01, 1980d.

American Society for Testing and Materials: Proposed standard practice for conducting chronic toxicity tests with the early life stages of fishes. In subcommittee E47.01, 1980e.

American Society for Testing and Materials: Proposed standard practice for conducting flow-through life cycle toxicity tests with *Daphnia magna*. In subcommittee E47.01, 1980f.

American Society for Testing and Materials: Proposed standard practice for conducting life cycle toxicity tests with mysid shrimp. In subcommittee E47.01, 1980g.

American Society for Testing and Materials: Proposed standard practice for conducting renewal life cycle toxicity tests with *Daphnia magna*. In subcommittee E47.01, 1980h.

American Society for Testing and Materials: Proposed standard practice for conducting static acute toxicity tests on wastewaters with *Daphnia*. In subcommittee D-19, 1980i.

American Society for Testing and Materials: Proposed standard practice for conducting tests with freshwater and saltwater algae. In subcommittee E47.01, 1980j.

American Society for Testing and Materials: Proposed standard practice for measuring the acute toxicity of effluents to fishes and macroinvertebrates. In subcommittee E47.01, 1980k.

APHA, AWWA, and WPCF: Standard Methods for the Examination of Water and Wastewater, 15th ed. Washington, D.C., 1981. American Public Health Association, American Water Works Association, and Water Pollution Control Federation.

Bliss CI: The method of probits. Science 79:38–39, 1934a.

Bliss CI: The method of probits—A correction. Science 79:409–410, 1934b.

Brusick DJ, Young RR, Hutchinson C, Vilkas AG, Gezo TA: Ecological assays. In: IERL–RTP Procedures Manual: Level 1 Environmental Assessment Biological Tests, pp. 69–112. EPA 68-02-2681. Washington, D.C.: U.S. EPA, Office of Research and Development, 1980.

Buikema AL, Jr, Niederlehner BR, Cairns J, Jr: Biological monitoring. IV. Toxicity testing. Water Res 16:239–262, 1982.

Cairns J, Jr, Thompson KW: A computer interfaced toxicity testing system for simulating variable effluent loading. In: Second Symposium on Process Measurements for Environmental Assessment, edited by PL Levin, JC Harris, KD Drewitz, pp. 183–198. Cambridge, Mass.: Arthur D. Little, 1980.

Committee on Methods for Acute Toxicity Tests with Aquatic Organisms: Methods for Acute Toxicity Tests with Fish, Macroinvertebrates and Amphibians. EPA-660/3-75-009. Washington, D.C.: U.S. EPA, 1975.

Davis JC, Hoos RAW: Use of sodium pentachlorophenate and dehydroabietic acid as reference toxicants for salmonid bioassays. J Fish Res Bd Can 32:411–416, 1975.

Davis JC: Standardization and protocols of bioassays—their role and significance for monitoring, research and regulatory usage. In: Proceedings of the 3rd Aquatic Toxicity Workshop, Halifax, Nova Scotia, November 2–3, 1976, edited by WR Parker, E Pessah, PG Wells, GF Westlake, pp. 1–14. EPS-5-AR-77-1, 1977.

Doudoroff P, Anderson BG, Burdick GE, Galtsoff PS, Hart WB, Pattrick R, Stronge ER, Surber EW, Van Horn WM: Bio-assay for the evaluation of acute toxicity of industrial wastes to fish. Sew Ind Wastes 23:1380–1397, 1951.

Duke KM, Davis ME, Dennis AJ: Ecological effects tests. In: IERL–RTP Procedures Manual: Level 1 Environmental Assessment Biological Tests for Pilot Studies, pp. 40–76. EPA-600/7-77-043. Washington, D.C.: U.S. EPA, Office of Research and Development, 1977.

Gaddum JH: Reports on biological standards. III. Methods of biological assay depending on quantal response. Medical Research Council Special Report Series 183. London: H.M.S.O., 1933.

Hunn JB, Schoettger RA, Wealdon E: Observations on the handling and maintenance of bioassay fish. Prog Fish Cult 30:164–167, 1968.

Klaverkamp JF, Kenney A, Harrison SE, Danell R: An evaluation of phenol and sodium azide as reference toxicants in rainbow trout. In: Second Annual Aquatic Toxicity Workshop 1975 Proceedings, Toronto, Ontario, November 4–5, 1975, edited by GR Craig, pp. 73–92, 1975.

Krogh A, Hemmingsen AM: The assay of insulin on rabbits and mice. Det Kgl Danske Videnskebernes Selskab Biol. VIII, 1928.

LaRoche E, Eisler R, Tarzwell CM: Bioassay procedures for oil and oil dispersant toxicity evaluation. J Water Pollut Control Fed 42:1982–1989, 1970.

Lee DR: Reference toxicants in quality control of aquatic bioassays. In: Aquatic Invertebrate Bioassays, edited by AL Buikema, Jr, JR Cairns, Jr, pp. 188–199. ASTM STP 715. Philadelphia: American Society for Testing and Materials, 1980.

Marking LL: Evaluation of p,p'-DDT as a reference toxicant in bioassays. Investigations in fish control. U.S. Dept Inter Fish Wildl Serv Resour Publ 14, 1966.

Miller WE, Greene JC, Shiroyama J: *Selenastrum capricornutum* Printz algal assay bottle test: Experimental design, application, and data interpretation protocol. EPA-600/9-78-018. Corvallis, Ore.: U.S. EPA, 1978.

Mount DI: Quarterly Report. Environmental Research Laboratory, Duluth, Minn.: U.S. EPA, 1976.

Mount DI, Stephan CE: A method of establishing acceptable toxicant limits for fish—malathion and the butoxyethanol ester of 2,4-D. Trans Am Fish Soc 96:185–193, 1967.

Organization for Economic Cooperation and Development: OECD Guidelines for Testing of Chemicals. Paris: OECD, 1981.

Peltier W: Methods for measuring the acute toxicity of effluents to aquatic organisms. EPA-600/4-78-012. Washington, D.C.: U.S. EPA, 1978.

Pessah E, Wells PG, Schneider JR: Dodecyl sodium sulfate (DSS) as an intralaboratory reference toxicant in fish bioassays. In: Second Annual Aquatic Toxicity Workshop 1975 Proceedings, Toronto, Ontario, November 4–5, 1975, edited by GR Craig, pp. 93–114.

Sprague JB: Measurement of pollutant toxicity to fish. I. Bioassay methods for acute toxicity. Water Res 3:793–821, 1969.

U.S. Department of Health, Education and Welfare, Food and Drug Administration: Nonclinical laboratory studies. Good laboratory practice regulations. Fed Regist 43:59986–60025, 1978.

U.S. Environmental Protection Agency: Proposed environmental standards and proposed good laboratory practice standards for physical, chemicals, persistence, and ecological effects testing. Fed Regist 45:77332–77365, 1980.

U.S. Environmental Protection Agency, Corps of Engineers, Technical Committee on Criteria for Dredged and Fill Material: Ecological evaluation of proposed discharge of dredged material into ocean waters. Vicksburg, Miss.: Environmental Effects Laboratory, U.S. Army Engineer Waterways Experiment Station, 1977.

U.S. Environmental Protection Agency, Environmental Research Laboratory: Recommended bioassay procedure for bluegill, *Lepomis macrochirus*, partial chronic tests. Duluth, Minn.: U.S. EPA, 1972a.

U.S. Environmental Protection Agency, Environmental Research Laboratory: Recommended bioassay procedure for brook trout, *Salvelinus fontinalis* (Mitchell), partial chronic tests. Duluth, Minn.: U.S. EPA, 1972b.

U.S. Environmental Protection Agency, Environmental Research Laboratory: Recommended bioassay procedure for fathead minnow *Pimephales promelas* Rafinesque, chronic tests. Duluth, Minn.: U.S. EPA, 1972c.

U.S. Environmental Protection Agency, Environmental Research Laboratory: Recommended bioassay procedure for *Jordanella floridae* (Goode and Bean) chronic tests. Duluth, Minn.: U.S. EPA, no date.

U.S. Environmental Protection Agency, Environmental Research Laboratory, Office of Research and Development: Bioassay procedures for the ocean disposal permit program. EPA-600/9-76-010. Washington, D.C.: U.S. EPA, 1976.

U.S. Environmental Protection Agency, Environmental Research Laboratory, Office of Research and Development: Bioassay procedures for the ocean disposal permit program. EPA-600/9-78-010. Washington, D.C.: U.S. EPA, 1978.

U.S. Environmental Protection Agency, Environmental Research Laboratory: Tentative guidelines for flow-through early life stage toxicity tests with fathead minnows. Unpublished report. Duluth, Minn.: U.S. EPA, 1979.

U.S. Environmental Protection Agency, Pacific Northwest Environmental Research Laboratory: Algal assay procedure: Bottle test. Corvallis, Ore.: U.S. EPA, 1971.

U.S. Environmental Protection Agency, Pacific Northwest Environmental Research Laboratory: Marine algal assay procedure: Bottle test. Corvallis, Ore.: U.S. EPA, 1974.

Willford WA: Toxicity of dimethyl sulfoxide (DMSO) to fish. Bur Sport Fish Wildl Invest Fish Control 20:3–8, 1968.

SUPPLEMENTAL READING

Butler GC (ed): Principles of Ecotoxicology. New York: Wiley, 1978.

Cairns J, Jr, Dickson KL (eds): Biological Methods for the Assessment of Water Quality. ASTM STP 528. Philadelphia: American Society for Testing and Materials, 1973.

Cairns J, Jr, Dickson KL, Maki AW (eds): Estimating the Hazard of Chemical Substances to Aquatic Life. ASTM STP 657. Philadelphia:

American Society for Testing and Materials, 1978.

Committee to Review Methods for Ecotoxicology: Testing for Effects of Chemicals on Ecosystems. Washington, D.C.: National Academy of Sciences Press, 1981.

Cox GV (ed): Marine Bioassays Workshop Proceedings 1974. American Petroleum Institute, Environmental Protection Agency, Marine Technology Society. Washington, D.C.: Marine Technology Society, 1974.

Glass GE (ed): Bioassay Techniques and Environmental Chemistry. Ann Arbor, Mich.: Ann Arbor Science Publishers, 1973.

McLean MP, McNicol RE, Scherer E (eds): Bibliography of toxicity test methods for the aquatic environment. Can Spec Publ Fish Aquat Sci 50, 1980.

Scherer E (ed): Toxicity tests for freshwater organisms. Can Spec Publ Fish Aquat Sci 44, 1979.

Toxicity Testing

Chapter 2
Acute Toxicity Tests

P. R. Parrish

INTRODUCTION

In the period since World War II, acute toxicity tests have been used extensively to determine the effects of potentially toxic materials (e.g., pesticides, metals, and industrial effluents) on aquatic organisms during short-term (usually 4 d or less) exposure. Most of the earlier acute aquatic toxicity tests were conducted with freshwater organisms, especially fishes, but the requirement for assessing the impact of test materials in the estuarine and marine environment has provided the impetus for the development of test methods for saltwater organisms, both invertebrates and fishes. This development has been most pronounced during the past 10–15 yr.

Toxicity tests with unicellular algae (phytotoxicity tests) have also been widely employed to screen chemicals, especially chemicals known to be herbicides or suspected of having phytotoxic activity. Such tests have been conducted according to the same principles as invertebrate and fish tests. However, even a 4- or 5-d exposure represents a chronic exposure of the algal population because growth rate and cell density have probably reached their maximum during this time. Thus, although they are short-term tests, phytotoxicity tests are based on the life cycle of the test organism and will be discussed only briefly in this chapter. Appropriate references for algal test methods are cited in the supplemental reading section.

The trend toward conducting acute toxicity tests according to uniform, detailed methods is relatively new, having been promoted most vigorously by the Committee on Methods for Toxicity Tests with Aquatic Organisms. The committee was formed in 1971, and the result of its efforts was a

U.S. Environmental Protection Agency (U.S. EPA) publication on acute toxicity tests (Committee on Methods for Toxicity Tests with Aquatic Organisms, 1975). The committee was dissolved because it was logical that the movement toward standardization of toxicity test methods be brought under the auspices of a consensus-type organization. Thus, the American Society for Testing and Materials (ASTM) has been the most recent focal point for test method standardization. At the time of this writing, two "standard practices" on acute test methods have been published (ASTM, 1980a,b), and several other standard practices on long-term test methods are near completion. A second contribution to the standardization of test methods has been the publication of Standard Methods for the Examination of Water and Wastewater by the American Public Health Association, American Water Works Association, and Water Pollution Control Federation (APHA, AWWA, and WPCF, 1981).

The application of routine acute toxicity test methods to evaluate the effects of test materials other than individual chemicals is valid. Tests have been conducted with industrial effluents for more than 35 yr, and more recently tests with dredged materials, drilling muds, and mine tailings have been conducted.

Because the principles for conducting acute toxicity tests with freshwater and saltwater organisms are essentially the same, the basic methods for testing will be discussed in this chapter with appropriate consideration given to special conditions for each aquatic medium.

GENERAL PRINCIPLES OF ACUTE TOXICITY TESTS

The objective of an acute aquatic toxicity test is to determine the concentration of a test material (e.g., a chemical or effluent) or the level of an agent (e.g., temperature or pH) that produces a deleterious effect on a group of test organisms during a short-term exposure under controlled conditions. Although toxicity tests with aquatic

organisms can be conducted by administering the material directly by injection or incorporating it into food, most tests are conducted by exposing groups of organisms to several treatments in which different concentrations of the material are mixed in water. Because death is an easily detected deleterious response, the most common acute toxicity test is the acute lethality test. The criteria for death are usually lack of movement (especially gill movement in fishes) and lack of reaction to gentle prodding. Experimentally, a 50% response is the most reproducible measure of the toxicity of a test material, and 96 h (or less) is the standard exposure time because it usually covers the period of acute lethal action. Therefore, the measure of acute toxicity most frequently used with fish and macroinvertebrates is the 96-h median lethal concentration (96-h LC50). However, because death is not easily determined for some invertebrates, an EC50 (median effective concentration) is estimated rather than an LC50. The effect used for estimating the EC50 with some invertebrates (e.g., daphnids and midge larvae) is immobilization, which is defined as lack of movement. The effects generally used for estimating the EC50 with crabs, crayfish, and shrimp are immobilization and loss of equilibrium, defined as inability to maintain normal posture.

A common acute testing approach is to structure a test so that a quantal response (i.e., an all-or-none response: dead or alive) is elicited. The relation between test material concentration and the percentage of exposed organisms affected can then be determined and a concentration-mortality curve plotted. Results of short-term tests have generally been expressed as (1) the percentage of organisms killed or immobilized in each test concentration, and (2) the LC50 or EC50 derived by observation (i.e., where 50% of the test organisms were killed in a concentration), interpolation, or calculation. When the median lethal concentration is calculated, the 95% confidence limits associated with that value are usually also reported.

Test organisms in acute toxicity tests may be exposed to the test materials by one of four tech-

ave. toxicity in a variable effluent is not as important as: 1) max. toxicity 2) freq. of occurance

niques—static, recirculation, renewal, or flow-through—as described in Chapter 1.

Acute lethality tests have been useful in providing rapid estimates of the concentrations of test materials that cause direct, irreversible harm to the test organism. The static and flow-through techniques are the most widely used in acute toxicity tests. As stated by Macek et al. (1978), static acute tests provide practical means for (1) deriving estimates of the upper limit of concentrations that produce toxic effects, (2) evaluating the relative toxicity of large numbers of test materials, (3) evaluating the relative sensitivity of different aquatic organisms to test materials, (4) evaluating the effects of water quality (e.g., dissolved oxygen concentration, pH, salinity, hardness, suspended particulates) on the toxicity of the test materials, and (5) developing an understanding of the concentration-response relationship and of the significance of duration of exposure to the test material. Flow-through acute tests enhance the ability to maintain satisfactory test conditions and are not limited in duration; thus they allow a more complete assessment of the relationship between exposure duration and effect.

METHODOLOGY FOR FISH AND INVERTEBRATES

Test Material

The test material may be one or more pure chemical compounds or a complex mixture such as an effluent or formulation. It should be representative of the material as it is used or as it enters the aquatic environment. The sample of test material may be collected by a single "grab" if the composition of the material remains relatively constant. Composite grab sampling is recommended for static tests with effluents whose composition is relatively constant. A composite effluent sample consisting of grab samples collected at each of four consecutive 6-h intervals is recommended. For effluents that are not constant in composition, samples should be collected at different times.

They should not be combined because knowledge of the maximum toxicity level and its potential frequency of occurrence is more important than knowledge of the average toxicity of a variable effluent. With an effluent of variable quality it is better to conduct a flow-through toxicity test, if possible. If a flow-through test is conducted and continuous sampling is impractical, a composite sample should be collected and transported to the effluent delivery system at least every 6 h. Each new sample should be used only during the time until the next sample delivery. An effluent sample should completely fill the sample container to exclude as much air space as possible, and the container should be sealed.

Test materials that are stable can be transported and stored in appropriate containers for reasonable periods. Test materials other than effluents should be stored in a place that is cool (to minimize chemical or biochemical degradation) and dark (to minimize photodegradation). Volatile test materials should be kept in tightly sealed, refrigerated containers (to minimize loss to atmosphere), but allowed to come to room temperature before testing. Effluents should be transported at a low (but above freezing) temperature and delivered to the testing facility within 24 h after collection. Effluents, especially those containing organic matter subject to bacterial decomposition, should be refrigerated at approximately 4°C but should never be frozen.

If required, stock solutions of the test material should be prepared in advance so that the appropriate volume can be easily added to the dilution water (directly in static tests or via some delivery system in flow-through tests) to obtain the different test concentrations. All solutions needed for a toxicity test should be prepared from the same sample of test material. Any undissolved material should be uniformly dispersed by shaking or mixing the stock solution before a sample is withdrawn and added to dilution water in the test containers. If possible, the test material should be added directly to the dilution water, without the use of any solvent or carrier other than water. If a solvent/carrier is necessary, the organic chemicals triethylene glycol (TEG) and dimethyl formamide (DMF) are preferred because of their low toxicity to aquatic organisms, low volatility, and ability to dissolve many organic materials. However, other solvent/carriers such as acetone, methanol, and ethanol may be used. When a solvent/carrier other than water is used, it is recommended that its concentration in the test solution be kept at a minimum and not exceed 0.5 ml/l. There may be tests in which this limit cannot be met, and in those tests higher concentrations are permitted as long as an appropriate solvent/carrier control is used and the test organisms show no sign of stress or toxicity in the solvent/carrier control.

Effluent tests should be conducted with a sample that has not been aerated or altered in any way. Undissolved materials should be dispersed by gentle agitation immediately before removal of a subsample and addition to dilution water. In flow-through tests, undissolved material may be kept in suspension by using a stirring device. The effluent sample should be used directly as a stock solution, but it may be necessary to prepare a stock solution by diluting the effluent with filtered freshwater or saltwater to obtain the desired concentration and volume for mixing with the dilution water. Stock solutions or test solutions should be prepared as a volume-to-volume ratio of dilution water and liquid effluent so that the percentage of effluent in each of the test solutions can be calculated. If the effluent is a solid waste, dilution should be on a weight-to-volume basis. If a volume-to-volume basis is used and the concentration is to be expressed as weight per unit volume, a correction should be made for specific gravity.

Dilution Water

Adequate dilution water for the test organisms and for the purpose of the test must be available. For an acute toxicity test, the minimal criterion for acceptable dilution water is that test organisms will live in it during acclimation to test conditions and testing without being stressed. Dilution water

should be well aerated before organisms or test material are added in order to bring the pH and concentrations of dissolved oxygen and other gases into equilibrium with the ambient air and thus minimize oxygen demand and concentration of volatiles. The initial concentration of dissolved oxygen in the dilution water should be greater than 90% of the saturation value. Dilution water that may contain undesirable microorganisms should be passed through a properly maintained ultraviolet sterilizer.

For effluent tests, the dilution water should be representative of the receiving water and should be obtained as close to the point of effluent discharge as possible, but upstream from the point of discharge or outside the zone of influence of the effluent. If acceptable dilution water cannot be obtained from the receiving water, some other uncontaminated surface, ground, or reconstituted water may be used; however, the water quality characteristics (e.g., hardness, alkalinity, salinity, and specific conductance) should be within approximately 25% and 0.2 pH unit of those of the receiving water at the time of the test. The dilution water should be uncontaminated, of constant quality, and should meet the specifications outlined by the ASTM (1980a).

Dilution water for tests with freshwater organisms should be obtained from an uncontaminated well or spring, if possible. Dechlorinated tap water should be used only if no other water supply is available. Whenever possible, dilution water with a hardness of 40–48 mg/l as $CaCO_3$ should be used for acute tests (ASTM, 1980a).

Dilution water for tests with saltwater organisms should be obtained from an uncontaminated natural body of water and filtered through a non-contaminating filter of 5-μm porosity before use. Reconstituted saltwater (ASTM, 1980a) or commercial sea salts may also be used for acute toxicity tests. Whenever possible, water of higher salinity—30–34 parts per thousand (ppt)—should be used when testing stenohaline species, and water of lower salinity (20–25 ppt) when testing euryhaline species.

Test Animals

Test animals should be sensitive, important species indigenous to the area of impact of a test material. They can be collected from wild populations in relatively unpolluted areas, purchased from commercial suppliers, or amenable to culture in the laboratory. Animals should not be collected by electroshocking or use of chemicals because of the physiological stress induced by these methods. All animals in a test should be from the same source. Test species may also be selected on the basis of availability and commercial, recreational, and ecological importance. The most commonly used species in acute aquatic toxicity tests are listed in Table 1.

Collecting, transporting, and handling animals should be done in a manner that minimizes injury and physiological stress. For example, many invertebrates and fishes can be collected by seining. It is far less harmful to the animals to scoop them from the water with a soft net and place them in a water-filled container while they are still within the enclosed seine in shallow water than to beach the seine. Also, slow tows of very short duration are recommended when trawls or other towed devices must be used to collect animals.

Containers for transporting animals should be circular or elliptical to prevent the animals from crowding in corners or damaging themselves by striking the walls (Cox, 1974), but conventional styrofoam coolers have proved acceptable. Other arrangements, such as the use of water-filled plastic bags inside the container, have also been successful. The density of animals in a container will vary according to the kind of animal, but it should never be great enough to stress the animals. When temporary containment and transportation time will be more than 30 min, additional measures should be taken to promote optimal conditions. For example, it may be necessary to shield the animals from sunlight, to protect them from extreme heat or cold, or to aerate water in order to maintain dissolved oxygen concentrations. For some sessile or slow-moving animals, large volumes of

Table 1 Fish and Invertebrate Species Commonly Used for Acute Toxicity Tests

Freshwater
  Vertebrates
    Rainbow trout, *Salmo gairdneri*
    Brook trout, *Salvelinus fontinalis*
    Fathead minnow, *Pimephales promelas*
    Channel catfish, *Ictalurus punctatus*
    Bluegill, *Lepomis macrochirus*
  Invertebrates
    Daphnids, *Daphnia magna, D. pulex, D. pulicaria*
    Amphipods, *Gammarus lacustris, G. fasciatus,*
      G. pseudolimnaeus
    Crayfish, *Orconectes* sp., *Cambarus* sp., *Procambarus*
      sp., or *Pacifastacus leniusculus*
    Midges, *Chironomus* sp.
    Snails, *Physa integra*
Saltwater
  Vertebrates
    Sheepshead minnow, *Cyprinodon variegatus*
    Mummichog, *Fundulus heteroclitus*
    Longnose killifish, *Fundulus similis*
    Silverside, *Menidia* sp.
    Threespine stickleback, *Gasterosteus aculeatus*
    Pinfish, *Lagodon rhomboides*
    Spot, *Leiostomus xanthurus*
    Sand dab, *Citharichthys stigmaeus*
  Invertebrates
    Copepods, *Acartia tonsa, Acartia clausi*
    Shrimp, *Penaeus setiferus, P. duorarum, P. aztecus*
    Grass shrimp, *Palaemonetes pugio, P. vulgaris*
    Sand shrimp, *Crangon septemspinosa*
    Mysid shrimp, *Mysidopsis bahia*
    Blue crab, *Callinectes sapidus*
    Fiddler crab, *Uca* sp.
    Oyster, *Crassostrea virginica, C. gigas*
    Polychaetes, *Capitella capitata, Neanthes* sp.

water may not be needed and materials such as wet seaweed or cloth may be used to provide moisture during transportation.

A separate, uncontaminated area at the testing facility should be set aside for maintaining test animals. When organisms are brought there, they should be quarantined at least until it is apparent that they are disease-free. Animals should be maintained in good condition, that is, without crowding and with adequate dissolved oxygen concentrations. To minimize stress, organisms should not be subjected to rapid changes in temperature or water quality. As a rule, organisms should not be subjected to more than 5°C gradual change in water temperature in any 24-h period, and saltwater organisms should not be subjected to more than a 5 ppt gradual salinity change in 24 h. Organisms should be fed at least once a day and tanks cleaned as needed. Recently collected animals may not eat, but this initial nonfeeding period may be shortened by "social facilitation," that is, by adding animals of the same species which are already feeding to the holding tank. One must not indiscriminately mix animals from different lots because of possible differences in age, condition, and stage of acclimation. When animals do not begin to eat, or stop eating after having begun, unhealthy conditions may be indicated. Animals should be carefully observed for signs of disease, stress, physical damage, and mortality. Dead, diseased, and abnormal individuals must be discarded.

During collection, transportation, and maintenance, organisms must be handled as little as possible. When necessary, transferring animals from one container to another should be accomplished gently and quickly. Small, soft nylon dipnets are generally best for moving larger organisms. Such nets are commercially available, or can be made from small-mesh nylon netting, nylon or silk bolting cloth, plankton netting, or similar material. Smooth-bore glass tubes with fire-polished ends and rubber bulbs should be used for transferring smaller organisms such as daphnids, midge larvae, copepods, and mysid shrimp.

It is generally recommended that fish be maintained for 7–14 d and invertebrates for 2–4 d after collection or transportation. All animals should be held in uncontaminated dilution water under stable conditions of temperature and water quality in a flow-through system with a flow rate of at least two water volume additions per day, or in a recirculating system in which the water flows through an appropriate filter.

Test organisms amenable to laboratory culture should be reared in dilution water at test temperature. Other animals should be acclimated simultaneously to the dilution water and test tempera-

ture in a flow-through system after transferring an appropriate number of similar sized animals to an acclimation tank by (1) gradually changing the water in the acclimation tank from 100% holding water to 100% dilution water over a period of 2 or more days, and (2) changing the water temperature at a gradual rate (not more than 5°C in 24 h) until the test temperature range is reached. Animals should be maintained for at least 2 d in the dilution water at the test temperature before a test is begun. Longer acclimation is generally desirable for fishes but may be unnecessary for invertebrates (Tatem et al., 1976).

In view of the importance of beginning a toxicity test with healthy organisms, a group of test animals must not be used for a test if they appear to be diseased or otherwise stressed or if more than 10% died during the 48 h immediately before the test. If a group fails to meet these criteria, it must be either discarded or treated for disease and reacclimated as described above.

Organisms should be uniform in size, age, and physiological condition to minimize variability of response to the test material. The small, early life stages of invertebrates and fishes (approximately 0.5 g each) and invertebrates with relatively short life cycles (approximately 60 d or less) must be fed up to the beginning of the test. Other organisms should not be fed for 24 h before the beginning of the test, nor should they be fed during the test to minimize variability due to nutritional and metabolic condition.

Most freshwater and some saltwater fishes may be chemically treated to prevent or cure diseases by using recommended treatments (ASTM, 1980a). If the fishes are severely diseased, however, it is often better to destroy the entire group. All diseased animals other than fishes should be discarded unless effective treatment is available. Since fishes have probably been stressed during collection or transportation (and because some are treated during transit), they should not be treated during the first 12–24 h after they arrive at the facility. Further, treated animals should be maintained for at least 4 d after treatment before they are used in a test.

If diseases occur among animal populations in a facility, care should be taken to isolate the diseased populations and to adequately clean the containers in which the diseased animals were maintained.

Exposure Apparatus

Static Acute Tests

The equipment necessary to conduct static acute toxicity tests includes a constant-temperature room or temperature-controlled water bath in which to place the test chambers, as well as an appropriate number of test chambers. The size and configuration of test chambers will vary according to the size of the test animals; the chambers can be glass finger bowls, jars, tanks, aquaria, beakers, crystallizing dishes, and so on. If the test containers are constructed in the testing facility, they should be made from materials that do not contain any substances that can leach or dissolve in the water and adversely affect the test animals. Likewise, materials and equipment that come in contact with stock solutions of test material should be chosen to minimize sorption of the test material. To minimize leaching, dissolution, and sorption, containers made of glass, no. 316 stainless steel, or perfluorocarbon plastics (e.g., Teflon) should be used whenever possible. Plasticized materials (nonrigid, soft plastics), rubber, copper, brass, or lead should not be used in any water delivery system as a test chamber, or in any exposure apparatus.

Flow-through Acute Tests

As with static tests, a constant-temperature room or temperature-controlled water bath is necessary to hold test chambers. There should also be a dilution water tank placed so that dilution water can flow into the test material delivery system. Temperature control and aeration for the dilution water tank are desirable. The heating/chilling device should be impervious to corrosion by the dilution water and the air used for aeration should

be free of oil and fumes. Filters to remove oil and water are also desirable. Materials for construction of other flow-through test system parts should be the same as described above.

Although many toxicant delivery systems have been used successfully, the proportional diluter (Mount and Brungs, 1967; Lemke et al., 1978) is probably best for routine use. Diluters can be constructed in the testing facility or can be purchased from a commercial source. A diluter consists of water cells of known volume which receive various volumes of uncontaminated dilution water and chemical cells of known volume which receive various volumes of test solution. Water from the various dilution water cells siphons down and mixes with the test solution from the various chemical cells to produce the test material concentrations. Chambers to promote mixing of the test solution and the dilution water are located between the diluter and the test chambers (Fig. 1).

The proportional diluter can generally deliver five to seven different test concentrations and uncontaminated water for a control at any desired flow rate up to 400 ml/min and with dilution factors from 0.75 to 0.50. If necessary, metering cells can be exchanged to provide dilution factors outside this range. The flow rates through the test chambers should be at least five tank volume additions per 24 h, but the size of the test animals, the size of the test chambers, and the loading (ratio of test animal biomass to total volume of test water in the chamber) should also be considered. The rates should be able to maintain desirable temperatures, oxygen concentrations, and safe concentrations of metabolites.

For effluent tests in which the highest test concentration might be nearly 100% effluent, the proportional diluter can be modified by introducing 100% effluent directly into the chemical cells and eliminating the first water and mixing cells (Fig. 2). A gradient of effluent concentrations, based on the dilution factor of the system, results.

The calibration of the toxicant delivery system should be checked before each test. This includes

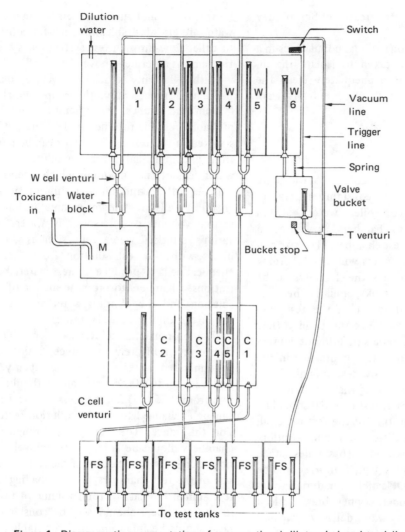

Figure 1 Diagrammatic representation of a proportional diluter designed to deliver serial concentrations of a chemical in clean dilution water to replicate test aquaria. Abbreviations: W1–W6, dilution water cells; M, mixing chamber in which the chemical is mixed with dilution water to produce a concentration equivalent to the highest to be tested; C1–C5, chemical cells, each of which contains the same concentration of the chemical as the other cells and the chemical mixing chamber; FS, flow-splitting cells, which divide the combined volume from the complementary water and chemical cells (e.g., W2 + C2) into two or more equal flows to the replicate test aquaria. *[Modified from Lemke et al. (1978).]*

the determination of the flow rate through each test chamber and measurement of either the concentration of toxicant in each test chamber or the volume of solution used in each portion of the delivery system. The general operation of the system should be checked at least daily during a test.

Experimental Design

The minimum number of test animals to be exposed to each treatment is 10 for a static test and 20 for a flow-through test. Depending on size and requirements of the test species, animals may be divided between two or more test chambers. Use of more organisms and replicate test chambers for each treatment is generally recommended, but the effort (and cost) necessary to test extremely large numbers of animals may not be worth the diminishing confidence in the data obtained (Jensen, 1972).

Distribution of test animals in the test chambers is important. A representative subsample of the test organism population should be impartially distributed, by adding either 2 animals (if there are to be 10 or fewer animals per chamber) or 4 animals (if there are to be more than 10 animals per chamber) to each chamber, and then adding 2 or 4 more, and repeating the process until each chamber has the correct number of test organisms in it. For very small organisms (e.g., daphnids or copepods) it is often convenient to place animals

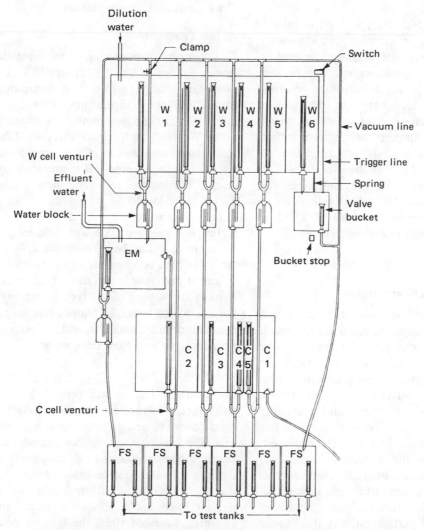

Figure 2 Diagrammatic representation of a proportional diluter designed to deliver serial concentrations of an effluent in clean dilution water to replicate test aquaria. Abbreviations: W1–W6, dilution water cells; EM, effluent mixing chamber; C1–C5, effluent cells; FS, flow-splitting cells. *[Modified from Lemke et al. (1978)]*

in interim containers during the distribution process and then gently add them to the test chambers as a group.

Weights and lengths or widths of test animals should be determined by measuring a group of representative animals from the test population immediately before the test or by measuring the control animals immediately after the test. If the former practice is followed, the animals that were weighed and measured should not be used in the test.

Every test requires a control. The control is a treatment consisting of the same dilution water, conditions, procedures, and organisms as used in the remainder of the test, except that no test material is added. If a solvent/carrier or other additive is used, a solvent/carrier or additive control should be maintained. This additional control is the same as the dilution water control except that the greatest volume of solvent/carrier or additive present in any other test chamber is added to this treatment. A test is generally not considered acceptable if more than 10% of the animals die in any control in a test to determine an LC50 or show the effect in a test to determine an EC50.

Test Conditions

Dissolved Oxygen Concentration

Test solutions in the test chambers or in the test material delivery system should not be aerated. If the dilution water is aerated before it enters the test chamber or delivery system (static or flow-through) and proper loading is ensured (discussed below), the dissolved oxygen concentration should remain ⩾60% of saturation during an entire flow-through test and the first 48 h of a static test and ⩾40% of saturation after 48 h in a static test. In situations where the dissolved oxygen concentration decreases substantially, test animals should be carefully observed for signs of stress. In tests with materials of known high biochemical oxygen demand (e.g., effluents), it is often useful to set up an additional test chamber containing the highest concentration of test material but no test

animals. The effect of the test material alone on the dissolved oxygen concentration can be monitored in this treatment and a judgment can be made at the conclusion of the test about the relative contribution of low dissolved oxygen concentration to toxicity. Alternatively, one can test materials known to deplete the dissolved oxygen concentration under both aerated and unaerated conditions in order to determine the toxicity of the test material in adequate and low dissolved oxygen concentrations.

Test Temperature

Test temperatures generally recommended are from the series 7, 12, 17, 22, and 27°C. The derivation of these increments is interesting—they come from the temperatures of well water at major industry and government freshwater laboratories. Whatever temperature is chosen, the actual test temperature should not instantaneously deviate from the selected test temperature by more than 2° during the test. The mean temperature during the test should be within ±1° of the selected temperature.

For flow-through tests with effluents, the test temperature should be between the daily low and the daily high temperature of the receiving water measured just outside the zone of influence of the effluent at the time of the test. Depending on the purpose of the tests, the temperature may remain constant or may fluctuate within the same temperature range as the receiving water.

Loading

The grams of test animals (biomass) per liter of test solution in the test chambers should not be great enough to unduly influence the results of the test. The loading must be low enough to ensure that the concentrations of dissolved oxygen and toxicant are not decreased below acceptable limits, that the concentrations of metabolic products are not increased above acceptable limits, and that crowding does not stress the test animals. Maximum recommended loading is generally 0.5–0.8 g/l for static tests and 1–10 g/l of test solution passing through the test chamber in 24 h for flow-through tests, based on the test temperature (ASTM, 1980a).

Test Procedures

Range-finding Test (precedes definitive test)

When test materials of unknown toxicity are tested, it is almost always necessary to conduct a range-finding test to determine the concentrations of test material that should be used in the full-scale definitive test. A range-finding test requires less effort than a definitive test, but the results of a good range-finding test go far toward ensuring success in the definitive test. Generally, groups of 3–5 animals are exposed to at least three test material concentrations spaced at order-of-magnitude intervals based on a logarithmic ratio (e.g., 0.01, 0.1, 1, 10, and 100 mg/l or ppm); a control is maintained concurrently. If the material is an effluent, the test concentrations are set up as a percentage of the effluent in the test concentration by volume (e.g., 0.01, 0.1, 1, 10, and 100%). Ideally, the duration of the range-finding test is the same as that planned for the definitive test, but in certain instances (if all acute toxic effect has been exerted) the test may be terminated. It is emphasized, however, that the range-finding test serves its function best when it most closely follows the conditions planned for the definitive test.

Definitive Test

For the determination of an LC50 or an EC50, the appropriate number of test animals should be exposed to at least five concentrations of test material or effluent in a geometric progression (that is, the sequence of concentrations should be such that the ratio of a concentration to its predecessor is always the same, as in 10, 5, 2.5, 1.25, and 0.62 ppm). Use of more than five concentrations may provide additional data and allow calculation of narrower confidence limits around the median effect concentration, but the effort (cost) to set up and monitor the extra concentrations should be weighed against the potential gain.

Ideally, a definitive test should meet the following criteria so that an LC50 or EC50 and reasonable confidence limits can be calculated:

- Each test material concentration should be at least 50% of the next higher test material concentration (for example, 60, 30, 15, 7.5, and 3.75 ppb).
- Fewer than 35% of the test animals in one treatment (other than the control) should have been killed or affected, and more than 65% of the test animals in one treatment should have been killed or affected. It is best to have several test concentrations in which some animals are killed or affected (ASTM, 1980a). Obviously, the effect should be related to the concentration of test material.

Beginning a Test

Static tests are begun by (1) adding the appropriate amount or volume of test material to the dilution water in the test chambers, (2) stirring the mixture, (3) making necessary chemical and physical measurements (discussed in detail below), and (4) adding the test animals. The animals should be placed in the test chambers within 1 h after addition of the test material.

Flow-through tests are begun by following essentially the same procedure, except that the test animals are placed in the chambers after the test solutions have been flowing through the exposure apparatus long enough to ensure equilibrium within the system and relatively constant concentrations of test material. Equilibrium can be verified by chemical analyses of test material in water samples from test chambers, if methods are available.

Feeding

Test organisms should not usually be fed while in the test chambers. Minimal feeding may be necessary, however, if (1) cannibalistic animals cannot be separated or restrained, or (2) the test duration constitutes a relatively large portion of the organism's life span. If feeding is necessary, all uneaten food should be removed so that dissolved oxygen and test material concentrations will not be reduced.

Duration

A test begins at the time the test animals are first placed in the test material or control. The normal duration of the acute toxicity test is 96 h, but some animals (daphnids, oyster larvae, and others) are exposed for only 48 h because of problems associated with longer exposure times or because the intent is to test up to a specific point in the developmental process of the animal.

Biological Data

The number of dead or affected animals in each test chamber should be counted every 24 ± 1 h from the beginning of the test until the termination. Death is the criterion for effect most often used in acute toxicity tests to estimate the LC50. The criteria for death are usually lack of movement and lack of reaction to gentle prodding. Since death is not easily determined for some invertebrates, effects such as immobilization and loss of equilibrium are used to estimate the EC50. Other effects can be used to determine an EC50, but the effect and its definition must always be reported. During all tests, general observations of erratic swimming, loss of reflex, discoloration, changes in behavior, excessive mucus production, hyperventilation, opaque eyes, curved spine, hemorrhaging, molting, and cannibalism should be quantified and reported.

Chemical and Physical Data

If a freshwater dilution water is used, the hardness, alkalinity, pH, suspended particulate matter, and specific conductance should be measured. If a saltwater dilution water is used, its salinity, suspended particulate matter, and pH should be measured. The dissolved oxygen concentration should be measured at the beginning of the test and every 24 ± 1 h thereafter until the end of the test in all treatments in which there are living test animals. The pH should be measured at least at the

beginning and end of the test in all treatments. Temperature, salinity or hardness, alkalinity, and specific conductance in the control should be measured and recorded daily.

If possible (if methods are available and costs are not prohibitive), the concentration of test material should be measured at least at the beginning and end of the test in all test chambers, especially in flow-through toxicity tests. Measurements at 24-h intervals are recommended. When test material concentrations are not measured in flow-through tests, the usefulness of the technique may be greatly diminished because the results of this test may lead to a need for further testing. The analytical method for measuring test material concentrations should be validated before the test. The accuracy of the method can be determined by the method of known additions, using dilution water from the tanks that contain test organisms or from the diluter. An analytical chemist should provide detailed information about the efficiency of the method. It is recommended, however, that standard solutions corresponding to the low, middle, and high concentrations plus a control (blank) be analyzed in determining percentage recovery of a method. This procedure allows quantification of the efficiency of the analytical method and the results assist in interpreting biological results. Generally, atomic absorption spectrophotometric methods are used for metals and gas chromatographic methods for organic test materials; colorimetric methods are not usually recommended (ASTM, 1980a). Techniques for chemical analyses are discussed in Chapter 16.

When water samples are taken from test chambers for chemical analyses, it is important that they be representative of the concentration to which the test animals are being exposed. Samples should be taken midway between the top, bottom, and sides of the test chambers and should not include surface scum or material stirred up from the bottom or sides. Samples should be treated immediately and appropriately to preserve the material being tested and the analytical method being used.

Data Analysis and Interpretation

Calculations

Based on the data from a test, time-dependent LC50s or EC50s and their 95% confidence limits should be calculated for each 24-h period by using the average measured concentrations of test material for flow-through tests, if concentrations are measured. If test material concentrations are not measured, the nominal (intended) initial concentrations should be used. For effluents, the calculated initial volume percentage of the effluent in the dilution water should be used. A variety of statistical methods can be used to calculate an LC50 or EC50, but the most widely used are the probit (Finney, 1971), logit, moving average, and Litchfield-Wilcoxon (Litchfield and Wilcoxon, 1949) methods. Some of these methods are discussed in Chapter 5. The percentage of test organisms that die or display the effect in the control treatment must not be used in calculating the results. It is not recommended that corrections be made for control mortality or control effect, but Abbott's formula (Abbott, 1925) may be used to do so, if necessary.

According to Stephan (1977), almost all concentration-mortality data generated during acute tests can be analyzed to produce a statistical "best estimate" of the LC50 and its 95% confidence limits by using the moving average method and logarithmic transformation of the concentration data. The exception is when there are no so-called partial kills—that is, when none of the test concentrations have test animal mortality $> 0 < 100\%$. The binomial method can be used in such cases to estimate the LC50 as follows: LC50 $= (AB)^{1/2}$, where A is the highest test material concentration in which none of the test animals were killed and B is the lowest concentration in which all the animals were killed. If a logarithmic transformation is not used, the formula LC50 $= (A + B)/2$ will give the same result as the moving average. Although the 95% confidence limits cannot be calculated in the absence of test material concentrations in which test animal mortality was $> 0 < 100\%$, the confidence limits are generally between A and B. The level of confidence associated with these limits depends on the number of animals in each treatment and can be calculated from the formula: confidence level $= 100[1 - 2(\frac{1}{2})N]$, where N is the number of animals. Thus, if five or fewer animals are used in each treatment the confidence level is less than 95%, but if six or more animals are used per treatment the confidence level represented by A and B is always greater than 95%.

Ecological Significance of Test Results

Although laboratory toxicity tests are conducted under "unnatural" conditions, the results are generally accepted as a conservative estimate of the potential effects of test materials in the field. Laboratory tests may give conservative estimates of field effects because of the absence of mitigating factors (sunlight, sediment, microbes) that would decrease the toxicity of the test material under "natural" conditions. There is great interest in conducting more environmentally realistic tests in the laboratory, and the ultimate goal is to conduct tests in the field to validate the results of laboratory tests.

As stated by Butler et al. (1977), any detectable and measurable response of organisms in a toxicity test should not be interpreted as an ecologically significant event. The effect must be related to the expected environmental concentration (Cairns et al., 1978) if one is to make a judgment about the risk posed by a material in the environment and thus estimate its ecological significance.

EXAMPLES OF TEST DATA

It is essential in any acute toxicity test that orderly, legible, and complete records be maintained. Information about the test material, test conditions, test animals, test procedures, physical and chemical measurements, biological results, date(s) of testing, and person(s) who performed the test should be permanently recorded, either in a laboratory notebook or on looseleaf sheets that are assembled into a project or test file. Toxicity test data sheets such as the ones shown in Figs. 3 and 4 have proved effective in data recording for static acute tests. They "force" the experimenter to provide all the information about the test because all blanks must be completed. Such a format is highly recommended. These forms are only one example of the types of forms that should comprise a complete quality assurance (QA) package for any aquatic toxicity test. Data sheets for flow-through acute tests are similar, except that additional information is included on the functioning and operation of the flow-through system.

After a test has been completed, it is important to present the data in tabular form. The data in Table 2 are the results of chemical analyses performed during a 96-h flow-through acute test in which sheepshead minnows (*Cyprinodon variegatus*) were exposed to sodium selenite. Similarly, the mortality (or other effect criterion) data can be grouped as shown in Table 3. Based on the mortality data, time-dependent LC50s can be calculated by one of the statistical methods previously described (see Table 4). Finally, physical or chemical data can be assembled as shown in Tables 5 and 6.

In the absence of a calculator or computer program to statistically estimate the LC50 (or EC50) value and confidence limits, the LC50 can be determined by graphical interpolation (APHA, AWWA, and WPCF, 1981). The mortality data from Table 3 have been used to plot the graph in Fig. 5. The LC50 value can be interpolated from the percentages of test organisms dying in two or more concentrations—in one less than 50% mortality and in another more than 50% mortality. Estimation of the LC50 by interpolation involves plotting the mortality data on semilogarithmic coordinate paper with concentrations (average measured) of sodium selenite on the log scale and percent mortality on the arithmetic scale. A straight line may be drawn between the two points that represent the percent mortality at the two successive concentrations that were lethal to more

than 50% and less than 50% of the test organisms. The point at which the line crosses the 50% mortality line is the LC50 value for the test. Figure 5 illustrates the use of this procedure (straight-line graphical interpolation) to determine the LC50s for the 48-, 72-, and 96-h exposures of sheepshead minnows to sodium selenite. The LC50 values for these exposures are 18, 11, and 8 ppm, respectively. The 72- and 96-h LC50s are different from the calculated values but within the 95% confidence limits. The graphically interpolated 48-h LC50 does not fall within the calculated 95% confidence limits. This can be explained by the fact that only two data points were used in the graphical interpolation but all five data points were used to statistically calculate the LC50s. An alternative to graphical interpolation is to plot the data on logarithmic-probability paper with toxicant concentrations on the logarithmic scale and percent mortality on the probability (probit) scale.

METHODOLOGY FOR PHYTOPLANKTON

Phytoplankton (microalgae) form the basis of food chains in the aquatic environment. These organisms store energy through photosynthesis and thus are the primary producers for the food webs in the aquatic environment. It is important that optimum conditions exist for their growth and reproduction because changes in abundance or diversity may affect the animals that use algae as a primary source of food. Furthermore, algal density and condition can affect the dissolved oxygen concentration, pH, color, alkalinity, clarity, and taste of surface waters. Therefore, the effects of potentially toxic test materials on algal cells should be of interest.

Since algal species and communities are sensitive to environmental changes, growth may be either inhibited or stimulated by the presence of various chemicals. Therefore, the response of algae must be considered when assessing the potential ecological effects of chemicals and other toxic agents on the aquatic environment.

The purpose of an algal toxicity test is to

QUALITY ASSURANCE FORM

| NO. BW-QAF-001 |
| PAGE   SIDE 1 |
| REVISION   #3 |

SUBJECT: STATIC ACUTE TOXICITY TEST DATA SHEET

EFFECTIVE 10 June 1981

FISH SPECIES	FISH SOURCE	LENGTH AND WEIGHT	IN THE 48 HOURS PRIOR TO TESTING

MEAN   RANGE

TANK _____
LOT NO. _____
STATE _____

L. _____ (mm)
W. _____ (g)

DATA FOUND ON PAGE _____   VOL: _____

DATE MEAN DETERMINED

1. % MORTALITY WAS _____
2. FISH WERE ☐ NOT FED   ☐ FED
3. TEMPERATURE RANGE IN TANK WAS:

DATA TAKEN FROM MONTHLY FISH CULTURE SHEET

REFERENCE TEST DATA   DATA IN REFERENCE TEST LOG

WATER BATH ID

CLIENT STUDY NO. _____ LC50 _____ mg/l DATE _____

SIGNATURE   INITIALS

COMMENTS:

pH METER USED: D.O. METER USED:

OBSERVATION KEY

NONE	:- OBSERVATION WAS MADE AND NOTHING OUT OF THE ORDINARY WAS OBSERVED				
	GENERAL BEHAVIOR		SWIMMING		RESPIRATION
AS	AT THE SURFACE	ERR	ERRATIC	RA	RAPID
MSP	MUSCLE SPASM		PIGMENTATION	RE	REDUCED
CLE	COMPLETE LOSS OF EQUILIBRIUM	LT	LIGHT		SOLUTION
PLE	PARTIAL LOSS OF EQUILIBRIUM	DRK	DARK	CLDY	CLOUDY
LETH	LETHARGIC		INTEGUMENT	PRE	PRECIPITATE
PFAE	PECTORAL FINS ANTERIORLY EXTENDED	EMP	EXCESSIVE MUCUS	FOS	FILM ON SURFACE
EXO	EXOPHTHALMUS	HEM	HEMORRHAGIC	UN	UNDISSOLVED CHEMICAL
EA	EXTENDED ABDOMEN			PM	PARTICULATE MATTER
HYP	HYPERACTIVE				

(a)

Figure 3 Quality assurance form for static acute toxicity tests with fish. This is one of the series of 10–15 forms that comprise a typical QA package for any test. (a) Species identification, source and measurements of test fish and general observations. [Courtesy of EG&G Bionomics Aquatic Toxicology Laboratory (1981)]

SAMPLE IDENTIFICATION	SPONSOR	SAMPLE LOT. NO.	TIME: CHEMICAL/FISH ADDED	% ACTIVITY	PRINCIPAL INVESTIGATOR

PROJECT NO.

DILUTION WATER: INFO BELOW NOT RAW DATA

TEST SYSTEM
☐ OPEN ☐ CLOSED

FOUND IN: RECON WATER QUALITY NOTEBOOK
VOL:___ PG: ___

SOURCE	pH	TOTAL ALKALINITY (mg/1 CaCO₃)
BATCH NO.	SALINITY °/oo	CONDUCTIVITY (µmhos/cm)
		TOTAL HARDNESS (mg/1 CaCO₃)

TYPE TEST PERFORMED
☐ PRELIMINARY ☐ DEFINITIVE

NUMBER OF ANIMALS PER JAR
3 5 10 20

NUMBER OF REPLICATES PER CONC.
0 2 4   THIS IS REP. ___

STOCK CONC   SOLVENT USED

TEST CONCENTRATIONS
% mg/1 µg/1 HIGH→LOW

TEST CHAMBER VOLUME (LITERS)
3.8 19.6

DILUENT VOLUME (LITERS)
3 15

PREPARED BY   DATE PREP.

CALCULATION APPROVED BY   DATE

AMOUNT OF CHEMICAL/STOCK ADDED ( ) CONT SOLV. CONT
AMOUNT OF SOLVENT ADDED (ml) N.A. N.A.

N.A. N.A. N.A. N.A.
96 HOUR NO DISCERNIBLE EFFECT CONC. ___

CIRCLE ONE: BG, CCF, Fhm, RBT

	0-HOUR		24-HOUR		48-HOUR		72-HOUR		96-HOUR	

DATE

TIME

DATA BY

	CONT. TEMP. °C	pH	DO	CONT. TEMP. °C	pH	DO	CONT. TEMP. °C	pH	DO	CONT. TEMP. °C	pH	DO	CONT. TEMP. °C	pH	DO
TEST CONC. % mg/1 µg/1	OBSERVATION	NO. DEAD		OBSERVATION	NO. DEAD CUM		OBSERVATION	NO. DEAD CUM		OBSERVATION	NO. DEAD CUM		OBSERVATION	NO. DEAD CUM	
CONTROL															
SOLV. CONT.															

(b)

Figure 3 Quality assurance form for static acute toxicity tests with fish. This is one of the series of 10–15 forms that comprise a typical QA package for any test. (*Continued*) (*b*) Characteristics of dilution water quality, verification of test chemical solution preparation, observations of fish mortality, and water quality measurements (temperature, pH, and dissolved oxygen) made during the toxicity test. [*Courtesy of EG&G Bionomics Aquatic Toxicology Laboratory (1981)*]

EG&G BIONOMICS

QUALITY ASSURANCE FORM

NO:	BW-QAF-I001
PAGE	Side 1
REVISION	Original
EFFECTIVE	October 1, 1978

SUBJECT: STATIC ACUTE TOXICITY TEST DATA SHEET — INVERTEBRATE LABORATORY

SAMPLE IDENTIFICATION: _____   SPONSOR: _____

SAMPLE LOT NO. _____   % ACTIVITY _____   JOB NO. _____

DENSITY gram/ml _____

PRINCIPAL INVESTIGATORS: _____

TIME ADDED CHEMICAL/ANIMALS	NO. OF ANIMALS PER JAR	NO. OF REPLICATES PER CONCENTRATION	TYPE TEST VESSEL	TEST SYSTEM USED
	5, 15, _____	0, 3, _____		open closed

TEST CHAMBER VOLUME (Liters)	TOTAL SOLUTION VOLUME (ml)	SPECIES	SOLUTION VOLUME PER CHAMBER (Liters)	AGE/SIZE
0.25, 1, 2, _____	500, _____		0.15, 0.5, _____	

CHEMICAL QUALITY OF DILUTION WATER: Information below is not raw data

DATA TRANSCRIBED NOTEBOOK _____	SOURCE _____ BATCH NO. _____	TOTAL ALKALINITY (mg/1 $CaCO_3$)
PAGE NO. _____	pH _____	TOTAL HARDNESS (mg/1 $CaCO_3$)
LOCATION _____	SALINITY _____	CONDUCTIVITY (μmhos/cm)

COMMENTS _____

_____

_____

_____

NO DISCERNIBLE EFFECT LEVEL AT 96 HOURS IS _____. DETERMINED BY:

OBSERVATIONS KEY		SIGNATURE	INITIAL
D - Daphnia magna	CO - CAUGHT ON		
OS - ON SURFACE	CLDY - CLOUDY SOLUTION		
OB - ON BOTTOM	PRE - PRECIPITATE		
LETH - LETHARGIC	UM - UNDISSOLVED MATERIAL		
ERR - ERRATIC SWIMMING	PM - PARTICIPATE MATTER		
FC - FLARED CARAPACE	(EFFLUENTS)		
SC - SWIMMING, CARRYING	F - FILM		

(a)

Figure 4 Quality assurance form for static acute toxicity tests with aquatic macroinvertebrates. This is one of the series of 10–15 forms that comprise a typical QA package for any test. (a) Test chemical characteristics, test design, dilution water quality characteristics, and general observations. [Courtesy of EG&G Bionomics Aquatic Toxicology Laboratory, 1978.]

SAMPLE ID

PRELIMINARY/DEFINITIVE TEST (circle one)

STOCK CONCENTRATION: _____ SOLVENT: _____
PREPARED BY: _____ DATE PREPARED: _____

TEST CONCENTRATIONS

mg/1 μg/1 %

	CONT	S. CONT		HIGH			LOW	
AMOUNT OF ( ) STOCK/CHEM ADDED	NA	NA		NA	NA	NA	NA	NA
AMOUNT OF (ml) SOLVENT ADDED	NA	NA		NA	NA	NA	NA	NA

0 HOUR   **48 HOUR**

	DATE							
	TIME							
	DATA BY							
	REP	CONC	DO	pH	TEMP	DO	pH	TEMP
CONTROL	A							
SOL. CONT.	A				NA			NA
HIGH	A				NA			NA
MIDDLE	A				NA			NA
LOW	A				NA			NA

0 HOUR

DATE
TIME
DATA BY

REPLICATE	A	B	C	A	B	C	A	B	C	CUM NO. DEAD
CONC. % mg/T μg/1	OBSER.	OBSER.	OBSER.	OBSER. NO. DEAD	OBSER. NO. DEAD	OBSER. NO. DEAD	OBSER. NO. DEAD	OBSER. NO. DEAD	OBSER. NO. DEAD	
CONTROL										
SOL. CONT.										

24 HOUR   **48 HOUR**

(b)

Figure 4 Quality assurance form for static acute toxicity tests with aquatic macroinvertebrates. This is one of the series of 10–15 forms that comprise a typical QA package for any test. (b) Observations of invertebrate mortality and water quality measurements (temperature, pH, and dissolved oxygen) made during the toxicity test. [Courtesy of EG&G Bionomics Aquatic Toxicology Laboratory, 1978.]

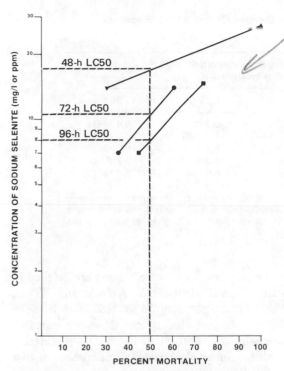

Figure 5 Estimation of time-dependent LC50s for sodium selenite by the graphical interpolation method.

Table 3 Test Concentrations and Mortality of Sheepshead Minnows ($n = 20$) Exposed to Sodium Selenite in Flowing, Natural Seawater[a]

Average measured concentration (mg/l)	Mortality (%)			
	24-h	48-h	72-h	96-h
Control	0	0	0	0
2.0	0	0	0	0
3.6	0	5	10	20
7.1	0	25	35	45
14	10	30	60	75
27	40	100	100	100

[a]Salinity was 25 ppt and temperature was 20°C. Concentrations are given as selenium ion (Se^{2+}) in seawater.

determine the relative toxicity of test materials to representative algal species. Algal toxicity may be expressed in terms of a broad range of responses, encompassing those that are inhibitory (50% reduction in cell numbers at specified time intervals), algistatic (halting of cell division), and algicidal (cell death). All three degrees of algal toxicity can be determined by the algal toxicity test.

General Methods

Algal toxicity tests are conducted according to the same general principles discussed earlier for fish and invertebrate testing. Cultures of a unicellular alga of known age and density are exposed to a range of test material concentrations in flasks

Table 2 Nominal and Measured Selenium Ion (Se^{2+}) Concentrations during a 96-h Exposure of Sheepshead Minnows to Sodium Selenite ($Na_2 Se_3 \cdot 5H_2O$) in Flowing, Natural Seawater[a]

Nominal concentration (mg/l)	Measured concentration (mg/l)			Percent of nominal
	0-h	96-h	Average	
Control	ND[b]	0.17	ND	—
1.9	1.9	2.1	2.0	105
3.8	4.0	3.3	3.6	95
7.5	6.6	7.6	7.1	95
15	15	13	14	93
30	26	28	27	90

[a]Salinity was 25 ppt and temperature was 20°C.
[b]None detected.

Table 4 Calculated LC50s of Sodium Selenite to Sheepshead Minnows Exposed in Flowing, Natural Seawater[a]

Time (h)	LC50 (mg/l)	95% confidence limits (mg/l)
24	>27	—
48	8.4	5.2–14
72	7.7	5.4–11
96	7.0	5.2–9.5

[a]Salinity was 25 ppt and temperature was 20°C. Calculations were based on measured concentrations of selenium ion (Se^{2+}) in seawater.

Table 5   Measured Concentrations of Dissolved Oxygen During a 96-h Exposure of Sheepshead Minnows to Sodium Selenite in Flowing, Natural Seawater[a]

Mean measured concentration (mg/l; ppm)	Dissolved oxygen concentration, mg/l (% of saturation)			
	24-h	48-h	72-h	96-h
Control	5.4 (83)	5.4 (83)	5.2 (80)	6.4 (98)
2.0	5.6 (86)	5.4 (83)	5.5 (85)	6.2 (95)
3.6	5.7 (88)	5.4 (83)	5.4 (83)	6.3 (97)
7.1	5.7 (88)	5.5 (85)	5.3 (82)	6.2 (95)
14	5.8 (89)	5.6 (86)	5.6 (86)	6.4 (98)
27	5.9 (91)	5.5 (86)	—[b]	—

[a]Salinity was 25 ppt and temperature was 20°C. Dissolved oxygen concentrations are averages of measurements in replicate test chambers A and B. Concentrations are given as selenium ion (Se^{2+}) in seawater.
[b]No measurement because all fish had died.

under defined static conditions in a temperature- and photoperiod-controlled environment. An untreated control flask (and/or solvent control) is maintained to measure the normal growth of the alga. The effects of the test materials are evaluated by measuring the growth of treated and untreated cultures and comparing the results. Because of the inherent variability of the test, the experimental design should include sufficient replication to permit statistical evaluation of the results.

General algal culture and exposure conditions including light intensity, photoperiod, temperature, pH, growth medium composition, and incu-

bation are carefully controlled and are detailed in standard methods (APHA, AWWA, and WPCF, 1981). Test algae may be selected from those in Table 7. Several algal species should be tested to determine the relative toxicity of the test material. Initiation of an algal toxicity test consists of two major phases, the preparation of the inoculum in the log growth phase and the preparation of test solutions.

Inoculum

Stock cultures of algal test species should be grown on suitable culture medium through at least

Table 6   Measured pH of Test Solutions during a 96-h Exposure of Sheepshead Minnows to Sodium Selenite in Flowing, Natural Seawater[a]

Mean measured concentration (mg/l)	pH							
	24-h		48-h		72-h		96-h	
	A	B	A	B	A	B	A	B
Control	8.0	8.1	8.2	8.1	8.1	8.1	8.2	8.2
2.0	8.1	8.2	8.1	8.2	8.1	8.2	8.2	8.2
3.6	8.1	8.2	8.2	8.2	8.1	8.2	8.2	8.2
7.1	8.2	8.2	8.3	8.2	8.2	8.3	8.2	8.2
14	8.2	8.2	8.3	8.3	8.3	8.3	8.3	8.3
27	8.3	8.3	8.2	8.3	—[b]	—	—	—

[a]Salinity was 25 ppt and temperature was 20°C. Concentrations are given as selenium ion (Se^{2+}) in seawater.
[b]No measurement because all fish had died.

Table 7 Recommended Algae Species for Toxicity Tests

Freshwater
  Chlorophyta (green algae)
    Selenastrum capricornutum
  Cyanophyta (blue-green algae)
    Anabaena flos-aquae
    Microcystis aeruginosa
  Chrysophyta (brown algae and diatoms)
    Navicula pelliculosa
    Cyclotella sp.
    Synura petersenii
Saltwater
  Chlorophyta (green algae)
    Chlorella sp.
    Chlorococcum sp.
    Dunaliella tertiolecta
  Chrysophyta (brown algae and diatoms)
    Isochrysis galbana
    Nitzschia closterium
    Pyrmnesium parvum
    Skeletonema costatum
    Thalassiosira pseudonana
  Rhodophyta (red algae)
    Porphyridium cruentum

two complete growth cycles before use as a source of inoculum for the toxicity test. This is necessary since the nutritional history of the culture can have marked effects on growth responses.

The inoculum is usually prepared by transferring between 0.1 and 1.0 ml of the stock algal culture into triplicate flasks containing nutrient-enriched saltwater or freshwater, depending on the species being tested. Three new flasks should be inoculated at the point of inflection of the growth curve, that is, at the start of the log growth phase. The second growth curve should be followed and cells from the second or later transfers can be used for the toxicity test because they have become adapted to the ambient nutrient levels. Algae acclimated in this manner will tend to give more reproducible results in toxicity tests. The algal cultures should also be checked to make sure the stock cultures are axenic (unispecies).

Test Solutions

Filter-sterilized, nutrient-enriched water is dispensed into presterilized flasks. An inoculum of alga is added to yield a specific cell density or concentration (number of cells per milliliter). Initial cell density or biomass (dry weight) is measured in an aliquot.

Test material stock solutions are prepared in water, or in solvents if the material is insoluble in water. Stock solutions should be prepared to ensure that the same volume is added to all treatments. Test material is added to the flasks containing the inoculated enriched water and the flasks are placed in an incubator.

Test Design

The general test design is similar to that for fish and invertebrates in that it includes a preliminary range-finding test to select concentrations for the final definitive test. The preliminary test should include concentrations of several orders of magnitude (e.g., 0.1, 1.0, 10, 100, and 1000 mg/l) and duplicate culture flasks should be used at each concentration. The flasks are first inoculated with a unialgal culture and then incubated under standard conditions. Typically, algal toxicity tests are conducted for 96 h. However, protocols are available for evaluations of longer duration. Biomass is determined in each flask and compared with that of the untreated controls. These results are used to determine the test concentrations for the definitive test. The criteria for selecting these concentrations are described in standard methods (APHA, AWWA, and WPCF, 1981) and are similar to those used for fish and invertebrates. The definitive toxicity test should include five or six test material concentrations and an untreated control, with three or four replicates of each. Three replicates may be inoculated with algae while the fourth serves as a blank. Three replicates are needed for statistical analysis, and the blank may be used, if necessary, to correct biomass measurements for particulates present in the treatments. If possible, the five or six test concentrations should include an algicidal concentration, an algistatic concentration, a slightly inhibitory concentration, and a concentration in which growth is similar to that of the control (no observed effect concentration). The flasks should be incubated for 4 d.

Growth should be monitored and measured once every 24 h for the duration of the study to determine the effects of the test material. Ideally, the experiment should continue until the control population of algae can complete its logarithmic growth phase (maximum standing crop) and reach a stationary growth rate (Fig. 6); however, the duration of these tests is usually predetermined to be 96 h.

Some test methods (ASTM, 1981) include a postexposure observation period in which living cells from each test concentration are transferred to growth medium without test material and the rate of their growth is measured. The purpose of the recovery period is to determine the ability of the previously exposed cultures to regain their normal rate of growth.

Criteria for Effect

There are a variety of parameters that characterize the growth response of algal cultures. These parameters are measures (or estimates) of biomass of treated and untreated cultures which, when plotted against time, produce a growth response curve (Fig. 6). This curve can be used to determine the rate of log growth and a maximum population density for control and exposed cultures.

Cell Counts   (flow cytometer)

Microscopic measurements of cell numbers can be made with a hemacytometer, Palmer-Maloney chamber, Sedgewick-Rafter plankton counting chamber, or inverted microscope. Some of these methods are discussed by Lund et al. (1958) and Palmer and Maloney (1954).

Direct counting methods are time-consuming and their statistical significance decreases at low cell densities ($<1 \times 10^4$). If large numbers of tests and replicates are needed, it becomes highly impractical to use cell counts for growth assessment of algae. In this case, it is rapid, practical, and reasonably accurate to use an electronic particle counter.

Chlorophyll

All algae contain chlorophyll *a,* and measuring the amount of this pigment can give some insight into the relative amount of algal biomass present. Chlorophyll may be measured *in vivo* or *in vitro* by fluorescence or spectrophotometric techniques. Fluorescent systems are more sensitive and can be used at cell densities $<1 \times 10^4$ cells/ml. Furthermore, the *in vivo* technique is sensitive, accurate and does not require pre-analysis extraction. A limitation of the chlorophyll *a* measurement is that it varies as a function of nutrition and environmental variables. For additional information on this method, see Forenzen (1966, 1967), Moss (1967), Odum et al. (1959), Yentsch and Ryther (1957), and Yentsch and Menzel (1963).

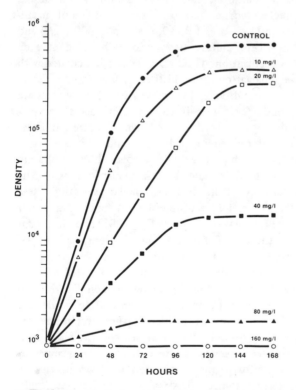

Figure 6 Hypothetical relationship between time-dependent algal growth measured as cell density and concentrations of test chemical to which algal cultures are exposed.

Carbon-14 Assimilation

The method based on carbon-14 assimilation is used for productivity measurements for freshwater and marine algae. It is used as a measure of photosynthetic activity, and it yields a biomass index that correlates well with growth rates. For more information on this technique, see Jenkins (1965), Jitts (1963), and McAllister (1961).

Adenosine Triphosphate Concentration

Adenosine triphosphate (ATP) measurements are a sensitive indicator of living biomass because of the constancy of the cellular ATP/carbon ratio. There is a good correlation between ATP and direct measures of biomass (counting) and labeling with carbon-14. Since ATP is a measure of living biomass, it may not be appropriate for contaminated wastes (e.g., sludge), which may provide interference. For more information on this method, see Hamilton and Holm-Hansen (1967), Holm-Hansen and Booth (1966), and Holm-Hansen (1969).

All the above techniques have certain advantages and disadvantages that depend on the test design, type of test material, and facilities.

Biological Data

Growth effects are most often used to define the toxicity of test materials to algae. Since growth is being measured rather than death, an EC50 is calculated. The EC50 is the test material concentration estimated to cause a 50% reduction in number of cells or chlorophyll a concentration relative to the control. Biomass measurements may be estimated after 24, 48, 72, 96, and 120 h of exposure by one or two of the techniques previously discussed (e.g., cell count, chlorophyll a). If the range of concentrations of the chemical tested results in average algal cell counts that bracket the 50% response level as compared with the controls, an EC50 value can be estimated. Semilogarithmic coordinate paper can be used to plot the average cell count for a concentration that yielded more than 50% and one that yielded less than 50% of the average cell count of control flasks (Fig. 7).

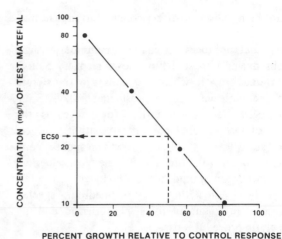

Figure 7 Estimation of EC50 for a chemical based on the degree of growth inhibition of exposed cultures relative to the growth of control culture.

The concentration should be plotted on the logarithmic axis and the percentage of growth in relation to the control on the arithmetic axis. A straight line should be drawn between these two points. The EC50 can be interpolated from the graph by determining the concentration at which this line crosses the 50% point on the percent growth response axis.

Data Analysis and Interpretation

Based on the data from a test, time-dependent EC50s and their 95% confidence limits should be calculated for each 24-h period through test termination. The statistical methods used are similar to those for fish and invertebrates. In some tests, stimulation of algal biomass to levels greater than that of controls may result from exposure to one or more concentrations of a chemical that can serve as a carbon source for the algae. Generally, these stimulatory effects are not used in the calculation of an EC50 since the purpose of the test is to estimate the median adverse effect (i.e., producing a decrease in biomass relative to controls) rather than a median change relative to controls. The results of each test can also include the algistatic concentration with its confidence intervals and the no observed effect concentration. The algistatic concentration is the test material concentration that produces no change in number of algal cells during exposure but allows recovery to logarithmic growth when the cells are transferred to medium without the test material. The noobserved effect concentration (or range) is the highest test material concentration that produces no statistically different growth response compared to controls throughout the exposure period. A description should also be included of the test conditions, including culture medium, species, temperature, light intensity, photoperiod, and any analytic procedures used.

SPECIAL CONSIDERATIONS

Safety

Many test materials used in aquatic toxicity tests are biocides. They are intended to kill microbes, plants, insects, rodents, birds, and other organisms. It is extremely important, therefore, to treat all test materials with care. Before any testing is begun, the testing facility should have information on safe handling of the test material, on its known toxicity, and on proper cleanup and disposal methods. This information should be used to decide whether the testing facility is able to test the material safely. It may also provide for the assignment of a hazard rating and for the stipulation of special precautions necessary to handle or test the material (e.g., wearing a respirator while working with the technical chemical). Finally, and most important, these safety data must be conveyed to the scientists or technicians who will perform the test.

Disposal

Closely related to safe handling of test material in the laboratory is proper disposal of the unused material and stock solutions and the contaminated animals and water. A testing facility must meet legal requirements for discharge of test materials into sewers, on-site waste treatment systems, deep wells, or surface waters. Fortunately, because of the recent emphasis on "cradle-to-grave" custody of chemicals, commercial waste handling and storage contractors are becoming more plentiful and, we hope, reliable. Such services may be considered for use by the testing facility.

Exotic Organisms

Control of test animals not indigenous to the geographic area of the testing facility is essential. Exotic or nonstandard test animals may be shipped to a facility from another area or even another country. The testing facility must prevent the escape of any living exotic animals. Instances of harm from the importation of plants and animals are numerous.

Good Laboratory Practices and Quality Assurance

No matter how well qualified the scientists and technicians who perform a test, the work will be meaningless if the conditions and results of testing cannot be reconstructed and verified in the future. Thus, the testing facility should be aware of requirements for standard operating procedures, test protocols, record retention, sample custody, and other basics of good laboratory practices and quality assurance. Good laboratory practice regulations for nonclinical laboratory studies have been published by the U.S. Department of Health, Education and Welfare (1978), and requirements for aquatic and environmental toxicity testing have been published (as proposed standards) by the U.S. Environmental Protection Agency (1980).

SUMMARY

Acute toxicity tests constitute only one of the many tools available to the aquatic toxicologist, but they are the basic means of providing a quick, relatively inexpensive, and reproducible estimate of the toxic effects of a test material. They are an indispensable "first-look" method, at least at this point in the development of the science of aquatic toxicology.

Acute tests are also useful in screening large

numbers of chemicals and in evaluating the relative sensitivity of different organisms to the same chemical. Thus they have been highly rated in "their present utility for use in assessing the hazard to aquatic environments" (Macek et al., 1978). They are the first step toward understanding the toxic effects of materials in aquatic systems.

There are limitations of acute tests that should be recognized. The results of acute toxicity tests usually do not provide substantive information about the sublethal or cumulative effects of a test material. Furthermore, these tests are not predictive of potential chronic toxicity (Macek et al., 1978). These limitations should be considered when planning testing programs for specific test materials. The chapters of this book are intended to inform and assist the reader in understanding such testing programs.

LITERATURE CITED

Abbott WS: A method of computing the effectiveness of an insecticide. J Econ Entomol 18:265–267, 1925.

APHA, AWWA, and WPCF: Standard Methods for the Examination of Water and Wastewater, 15th ed. Washington, D.C., 1981.

American Society for Testing and Materials: Standard practice for conducting toxicity tests with fishes, macroinvertebrates, and amphibians. ASTM E 729-80. Philadelphia: ASTM, 1980a.

American Society for Testing and Materials: Standard practice for conducting toxicity tests with larvae of four species of bivalve molluscs. ASTM E 724-80. Philadelphia: ASTM, 1980b.

American Society for Testing and Materials: Proposed standard practice for conducting toxicity tests with freshwater and saltwater algae. ASTM E47.01, Draft. Philadelphia: ASTM, 1981.

Brown VW: Concepts and outlooks in testing the toxicity of substances to fish. In: Bioassay Techniques and Environmental Chemistry, edited by GE Glass, pp. 73–96. Ann Arbor, Mich.: Ann Arbor Science, 1973.

Butler PA, Doudoroff P, Fontaine MA, Fujiya M, Lange R, Lloyd R, Reish DJ, Sprague JB, Swedmark M: Manual of Methods in Aquatic Environment Research. Part 4: Bases for Selecting Biological Tests to Evaluate Marine Pollution. Rome, Italy: U.N. Food and Agricultural Organization, 1977.

Cairns J, Jr, Dickson KL, Maki AW (eds): Estimating the hazard of chemical substances to aquatic life. ASTM STP 657. Philadelphia: American Society for Testing and Materials, 1978.

Committee on Methods for Acute Toxicity Tests with Aquatic Organisms: Methods for Acute Toxicity Tests with Fish, Macroinvertebrates, and Amphibians. EPA-660/3-75-009, 1975.

Cox, GV (ed): Marine Bioassays Workshop Proceedings 1974. American Petroleum Institute, Environmental Protection Agency, Marine Technology Society. Washington, D.C.: Marine Technology Society, 1974.

Finney DJ: Probit Analyses. London: Cambridge Univ. Press, 1971.

Hamilton RD, Holm-Hansen O: Adenosine triphosphate content of marine bacteria. Limnol Oceanogr 12:319–324, 1967.

Holm-Hansen O, Booth CR: The measurement of adenosine triphosphate in the ocean and its ecological significance. Limnol Oceanogr 11:510–519, 1966.

Holm-Hansen O: Determination of microbial biomass in ocean profiles. Limnol Oceanogr 14:740–747, 1969.

Jenkins D: Determination of primary productivity of turbid waters with carbon-14. J Water Pollut Control Fed 37:1281–1288, 1965.

Jensen AL: Standard error of LC50 and sample size in fish bioassays. Water Res 6:85–89, 1972.

Jitts HR: The standardization and comparison of measurements of primary production by the carbon-14 technique. In: Proceedings of a Conference on Primary Productivity Measurement, Marine and Fresh Water, Univ. of Hawaii, Aug-Sept 1961, edited by MS Doty, pp. 103–113. U.S. AEC Div Tech Inf TID 7633, 1963.

Lemke AE, Brungs WA, Halligan BJ: Manual for Construction and Operation of Toxicity-Testing Proportional Diluters. EPA-600/3-78-072, 1978.

Litchfield JT, Jr, Wilcoxon F: A simplified method of evaluating dose-effect experiments. J Pharmacol Exp Ther 96:99–113, 1949.

Lorenzen CJ: A method for the continuous measurement of *in vivo* chlorophyll concentration. Deep Sea Res 13:223–227, 1966.

Lorenzen CJ: Determination of chlorophyll and pheopigments: Spectrophotometric equations. Limnol Oceanogr 12:343–346, 1967.

Lund JW, Kipling C, Lecren ED: The inverted microscope method of estimating algae numbers and the statistical basis of estimations by counting. Hydrobiologia 11:143–170, 1958.

Macek K, Birge W, Mayer FL, Buikema AL, Jr, Maki AW: Toxicological effects. In: Estimating the Hazard of Chemical Substances to Aquatic Life, edited by J Cairns, Jr, KL Dickson, AW Maki, pp. 27–32. ASTM STP 657. Philadelphia: American Society for Testing and Materials, 1978.

McAllister CD: Decontamination of filters in the C-14 method of measuring marine photosynthesis. Limnol Oceanogr 6:447–450, 1961.

Moss B: A spectrophotometric method for the estimation of percentage degradation of chlorophylls to pheopigments in extracts of algae. Limnol Oceanogr 12:335–340, 1967.

Mount DI, Brungs WA: A simplified dosing apparatus for fish toxicological studies. Water Res 1: 21–29, 1967.

Odum HT, McConnel W, Abbot W: The chlorophyll "a" of communities. Publ Texas Inst Mar Sci 5:65–95, 1959.

Palmer CM, Maloney TE: A new counting slide for nannoplankton. Am Soc Limnol Oceanogr Spec Publ No 21, 1954.

Stephan CE: Methods for Calculating an LC50. In: Aquatic Toxicology and Hazard Evaluation, Proceedings of the First Annual Symposium on Aquatic Toxicology, edited by FL Mayer and JL Hamelink, pp. 65–84. ASTM STP 634. Philadelphia: American Society for Testing and Materials, 1977.

Tatem HE, Anderson, JW, Neff JM: Seasonal and laboratory variations in the health of grass shrimp *Palaemonetes pugio:* Dodecyl sodium sulfate bioassay. Bull Environ Contam Toxicol 16:368–375, 1976.

U.S. Environmental Protection Agency: Proposed environmental standards; and proposed good laboratory practice standards for physical, chemicals, persistence, and ecological effects testing. Fed Regist 45:77332–77365, 1980.

U.S. Department of Health, Education and Welfare, Food and Drug Administration: Nonclinical laboratory studies. Good laboratory practice regulations. Fed Regist 43:59986–60025, 1978.

Yentsch CS and Ryther JH: Short-term variations in phytoplankton chlorophyll and their significance. Limnol Oceanogr 2:140–142, 1957.

Yentsch CS and Menzel DW: A method for the determination of phytoplankton chlorophyll and phaeophytin by fluorescence. Deep Sea Res 10: 221–231, 1963.

SUPPLEMENTAL READING

Brungs WA: Continuous-Flow Bioassays with Aquatic Organisms: Procedures and Applications. In: Biological Methods for the Assessment of Water Quality, edited by J Cairns, Jr, KL Dickson, pp. 117–126. ASTM STP 528. Philadelphia: American Society for Testing and Materials, 1973.

Brusick DJ, Young RR, Hutchinson C, Vilkas, AG, Gezo TA: Aquatic ecological assays. In: IERL-RTP Procedures Manual: Level 1 Environmental Assessment Biological Tests, pp. 69–112. EPA 68-02-2681. U.S. EPA Office of Research and Development, 1980.

David HS: Culture and Diseases of Game Fishes. Berkeley: Univ. of California Press, 1953.

Duke KM, Davis ME, Dennis AJ: Ecological effects tests. In: IERL-RTP Procedures Manual: Level 1 Environmental Assessment Biological Tests for Pilot Studies. pp. 40–76. EPA-600/7-77-043. Washington, D.C.: U.S. EPA, Office of Research and Development, 1977.

Hoffman GL, Meyer FP: Parasites of Freshwater Fishes. Neptune City, N.J.: TFH Publications, 1974.

Kester E, Dredall I, Conners D, Pytowicz R: Preparation of artificial seawater. Limnol Oceanogr 12:176–178, 1967.

Miller WE, Greene JC, Shiroyama T: *Selenastrum capricornutum* Printz Algal Assay Bottle Test: Experimental Design, Application, and Data Interpretation Protocol. EPA-600/9-78-018. Corvallis, Ore.: U.S. EPA, 1978.

Organization for Economic Cooperation and Development: OECD Guidelines for Testing of Chemicals. Paris: OECD, 1981.

Payne AG, Hall RH: A method for measuring algal toxicity and its application to the safety assessment of new chemicals. In: Aquatic Toxicology, Proceedings of the Second Annual Symposium on Aquatic Toxicity, edited by LL Marking, RA Kimerle, pp. 171–180. ASTM STP 667. Philadelphia: American Society for Testing and Materials, 1979.

Peltier W: Methods for Measuring the Acute Toxicity of Effluents to Aquatic Organisms. EPA-600/4-78-012, 1978.

Reichenbach-Klinke H, Elkan E: The Principal Diseases of Lower Vertebrates. New York: Academic, 1965.

Snieszko SF (ed): A Symposium on Diseases of Fish and Shellfishes. Washington, D.C.: American Fisheries Society, 1970.

Sprague JB: Measurement of pollutant toxicity to fish. I. Bioassay methods for acute toxicity. Water Res 3:793–821, 1969.

Sprague JB: Measurement of pollutant toxicity to fish. II. Utilizing and applying bioassay results. Water Res 4:3–32, 1970.

Sprague JB: Measurement of pollutant toxicity to fish. III. Sublethal effects and "safe" concentrations. Water Res 5:245–266, 1971.

Sprague JB: The ABC's of pollutant bioassay using fish. In: Biological Methods for the Assessment of Water Quality, edited by J Cairns, Jr, KL Dickson, pp. 6–30. ASTM STP 528. Philadelphia: American Society for Testing and Materials, 1973.

Steel RGD, Torrie JH: Principles and Procedures of Statistics. New York: McGraw-Hill, 1960.

U.S. Environmental Protection Agency, Corps of Engineers, Technical Committee on Criteria for Dredged and Fill Material: Ecological Evaluation of Proposed Discharge of Dredged Material into Ocean Waters. Vicksburg, Miss.: Environmental Effects Laboratory, U.S. Army Engineer Waterways Experiment Station, 1977.

U.S. Environmental Protection Agency, Environmental Research Laboratory, Office of Research and Development: Bioassay Procedures for the Ocean Disposal Permit Program. EPA-600/9-78-010, 1978.

Van Duijn C, Jr: Diseases of Fishes, 3rd ed. Springfield, Ill.: Thomas, 1973.

Chapter 3

Early Life Stage Toxicity Tests

J. M. McKim

INTRODUCTION

The life cycle toxicity test is considered by most aquatic toxicologists to be the ultimate test in establishing long-term "safe" environmental concentrations of toxic chemicals for both vertebrate and invertebrate aquatic populations.

The first aquatic vertebrate life cycle toxicity study with fish was performed with the fathead minnow, *Pimephales promelas*, by Mount and Stephan (1967); this was followed by studies with the bluegill, *Lepomis macrochirus* (Eaton, 1970); the brook trout, *Salvelinus fontinalis* (McKim and Benoit, 1971, 1974); the flagfish, *Jordanella floridae* (Smith, 1973); and the only saltwater species to date, the sheepshead minnow, *Cyprinodon variegatus* (Hansen et al., 1977; Hansen and Parrish, 1977). The development of life cycle toxicity tests for invertebrates has fallen behind

that for fish, mainly because of lack of emphasis and low research funding. However, a number of important invertebrates can be used in life cycle toxicity tests (Buikema and Cairns, 1980). These include the water flea, *Daphnia magna* (Biesinger and Christensen, 1972); the amphipod *Gammarus pseudolimnaeus* (Arthur, 1970); the gastropods *Physa integra* and *Campeloma* sp. (Arthur, 1970); and the midges *Chironomus tentans* (Derr and Zabik, 1972a,b) and *Tanytarsus dissimilis* (Nebeker, 1973). Saltwater invertebrates are represented by the opossum shrimp, *Mysidopsis bahia* (Nimmo et al., 1977); the grass shrimp, *Palaemonetes pugio* (Tyler-Schroeder, 1979); and the polychaetous annelids *Neanthes arenaceodentata, Capitella capitata,* and *Ctenodrilus serratus* (Reish, 1980).

A life cycle test demands a minimum laboratory exposure of the animal from "embryo to embryo," which for many animals, especially vertebrates (fish), requires a minimum of 6-12 mo of concentrated effort. The Toxic Substances Control Act of 1976, which required the Environmental Protection Agency (EPA) and industry to evaluate the environmental impact of new chemicals before commercial production, and the manufacture or marketing of an estimated 1000 new chemicals each year created the need for a more rapid, less costly, and less risky vertebrate test than the fish life cycle test for determining safe environmental concentrations of toxic chemicals.

During life cycle tests with several species of fish and a variety of toxicants, certain developmental stages have consistently been more sensitive than others. The possibility of focusing research efforts on these more sensitive stages promises success in searching for quicker and less costly ways of predicting chronic toxicity of chemicals to fish. Several investigators proposed that chronic toxicity to fish might be predicted by use of shorter tests with early developmental stages. In studies with selected toxicants, these early stages were shown to be among the most sensitive in the life cycle (Pickering and Thatcher, 1970; Pickering and Gast, 1972; McKim et al., 1975, 1978; Eaton et al., 1978; Sauter et al., 1976). It was emphasized that, with a relatively short exposure (several months) of the embryo-larval and early juvenile stages of fish to a toxicant, an estimate of the maximum acceptable toxicant concentration (MATC) could be obtained without a complete life cycle test.

The need for toxicity tests of short duration was not as great for the more routinely tested invertebrates (daphnids and mysids), since most invertebrate life cycle tests require only 1-2 mo. Shorter, partial life cycle tests with certain invertebrates have, in some cases, resulted in less sensitive responses than the complete life cycle or lifetime test (Buikema and Cairns, 1980).

Reviews of life cycle toxicity test data on freshwater fish, from more than 60 chronic tests with more than 40 organic and inorganic chemicals, show that tests with early life stages of four species of fish can be used to estimate the MATC

within a factor of 2 in most cases (McKim, 1977; Macek and Sleight, 1977). A comparison of chronic toxicity data for saltwater fish also indicates that early life stage exposures provide a close estimate of the MATC (Ward and Parrish, 1980; D. I. Mount, personal communication). The greater sensitivity of the early life stages compared to the later stages provides aquatic toxicologists with an accurate, efficient tool for predicting chronic effects of environmental pollutants in 1-2 mo of testing. It also makes it feasible to test other important fish species that cannot be studied in life cycle tests because of size or age at maturity, spawning requirements, or other factors inconducive to laboratory culture.

This chapter will provide more details on terminology, fish developmental events, end points used in determining effects, general methodologies employed, and the interpretation and utility of early life stage (ELS) tests with aquatic animals.

TERMINOLOGY

The terminology used in life cycle, partial life cycle, and early life stage aquatic toxicology and in developmental fish biology is reviewed below. For more general aquatic toxicology terminology, the reader is referred to the glossary in this book and to ASTM (1980a).

Aquatic Toxicology

Fish Life Cycle Toxicity Test

Each of several groups of individuals of one species is exposed to a different concentration of a toxicant throughout a life cycle in order to study the effect of the toxicant on the survival, growth, and reproduction of the species. To ensure that all life stages and life processes are exposed, the test begins with embryos or newly hatched young fish less than 8 h old, continues through maturation and reproduction, and ends not less than 28 d (60 d for salmonids) after the hatching of the next generation. Figure 1 shows the chronology of a life cycle test with brook trout which began with

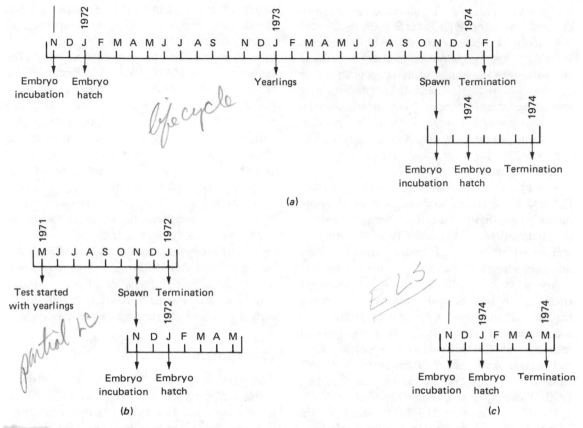

Figure 1 Chronology for (a) brook trout life cycle toxicity test; (b) partial life cycle toxicity test; and (c) early life stage (ELS) toxicity test. [Modified from Holcombe et al. (1979)]

embryo incubation in November 1971 and terminated 60 d after embryo hatch in May 1974. The trout requires 30 mo for a life cycle test, while the fathead minnow requires 12 mo.

Fish Partial Life Cycle Toxicity Test

Each of several groups of individuals of one species is exposed to a different concentration of a toxicant through part of a life cycle, which includes life stages observed to be especially sensitive to chemical exposure. Partial life cycle tests are conducted with fish species that require more than 1 yr to reach sexual maturity (e.g., brook trout and bluegills). The test can be completed in less than 15 mo and all major life stages are still exposed to the toxicant. With fish, exposure to the

toxic agent begins with immature juveniles at least 2 mo before active gonad development, continues through maturation and reproduction, and ends not less than 30 d (60 d for salmonids) after the hatching of the next generation. The chronology of a partial life cycle test with brook trout is also illustrated in Fig. 1. The exposure began in May 1971 with first-generation yearlings and ended in May 1972 with second-generation offspring.

Fish Early Life Stage (ELS) Toxicity Test

The early life stages of a species of fish are exposed for 28–32 d (60 d posthatch for salmonids), from ova fertilization through embryonic, larval, and early juvenile development. The major toxic effects measured are on survival and growth. The time intervals involved in a brook trout ELS toxicity test are also illustrated in Fig. 1.

Teleost Early Life Stage Development

The following terms describe the anatomy, developmental periods, and developmental phases of a typical teleost which are essential in ELS toxicity tests. The major anatomic features clearly recognizable at various stages of fish embryonic and larval development are illustrated in Fig. 2. Those not familiar with these fish embryological terms may consult the glossary in Jones et al. (1978). The description of periods and phases presented here is drawn in part from Balon (1975) and Snyder et al. (1977).

Embryonic Period

Begins with fertilization or union of the gametes and is characterized by an endogenous food source or yolk. The period ends at hatching. The embryonic period is divided into two phases:

1 The cleavage phase involves the first interval of development within the egg membranes, from the beginning of development to organogenesis. Most ELS toxicity tests begin early in this phase, although some begin at fertilization. The start of this phase corresponds to the early cleavage stage in Fig. 2.

2 The embryonic phase involves the interval of intense organogenesis within the egg membranes and continues until hatching is completed. The start of this phase corresponds to the early embryo stage illustrated in Fig. 2.

Larval Period

Begins with hatching of the egg and lasts until the disappearance of the last vestige of the embryonic median fin fold and the appearance of a full complement of fin rays and spines. This period is divided into three phases (Fig. 3):

1 Protolarva is the larval phase with no dorsal, anal, or caudal spines or rays apparent. The only median fin elements present are the dorsal and ventral fin folds.

2 Mesolarva is the larval phase where at least one of the principal rays is apparent in the median fin (see incipient rays of dorsal and anal fins in Fig. 3, mesolarva) or, if all fin rays are present in the median fin and the adult has pelvic fins, the pelvic buds or fins are not yet apparent.

3 Metalarva is the larval phase where all principal median fin rays are apparent. If the adult has pelvic fins, the pelvic buds or fins are apparent.

The salmonids do not go through the three phases described above. Their larval period is represented by the yolk-sac or alevin period, which begins at hatching and ends, after complete absorption of the yolk, with the juvenile.

Juvenile Period

Begins when all fins are fully differentiated and no median fin fold is apparent. The body is entirely scaled. The juvenile at this point is a miniature adult from all outward appearances (Fig. 3, juvenile). Most ELS toxicity tests with fish end shortly after metamorphosis from the larval to the juvenile period.

Adult Period

Commences with the first maturation of the gamete and is accompanied by secondary sexual characteristics and spawning behavior.

Senescent Period

Old age, accompanied by slow to no growth and few to no gametes.

END POINTS FOR FISH EARLY LIFE STAGE TOXICITY

Early life stages are sensitive parts of the life cycle of a fish because of the many critical events that take place in a very short span of time. For example, in a period of 7–8 d from fertilization through hatching to the first exogenous food consumption, the fathead minnow goes from an initial two cells to a swimming, feeding, functional animal with well-developed organ systems. If at

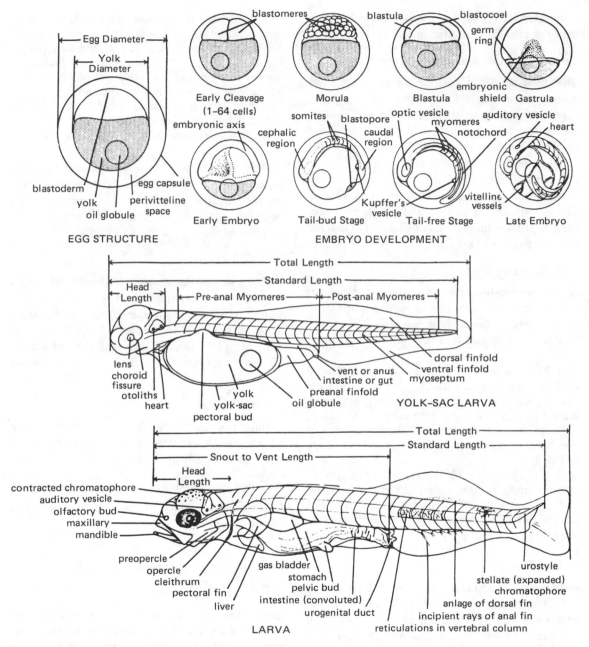

Figure 2 Diagrammatic representation of morphology and development of embryonic and larval periods of a typical teleost. *[Modified from Jones et al. (1978),]*

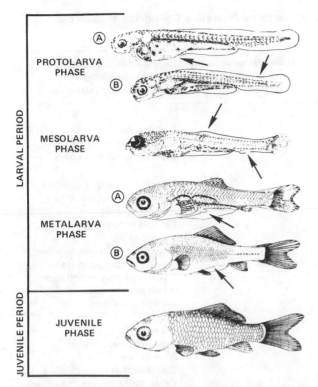

Figure 3 Sequence showing morphological changes separating larval fish into phases. *[Drawings from Jones et al. (1978).]* Protolarva: (*a*) Just hatched with large yolk sac and complete median fin fold; (*b*) yolk almost gone approaching shift to exogenous food, median fin fold still complete. Mesolarva: Feeding on exogenous food and distinct fin rays apparent in median fin folds. Metalarva: (*a*) Rays in median fins well developed and pelvic fin bud just apparent; (*b*) fins well developed, but preanal median fin fold still present. Juvenile: Full complement of fins and no median fin folds remaining.

any point during this period an environmental stress induces a change in the timing of these developmental events, the animal's chances of survival are reduced. For example, if the biochemistry for digesting exogenous food is not in place when the yolk is gone, the animal will starve. Or if the development of the eye is abnormal and sight is imperative for feeding at swim-up, again the animal is doomed.

The rapidity of growth and morphological changes during early fish development is a prime factor in the usefulness of these early life stage

tests to the aquatic toxicologist seeking a short, sensitive, predictive toxicity test. At present, standardized ELS toxicity tests deal primarily with survival and growth. However, there are many possible toxic end points available for estimating the chronic toxicity of chemicals in the aquatic environment (see Table 1).

Rosenthal and Alderdice (1976) used an ontogenetic sequence to group and discuss the sublethal effects of toxic chemicals on the early life stages of marine fish. The sequence included fertilization, embryonic development, hatching, larval development, and morphogenesis. Effects on gonadal tissue were also considered. Since sublethal effects by definition do not cause mortality, the sublethal effect of a stress on a particular early life stage will not be seen in that life stage. Instead, the effect will show up at some later stage of development, either in behavioral impairment, poor growth, or death. Rosenthal and Alderdice related this altered structure-function to stage of development and to the observed or suspected detrimental effects on the individual and/or population. Table 1 shows sublethal effects (toxic end points) according to stage of development; the last column gives the observed or suspected consequences of the effects or responses to stress. This list of observed effects at different stages of development was included to show that there are many possible adverse effects other than decreases in survival and growth. Many of the effects in Table 1 were observed at much higher water concentrations than would be tolerated in an exposure of 30–90 d, such as required in an ELS toxicity test with fish. However, many of the responses are commonly seen in ELS toxicity tests, as indicated in the third column of Table 1. The toxic effects most readily observed in ELS toxicity tests occur at hatching and/or during larval and early juvenile development. There are several reasons for this. First, most investigators do not make detailed examinations of embryonic development, and record gross abnormalities only after hatching. Second, the chorion (eggshell) in most cases provides some protection to the developing embryo;

Table 1   Summary of Some Observed Responses to Environmental Alteration Considered as Sublethal Effects[a]

Stage of organization where stress is imposed or recognized	Observed or deduced response to stress (altered structure or function)	Toxic effects/observed in 30–90 d ELS toxicity tests[b]	Observed or suspected consequences of response to stress
Sex products:			
Sperm (prior to fertilization)	Reduction in motility		Reduced fertility
	Reduced fertility		Reduced rate of fertilization
	Gene damage		Embryonic malformations
Eggs (unfertilized and during fertilization)	Changes in properties of egg:		
	Membranes, related to surface structure capsule	x	Reduced strength of chorion
			Reduced rates of gas diffusion, respiration
	Water uptake during and after fertilization	x	Changes in osmoregulatory capacity
			Changes in buoyancy of pelagic eggs (changes in transport, distribution and location in water column)
	Rate of fertilization		Reproductive success
Embryonic development (early and advanced)	Biochemical effects:		
	Changes in ATP levels		Energy deficit
			Retarded development
			Necrotic tissue
			Dedifferentiation
			Organ malformation
	Changes in enzyme activity		Interference with general metabolism and biosynthetic processes, retarded development, reduced yolk energy conversion, smaller larval size at hatching, reduced hatching success
	Physiological effects:		
	Respiration changes		Changes in embryonic growth rates
			Changes in incubation rate
	Embryonic heart rate		Retarded development
	Morphological effects:		
	Unusual shape of blastodisc		Embryonic malformations(?)
	Deformation of blastomeres		Embryonic malformations(?)
	Irregular cleavage of blastomeres		Embryonic malformations(?)
	Amorphous embryonic tissue (no definite embryo formed)	x	No visible hatch
	Yolk deformation		Impaired yolk utilization, respiration(?)

Note: See footnotes on page 66.

Table 1 Summary of Some Observed Responses to Environmental Alteration Considered as Sublethal Effects[a] (Continued)

Stage of organization where stress is imposed or recognized	Observed or deduced response to stress (altered structure or function)	Toxic effects/observed in 30–90 d ELS toxicity tests[b]	Observed or suspected consequences of response to stress
	Yolk-sac blood circulation not well developed		Impaired yolk utilization(?) respiration(?)
	Organ malformations		
	Bent body axis		Impaired swimming, feeding, escape reactions
	Elongated heart tube	x	Impaired blood circulation(?)
	Eye malformations (see also yolk sac larvae)	x	Impaired vision, prey hunting, photoaxis
	Malformed otoliths and/or otic capsules		Impaired equilibrium, swimming, prey hunting
	Behavioral effects:		
	Embryonic activity reduced		Reduced mixing of perivitelline fluid affecting respiration, distribution of hatching enzyme; retarded development, abnormal hatching process
	Pectoral fin movements reduced		As above (embryonic activity)
Larvae at hatching	Altered hatching parameters:		
	Change in duration of hatching period	x	Altered distribution, density of larvae in time and space
	Increased or decreased incubation time	x	Desynchronizing of food availability at time of first feeding
	Reduced viable hatch	x	Reduced survival potential at population level
	Smaller larval size at hatching	x	Reduced biomass, increased susceptibility to predation
	Head first hatching	x	
Yolk-sac larvae (protolarvae)	Buoyancy anomalies		Difficulty in maintaining position in water column
	Swimming behavior:		
	Inability to swim		Impaired ability to maintain position in water column
	Equilibrium anomalies	x	Inability to capture food
	Loss of avoidance reaction		Reduced escape reaction, increased susceptibility to predation
	Altered yolk utilization:		
	Reduced conversion efficiency	x	Reduced biomass production, reduced larval size at time of first food intake, increased susceptibility to predation

Note: See footnotes on page 66.

Table 1 Summary of Some Observed Responses to Environmental Alteration Considered as Sublethal Effects[a] (Continued)

Stage of organization where stress is imposed or recognized	Observed or deduced response to stress (altered structure or function)	Toxic effects/observed in 30–90 d ELS toxicity tests[b]	Observed or suspected consequences of response to stress
	Changed rate of yolk utilization	x	Shift in timing to first food intake
	Malformations:		
	Serrated fins	x	Altered dermal respiration, swimming ability, susceptibility to disease
	Eye defects (anophthalmia, microphthalmia, monophthalmia, cyclopia)	x	Reduced visual perception, phototaxis, prey hunting ability
	Mouth, lower jaw, branchial apparatus	x	Impaired respiration, feeding success
	Vertebral column	x	Impaired swimming ability, escape reaction, prey hunting
Larvae (post yolk sac) (meso–meta larvae and early juvenile)	Altered food relations:		
	Reduced food availability, conversion efficiency, growth		Starvation; increased susceptibility to disease, predation; reduced survival potential at population level
	Reduced swimming capacity	x	Increased susceptibility to predation
	Behavioral effects:		
	Changes in opercular rates coughing response		Impaired gill function, respiration
Gonadal tissue (adult)	Success and timing of gamete production:		Desynchronization of spawning, larval production, and food supply
	Reduced fecundity		Impaired reproductive success
	Inhibition of maturation of ova		Impaired reproductive success
	Destruction of male germinal tissue		Impaired reproductive success
	Passage of contaminants through eggs to next generation		Deleterious effects on offspring

[a]These are shown in relation to ontogenetic stages of development in which they are observed and to known or possible consequences at later stages of development. For example, response to stress imposed at fertilization may be observed first as tissue anomalies in advanced embryos, whose significance to survival is expressed later as altered behavior in hatched larvae [modified from Rosenthal and Alderdice (1976), reproduced by permission of the Ministry of Supply and Services Canada].

[b]The effects listed in this column were taken from the references listed in Table 6 of this chapter.

this is lost at hatching, exposing the larval fish to the full impact of the toxic chemical. Third, subtle alterations of the embryo are often missed by the untrained eye and show up later as gross abnormalities. Several examples of the toxic effects listed in Table 1 are given in Tables 2 and 3 and Figs. 4–14.

Tables 2 and 3 represent effects caused by zinc at fertilization and during early developmental changes in the membranes involved in the surface structure of the chorion (Benoit and Holcombe, 1978; Holcombe et al., 1979). Similar changes in chorion structure occurred in marine fish exposed to cadmium (Rosenthal and Alderdice, 1976) and freshwater fish exposed to copper and nickel (J. M. McKim, unpublished data). This is a very sensitive end point, which develops quickly and can in most cases be related to sublethal or chronic effects seen later in the life cycle. The effects on chorion structure and the force required to rupture the chorion seem to be more severe if embryos are exposed before water hardening (Table 2). The force required to rupture the chorion also seems to be inversely related to the toxicant exposure concentration (Table 3).

Both gross and microscopic abnormalities are useful in determining the sublethal effects of toxicants on embryonic development. Figure 4 shows the teratogenic effect of low concentrations of methyl mercury on eye development in *Fundulus* sp. shortly before hatching. Further teratogenic effects of methyl mercury are seen after hatching (Fig. 5) and consist of severe scoliosis and jaw abnormalities, which preclude feeding or swimming. Newly hatched pike larvae exposed to extremely low concentrations of 2,3,7,8-tetrachlorodibenzo-*p*-dioxin (TCDD) show reduced size at hatching and edema in the heart area (Fig. 6). The intensity of these effects is directly related to the toxicant concentration. Photomicrographs of 6-d-old bluegill larvae exposed to cadmium (Fig. 7) showed pericardial and abdominal edema. In addition, they showed lordosis dorsally of more than $90°$ from normal and delayed yolk sorption. Other sublethal effects of cadmium on embryonic development are seen in Fig. 8, which shows the serrated caudal fins of newly hatched garpike larvae.

Other common effects seen after hatching, during the larval phases of development, are reduced growth and poor yolk utilization (Fig. 9). The copper-exposed brook trout alevins are twice as old as the controls, yet have used almost no yolk and are half as large. These gross effects are indicative of subtle effects on metabolism, possibly on

Table 2   Fathead Minnow Embryos Spawned in Control Water and Transferred Intact (Attached to the Substrate) before and after Water Hardening to Water Containing Zn at 295 μg/l[a]

Item	Before water hardening				After water hardening[b]	
Eggs spawned on substrate and transferred intact	14	20	39	68	54	17
Hours incubated after transfer	4	4	4	24	4	24
Chorions ruptured during removal from substrate (%)	21[c]	30[c]	15[c]	13[c]	0[d]	6[d]

[a]With permission from Benoit and Holcombe (1978); copyright the Fisheries Society of the British Isles.

[b]Embryos transferred were approximately 25–35 min old. At 25°C embryos became water-hardened approximately 20 min after they were spawned.

[c]Embryos adhered poorly to spawning substrate and fell off at the slightest touch.

[d]Embryos adhered normally to spawning substrate.

Table 3 Force Required to Burst Brook Trout Chorions Exposed to Various Concentrations of Zinc Prior to Water Hardening[a]

Mean total zinc concentration (μg/l)	Duplicates	Mean weight required to rupture the chorion after 11 d exposure to zinc (g)[b]
1360	A	182 ± 121 (6)
	B	
534	A	971 ± 111 (15)
	B	
266	A	993 ± 179 (7)
	B	
144	A	1155 ± 64 (2)
	B	
69	A	
	B	
39	A	
	B	
Control 2.6	A	1223 ± 107 (11)
	B	

[a]Modified from Holcombe et al. (1979).

[b]Mean in grams ±95% confidence interval. Numbers of groups of five embryos examined are in parentheses. Missing entries indicate that fragility was not measured.

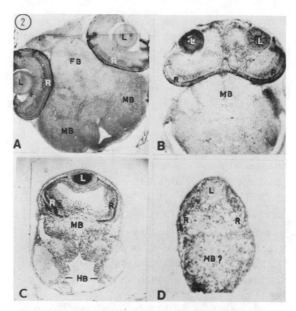

Figure 4 Photomicrographs of *Fundulus* embryos fixed near time of hatching (stage 34.14 d), sectioned coronally and stained with toluidine blue. (a) Control embryo; (b) third-degree (partially fused) synophthalmic embryo; (c) cyclopic embryo; (d) severely retarded and cyclopic embryo. Key: L, lens; R, retina; FB, MB, and HB, forebrain, midbrain, and hindbrain, respectively. Magnifications: (a–c) ×60; (d) ×100. *[From Weis and Weis (1977).]*

specific enzyme or hormonal systems. They are commonly seen in ELS toxicity tests. Another common anomaly is scoliosis or the broken back syndrome (Figs. 10 and 11), which occurs at different stages of development, depending on the chemical used and the exposure regime. Again, these abnormalities are probably tied to metabolic disruption.

Enzymatic and hormonal monitoring, which has received little attention in ELS testing, would provide a measure of the disruption of normal enzyme and/or hormone development during organogenesis in the growing embryo and larval fish. Figures 12, 13, and 14 show the normal development of three essential biochemicals in fish embryos and larvae. Alteration of these development patterns and timing sequences by low concentrations of toxic chemicals could greatly reduce the survival potential of rapidly growing fish. Future research should be aimed at studying changes in

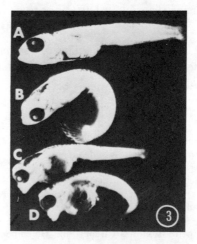

Figure 5 One-day posthatch larval *Fundulus,* approximately ×13. (a) Control; (b–d) treated with 0.02 mg/l methyl mercury *in ovo,* showing that inability to uncurl after hatching (b and d) can occur independently of craniofacial anomalies (c and d). *[Modified from Weis and Weis (1977).]*

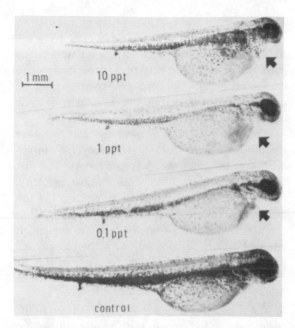

Figure 6 Appearance of pike yolk-sac fry exposed to different concentrations of TCDD, 11 d after fertilization. Arrows indicate the onset of edema. *[From Helder (1980).]*

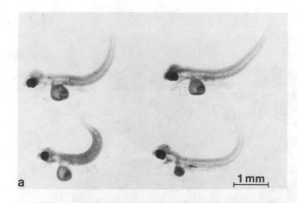

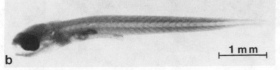

Figure 7 Photomicrographs of (a) crippled and (b) normal 6-d-old bluegill larvae from the 239 μg/l cadmium and control tanks, respectively. *[From Eaton (1974).]*

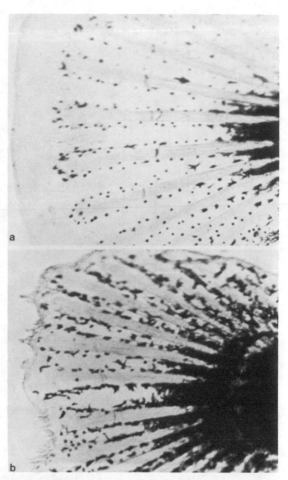

Figure 8 Serrated caudal fin of a newly hatched larva incubated in cadmium-contaminated seawater (b) compared to the undamaged primordial fin of a control specimen (a). *[From Von Westernhagen et al. (1975).]*

hormonal and enzymatic development at low levels of toxic chemicals.

Effects used as critical end points in life cycle and ELS toxicity tests to establish MATCs are discussed further in a later section.

METHODOLOGY FOR EARLY LIFE STAGE TOXICITY TESTS IN FISH

The methodology for acute and chronic toxicity tests in fish has developed rapidly over the past decade. Protocols for both types of tests are presented in Chapters 2 and 4. A few points related to

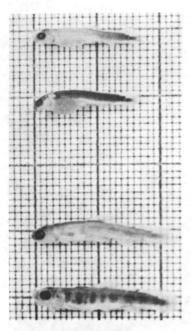

Figure 9 Copper effects on brook trout development and yolk sac absorption: (top) 32.5 µg/l copper, 553 degree-days after hatch; (bottom) control (1.9 µg/l copper), 276 degree-days after hatch (each division equals 1 mm) (degree-days = mean daily temperature × number of days). *[From McKim and Benoit (1971); reproduced by permission of the Ministry of Supply and Services Canada.]*

chronic testing are mentioned here as a lead-in to ELS tests. Fish life cycle toxicity tests were initially performed only with fathead minnows. The need for partial life cycle tests arose in order to test more species, so that sensitivities could be compared with those found in the earlier life cycle tests with fathead minnows.

The fish selected for these comparisons were the brook trout, a salmonid, the bluegill, a centrarchid, and the flagfish, a cyprinodontid. The first two species require 2 yr to reach sexual maturity, but this period was shortened by starting the fish as yearlings just prior to gonad development. Thus the partial life cycle toxicity test was created. It required 12 mo to complete with the bluegill and the brook trout. All important aspects of the life cycle, including reproduction, were exposed to the toxicant.

The similarity in sensitivity between partial life cycle tests and life cycle tests was established for four toxicants (copper, methyl mercury, cadmium, and lead) by conducting both types of tests with brook trout (McKim and Benoit, 1971, 1974; McKim et al., 1976; Benoit et al., 1976; Holcombe et al., 1976) and fathead minnows (Pickering et al., 1977). Partial life cycle tests were considered

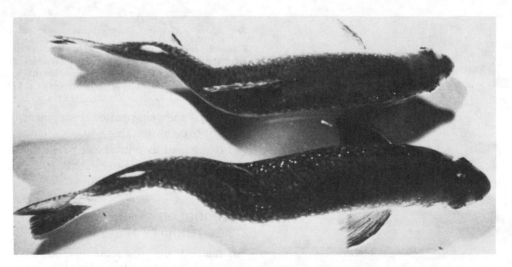

Figure 10 Deformed 65-wk-old second-generation brook trout exposed to 125 µg/l lead. *[From Holcombe et al. (1976); reproduced by permission of the Ministry of Supply and Services Canada.]*

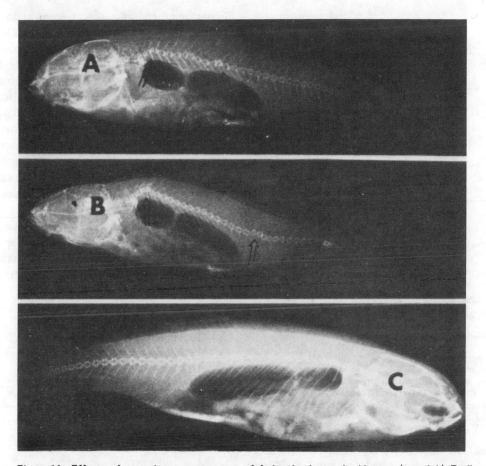

Figure 11 Effects of toxaphene on structure of fathead minnow backbones. (*a* and *b*) Radiographs representative of fish exposed to 55 ng/l toxaphene; (*c*) control fish. Arrows point to areas of backbone affected. *[From Mehrle and Mayer (1975); reproduced by permission of the Ministry of Supply and Services Canada.]*

equivalent to life cycle tests in the development of water quality criteria for aquatic animals. The desire to have even shorter tests for predicting the chronic toxicity of chemicals to fish led to the development of ELS toxicity tests over the past decade. This evolution was a logical outgrowth of life cycle and partial life cycle testing, which showed the great sensitivity of these stages in the life cycle.

Specific methodologies for conducting ELS tests with fish are documented in the references cited at the end of this chapter, which should be consulted for detailed information on culture

techniques for selected species. References of particular interest are ASTM (1981) and USEPA (1981b). The rest of this section describes the general methods used at present and some innovations available for conducting ELS toxicity tests with fish.

GENERAL METHODS

Physical-Chemical System

Exposure System

Various designs have been used for toxicant delivery systems, but all of them are offshoots of the serial diluter (Mount and Brungs, 1967) and the

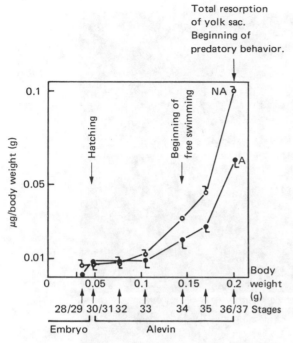

Figure 12 Adrenalin (A) and noradrenalin (NA) contents in embryos and larvae of rainbow trout in relation to body weight (wet). Each point represents the average for 6–12 animals. *[From Meyer and Sauerbier (1977) with permission; copyright 1977 Fisheries Society of the British Isles.]*

continuous flow diluter (Warner, 1964). Complete design and construction details are available for diluters (Lemke et al., 1978), and these diluter systems can be adapted for ELS toxicity studies with fish. They are discussed in detail in Chapters 2 and 4.

Recently, an integrated system designed especially for use in ELS tests with fish and invertebrates was built and evaluated for use both in the laboratory and in the field (Benoit et al., 1981a,b). This is a relatively small, space-saving, portable, flow-through diluter. It is adaptable for use with either single toxicants or complex effluents and requires only 24 l of test water per hour (Figs. 15 and 16). The system handles water containing suspended solids. It continues normal operation for 10 h if the effluent supply is cut off and up to 4 h if the diluent water is cut off. The smaller

volumes required with this system allow easier shipment of effluent samples for testing. They also facilitate the removal of hazardous chemicals from test water by laboratory filtration prior to discharge into the sewer system. Although this minidiluter system was designed primarily for ELS studies with fathead minnows, it would perform equally well with other fish species routinely used in ELS studies except salmonids. Salmonids are too large and active 60 d after hatching for the small exposure chambers of the minidiluter (Fig. 17). The system has also been used successfully with invertebrates (insects and amphipods).

In addition, Benoit et al. (1981a) designed a stationary vented exposure system for containing and exhausting the fumes of hazardous volatile chemicals used in ELS tests (Figs. 18 and 19).

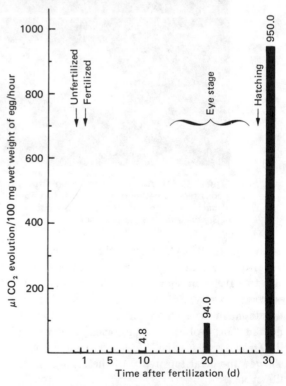

Figure 13 Acetylcholinesterase activity of rainbow trout embryo homogenate during development. Activity is expressed as microliters of CO_2 evolved per 100 mg of egg (wet weight) per hour. *[From Uesugi and Yamazoe (1964).]*

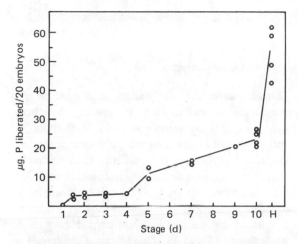

Figure 14 Change in adenosinetriphosphatase activity of fish embryos during embryonic development. Conditions: 0.05 *M* histidine buffer, 1 m*M* ATP, 0.1 *M* KCl. Activity is expressed as micrograms of P split per 20 embryos in 15 min at pH 9.1 and 37°C. *[From Ishida et al. (1959).]*

The diluter system is the same minidiluter just described hung inside an enclosure that has ample viewing and sampling ports, a lower watertight shelf for saturators (Veith and Comstock, 1975; Gingerich et al., 1979), metering pumps, and a carbon filtration device for waste water before it enters the sanitary sewer. The lower portion of the unit is watertight and can hold up to 100 l of water—enough to protect the room from contamination in case a leak develops in the system. To date, 32 ELS studies with fathead minnows and several invertebrates have been performed with this system.

The toxicant delivery system selected should be designed to accommodate a minimum of five exposure concentrations plus controls. A dilution factor not greater than 50% between concentrations should be used. There must be at least two separate exposure chambers for each toxicant concentration, and the test water delivery tubes from the toxicant delivery system to these individual exposure chambers should be positioned by stratified random assignment (Fig. 20). A minimum of 5–10 water volume turnovers per 24 h in

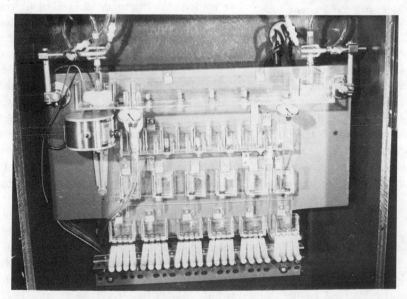

Figure 15 Continuous flow minidiluter for use with either single chemicals or treated complex effluents. *[Reprinted with permission from Benoit et al. (1981a); copyright 1981, Pergamon Press, Ltd.]*

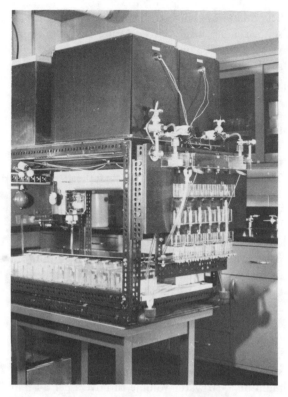

Figure 16 Portable early life stage exposure system. *[Reprinted with permission from Benoit et al. (1981a); copyright 1981, Pergamon Press, Ltd.]*

each exposure chamber is usually required to maintain proper toxicant concentrations, dissolved oxygen concentrations above 60% of saturation, and test temperatures within ±1°C, and to prevent the buildup of dissolved waste materials, such as ammonia, in the experimental chambers. Once daily feeding of larval fish begins, all exposure chambers should be siphoned daily to remove solid waste materials and uneaten food. The photoperiod should be held constant throughout the test at 16 h light and 8 h dark, while light intensity at the water surface should be 30–60 lumens.

Before starting an ELS study, the system should be calibrated and run without animals for several days to check toxicant delivery. It should

be checked daily during a test and recalibrated if necessary.

Water Characteristics

Dilution water used in toxicity tests must be uncontaminated and of constant quality. The best source of dilution water for freshwater studies is spring or well water. The second choice is uncontaminated surface water; and the least desirable source is dechlorinated city water, which contains small amounts of residual chlorine that are very difficult to remove. For saltwater tests, an uncontaminated surface source of constant salinity ranging between 15 and 35 g/kg (parts per thousand) is recommended. Saltwater from a natural source must be filtered through a filter with a pore size <10 μm to remove the larval stages of predators. Dilution water for both freshwater and saltwater studies should be filtered, ultraviolet-sterilized, brought to the desired test temperature, and vigorously aerated to stabilize oxygen and pH before use.

Certain water chemistry measurements should be made at the beginning and end of all freshwater and saltwater tests to make sure the quality of the dilution water remains constant. Total hardness, alkalinity, pH, conductivity, total organic carbon, and particulate matter should be measured for freshwater. If possible, calcium, magnesium, sodium, potassium, chloride, and sulfate should be determined. Salinity, pH, and particulate matter (total suspended solids) should be measured for saltwater. For both saltwater and freshwater tests, dissolved oxygen should be measured at least twice a week in all test concentrations throughout the test period. Temperature and salinity should be recorded continuously for the dilution water, and temperatures at each exposure concentration should be taken at least twice a week. All chemical measurements should be performed as described by the ASTM (1980b), American Public Health Association (APHA) et al. (1975), and Strickland and Parsons (1968).

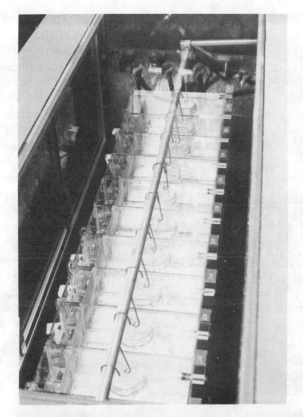

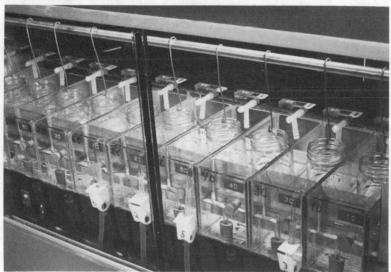

Figure 17 Exposure chambers with egg cups on rocker arm. *[From Benoit et al. (1981c).]*

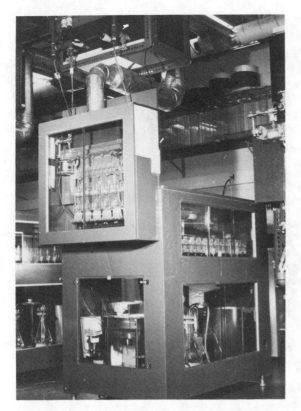

Figure 18 Stationary vented early life stage exposure system. *[Reprinted with permission from Benoit et al. (1981a); copyright 1981, Pergamon Press, Ltd.]*

Toxicant Solutions

Stock solutions of test chemicals to be metered into the dilution water in a toxicity test are at best saturated water solutions of the test chemical. Use of water as the solvent avoids the possible toxic effects of an organic carrier and is generally more realistic. Several excellent devices for saturating water with chemicals have been designed by Veith and Comstock (1975) and Gingerich et al. (1979). If solvents (carriers) other than water must be used, dimethyl formamide and triethylene glycol are preferred. No organic carrier should exceed 0.5 ml/l in the test water. If an organic carrier is used, it is usually necessary to run a separate carrier control along with the regular (negative) control to make sure there are no effects of the

carrier on the test animals. The amount of carrier added should be the same at all toxicant concentrations tested. Metering pumps, mechanical injectors, and Mariotte bottles are commonly used to deliver the toxicant stock solution to the diluter system (Mount and Brungs, 1967; Warner, 1964; Benoit et al., 1981a). Exposure concentrations are assigned in a stratified random manner to the exposure chambers in order to eliminate position effects. In starting a new toxicity test, the exposure concentrations should be checked immediately before placing animals in the system. Exposure concentrations are routinely monitored twice a week in alternate replicate exposure chambers.

Analytical methods should be standardized accepted procedures such as those found in the Annual Book of ASTM Standards (ASTM, 1980b),

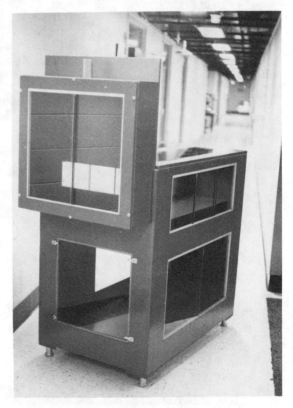

Figure 19 Vented enclosure for testing hazardous volatile chemicals. *[Reprinted with permission from Benoit et al. (1981a); copyright 1981, Pergamon Press, Ltd.]*

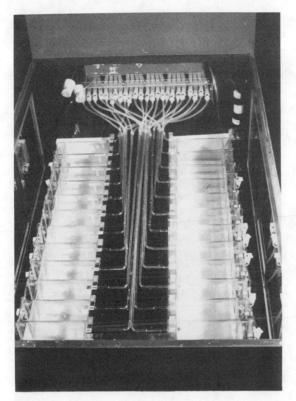

Figure 20 Delivery tubes showing stratified random assignment. *[From Benoit et al. (1981c).]*

Methods for Chemical Analysis of Water and Wastes (USEPA, 1979), and Manual of Analytical Methods for the Analysis of Pesticides in Human and Environmental Samples (USEPA, 1980). All analytical methods must be validated before animals are placed in the system. As a minimum, accuracy should be checked by the method of known additions, using dilution water from the diluter apparatus. Precision should be evaluated by analyzing three samples collected on two separate days from one of the lower exposure concentrations. The analytical method should be further checked against reference or split samples and, if possible, against other methods.

Biological System

A number of freshwater fish species and several saltwater fish species (Table 4) have been used in life cycle or ELS toxicity tests (Eaton et al., 1978; Nebeker et al., 1977; Chapman and Shumway, 1977; McKim et al., 1975, 1978; Hokanson et al., 1973a,b; Benoit et al., 1981b; McCormick et al., 1977; Eaton, 1970; Mayer et al., 1977; Schimmel and Hansen, 1974; Hansen and Parrish, 1977; Goodman et al., 1976; Parrish et al., 1978; Middaugh and Lempesis, 1976; Middaugh and Dean, 1977). The species listed in Table 4 were selected on the basis of availability; commercial, recreational, and ecological importance; and past successful use or ease of culture in the laboratory. Test temperatures were taken from the references cited above or from Brungs and Jones (1977). The duration of ELS tests is 28 d posthatch for all the species in Table 4 except the salmonids, which require 60 d, and the sheepshead minnow, which require 24 d. These periods allow exposure from fertilization through embryonic, larval, and early juvenile stages of development.

Before performing an ELS toxicity test with a particular species, a 6–10 d range-finding test should be conducted with 24-h-old (newly hatched) larvae. The lowest concentration that has obvious effects on the larvae should be used as the high exposure concentration in the final definitive test. All other exposure concentrations should be diluted downward from this concentration by using a set dilution factor of not less than 0.5.

Embryonic Period

Stop 9/17

The initial step in setting up an ELS toxicity test is obtaining high-quality test animals. Fish embryos can generally be obtained by (1) collecting mature, ripe adults in the field and stripping gametes, (2) buying mature, ripe adults from a commercial hatchery and stripping gametes, (3) obtaining, as needed, newly fertilized embryos from a laboratory stock culture unit, or (4) buying disease-free embryos from a commercial hatchery or another laboratory. The species to be tested will in many cases dictate the method used to obtain embryos.

The ELS test is started by impartially placing 50–100 newly fertilized (<8 h old) embryos into

Table 4   Recommended Species, Test Temperature, Salinity, Duration, and Photoperiod for the Testing of Fish Early Life Stages[a]

Species[b]	Temperature (°C)	Salinity (ppt)	Duration (d)
Freshwater:			
Coho salmon, *Oncorhynchus kisutch*	10, 12[c]	NA[d]	60[e]
Chinook salmon, *O. tshawytscha*	10, 12	NA	60
Rainbow trout, *Salmo gairdneri*	10, 12	NA	60
Brown trout, *S. trutta*	10	NA	60
Brook trout, *Salvelinus fontinalis*	10	NA	60
Lake trout, *S. namaycush*	7	NA	60
Northern pike, *Esox lucius*	12, 18	NA	28
Fathead minnow, *Pimephales promelas*	25	NA	28
White sucker, *Catostomus commersoni*	15	NA	28
Bluegill, *Lepomis macrochirus*	28	NA	28
Channel catfish, *Ictalurus punctatus*	26	NA	28
Saltwater:			
Sheepshead minnow, *Cyprinodon variegatus*	30	15-30	28[f]
Silversides, *Menidia* spp.	25	15-35	28

[a]Modified from ASTM (1981); copyright American Society for Testing and Materials; adapted with permission.
[b]Scientific name must be verified.
[c]10°C refers to embryo test temperature, 12°C to larval test temperature.
[d]Not applicable.
[e]Posthatch exposure duration.
[f]Includes incubation.

the incubation chambers in each exposure chamber. An alternative procedure involves mixing the gametes together and fertilizing the eggs in the exposure water before placing the embryos in the incubation chambers. The latter method is preferred since effects on fertilization and water hardening of the eggs are included in the same test. If the first method is used, the exact stage of embryo development should be recorded (see Figure 2 and Lagler et al., 1977, pp. 302–323). The embryos are incubated in vertically oscillating 120-ml glass jars with 40-mesh nylon screen bottoms similar to those of Mount (1968) or in stationary incubation containers with fluctuating water levels controlled by self-starting siphons. The embryo incubation chambers are randomly placed in the exposure chambers. Salmonid embryos are sensitive to light and must be incubated in the dark from fertilization to 1 wk after hatching. During incuba-

tion, dead embryos must be removed daily to prevent the spread of fungal infections. Dead embryos usually appear opaque and are easily distinguished from living ones.

Larval Period

This phase begins with hatching. An accurate daily record of abnormal larvae, with descriptions of abnormalities, should be kept. Except for salmonids, release from the incubation cup should occur when hatching is 90% complete or 48 h after the first hatch in that incubation cup. Unhatched embryos should remain in the cup, and larvae should be allowed to swim out of the cup into the exposure chamber. If more embryos were used for hatchability than are to be used for the larval portion of the test, the fish retained to complete the test should be randomly selected from all larvae hatched, both normal and abnormal. Salmonids are released from the incubation cups 21 d after hatching or at swim-up and are handled as described above.

Food should be provided to the growing larvae as the larvae absorb the yolk and begin to swim up off the bottom of the exposure tank. The interval between hatching and swim-up varies greatly. For example, it is 2–3 d for fathead minnows at 25°C and 21–28 d for brook trout at 10°C. Newly hatched brine shrimp nauplii are the food of choice for the fish listed in Table 4 except channel catfish and salmonids, which require a commercially prepared starter food, and silversides, which require a rotifer (*Brachionus* sp.). Feeding should take place at least three times a day and be spaced so that food is present in the water continously during daylight. A weight or volume system should be used to quantitate the food placed in the exposure chambers so that the amounts fed are equal. The amounts should be reduced on a percentage basis as larvae die in the higher concentrations.

Survival is determined daily for larval fish in each exposure chamber. This is best done by counting live larvae in each exposure chamber, because during the first few weeks many newly hatched species deteriorate rapidly after death. Behavior (feeding, sluggish movement, loss of equilibrium, and so on) should be observed. The development and number of morphological abnormalities should also be recorded.

Early Juvenile Period

At the end of the ELS test the number of surviving juveniles at each exposure is recorded, weights and lengths are recorded for growth, and all deformities are described (with photographs if possible) and quantitated.

Biological Data

The following biological data should be collected during a typical ELS toxicity test for each developmental period.

Embryonic period:

1 Incubation period, the time from fertilization to complete hatching.
2 Hatching time, the time required for all embryos to hatch at a given exposure concentration once the first one hatches.
3 Time from complete hatch to first feeding.
4 Percent of normal and abnormal larvae at complete hatch.
5 Weight of larvae at complete hatch.

Larval and early juvenile periods:

1 Abnormal behavior.
2 Total percent of deformed fish at the end of the test.
3 Percent survival of fish at the end of the test.
4 Weights and lengths of all fish at the end of the test.
5 Occurrence of normal metamorphosis from the metalarval phase to the juvenile phase as compared to controls.

Special Examinations

Restart 9/17

This category can always be expanded and can result in the generation of useful end points for future ELS tests. Examples of the kinds of measurements that can be made are shown in Table 1. These include embryological, physiological, biochemical, histological, and behavioral observations.

Conclusions and Interpretation of Data

Once the data have been collected, evaluated, and categorized (for example, see Table 5), they must be analyzed statistically to determine whether there are significant effects of the toxicant.

If an organic carrier is used to introduce the toxicant, a t-test (Steel and Torrie, 1960) must be performed to determine the differences (if any) between the regular control and the carrier control. If differences exist, the results are questionable. If both controls are the same, then all the control data can be combined for the remaining statistical analyses.

Once the controls have been analyzed, the question is whether significant differences exist in each data set (items in Table 5) collected during the ELS

Table 5   Hatchability of Embryos, Normal Larvae at Hatch, and Survival and Weight of 28-d-old Fathead Minnows Exposed to Various 1,2-Dichloropropane Concentrations[a]

Item	1,2-Dichloropropane (mg/l)					Control[b] (0.1 ± 0.02)
	110 ± 3[c]	51 ± 2	25 ± 1	11 ± 2	6 ± 1	
Hatchability of embryos (%)[d]	96 (90–100)	96 (93–100)	98 (93–100)	98 (93–100)	96 (93–100)	97 (97)
Normal larvae at hatch (%)	0	67[f] (53–80)	100	100	100	100
Survival of 28-d-old fish (%)[e]	0	27[f] (0–40)	58[f] (0–93)	95 (87–100)	92 (87–100)	95 (93–100)
Weight of 28-d-old fish (mg)	—	18[f] ±6	79[f] ±20	126[f] ±33	140 ±29	145 ±45

[a] Each entry represents the mean of four replicates per treatment and numbers in parentheses denote replicate range. From Benoit et al. (1981b).
[b] Slight contamination of control water was from air inside vented enclosure.
[c] Mean and standard deviation.
[d] Thirty 2–5-h-old embryos exposed per replicate.
[e] Fifteen fish exposed per replicate.
[f] Significantly different from control, $P = 0.05$ (analysis of variance with Dunnett's test).

test. Therefore an analysis of variance (ANOVA) F-test is run on each data set (Steel and Torrie, 1960; McClave et al., 1981; Sokal and Rohlf, 1969; Box et al., 1978). For data sets or items showing significant differences ($P = 0.05$), all exposure concentration measurements are compared with the control measurements by an appropriate multiple comparison test, such as Dunnett's procedure (Dunnett, 1955, 1964) and Williams' procedure (Williams, 1971, 1972). Significant differences from the controls ($P = 0.05$) are then used to establish the *lowest observed effect concentration* (LOEC) and the highest *no observed effect concentration* (NOEC), or the MATC range. In the example in Table 5, the LOEC and NOEC were 11 and 6 mg/l, respectively, based on the most sensitive effects in the test. With 1,2-dichloropropane that effect was 28-d growth (Benoit et al., 1981b). Therefore, the estimated MATC of 1,2-dichloropropane for fathead minnows can be reported as >6 < 11 mg/l based on 28-d growth.

The sublethal effects used to establish the NOEC (growth in the example above) are assumed to be important for the individuals' well-being and

the maintenance of a healthy population. Decisions about the importance of specific effects must be made by the researcher. The validity of such decisions in most cases depends on the experience and biological expertise of the individual. The importance of selected sublethal effects was discussed in the earlier section on end points.

INVERTEBRATE EARLY LIFE STAGE TOXICITY TESTS

Freshwater and saltwater aquatic invertebrates have become very important in aquatic toxicology in recent years because of (1) the speed with which an invertebrate life cycle test can be performed (1–5 mo compared to 12–24 mo for a fish life cycle test) and (2) the similar sensitivities of the two groups. The latter fact has enhanced the development of fish partial life cycle and ELS toxicity tests, while little need existed for the development of shorter predictive invertebrate tests.

Daphnia magna is the best known and most used invertebrate test species in freshwater toxicology. Life cycle toxicity tests with this species range from 21–28 d to lifetime studies requiring several months. The 21–28 d studies have been more or less standardized for use in long-term toxicity testing. There is some evidence, however, that lifetime studies with *Daphnia* are more sensitive than the 21–28 d exposures (Winner and Farrell, 1976; Buikema et al., 1980). Buikema et al. (1980) reported that with the water-soluble fractions of hydrocarbons the 21-d daphnid test measuring growth and reproduction was predictive for lifetime studies only 56% of the time. Some work on the development of short predictive tests for the 21–28 d daphnid life cycle tests (e.g., Geiger et al., 1980) indicated that the size of daphnid preadults after 7 d of exposure to the water-soluble fraction of hydrocarbons gave the same toxic effect values as the 21-d exposures. There are enough chronic toxicity data for daphnids to evaluate new predictive methods, but a standardized short predictor of chronic toxicity does not yet exist and the standard daphnid 21–28 d chronic toxicity test continues to be the major freshwater invertebrate test (see Chapter 4 for details on chronic daphnid tests). At present, the only short predictive test with an invertebrate on a par with the fish ELS toxicity test is that with *Daphnia magna.*

Review articles on two other less tested freshwater invertebrates, the chironomids (Anderson, 1980) and the amphipods (Arthur, 1980), show considerable progress in life cycle and partial life cycle test development. However, the already short duration of the life cycle tests and lack of life cycle data for evaluating the predictive capabilities of shorter tests inhibit the development of short predictive tests. Therefore, as with *Daphnia,* no standardized short tests for predicting chronic toxicity have been established and life cycle tests with these species continue to be important.

Essentially, the same arguments hold for saltwater invertebrates. Mysids (Nimmo et al., 1977), grass shrimp (Tyler-Schoeder, 1979) and polychaete annelids (Reish, 1980) are used in life cycle tests that require 1–2 mo. Until more data on life cycle tests with these animals are available for evaluating new shorter predictive tests, and until more is known about the biology and sensitivity of the developmental stages of each life cycle, few useful predictive tests will be developed with these saltwater invertebrates. Other saltwater invertebrates used in toxicity tests are larvae of the oyster (Calabrese et al., 1973; Roberts, 1980) and larvae of the crab and lobster (APHA et al., 1975). The time intervals and culturing difficulties with these species make routine life cycle tests nearly impossible at this time.

Invertebrates have an excellent potential as rapid (a few days or weeks), sensitive predictors of long-term toxicity because of their diversity and short, sensitive life cycles. However, the biology of each species must be better known and a chronic data base made available in order to evaluate the usefulness of new short-term predictive tests.

EXTRAPOLATION FROM EARLY LIFE STAGE TOXICITY TESTS TO LIFE CYCLE TOXICITY TESTS

Evaluation of the usefulness of ELS toxicity tests with fish has been made possible by the large data base from life cycle toxicity tests generated over the past decade. In addition, several investigators have shown that the ELS portions of life cycle tests are the most sensitive to single toxicants. However, acceptance of the ELS toxicity test approach and its widespread use came only after comprehensive reviews of all existing data from freshwater life cycle toxicity tests (Macek and Sleight, 1977; McKim, 1977). Table 6 gives a summary of these data, as well as recent life cycle test data from freshwater and saltwater laboratories. The new data presented here were subjected to the same rigorous criteria for inclusion that were used previously. These data confirm that the embryo-larval, early juvenile portion of the life cycle is the most, or one of the most, sensitive in the life cycle of both freshwater and saltwater fish. This updated evaluation is based on 72 life cycle

Table 6 Results of Partial (P) and Complete (C) Life Cycle Toxicity Tests with Fish Including the MATC Established by Each Life Cycle Test and an MATC Estimated by Embryo, Larval, and Early Juvenile (ELEJ) Exposures Conducted as Part of Each Life Cycle Test[a]

Toxicant	Species	Type of life cycle test	Critical life stage end points
Freshwater			
Metals			
1. Cadmium	Fathead minnow	P	ELEJ–J
2. Cadmium	Bluegill	P	ELEJ–M, G
3. Cadmium	Flagfish	C	A–S
4. Cadmium	Flagfish	C	ELEJ–M
5. Cadmium	Flagfish	C	ELEJ–M
6. Cadmium	Flagfish	C	ELEJ–M
7. Cadmium	Brook trout	C	ELEJ–G
8. Copper	Fathead minnow	P	ELEJ–M; A–S
9. Copper	Brook trout	P	ELEJ–G
10. Copper	Brook trout	C	ELEJ–G
11. Copper	Bluegill	P	ELEJ–M
12. Chromium	Fathead minnow	P	ELEJ–M, G
13. Chromium	Brook trout	C	ELEJ–M
14. Lead	Brook trout	C	ELEJ–D
15. Lead	Flagfish	C	A–S
16. Mercury	Fathead minnow	C	ELEJ–G
17. Nickel	Fathead minnow	P	ELEJ–H
18. Zinc	Fathead minnow	P	ELEJ–F
19. Zinc	Flagfish	C	A–G
20. Zinc	Flagfish	C	A–G
21. Zinc	Brook trout	P	ELEJ–F
22. Zinc	Fathead minnow	C	ELEJ–F
Trimetallic			
23. Mixture: zinc + cadmium + copper	Fathead minnow	P	ELEJ–F
Organometallics			
24. Methylmercury	Fathead minnow	C	A–M, S
25. Methylmercury	Flagfish	P	ELEJ–G; A–S
26. Methylmercury	Brook trout	C	ELEJ–M, G
Halogens			
27. Chlorine	Fathead minnow	P	ELEJ–M
28. Chloramine	Fathead minnow	P	A–S
29. Fluoride	Fathead minnow	P	ELEJ–M
Polychlorinated biphenyls			
30. PCB-1254	Fathead minnow	C	ELEJ–M
31. PCB-1242	Fathead minnow	C	ELEJ–M
32. PCB-1248	Fathead minnow	C	ELEJ–M
33. PCB-1260	Fathead minnow	C	ELEJ–M
Pesticides			
34. Acrolein	Fathead minnow	P	ELEJ–M
35. Atrazine	Brook trout	P	A–G
36. Captan	Fathead minnow	P	ELEJ–M, G

Note: See page 84 for footnotes.

MATC (µg/l)	Estimated MATC (µg/l)	Type of embryolarval test (d)	Reference
		Freshwater	
37.0–57.0	37.0–57.0	60 (Pue) (Pe)[b]	Pickering and Gast (1972)
31.0–80.0	31.0–80.0	60 (Pe)	Eaton (1974)
4.1–8.1	8.1–16.0	60 (Pue)	Spehar (1976)
7.4–16.9	7.4–16.9	30 (Pue) (Pe)[b]	A. R. Carlson and J. H. Tucker[c]
3.0–6.5	3.0–6.5	30 (Pue) (Pe)	A. R. Carlson and J. H. Tucker[c]
3.4–7.3	3.4–7.3	30 (Pue) (Pe)	A. R. Carlson and J. H. Tucker[c]
1.7–3.4	1.7–3.4	90 (Pe) (Pe$_1$)	Benoit et al. (1976)
10.6–18.4	10.6–18.4	120 (Pue) (Pe)[b]	Mount and Stephan (1969)
9.5–17.4	9.5–17.4	90 (Pe)	McKim and Benoit (1971)
9.5–17.4	9.5–17.4	90 (Pue) (Pe) (Pe$_1$)[b]	McKim and Benoit (1974)
21.0–40.0	21.0–40.0	90 (Pue)	Benoit (1975)
1000.0–3950.0	1000.0–3950.0	30 (Pue)	Q. H. Pickering[c]
200.0–350.0	200.0–350.0	90 (Pue) (Pe)[b]	Benoit (1976)
58.0–119.0	58.0–119.0	120 (Pe) (Pe$_1$)	Holcombe et al. (1976)
31.3–62.5	62.5–125.0	120 (Pue) (Pe)[b]	R. L. Anderson[c]
<0.26	<0.26	30 (Pe)	V. M. Snarski and G. F. Olson (1981)[c]
380.0–730.0	380.0–730.0	30 (Pe)	Pickering (1974)
30.0–180.0	30.0–180.0	30 (Pe)	Brungs (1969)
26.0–51.0	51.0–85.0	30 (Pue)	Spehar (1976)
75.0–1239.0	139.0–267.0	30 (Pue)	Spehar (1976)
532.0–1368.0	532.0–1368.0	90 (Pue) (Pe) (Pe$_1$)[b]	Holcombe et al. (1979)
78.0–145.0	78.0–145.0	90 (Pue) (Pe)[b]	Benoit and Holcombe (1978)
27.3–42.3	27.3–42.3	30 (Pe)	Eaton (1973)
3.9–7.1	3.9–7.1		
5.3–6.7	5.3–6.7		
0.07–0.13	0.13–0.23	60 (Pue)	D. I. Mount and G. F. Olson[c]
0.17–0.33	0.17–0.33	30 (Pue)	W. E. Smith[c]
0.29–0.93	0.29–0.93	90 (Pe) (Pe$_1$)	McKim et al. (1976)
14.0–42.0	14.0–42.0	60 (Pe)	Arthur et al. (1975)
16.0–43.0	43.0–108.0	30 (Pe)	Arthur and Eaton (1971)
6800.0–13,600.0	6800.0–13,600.0	30 (Pe)	D. Olson[c]
1.8–4.6	1.8–4.6	90 (Pue) (Pe)	Nebeker et al. (1974)
5.4–15.0	5.4–15.0	90 (Pue) (Pe)	Nebeker et al. (1974)
1.1–3.0	1.1–4.4	60 (Pue) (Pe)	DeFoe et al. (1978)
2.1–4.0	2.1–4.0	60 (Pue) (Pe)	DeFoe et al. (1978)
11.4–41.7	11.4–41.7	30 (Pe)	Macek et al. (1976c)
60.0–120.0	120.0–240.0	90 (Pue) (Pe)[b]	Macek et al. (1976b)
16.5–39.5	16.5–39.5	30 (Pe)	Hermanutz et al. (1973)

Table 6 Results of Partial (P) and Complete (C) Life Cycle Toxicity Tests with Fish Including the MATC Established by Each Life Cycle Test and an MATC Estimated by Embryo, Larval, and Early Juvenile (ELEJ) Exposures Conducted as Part of Each Life Cycle Test[a] *(Continued)*

Toxicant	Species	Type of life cycle test	Critical life stage end points
37. Carbaryl	Fathead minnow	C	ELEJ–M
38. DDT	Fathead minnow	C	ELEJ–H, M
39. Diazinon	Flagfish	C	ELEJ–H
40. Diazinon	Fathead minnow	P	ELEJ–M, G
41. Diazinon	Brook trout	P	ELEJ–G
42. Endosulfan	Fathead minnow	P	ELEJ–H
43. Endrin	Flagfish	C	ELEJ–G
44. Endrin	Fathead minnow	C	ELEJ–M
45. Guthion®	Fathead minnow	C	A–S
46. Heptachlor	Fathead minnow	C	ELEJ–M
47. Lindane	Fathead minnow	C	A–G
48. Malathion	Flagfish	C	ELEJ–G
49. Trifluralin	Fathead minnow	P	A–M
50. Toxaphene	Brook trout	P	ELEJ–M, G
51. Toxaphene	Fathead minnow	C	ELEJ–G
52. Toxaphene	Channel catfish	P	ELEJ–G, M
Sewage			
53. Nondisinfected	Fathead minnow	C	ELEJ–M, G
54. Chlorinated	Fathead minnow	C	ELEJ–G
55. Dechlorinated	Fathead minnow	C	ELEJ–M
56. Chlorobrominated	Fathead minnow	C	ELEJ–M
Other			
57. Linear alkylate sulfonate	Fathead minnow	P	ELEJ–M
58. pH	Fathead minnow	C	ELEJ–H
59. pH	Brook trout	P	ELEJ–M, G
60. NTA	Fathead minnow	P	A–M
61. Oxygen	Fathead minnow	P	ELEJ–M
Saltwater			
1. Carbofuran	Sheepshead minnow	C	ELEJ–M
2. Caustic waste	Sheepshead minnow	C	ELEJ–M
3. Chlordane	Sheepshead minnow	C	ELEJ–H
4. Endrin	Sheepshead minnow	C	ELEJ–H, M
5. EPN	Sheepshead minnow	C	ELEJ–G
6. Kepone	Sheepshead minnow	C	ELEJ–G
7. Malathion	Sheepshead minnow	C	ELEJ–M
8. Methoxychlor	Sheepshead minnow	C	ELEJ–H, M
9. Pentachlorophenol	Sheepshead minnow	C	A–M
10. Tributyltin oxide	Sheepshead minnow	C	ELEJ–M
11. Trifluralin	Sheepshead minnow	C	A–S, ELEJ–M

[a]Pue, embryos, and larvae from previously unexposed parents; Pe, from previously exposed parents; Pe_1, from previously exposed first-generation parents; A, adult; M, mortality; G, growth; F, egg fragility; H, hatchability; D, deformities; S, spawning.

[b]No difference in sensitivity between embryos and larvae from previously exposed (Pe) and unexposed (Pue) parents [*modified from McKim (1977); reproduced by permission of the Ministry of Supply and Services Canada*].

[c]Personal communication, Environmental Research Laboratory, Duluth, Minn.

[d]Author states value may be high by 50%.

MATC (μg/l)	Estimated MATC (μg/l)	Type of embryolarval test (d)	Reference
210.0–680.0	210.0–680.0	60 (Pue) (Pe)[b]	Carlson (1971)
0.36–1.5	0.36–1.5	30 (Pe)	Jarvinen et al. (1977)
54.0–88.0	54.0–88.0	60 (Pue) (Pe)[b]	Allison (1977)
6.8–13.5	6.8–13.5	60 (Pue) (Pe)	Allison and Hermanutz (1977)
<0.80	<0.80	120 (Pue) (Pe)	Allison and Hermanutz (1977)
0.20–0.40	0.20–0.40	30 (Pue)	Macek et al. (1976c)
0.22–30	0.22–0.30	30 (Pue) (Pe)	Hermanutz (1978)
<0.14	<0.14	30 (Pe)	Jarvinen and Tyo (1978)
0.33–0.51	0.7–1.8[d]	50 (Pue) (Pe)[b]	Adelman et al. (1976)
0.86–1.84	0.86–1.84	60 (Pue) (Pe)[b]	Macek et al. (1976c)
9.1–23.5	No effect	60 (Pe)	Macek et al. (1976a)
8.6–10.9	8.6–10.9	30 (Pue) (Pe)	Hermanutz (1978)
1.95–5.1	5.1–8.2	60 (Pe)	Macek et al. (1976c)
<0.039	<0.039	60 (Pue)	Mayer et al. (1975)
0.025–0.054	0.025–0.054	30 (Pe)	Mayer et al. (1977)
0.129–0.299	0.129–0.299	30 (Pe)	Mayer et al. (1977)
25–50%	25–50%	30 (Pue) (Pe)[b]	Ward et al. (1976)
7–14%	7–14%	30 (Pue) (Pe)[b]	Ward et al. (1976)
50–100%	50–100%	30 (Pue) (Pe)[b]	Ward et al. (1976)
50–100%	50–100%	30 (Pue) (Pe)[b]	Ward et al. (1976)
630.0–1200.0	630.0–1200.0	30 (Pe)	Pickering and Thatcher (1970)
6.6–5.9 (pH)	6.6–5.9 (pH)	30 (Pue) (Pe)[b]	Mount (1973)
6.5–6.1 (pH)	6.5–6.1 (pH)	90 (Pue) (Pe)[b]	Menendez (1976)
54,000.0–114,000.0	54,000.0–114,000.0	—	Arthur et al. (1974)
5.01–4.02 (mg/l)	5.01–4.02 (mg/l)	30 (Pe)	Brungs (1971)
Saltwater			
15.0–23.0	15.0–23.0	30 (Pe) (Pue)	Parrish et al. (1977)
1500.0–3000.0	1500.0–3000.0	30 (Pue) (Pe)	Hollister et al. (1980)
0.5–0.8	0.5–0.8	30 (Pe) (Pue)	Parrish et al. (1976, 1978)
0.12–0.31	0.12–0.31	30 (Pe) (Pue)[b]	Hansen et al. (1977)
4.1–7.9	4.1–7.9	30 (Pue) (Pe)	U.S. EPA (1981a)
0.074–0.12	0.074–0.12	30 (Pe) (Pue)	Goodman et al. (1981)
4.0–9.0	4.0–9.0	30 (Pe) (Pue)	Parrish et al. (1977)
12.0–23.0	12.0–23.0	30 (Pe) (Pue)[b]	Parrish et al. (1977)
47.0–88.0	88.0–195.0	30 (Pe) (Pue)	Parrish et al. (1978)
1.0–4.8	1.0–4.8	30 (Pe) (Pue)[b]	Ward and Parrish (1980)
1.3–4.8	1.3–4.8	30 (Pe) (Pue)[b]	Parrish et al. (1978)

tests with 4 freshwater species and 37 organic and inorganic chemicals plus 1 saltwater species and 11 organic chemicals. In 83% of these tests the ELS portion of the life cycle gave the same MATC as the full life cycle, while the remaining 17% of the ELS tests showed more or less sensitivity than the life cycle test by a factor of 2. However, a factor of 2 variation is almost meaningless, since the MATCs for specific toxicants, species, and water combinations can easily vary by a factor of 2. Data for flagfish exposed to cadmium in soft water (Table 6, tests 3, 4, 5, and 6) and to zinc in soft water (Table 6, tests 19 and 20) illustrate this.

McKim (1977) showed that the sensitivity of embryo-larval, early juvenile stages was usually the same when embryos from exposed and unexposed parents were compared. There still seems to be considerable variation in the data (Table 6), but in general the determination of freshwater MATCs does not seem to be drastically affected by parental exposure. This is due in part to the variability and insensitivity of the ELS and life cycle test designs as well as the mode of action of the chemical. Saltwater ELS exposures started with embryos from exposed (Pe) or unexposed (Pue) parents show essentially the same variability as the freshwater studies. Specifically, 4 of the 11 saltwater studies showed no differences in sensitivity between Pue and Pe embryos (tests 4, 8, 10, and 11), 2 studies showed Pue embryos to be more sensitive (tests 2 and 5), and 5 studies showed Pe embryos to be more sensitive (tests 1, 3, 6, 7, and 9). Again, a combination of variations in experimental design and toxicant mode of action seems to make this difficult to evaluate. These variations usually make at most a twofold difference in the MATC.

The critical life stage effects listed for each toxicant in Table 6 are representative of the toxic effects used to determine the MATC in each case. In cases where the MATC was determined by the ELS portion of the life cycle test, growth and mortality of larval and early juvenile fish were the major effects observed. Embryo hatchability was next, followed by chorion fragility and deformities. Other symptomatologies of toxic effect were

noted in most of these studies and are described in the references cited. These symptomatologies (ELS effects), shown in column 3 of Table 1, are manifested later in development through growth and mortality. These later manifestations are the major effects used to establish the statistically significant effect levels (MATCs) listed in Table 6. Ward and Parrish (1980) found that in 90% of their ELS studies with sheepshead minnows (saltwater fish), mortality was the most sensitive indicator of effect. In only one case was growth the most sensitive indicator. This was not the case in freshwater fish or several saltwater studies listed in Table 6, although most of the sheepshead minnow effects were mortality.

Data on the sensitivity of various species to single toxicants in the same water are summarized in Table 7. With some toxicants, species differences in sensitivity were not very great, while with other toxicants sensitivity varied considerably among species. Thus the most important species or the most sensitive, if known, should be tested in a particular situation. For screening large numbers of chemicals, one or two consistently sensitive species (e.g., fathead minnows and sheepshead minnows) will suffice until more is known about species sensitivity to specific types or classes of compounds. The ELS toxicity test should prove effective for rapidly testing the sensitivity of selected species to specific classes of chemicals in order to help determine the minimum number of species required in developing criteria for safe environmental concentrations.

CONCLUSIONS

Early life stage toxicity tests with fish have developed rapidly and can be used to estimate the MATC within a factor of 2 for most freshwater and saltwater fish. Eighty-three percent of the time the MATC estimated from ELS effects was identical to that established by the longer, more involved, and more costly partial or complete life cycle toxicity test. Water quality, species, type of

Table 7 Estimated MATC for 12 Species of Fish Established By Embryo, Larval, and Early Juvenile Tests and Grouped According to Quality of Diluent Water Used[a]

Water type and test location	Species	Estimated MATC (μg/l)	Type of embryo, larval test	Reference
		Cadmium		
Soft water	Flagfish	8.1–16.0	60-d (Pue) 25°C	Spehar (1976)
(45 mg/l as CaCO$_3$)	Flagfish	7.4–16.9	30-d (Pue) (Pe) 25°C	A. R. Carlson and J. H. Tucker[b]
Duluth, Minn.	Flagfish	3.0–6.5	30-d (Pue) (Pe) 25°C	A. R. Carlson and J. H. Tucker[b]
	Flagfish	3.4–7.3	30-d (Pue) (Pe) 25°C	A. R. Carlson and J. H. Tucker[b]
	Brook trout	1.7–3.4	90-d (Pe) 9°C	Benoit et al. (1976)
	Brook trout	1.1–3.8	90-d (Pue) 10°C	Eaton et al. (1978)
	Brown trout	3.8–11.7	60-d (Pue) 10°C	Eaton et al. (1978)
	Lake trout	4.4–12.3	60-d (Pue) 10°C	Eaton et al. (1978)
	Coho salmon	4.1–12.5	60-d (Pue) 10°C	Eaton et al. (1978)
	Northern pike	4.0–12.9	30-d (Pue) 16°C	Eaton et al. (1978)
	Smallmouth bass	4.3–12.7	30-d (Pue) 20°C	Eaton et al. (1978)
	White sucker	4.2–12.0	30-d (Pue) 18°C	Eaton et al. (1978)
Soft water	Brook trout	1.0–3.0	60-d (Pue) 10°C	Sauter et al. (1978)
(36 mg/l as CaCO$_3$) Wareham, Mass.	Channel catfish	11.0–17.0	60-d (Pue) 22°C	Sauter et al. (1978)
Hard water	Fathead minnow	37.0–57.0	60-d (Pue) (Pe) 24°C	Pickering and Gast (1972)
(200 mg/l as CaCO$_3$) Newtown, Ohio	Bluegill	31.0–80.0	60-d (Pe) 26°C	Eaton (1974)
Hard water	Brook trout	7.0–12.0	60-d (Pue) 10°C	Sauter et al. (1976)
(187 mg/l as CaCO$_3$) Wareham, Mass.	Channel catfish	12.0–17.0	60-d (Pue) 22°C	Sauter et al. (1976)
		Chromium		
Soft water	Rainbow trout	51.0–105.0	60-d (Pue) 10°C	Sauter et al. (1976)
(36 mg/l as CaCO$_3$)	Lake trout	105.0–194.0	60-d (Pue) 10°C	Sauter et al. (1976)
Wareham, Mass.	Channel catfish	150.0–305.0	60-d (Pue) 22°C	Sauter et al. (1976)
	Bluegill	522.0–1122.0	60-d (Pue) 25°C	Sauter et al. (1976)
	White sucker	290.0–538.0	60-d (Pue) 17°C	Sauter et al. (1976)
Soft water	Rainbow trout	200.0–350.0	90-d (Pue) 10°C	Benoit (1976)
(45 mg/l as CaCO$_3$) Duluth, Minn.	Brook trout	200.0–350.0	90-d (Pue) 9°C	Benoit (1976)
		Copper		
Soft water (40 mg/l as CaCO$_3$) Newtown, Ohio	Fathead minnow	10.6–18.4	90-d (Pue) (Pe) 24°C	Mount and Stephan (1969)
Soft water	Brook trout	9.5–17.4	90-d (Pe) 9°C	McKim and Benoit (1971)
(45 mg/l as CaCO$_3$)	Brook trout	9.5–17.4	90-d (Pue) (Pe) 9°C	McKim and Benoit (1974)
Duluth, Minn.	Bluegill	21.0–40.0	90-d (Pue) 27°C	Benoit (1975)
	Brook trout	22.3–43.5	60-d (Pue) 6°C	McKim et al. (1978)
	Lake trout	22.0–42.3	60-d (Pue) 6°C	McKim et al. (1978)
	Brown trout	22.0–43.2	60-d (Pue) 6°C	McKim et al. (1978)

Note: See page 88 for footnotes.

Table 7   Estimated MATC for 12 Species of Fish Established by Embryo, Larval, and Early Juvenile Tests and Grouped According to Quality of Diluent Water Used[a] (Continued)

Water type and test location	Species	Estimated MATC (μg/l)	Type of embryo, larval test	Reference
	Rainbow trout	11.4–31.7	30-d (Pue) 11°C	McKim et al. (1978)
	White sucker	12.9–33.8	30-d (Pue) 15°C	McKim et al. (1978)
	Northern pike	34.9–104.4	30-d (Pue) 16°C	McKim et al. (1978)
Soft water	Brook trout	5.0–7.0	60-d (Pue) 10°C	Sauter et al. (1976)
(36 mg/l as $CaCO_3$)	Channel catfish	12.0–18.0	60-d (Pue) 22°C	Sauter et al. (1976)
Wareham, Mass.				
Hard water	Brook trout	5.0–8.0	60-d (Pue) 10°C	Sauter et al. (1976)
(187 mg/l as $CaCO_3$)	Channel catfish	13.0–19.0	60-d (Pue) 22°C	Sauter et al. (1976)
Wareham, Mass.				
		Lead		
Soft water	Brook trout	58.0–119.0	(Pe) 9°C	Holcombe et al. (1976)
(45 mg/l as $CaCO_3$)	Flagfish	60.0–125.0	(Pue) 27°C	L. E. Anderson et al.[b]
Duluth, Minn.				
Soft water	Rainbow trout	71.0–146.0	60-d (Pue) 10°C	Sauter et al. (1976)
(36 mg/l as $CaCO_3$)	Lake trout	48.0–83.0	60-d (Pue) 10°C	Sauter et al. (1976)
Wareham, Mass.	Channel catfish	75.0–136.0	60-d (Pue) 22°C	Sauter et al. (1976)
	Bluegill	70.0–120.0	60-d (Pue) 25°C	Sauter et al. (1976)
	White sucker	119.0–253.0	60-d (Pue) 17°C	Sauter et al. (1976)
		Zinc		
Soft water	Flagfish	51.0–85.0	30-d (Pue) 25°C	Spehar (1976)
(45 mg/l as $CaCO_3$)	Flagfish	139.0–267.0	30-d (Pue) 25°C	Spehar (1976)
Duluth, Minn.	Brook trout	532.0–1368.0	90-d (Pue) (Pe) 9°C	Holcombe and Benoit (1979)
	Fathead minnow	78.0–145.0	90-d (Pue) (Pe) 23°C	Benoit and Holcombe (1978)
		Organometallics **methylmercuric chloride**		
Soft water	Fathead minnow	0.13–0.23	60-d (Pue) 23°C	D. I. Mount and G. F. Olson[b]
(45 mg/l as $CaCO_3$)	Flagfish	0.17–0.33	30-d (Pue) 25°C	W. E. Smith[b]
Duluth, Minn.	Brook trout	0.29–0.93	90-d (Pe) 9°C	McKim et al. (1976)
		Linear alkylate sulfate (LAS)		
Soft water	Fathead minnow	1100.0	30-d (Pue) 23°C	McKim et al. (1975)
(45 mg/l as $CaCO_3$)	Northern pike	1200.0	30-d (Pue) 15°C	McKim et al. (1975)
Duluth, Minn.	Smallmouth bass	5800.0	30-d (Pue) 15°C	McKim et al. (1975)
	White sucker	500.0	30-d (Pue) 15°C	McKim et al. (1975)

[a]From McKim (1977); reproduced by permission of the Ministry of Supply and Services Canada.
[b]Personal communication, Environmental Research Laboratory, Duluth, Minn.

toxicant, and parental exposure had little effect on these conclusions.

These conclusions for individual toxicants are probably also true for toxicant mixtures or complex effluents. Little information is available on life cycle toxicity tests with complex effluents or mixtures, but the work cited in Table 6 on sewage (tests 53 to 56) and metal mixtures (test 23) supports this assumption to some degree. Laboratory and field methods now available for ELS tests allow relatively rapid screening of single chemicals and complex effluents with selected species both in the laboratory and on site (field testing). Further development of these tests is under way; the major emphasis is on reducing the duration of exposure through the development of new and more sophisticated toxicity end points by embryological, physiological, and biochemical approaches.

Muul et al. (1976) described the need in mammalian toxicology for faster, less costly tests to screen out potentially carcinogenic and toxic chemicals from the ever-expanding list of potentially useful chemicals. Faster, less costly testing procedures are also of extreme importance in aquatic toxicology. In the United States these procedures are especially desirable for the implementation of the Federal Insecticide, Fungicide, and Rodenticide Act of 1972 and the Toxic Substances Control Act of 1976. These laws require prescreening by industry of some chemicals before commercial production. The use of ELS fish toxicity tests permits testing with species which, because of their extensive life cycle requirements, could not be used in a life cycle test. In addition, these tests provide the opportunity to screen large numbers of chemicals rapidly at a far lower cost per test than a life cycle toxicity test.

Life cycle tests with aquatic invertebrates will continue to be important for evaluating chemical impacts on the aquatic environment. However, the development of standardized predictive tests is less important than with fish because of the short time period required for definitive invertebrate life cycle tests.

LITERATURE CITED

Adelman IR, Smith LL, Jr, Siesennop GD: Chronic toxicity of guthion to the fathead minnow (Pimephales promelas Rafinesque). Bull Environ Contam Toxicol 15:726–733, 1976.

Allison DT: Use of exposure units for estimating aquatic toxicity of organophosphate pesticides. EPA-600/3-77-077. Duluth, Minn.: U.S. EPA, 1977.

Allison DT, Hermanutz RO: Toxicity of diazinon to brook trout and fathead minnows. EPA-600/3-77-060. Duluth, Minn.: U.S. EPA, 1977.

American Public Health Association, American Water Works Association, and Water Pollution Control Federation: Standard Methods for the Examination of Water and Wastewater, 14th ed. Washington, D.C.: American Public Health Association, 1975.

American Society for Testing and Materials: Standard practice for conducting acute toxicity tests with fishes, macroinvertebrates, and amphibians. ASTM E729-80. Philadelphia: ASTM, 1980a.

American Society for Testing and Materials: Annual Book of ASTM Standards. Part 31: Water. Philadelphia: ASTM, 1980b.

American Society for Testing and Materials: Standard practice for conducting chronic toxicity tests with the early life stages of fish. ASTM E-47.01. Philadelphia: ASTM, 1981 (draft).

Anderson RL: Chironomidae toxicity tests— Biological background and procedures. In: Aquatic Invertebrates Bioassays, edited by AL Buikema Jr., J Cairns Jr., pp. 70–80. ASTM STP 715. Philadelphia: ASTM, 1980.

Arthur JW: Chronic effects of linear alkylate sulfonate detergent on Gammarus pseudolimnaeus, Campeloma decisum, and Physa integra. Water Res 4:251–257, 1970.

Arthur JW: Review of freshwater bioassay procedure for selected amphipods. In: Aquatic Invertebrates Bioassays, edited by AL Buikema Jr., J Cairns Jr., pp. 98–108. ASTM STP 715. Philadelphia: ASTM, 1980.

Arthur JW, Eaton JG: Chloramine toxicity to the amphipod Gammarus pseudolimnaeus and the fathead minnow (Pimephales promelas). J Fish Res Bd Can 28:1841–1845, 1971.

Arthur JW, Lemke AE, Mattson VR, Halligan BJ: Toxicity of sodium nitrilotriacetate (NTA) to the fathead minnow and an amphipod in soft water. Water Res 8:187–193, 1974.

Arthur JW, Andrew RW, Mattson VR, Olson DT, Glass GE, Halligan BJ, Walbridge CT: Comparative toxicity of sewage-effluent disinfectants to freshwater aquatic life. EPA-600/3-75-012. U.S. EPA, 1975.

Balon EK: Terminology of intervals in fish development. J Fish Res Bd Can 32:1663–1670, 1975.

Benoit DA: Chronic effects of copper on survival, growth, and reproduction of the bluegill (*Lepomis macrochirus*). Trans Am Fish Soc 104:353–358, 1975.

Benoit DA: Toxic effects of hexavalent chromium on brook trout (*Salvelinus fontinalis*) and rainbow trout (*Salmo gairdneri*). Water Res 10:497–500, 1976.

Benoit DA, Holcombe GW: Toxic effects of zinc on fathead minnows (*Pimephales promelas*) in soft water. J Fish Biol 13:701–708, 1978.

Benoit DA, Leonard EN, Christensen GM, Hunt EP: Toxic effects of cadmium on three generations of brook trout (*Salvelinus fontinalis*). Trans Am Fish Soc 105:550–560, 1976.

Benoit DA, Mattson VR, Olson DL: A compact continuous flow mini-diluter exposure system for testing early life stages of fish and invertebrates in single chemicals and complex effluents. Water Res, 1981a, in press.

Benoit DA, Puglisi FA, Olson DL: A fathead minnow (*Pimephales promelas*) early life stage toxicity test method evaluation and exposure to four organic chemicals. Environ Pollut, 1981b, in press.

Benoit DA, Syrett RF, Freeman FB: Design manual for construction of a continuous flow mini-diluter exposure system. Duluth, Minn.: U.S. EPA, 1981c (unpublished report).

Biesinger KE, Christensen GM: Effects of various metals on survival, growth, reproduction, and metabolism of *Daphnia magna*. J Fish Res Bd Can 29:1691–1700, 1972.

Box GEP, Hunter WG, Hunter JS: Statistics for Experimenters. New York: Wiley-Interscience, 1978.

Brungs WA: Chronic toxicity of zinc to the fathead minnow, *Pimephales promelas* Rafinesque. Trans Am Fish Soc 98:272–279, 1969.

Brungs WA: Chronic effects of low dissolved oxygen concentrations on the fathead minnow (*Pimephales promelas*). J Fish Res Bd Can 28:1119–1123, 1971.

Brungs WA, Jones BR: Temperature criteria for freshwater fish: Protocol and procedures. EPA-600/3-77-061. Duluth, Minn.: U.S. EPA, 1977.

Buikema AL Jr., Cairns J Jr. (eds): Aquatic invertebrate bioassays, pp. 1–209. ASTM STP 715. Philadelphia: ASTM, 1980.

Buikema AL Jr., Geiger JG, Lee DR: *Daphnia* toxicity tests. In: Aquatic Invertebrate Bioassays, edited by AL Buikema Jr., J Cairns Jr., pp. 48–69. ASTM STP 715. Philadelphia: ASTM, 1980.

Calabrese A, Collier RS, Nelson DA, MacInnes JR: The toxicity of heavy metals to embryos of the American oyster (*Crassostrea virginica*). Mar Biol 18:162–166, 1973.

Carlson AR: Effects of long-term exposure of carbaryl (sevin) on survival, growth, and reproduction of the fathead minnow (*Pimephales promelas*). J Fish Res Bd Can 29:583–587, 1971.

Chapman GA, Shumway DL: Effects of sodium pentachlorophenate on survival and energy metabolism of embryonic and larval steelhead trout. In: Pentachlorophenol, edited by RK Rao, pp. 285–299. New York: Plenum, 1977.

Derr SK, Zabik MJ: Biologically active compounds in the aquatic environment: The effect of DDE on the egg viability of *Chironomus tentans*. Bull Environ Contam Toxicol 7:366–368, 1972a.

Derr SK, Zabik MJ: Biologically active compounds in the aquatic environment: The uptake and distribution of [1,1-dichloro-2,2-bis(*p*-chlorophenyl) ethylene], DDE by *Chironomus tentans* Fabricius (Diptera: Chiromonidae). Trans Am Fish Soc 101:323–329, 1972b.

DeFoe DL, Veith GD, Carlson RW: Effects of Aroclor 1248 and 1260 on the fathead minnow (*Pimephales promelas*). J Fish Res Bd Can 35:997–1002, 1978.

Dunnett CW: A multiple comparisons procedure for comparing several treatments with a control. J Am Stat Assoc 50:1096–1121, 1955.

Dunnett CW: New tables for multiple comparisons with a control. Biometrics 20:482–491, 1964.

Eaton JG: Chronic malathion toxicity to the bluegill (*Lepomis macrochirus* Rafinesque). Water Res 4:673–684, 1970.

Eaton JG: Chronic toxicity of copper, cadmium, and zinc mixture to the fathead minnow (*Pimephales promelas*). Water Res 7:1723–1736, 1973.

Eaton JG: Chronic cadmium toxicity to the bluegill (*Lepomis macrochirus* Rafinesque). Trans Am Fish Soc 103:729–735, 1974.

Eaton JG, McKim JM, Holcombe GW: Metal toxicity to embryos and larvae of seven freshwater fish species. I: Cadmium. Bull Environ Contam Toxicol 19:95–103, 1978.

Geiger JG, Buikema AL Jr., Cairns J Jr.: A tentative seven-day test for predicting effects of stress on populations of *Daphnia pulex*. In: Aquatic Toxicology, edited by JG Eaton, PR Parrish, AC Hendricks, pp. 13–26. ASTM STP 707. Philadelphia: ASTM, 1980.

Gingerich WH, Seim WK, Schonbrod RD: An apparatus for the continuous generation of stock solutions of hydrophobic chemicals. Bull Environ Contam Toxicol 23:685–689, 1979.

Goodman LR, Hansen DJ, Couch JA, Forester J: Effects of heptachlor toxaphene on laboratory-reared embryos and fry of the sheepshead minnow. 13th Annu Conf Southeast Assoc Game Fish Comm, pp. 192–202, 1976.

Goodman LR, Hansen DJ, Manning CS, Faas LF: Effects of Kepone on the sheepshead minnow in an entire life-cycle toxicity test. Arch Environ Contam Toxicol 11:335–342, 1982.

Hansen DJ, Parrish PR: Suitability of sheepshead minnows (*Cyprinodon variegatus*) for life-cycle toxicity tests. In: Aquatic Toxicology and Hazard Evaluation, edited by FL Mayer, JL Hamelink, pp. 117–126. ASTM STP 634. Philadelphia: ASTM, 1977a.

Hansen DJ, Schimmel SC, Forester J: Endrin: Effects on the entire life-cycle of saltwater fish, *Cyprinodon variegatus*. J Toxicol Environ Health 3:721–726, 1977b.

Helder T: Effects of 2,3,7,8-tetrachlorodibenzo-*p*-dioxin (TCDD) on early life stages of the pike (*Esox lucius* L.). Sci Total Environ 14:255–264, 1980.

Hermanutz R: Endrin and malathion toxicity to flagfish (*Jordanella floridae*). Arch Environ Contam Toxicol 7:159–168, 1978.

Hermanutz RO, Mueller LH, Kempfert KD: Captan toxicity to fathead minnows (*Pimephales promelas*), bluegills (*Lepomis macrochirus*), and brook trout (*Salvelinus fontinalis*). J Fish Res Bd Can 30:1811–1817, 1973.

Hokanson KEF, McCormick JH, Jones BR, Tucker JH: Thermal requirements for maturation, spawning, and embryo survival of the brook trout (*Salvelinus fontinalis*). J Fish Res Bd Can 30:975–984, 1973a.

Hokanson KEF, McCormick JH, Jones BR: Temperature requirements for embryos and larvae of the northern pike, *Esox lucius* (Linnaeus). Trans Am Fish Soc 102:89–100, 1973b.

Holcombe GW, Benoit DA, Leonard EN, McKim JM: Long-term effects of lead exposure on three generations of brook trout (*Salvelinus fontinalis*). J Fish Res Bd Can 33:1731–1741, 1976.

Holcombe GW, Benoit DA, Leonard EN: Long-term effects of zinc exposures on brook trout (*Salvelinus fontinalis*). Trans Am Fish Soc 108:76–87, 1979.

Hollister TA, Heitmuller PT, Parrish PR, and Dyar EE: Studies to determine relationships between time and toxicity of an acidic effluent and an alkaline effluent to two estuarine species. In: Aquatic Toxicology, edited by JG Eaton, PR Parrish, AC Hendricks, pp. 251–265. ASTM STP 707. Philadelphia: ASTM, 1980.

Ishida J, Tagushi S, Maruyama K: ATP content and ATPase activity in developing embryos of the teleost (*Oryzias latipes*). Annot Zool Jpn 32:1–5, 1959.

Jarvinen AW, Tyo RM: Toxicity to fathead minnows of endrin in food and water. Arch Environ Contam Toxicol 7:409–421, 1978.

Jarvinen AW, Hoffman MJ, Thorslund TW: Long-term toxic effects of DDT food and water exposure on fathead minnows (*Pimephales promelas*). J Fish Res Bd Can 34:2089–2103, 1977.

Jones PW, Martin FD, Hardy JD Jr.: Development

of fishes of the mid-Atlantic bight: An atlas of egg, larval and juvenile stages, vol. 1. Biol Serv Prog US Dept Inter Publ FWS/OBS-78/12, 1978.

Lagler KF, Bardach JE, Miller RM, Passino DM: Ichthyology, 2d ed. New York: Wiley, 1977.

Lemke AE, Brungs WA, Halligan BJ: Manual for construction and operation of toxicity-testing proportional diluters. EPA-600/3-78-072. Duluth, Minn.: U.S. EPA, 1978.

Macek KJ, Sleight BH: Utility of toxicity tests with embryos and fry of fish in evaluating hazards associated with the chronic toxicity of chemicals to fishes. In: Aquatic Toxicology and Hazard Evaluation, edited by FL Mayer, JL Hamelink, pp. 137–146. ASTM STP 634. Philadelphia: ASTM, 1977.

Macek KJ, Buxton KS, Derr SK, Dean JW, Sauter S: Chronic toxicity of lindane to selected aquatic invertebrates and fishes. EPA-600/3-76-046. U.S. EPA, 1976a.

Macek KJ, Buxton KS, Sauter S, Gnilka S, Dean JW: Chronic toxicity of atrazine to selected invertebrates and fishes. EPA-600/3-76-047. U.S. EPA, 1976b.

Macek KJ, Lindberg MA, Sauter S, Buxton KS, Costa PA: Toxicity of four pesticides to water fleas and fathead minnows. Acute and chronic toxicity to acrolein, heptachlor, endosulfan, and trifluralin to the water flea (Daphnia magna) and the fathead minnow (Pimephales promelas), EPA-600/3-76-099. U.S. EPA, 1976c.

Mayer FL Jr., Mehrle PM Jr., Dwyer WP: Toxaphene effects on reproduction, growth, and mortality of brook trout. EPA-600/3-075-013. Duluth, Minn.: U.S. EPA, 1975.

Mayer FL Jr., Mehrle PM Jr., Dwyer WP: Toxaphene: Chronic toxicity to fathead minnows and channel catfish. EPA-600/3-77-069. Duluth, Minn.: U.S. EPA, 1977.

McClave JT, Sullivan JH, Pearson JG: Statistical analysis of fish chronic toxicity. In: Aquatic Toxicology and Hazard Evaluation, edited by DR Branson and KL Dickson, pp. 359–376. ASTM STP 737. Philadelphia: ASTM, 1981.

McCormick JH, Jones BR, and Hokanson KEF: White sucker (Catostomus commersoni) em-

bryo development, and early growth and survival at different temperatures. J Fish Res Bd Can 34:1019–1025, 1977.

McKim JM: Evaluation of tests with early life stages of fish for predicting long-term toxicity. J Fish Res Bd Can 34:1148–1154, 1977.

McKim JM, Benoit DA: Effects of long-term exposures to copper on the survival, growth, and reproduction of brook trout. J Fish Res Bd Can 28:655–662, 1971.

McKim JM, Benoit DA: Duration of toxicity tests for establishing "no effect" concentrations for copper with brook trout. J Fish Res Bd Can 31: 449–452, 1974.

McKim JM, Arthur JW, Thorslund TW: Toxicity of a linear alkylate sulfonate detergent to larvae of four species of freshwater fish. Bull Environ Contam Toxicol 14:1–7, 1975.

McKim JM, Holcombe GW, Olson GF, Hunt EP: Long-term effects of methylmercuric chloride on three generations of brook trout (Salvelinus fontinalis): Toxicity, accumulation, distribution, and elimination. J Fish Res Bd Can 33: 2726–2739, 1976.

McKim JM, Eaton JG, Holcombe GW: Metal toxicity to embryos and larvae of eight species of freshwater fish. II: Copper. Bull Environ Contam Toxicol 19:608–616, 1978.

Mehrle PM, Mayer FL Jr.: Toxaphene effects on growth and bone composition of fathead minnows, Pimephales promelas. J Fish Res Bd Can 32:593–598, 1975.

Menendez R: Chronic effects of reduced pH on brook trout (Salvelinus fontinalis). J Fish Res Bd Can 33:118–123, 1976.

Meyer W, Sauerbier I: The development of catecholamines in embryos and larvae of the rainbow trout (Salmo gairdneri Rich.). J Fish Biol 10:431–435, 1977.

Middaugh DP, Dean JM: Comparative sensitivity of eggs, larvae, and adults of the estuarine teleosts, Fundulus heteroclitus and Menidia menidia to cadmium. Bull Environ Contam Toxicol 17:645–651, 1977.

Middaugh DP, Lempesis PW: Laboratory spawning and rearing of a marine fish, the silverside Menidia menidia menidia. Mar Biol 35:295–300, 1976.

Mount DI: Chronic toxicity of copper to fathead minnows. Water Res 2:215–223, 1968.

Mount DI: Chronic effect of low pH on fathead minnow survival, growth, and reproduction. Water Res 7:987–993, 1973.

Mount DI: An assessment of application factors in aquatic toxicology. In: Recent Advances in Fish Toxicology—A Symposium, edited by RA Tubb, pp. 183–189. EPA-600/3-77-085. U.S. EPA, 1977.

Mount DI, Brungs WA: A simplified dosing apparatus for fish toxicology studies. Water Res 1:21–29, 1967.

Mount DI, Stephan CE: A method for establishing acceptable limits for fish—Malathion and the butoxyethanol ester of 2,4-D. Trans Am Fish Soc 96:185–193, 1967.

Mount DI, Stephan CE: Chronic toxicity of copper to the fathead minnow (Pimephales promelas) in soft water. J Fish Res Bd Can 26:2449–2457, 1969.

Muul I, Hegyeli AF, Dacre J, Woodard G: Toxicological testing dilemma. Science 193:834, 1976.

Nebeker AV: Temperature requirements and life cycle of the midge Tanytarsus dissimilis. J Kans Entomol Soc 46:160–165, 1973.

Nebeker AV, Puglisi FA, DeFoe DL: Effect of polychlorinated biphenyl compounds on survival and reproduction of the fathead minnow and flagfish. Trans Am Fish Soc 103:562–568, 1974.

Nebeker AV, Andros JD, McCrady JK, Stevens DG: Survival of steelhead trout (Salmo gairdneri) eggs, embryos, and fry in air-supersaturated water. J Fish Res Bd Can 35:261–264, 1977.

Nimmo DR, Bahner LH, Rigby RA, Sheppard JM, Wilson AJ Jr.: Mysidopsis bahia: An estuarine species suitable for life-cycle toxicity tests to determine the effects of a pollutant. In: Aquatic Toxicology and Hazard Evaluation, edited by FL Mayer, JL Hamelink, pp. 109–116. ASTM STP 634. Philadelphia: ASTM, 1977.

Parrish PR, Schimmel SC, Hansen DJ, Patrick JM Jr., Forester J: Chlordane: Effects on several estuarine organisms. J Toxicol Environ Health 1:485–494, 1976.

Parrish PR, Dyar EE, Lindberg MA, Shanike CM, Enos JM: Chronic toxicity of methoxychlor, malathion, and carbofuran to sheepshead minnows (Cyprinodon variegatus). EPA-600/3-77-059. U.S. EPA, 1977.

Parrish PR, Dyar EE, Enos JM, Wilson WG: Chronic toxicity of chlordane, trifluralin, and pentachlorophenol to sheepshead minnows (Cyprinodon variegatus). EPA-600/3-78-010. U.S. EPA, 1978.

Pickering QH: Chronic toxicity of nickel to the fathead minnow. J Water Pollut Control Fed 46:760–765, 1974.

Pickering QH, Gast MH: Acute and chronic toxicity of cadmium to the fathead minnow Pimephales promelas. J Fish Res Bd Can 29:1099–1106, 1972.

Pickering QH, Thatcher TO: The chronic toxicity of linear alkylate sulfonate (LAS) to Pimephales promelas Rafinesque. J Water Pollut Control Fed 42:243–254, 1970.

Pickering QH, Brungs W, Gast M: Effect of exposure time and copper concentration on reproduction of the fathead minnow (Pimephales promelas). Water Res 11:1079–1083, 1977.

Reish DJ: Use of polychaetous annelids as test organisms for marine bioassay experiments. In: Aquatic Invertebrate Bioassays, edited by AL Buikema Jr., J Cairns Jr., pp. 140–154. ASTM STP 715. Philadelphia: ASTM, 1980.

Roberts MH Jr.: Flow-through toxicity testing system for molluscan larvae as applied to halogen toxicity in estuarine water. In: Aquatic Invertebrate Bioassays, edited by AL Buikema Jr., J Cairns Jr., pp. 131–139. ASTM STP 715. Philadelphia: ASTM, 1980.

Rosenthal H, Alderdice DF: Sublethal effects of environmental stressors, natural and pollutional, on marine fish eggs and larvae. J Fish Res Bd Can 33:2047–2065, 1976.

Sauter S, Buxton KS, Macek KJ, Petrocelli SR: Effects of exposure to heavy metals on selected freshwater fish. EPA-600/3-76-105. U.S. EPA, 1976.

Schimmel SC, Hansen DJ: Sheepshead minnow (Cyprinodon variegatus): An estuarine fish suitable for chronic (entire life-cycle) bioassays.

Proc 28th Am Conf Southeast Game Fish Comm, pp. 392–398, 1974.

Smith, WE: A cyprinodontid fish, *Jordanella floridae*, as reference animals for rapid chronic bioassays. J Fish Res Bd Can 39:329–330, 1973.

Snyder DE, Snyder MBM, Douglas SC: Identification of golden shiner, *Notemigonus crysoleucas*, spotfin shiner, *Notropis spilopterus*, and fathead minnow, *Pimephales promelas*, larvae. J Fish Res Bd Can 34:1397–1409, 1977.

Sokal RR, Rohlf FJ: Biometry. San Francisco: Freeman, 1969.

Spehar RL: Cadmium and zinc toxicity to *Jordanella floridae*. J Fish Res Bd Can 33:1939–1945, 1976.

Steel RG, Torrie JH: Principles and Procedures of Statistics with Special Reference to Biological Sciences. New York: McGraw-Hill, 1960.

Strickland JDG, Parsons TR: A practical handbook of seawater analysis. Fish Res Bd Can Bull 167:21–26, 1968.

Tyler-Schroeder DB: Use of the grass shrimp (*Palaemonetes pugio*) in a life-cycle toxicity test. In: Aquatic Toxicology, edited by LL Marking, AA Kimerle, pp. 159–170. ASTM STP 667. Philadelphia: ASTM, 1979.

Uesugi S, Yamazoe S: Acetyl cholinesterase activity during the development of rainbow trout eggs. Gunma J Med Sci 13:91–93, 1964.

U.S. Environmental Protection Agency: Methods for chemical analysis of water and wastes. EPA-600/4-79-020. U.S. EPA, 1979.

U.S. Environmental Protection Agency: Manual of analytical methods for the analysis of pesticides in humans and environmental samples. EPA-600/8-80-038. U.S. EPA, 1980.

U.S. Environmental Protection Agency: Acephate, aldicarb, carbophenothion, DEF, EPN, ethoprop, methyl parathion, and phorate: Their acute and chronic toxicity, bioconcentration potential, and persistence as related to marine environments. EPA-600/4-81-023. Gulf Breeze, Fla.: U.S. EPA, 1981a.

U.S. Environmental Protection Agency: Test standard for conducting an early life stage toxicity test using the fathead minnow, sheepshead minnow, and brook trout or rainbow trout. Washington, D.C.: U.S. EPA, Health and Environmental Review Division (TS-792), 1981b (draft).

Veith GD, Comstock VM: Apparatus for continuously saturating water with hydrophobic organic chemicals. J Fish Res Bd Can 32:1849–1851, 1975.

Von Westernhagen H, Dethlefsen V, Rosenthal H: Combined effects of cadmium and salinity on development and survival of garpike eggs. Helgol Wiss Meeresunters 27:268–282, 1975.

Ward GS, Parrish PR: Evaluation of early life-stage toxicity tests with embryos and juveniles of sheepshead minnows (*Cyprinodon variegatus*). In: Aquatic Toxicology, edited by JG Eaton, PR Parrish, AC Hendricks, pp. 243–247. ASTM STP 707. Philadelphia: ASTM, 1980.

Ward RW, Griffin RD, DeGraeve GM, Stone RA: Disinfection efficiency and residual toxicity of several wastewater disinfectants, vol. 1. EPA-600/2-76-156. Grandville, Mich.: U.S. EPA, 1976.

Warner RE: Toxicant-induced behavioral and histological pathology: A quantitative study of sublethal toxication in the aquatic environment. Contract PH 66-63-72. U.S. Public Health Service, 1964.

Weis P, Weis JS: Methylmercury teratogenesis in the killifish, *Fundulus heteroclitus*. Teratology 16:321–324, 1977.

Williams DA: A test for differences between treatment means when several dose levels are compared with a zero dose control. Biometrics 27:103–117, 1971.

Williams DA: The comparison of several dose levels with a zero dose control. Biometrics 28:519–531, 1972.

Winner RW, Farell MP: Acute and chronic toxicity of copper to four species of *Daphnia*. J Fish Res Bd Can 33:1685–1691, 1976.

SUPPLEMENTAL READING

Blaxter JHS: Fish Physiology, chapter 4, Development: Eggs and Larvae. New York: Academic, 1969.

Blaxter JHS: The Early Life History of Fish, Proceedings of an International Symposium held at

Dunstaffnage Marine Research Laboratory of the Scottish Marine Biological Association at Oban, Scotland, March 17–23, 1973. New York: Springer-Verlag, 1974.

Buikema AL Jr., Cairns J Jr. (eds): Aquatic Invertebrate Bioassays, pp. 1–209, ASTM STP 715. Philadelphia: ASTM, 1980.

Lagler KF, Bardach JE, Miller RM, Passino DM: Icthyology, 2d ed. New York: Wiley, 1977.

Mansueti A, Hardy JD Jr.: Development of Fishes of the Chesapeake Bay Region: An Atlas of Egg, Larval and Juvenile Stages. College Park, Md.: Natural Resources Institute, University of Maryland, 1967.

New DAT: The Culture of Vertebrate Embryos, chapter 6, Fish. New York: Academic, 1966.

Yamamoto T: Medaka (Killifish): Biology and Strains. Tokyo: Yugaku-sha, 1975.

Chapter 4

Chronic Toxicity Tests

S. R. Petrocelli

INTRODUCTION

An important tool for understanding and evaluating the potential hazard of chemicals to aquatic organisms is the chronic or full life cycle toxicity test. Data from this test can be used to estimate the effect and no-effect concentrations of a chemical to which aquatic organisms are exposed continuously during an entire reproductive life cycle. A chronic toxicity test can indicate the concentrations of a chemical that will interfere with normal growth, development, and attainment of reproductive potential of an aquatic organism. Generally, concentrations that produce chronic effects are lower than those that produce more readily observable acute effects such as mortality. Therefore, chronic toxicity tests can provide a more sensitive measure of chemical toxicity than acute toxicity tests.

A chronic toxicity test is designed to expose all life stages of the test animal—viable gametes, newly fertilized ova, early stages of developing embryos, or newly hatched larvae—to a range of chemical concentrations estimated (from acute toxicity test exposures) to bracket the threshold for significant deleterious effects. If appropriate test concentrations have been selected, the populations exposed to the higher concentrations in this test will be adversely affected, as judged by standard criteria, while those exposed to the lower concentrations will not be adversely affected as compared with unexposed populations (controls).

In a chronic toxicity test all test populations, except controls, are exposed continuously to the chemical for a period of time sufficient for the controls to grow, develop, become sexually mature, and produce offspring (F_1, first filial generation). Each population exposed to a different

Application Factor

chemical concentration is observed at regular intervals for an assessment of mortality, normal growth, and development to sexual maturity and fecundity as compared with control populations.

Specific criteria for effect in chronic toxicity tests depend on the species tested and may include the number and percent of embryos that complete development and hatch normally; larvae and juveniles that survive and grow normally as measured by incremental increases in length and weight, through distinct stages of development including sexual maturity; viable eggs and subsequent F_1 produced by these sexually mature animals; and survival, growth, and development of the F_1 for a predetermined period of time (e.g., 30 d after hatching for certain fish).

When these quantitative biological data have been compiled, statistical analyses are used to identify and describe significant differences between observed responses from exposed populations and controls. Measurements that are statistically different ($P \leq 0.05$) from those of the control populations are generally considered to be significant and are designated as an effect. Chemical concentrations at which a statistically significant deleterious effect is observed are considered effect concentrations. Concentrations at which no statistically significant deleterious effect is observed are considered no-effect concentrations.

The threshold concentration that produces statistically significant deleterious effects is commonly expressed as the maximum acceptable toxicant concentration (MATC) (Mount and Stephan, 1967). The MATC is a hypothetical concentration and is in a range bounded at the lower end by the highest concentration in the chronic test that produced no effect (NOEC, no observed effect concentration) and at the higher end by the lowest concentration tested that produced a statistically significant effect (LOEC, lowest observed effect concentration). Therefore, the MATC can be represented as NOEC < MATC < LOEC.

In attempting to relate the acute toxicity and chronic toxicity of chemicals to aquatic organisms, the application factor (AF) concept was proposed

(Mount and Stephan, 1967). The AF is a unitless, chemical-specific measure calculated as the threshold chronically toxic concentration of a chemical divided by its acutely toxic concentration. In practice, the AF is calculated by dividing the limits (NOEC and LOEC) of the MATC by the time-independent or incipient LC50 (see Chapter 1) or, if that value is not available, by the 96-h LC50 (or 48-h LC50 for daphnids) from a flow-through acute toxicity test. The AF is reported as a concentration range. For example, if the MATC is $>0.5 < 1.0$ mg/l and the LC50 is 10 mg/l, then

$$AF = \frac{MATC}{LC50 \text{ (acute)}} = \frac{>0.5 < 1.0 \text{ mg/l}}{10 \text{ mg/l}} = 0.05\text{--}0.1 \text{ conc. range}$$

In concept, the AF would be relatively constant for a specific chemical. Thus, if the AF for a chemical was empirically determined with one aquatic species, it could be applied to other aquatic species. This hypothesis was considered very useful. It decreased the reliance on arbitrary application of safety factors, and it provided an estimate of chronically toxic concentrations of a chemical for species that could not be tested under chronic conditions because not enough was known about the requirements for sustaining the animal's life.

In some cases, the AF was used to provide an estimate of chronic toxicity without a chronic test, even if the test was possible with that species. This saved the time and costs associated with the chronic test. The investigator would estimate the AF for a chemical with one organism and then apply the AF to the acutely toxic concentration for the second organism. That is, if the AF for a chemical was estimated as 0.05–0.1 based on acute and chronic toxicity tests with a fish, this AF would be applied to the acutely toxic concentration for a crustacean to estimate the limits (MATC) of the chronically toxic concentration for that crustacean. For example, if the LC50 of a chemical to shrimp was 1.0 mg/l and the AF for the chemical was 0.05–0.1 based on tests with a fish, the MATC of this chemical to shrimp would be calculated as

$$MATC = AF \times LC50 = 0.05\text{--}0.1 \times 1.0 \text{ mg/l}$$
$$= >0.05 <0.1 \text{ mg/l}$$

More recently, however, the AF concept has been replaced by the use of shorter term, early life stage or most sensitive life stage tests, which empirically estimate the chronic toxicity of a chemical without performing a full chronic exposure. These early life stage tests have proved to be effective predictors of chronic toxicity for a wide variety and number of chemicals (Macek and Sleight, 1977; McKim, 1977). Early life stage tests and their utility for estimating chronic effect concentrations are described in detail in Chapter 3.

Finally, a comparison of the chemical concentrations that caused significant deleterious effects in a chronic study with the chemical concentrations that can reasonably be expected to occur in the aquatic environment (estimated environmental concentration, EEC) permits an evaluation of the potential hazard that the chemical poses to aquatic organisms.

TEST SPECIES

A major limitation to the use of chronic toxicity tests to estimate effects of long-term exposures of aquatic organisms to chemicals is the availability of suitable test species. The normal physiological requirements of relatively few aquatic species are known and understood well enough to permit the use of these species in chronic toxicity tests. Obviously, in order to evaluate the effects of a chemical on normal reproduction, growth, and development of an organism, a good understanding of what is normal is necessary.

Since only a handful of aquatic species can be routinely tested under chronic conditions, most investigators generally work with a total of only two to four species of invertebrates (generally crustaceans) and vertebrates (almost exclusively fish).

The most commonly used vertebrates are the freshwater fathead minnow, *Pimephales promelas* (Mount and Stephan, 1967), and the saltwater sheepshead minnow, *Cyprinodon variegatus* (Hansen and Parrish, 1977; Hansen et al., 1977; Schimmel and Hansen, 1974), the only saltwater fish species routinely used in chronic toxicity tests. Other fish that have been used in chronic toxicity tests include the freshwater flagfish, *Jordanella floridae* (Smith, 1974), brook trout, *Salvelinus fontinalis* (McKim and Benoit, 1971, 1974), and bluegill sunfish, *Lepomis macrochirus* (Eaton, 1970).

The most commonly used invertebrates are the freshwater water flea, *Daphnia magna* (Biesinger and Christensen, 1972), and the saltwater mysid shrimp, *Mysidopsis bahia* (Nimmo et al., 1977). Compared with fish, there is a greater number and taxonomic diversity of invertebrate species that can be used in chronic toxicity tests. Other invertebrates include crustaceans: the saltwater calanoid copepod, *Acartia tonsa* (Sosnowski and Gentile, 1978), the grass shrimp, *Palaemonetes pugio* (Tyler-Schroeder, 1979), and the freshwater amphipod, *Gammarus pseudolimnaeus* (Arthur, 1970); insects: the freshwater midges, *Chironomus tentans* (Derr and Zabik, 1972a,b) and *Tanytarsus dissimilis* (Nebeker, 1973); and annelids: the saltwater polychaetes, *Neanthes arenaceodentata* and *Capitella capitata* (Reish, 1974; Reish et al., 1976; Grassle and Grassle, 1976).

The second significant problem with chronic toxicity testing is the length of time required to complete the test. Chronic toxicity tests with the fish species above require a minimum exposure period of 6–12 mo or more. Even with invertebrate species, chronic tests take 3–4 wk or more. Therefore, the success of these tests is critically dependent on the investigator's ability to closely control experimental conditions during the entire exposure period.

As a result of constraining factors such as test duration, cost, and lack of a broad range of suitable species associated with chronic toxicity testing, emphasis has been placed recently on the use of early life stage tests (see Chapter 3) to estimate chronic toxicity. However, for chemicals that are cumulatively toxic or that affect physiological processes not adequately studied in early life stage tests, chronic toxicity testing is the best means of making an evaluation of chronic toxicity.

METHODOLOGY

Methodology for chronic toxicity testing varies somewhat with the test species selected. The species most commonly used are the fathead and sheepshead minnows and the water flea and mysid shrimp. Most chronic toxicity data for xenobiotics have been developed with one or more of these species. Generally, a chronic toxicity test involves the exposure of populations of the species to six or seven test concentrations for the entire reproductive life cycle of the animal. Controls that duplicate the conditions of exposure except for the test chemical are maintained concurrently. Each treatment and control is duplicated for fish and may be quadruplicated for water fleas to ensure statistical confidence in the data. Several standard protocols for chronic toxicity tests with aquatic species have been published (U.S. EPA, 1978) and others are being developed (ASTM Special Task Groups).

Preparation and delivery of test concentrations to exposure aquaria in a chronic test should be as precise and consistent as possible. It is important in exposing test populations to a range of concentrations in a chronic test to maintain each concentration at a consistent level for the duration of the test—12 mo or longer, if necessary—and to maintain consistent relationships among all the concentrations tested. It is desirable that measured concentrations be related as closely as possible to nominal concentrations. The physical-chemical properties of the test material and the quality of the test concentration preparation and delivery system affect the relationship between measured and nominal concentrations. When a chemical is insoluble or only slightly soluble in the diluent water, organic solvents may be used to make the chemical more miscible in the diluent. If a solvent is used to prepare the test concentrations, then a solvent control—a treatment that contains the maximum concentration of the solvent present in any test concentration but contains no test chemical—must be maintained concurrently with the other treatments. The solvent control is used to evaluate the possible effects on the test animals of chronic exposure to the solvent.

Analytical methods for determining the actual concentrations to which test animals are exposed must be developed, if they are not available, before the chronic test is initiated. Analyses generally involve extraction and concentration of the test chemical from the diluent water, followed by cleanup to remove interfering compounds and then measurement. Gas-liquid chromatography with electron capture or flame ionization detectors is used to measure organic chemicals, and atomic absorption spectrophotometry is used for elemental metals (see Chapter 16). The analytical techniques used depend on the investigator's preference and resources and on the nature of the test chemical. Test concentrations should be sampled frequently enough—at least weekly—to ensure desired exposure concentrations and confirm that no contamination has occurred.

Test animals should be observed as often as possible—daily or more frequently—especially at significant milestones during the developmental period such as egg hatching, attainment of identifiable life stages, appearance of secondary sexual characteristics, and egg production. These observations show how well the population is progressing in normal development to maturity and can identify physical abnormalities or anomalous behavior. For example, observations for fish include, but are not necessarily limited to, the number of viable fertilized eggs, number of eggs that hatch normally, number of larvae that survive hatching, growth measured as length and weight of larvae, number of larvae that successfully develop to juveniles, length and weight of juveniles, number of juveniles that develop to sexual maturity as indicated by development of secondary sexual characteristics and stereotypic reproductive behavior, number of eggs produced by sexually mature fish, number of viable F_1 embryos, and hatching, survival, and growth of F_1 larvae.

Statistical analyses of the data for exposed and control populations show which measurements, if any, are significantly different. The concentrations that produce statistically significant adverse effects on test populations are considered effect concentrations. Those that do not produce statistically significant adverse effects are considered no-effect concentrations. The data should also be evaluated for biological significance, since statistically significant differences are not necessarily biologically significant. Furthermore, if there are no statistically significant differences in a well-controlled study, it is unlikely that there will be any significant biologically adverse effects at the concentrations tested. The subjective judgment of an experienced investigator is required to make these data evaluations.

Test Design

In describing the design of chronic toxicity tests with aquatic animals, it is appropriate to begin with standard test procedures used for flow-through, complete reproductive life cycle tests with the fathead minnow (*Pimephales promelas*), as this was the first aquatic vertebrate to be tested in this manner (Mount and Stephan, 1967). The procedures described and based on *Recommended Bioassay Procedures for Fathead Minnow (Pimephales promelas Rafinesque) Chronic Tests* (Bioassay Committee, 1971). General information about test systems, dilution water characteristics, procedures for flow-through testing, and reporting has been presented by the U.S. EPA (1975).

Physical System

The exposure system used in the test should be capable of establishing a minimum of five chemical concentrations, a negative control, and (if appropriate) a solvent control, in duplicate. Flow rate through the system should provide a minimum of five aquarium volumes per day. A proportional

diluter or mechanical pumping system may be used if its long-term reliability can be confirmed. The system should be constructed of materials, such as glass or stainless steel, that will not add contaminants. No plastic, rubber, or metals such as copper should be used in the system. The test chemical can be introduced by mechanical devices, siphons, pumping systems, or other means that can be shown to be reliable, accurate, and precise. Sizes of exposure chambers should be appropriate for the sizes of the various life stages that will develop in the system. For example, containers for egg incubation can be glass jars approximately 120 ml in volume with an outside diameter of 5 cm and a height of 12 cm. The bottoms of the jars are removed and replaced with a piece of nylon or stainless steel screen (100 mesh/cm). Larval growth and development chambers can be 40 × 21 × 27 cm and adult spawning chambers 60 × 30 × 30 cm.

Dilution Water

The dilution water (diluent) used in the test should be from a deep well or other source not subjected to surface runoff or other contamination. Chlorinated water should not be used if another water source is available. The water quality characteristics (pH, hardness, alkalinity, and specific conductance) of the diluent should be measured weekly and recorded. Other diluent characteristics such as ionic content (Ca^{2+}, Mg^{2+}, Na^+, K^+, Cl^-, SO_4^{2-}, etc.), total solids, and total dissolved solids should be measured at least at the initiation and termination of the test.

The system should provide water temperature control to maintain the desired test temperature ±1.0°C and dissolved oxygen levels of 60% saturation or more for the duration of the test. Artificial light simulating as closely as possible the wavelengths of natural sunlight should be provided on a constant photoperiod such as 12 h on and 12 h off except during the spawning period. During the spawning period, the photoperiod should be adjusted to be appropriate for the species being tested.

Chemical System

Test concentrations should be selected on the basis of previously developed toxicity test data, as described earlier. If possible, the test chemical should be added directly to the dilution water to establish the test concentrations. If it is necessary to use an organic solvent to facilitate miscibility of the test chemical with the diluent, the maximum concentration of solvent in exposure aquaria should be less than 1/1000 of the 96-h LC50 of that solvent with juvenile fathead minnow and should not exceed 0.5 ml per liter of diluent. Typical solvents used in chronic toxicity tests and their LC50s are as follows. TEG and DMF are preferred solvents for aquatic toxicity testing.

Solvent	LC50	Reference
Triethylene glycol (TEG)	92,500 mg/l	Stephan (1979) U.S.EPA (personal communication)
Dimethyl formamide (DMF)	10,410 mg/l	
Acetone	9,100 mg/l	
Dimethyl sulfoxide (DMSO)	33,500 mg/l	Willford (1968)

Stock solutions and samples of the exposure solutions should be chemically analyzed to confirm intended concentrations prior to the addition of test animals to initiate the study.

During a chronic toxicity test, weekly sampling of each replicate of each test concentration and analysis of these samples should confirm the desired exposure concentrations and their stability over time. Measured concentrations should be $\geqslant$50% of nominal at a minimum and should remain within 20% of the mean for the duration of the test. Analysis of water samples from controls should confirm that there has been no contamination by the test material. Temperature and dissolved oxygen concentration should be measured daily, and pH, hardness, alkalinity, acidity, and specific conductance should be measured weekly. If any of these characteristics seem to be affected by the test material, measure-

ments should be made more frequently to characterize the variability.

Biological System

The most desirable source of eggs for a chronic test is a well-established brood unit in the laboratory where the test is performed. Fish from this unit should have a good history of reproductive success, growth, and normal development and be free of disease or abnormalities.

Eggs used to initiate the test should be <48 h old. A minimum of 60 eggs should be distributed to each exposure tank and control, thus providing 120 eggs between the duplicate tanks at each exposure concentration and control. Tanks should be observed daily.

Hatching should occur by the time the eggs are 4 d old. The minimum acceptable successful egg hatch in each control tank should be 60%. The times when hatching begins and ends should be noted for each tank. The number and percent of eggs that successfully hatch viable larvae should be recorded for each tank. Newly hatched fish can be fed brine shrimp (*Artemia salina*) nauplii for the first 20 d and frozen brine shrimp for the remainder of the test. Feeding should be *ad libitum* at least once daily. Observations of normal or abnormal feeding responses should be recorded. Survival of juvenile fish and measurements of total length and wet weight should be recorded 30 and 60 d after hatching. If little mortality has occurred by d 60, the fish population in each tank should be thinned to provide space for growth and diminish competition for food.

After observation of the appearance of secondary sexual characteristics such as development of urogenital papilla in females and display of dark coloration and territorial behavior by males, the population in each tank should be further thinned to three dominant males and seven females for optimal reproductive potential. Each tank should be provided with several suitable spawning substrates, such as cylindrical water drain pipes that are split in half and placed in the tanks with their concave surface facing downward. Eggs will be deposited on the undersurface of the pipes. Pipes should be observed daily for the presence of eggs and the numbers found should be recorded. Parental fish will be sacrificed at the end of a 1-wk period during which no additional spawning has occurred. Several (at least 10) batches of eggs should be incubated in each tank, and, upon hatching, a minimum of 40 larval fish should be selected randomly and transferred into larval growth chambers. These F_1 fish should be observed for 30 d after hatching to evaluate survival, growth (length and weight), and development. At the end of this period, the study can be terminated and fish can be preserved for subsequent chemical analysis to determine tissue residues or for histopathological investigation.

Data Collected

Data developed as a result of this chronic toxicity test include:

1 Actual chemical concentrations to which eggs and fish were exposed;

2 Results of water quality analyses;

3 Number and percent of eggs used to begin the test which hatched viable larvae;

4 Number and percent of juveniles surviving through 30 d of exposure;

5 Total length and wet weight of these fish;

6 Physical or behavioral abnormalities;

7 Items described in 4–6 for 60- and 160-d-old fish and at test termination;

8 Time to egg production;

9 Number of spawns, eggs per spawn, spawns per female, and eggs per female;

10 Number and percent hatch of F_1 eggs;

11 Survival, length, and weight of 30-d post-hatch F_1 fish; and

12 Any other observations that the investigator believes might indicate effects of the test material.

Data Analysis

These data are collated and analyzed by standard statistical tests that compare results from exposed and control populations for statistically significant differences (for details, see the data analysis meth-

ods section of this chapter and Chapter 5). Establishment of effect and no-effect concentrations permits estimation of the MATC, which is the end product of the chronic toxicity test.

As mentioned previously, the other species commonly used in chronic toxicity tests are the freshwater crustacean *Daphnia magna,* (water flea), the saltwater fish *Cyprinodon variegatus* (sheepshead minnow), and the saltwater crustacean *Mysidopsis bahia* (mysid shrimp).

The protocol for chronic toxicity tests with the sheepshead minnow is similar to that just described for tests with the fathead minnow; the major exceptions are related to the saltwater medium in which sheepshead minnow tests are conducted (Hansen et al., 1974; Schimmel and Hansen, 1974). For example, one of the water quality characteristics that is measured is salinity, replacing the hardness and alkalinity measurements in the freshwater chronic test. The experimental design is comparable for the sheepshead and fathead minnows, as are the type of data collected and methods of data analysis. The results of a sheepshead minnow chronic test are also reported as the MATC.

Chronic toxicity tests with the water flea and the mysid shrimp are designed with consideration of the size, life cycle duration, habitats, and behavior of these species.

Water flea are unique in that they reproduce parthenogenetically when maintained under favorable culture conditions. Under unfavorable conditions, reproduction ceases and the animals produce ephippia, a protected dormant stage of the daphnid life cycle. The presence of ephippia in a culture indicates unfavorable conditions and an unhealthy population. Daphnids from a population containing ephippia should not be used for toxicity testing.

Water flea chronic tests are generally conducted in a proportional diluter system with four replicate exposure containers (2-l battery jars) for each concentration and control. The other physical and chemical system conditions are similar to those previously described. The tests are begun with animals <24 h old obtained from a well-established brood unit. Each of the four replicate test containers receives 20 daphnids, resulting in the exposure of 80 water flea per exposure concentration. Water quality characteristics are monitored as described for fathead minnow tests. Daphnids are fed a mixture of trout food and algae, which is introduced several times per day into the test containers. Daily observations are made to detect apparent stress, abnormal behavior, or immobilization. From exposure d 7 through 21, survival of adults and production of young are observed daily. Statistical analyses of the data indicate effect and no-effect concentrations and permit the estimation of an MATC for the test chemical. This test can be extended to a second generation by selecting 20 progeny from each exposure container on d 21 and eliminating the remaining animals.

Chronic toxicity tests with mysid shrimp are generally conducted in a proportional diluter system similar to those used for other aquatic chronic toxicity tests. However, because of the size and jumping ability of these animals, exposure containers are constructed of standard glass Petri dishes (of the type used for bacterial colonization studies) to which a nylon screen collar approximately 15 cm high is attached. Four replicate containers with 5 juvenile mysids each are placed in each glass aquarium, which contains 15 l of the appropriate concentration of the test chemical. A minimum of five test concentrations and appropriate controls are maintained concurrently. Daily observations of shrimp mortality and production of young are made by lifting the exposure containers from the aquaria and permitting the test solution volume in the containers to drain through the screen down to the level of the top of the Petri dish. Placing the dish on a backlighted counter facilitates these observations, which include counts of the number of living animals, the number of females with brood pouches, and the number of young produced. Control adult mysids should release young after test d 10. Mysids exposed to a chemical may require additional time for produc-

tion of young if the chemical adversely affects reproduction. Young shrimp will be observed for approximately 1 wk following release. Data from a mysid chronic test include number of live adult mysids, time to brood pouch formation, time to release of young, number of young produced per female, and survival of young. Significant differences between exposed populations and controls indicate effect and no-effect concentrations, from which an MATC can be estimated for the test chemical.

Other aquatic species have been used in chronic toxicity testing, but the test protocols are less standardized than those for the four species discussed above. The reader is advised to consult the specific references cited in the section of this chapter on test species for details of those methodologies.

Apparatus

The apparatus used for chronic toxicity tests should be capable of producing and delivering, on a flowing, once-through basis, five or more test concentrations that encompass a reasonably wide range, are consistent over the duration of the test (12 mo or longer, if necessary), are reproducible between and among replicate exposure aquaria, and closely represent nominal concentrations. The system should be adjustable and easily calibrated to deliver these concentrations while maintaining acceptable water quality conditions (dissolved oxygen, pH, and organic waste concentrations) and should be designed to minimize the possibility of over- or underdosing. The apparatus should be constructed of inexpensive, readily available materials that will not contaminate test waters and are relatively easy to clean.

Various types of pumping systems were used in the past. These systems generally suffered from a dependence on electrical power, varied greatly in accuracy, precision, and longevity, and were susceptible to gross over- and underdosing. The serial diluter (Mount and Brungs, 1967) was developed to provide the aquatic toxicologist with a more useful dosing apparatus. Its evolution has resulted in the present proportional diluter (Lemke et al., 1978; also see Figs. 1 and 2 in Chapter 2), which is used extensively for chronic toxicity tests as well as flow-through acute toxicity tests and early life stage tests. Other special-purpose diluters have been developed and are described in Chapter 3.

The diluter functions by mixing the test material into diluent water in the mixing chamber and distributing this single concentration to each of the chemical cells. When the diluter cycles, a specific volume of clean water from the diluent water cells combines with the calibrated volume of chemical-containing water from the chemical cells to produce the desired exposure concentration. This total volume from each pair of complementary cells (water plus chemical cells) is delivered to a flow-splitting chamber, which divides the volume equally and delivers the divided volumes to the replicate exposure aquaria. The total volume is the same for each concentration, but the proportions of clean and chemical-containing water are different, thus producing the desired concentrations. This system satisfies the requirements described previously and is the most frequently used system for aquatic toxicity testing in the United States.

Selection of Test Concentrations

Selection of appropriate concentrations is critical for the success of a chronic toxicity test. Ideally, at the termination of the test, one or more of the highest test concentrations should have had an unequivocal adverse effect on the exposed population and one or more of the lowest concentrations should have had no effect. In that way, effect and no-effect concentrations can be clearly identified. If the test concentrations are too high, all the exposed populations may show adverse effects and a no-effect concentration cannot be determined. If they are too low, none of the exposed populations may be adversely affected and the effect concentration will not be determined. In either case, the study should be rerun with a new range of test concentrations. Obviously, this greatly in-

creases the cost and time required to develop the data necessary for a hazard evaluation.

Chronic test concentrations are generally based on the results from a flow-through acute toxicity test performed immediately before the chronic test. In extrapolating from acute to chronic test concentrations, the concentration-response relationship, including time to mortality, degree of mortality, and general mortality patterns, must be considered. In addition, physical-chemical characteristics of the compound can indicate whether it will be soluble in diluent water, degrade in the test system, or otherwise have its biological activity altered under chronic exposure conditions.

In most cases, the concentration range selected for the chronic test will be lower than that for the acute test, but how much lower is a decision that requires the attention of an experienced investigator with a knowledge of the test species and its response to xenobiotics as well as the properties of the chemical being tested. Historically, various application factors have been used to estimate chronic toxicity concentrations from acute toxicity test data. Hypothetical factors such as 0.01, 0.05, and 0.1 have been used for this purpose. Factors empirically determined from full chronic studies with fish have ranged from 0.01 to 0.50 for many xenobiotics, but have been estimated to be as low as 0.003 for lead and chromium and even lower for some pesticides (Macek and Sleight, 1977).

Since a chronic study should include both effect and no-effect concentrations, the range of concentrations tested must be wide enough to produce this information but not too wide for the MATC range to be useful. In many chronic studies a proportional diluter is used to prepare and deliver the desired concentrations to the exposure aquaria. Typical dilution factors used are 50, 65, and 75%. The ranges of test concentrations produced from these dilution factors differ greatly (Table 1). For example, a 50% diluter with six test concentrations produces concentrations that encompass a range of 1.00 to 0.0312, a factor of

Table 1 Range of Test Concentrations Produced by Proportional Diluters with Typical Dilution Factors[a]

Typical dilution factor (%)	Ratio of high to low concentration	Range of test concentrations	Example of typical test concentration series ($X = 1.00$)
50	32	X–0.0312X	1.00, 0.500, 0.250, 0.125, 0.0625, 0.0312
65	8.6	X–0.116X	1.00, 0.650, 0.422, 0.275, 0.178, 0.116
75	4.2	X–0.237X	1.00, 0.750, 0.562, 0.422, 0.316, 0.237

[a]It is assumed that there are six test concentrations.

approximately 32. A similar 75% diluter produces a range of 1.00 to 0.237, a factor of approximately 4.2. Therefore, the investigator should be familiar with the test species, the chemical to be tested, and its concentration-response relationship before selecting the exposure apparatus.

Controls

In evaluating chronic toxicity of a chemical to aquatic organisms, the results for the exposed populations are compared with those for the control populations. That is, the determination of significant adverse effects due to chemical exposure is made relative to the control populations. Therefore, adequate controls are essential in the chronic test design. The minimum acceptable control in a chronic test with a chemical that is soluble in diluent water involves the maintenance, under conditions identical to those of the exposed populations but without exposure to the chemical, of a subpopulation of animals selected randomly from the main population used to conduct the test. The control population should exhibit little or no mortality and should develop, mature, and reproduce in a predictable manner; this indicates the basic good quality of the main population and provides a basis for judging adverse effects of the test chemical on the exposed populations. The investigator experienced with animals used in chronic toxicity tests and familiar with the literature has the background necessary for evaluating the acceptability of the response of control animals. If the performance of control animals during the chronic test is below acceptable levels, it may be necessary to repeat the test.

If solvents are used to make the test chemical more miscible with diluent water, a solvent control must be maintained concurrently with the regular ("negative" or "zero") control. In this case, the population exposed to the solvent must also show acceptable performance and, ideally, should respond in a manner similar to that of the negative controls. If statistical analyses show no significant differences between measurements for the solvent and negative controls, the measurements for the two groups can be combined and averaged and the average used for statistical comparisons with the results for chemical-exposed populations. This combined average provides more powerful statistical discrimination between exposed and control populations and can facilitate the identification of effect and no-effect concentrations.

Typical Measurements

Both chemical and biological measurements are made during a chronic toxicity test. Chemical measurements include dissolved oxygen concentration, pH, temperature, and test chemical concentrations. The first three indicate the water quality maintained during the test and the last one shows the actual concentrations of the chemical to which test animals are exposed. The dissolved oxygen concentration should be ⩾60% of saturation for the duration of the test; the pH should not vary by more than 1.0 unit; the temperature—which is selected, depending on the species being tested, from the series 7, 12, 17, 22, and 27°C—should not instantaneously deviate by more than 2° during the test and its mean during the test should remain within 1° of the selected temperature (U.S. EPA, 1975); and the measured concentrations should be ⩾50% of nominal and should not vary by more than ±20% from the overall mean during the test. If any of the measurements fall outside these acceptable ranges, the test may have to be repeated unless it can be shown that the variation had no adverse effect on the test results.

[handwritten margin note: 0.2 units for acute tests]

Biological measurements from fish chronic toxicity tests include those described in the general methodology section and are generally related to survival, growth, development, and reproductive potential of the test animals. Experience since the mid-1970s with chronic toxicity testing has indicated that the early life stages of aquatic animals are most severely affected (Macek and Sleight, 1977; McKim, 1977). These are generally the stages that are most sensitive to xenobiotic exposure. The adverse effects include decreased survival during the first 2–4 wk after hatching and less than normal growth during the same period. Only rarely have chemicals been shown to adversely affect embryo development and egg hatching (it appears that the chorion is impervious to many waterborne chemicals) at concentrations lower than those that affect the larvae. Furthermore, adverse effects are not typically observed at lower concentrations over the duration of a chronic test except for cumulatively toxic materials such as hexavalent chromium (Benoit, 1976), lead (Davies et al., 1976), and a few others. Most chemicals tested under chronic conditions have not been cumulatively toxic.

Data Analysis Methods

The methods used to evaluate the results of chronic toxicity tests are basically tests that compare the responses of exposed populations with those of controls to determine whether these responses are significantly different and whether the adverse responses are due to chemical exposure or simply to random biological variation. Details of this approach are presented in Chapter 5. In practice, statistical analysis of chronic test data frequently begins with a consideration of the response of control populations. Initially, a comparison is made between or among the replicated negative controls and the replicated solvent controls, if any, to determine whether there are any significant differences. If a statistically significant difference is observed, the validity of the entire test may be questionable and it may be necessary to repeat the test. If there is no significant difference between the controls, all the control data can be pooled and compared with the data for exposed populations, using analysis of variance (ANOVA) (Steel and Torrie, 1960; Sokol and Rohlf, 1973). When significant ($P \leqslant 0.05$) differences are indicated, the mean values for exposed populations are compared with those for controls by appropriate multiple comparison tests (Duncan, 1955; Dunnett, 1955, 1964; Keuls, 1952; Williams, 1971, 1972). From these analyses, the effect and no-effect concentrations are identified and used to designate the NOEC and LOEC. The MATC for the test is reported and the criterion (survival, growth, reproduction, etc.) that was adversely affected is specified. A sample analysis with hypothetical chronic toxicity test data is presented in detail in Chapter 5.

Data Interpretation

Criteria of effect in chronic toxicity tests can include both lethal and sublethal measures. However, in practice, chronically toxic effects are manifested by relatively few quantifiable criteria. Generally, the MATC is based on survival of newly hatched animals, growth of those animals, or numbers of offspring they produce. While the investigator can be relatively confident in ascribing significant adverse effects to a concentration that produces significantly greater mortality in the exposed population, there is less confidence in ascribing the same level of significance to a concentration in which the exposed population is 2 mm smaller or 50 mg lighter than the controls. However, in experiments with good correspondence between replicates, use of the statistical tests described above and selection of $P \leqslant 0.05$ as the level of significance can result in the designation of effect concentrations on the basis of these small incremental differences. At these times the investigator's experience and judgment must be used to designate the effect and no-effect concentrations. For example, it may not be reasonable to ascribe toxicological significance to a concentration that produces statistically significant effects only on total length of the animals and not on

survival, weight, or reproduction, especially if this concentration is two or more dilutions below the next highest effect concentration. Conversely, if there is general corroboration of effects at a concentration, or if the pattern observed is such that there are adverse effects at sequentially lower concentrations as the duration of exposure increases (indicating potential cumulative toxicity of the chemical; see Table 2), then the lowest observed effect concentration should be so identified. The MATC for the hypothetical data set in Table 2 would be $>0.049 < 0.096$ mg/l based on the average wet weight of fry. These data also indicate that compound X has a cumulatively toxic effect on the fish. This effect might be ob-

Table 2 Biological Measurements from a Chronic Toxicity Test in Which Fish Were Exposed to Chemical X

Mean measured concentration of of chemical X (mg/l)	Replicate	Egg hatch (%)	At 30 d		At 60 d		
			Survival (%)	Length (mm)	Survival (%)	Length (mm)	Weight (mg)
27	A	0	—	—	—	—	—
	B	0[a]	—	—	—	—	—
12	A	0	—	—	—	—	—
	B	10[a]	2[a]	19[a]	0	—	—
6.2	A	55	0	—	—	—	—
	B	60[a]	5[a]	21[a]	0	—	—
3.3	A	83	10	21	0	—	—
	B	85	5[a]	19[a]	0	—	—
1.6	A	80	86	20	10	21	180
	B	87	88	21	6[a]	22[a]	195[a]
0.81	A	76	90	22	23	25	245
	B	71	89	21[a]	21[a]	24[a]	240[a]
0.43	A	72	91	27	80	28	265
	B	78	90	26	85	31[a]	290[a]
0.19	A	70	93	26	89	38	300
	B	69	100	28	90	36	310[a]
0.096	A	68	99	28	91	36	435
	B	66	97	28	89	37	450[a]
0.049	A	65	96	27	88	35	515
	B	67	97	29	91	37	525
Solvent control	A	71	98	27	90	38	550
	B	74	98	28	88	36	540
Control	A	70	97	28	89	37	545
	B	73	99	27	91	39	540

[a]Indicates that average measurements of replicates A and B are significantly ($P \leqslant 0.05$) lower than controls.

served at the 0.049 mg/l concentration at the next measurement interval.

In interpreting the significance of data from a chronic toxicity test, it should be recognized that these data represent the effects on test animals of exposure to relatively constant concentrations of the test chemical under laboratory-controlled, clean water conditions. The laboratory chronic toxicity test does not attempt to simulate field conditions, but rather to evaluate a chemical under controlled conditions to develop an understanding of causal relationships.

CONCLUSION

Chronic toxicity tests provide a useful tool for estimating the potential adverse effects of chemicals on aquatic organisms under carefully controlled conditions in a manner that permits an evaluation of causal relationships. However, it should be recognized that chronic toxicity tests are laboratory studies and the results obtained cannot necessarily be extrapolated directly to the aquatic environment. Therefore, natural environmental factors that can affect the concentration, bioavailability, distribution, and fate of a chemical should be understood and carefully considered when making a judgment about the hazard posed by a chemical in the aquatic environment.

LITERATURE CITED

Arthur JW: Chronic effects of linear alkylate sulfonate detergent on *Gammarus pseudolimnaeus, Campeloma decisum,* and *Physa integra.* Water Res 4:251–257, 1970.

Benoit DA: Toxic effects of hexavalent chromium on brook trout (*Salvelinus fontinalis*) and rainbow trout (*Salmo gairdneri*). Water Res 10:497–500, 1976.

Biesinger KE, Christensen GM: Effects of various metals on survival, growth, reproduction, and metabolism of *Daphnia magna.* J Fish Res Bd Can 29:1691–1700, 1972.

Bioassay Committee: Recommended bioassay procedures for fathead minnow (*Pimephales pro-*

melas Rafinesque) chronic tests. Duluth, Minn.: National Water Quality Laboratory, 1971.

Davies PH, Goettl JP, Jr., Sinley JR, Smith NF: Acute and chronic toxicity of lead to rainbow trout *Salmo gairdneri,* in hard and soft water. Water Res 10:199–206, 1976.

Derr SK, Zabik MJ: Biologically active compounds in the aquatic environment: The effect of DDE on the egg viability of *Chironomus tentans.* Bull Environ Contam Toxicol 7:366–368, 1972a.

Derr SK, Zabik MJ: Biologically active compounds in the aquatic environment: The uptake and distribution of {1,1-dichloro-2,2-bis (*p*-chlorophenyl) ethylene}, DDE, by *Chironomus tentans* Fabricius (Diptera: Chironomidae). Trans Am Fish Soc 101:323–329, 1972b.

Duncan DB: Multiple range and multiple F-tests. Biometrics 11:1–42, 1955.

Dunnett DW: A multiple comparisons procedure for comparing several treatments with a control. J Am Stat Assoc 50:1096–1121, 1955.

Dunnett DW: New tables for multiple comparison with a control. Biometrics 20:482–491, 1964.

Eaton JG: Chronic malathion toxicity to the bluegill (*Lepomis macrochirus* Rafinesque). Water Res 4:673–684, 1970.

Grassle JP, Grassle JF: Sibling species in the marine pollution indicator *Capitella* (polychaete). Science 192:567–569, 1976.

Hansen DJ, Parrish PR: Suitability of sheepshead minnows (*Cyprinodon variegatus*) for life-cycle toxicity tests. In: Aquatic Toxicology and Hazard Evaluation, edited by FL Mayer, JL Hamelink, pp. 117–126. ASTM STP 634. Philadelphia: ASTM, 1977.

Hansen DJ, Parrish PR, Forester J: Aroclor 1016: Toxicity to and uptake by estuarine animals. Environ Res 7:363–373, 1974.

Hansen DJ, Schimmel SC, Forester J: Endrin: Effects on the entire life-cycle of saltwater fish, *Cyprinodon variegatus.* J Toxicol Environ Health 3:721, 1977.

Keuls M: The use of the studentized range in connection with an analysis of variance. Euphytica 1:112–122, 1952.

Lemke AE, Brungs WA, Halligan BJ: Manual for construction and operation of toxicity-testing proportional diluters. EPA-600/3-78-072, 1978.

Macek KJ, Sleight BH: Utility of toxicity tests

with embryos and fry of fish in evaluating hazards associated with the chronic toxicity of chemicals to fishes. In: Aquatic Toxicology and Hazard Evaluation, edited by FL Mayer, JL Hamelink, pp. 137–146. ASTM STP 634. Philadelphia: ASTM, 1977.

McKim JM: Evaluation of tests with early life stages of fish for predicting long-term toxicity. J Fish Res Bd Can 34:1148–1154, 1977.

McKim JM, Benoit DA: Effects of long-term exposures to copper on the survival, growth, and reproduction of brook trout. J Fish Res Bd Can 28:655–662, 1971.

McKim JM, Benoit DA: Duration of toxicity tests for establishing "no effect" concentrations for copper with brook trout. J Fish Res Bd Can 31:449–452, 1974.

Mount DI, Brungs WA: A simplified dosing apparatus for fish toxicology studies. Water Res 1:21–29, 1967.

Mount DI, Stephan CE: A method for establishing acceptable limits for fish—malathion and the butoxyethanol ester of 2,4-D. Trans Am Fish Soc 96:185–193, 1967.

Nebeker AV: Temperature requirements and life cycle of the midge Tanytarsus dissimilis. J Kans Entomol Soc 46:160–165, 1973.

Nimmo DR, Bahner LH, Rigby RA, Sheppard JM, Wilson AJ, Jr.: Mysidopsis bahia: An estuarine species suitable for life-cycle toxicity tests to determine the effects of a pollutant. In: Aquatic Toxicology and Hazard Evaluation, edited by FL Mayer, JL Hamelink, pp. 109–116. ASTM STP 634. Philadelphia: ASTM, 1977.

Reish DJ: The sublethal effects of environmental variables on polychaetous annelids. Rev Int Oceanogr Med 33:1–8, 1974.

Reish DJ, Piltz F, Martin JM, Word JQ: The effect of heavy metals on laboratory populations of the marine polychaetes Neanthes arenaceodentata and Capitella capitata. Water Res 10:299–302, 1976.

Schimmel SC, Hansen DJ: Sheepshead minnow (Cyprinodon variegatus). An estuarine fish suitable for chronic (entire life-cycle) bioassays. Proc 28th Am Conf Southeast Game Fish Comm 392–398, 1974.

Smith WE: A cyprinodontid fish, Jordanella floridae, as reference animals for rapid chronic bioassays. J Fish Res Bd Can 39:329–330, 1974.

Sokol RR, Rohlf FJ: Introduction to Biostatistics. San Francisco: Freeman, 1973.

Sosnowski SL, Gentile JH: Toxicological comparison of natural and cultured populations of Acartia tonsa to cadmium, copper, and mercury. J Fish Res Bd Can 35:1366–1369, 1978.

Steel RGD, Torrie JH: Principles and Procedures of Statistics with Special Reference to Biological Sciences. New York: McGraw-Hill, 1960.

Stephan CE: U.S. Environmental Protection Agency, personal communication.

Tyler-Schroeder DB: Use of the grass shrimp (Palaemonetes pugio) in a life-cycle toxicity test. In: Aquatic Toxicology, edited by LL Marking, RA Kimerle, pp. 159–170. ASTM STP 667. Philadelphia: ASTM, 1979.

U.S. Environmental Protection Agency: Methods for acute toxicity tests with fish, macroinvertebrates, and amphibians. EPA-660/3-75-009, Washington, D.C., 1975.

U.S. Environmental Protection Agency: Bioassay procedures for the ocean disposal permit program. EPA-600/9-78-010, Washington, D.C., 1978.

Willford WA: Toxicity of dimethyl sulfoxide (DMSO) to fish. Bur Sport Fish Wildl Invest Fish Control 20:3–8, 1968.

Williams DA: A test for differences between treatment means when survival dose levels are compared with a zero dose control. Biometrics 27:103–117, 1971.

Williams DA: A comparison of several dose levels with a zero dose control. Biometrics 28:519–531, 1972.

Chapter 5

Statistical Analysis

R. D. Gelber, P. T. Lavin, C. R. Mehta, and D. A. Schoenfeld

INTRODUCTION

This chapter describes statistical concepts for the analysis of data from acute and chronic aquatic toxicity experiments. It is intended to present the methods of analysis that are currently being used, the drawbacks of these methods, and methods that may be better than those now in use. The chapter is divided into two subsections corresponding to acute and chronic tests.

ACUTE TOXICITY TESTS

In an acute toxicity test (see Chapter 2), groups of aquatic animals are exposed to progressively increasing concentrations of a toxicant. The primary purpose of the test is to estimate the concentration of the test material that is lethal to 50% of the animals of a given species within a specific length of time (usually 24, 48, 72, or 96 h). This concentration is referred to as the median lethal concentration (LC50). The use of the LC50 to characterize the potency of a toxicant is arbitrary. In some situations the LC95 or some other LC value, analogously defined, might be of greater interest. The LC50 is chosen in most acute toxicity tests because, for a fixed sample size, an estimate of the median tolerance (50% kill) has less sampling variance (is more reproducible) than an estimate of any other quantile.

It is reasonable to expect that the percentage of animal deaths will increase monotonically with the concentration of the toxicant. It is, however, highly unlikely that one of the concentrations selected in the experiment will kill exactly 50% of the exposed animals. Therefore, the LC50 is esti-

Partial support for this work was provided by Grants CA-23415, CA-06516, CA-25162, and CA-33019 awarded by the National Cancer Institute, DHHS, and by Faculty Development Grants from the Mellon Foundation.

ACUTE (handwritten)

mated either by fitting a smooth parametric function to the observed data or by numerical interpolation. Since the estimated LC50 is based on data from only a sample of a particular aquatic species, it does not coincide with the *true* LC50, which is the concentration that would be lethal to exactly 50% of the entire species. Thus, a confidence interval for the true LC50 is usually computed along with its point estimate. It can be asserted with a prespecified level of confidence that this interval contains the true LC50. Typically, it is the 95% confidence interval that is computed.

Several methods for estimating the LC50 and its associated confidence interval have been proposed in the statistical and biological literature. Early approximate techniques were developed by Behrens (1929), Kärber (1931), and Gaddum (1933). Subsequently, three independent approaches for estimating the LC50 evolved. They are referred to here as the parametric, the moving average, and the nonparametric methods, respectively. The parametric method is based on transforming the concentration levels so that the transformed concentration-mortality relationship has a known functional form. Since this method involves the entire concentration-mortality curve, and not merely a single point on it (such as the LC50), it is applicable to bioassay as well as to acute toxicity testing. The moving average method is based on numerical interpolation and is applicable only to LC50 estimates from acute toxicity tests. The nonparametric methods use the monotonicity of the concentration-mortality curve to generate an empirical curve from which LC50 estimates are obtained.

Among parametric methods, the use of the probit transformation for the analysis of quantal assay data can be first attributed to Bliss (1934). The probit transformation maps an outcome between 0 and 100% (mortality data) into a full range of values from $-\infty$ to $+\infty$ (probit values) to generate a sigmoid-shaped curve when plotted against the logarithm of the concentration. Empirical studies suggest that the probit transformation is reasonably accurate, but not always optimal. Finney (1971) presented a systematic

Probit (handwritten)

account of probit analysis in his classic textbook. The probit method has the disadvantage of requiring laborious, time-consuming calculations for the maximum likelihood estimation of the unknown parameters. Modifications of the probit method, using nomograms to simplify the calculations, were proposed by De Beer (1945) and by Litchfield and Wilcoxon (1949). In the meantime, alternative parametric representations of quantal data were being investigated. The logistic function was proposed by Wilson and Worcester (1943) and by Berkson (1944) as a competitor of the probit. Another technique, the angular arc-sine transformation of the percent mortalities, was developed by Knudsen and Curtis (1947) because of its variance-stabilizing properties. Moving average interpolation for estimating the LC50 was proposed by Thompson (1947) and Bennett (1952). Bennett also proposed combining the moving average interpolation with an angular transformation of the mortality percentages. Hamilton et al. (1977) suggested use of a nonparametric technique, the trimmed Spearman-Karber method, which produces fail-safe LC50 estimates.

None of the methods above are applicable in their original form if the acute toxicity test yields concentration levels with no partial kills. For this special case, the LC50 is computed as the arithmetic mean of the highest toxicant concentration in which there was 0% mortality and the lowest toxicant concentration in which there was 100% mortality. A simple binomial calculation can be used to evaluate the confidence interval, as discussed by Stephan (1977). There are, in addition, various ways of adjusting the observed data so that the parametric methods or the moving average interpolation method may be applied to the special case of no partial kill. Berkson's adjustment (Finney, 1971) is the most widely accepted one. However, these adjustments are not commonly used in routine aquatic toxicity testing.

In the next section, the principles underlying the parametric methods, the moving average interpolation method, and a nonparametric method for estimating the LC50 are discussed. Binomial confidence intervals for the special case of no partial kill are also discussed. The section concludes with a comparison of LC50 estimates obtained by the probit, moving average, and nonparametric methods for a few typical data sets. Some guidelines for choosing among the methods are then provided.

Methods of Estimating the LC50

Parametric methods, moving average interpolation methods, nonparametric methods, and the binomial method are considered. Unless Berkson's adjustment is first applied to the data, parametric methods are applicable only when there are partial kills at two or more concentration levels. Moving average interpolation requires that at least one concentration level have a partial kill. The nonparametric methods exploit the monotonic behavior of increased mortality associated with increased concentration. Finally, the binomial method has been developed for the special case of no partial kill.

Parametric Methods

The original data consist of a series of concentration levels and a series of corresponding mortality rates. One way to estimate the LC50 is to first transform the concentration levels to a suitable scale whereon the transformed concentration-mortality relationship has a known parametric form. There are sound biological reasons for asserting that when the concentration levels are expressed in logarithmic units, the curve of concentration versus mortality is sigmoid-shaped. Two popular sigmoid-shaped functions are the probit and the logistic. Either of these functions may be fitted to the transformed data and its parameters may be estimated by the maximum likelihood method. The LC50 and its confidence interval are then deduced from the maximum likelihood estimates.

Consider the probit method as a specific example of the technique. Suppose that the logarithms of the concentration levels are x_1, x_2, ..., x_k. For $i = 1, 2, \ldots, k$, let n_i be the size of the batch treated at concentration level x_i and let P_i be the proportion of deaths observed in this batch. The underlying concentration-mortality relation is explained by:

$$P = \Phi(\alpha + \beta x)$$

where P is the probability of death at concentration level x, Φ is the standard normal distribution function, and α and β are unknown parameters that define the concentration-mortality relationship. Maximum likelihood estimates of α and β are computed as functions of the observed data (x_i, p_i, $i = 1, 2, \ldots, k$). The value of x corresponding to $P = 0.5$ is then deduced from these estimates. This is the LC50 estimate. The maximum likelihood equations for estimating the LC50 and its confidence interval are fairly complicated and must be solved iteratively. This is no longer a serious limitation because of the availability of high-speed computers. However, during the early days of probit analysis, the computational complexities of the problem were resolved by various approximations with the help of nomograms. Even today, circumstances might arise which necessitate estimating the LC50 without the use of a computer. A rapid and easy graphical approach is to plot the logarithms of the concentration levels against the mortalities on probit paper. (The ordinates of this paper are measured on a linear scale of probits instead of percentages.) A straight line is then fitted by eye to the plotted points and the LC50 is read off the graph. Note that this graphical technique will not provide confidence intervals for the LC50.

Parametric methods have several undesirable properties if the data do not conform to the assumed model. The maximum likelihood iterative procedures may not converge at all or may converge to different estimates of LC50 depending on the initial guesses used to start the procedure. Furthermore, in duplicate experiments with two toxicants, if one assay yields greater mortality at each concentration, one would want the LC50 estimate for that assay to be no greater than the LC50 estimate for the other. However, with parametric methods it is possible that the assay with the greater mortality will yield the higher LC50 estimate (Hamilton et al., 1977). These difficulties do not arise when the nonparametric procedures discussed later are used.

Moving Average Interpolation

Suppose once more that for $i = 1, 2, \ldots, k$, the percentage mortality is P_i at concentration level x_i. The formulas for the LC50 and its confidence interval are considerably simplified if the concentration levels form a geometric series, so that by transforming them to the logarithmic scale we achieve the necessary uniform spacing. A moving mortality rate of span $s + 1$ (where s is even) is obtained by calculating the weighted sum

$$\hat{P}_i = \sum_{j=i-s/2}^{i+s/2} w_j P_j$$

for each concentration x_i. One then interpolates linearly between consecutive values of the moving average $\hat{P}_i$ on either side of 0.5. The weights w_j are obtained by least-squares techniques, as shown in Bennett (1952), for spans 3 and 5. The variance of the LC50 has also been computed by Bennett. However, this variance estimate does not apply unless the concentration levels are equally spaced. This currently limits the applicability of the moving average method relative to the probit method, although more complicated variance formulas for unequally spaced concentration levels can be derived if necessary. The resulting formulas would, however, be exceedingly complicated. Another limitation of the moving average method is that it cannot be used to estimate any other quantile of the tolerance distribution. If the LC95 is of interest, the moving average method cannot be used.

Bennett also suggested applying the arc-sine transformation to the percent mortalities before using the moving average interpolation. This is referred to as moving average angle interpolation. No justification for applying the angular transformation has been provided. The variance-stabilizing properties of this transformation do not simplify the variance calculations of the LC50, nor is there any evidence that the angular transformation linearizes the concentration-mortality relationship. Nevertheless, moving average angle interpolation is currently recommended as the method of choice for a standardized determination of the LC50 (Stephan, 1977).

Trimmed Spearman-Karber Method

Suppose that for $i = 1, \ldots, k$ the percentage mortality is P_i at log concentration level x_i. Let x_l be the lowest concentration producing 100% mortality and x_h be the highest concentration producing 0% mortality. The Spearman-Karber method for estimating the LC50 is model-free, requiring only symmetry of the tolerance distribution. Finney (1964) describes the conventional method, while Hamilton et al. (1977) describe the trimmed Spearman-Karber method. For the trimmed method, the experimenter must choose a value α in the range $0 \leqslant \alpha \leqslant 50$ which is the percent of extreme values to be trimmed from each tail of the tolerance distribution before calculating the LC50 estimate. (For example, if $\alpha = 10$, only the central 80% of the estimated tolerance distribution would be used to estimate the LC50; note that $\alpha = 0$ yields the conventional method.) The trimmed estimate is robust in the sense that its value relies on the values in the central, more stable portion of the tolerance distribution. The four-step procedure for estimating the LC50 is as follows:

Step 1. Adjust $P_1, \ldots, P_k$. Successive P_i should satisfy $P_h \leqslant P_{h+1} \leqslant \ldots \leqslant P_l$. Adjacent P_i violating this rule should be pooled (replaced by their average value) to obtain a monotone nondecreasing sequence $\bar{P}_h, \bar{P}_{h+1}, \ldots, \bar{P}_l$.

Step 2. Plot $(x_i, \bar{P}_i)$. A polygonal figure is constructed by plotting the $(x_i, \bar{P}_i)$ pairs and connecting the points. This figure estimates the cumulative relative frequency curve for the tolerance distribution.

Step 3. Trim off the upper and lower α percentiles. Change the ordinate scale by replacing $\bar{P}_i$ by $_\alpha \bar{P}_i = (\bar{P}_i - \alpha/100) \div (1 - 2\alpha/100)$. Ignore

$_{\alpha}\bar{P}_i$ values that are less than zero or greater than one. The resulting polygon is an estimate of the trimmed cumulative relative frequency curve for the central $(100 - 2\alpha)$ percent of the tolerance distribution.

Step 4. Calculate the LC50 estimate. The mean associated with the cumulative relative frequency polygon formed in step 3 is the α%-trimmed Spearman-Karber estimate of log LC50. For each interval (x_{i-1}, x_i) calculate the product of the interval midpoints $[(x_{i-1} + x_i)/2]$ times the estimated proportion of population tolerance log concentrations that are in the interval $(_{\alpha}\bar{P}_i - _{\alpha}\bar{P}_{i-1})$. The sum of these products is the mean associated with the polygon, and the antilog is the LC50 estimate.

The nonparametric Spearman-Karber method has several advantages over the parametric probit and logit models described earlier. The method never fails to produce an LC50 estimate provided α is chosen to satisfy $\alpha \geqslant 100\bar{P}_1$ and $\alpha \geqslant 100(1 - \bar{P}_k)$ and $\bar{P}_1 \leqslant 0.5 \leqslant \bar{P}_k$ (i.e., at least one concentration with mortality above 50% and one with mortality below 50%). In addition, the calculations can be performed easily by hand or on a desk calculator. Finally, the method always yields estimates that satisfy the monotone relationship between concentration and mortality. In duplicate experiments, the assay having greater mortality proportions at each concentration always yields the lower estimated LC50. Hamilton (1979) reports the results of Monte Carlo simulation studies and concludes that, in terms of the sensitivity of the estimate to an anomalous response and the possibility that the estimate is incalculable, the Spearman-Karber estimator is especially reliable when compared to five other LC50 estimation procedures.

Binomial Confidence Intervals

Suppose we have observed 0% mortality at concentration level x_1 and 100% mortality at concentration level x_2. Let n_i be the number of animals treated at level x_i, and suppose that no animals were treated at concentration levels between x_1 and x_2. The LC50 is estimated as the arithmetic mean of x_1 and x_2. The confidence interval for the LC50 is the interval (x_1, x_2) and its confidence coefficient is computed from the formula

$$1 - (\tfrac{1}{2})^{n_1} - (\tfrac{1}{2})^{n_2}$$

If both n_1 and n_2 equal 6 or more, the above confidence coefficient will always exceed 95%.

Guidelines for Selecting the Appropriate Method of Estimating the LC50

From the preceding section it is apparent that point and interval estimates of the LC50 can be made by several methods. If there are fewer than two concentration levels with partial kills, Berkson's adjustment should be applied to the data before proceeding with parametric estimation. For the special case of no partial kill, binomial confidence intervals may be used.

From a practical point of view, it is not crucial that rigid guidelines be established for selecting among the different available procedures. For most types of data the estimate of the LC50 and its confidence interval will not vary significantly if different methods are used, especially considering the normal biological and test condition variability that can occur from test to test. Ultimately, all these methods are alternative ways of smoothing the data and then estimating the median effect value. Stephan's (1977) computations clearly demonstrate that one estimation technique is practically equivalent to another from the point of view of numerical results. Hamilton et al. (1977) estimate the LC50 and its 95% upper and lower confidence limits for five data sets, using the probit, logit, and trimmed Spearman-Karber methods. Table 1 summarizes these calculations. The results in Table 1 look similar irrespective of the method of calculation used. However, Hamilton et al. caution that estimation of the 95% confidence limits was not possible for data sets 4A and 4B with the probit technique. This is due either to failure of convergence of the estimation procedure or to the occurrence of negative variance estimates. Although the LC50 estimates are

ACUTE

Table 1 Results of Hypothetical Acute Toxicity Tests (10 Organisms per Concentration)[a]

Tank	1	2	3	4	5	6	C
Concentration (μg/l)	7.8	13	22	36	60	100	Control
No. of test fish	10	10	10	10	10	10	10
Data set							
4A	0	0	10	100	100	100	0
4B	0	0	70	100	100	100	0
4C	0	0	10	40	100	100	0
4D	0	0	20	70	100	100	0
4E	0	0	20	30	100	100	0

Hypothetical sets of data and acceptable results—percent mortality

Results calculated by different methods

Data set	Value	Acceptable values	Probit Daum[b]	BMD[c]	Logit[d]	Spearman-Karber[e] (%) 0	5	10	20
4A	LC50	25.5–27.5	26.4[f]	24.1[g]	26.2	26.7	27.2	27.4	27.4
	Lower[h]	21.1–24.0	NC[i]	NC	20.3	22.6	22.5	22.0	22.0
	Upper[h]	28.6–30.8	NC	NC	33.6	31.7	32.8	36.0	36.0
4B	LC50	19.0–21.5	20.0[f]	21.0	20.0	19.7	19.5	19.4	19.1
	Lower	14.7–19.4	NC	NC	16.6	15.2	14.7	14.3	13.8
	Upper	22.9–24.5	NC	NC	24.1	25.5	25.9	26.2	26.4
4C	LC50	35.5–37.2	35.5	35.5	36.4	36.1	37.0	37.5[g]	38.2[g]
	Lower	26.1–30.7	28.8	26.1	27.7	28.7	29.0	29.3	28.1
	Upper	43.4–45.3	44.1	48.4	47.8	45.5	47.2	48.0	51.8
4D	LC50	29.4–30.0	29.5	29.5	29.4	29.5	29.7	29.8	29.7
	Lower	23.5–23.9	23.8	24.3	23.8	23.2	22.8	22.7	23.3
	Upper	36.3–37.4	36.6	35.8	36.5	37.7	38.6	39.1	38.0
4E	LC50	35.4–40.5	35.4	35.4	37.5	36.1	37.1	38.1	40.2
	Lower	28.1–30.8	28.2	26.2	26.5	28.3	28.4	28.7	29.6
	Upper	44.5–46.0	44.5	47.7	52.9	46.1	48.3	50.5	54.7

[a]Reprinted with permission from Hamilton et al. (1977); copyright 1977, American Chemical Society.

[b]Maximum likelihood estimate based on the probit model; confidence interval using the Fieller procedure.

[c]Maximum likelihood estimate based on the probit model; confidence interval end points from $\log_e(LC50) \pm 2 \times SE[\log_e(LC50)]$.

[d]Minimum transform chi-square estimate based on the logit model. The logit transform suggested by Anscombe was used.

[e]α%-Trimmed Spearman-Karber estimates: $\alpha = 0, 5, 10, 20$.

[f]Probit method did not converge.

[g]Indicates point estimates of LC50 that are not in the range of acceptable values.

[h]Lower and upper 95% confidence interval end points.

[i]NC indicates 95% confidence interval end points are not calculable.

similar for the various procedures, the 95% confidence limits can vary considerably depending on the procedure used. Notice that the choice between the two probit procedures and the choice of the percent trimming (α) for the Spearman-Karber method can produce different 95% confidence limits.

There are, however, certain guidelines that should be followed to use the data to maximum advantage:

1 If there are biological grounds for believing that the distribution of tolerance to log concentrations of the toxicant is normal, the probit method is the most efficient one to use.

2 The Spearman-Karber method provides failsafe LC50 estimates even when normality does not hold. These estimates are resistant to anomalies in the data and exploit the monotone relationship between concentration and mortality.

3 The technique of adjusting data as proposed by Berkson is not very intuitive and does not appeal to most toxicologists. If possible, it should be avoided, even though its use will not affect the numerical results to any significant degree. Accordingly, the moving average method, with unadjusted data, may be used if there is only one concentration level at which a partial kill is observed. The binomial method may be used when there are no partial kills.

4 The moving average method in its present form is not applicable unless the concentration levels (appropriately transformed) are equally spaced.

5 The moving average method is not applicable for estimating any quantile other than the LC50.

6 There is little or no advantage to using the moving average angle method in preference to the moving average method with untransformed mortality rates.

CHRONIC TOXICITY TESTS

The background, rationale, techniques, and end points for chronic and partial life cycle tests were presented in Chapters 3 and 4. References were made to the statistical analyses that are often used to analyze data from chronic toxicity tests. Techniques such as analysis of variance (ANOVA) and Dunnett's procedure were mentioned (Snedecor and Cochran, 1967; Steele and Torrie, 1960; Dunnett, 1955, 1964). In this section some of the rationale behind the use of these procedures is discussed and some of the potential difficulties of the currently accepted methods (ASTM, 1981; U.S. EPA, 1981) are highlighted. In particular, it is indicated that the results of Dunnett's procedure may contradict those of the ANOVA F-test. Furthermore, Dunnett's procedure is inefficient when a nondecreasing concentration-response relationship is assumed. Some statistical procedures are suggested that do not have these difficulties. A numerical example is presented.

Objectives of Chronic Toxicity Tests

The objective of the chronic toxicity experiment is to determine the effects of a toxicant on the viability of a species exposed for an extended period of time. In a typical experiment, fish are placed in tanks containing various concentrations of the toxicant, with each concentration being replicated in several tanks. In addition, several tanks contain no toxicant and provide zero-concentration control data. Tank concentrations are maintained by either static or dynamic volume exchange. After the experiment has proceeded for a predetermined amount of time (which depends on the species, i.e., the length of its reproductive life cycle), data on various end points are recorded for the populations in each of the tanks and results are summarized for each toxicant concentration and for the control. The results for the various toxicant concentrations are compared to those for the control by performing statistical tests of significance. The outcome of these experiments is summarized by the range of the MATC (maximum acceptable toxicant concentration). The upper end of the MATC range is represented by the lowest test concentration that shows a statistically significant effect (lowest observed effect concentration, LOEC). The lower end of the MATC range is represented by the highest test concentration that shows no statistically significant difference from the control (highest no observed effect concentration, NOEC). Several response end points are analyzed, including survival percent, percent egg hatchability, fish length, and fish weight. The experiment-wide range of the MATC is often taken as the lowest concentrations that demonstrate an effect on any of the specified response end points of interest. Since the concept of statistically significant effect is so crucial to the determination of the MATC, this concept is discussed more carefully below.

The Concept of Statistical Significance

A basic hypothesis is that a given concentration of toxicant will have a certain effect on the species of fish under study. Very low concentrations will have little or no effect on the end point being studied, while very high concentrations will have a major effect. Concentrations between these extremes are expected to produce adverse effect responses that are directly proportional to the exposure concentration (concentration-response relationship). The data obtained from chronic toxicity experiments are used to estimate the underlying effects of several concentrations of toxicant. However, these observations are subject to biological and experimental variability. As a result, observed differences between effects at various concentrations and those of the control may be due to random variation rather than to any real differences. A statistical hypothesis test is a method that indicates whether the observed differences were likely to have occurred by random variation alone rather than as a direct result of chemical exposure. If it is unlikely that the observed differences could have occurred by chance alone, it can be concluded from the experimental evidence that the underlying effect of the toxicant concentration is different from that of the control. The observed effects are then referred to as statistically significant effects.

In practice, the data from the experiment are summarized in the form of a test statistic. This test statistic obeys a known probability distribution if the null hypothesis is true. The summary statistic is specially selected to be sensitive to alternative hypotheses that are of interest. By assuming that the null hypothesis is true, it is possible to determine a range of values (rejection region) of the test statistic that would be unlikely to occur if the null hypothesis were true. Historically, the rejection region is determined so that there is less than a 5% chance of the statistic having a value in the region if the null hypothesis is true. Such tests are said to be conducted at the 5% level of significance. If the observed value for the test statistic exceeds the critical value for the test (i.e., falls in the rejection region), then one of the following situations exists. Either

1 The null hypothesis is true, but a rare event has been observed (one that would occur less than 1 time in 20), or
2 The null hypothesis is not true.

Since the chance of obtaining the experimental results by random fluctuation alone is small, values of the test statistic in the rejection region are considered to provide evidence against the null hypothesis that the underlying effects do not differ. With this test procedure, the error of rejecting the null hypothesis when it is true occurs less than 5% of the time. The P value is the probability of obtaining observed experimental results by chance alone, assuming the null hypothesis to be true. Thus, observed effects that yield test statistics in the rejection region are associated with a P value $\leqslant 0.05$ and are considered statistically significant effects.

Current Statistical Practice

The usual statistical techniques currently applied for the analysis of data from chronic toxicity experiments proceed in four steps. These steps are transformation of the data, testing for equivalence of the regular control and the carrier control, using an ANOVA F-test to test for equality of concentration effects, and using a multiple comparison test (e.g., Dunnett's procedure) to determine which of several concentrations produced a statistically significant effect. The data transformation step is applicable only for estimates of percentages, and the test for equivalent controls is used only when an active (solvent) control is available.

Transforming the Data

It is often convenient to transform the observed data before an analysis. In the acute experiment, probit transformations were performed prior to the linear fit of the concentration-response curve. In chronic toxicity experiments, many of the end point estimates are obtained as a proportion. For example, we report the hatchability of embryos (%), normal larvae at hatch (%), and survival of 28-d-old fish (%). Prior to analyzing data of this type, the observed proportion in each tank is transformed by using the arc-sine square root transformation (Snedecor and Cochran, 1967). The rationale for using the arc-sine square root transformation is as follows for the analysis of observed proportion surviving.

The observed survival proportions represent estimates of the underlying survival probability for each of the concentration-tank combinations. Although the same number of fish are tested within each tank, the estimated survival proportions will have different variances that depend on the underlying survival probabilities. This dependence makes it difficult to accurately assess the significance of differences among the observed survival proportions, since the underlying survival probabilities are unknown. By considering the arc-sine square root of the observed proportions, estimates of treatment effect are obtained that have a common variance independent of these treatment effects. In addition to stabilizing the variance of the estimates, the distribution of the transformed estimates is more closely approximated by a normal distribution than are the original observed survival proportions. Thus, use of the transformed estimates enables the application of standard normal theory procedures (e.g., ANOVA) for the analysis.

Equality of Active and Passive Controls

If an organic solvent is used to introduce a toxicant, it must first be determined whether the solvent itself has any effect. A t-test (Steele and Torrie, 1960) is used to compare the effects of the untreated (nonactive or zero) control to that of the solvent control. If differences exist, then the solvent control must be used for the remaining analyses. In this case, subsequent analyses reflect effects of toxicant over and above the effects of the organic solvent. If the difference between controls is not statistically significant, then all control data can be combined for the remaining analyses.

Analysis of Variance

The next step in the analysis is to determine whether any of the observed differences among the concentrations are statistically significant. The standard procedure is to perform an ANOVA F-test with the transformed data. This is a test of the null hypothesis that the effect at all of the concentrations and at the control are the same. The test is likely to indicate significance in any situation other than that in which strict equality of the effects holds over all toxicant concentrations. If the F-test is not statistically significant ($P > 0.05$), it can be concluded that the effects observed in the toxicant treatments are all the same and not different from the control. The NOEC based on this end point is then taken to be the highest test concentration analyzed. Other end points of interest are then evaluated to determine whether any significant effects are detected. If the F-test is statistically significant, the next phase of the analysis is utilized.

Multiple Comparison Test

Following a significant F-test result, all exposure concentration responses are compared with the control response by using a Dunnett's procedure. Dunnett's procedure is a multiple comparison test specifically designed to compare several experimental samples to the concurrent control. A multiple comparison test is a technique that accounts for the fact that several comparisons are being made simultaneously. If each of the separate comparisons in the experiment was conducted at the $P = 0.05$ level with the usual t-test, the experimentwide P value can be substantially greater than 0.05. That is, the chance that at least one of the comparisons is statistically significant will be greater than 0.05 even when the underlying effects are not different. For example, consider the situation in which 100 tests of significance, each at the 0.05 level, are conducted. On the average, by chance alone, it is expected that five of these tests will be statistically significant, even when there is no underlying toxicant effect. Dunnett's procedure accounts for the fact that multiple comparisons are being conducted. It adjusts the rejection region so that over the entire experiment the probability of finding a statistically significant difference between an experimental concentration and a control is less than 0.05 when no underlying differences exist.

Dunnett's procedure provides a cutoff value for the difference in response between a test concentration and the control. The lowest concentration for which the difference in observed response exceeds the cutoff value is defined as the LOEC for that end point. The highest concentration for which the difference in response is not greater than the cutoff value is defined as the NOEC for that end point.

Determining the MATC

Several end points are measured in a chronic toxicity experiment. Survival percentage, hatchability, normal larvae, weight, and length are considered important end points for the maintenance of a healthy population. Data for each of these end points are analyzed by the procedures discussed above. The most sensitive end point, that for which significant effects are observed at the lowest concentration, is then used to define the MATC. The estimated MATC for the given toxicant and test species is reported as "> NOEC < LOEC" based on the most sensitive end point. This gives the experimentwide MATC range.

Suggested Improvements

The preliminary F-test is unnecessary. In current practice Dunnett's procedure is used to refine the result of the ANOVA F-test. A significant F-test is followed by a Dunnett's procedure so that it can be determined which toxicant concentrations have produced results that are significantly different from the control. However, it is possible for the F-test to be statistically significant while none of the comparisons in the Dunnett's procedure are statistically significant. Conversely, it is possible for the F-test to show no significant effect, while the Dunnett's procedure indicates that a concentration effect is significantly different from the control.

Use of the preliminary F-test is unnecessary since Dunnett's procedure has exactly a 5% chance of showing significant results if all the concentrations have the same effect as the control. The preliminary test reduces this probability below 5% and thereby reduces the sensitivity of the experiment. Thus, the preliminary F-test should not be performed.

Dunnett's procedure is not the most powerful test available; Williams' test is preferable. The power of a statistical test is a measure of how well the test is able to detect alternatives to the null hypothesis. It is the probability that the null hypothesis will be rejected when the null hypothesis is not true. The power of a given test depends on the true underlying alternative hypothesis. In the chronic experiment, the alternative hypothesis is that higher concentrations are associated with increased morbidity and mortality. Dunnett's procedure does not make use of the fact that underlying toxicant effects are ordered by increasing concentration. Instead, it considers each comparison of a concentration with the control separately, without regard to the concentration-response ordering of the effects. Failure to consider the logical ordering of the responses in the alternative hypothesis results in loss of power to detect such alternatives.

Williams' test (Williams, 1971, 1972) is specifically designed to detect an increasing concentration-response. It is more powerful than Dunnett's test for the type of data generated by aquatic toxicology experiments. The presence of very toxic levels in an experiment will not affect the ability to detect moderate levels of toxicity if this procedure is used.

The following procedure should be used to establish the LOEC and the NOEC. First, test whether the highest concentration is more toxic than the control by using Williams' procedure. If the hypothesis that this concentration is nontoxic is accepted, the highest concentration is the NOEC. However, if the hypothesis of no effect at this concentration is rejected, then test whether the next lower concentration is toxic. Proceed in this way until the first time the hypothesis of a nontoxic effect is accepted. This nontoxic concentration is the NOEC. The error rate of this sequential procedure is 5% even though the individual tests are not corrected for multiple comparisons (Marcus et al., 1976).

Tests of length and weight are invalid when there are survival differences. When length and weight of surviving fish are compared, the average length of the surviving fish is often used as a measure of toxic effect. However, this can be a biased measure because the toxin may selectively kill smaller fish and thus increase the average weight or length of the surviving fish in that group. Furthermore, the test that is often used assumes an equal number of experimental units in each experimental group. If there are survival differences, the numbers of surviving fish in individual tanks may differ widely. Weight and length differences should be tested only at concentrations that are at or below the NOEC for survival. In this way, mortality will not affect the average length and weight differently for different toxicant concentrations. Furthermore, there will be roughly the same number of fish in each tank, ensuring the validity of the test statistics. This procedure does not severely restrict the ability to make inferences about toxicity, because if a concentration affects fish survival, its effect on fish length and weight is of minor interest.

Testing procedures underestimate the maximum safe concentration. The NOEC should not be considered the maximum safe concentration of a toxicant. The power of a statistical test to detect a toxic effect is dependent on the number of fish in each tank and on the number of tanks. Thus serious environmental effects that were not detected by the experiment could occur at concentrations below the NOEC. A better method of determining a maximum safe concentration would be to construct a confidence interval on the LC10. That is, determine the concentration that one is 95% confident will produce 10% or less mortality. Parametric methods of performing this estimation are available but have not been applied to aquatic toxicology data. Nonparametric methods should also be developed for this application.

Other Considerations

When the mortality in a tank is less than 5%, the arc-sine square root transformation will not yield normally distributed data points, and the resulting P value may not be accurate. Other methods for testing for concentration effects should be developed that do not depend on this approximation.

All the methods that have been discussed assume that the survival of fish in each tank may be correlated. In this case the variability of test statistics must be estimated from the data. If each animal's survival depended only on the concentration and was independent of the tank, the variability of the test would be known exactly and much more powerful statistical tests could be used. The existence of this "tank effect" should be investigated to determine whether this more powerful analysis is appropriate (Schoenfeld and Gelber, 1980).

Example of a Chronic Toxicity Experiment

The following example illustrates current practices as well as new recommendations for the analysis of chronic test data. Table 2 presents the data from a chronic test with four active concentrations and two replicate tanks. The data include corresponding 28-d survival percentages, transformed survival

Table 2 Results of Hypothetical Chronic Toxicity Test (40 Organisms per Concentration)

A. Data set

Concentration (μg/l)	Percentage alive within replicates		Transformed percentage [arc sine $\sqrt{\hat{p}}$]		Replicate average $[(\hat{z}_{i_1} + \hat{z}_{i_2})/2]$
	$\hat{P}_{i_1}$	$\hat{P}_{i_2}$	$\hat{Z}_{i_1}$	$\hat{Z}_{i_2}$	$\hat{Z}_i$
100	32.5	22.5	.61	.49	0.55
50	85	90	1.17	1.25	1.21
25	90	97.5	1.25	1.41	1.33
12.5	95	87.5	1.35	1.21	1.28
Control	87.5	95	1.21	1.35	1.28

B. Standard approach

Step 1. *Analysis of variance test for concentration effects*

ANOVA 5% critical value = $F_{4,5}(0.95) = 5.19$

Sum of squares between concentrations   0.8556

Sum of squares within concentrations   0.0428

F-ratio $(0.8556/4)/(0.0428/5) = 24.99$

Reject hypothesis of no concentration effect since $24.99 > 5.19$

Step 2. *Dunnett's procedure for differences from control (Dunnett, 1955)*

Dunnett's 5% critical value = $D_{5,4}(0.95) = 3.66$

Estimated standard deviation of $\hat{Z}_{ij} = s =$ root mean sum of squares within concentration $= \sqrt{0.0428/5} = 0.0925$

A. $(\hat{Z}_{\text{control}} - \hat{Z}_{100\mu g/l})/\sqrt{2\,s^2/2} = 0.73/0.0925 = 7.89 > 3.66$

     Difference is statistically significant.

B. $(\hat{Z}_{\text{control}} - \hat{Z}_{50\mu g/l})/\sqrt{2\,s^2/2} = 0.07/0.0925 = 0.757 < 3.66$

     Difference is not statistically significant. Hence, LOEC = 100 μg/l, NOEC = 50 μg/l.

C. Recommended approach

Step 1. *Williams' test for differences from control (isotonic regression model)*

A. Pool adjacent violators to form a decreasing Z_i sequence.

	Control	12.5	25	50	100
Original $\hat{Z}_i$	1.28	1.28	1.33	1.21	0.55
Isotonized $\hat{Z}_i^*$	1.297	1.297	1.297	1.21	0.55

     Estimate standard deviation of $(s) = 0.0925$

B. Williams' 5% critical value (4 concentrations)

$t_{4,5}(0.95) = 2.21$

$(\hat{Z}_{\text{control}} - \hat{Z}_{100\mu g/l}^*)/\sqrt{2\,s^2/2} = 0.73/0.0925 = 7.89 > 2.21$

     Difference is statistically significant. Therefore, test further.

C. Williams' 5% critical value (3 concentrations)

$t_{3,5}(0.95) = 2.19$

$(\hat{Z}_{\text{control}} - \hat{Z}_{50\mu g/l}^*)/\sqrt{2\,s^2/2} = 0.07/0.0925$

$$= 0.757 < 2.19$$

     Difference is not statistically significant. Hence, LOEC = 100 μg/l, NOEC = 50 μg/l.

percentages for each tank, and tank averages of the transformed survival percentages.

The standard approach begins with a test for differences in survival among concentrations. The F-test (step 1) is significant ($P < 0.01$), suggesting that concentration is associated with 28-d survival. Dunnett's procedure is used to locate the concentrations for which survival is significantly different from the control (step 2). The NOEC is 50 $\mu g/l$ and the LOEC is 100 $\mu g/l$.

The recommended approach is to use Williams' test only to locate the NOEC and LOEC. The first step in this analysis is to obtain smoothed estimates for the survival percentages, using isotonic regression techniques (Barlow et al., 1972; Williams, 1971, 1972). Using Williams' test, the isotonized estimate for 100 $\mu g/l$ is compared to the estimate for the control. Since this comparison is statistically significant, Williams' test is repeated at 50 $\mu g/l$. This difference is not statistically significant. Consequently, the NOEC is 50 $\mu g/l$ and the LOEC is 100 $\mu g/l$. In this example, the results are the same as those obtained with the standard approach.

SUMMARY

In this chapter current practices for the analysis of data from acute and chronic tests have been presented and critically evaluated. For the acute test, most methods currently used yield comparable estimates for the LC50. The probit method is optimal when the tolerances to log concentrations of the toxicant are normally distributed. For the chronic test, the current practice of performing an F-test among all concentrations, followed by Dunnett's procedure, is statistically inefficient for a variety of reasons. It does not allow for data pooling or exploitation of the expected concentration-response relationship. It can lead to misleading situations where the global F-test is significant while Dunnett's procedures do not identify any significant control-concentration differences. Existing statistical procedures, namely

those for data pooling and isotonic regression, provide the toxicologist with improved procedures for MATC determination.

LITERATURE CITED

American Society for Testing and Materials: Standard practice for conducting chronic toxicity tests with early life stages of fish. ASTM E-47.01. Philadelphia: ASTM, 1981 (draft).

Barlow RE, Bartholomew DJ, Bremner JM, Brunk HD: Statistical Inference under Order Restrictions. London: Wiley, 1972.

Behrens B: Zur Auswertung der Digitalisblätter in Froschversuch. Arch Exp Pathol Pharmakol 140:237–256, 1929.

Bennett BM: Estimation of LD50 by moving averages. J Hyg 50:157–164, 1952.

Berkson J: Application of the logistic function to bioassay. J Am Stat Assoc 39:357–365, 1944.

Bliss CI: The method of probits. Science 79:38–39, 1934.

De Beer EJ: The calculation of biological assay results by graphic methods. The all or none type of response. J Pharmacol Exp Ther 85:1–13, 1945.

Dunnett CW: A multiple comparisons procedure for comparing several treatments with a control. J Am Stat Assoc 50:1096–1121, 1955.

Dunnett CW: New tables for multiple comparisons with a control. Biometrics 20:482–491, 1964.

Finney DJ: Statistical Methods in Biological Assay. 2nd ed. London: Griffin, 1964.

Finney DJ: Probit Analysis, 3rd ed. Cambridge: Cambridge Univ. Press, 1971.

Gaddum JH: Reports on biological standards. III. Methods of biological assay depending on a quantal response. Spec Rep Ser Med Res Coun London, no. 183, 1933.

Hamilton MA: Robust estimates of the ED50. J Am Stat Assoc 74:344–354, 1979.

Hamilton MA, Russo R, Thurston RV: Trimmed Spearman-Karber method for estimating median lethal concentrations in toxicity bioassays. Environ Sci Technol 11:714–718, 1977.

Kärber G: Beitrag zur kollektiven Behandlung Pharmakologischer Reihenversuche. Arch Exp Pathol Pharmakol 162:480–487, 1931.

Knudsen LF, Curtis J: The use of angular transformation in biological arrays. J Am Stat Assoc 42:282–296, 1947.

Litchfield JT, Wilcoxon F: A simplified method of evaluating dose/effect experiments. J Pharmacol Exp Ther 96:99–113, 1949.

Marcus R, Peritz E, Gabriel DR: On closed testing procedures with special reference to ordered analysis of variance. Biometrika 63:655–660, 1976.

Schoenfeld DA, Gelber RD: Lectures on the Analysis of Aquatic Toxicity Data Presented at E.G.&G. Wareham, Mass.: Bionomics Aquatic Toxicity Laboratory, 1980.

Snedecor GW, Cochran WG: Statistical Methods, 6th ed., pp. 327–329. Ames, Iowa: Iowa State University Press, 1967.

Steele RG, Torrie JH: Principles and Procedures of Statistics with Special Reference to Biological Sciences. New York: McGraw-Hill, 1960.

Stephan CE: Methods for calculating an LC50. In: Aquatic Toxicology and Hazard Evaluation, edited by FL Mayer, JL Hamelink, pp. 65–84. ASTM STP 634. Philadelphia: American Society for Testing and Materials, 1977.

Thompson WR: Use of moving averages and interpolation to estimate median effective dose. Bacteriol Rev 11:115–145, 1947.

U.S. Environmental Protection Agency: Test standard for conducting an early life stage toxicity test using the fathead minnow, sheepshead minnow, and brook trout or rainbow trout. Washington, D.C.: U.S. Environmental Protection Agency, Health and Environmental Review Division (TS-792), 1981 (draft).

Williams DA: A test for differences between treatment means when survival dose levels are compared with a zero dose control. Biometrics 27:103–117, 1971.

Williams DA: A comparison of several dose levels with a zero dose control. Biometrics 28:519–531, 1972.

Wilson EB, Worcester J: The determination of LC50 and its sampling error in bioassay. Proc Natl Acad Sci USA 28:79–85, 1943.

Chapter 6

Factors that Modify Toxicity

J. B. Sprague

INTRODUCTION

Various characteristics of water and of organisms that may change the toxicity of water pollutants are considered in this chapter. The preceding chapters on test methods placed considerable emphasis on standard procedures and control of test conditions, and the reader may occasionally have wondered whether it was necessary to be so careful about them. Here the reasons for the recommended procedures will become evident—they are largely an attempt to eliminate extraneous factors that may affect results of the toxicity test. For example, it will be seen below that poor control of pH during a test could have an enormous influence on the estimated toxicity of some pollutants. Thus, control of conditions in toxicity tests is simply an application of a basic scientific procedure: eliminating all the variables in an experiment except the one of interest. In this case, the series of concentrations of the toxicant is the variable of interest.

It may seem a little surprising that a chapter of this book emphasizes the variation in toxicity that is sometimes encountered. At times the reader may even be discouraged about the accuracy and value of toxicity testing, but this is not the intention. In some cases the modifying effects are surprisingly small, and the reader may then assimilate the interpretations and principles of other chapters. On the other hand, some major changes in toxicant potency are caused by modifying characteristics of the dilution water, and it is important to keep these in mind when considering the information in the rest of the book. Awareness of possible variations may help one to ignore some of the less important minor differences in toxicity data and instead look for broader and more useful generalizations.

A section on unanticipated variation has been placed near the beginning of the chapter. Some examples are reassuringly precise, and others show rather shocking scatter of data. Some of this unexplained variation must make us uncomfortable as scientists, but it must not be ignored. Awareness of the background variation explains why a twofold difference in toxicity may sometimes be described here as a modest one. Perhaps it should be repeated that the intention is not to cast doubt on aquatic toxicology as a field of science, but to focus in a realistic way on the more important major effects of modifying factors.

Both biotic and abiotic characteristics may act as modifying factors. The biotic ones include all the features that are within the organism. Primary features are the type of organism—alga, insect, or fish—and beyond that the particular species, since one species may respond to pollutants in a different way than others in the same general group. Other biotic features are stage of life (larva, juvenile, adult), size of individual, nutritional status and health, seasonal changes in physiological state, and degree of acclimation to natural environmental conditions or to a pollutant. The abiotic conditions that can act as modifying factors are the multitude of physicochemical characteristics of the water surrounding an organism. Obvious ones are water temperature, pH, dissolved oxygen content, salinity or hardness, and the extent of fluctuation of each of these in a particular body of water. Other abiotic conditions could include suspended materials, organic or inorganic; dissolved salts or nutrients and their relative proportions; dissolved CO_2 and other gases; intensity of light and photoperiod; water movements and their velocity; and binding or chelating action of substances in the water.

A complete review of the literature on modifying factors is not attempted; that would expand this chapter to a book. However, the major effects are covered and illustrated by specific examples.

Some items have been left out; an example is the sex of test organisms, since it usually has only a slight effect on reactions to pollutants. In any case, tests are often performed with sexually immature individuals, which are usually more sensitive than adults. The presence of another toxicant could obviously affect the action of a given pollutant, and this topic is covered in Chapter 7 by Marking. Information on how survival times are affected by modifying factors has been largely omitted. It often happens that there are differences in short-term survival, say in the first 24 h of an experiment, and yet the threshold of lethal effect is much the same if the experiment is continued long enough to determine that parameter.

TERMINOLOGY

Modifying factor. Any characteristic of the organism or the surrounding water that affects toxicity of a pollutant is considered to act as a modifying factor. Thus the size or species of the organism reacting to the toxicant could be a biotic modifying factor. Physicochemical entities such as pH or temperature of the water could be abiotic modifying factors. The environmental or abiotic entities should probably be called *masking factors,* following F. E. J. Fry's well-known classification of the environment according to the ways in which such entities act on an organism. By his definition, "A masking factor is an identity which modifies the operation of a second identity on the organism" (Fry, 1971). However, the term is not used here, because Fry's examples of the action of masking factors concern interactive effects within the organism, that is, physiological actions and the regulatory systems of the organism. In aquatic toxicology we are often still at the stage of observing a changed response without understanding the mechanism. Indeed, in many cases the modifying entity has a purely chemical effect on the toxic material, not within the organism but in the water. For example, pH can affect the chemical forms of metals, ammonia, and cyanide present in water. Use of the more general term, modifying factor, also allows inclusion of biotic characteristics that affect toxicity.

Resistance. Ability of an organism or species to resist a condition (e.g., a toxicant) which is at a level that will ultimately be lethal. Thus the description should ordinarily be accompanied by an indication of the time of exposure, and *median resistance times* (*median lethal times* or *median survival times*) are often used.

Tolerance. Ability of an organism to tolerate a condition for an indefinitely long exposure without dying. For toxicants, an organism is tolerant of concentrations at or below the incipient lethal level.

Isosmotic. Of equal osmotic pressure. Applicable when the dissolved materials in the body fluids of an organism exert an osmotic pressure equal to that of substances dissolved in the surrounding water. Thus there would be no tendency for the fish to gain or lose water.

Hyperosmotic. Having greater osmotic pressure than another fluid system. For example, a fish in fresh water would have body fluids with a greater concentration of dissolved materials than the concentration in the water, and the fish would tend to take in water. A *hypoosmotic* organism (most fish in the sea) would tend to lose water to the environment. In each case, the organisms would need regulatory systems to control the flux of water.

Euryhaline. Having a wide range of tolerance for salinity. For example, some estuarine organisms can exist in full-strength seawater or in low salinities approaching those of fresh water.

Stenohaline. Restricted to a narrow and constant range of salinity.

UNANTICIPATED VARIATION

When toxicity tests are repeated, results may not coincide exactly. A small part of such variation is due to truly random factors such as individual differences in resistance within any group of organisms. At present, however, large portions of the variation often cannot be explained; they could result from unrecognized changes in the organisms or in the test conditions.

The extremes of such variation may be illustrated by the experiences of three researchers in my laboratory. The least variation, comparing favorably with anything in the literature, was in the following series of 25 tests on copper lethality, carried out periodically during 2 yr as controls in an acclimation experiment with rainbow trout in very hard water (Dixon and Sprague, 1981b). The LC50s (μg/l) are listed in order of magnitude, not time of occurrence.

381	367	329	320	302
374	365	328	316	299
371	360	328	311	298
371	335	324	305	294
369	333	320	304	274

The geometric mean value was 330 μg/l and the highest and lowest values differed by only a factor of 1.39.

At the opposite extreme were two sets of results obtained about 3 yr earlier. These LC50s were obtained in adjacent parts of the laboratory with rainbow trout from the same stock, the same hard well-water mentioned above, measured concentrations of dissolved copper, and a flow-through apparatus but somewhat different flow rates. The LC50s were 94 μg/l (Fogels and Sprague, 1977) and 520 μg/l (Howarth and Sprague, 1978), different by a factor of 5.5 and different from the results given above. No explanation was evident to any of the researchers, and each result appears valid.

The situation is not unique to one laboratory. Brown (1968) reported that "the 48-hour LC50 values obtained for ammonia, phenol, and zinc in successive tests on a stock of rainbow trout over a period of 9 months varied by a factor of 2.5. The causes of this variation have not been identified." Adelman and Smith (1976) conducted eight sets of acute toxicity tests over 2 yr, using four different toxicants. They reported a coefficient of variation for NaCl of 6, a very low value which suggests that the ratio of the highest and lowest LC50s was about 1.3. Coefficients for the organophosphate insecticide Guthion were 29 and 39 for two species of fish, suggesting that the high and low LC50s differed by factors of about 5 or more.

Aquatic toxicologists may be uncomfortable about revealing such information, but it should not be hidden. Fogels and Sprague (1977) review the subject and conclude that between-laboratory differences in LC50 may approach a factor of 10.

An example of between-laboratory variability is a "ring test" or "round-robin" test, using the insecticide endosulfan against fish with a standard test procedure (EPA, 1979). LC50s in duplicate from four laboratories were as follows:

(Lab 1)	(Lab 2)	(Lab 3)	(Lab 4)
3.30	1.88	1.08	0.96
2.10	1.25	0.89	0.68

The geometric mean was 1.34, and the lowest and highest values differed by a factor of 4.9.

Some extremely variable examples were chosen above in order to make a point, but often results will be much closer. For example, there was only a twofold variation in an interlaboratory comparison of the lethality of sodium pentachlorophenate (Davis and Hoos, 1975). In a European ring test of 11 detergents, each laboratory used its particular standard method and species of fish, which varied from brown trout to the tropical harlequin fish. Eleven laboratories conducted either 2-d or 4-d tests. For the detergent showing the least interlaboratory variation, the factor between high and low LC50s was only 2.2—remarkably close considering the variety of approaches. For the most variable detergent the factor was 12, and the median of the factors was 6.8. The authors concluded that "a reliable order of magnitude for the acute toxicity to fish of the group of detergents tested can be obtained by a variety of test fish and by a variety of test procedures" (Reiff et al., 1979).

This section was begun with an example of good agreement among toxicity tests, and perhaps it would be well to end it with a similar example. Lloyd (1961b) published a guide for estimating the lethal level of ammonia, based on his research with rainbow trout and the chemical behavior of ammonia in water. In using the guide, an LC50 is read from a graph according to the pH and alkalinity of the water. Correction factors are applied for water temperature and for amounts of dissolved oxygen and carbon dioxide. The system may be used to predict LC50s for the water characteristics used in a recent study of ammonia toxicity to rainbow trout (Thurston et al., 1981). Over the usable ranges given by Lloyd the agreement with actual LC50s (total ammonia as milligrams of N per liter) is very good, as shown in Table 1. The greatest difference is a factor of 1.14, rather satisfactory since the two pieces of research span 20 yr and the Atlantic Ocean, and involve five chemical characteristics of the water which act as modifying factors.

TEST CONDITIONS

Here we consider more subtle things than test temperature or basic type of water. Obvious conditions such as having enough test solution per gram of fish fall in the category of good practice; these are fairly well established and are covered in other parts of this book.

An assortment of biotic and abiotic components of test procedure may affect results, although usually not in a major way. Seasonal

Table 1 Predicted and Measured LC50s
for Ammonia in Rainbow Trout

Oxygen in test (% saturation)	LC50 (total ammonia as mg N/l)	
	Predicted (Lloyd, 1961b)	Actual (Thurston et al., 1981)
81	42	45
62	34	38
41	25	24
30	21	24

variation is a possibility, and may have contributed to the 2.5-fold variation in response to ammonia, phenol, and zinc over 9 mo mentioned above (Brown, 1968). However, trout showed the same LC50s for pulp mill effluent whether acclimated to summer or winter photoperiod (McLeay and Gordon, 1978). In another test with zinc, a significant change in resistance time was associated with photoperiod acclimation and the time of day for starting a test of acute lethality, but the changes were not great, all values being in the range 160–230 min (McLeay and Munro, 1979). Both of the papers cited above review other work on these topics.

The activity of a fish in a test tank would not seem to bear much relation to its behavior in a natural habitat. However, one of the most obvious differences, the physical activity of fish, has less effect on resistance than might be thought. Trout forced to swim at 55% of their maximum sustainable velocity showed no increase in susceptibility to ammonia or zinc (Herbert and Shurben, 1963). Even at 85% of maximum cruising speed, lethal concentrations dropped only to 0.8 and 0.7 of the values for still water. The differences were a little less than might be expected from the increased irrigation of gills (see the section on dissolved oxygen, below).

The artificial nature of the exposure tank is usually ignored as a factor, but it may have small effects on estimates of tolerance, or at least on the variability of fish response. Sparks et al. (1972) are among the few people to assess this. They kept pairs of bluegills in bare aquaria and found that one fish became dominant over the other. When exposed to zinc, the dominant fish survived significantly longer (e.g., 20 compared to 9.5 h). Most interestingly, when the experiment was done with a flowerpot in the tank for shelter, there were no significant differences in survival time between dominant and submissive fish. Some unusual results related to aggression were obtained by Sprague et al. (1978). During a 2-yr project on sublethal effects, 90 screening tests were conducted to assess the lethality of batches of ef-

fluent. Most of the batches gave standard and satisfactory results, but during two periods there was extreme aggression between fish after they were removed from the holding tank and put into the test tanks. There were odd results for four batches of effluent in particular; the numbers of dead fish are shown in Table 2. It was obvious from looking into the tanks that fish were killing each other, and the results were interpreted as follows. In tests 38 and 39, 100% effluent was lethal to some or all fish, while in the control and low concentration, fish were being killed by aggression. In the middle concentrations fish were pacified by the effluent, which was apparently not lethal at concentrations of 50% or less. In tests 15 and 41 the effluent had little or no lethality, but high concentrations dampened the aggression. Test 41 must be some sort of classic for reversal of results in an acute toxicity test. These results demonstrate that biotic factors may sometimes be of importance in toxicology.

If invertebrate animals are being tested, some, such as *Daphnia,* may be quite at home in an ordinary container of water, but others have special habitat requirements that may be important for applying laboratory results to the real world. Pesch and Morgan (1978) demonstrated this for a marine polychaete worm. When the worms were provided with sand and made burrows, as in nature, the long-term LC50 for copper was four times the value for worms in bare tanks. Those in sand had lower body levels of copper, and it ap-

Table 2 Effects of Aggression between Fish on Mortality in Different Batches of Refinery Effluent

Batch and test number	Control	Fish mortality out of 10 (% effluent)			
		12	25	50	100
15	5	5	8	6	1
38	5	2	0	0	6
39	4	3	0	0	10
41	4	2	3	1	0

peared that they had reduced their exposure by circulating only small amounts of water through their burrows.

The keys to reducing such variation from miscellaneous causes would be to follow good laboratory practice and to standardize everything except the variable being studied, that is, concentration of toxicant. If it is suspected that an aspect of the test procedure, such as the habitat provided for an invertebrate, is important and of interest, then this aspect should also be singled out as a variable in a suitably designed experiment. It is therefore important that the investigator be familiar with the life history and general requirements of organisms used in testing. The alternative is to use the standard test species, whose requirements are well known.

BIOTIC CHARACTERISTICS AS MODIFYING FACTORS

This topic has received considerably less attention than the abiotic modifying conditions described below, but recent work shows that it should not be ignored. Such variation as is described here should be kept in mind when considering the overall significance of differences caused by all the abiotic modifying factors.

Test Species

There are real differences among different groups of organisms, and many authors have suggested that pollutants should be tested against an alga and one or more invertebrates, as well as fish, to obtain a more complete picture of toxicity. For example, crustaceans seem to be particularly susceptible to metals, pesticides, and many other pollutants. This is usually taken into consideration in modern criteria for natural waters.

A general idea of species variability is provided by the comparison of data in a literature review by Klapow and Lewis (1979). Some impressions are provided by Fig. 3, discussed in the salinity section below, but Klapow and Lewis made a more precise comparison by collecting results for various kinds of organisms and life stages tested under similar conditions. One kind of comparison involved tests by different investigators with the same species and toxicants. In 21 of 36 cases, the highest LC50 was within an order of magnitude of the lowest LC50, and the remainder were within two orders of magnitude. Differences were much greater in the second kind of comparison, between results for different kinds of organisms tested against a given toxicant in single studies. When the highest LC50 was divided by the lowest LC50 in the same study, there were 47 cases in which the spread was an order of magnitude or less (i.e., ratio of 10 or less), 16 cases with the spread ranging up to two orders of magnitude, and 11 cases with the spread mostly within three orders of magnitude. From the two comparisons it is evident that much greater variability is associated with the kind of test organism used than with test conditions and techniques. It should be kept in mind, however, that Klapow and Lewis placed no restrictions on the data used in their comparisons. For a given toxicant, they could have accepted results for fish, algae, sensitive microcrustacean larvae, or notoriously resistant invertebrates.

There are some differences even within one group, fishes. For example, the careful review of data by Spear and Pierce (1979) indicates that sunfishes (Centrarchidae) are about 15 times more tolerant of copper than are salmonids and minnows. Organophosphate insecticides also provide an extreme example of differences between species. Thirteen insecticides produced differences that ranged from 4- to 900-fold between bluegills and guppies, which were sensitive, and goldfish and fathead minnows, which were generally tolerant of the chemicals (Pickering et al., 1962). Results were also compared for different species with chlorinated hydrocarbons, cyanides, organic solvents, metals, detergents, and other chemicals, and the authors concluded, for their organophosphate results, that "In no other group of compounds that have been tested in our laboratories have the differences in species sensitivity been so great . . . the range . . . has generally been less than 10" (Pickering et al., 1962).

Organophosphates may be unusual in this respect; there often seems to be more concern than is warranted about possible differences between species of fish. For example, the small tropical flagfish and zebra fish averaged only 4.2 and 2.6 times the tolerance of rainbow trout for five representative toxicants, and it was concluded that this was not a major difference compared to within- and between-laboratory variation (Fogels and Sprague, 1977). Comparing trout with three species of "coarse" fish, Ball (1967) found that the lethal thresholds were almost identical for ammonia. When oil refinery waste was tested against 57 species of fish, there was only a fivefold difference between gizzard shad, the most sensitive species, and the guppy, which was the most resistant (Irwin, 1965). Similarly, the variation may not be large for closely related invertebrates. When 40 insecticides and herbicides were tested with two daphnids of different genera, 23 pairs of LC50s were not significantly different. The overall ratio of LC50s of the more resistant species to those of the more sensitive one was 1.8, a fairly modest difference (Sanders and Cope, 1966).

Life Stage and Size

For aquatic arthropods, the time of molting may be particularly susceptible and could appreciably affect results, even in acute toxicity tests. Lee and Buikema (1979) demonstrated this for *Daphnia pulex,* and recommended 48-h tests so that all or most of the animals will have molted during the exposure. They pointed out that there may be near-synchrony of molting in some populations, and 24-h tests might involve an all-or-none aspect of molting that would complicate comparisons.

For fish, the most sensitive life stages seem to be the embryo-larval and early juvenile stages, and advantage has been taken of this in designing chronic tests. McKim (1977) reviewed 56 life cycle tests and found that the estimated "no-effect" concentrations were virtually identical, in 80% of

the cases, for the short embryo-larval-juvenile phase and the lengthy life cycle test. In the rest of the cases the differences were factors of 2 or less.

Concerning size, larger fish might be expected to be more tolerant of a toxicant, and this is often the case. However, there is no overall relation that can be applied across species, toxicants, and size ranges. This is summed up succinctly by Anderson and Spear (1980): "The results of this study demonstrate that lethal tolerance to copper may or may not vary with fish size." They found that pumpkinseed sunfish weighing 1.2 g (wet) had an LC50 of 1.24 mg/l for copper, but resistance gradually increased with weight so that fish of 7.6 g had an LC50 of 1.94 mg/l. On the other hand, there was no change in the LC50 of rainbow trout over the size range 3.9–176 g. To add more confusion, Howarth and Sprague (1978) reported that copper resistance of rainbow trout gradually increased with size—in fact, by a factor of 2.5 in LC50 for 10-g fish over those weighing 0.7 g. It may be that there is a change with weight in the smaller trout which disappears when they reach the larger weight range studied by Anderson and Spear. Such a picture was recently presented for the insecticide Permethrin (Kumaraguru and Beamish, 1981). Tolerance of rainbow trout doubled between 1 and 5 g, increased regularly by a factor of 5 between 5 and 50 g, and then did not show any change between 50 and 200 g. The results seemed to fit a fairly standard explanation, inasmuch as the weight-specific metabolic rate of fish decreases in larger fish. It seems reasonable that the smaller fish, with higher metabolic rates, would take up more of the poison. In addition, hydrolytic breakdown of the poison by microsomal esterases in the liver would be more effective in the larger fish, because of the relatively larger ratio of enzyme to insecticide.

It is apparent that if size is a factor in toxicity studies, the effect must be determined empirically in each case. For tests of acute lethality, the standard relation used is

$$LC50 = aW^b$$

where W is the weight of the organism and a and b must be determined from the experiment. The value of b is the slope of the relation between LC50 and weight, more clearly seen if the equation above is put in the form log LC50 = log a + b log W. Although values of b are frequently around 0.7 (Anderson and Weber, 1975), b may have any value, such as 0.27 for the sunfish of Anderson and Spear, mentioned above, and 0.0 for their trout.

Nutrition, Health, and Parasitism

Most descriptions of standard methods for toxicity tests caution that only healthy stocks of fish must be used and that mortality during holding must be low. It would seem likely that any stress of disease would increase or enhance the stress from the toxicant and affect the results. However there is only slim evidence for this, and effects seem to be small.

Adelman and Smith (1976) compared "normal" goldfish with a stock that had been infested with skin flukes and probably with bacterial disease. The latter group had been heavily treated and had suffered 50% mortality during holding. The unhealthy fish were more sensitive to NaCl, with LC50s about 84% of the "normal" LC50 and outside the expected range of variation. They also seemed much more sensitive to Guthion (an organophosphate insecticide), but this could not be proved because of extreme variation in normal results. For chromium and pentachlorophenol, unhealthy fish showed LC50s within the range of normal values. It is possible, of course, that "weaker" diseased fish died during holding and that testing of "stronger" fish tended to balance the effects of disease. Small decreases in survival time have been reported for parasitized fish and snails exposed to zinc or cadmium, but effects on threshold tolerance, if any, were not included in the studies (Boyce and Yamada, 1977; Guth et al., 1977; Pascoe and Cram, 1977).

Nutrition of test animals has almost certainly received too little attention as a variable affecting toxicity results. In some cases the effect could be major. Wild populations of the marine copepod showed a sixfold variation in lethal levels of copper, being more resistant when food was more abundant (Sosnowski et al., 1979). That could have resulted, partly or wholly, from chelation by products of those food organisms, but copper resistance of trout is definitely affected by diet. As carbohydrate formed an increasing proportion of an equicaloric diet, trout became less tolerant of the metal. The LC50 increased by a factor of 1.7 in direct proportion to the percentage of protein in the liver (Dixon and Hilton, 1981). Apparently the high-carbohydrate diet brought about glycogen-filled livers, which were less effective in detoxifying copper. The finding is relevant inasmuch as wild carnivorous fish would receive a low-carbohydrate diet.

Susceptibility to pesticides seems particularly affected by diet. Increased protein in the food was associated with a six times greater tolerance of rainbow trout to lethal levels of chlordane. There was much more variability of response in the low-protein fish, and the type of protein also played a role (Mehrle et al., 1977). Diet (pellet versus worms) can also affect results of chronic tests, judged by growth of fish exposed to dieldrin (Phillips and Buhler, 1979). Fish exposed to toxaphene use vitamin C in its detoxification, resulting in deficiency symptoms in bones. Large increases of vitamin C in the diet can counteract this and raise the threshold for chronic effects of toxaphene by a factor of 2 to 4 (Mayer et al., 1978). However, a lack of vitamin C, or an excess, does not appear to change symptoms of lead toxicity, despite their similarity to the symptoms of vitamin C deficiency (Hodson et al., 1980).

Acclimation

It has long been known that aquatic animals can acclimate to temperature and to low oxygen. Fry (1947, 1971) provided comprehensive reviews showing that higher acclimation temperatures could raise the upper and lower lethal temperatures of fish by 3-10°C, and change other phenomena, such as temperature for maximum swim-

132

ming speed, by similar amounts. Fish also acclimate to low levels of dissolved oxygen. Shepard (1955) demonstrated that as the acclimation level in brook trout decreased from an oxygen saturation of 11 mg/l to 2.5 mg/l, the lethal level of oxygen also decreased from 1.8 to 1.0 mg/l. However, young salmonids apparently do not acclimate to low pH (Daye, 1980).

Many hints and incidental observations in the literature suggest that aquatic organisms may acclimate to some toxicants. Much of this information is based on changes in survival times, not threshold lethal concentrations, which would be more meaningful. It might be hypothesized that animals exposed to a sublethal level of a pollutant could become more tolerant or become weakened, depending on the mode of action of the poison and the type of detoxifying mechanism, if any, available to the animal. A recent series of papers show that both situations occur (Dixon and Sprague, 1981a,b,c). Trout were acclimated for 3 wk to constant sublethal levels of various pollutants, and their response to lethal levels of the same pollutant was used as a measure of acclimation. For acclimation to about 0.22 of the lethal level of arsenic, the threshold LC50 of arsenic in-

creased by a factor of 1.5, and acclimation to copper could double the tolerance for that metal. For acclimation at one-third of the lethal level of cyanide, fish became more sensitive by about one-third in the first week, then, with continued acclimation, their tolerance climbed back to the original level by the end of 3 wk.

A thorough study of the copper response showed that there was a greater increase in tolerance with higher preexposure concentrations up to about 0.6 of the lethal level, and also with time of preexposure over a 3-wk period (Fig. 1). When returned to clean water, trout lost their increased tolerance. Acclimation stimulated production of a liver protein, probably a metallothionein, the apparent defense mechanism. Acclimated fish were able to maintain their body burden of copper at a steady level, with no increase during subsequent exposures that should have been quickly lethal. Acclimation at 0.18 of the lethal level was about the threshold for triggering a strengthened defense mechanism, the ill effects of preexposure being just balanced by increased resistance to the subsequent lethal exposure. At a lower level of acclimation (0.09 of the lethal level), fish had an increased body burden of copper but apparently were not

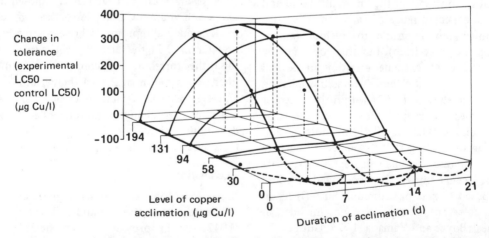

Figure 1 Change in incipient lethal levels of copper for rainbow trout following acclimation to different sublethal concentrations of copper for periods up to 3 wk. Points are observed LC50s; lines represent a fitted response surface. Average control LC50 was 330 μg/l; thus acclimation could double tolerance. Following acclimation to 30 μg/l (0.09 of the incipient lethal level), fish were more sensitive in the subsequent lethal exposures. *[From Dixon and Sprague (1981b).]*

"physiologically aware" of the copper and did not acclimate upward. They were, in fact, more sensitive than control fish to subsequent lethal exposure. The threshold of 0.18 of the LC50 for triggering the defense mechanism was apparently a meaningful one; above that there was reduced growth, and below it there was no effect on growth.

The effects of acclimation described above are not major, being twofold or less for these three toxicants, but they could be of some importance for aquatic organisms in waters that are mildly polluted over long periods. Also important could be genetic selection for increased tolerance. This appears to have occurred in polychaete worms from sediments that were high in metals (Bryan and Hummerstone, 1971, 1973) and in an isopod from rivers with a long history of pollution from metal-mining waste (Brown, 1976).

BACKGROUND ON ABIOTIC CHARACTERISTICS OF WATER

These are natural characteristics of water that may be influenced by human activity. Although this chapter emphasizes the ways in which they modify the potency of toxic substances, it must not be forgotten that each abiotic condition can be of fundamental importance by virtue of its direct action on aquatic organisms; for example, high temperature may act as a lethal factor. Because of this direct importance, the major physicochemical characteristics of water, and their actions on organisms, are briefly described below. There is a vast literature on effects of these natural characteristics, especially for fish. For more details, the reader may consult reviews of environmental factors by Fry (1971), of temperature, oxygen, pH, and suspended solids by Alabaster and Lloyd (1980), and of dissolved oxygen by Doudoroff and Shumway (1970) and Davis (1975).

For each of these natural characteristics, there will be a certain optimal level or zone for a given species; the organism functions most efficiently at that level. For example, there will be an optimum for temperature, and the "preferred temperature" of a fish will usually coincide. If the environmental condition changes to a less favorable level, the organism usually has physiological processes that allow it to partially compensate, but at some metabolic cost. The change within the organism may be semipermanent, in which case the animal has "acclimated" to the new condition. For example, fish held at an elevated temperature show an increase in upper lethal temperature and may, for a while, prefer a temperature above that normally selected. Near the outer limits of the biokinetic range, the metabolic loading on the organism becomes greater, and it will have less capacity to carry out normal activities such as feeding and reproduction. Such a situation is analogous to sublethal effects of a toxic substance. Eventually a limit is reached, beyond which the organism will die from the environmental condition, be it high temperature or pH or low dissolved oxygen.

The implications of the direct actions of many natural environmental entities for modifying pollutant toxicity are obvious. If an organism is already under stress or metabolic loading from such an environmental condition, then faced with the added complication of a toxic pollutant, it would probably be less capable of dealing with that pollutant, and indeed might show greatly increased susceptibility. The environmental entity would have acted as a factor modifying the toxicity of the pollutant.

Temperature

Temperatures in fresh surface waters of the temperate zone are usually within a range from the freezing point to 30°C; values to 35°C or even higher have been recorded—for example, in rivers near the Gulf of Mexico (Fry, 1960; Alabaster and Lloyd, 1980). Of course, there are streams in mountains or wooded regions where temperatures seldom exceed 20°C. Latitude governs not so much the maximum temperature attained as the length of time for which it prevails. The species present in a given aquatic community are largely determined by the temperature regime.

Most aquatic organisms are at the same temperature as the water, and there are upper and lower lethal temperatures beyond which they cannot survive. In various species of fish, these lethal levels may change by 3–10°C, depending on the temperature to which they are acclimated. Many fish seem to have an upper incipient lethal temperature that is at least 5°C higher than the maximum usually encountered in their habitat.

Within the lethal zone, temperature has profound effects on metabolic processes of poikilotherms, and indeed the metabolic rate may double for every 10° rise in temperature. There are optimal temperatures for such things as growth efficiency and performance of various activities. However, the favorable range can be modified to some extent; salmonids can give similar performance in spawning and growth over a 3 or 4° range if given a chance to acclimate, and goldfish can adapt over about 15° to show similar swimming speeds (Fry, 1971; NAS/NAE, 1974).

Water temperatures can be raised by discharge of cooling water, especially from power plants; diversion of watercourses for irrigation; and clearing of forest cover. Effects are greater in streams and rivers than in lakes or bays. To protect aquatic life against such changes, the all-pervading influence of temperature requires complex criteria. Modern ones (EPA, 1976) are individually designed for each species, and include at least: (1) a temperature that will not cause lethality in short exposures, (2) a maximum during the cold season that protects against lethality from sudden drops in temperature, (3) a weekly average in the warm season that protects against sublethal metabolic loading, and (4) specific requirements for successful reproduction.

Increased water temperature also increases the solubility of many substances, influences the chemical form of some, and governs the amount of oxygen that dissolves in water. Such changes can interact with the direct deleterious effects of elevated temperature.

Dissolved Oxygen Content

The dissolved oxygen content of fresh water is about 14.6 mg/l for saturation at 0°C and decreases gradually with temperature to 9.1 mg/l at 20°C and 7.5 mg/l at 30°C. In full-strength seawater the corresponding values range from 11.4 to 6.2 mg/l. Natural oxygen levels are often below saturation, particularly in the bottom layer of lakes. They may fluctuate because of algal activity, being below saturation at night and near saturation or even supersaturated during the day, when photosynthesis takes place.

One of the most studied effects of pollution is the lowering of dissolved oxygen caused by organic wastes; this occurs because oxygen is used in the decomposition process. From the literature of the first half of the century, one would almost gather that this was the only kind of pollution. Much fieldwork was done; systems of "indicator species" were developed to classify the degree of pollution, and these continue to be useful. There is a dramatic decrease and change of species in waters deoxygenated by heavy sewage pollution, the normal mixed assemblages of bottom-living invertebrates being replaced in extreme cases by vast numbers of red (hemoglobin-containing) midge larvae or red oligochaete worms.

Since oxygen is required for respiration, decreased levels can be effective as a limiting factor for aquatic organisms. Lethal levels are surprisingly low, most fish showing incipient values in the vicinity of 2 mg/l (Doudoroff and Shumway, 1970). However, these values are mostly from the laboratory, where fish are not required to pursue the activities that would be normal in a natural habitat. Such activities are hampered at much higher levels of oxygen. For example, the swimming speed of fish is directly related to the concentration of dissolved oxygen, and they can improve their performance above expected levels if the water is supersaturated (Fry, 1971). Modern water quality criteria recognize that any reduction of oxygen below natural levels will have some deleterious effect on organisms (Doudoroff and Shumway, 1970; Davis, 1975), and there is no single "magic number" that can be used as a criterion of acceptable levels. Rather, a series of levels of protection have been established for various degrees of impairment of the fauna, and a selection must be made of the desired level—that is, socioeconomic factors enter into the decision. For example, if the natural oxygen minimum of a stream was 9.1 mg/l in a particular season, the criterion of Doudoroff and Shumway (1970) for protection of important fisheries (an estimated 3% impairment) would be a minimum of 7.6 mg/l dissolved oxygen.

Hydrogen Ion Concentration

The hydrogen ion concentration is usually measured as pH, the logarithm of the reciprocal of hydrogen ion activity (the negative logarithm of $[H^+]$). Thus pH 7 represents 1×10^{-7} mole of H^+ per liter and, this being the point of neutrality, it is balanced by the same concentration of OH^- (hydroxyl ions). Most natural fresh waters are in the range of pH 5-9, soft waters often being pH 6-7 and hard waters 8-8.3. The oceans are relatively well buffered, usually in the pH range 8.0-8.2, although sometimes a little lower.

Related to pH is the buffering capacity of a water. *Acidity* is the ability of a water to resist a change in pH when a base is added. The acidity is largely caused by carbon dioxide, the salts of strong acids and weak bases, and other factors; above pH 8.3 there is considered to be no measurable acidity. *Alkalinity* in fresh water results chiefly from the carbonate-bicarbonate buffering system, and below pH 4.5 the alkalinity is zero. Fresh waters with high levels of calcium and magnesium (hard waters) have relatively high alkalinity, often in the vicinity of 60% of the total hardness when each is expressed as milligrams of $CaCO_3$ per liter.

Direct effects of pH on organisms are graded, becoming more severe as pH deviates either way from the neutral zone. Alabaster and Lloyd (1980; see also NAS/NAE, 1974) give a useful table summarizing these effects, with a middle range of pH 6.5-9.0 being considered "harmless to fish." A few fish such as perch and pike can acclimate to the acid pH range of 4.0-4.5, but most could not reproduce and only a few kinds of invertebrates would live in such waters. On the alkaline side, at pH 9.0-9.5 most invertebrates are not affected, but this range approaches the tolerance of many fish; pH 9.5-10.0 may be lethal to salmonids over a prolonged period.

Historically, major effects on pH due to human activity have come from acid runoff in coal and metal mining areas. This is chiefly caused by exposure of sulfide-containing minerals. In the past two decades, however, acid rain has dwarfed other types of pollution as a factor in pH. There has been catastrophic acidification of soft-water lakes and rivers by fallout of combustion products, chiefly oxides of sulfur and nitrogen. This has resulted in hundreds of fishless lakes in Scandinavia, Canada, and the northeast United States.

Some modern water quality criteria recognize the graded nature of pH effects. NAS/NAE proposed levels of protection with increasingly wider limits and a wider allowance of fluctuation. The highest level of protection for freshwater organisms specified pH in the range 6.5-8.5, with no change greater than 0.5 unit beyond the estimated natural limits.

Dissolved Salts

Calcium and, to a lesser extent, magnesium are the predominant dissolved cations in fresh water and are chiefly responsible for water hardness. A commonly used classification is: soft water, 0-75 mg/l expressed as $CaCO_3$; moderately hard, 75-150; hard, 150-300; and very hard, 300 mg/l and above (EPA, 1976). The mean hardness of the rivers of the world is about 50 mg/l, the median hardness of major U.S. municipal supplies about 90 mg/l, but all levels may be found in nature. Streams may consistently run at 20 mg/l or less in some forested, mountainous, or igneous areas. Generally, biological productivity is low in such waters, probably because of a concomitant lack of nutrient minerals for primary production. There is also some evidence that fish are under appreciable osmotic stress in such "pure" water. Ground water from wells in limestone areas often seems to emerge at 350–380 mg/l total hardness, about the maximum that is usually encountered, and a level that causes severe encrustation in water pipes of houses. Hard-water streams and lakes are productive ones; certainly these natural dissolved salts are not harmful to organisms.

Along with the cations go higher levels of carbonates, bicarbonates, and some sulfates. Their important role in complexing toxic metals is described in a later section.

Inert Suspended Solids

Here are included suspended particles such as silt which do not have a toxic action, but do have other effects on aquatic systems. Streams in forested areas have low levels of suspended solids, usually in the range 0–20 or 0–50 mg/l at all times. Some waters are naturally high in solids; the Mississippi is famous for this and may approach 300 mg/l in Louisiana, although present levels are partly due to human activity. However, even the Mackenzie River, which flows through pristine areas of subarctic Canada, may run at 200 mg/l of nonfilterable residue (suspended solids), reducing underwater vision to a meter or less. Anthropogenic causes of high levels in surface waters are erosion and direct discharge of wastes such as pulp mill effluent and tailings from mining and milling.

These particulate solids are commonly measured in milligrams per liter by drying those that are retained on a filter. However, they may also be assessed by their light-scattering effect in water (turbidity) or as the percent transmission of light at depth. There is no general way of converting from one measurement to another, since this will depend on the specific gravity of particles and their size, shape, and angularity.

Lack of light penetration into turbid lakes will reduce primary production and hence the produc-tion of the whole system. Solids that settle to the bottom can blanket the interstices and reduce numbers of benthic algae and invertebrates, and can drastically reduce survival of buried fish eggs by impeding flow through bottom gravel. Alabaster and Lloyd (1980) give the general conclusions of European experts concerning damaging levels of solids for aquatic life, and these have been widely adopted as water quality criteria. Again, there is a graded response. Less than 25 mg/l finely divided suspended solids seems to have no harmful effect on fisheries. From 25 to 80 mg/l may reduce fish production, waters of 80–400 mg/l are unlikely to support good fisheries, and poor fisheries are likely at levels above 400 mg/l. Extremely high levels of suspended solids can be acutely lethal to fish, presumably by clogging or abrading the gills. No single level can be specified as lethal, since it depends on the type of particle, but most reported values are in the tens or hundreds of thousands of milligrams per liter.

Some suspended materials, especially organic ones, can have a major detoxifying action on certain pollutants by sorbing or chelating them.

ABIOTIC CONDITIONS AS MODIFYING FACTORS

Water Temperature

There is no single pattern for effects of temperature on toxicity of pollutants to aquatic organisms. Temperature change in a given direction may increase, decrease, or cause no change in toxicity, depending on the toxicant, the species, and in many cases the experimenter who has selected a particular procedure and response. Limited evidence suggests that temperature may not have much effect on the chronic "no-effect" thresholds of pollutants, which are ultimately of most importance to aquatic organisms.

One statement that can be made is that the short resistance times caused by a severely lethal level of toxicant are changed by temperature roughly in accordance with van't Hoff's equation;

that is, survival time decreases by a factor of 2 or 3 for each rise of 10°C (Lloyd and Herbert, 1962; Hodson and Sprague, 1975; MacLeod and Pessah, 1973). This is interesting, since most physiological processes of poikilotherms show similar increases in rate with rising temperature, but it is not emphasized here because of the greater interest in *tolerance,* that is, the threshold LC50. Of even more importance is the effect on chronic sublethal toxicity, and it is unfortunate that there has been relatively little research on that topic.

Temperature effects on zinc toxicity are described first as an example of diversity in response; then some other examples are considered. It might be expected that zinc would be more lethal to a poikilothermic animal at high temperature, but this is far from true as a generalization. A good example is Atlantic salmon acclimated and tested at one of three temperatures: 3, 11, or 19°C (Hodson and Sprague, 1975). The lethal concentrations for 24-h exposures indicate that fish died more slowly of zinc poisoning in cold water. That is, they were more resistant, and the lethal concentration was higher by a factor of about 4 in cold water than in warm water, as shown in Table 3. At 96 h there was some evidence of a similar effect, but the overall picture was not clear. However, at 2 wk the threshold LC50 was higher in warm water; that is, salmon were more tolerant in warm water than in cold, the opposite of the usual expectation.

To explain this, it might be hypothesized that the "warm" fish, with their higher metabolic activity, were able to detoxify zinc more rapidly, perhaps by moving it out of the gills, the primary site of acutely lethal damage (Skidmore and Tovell, 1972; Burton et al., 1972). Hodson (1975) found the opposite when he pursued the mechanism of the temperature effect. Salmonids that died of zinc at 19°C had about 2.5 times *more* zinc in their gill tissue than those killed at 3 and 11°C.

This surprising result was not related to temperature-induced changes in lactate-glycogen metabolism (Hodson, 1976), which might have remedied tissue hypoxia, the secondary lethal effect of gill destruction (Skidmore, 1970). In fact, the warm-temperature salmonid gill tissue could accommodate more zinc before the cells broke down in the usual syndrome of zinc poisoning. The best-fit lines in Fig. 2 show that, in colder water, a given concentration of zinc caused more histological damage to the gills (Hodson, 1974). The damage was measured by four criteria: distance of delamination of epithelium from its basement membrane and from the gill filament, angle of bending of lamellae, and amount of cellular debris.

This example shows that temperature can indeed affect the actions of toxicants. It also shows that one should not prejudge the direction of temperature effects. An even stronger example of this unpredictability was shown in the same series of experiments with zinc and salmon (Hodson and Sprague, 1975). Fish tested at a temperature lower than their acclimation temperature (i.e., a cold stress) became less tolerant of zinc than they would have been at their acclimation temperature. The opposite might have been expected if one considered the slowing of metabolic rate when fish are moved to a lower temperature, with slower gill irrigation and a probable decrease in zinc uptake.

Results of other work add to the complexity. Rainbow trout have been reported to show no change in zinc tolerance between 13.5 and 21.5°C (Lloyd and Herbert, 1962) and also an increase of about 65% in tolerance at 3 compared to 20°C (Brown, 1968). Thus in the same genus we may quote all three possible results for the effect of temperature on zinc lethality.

Table 3 Effect of Temperature on Zinc Toxicity

Exposure	LC50 of zinc (mg/l) at different temperatures		
	3°C	11°C	19°C
24 h	20	8.4	5.4
96 h	7.2	3.6	5.4
2 wk (threshold)	3.5	3.6	5.4

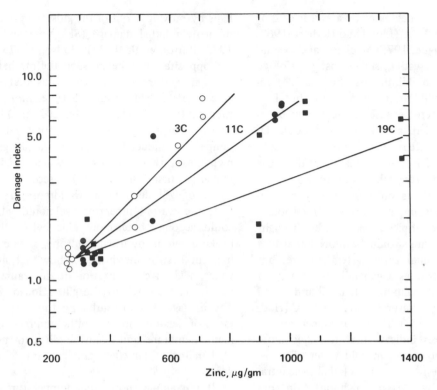

Figure 2 Amount of damage to gill tissue of salmonid fish related to amounts of zinc in that tissue. Fish were sampled at various stages of zinc intoxication, following acclimation and testing at 3, 11, or 19°C. Histological damage was assessed by a combination of four criteria from photographs of gill preparations, with a higher index for greater damage. *[From Hodson (1974).]*

Among other species, fathead minnows were three times more tolerant of zinc at 15 than at 25°C, yet bluegills showed no difference in threshold LC50 (Pickering and Henderson, 1966b). Several Hudson River fishes displayed no difference in tolerance to zinc at 15 and 28°C (Rehwoldt et al., 1972). (Nor were there differences for four other metals. Only for mercury was there decreased tolerance at the high temperature.) Various other reviewers also concluded that temperature has diverse effects on zinc toxicity to aquatic organisms (Alabaster and Lloyd, 1980; Cairns et al., 1975; Eedy, 1974).

Similar diverse effects on lethality are found for other pollutants. Some show a negligible temperature effect or become more toxic in cold water. Temperature has a profound but purely chemical influence on the proportion of ammonia present in the toxic unionized state, as discussed in the section on pH. However, when allowance is made for that chemical change, the threshold lethality of unionized ammonia per se does not change above 10°C, while at lower temperatures toxicity may increase by a factor of 2 or more (EIFAC, 1973b). Phenol is twice as lethal to trout at 6 as at 18°C (Brown et al., 1967). Similarly, naphthenic acids are twice as toxic to snails at 20 than at 30°C in soft water. Oddly enough, no difference with temperature has been reported for snails in hard water, and no differences for bluegills in either kind of water (Cairns and Scheier, 1962). Linear alkyl sulfonate (LAS), a component of detergents, is not appreciably different in lethality to bluegills at 15 and 25°C (Hokanson and Smith, 1971).

In contrast, some pollutants become more toxic at higher temperatures. An increase of about 40% was noted for cyanide between 18 and 30°C (Cairns and Sheier, 1963). Whole effluent from a pulp mill became more toxic over the range 8–19°C (Loch and MacLeod, 1974), but inspection of the data suggests a modest change in threshold LC50, perhaps only by a factor of 2. One of the largest temperature effects is for hydrogen sulfide. Adelman and Smith (1972) found that goldfish tested at 25°C were an order of magnitude less tolerant than those at 6.5°C (530 μg/l compared to 44 μg/l, the logarithm of LC50 showing a linear relation to temperature). These results were for 4-d exposures; 11-d LC50s were closer in warm and cool waters, but still different. The findings were based on toxic undissociated H_2S only, and so variation in proportions of ionic species was not a factor (see later section).

As a lethal agent, pH can be affected in either direction by temperature. Fingerling trout were more resistant to acid in cold water (LC50 at 10°C = pH 4.1, LC50 at 20°C = pH 4.3, representing a 60% increase in actual concentration of hydrogen ions resisted at the cooler temperature). However, trout eggs were less resistant to acid in cold water (LC50 at 5°C = pH 5.5, LC50 at 10°C = pH 4.8, a fivefold decrease in concentration resisted in colder water) (Kwain, 1975).

There have been many toxicity tests with pesticides at different temperatures, and in this group there is also a diversity of modifying effects. Many are more toxic in warm water, including endrin to five species of fish (Johnson, 1968), 14 of 15 pesticides tested against bluegills and rainbow trout (Macek et al., 1969), two herbicides (Woodward, 1976), and pentachlorophenol (Asano et al., 1969). Other pesticides showed stronger lethal action at low temperatures. This was true of several of the 22 chemicals tested against cladocerans by Sanders and Cope (1966); in particular, DDT was three times as toxic at 10 as at 27°C. A very large change occurred with Permethrin, a synthetic pyrethroid, which was an order of magnitude more toxic to rainbow trout at low tempera-

tures. The LC50 dropped from 6.4 μg/l at 20°C to 3.2 μg/l at 15°C, and 0.7 and 0.6 μg/l at 10 and 5°C (Kumaraguru and Beamish, 1981). Still other pesticides are little affected by temperature, including Zectran at 7 and 17°C (Mauck et al., 1977) and rotenone at 7 and 22°C (Marking and Bills, 1976). Two studies on toxaphene show the same picture—that is, differences in survival times but no effect on eventual lethal concentrations in long exposures (Johnson, 1961; Koeppe, 1961).

The preceding review shows that modifying effects of temperature on acute lethality are diverse, but for the most part they are only small or moderate. Whether temperature plays a major role in sublethal or chronic toxicity is a more important question for the well-being of organisms in their environment. On this topic there has been much less relevant research. One perceptive study of the toxicity of chromate and arsenate to a rotifer is particularly interesting. In the first part of their research, Schaefer and Pipes (1973) showed what was generalized above—that in short lethal exposures there was more apparent toxicity at high temperatures, but in long exposures the difference decreased to a factor of only about 2, between 5 and 30°C. The work then proceeded to a masterful study of life spans, which were, of course, much longer at cold temperatures in clean water (Table 4). Tests were then run to determine the median effective concentrations (EC50s) of added toxicants that allowed the same life spans as in clean water. One might attempt to see trends in their results, but in fact the variation in EC50 at any temperature is well within the confidence limits of EC50s at other temperatures (Table 4). The authors stated that at higher temperatures the EC50 for life span "may either increase or decrease; that is, no general pattern is evident . . . . The conclusion . . . is that temperature has no effect on the life span [EC50]."

This finding is an important one. If further studies resulted in similar findings, it would mean that we could use the same water quality criteria from the tropics to the Arctic. There would be no need for expensive repeated testing in warm, tem-

Table 4 Lack of Influence of Temperature on Effective Concentrations of Chromate and Arsenate that Resulted in No Change in Life Span, Compared to Controls, in the Rotifer *Philodina roseola*[a]

Temperature (°C)	Median life span, control conditions (d)	Concentration (and confidence limits) resulting in same median life span (mg/l)	
		Chromate	Arsenate
15	28	3.5 (2.2–5.6)	6.0 (3.8–9.5)
20	10	4.6 (2.8–7.7)	9.0 (5.0–16)
25	5.9	4.5 (3.1–6.4)	10 (7.8–13)
30	3.7	3.8 (2.5–5.9)	13 (7.1–23)
35	3.0	3.7 (2.7–5.0)	11 (7.2–18)

[a]Data reproduced with permission from Schaefer and Pipes (1973); copyright 1973, Pergamon Press, Ltd.

perate, and cold conditions. An important consideration is that the results are for one species of rotifer over a range of temperatures that includes the extremes of its spectrum (the species did not reproduce at 5°C). If there was no major effect of temperature in this case, there seems little reason to expect great differences in no-effect levels of pollutants between an arctic organism tested in cold water, to which it is adapted, and a similar tropical species tested in its native warm water.

In some studies temperature was a modifying factor in avoidance reactions of fish. Goldfish avoided low levels of copper in a particular experimental configuration with steep gradients (Kleerekoper et al., 1973). However, if the copper-containing water mass was warmer, fish were attracted to it more than to warm water alone. The situation is not simplified if we look at another side of it; fathead minnows selected a lower temperature if preexposed to a sublethal level of copper (Opuszyński, 1971). Like most avoidance work, this is difficult to extrapolate into field conditions. A simpler finding is lack of change in levels of hypochlorous acid avoided by fish at 6 and 30°C (Cherry et al., 1977).

A within-organism study showed a temperature difference in apparent physiological defense mechanism. *Fundulus* exposed to an aromatic hydrocarbon in cold water (6.5°C) showed no induction of cytochrome P-450 (Stegeman, 1979). Induction was found, however, after exposure at 16.5°C. The study did not actually show whether lack of this metabolic pathway would result in deleterious effects on the whole organism. Finally, there is an indirect but important effect of temperature on the activity of DDT within organisms, an effect that may exist for other toxicants which are stored in body fat. Salmonids accumulate more of the pesticide at a warm temperature (Reinert et al., 1974), but following such accumulation there can be near-complete mortality when the fish are subjected to a dropping temperature and their food intake decreases. The latter aspect has been demonstrated in a laboratory experiment (Macek, 1968) and also in wild fish from a sprayed stream (Elson and Kerswill, 1966). Presumably DDT is released from storage and becomes acutely toxic when body fats are mobilized by the fish at times of low food intake. Such delayed mortality could be of major significance in temperate climates, although it would not occur with pollutants that were not stored in body fat.

Dissolved Oxygen

It might be expected that stresses on aquatic organisms caused by a reduction in ambient dissolved oxygen would greatly increase the toxicity of a pollutant in the water. Effects of this kind exist, but often they are not major ones. Most findings show a change in toxicity by only a factor of 2 or less for tests conducted at low and high levels of dissolved oxygen.

The most general examination of the question goes back two decades to Lloyd (1961a). He showed very similar increases in lethality of copper, lead, zinc, and phenols in relation to degree of deoxygenation, and fitted a curve with values approximating those in Table 5. The values labeled "toxicity" were essentially ratios of near-threshold lethal concentrations, that is, the LC50 at full oxygen saturation divided by the LC50 at specified partial saturation. Lloyd advanced a convincing explanation of the increase in lethality, relating it to increased irrigation of the gills at reduced oxygen levels. The increased water flow was thought to bring about speedier laminar flow, causing higher concentrations of pollutants in the immediate vicinity of gill membranes and thus a higher rate of diffusion of toxicants into the gills. The explanation was supported by calculations based on known values for gill irrigation and gradients with such laminar flow. Lloyd concluded that the explanation

... implies that any environmental or physiological change which affects the rate of respiratory flow of a fish will also affect the concentration of poison at the surface of the gill epithelium, and that a known relation exists between these two factors. It also implies that

Table 5   Effect of Dissolved Oxygen on Toxicity

Oxygen (% saturation)	Toxicity
100	1.0
80	1.06
60	1.18
50	1.28
40	1.4
30	1.56

Table 6   Toxicity of Pulp Mill Effluent at Reduced Oxygen Levels

Oxygen (% saturation)	Toxicity
55	1.23
47	1.34
38	1.53

the relation between the increase in toxicity of poisons to fish and a reduced dissolved oxygen concentration of the water will be the same for all poisons except those whose toxicities are affected by the pH value of the water.

If toxicity of a substance depends on pH, it may change to a greater extent at reduced levels of oxygen. Ammonia behaved in this way, with up to 2.5-fold increases in toxicity (Lloyd 1961a). Briefly, the explanation was that lower dissolved oxygen meant greater irrigation and lower respiratory CO_2 near the gills, causing higher pH locally, an increase in the concentration of unionized ammonia, and greater toxicity (also see the section on pH). Recent work on ammonia toxicity is not in conflict with the hypothesis. Thurston et al. (1981) found that the toxicity of ammonia to rainbow trout increased by a factor of 1.9 when dissolved oxygen dropped from 80 to 30% saturation. This is close to the factor of 2.0 predicted by Lloyd (1961a), and greater than the factor of about 1.5 for other toxicants, as calculated in Table 5 for these oxygen saturations.

There has not been a great deal of additional research on the topic. Hicks and DeWitt (1971) measured 24-h LC50s of whole pulp mill effluent at reduced oxygen levels. The highest oxygen value was 79% saturation, and compared to this, toxicity factors at various oxygen levels were those shown in Table 6. These values do not appear to be greatly different in magnitude from those of Lloyd.

The 20-d LC50s of zinc to bluegills were similarly reduced by low oxygen (Pickering, 1968).

Average lethal concentrations of zinc at the various oxygen saturations are shown in Table 7. The LC50 at the lowest oxygen level was lower than the other two (statistically significant), and toxicity was increased by a factor of 1.5 over that at 67% saturation. Unfortunately, no test was done at full saturation, but the modifying effect of oxygen is similar to those described above.

The surfactant LAS appeared to be an order of magnitude more lethal to bluegills at low oxygen (22% saturation) than at near-saturation (Hokanson and Smith, 1971). However, the difference decreased to a factor of 1.7 if the fish were first given some acclimation to low oxygen and LAS. Further, tolerance to LAS by the most sensitive life stage (feeding sac fry) did not vary between 40% and full oxygen saturation. Hokanson and Smith concluded that the "acclimated" findings would be more relevant to field conditions, and that the lack of modifying effect on the most sensitive life stage was more important for establishing water quality criteria than were the variations found in other parts of the work.

Adelman and Smith (1972) found H_2S to be about 1.4 times as toxic to goldfish at 10% oxygen saturation as at 63% saturation. Cairns and Scheier (1958) cycled oxygen levels, with daily 8-h periods during which oxygen dropped to either 53 or 21% saturation. For the remainder of each day, the dissolved oxygen was at 95% saturation. For the more extreme depletion, toxicity was increased by factors of 4.5 for KCN, 2.8 for naphthenic acid, 1.6 for zinc, and 1.0 for potassium permanganate. The variation among toxicants is considerable and

cannot be related precisely to the results of experiments with constant levels of dissolved oxygen.

Some lethality results show no modifying effect of dissolved oxygen. No difference in 4-d LC50s of cadmium for a marine fish were found between 4 mg/l oxygen and saturation (Voyer, 1975). Oseid and Smith (1974) noted differences in survival times of invertebrates exposed to H_2S at various levels of oxygen, but the final LC50s of H_2S were not greatly different for 35 and 60% oxygen saturation.

Unfortunately, there appears to have been very little research on *sublethal* effects of toxicants, as influenced by reduced oxygen. Pickering (1968) assessed the growth of bluegills in a well-designed experiment, with three levels of zinc at each of three levels of dissolved oxygen (21, 38, and 67% saturation). Growth was reduced in the lower levels of oxygen, but zinc did not have a statistically significant effect on growth, nor was there a significant interactive effect of oxygen and zinc on growth (confirmed by reanalysis of Pickering's data). Even at the lowest oxygen level, and a very high measured concentration of 4.7 mg/l zinc (equivalent to 0.64 of the 20-d LC50), the reduced growth was statistically ascribable to low oxygen, not to zinc or the interaction of the two. This is an interesting experiment inasmuch as it is the same one mentioned four paragraphs above, in which 21% saturation of oxygen made the fish less tolerant to lethal levels of zinc, yet the same level of oxygen did not modify sublethal toxicity. Although such a modifying effect could have been hidden by random variability in the experimental design, it is clear that low oxygen was less important than might be expected as a modifier of sublethal toxicity. Similarly, eggs and fry of walleye and suckers showed little difference in deformities and mortality caused by H_2S at 28 and 56% oxygen saturation (Smith and Oseid, 1972). It might have been predicted that the sensitivity of these stages to low oxygen would result in major effects when a toxic compound was also present.

A major modifying effect of oxygen has, however, been documented for the respiratory be-

Table 7 LC50s of Zinc to Bluegills at Reduced Oxygen Levels

Oxygen (% saturation)	LC50 (mg/l)
67	11.3
38	10.6
21	7.3

havior of young Pacific salmon exposed to pulp mill effluent in about half-strength seawater. Alderdice and Brett (1957) estimated that at 72% oxygen saturation, respiratory distress (gasping at the surface) was caused in the salmon by 18% effluent. When oxygen was lowered, less effluent was required to cause the effect, so that at 36% oxygen saturation the critical level was only 2% pulp mill effluent. The change is almost an order of magnitude, a sharp contrast between this behavioral response and the other sublethal effects documented above which were not modified by oxygen level.

It is evident that there is not yet a comprehensive picture of the influence of reduced oxygen on chronic or sublethal actions of toxicants. However, the effects may be as small as, or even smaller than, the modest effects on acute lethality.

Hydrogen Ion Concentration

Major modifying effects of pH might be expected for toxicants that ionize under the influence of pH, and this is the case for some. Undissociated molecules may be more toxic since they penetrate cell membranes more easily.

A classic example is ammonia. Its toxic activity is now fairly well understood and can be predicted from characteristics of the water, as reviewed in Alabaster and Lloyd (1980), EIFAC (1973b), and NAS/NAE (1974). Ionized ammonia (NH_4^+) has little or no toxicity, but the unionized form (NH_3) is quite toxic, the LC50 for salmonids being in the range 0.2–0.7 mg/l as N. A rise of one pH unit, within the usual middle range of surface waters, increases the proportion of NH_3 about sixfold, with a concomitant increase in toxicity. Factors other than pH also affect the toxicity of ammonia. A second modifying factor is temperature, which also affects ionization. Lloyd (1961b) showed a 2.5-fold increase in toxicity for an increase in temperature from 7 to 20°C, and that factor has been confirmed by the dissociation constants of Emerson et al. (1975). For a temperature change from 0 to 30°C, the dissociation constants indicate an approximately ninefold increase in the proportion of NH_3 at a representative pH of 8.0. In most

waters alkalinity per se would not be a major factor in ammonia toxicity, but in unusual waters the interrelation of pH, alkalinity, and CO_2 could have an influence. Lowered alkalinity would be associated with higher CO_2 and lower pH, hence a lower proportion of NH_3 and reduced toxicity. In waters with an extremely low CO_2 content, respiratory CO_2 could reduce pH in the immediate vicinity of the fish's gill and thus diminish the apparent toxicity of ammonia [see the oxygen section above (Lloyd 1961a) or the review by Alabaster and Lloyd (1980)]. Thus the toxicity of ammonia is complex, but is primarily governed by pH-caused ionization and is thus predictable. Since only total ammonia can be measured in the water, the amount of NH_3 must be calculated from known dissociation constants (Emerson et al., 1975; NAS/NAE, 1974) or interpolated from graphs (Lloyd, 1961b). Sublethal effects of ammonia seem to follow the same pattern of toxicity, related to unionized ammonia.

Cyanide is another toxicant affected by pH. Molecular hydrogen cyanide (HCN) predominates in acid and middle pH values, but above pH 8.5 an appreciable proportion of CN^- is present. Apparent toxicity drops somewhat if calculated on the basis of total free cyanide, since the undissociated molecule (HCN) seems to be about twice as toxic as the ion (Broderius et al., 1977). Even more striking examples are provided by changes in toxicity of various complex metal cyanides. For instance, a change from pH 7.8 to 7.5 causes an apparent tenfold increase in toxicity of nickelocyanide. This has been convincingly explained by Doudoroff et al. (1966). The toxicity is related to the free cyanide, not to the metal complex, and dissociation is governed primarily by pH. The situation is similar for hydrogen sulfide, whose toxicity is chiefly due to H_2S, not dissociated ions. The effect of pH can be major, since undissociated H_2S forms only 4% of the total at pH 8.4 but more than 90% at pH 6 (NAS/NAE, 1974). The observed LC50 of total dissolved sulfide (i.e., $H_2S + SH^- + S^{2-}$) changed from 64 μg/l at pH 6.5 to 800 μg/l at pH 8.7, apparently because HCN is about 15 times as toxic as the ionized forms (Broderius et al., 1977).

Sulfite becomes more toxic at low pH because the predominant form is HSO_3^-, which is about an order of magnitude more toxic than the SO_3^{2-} ion (Sano, 1976). Nitrite can be 20 times as toxic at high pH, as HNO_2 becomes less predominant over NO_2^-, but both are toxic and whether one is more so is not evident (Russo et al., 1981).

In most of the cases above, the undissociated molecule, or the "less dissociated" ion, had greater toxicity. The situation is usually the opposite for metals; that is, the free or ionic form is thought to have relatively high toxicity (see separate section below).

For some biocides toxicity changes with pH and for some it does not. The lethality of a di-nitrophenol herbicide was about five times as great to fish at pH 6.9 as at pH 8 (Lipschuetz and Cooper, 1961). Holcombe et al. (1980) found that 2,4-dichlorophenol had somewhat less lethality at high pH and also caused much less disturbance of schooling behavior of fathead minnows. This was explained in terms of lower proportions of the un-dissociated form at higher pH. The same general result and explanation apply to the piscicide anti-mycin, for which there is much less toxicity above pH 8.5 (Marking, 1975). In fact, the toxicity results indicated that the previously estimated disso-ciation constant was erroneous. Similarly, the insecticide Zectran was 6–20 times as lethal to various fish at pH 9 as at near-neutrality (Mauck et al., 1977). However, the same explanation did not apply since the material was unionized at all tested pH values. Hydrolysis in alkaline water to more toxic products was the apparent explanation for Zectran and also for malathion (Bender, 1969). Among the biocides that are little affected by pH are rotenone (Marking and Bills, 1976) and three esters of 2,4-Dichlorophenoxyacetic acid (2,4-D) (Woodward and Mayer, 1978), which, unlike the amine form of 2,4-D, did not behave as weak acids and change in toxicity.

Some other substances do not change much in toxicity with pH—for example, phenols (EIFAC,

1973a) and the surfactant alkyl benzenesulfonate (ABS) (Marchetti, 1965). Probably this is the case for many other common pollutants. However, whole effluents may be expected to vary in tox-icity with pH if an active constituent is subject to ionization. Pulp mill effluents were about three times as lethal to rainbow trout at pH 9 as at pH 5 in both fresh and seawater dilutions (McLeay et al., 1979b). The explanation appeared to be in-creased toxicity of the resin acid component, which was much more toxic in the unionized form dominant at high pH (McLeay et al., 1979a).

Salinity

The greatest differences in chemical characteristics of surface waters are those between sea water and fresh waters. It might be expected that this could cause enormous differences in toxicity of pollu-tants to organisms, but this is not the case. The general picture is that marine organisms are similar in tolerance to their freshwater cousins, *when both are tested in their own environments.* Euryhaline organisms seem to be most resistant in about one-third seawater, close to the isosmotic level. Marine animals probably become less tolerant of other stresses if the salinity decreases appreciably.

An overall view of this similarity is presented by Klapow and Lewis (1979), who made a non-selective comparison of published acute lethality data for nine metals and six other pollutants to marine, estuarine, and freshwater organisms. In their figures (Fig. 3), results for a given toxicant are usually clustered over one or two orders of magnitude, with outlying values spreading the range to about four orders of magnitude. However, what is *not* seen in most of the figures is a spread of marine data at one end of the distribution and freshwater values at the other end. Instead the scatters seem similar, considering the larger num-ber of freshwater LC50s (e.g., chromium; Fig. 3). Klapow and Lewis tested median values for statis-tically significant differences, and found no differ-ences between marine and freshwater organisms for 14 of the pollutants, the only significant differ-ence being for cadmium. Inspection of their cadmium data (Fig. 3) shows a median LC50 of about 8 mg/l for marine and estuarine organisms and about 2 mg/l for freshwater ones. The similarity for most pollutants is perhaps surprising, particularly since there were so many metals included in the comparison and their toxicity may be greatly influenced by dissolved salts (see later section). From their overall comparisons, Klapow and Lewis concluded that, if there are influences of salinity on toxicity, they are obscured by "more important factors producing variation in bioassay results."

A similar indication of little difference between marine and freshwater species arises from tabulations by the U.S. EPA, presented in their proposed guidelines for processing diverse sets of toxicity data into unified water quality criteria (EPA, 1978). The document indicates that chronically toxic concentrations for saltwater fish and invertebrates were "in the same range" as those for freshwater fish and invertebrates. One of their tabulations compares lethal concentrations of many pollutants to a variety of fish. From the generalized presentation, a toxicant-by-toxicant comparison of saltwater and freshwater species cannot be made, but an overall comparison emerges. Tabula-

tions of LC50s of 62 toxicants for various freshwater fish yielded an average value of 0.83 for the logarithm to base e ($\log_e$) of standard deviations (SDs) among species. For 38 toxicants acting on various marine fish, the average of $\log_e$ SD was 0.79. This in itself indicates only that the degree of variability was similar in the two groups. However, when marine and freshwater fish were combined for the individual toxicants, the average $\log_e$ SD remained almost identical at 0.83. This indicates that the variability among all species was no greater than the variability within freshwater species or within marine species. If either group of fish had been more sensitive overall, there would have been increased variability in the combined data, that is, a larger value of average $\log_e$ SD.

From other chapters, it will become evident why logarithms were used by the EPA in the calculations above. Briefly, a logarithmic scale of concentration deals with proportional changes in concentration instead of absolute changes and thus gives a truer representation of fish response in different parts of a concentration range. It follows that averaging of concentrations is best done as the geometric mean, that is, the antilog of the average of logarithmic concentrations (or the nth root of the product of n concentrations). In the example above, basing calculations on the logarithms of individual LC50s and using the logarithms of SD meant that comparisons of variability were always made as proportions of the LC50s. This allowed comparison of variability among species, even for LC50s that had large differences in the absolute arithmetic values.

The two general comparisons above indicate that there is little difference in overall tolerance to pollutants between freshwater organisms in fresh water and marine organisms in the sea. However, a particular species of fish may show differences in tolerance if the salinity of the water is changed. This might be expected, since all fish in fresh water are hyperosmotic with respect to their environment and most fish in the sea are hypoosmotic. Different strategies are required to maintain osmotic balance, but in either case there is an

Chromium

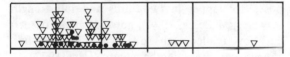

Cadmium

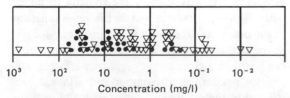

10^3 10^2 10   1 10^{-1} 10^{-2}

Concentration (mg/l)

Figure 3 Range of reported lethal concentrations of two toxicants for (●) marine and estuarine organisms and (▽) freshwater organisms. For chromium there was no significant difference in median LC50 between the two groups of organisms, but the median for marine organisms was higher for cadmium. *[Modified from Klapow and Lewis (1979).]*

imposed physiological load that could be considered a form of stress. If the fish is euryhaline, it would be in overall osmotic balance at an intermediate salinity, and it could be hypothesized that at this balance point the fish would be physiologically more effective. For example, *Cyprinodon macularius* shows better food conversion efficiency in half-strength sea water than in either fresh water or full-strength sea water (Kinne, 1966). Euryhaline fish may also be more effective in dealing with pollutants at their isosmotic point.

This was clearly demonstrated by Herbert and Wakeford (1964) and Herbert and Shurben (1965), who tested the tolerance of rainbow trout and Atlantic salmon smolts to various pollutants at different salinities. For zinc and ammonium chloride, tolerance increased from a minimum in fresh water to a peak in the isosmotic range of 30–40% seawater, then dropped off in higher salinities. For zinc there was a large change in tolerance, by a factor of about 14, and for ammonia a smaller change of 3. The authors advanced the explanation that there was decreased osmotic stress as salinity was increased toward the isosmotic point, with a decreased inward flow of water, which would presumably be accompanied by a reduced intake of toxic ions.

A similar relation was found for naphthalene toxicity to the euryhaline mummichog, with least mortality at isosmotic salinities (Levitan and Taylor, 1979). Less mortality occurred in low salinities than in high salinities, which were apparently associated with osmoregulatory dysfunction and increased uptake of naphthalene. Near the isosmotic point, mummichogs were twice as tolerant of cadmium as in 5% seawater (Voyer, 1975) and mummichogs and eels experienced minimum toxicity for a detergent (Eisler, 1965). Even lethal temperatures seem to follow the same pattern; Garside and Jordan (1968) found greatest tolerance of the mummichog and another cyprinodontid in isosmotic water, with decreases of 4.6° in lethal temperature in both fresh- and seawater. They again advanced the explanation of osmoregu-

latory stress and cited other work showing similar patterns.

Brackish-water clams (*Rangia cuneata*) were about equally tolerant to copper, chromium, and mercury in salinities equivalent to about 70 and 17% seawater (Olson and Harrel, 1973). They were an order of magnitude less tolerant to copper and cadmium at or somewhat below 3% seawater, the lower limit of their range, and slightly less tolerant of mercury. Work on whole effluents is less complete, but pulp mill effluent was equally toxic to coho salmon in fresh and salt water if the pH was the same and the fish were acclimated to the water (McLeay et al., 1979a).

Truly marine organisms seem fully adapted to seawater, and we might expect them to become less tolerant of other stresses if salinity were reduced. This was illustrated by the classic work of McLeese (1956) on the American lobster, an inhabitant of cool marine waters. In full seawater they could withstand very low levels of dissolved oxygen (about 1 mg/l) and high temperatures (around 30°C, depending on acclimation). Resistance to those variables dropped precipitously with any lowering of salinity, and osmotic stress became lethal at about 25% seawater. That pattern may or may not hold for toxic materials. There was no difference in survival times of lobsters exposed to copper in two-thirds and full-strength seawater (McLeese, 1974), nor did uptake of mercury by fiddler crabs differ at 17% and full-strength seawater (Vernberg and O'Hara, 1972).

From these examples it is clear that salinity per se does not greatly modify the toxicity of pollutants. The important aspect is the genetic nature of the organism, whether it is a marine, euryhaline, or freshwater organism. This determines whether it can adapt to a given salinity and thus affects tolerance to pollutants. Also important, although not stressed in the discussion, would be the immediate prehistory or acclimation of the organism with respect to salinity. Most other parts of this chapter will deal with modifying effects in fresh water, partly because most of the research has been done in fresh water but also because its variations are much greater than those in relatively uniform oceanic waters.

Water Hardness

The major effects of hardness on metal toxicity are covered in a separate section below. Other pollutants are covered in this section, and for them the hardness effect is small or negligible with few exceptions. For example, there are no differences in ammonia toxicity with hardness (EIFAC, 1973b) and little difference for phenols (EIFAC, 1973a).

Surfactant toxicity is less affected by water hardness than might be predicted. Alkyl benzene sulfonate was, on the average, 1.5 times more toxic in hard water than in soft water when tested with fathead minnows (Henderson et al., 1959a). A similar result was obtained for commercial detergent formulations. LAS was also 1.5 times as toxic to bluegills in hard water as in soft water (Hokanson and Smith, 1971). However, hardness caused no difference in ABS lethality to bluegills or to the snail *Physa;* an apparent difference for diatoms was confounded with variation in test species (Cairns et al., 1964). Lethal levels of sodium lauryl sulfate were the same in hard and soft water (Henderson et al., 1959a), and survival times did not change greatly in exposures of guppies to another nonionic detergent (Tovell et al., 1975). As might be expected, commercial soaps were one or two orders of magnitude more toxic in soft water, since they are deactivated by calcium and magnesium (Henderson et al., 1959a).

A comparison of the toxicity of 14 petrochemicals in hard and soft water showed significant differences for only 4 of them (Pickering and Henderson, 1966a). All were more toxic to fathead minnows in soft water, but only by a factor of 2 or less. A study of four hydrazines showed no differences for two of them in toxicity to guppies (Slonin, 1977). Hydrazine itself was six times more toxic in soft water, while dimethylhydrazine was 2.5 times more toxic in hard water. Part of the explanation for hydrazine was probably its rapid decomposition in hard water but not in soft water.

Pesticide toxicity seems little affected by water hardness. This was the case for lethality of 16 organophosphates and 12 chlorinated hydrocarbons tested with various fish (Henderson and Pickering, 1958; Henderson et al., 1959b; Pickering and Henderson, 1966c). It was also the case for four of six carbamates; the other two showed about a threefold difference, but in opposite directions, with respect to water hardness (Mauck et al., 1977; Pickering and Henderson, 1966c). For rotenone (Marking and Bills, 1976) and three herbicides (Woodward and Mayer, 1978), there was no difference in toxicity to fish in hard and soft water.

HARDNESS AND ASSOCIATED QUALITIES THAT MODIFY METAL TOXICITY

For a long time, it has been known that most heavy metals become less toxic in harder water. A general relation was developed by the British Water Pollution Research Laboratory (Fig. 4; from Brown, 1968) and this has often been reproduced and utilized (e.g., NAS/NAE, 1974). This empirical relation is useful, although it is now clear that hardness alone does not govern the potency of the metals. Copper will be used to illustrate the complexity of the situation, and similar pictures probably apply to most of the metals. For complete assessments of the wealth of information about copper, readers should consult the superb reviews of Alabaster and Lloyd (1980) or Spear and Pierce (1979). Much of the following is a condensed version of material covered in the latter review.

Spear and Pierce (1979) summarized the lethal levels of copper for fish, as determined by many investigators, and found a reassuringly consistent pattern with hardness. Results were divided according to four taxa of fish, with bluegills and their relatives being most tolerant of copper. The relation for most salmonid fish is shown in Fig. 5. This embodies results from 19 separate papers, with only a few estimates excluded as being atypic. For salmon and trout, the lethal level of copper could be predicted by the equation shown

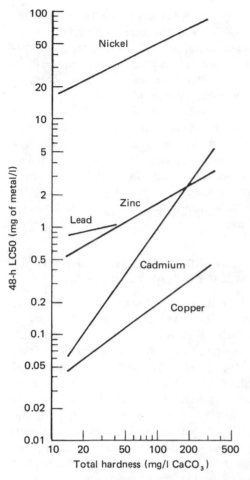

Figure 4 Relation between total hardness of water and 48-h LC50 to rainbow trout of nickel, lead, zinc, cadmium, and copper. *[Reprinted from Brown (1968) with permission from the Controller of Her Majesty's Stationery Office.]*

Beamish, 1978a,b). The generally consistent patterns in Fig. 5 enable an easy prediction of the effects of copper, at least in laboratory situations. There is an apparently straightforward relation with water hardness, and sublethal thresholds are in the vicinity of 0.1–0.3 of the lethal concentrations of copper.

It is generally considered that this sparing effect of increased hardness is a phenomenon within the fish. The usual explanation is that higher levels of calcium in the fish tissues make the cell membranes in the gills less permeable, so that less metal enters the fish. The calcium content of fish tissue does increase with that of the water (Houston, 1959), and fish reared in hard water apparently require several days to lose calcium before they become as sensitive to heavy metal intoxication as fish reared in soft water (Lloyd, 1965). Simply adding calcium or magnesium to test water has little effect on copper resistance of fish (Zitko and Carson, 1976). However, there do not appear to be any published measurements of the relative amounts of the metal entering gills in hard and soft water.

The simple empirical relation with hardness disappears if tests are done in unusual waters, in which pH and alkalinity are not associated with hardness in the usual way. The two factors, pH and alkalinity, in fact govern the forms of copper present in water (Spear and Pierce, 1979) and a typical array of "ionic species" is shown in Fig. 6. The picture would change slightly for different alkalinities. At pH 5, for example, a large proportion of the copper is present as Cu^{2+}, the free copper ion, but at higher pH there is a variety of hydroxides and carbonates.* It would stretch the imagination a little too far to assume that all these forms were equally toxic, and indeed they are not.

A number of investigations on the toxicity of "ionic species" have been carried out in the past

in Fig. 5. Fathead minnows and certain other members of the minnow family showed a lethality relation very close to the one in Fig. 5.

Even more important with respect to water quality criteria, the sublethal toxicity of copper shows a similar change with water hardness. Some results for growth are shown in Fig. 5. Other sublethal responses such as critical swimming speed and food conversion efficiency are also more affected by copper in soft water (Waiwood and

---

*Actually, free copper is thought to be present as the aquo ion $[Cu(H_2O)_6]^{2+}$ (Spear and Pierce, 1979). Some other hydroxides and carbonates precipitate, including $Cu(OH)_2$, malachite $Cu_2(OH)_2CO_3$, and azurite $Cu_3(OH)_2(CO_3)_2$ (Stiff, 1971b; Silva, 1976).

decade, and a toxicity picture is shown in Fig. 7 for diverse combinations of hardness and pH, with alkalinity allowed to find its own level. Some general effect of hardness may be seen. Several groups of investigators have shown that for fixed combinations of pH and alkalinity, increasing hardness causes a reduction in toxicity (Anderson et al., 1979; Chakoumakos et al., 1979; Inglis and Davis, 1972; Miller and MacKay, 1980). But it is clear from Fig. 7 that great changes in toxicity are also associated with pH. Here, again, there is ample documentation that at a fixed hardness, toxicity can be changed by alkalinity or pH changes (Andrew, 1976; Chakoumakos et al., 1979; Chapman and McCrady, 1977; Mancy and Allen, 1977; Pagenkopf et al., 1974; Sunda and Guillard, 1976). The general conclusion of these workers is that the toxicity to fish and phytoplankton is

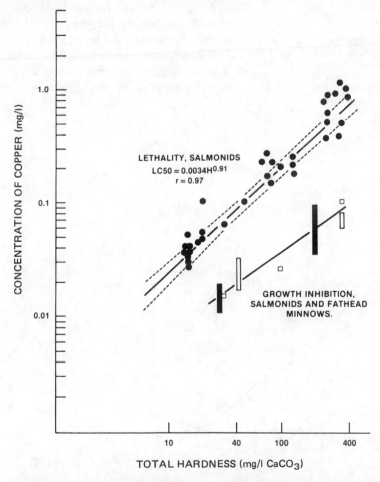

Figure 5 Empirical relation between copper toxicity and total hardness of fresh water. The upper line represents median lethal concentrations for most salmon and trout. The lower line represents thresholds for inhibition of growth. Growth results shown in darkened bars are for fathead minnows; those in open bars are for brook and rainbow trout in neutral or alkaline water. Modified from figures in Spear and Pierce (1979). Lethal data are from many reports in the literature. Growth results are from Lett et al. (1976), McKim and Benoit (1971), Mount (1968), Mount and Stephan (1969), and Waiwood and Beamish (1978b). In the formula for predicting lethal concentration, H is the total hardness of the water.

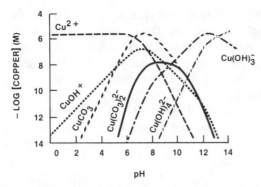

Figure 6 Comparison of log concentration of various forms of copper with pH for a total copper content of 2.4×10^{-6} M and a total carbonate content of 10^{-3} M. *[Reproduced with permission from Ernst et al. (1975); copyright 1975, Pergamon Press, Ltd.]*

due either to ionic copper or to that ion plus ionized hydroxides. The large hump at pH 8 in Fig. 7 represents high concentrations of copper carbonates and unionized hydroxides, which are not thought to be toxic. This suggestion was made a decade ago by Stiff (1971a) and is agreed with by most of the investigators listed above. When Fig. 7 was replotted, and the vertical axis displayed the concentration of supposedly toxic forms (Cu^{2+} and two ionized hydroxides) instead of total dissolved copper, the response surface lost its wild undulations and became fairly smooth.

However, the replotted response surface was far from flat, leading to a final complexity. The lethal concentrations of "toxic" forms were 200–2000

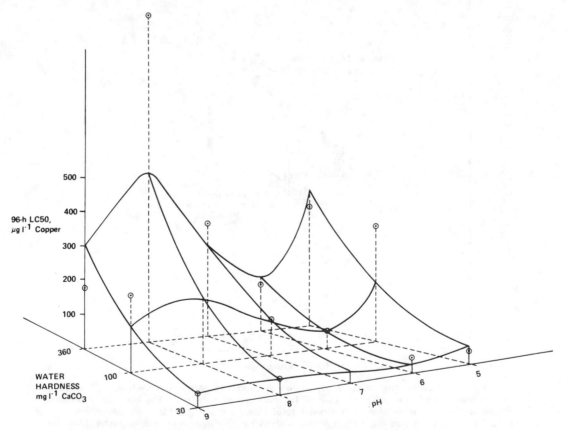

Figure 7 Lethal concentrations of total dissolved copper to 10-gram rainbow trout, at different combinations of water hardness and pH. Points show the LC50s obtained, the response surface was mathematically fitted. *[Reproduced with permission from Howarth and Sprague (1978); copyright 1978, Pergamon Press, Ltd.]*

times higher at pH 5 than at pH 9, depending on the hardness in a given set of tests. In other words, the active forms of copper were much more toxic at high pH. It is difficult to give credence to this variation, but it may exist.* Andrew (1976) suggests that the increasing toxicity of the cupric ion at high pH may result from interactions with sulfhydryl-containing proteins or enzymes. Other authors confirmed this change in toxicity with pH. When the LC50 of copper for guppies was calculated on the basis of labile copper (i.e., that measured by pulse polarography), it changed from 240 µg/l at pH 5.7 to 15 µg/l at pH 8.1, with the same hardness in each test—a 16-fold increase in toxicity at high pH (Mancy and Allen, 1977).

This research indicates that to predict copper lethality in unusual fresh waters, it will be necessary to take into account three modifying factors: hardness, alkalinity, and pH. Unfortunately, it requires fairly sophisticated chemical calculations to estimate the proportions of the various forms of copper, or else access to a good computer program to make these predictions. Even after that, there does not yet exist a single value for the toxicity of the apparently toxic forms of copper—it varies with water characteristics. Perhaps the working biologist will be able to use the empirical relation with hardness (Fig. 4), which will fit the usual conditions in surface waters. As partial justification, it may be considered that unusual combinations of pH, alkalinity, and hardness, perhaps brought about by acid or alkaline pollution, will change to the more usual combinations, given some time and the natural aeration that takes place in surface waters.

There are similar quandaries about the forms of other metals that should be measured in order to evaluate toxicity. For example, Davies et al.

(1976) found great differences in the toxicity of lead between soft and hard water when the metal was measured as total concentration. The differences were minor when only dissolved lead was considered. Their results are simplified in Table 8 by using geometric averages of their toxicity ranges. In this case it seems clear that dissolved lead is the active toxic agent. The chronic thresholds of dissolved lead almost exactly fit findings of Hodson et al. (1978), and it appears that the difference between 0.010 and 0.024 mg/l is not an effect of hardness but of pH. Hodson and colleagues showed that the level of lead in the blood of trout, which is directly related to sublethal toxicity, increases by a factor of 2.1 for a drop of one unit of pH. The soft water of Davies et al. was just about one unit lower in pH than their hard water, and the toxicity increase of 2.4 agrees rather well with the factor of Hodson et al.

Thus for some metals we are coming close to understanding which forms are the toxic ones, and the information should be utilized in evaluating pollution of natural waters. One note of caution might be added for such applied work. The total content of metal, such as the large amount of nontoxic lead in the hard water of Table 2, should not be ignored. If water conditions changed (say from acid pollution), the ionic species of a metal could change and previously nontoxic forms could become toxic.

Table 8 Differences in Lead Toxicity to Rainbow Trout in Soft and Hard Water (28 and 350 mg/l $CaCO_3$)[a]

Measurement	Soft (mg/l)	Hard (mg/l)
LC50		
Total lead	1.2	510
Dissolved lead	1.2	1.4
Chronic threshold		
Total lead	0.010	0.21
Dissolved lead	0.010	0.024

[a]Modified from Davies et al. (1976); copyright 1976, Pergamon Press, Ltd.

*Reexamination of the data of Howarth and Sprague (1978) suggests a way of decreasing the large variation in apparent toxicity. If one form of ionized carbonate $Cu(CO_3)_2^{3-}$ were also considered toxic and added in to the LC50 with the other three forms, the variation with pH would become only three- to eightfold. There would still be more toxicity in alkaline pH.

Most of the discussion above concerns lethality, but the influence of pH, alkalinity, and so on, on the sublethal action of metals has become much more important in recent years. Severe acidification of soft-water lakes is occurring in many parts of the world, and is accompanied by increased metal content of the waters. There is some evidence that the metals may play a primary role in the observed reproductive failure of fish in such lakes, which leads eventually to fishless lakes. Considerable research on this is under way, and any attempt to review it would be quickly out of date. However, it can be said that the knowledge about toxic forms of metal that has been gained from work on lethality should be most useful for designing the lengthier experiments needed to assess the modifying factors of sublethal metal toxicity.

Binding and Sorption

Suspended and dissolved materials in surface waters may partly detoxify some pollutants. This is true for many metals, particularly copper, and for some other toxicants. Metals in water are commonly analyzed by atomic absorption spectroscopy (see chapter 16), which includes all configurations of metal in the measurement. Such measurements may not agree with responses in biological tests, which may show toxicity that is equivalent to much lower concentrations. As mentioned above, there is some justification for thinking that all forms of metal should be included in pollution assessment or in setting water quality criteria, since nontoxic forms can change to toxic forms (e.g., NAS/NAE, 1974). However, at least for some metals, understanding has progressed to the point where more realistic assessments can be based on the active forms. The following discussion is based mainly on complexing of metals, particularly copper, since there has been considerable research on that metal.

One form of complexation is with natural inorganic ions in surface water such as carbonates and hydroxides. This was outlined in the section immediately above. Excellent discussions of copper complexation have been provided by Pagen-

kopf et al. (1974) and Andrew et al. (1977), who demonstrated that carbonate, orthophosphate, and pyrophosphate complexes of copper were nontoxic. Other types of complexation will be considered in this section.

Many field studies have shown that aquatic organisms may be unaffected by supposedly toxic levels of metals. An early example was a trial of lake poisoning which showed persistence of copper in the water, but in a nontoxic form (Smith, 1939). In upwelling deep oceanic water, copper seems to be about an order of magnitude more toxic to algae than in surface waters, because the deep waters apparently lack natural chelating agents (Steeman Neilsen and Wium-Andersen, 1970). In the water of a Newfoundland river, 125 μg/l copper was required for lethality to young salmon, instead of the expected level of about 30 μg/l (Wilson, 1972). Addition of spent sulfite liquor from a pulp mill raised the LC50 to more than 250 μg/l. In certain Norwegian rivers and lakes, healthy populations of salmonids existed in copper-zinc concentrations that exceeded the carefully established European criteria for "safe" levels by factors of 3–9 (EIFAC, 1977). Chemical examinations indicated that as much as 86% of the copper might be present as organometal complexes that were not toxic.

A massive field experiment in Ohio was designed to assess the validity of laboratory research on copper, when applied to surface waters (Geckler et al., 1976). An important finding was that lethal levels of total copper for fathead minnows averaged 12 times higher in the stream than in nearby laboratory water. The no observed effect level for reproduction was three to four times higher in stream water. Clearly, there was considerable complexing or other detoxification of copper in the stream water, which contained final products from an upstream sewage treatment plant. LC50s in the stream fluctuated greatly over 1.5 yr, from 1.6 to 21 mg/l based on a measure of *total* copper, but values were relatively constant at 0.60–0.98 mg/l when based on "dissolved" copper that passed a 0.45-μm membrane filter. It was concluded that predictive ability was much improved for several of the heavy metals if assessments were based on dissolved metal (Brungs et al., 1976).

Laboratory studies on complexing have further added to the understanding of these effects. As might be expected, certain organic chemicals designed to be chelators of cations are very good at making metals nontoxic to aquatic organisms. Nitrilotriacetic acid (NTA) effectively eliminates copper and zinc lethality to brook trout even when the metals are present at 33 times their usual threshold LC50 (Sprague, 1968). Similar findings are reported for guppies (Gudernatsch, 1970) and the crustacean *Daphnia magna* (Biesinger et al., 1974). Cadmium is also detoxified for *Daphnia* by EDTA, a comparable chelating agent (Teulin, 1978). The actions of the agents above are quite predictable; for example, NTA binds cations in a one-to-one molecular ratio, with a known order of priority for various cations.

Laboratory tests have documented similar actions for other, more natural organic molecules. Algae exude complexing ligands that can detoxify metals such as copper or bind essential micronutrients (Van den Berg et al., 1979). The amino acid glycine detoxified copper by an order of magnitude (Brown et al., 1974). Other amino acids and polypeptides can be expected to do so (Stiff, 1971b). Sewage plant effluents and suspended solids have a smaller effect (Brown et al., 1974), but colloids, clays, and soil particles can adsorb major proportions of copper in water, with largely unknown effects on toxicity. Between 10 and 80% of various metals were bound to suspended particles in Lake Ontario (Nriagu et al., 1981; Spear and Pierce, 1979). Finally, humic and fulvic acids, which darken streams in many forested areas, have a well-documented effect. Humic acid can cause an order-of-magnitude decrease in copper toxicity in very soft water, but its binding action falls off in harder water (Brown et al., 1974; Zitko et al., 1973). Fulvic acid is somewhat less effective, and neither of these agents has an appreciable effect in detoxifying zinc and cadmium (Zitko et al., 1973; Giesy et al., 1977). All the above findings concern

lethality, but Carson and Carson (1973) made the significant finding that avoidance reactions of Atlantic salmon to copper could be decreased by a factor of about 5 with respect to copper concentration if 20 mg/l humic acid was added to soft water. Such levels of humic acid could be found in natural waters.

It is clear that both inorganic and organic complexing can lower toxicity of metals, particularly copper. The problem is how to assess concentrations of the toxic fractions, and recent work brings us closer to satisfactory methods. Atomic absorption spectrometry, commonly used at present, measures all forms of metal in the sample—that is, total metal. A relevant comment is that of Andrew (1976) about the "futility of basing the results of toxicity bioassays on total metal analyses. . . . Such data are not useful to any extent." Earlier in this chapter, reference was made to the use of chemical equilibrium calculations to distinguish between toxic forms such as ions and apparently nontoxic inorganic complexes. These calculations can be useful; however, they are not a direct measurement but a prediction based on equilibrium constants and the chemical characteristics of the dilution water. McCrady and Chapman (1979) urged that such predictions "be used with caution, realizing that at best, quantitative results might be obtained at higher concentrations."

It was also mentioned above that measurements of so-called dissolved metal, which passes a 0.45-μm filter, can give better estimates of concentrations of the toxic forms than measurements of total metal. This, too, can be deceptive, since many organic ligands would pass such a filter (Giesy et al., 1977). Most "nontoxic" suspended precipitates would be expected to stay on the filter, but some may pass, and some dissolved molecules may be taken up by the filter.

A closer approach to measuring concentrations of toxic forms of metals would be provided by differential pulse polarography, which is said to measure "labile" forms. These include the free ion and other ions that are easily dissociated; obviously, this is another operational division of forms of metals rather than an absolute one. Polarography has the advantage of detecting very low concentrations—for example, 0.2–0.7 μg/l for some common metals in water (Chau and Lum-Shue-Chan, 1974).

Finally, a technique that is receiving a great deal of attention in recent literature involves ion-selective electrodes, which are more or less specific for measurement of one metallic ion (or its hydrated form). Detection of low concentrations is not as satisfactory as with polarography. McCrady and Chapman (1979) reported reasonable agreement between cupric ion concentrations measured with such an electrode and concentrations predicted from a chemical equilibrium model. However, measured concentrations in natural waters were lower than predicted, presumably because of complexing by organic ligands and other materials in the water. Specific ion electrodes have been used with success to measure proportions of metals not bound by humic acid (Zitko et al., 1973) and to assess which species of algae are primarily responsible for binding heavy metals in natural waters (Briand et al., 1978).

Thus, for the complicated subject of toxic species of metals and their chelation in natural waters, a good deal of progress has been made in the past decade. By applying recent technology, admittedly rather sophisticated technology, a reasonable picture can be obtained of the true toxicity of metals in water, and fairly accurate predictions can be made.

The effect of binding and sorption on other, nonmetallic pollutants appears to have been studied very little and, for the most part, strong modifying effects have not been noted. Toxicity of the insecticide endrin to fathead minnows was not reduced when it was added to suspensions of clay (Brungs and Bailey, 1966). In contrast, addition of a soil suspension to endrin solutions seemed to moderate its toxicity somewhat, and endrin already sorbed onto runoff sediments was not released into water in sufficient amounts to be lethal to fish (Ferguson et al., 1965). Clay suspensions at levels that might be found in nature had little influence on the toxicity of the surfactant LAS (Hokanson and Smith, 1971). Very strong suspensions (about 20,000 mg/l) of drilling fluid, mostly a mixture of inert barium sulfate and clay, reduced the toxicity of three surfactants but not of two others, and also reduced toxicity of paraformaldehyde and capryl alcohol (Sprague and Logan, 1979). Reductions were only by factors of 1.5–2.0, not very large considering the large amount of suspended matter, including the clay bentonite, which has a relatively high cation exchange capacity. It may be that the lack of such research on complexing of nonmetallic pollutants is an indication that effects are not major.

SUMMARY

1 Factors that modify the toxicity of pollutants to aquatic organisms, including biotic variables such as species and abiotic variables such as water temperature, have been considered in this chapter.

2 Effects of modifying factors must be cautiously interpreted within experiments and not between them, bearing in mind that even repeated toxicity tests in the same laboratory will not give identical results. Some within-laboratory variation is difficult or impossible to explain. A careful investigator may obtain a series of LC50s with a range of only ±20% of the median value. On the other hand, LC50s from the same laboratory have been known to vary by a factor of 5. Interlaboratory comparisons may show variation by a factor of only 1.2 or differences as great as 10-fold.

3 If good basic procedures are followed in acute lethality tests, other differences in test procedure do not affect results greatly. For example, when trout were tested at their maximum cruising speed, their LC50s dropped to only 0.7 or 0.8 of the values for unexercised fish.

4 The kind of test organism has a major influence on toxicity data, but perhaps less than might be expected. A literature review with individiual comparisons of 15 pollutants tested under similar conditions, with results accepted for all

types of organisms, showed that well over half of the lethal levels fell within one order of magnitude. The range was spread over three orders of magnitude because of variation in only 15% of the observed LC50s. Within one group such as fish, lethal levels for a given pollutant would generally fall within an order of magnitude. For example, oil refinery waste showed only a fivefold variation in LC50s between the most and least sensitive of 57 species. Some heavy metals and organophosphate insecticides are exceptions, with extreme variation between species of fish. However, bluegills are tolerant of the former and sensitive to the latter, which suggests that caution should be used in generalizing about "tolerant species."

5 In the life cycle of fish, the egg, larval, and early juvenile stages are most sensitive in chronic exposures. Large fish are not necessarily more tolerant than small juveniles; the effect of size on LC50 may go either way, or may be absent.

6 There is only slim evidence that diseased stocks of fish are less tolerant of toxicants. On the other hand, nutrition of test organisms can be quite important. Fish on a low-protein diet may be two to six times less tolerant of some pollutants. Acclimation of fish to a toxicant may result in a doubling of tolerance or in no increase, depending on the substance involved and whether a defense mechanism is stimulated.

7 There is no general effect of temperature on toxicity. Depending on the species and pollutant, fish in warmer water may be more, less, or equally tolerant. Limited evidence suggests that thresholds of sublethal effect may be about the same at all water temperatures.

8 Dissolved oxygen concentrations in the vicinity of 20–30% of saturation seem to cause an increase of only about 1.5-fold in lethality of toxicants to fish. Some experimental results indicate that sublethal effects of a toxicant are not greatly modified by low oxygen, even when the reduced oxygen itself has such sublethal action.

9 Some pollutants show large changes in toxicity with pH of the water if they are ionized under the influence of that variable. Usually it is the undissociated or less dissociated form that is most toxic, and the change may be an order of magnitude for a difference of one pH unit or less.

Ammonia, cyanide, and hydrogen sulfide show such changes, and their lethality can be predicted accurately on the basis of the chemical transformations. Most metals act in the opposite way, with the free ionic species being more toxic than the undissociated compounds. Changes in sublethal toxicity appear to parallel changes in chemical behavior and lethality.

10 Salinity is a major variable among the characteristics of surface water, but its influence on toxicity is not so important. Marine organisms in seawater and freshwater organisms in their environment seems to be about equally tolerant of a given pollutant. Euryhaline organisms, which are less common, attain maximum tolerance in isosmotic water—that is, about 30–40% seawater—and the increase in tolerance may be an order of magnitude. Modification of sublethal effects by salinity has been less studied.

11 Total hardness of fresh water has little effect on the potency of most pollutants (except metals). A few substances change their toxicity up to two- or threefold, but the direction of change with hardness varies.

12 Many heavy metals become an order of magnitude more lethal in very soft water than in very hard water, and sublethal changes are roughly parallel. This is thought to result from changes in gill permeability caused by calcium content of the fish. For peculiar waters in which pH and alkalinity do not follow the usual relations with hardness, the importance of those two variables becomes more obvious. They may partially or wholly govern the proportions of various ionic species of metal that are present, and these differ in toxicity. To generalize from knowledge of copper, it appears that the free or ionic metal is very toxic. Ionized hydroxides of metal may also be toxic, but unionized carbonates are probably not. Furthermore, for copper at least, toxicity changes when alkalinity is varied but hardness kept constant, and there is much higher potency of the toxic forms of metal at high pH than at low pH, again for the same hardness.

13 Natural waters often contain suspended and dissolved matter including organic ligands or chelators. Metals are the chief examples of pollutants that may be detoxified because of sorption

or binding by these materials; most other pollutants seem much less affected. Among the metals copper is particularly affected, and binding and sorption may decrease its lethal and sublethal toxic effects by an order of magnitude.

14 Because of the extreme effects of modifying factors on metal toxicity described in items 12 and 13, a number of approaches to chemical measurement of metallic pollutants should be considered. Measurement of toxic forms of metal is better approximated by the "dissolved" metal (i.e., the metal able to pass through a 0.45-μm filter) than by the total metal (atomic absorption spectrometry). The empirical relation between toxicity of total dissolved metal and water hardness may suffice for routine use in many natural waters. It is conceivable that the nontoxic ionic forms included with total dissolved metal could change to toxic forms following an event such as acid pollution. The proportions of supposedly toxic ionic forms, present as parts of the total dissolved metal, could be predicted from models using chemical equilibrium constants, although this requires effective use of computer programs. None of the methods above adequately allows for metals detoxified by binding to dissolved or suspended materials. A closer approximation of toxic species can be made by polarography, which detects ionic or free metals plus easily dissociating forms. Specific ion electrodes can measure the free forms only for certain metals, but with less sensitivity to low concentrations than is obtained by polarography.

15 It is difficult to sift out "concepts of aquatic toxicology" from this review of modifying factors. They will have to be particular relations rather than sweeping principles. First, we must expect an order-of-magnitude variation in toxicity data gathered from a number of laboratories. Second, biotic variables seem to have generally more important modifying effects than do abiotic ones, and the principal one is the kind of organism. Although most kinds would show tolerances within an order-of-magnitude range, some groups are sensitive and total variation is often about three orders of magnitude. Nutritional status of test organisms appears to be another important biotic modifier. Third, the pollutants most affected by abiotic modification are those

that ionize, and the most important modifying entities are pH and alkalinity. Fourth, metals are subject to large changes in toxicity, not only through ionization but through precipitation, sorption, and binding to suspended and dissolved matter. Finally, temperature, low dissolved oxygen, saltwater versus freshwater medium, and hardness of fresh water are not generally *major* modifying entities. Their effects are often only two- or threefold or much less, with some exceptions, including a hardness effect on metals.

LITERATURE CITED

Adelman IR, Smith LL, Jr: Toxicity of hydrogen sulfide to goldfish (*Carassius auratus*) as influenced by temperature, oxygen, and bioassay techniques. J Fish Res Bd Can 29:1309–1317, 1972.

Adelman IR, Smith LL, Jr: Fathead minnows (*Pimephales promelas*) and goldfish (*Carassius auratus*) as standard fish in bioassays and their reaction to potential reference toxicants. J Fish Res Bd Can 33:209–214, 1976.

Alabaster JS, Lloyd R: Water Quality Criteria for Freshwater Fish. London: Butterworths, 1980.

Alderdice DF, Brett JR: Some effects of kraft mill effluent on young Pacific salmon. J Fish Res Bd Can 14:783–795, 1957.

Anderson PD, Spear PA: Copper pharmacokinetics in fish gills. II. Body size relationships for accumulation and tolerance. Water Res 14:1107–1111, 1980.

Anderson PD, Weber LJ: Toxic response as a quantitative function of body size. Toxicol Appl Pharmacol 33:471–483, 1975.

Anderson PD, Horovitch H, Weinstein NL: Pollutant mixtures in the aquatic environment: A complex problem in toxic hazard assessment. Proc 5th Ann Aquatic Toxicity Workshop, Hamilton, Ont, Nov 7–9, 1978. Can Fish Mar Serv Tech Rept 862, pp. 100–114, 1979.

Andrew RW: Toxicity relationships to copper forms in natural waters. In: Toxicity to Biota of Metal Forms in Natural Water. Proc Workshop, Duluth, Minn, Oct 7–8, 1975, edited by RW Andrew, PV Hodson, DE Konasewich, pp. 127–143. Windsor, Ont: International Joint Commission, 1976.

Andrew RW, Biesinger KE, Glass GE: Effects of inorganic complexing on the toxicity of copper to *Daphnia magna*. Water Res 11:309–315, 1977.

Asano S, Nagasawa S, Fushimi S: Biological trials of chemicals on fish. VI. Relation between temperature and the toxicity of pentachlorophenol (PCP) to carp. Bochu-Kagaku 34:13–21, 1969; Chem Abstr 71(11):260, 1969.

Ball IR: The relative susceptibilities of some species of fresh-water fish to poisons. I. Ammonia. Water Res 1:767–775, 1967.

Bender ME: The toxicity of the hydrolysis and breakdown products of malathion to the fathead minnow (*Pimephales promelas* Rafinesque). Water Res 3:571–582, 1969.

Biesinger KE, Andrew RW, Arthur JW: Chronic toxicity of NTA (nitrilotriacetate) and metal-NTA complexes to *Daphnia magna*. J Fish Res Bd Can 31:486–490, 1974.

Boyce NP, Yamada SB: Effects of a parasite, *Eubothrium salvelini* (Cestoda; Pseudophyllidea), on the resistance of juvenile sockeye salmon (*Oncorhynchus nerka*) to zinc. J Fish Res Bd Can 34:706–709, 1977.

Briand F, Trucco R, Ramamoorthy S: Correlations between specific algae and heavy metal binding in lakes. J Fish Res Bd Can 35:1482–1485, 1978.

Broderius SJ, Smith LL, Jr, Lind DT: Relative toxicity of free cyanide and dissolved sulfide forms to the fathead minnow (*Pimephales promelas*). J Fish Res Bd Can 34.2323–2332, 1977.

Brown BE: Observations on the tolerance of the isopod *Asellus meridianus* Rac. to copper and lead. Water Res 10:555–559, 1976.

Brown VM: The calculation of the acute toxicity of mixtures of poisons to rainbow trout. Water Res 2:723–733, 1968.

Brown VM, Jordan DHM, Tiller BA: The effect of temperature on the acute toxicity of phenol to rainbow trout in hard water. Water Res 1:587–594, 1967.

Brown VM, Shaw TL, Shurben DG: Aspects of water quality and the toxicity of copper to rainbow trout. Water Res 8:797–803, 1974.

Brungs WA, Bailey GW: Influence of suspended solids on the acute toxicity of endrin to fathead minnows. Proc 21st Ind Waste Conf Purdue Univ Eng Extn Ser No 121, part 1, 50(2):4–12, 1967.

Brungs WA, Geckler JR, Gast M: Acute and chronic toxicity of copper to the fathead minnow in a surface water of variable quality. Water Res 10:37–43, 1976.

Bryan GW, Hummerstone LG: Adaptation of the polychaete *Nereis diversicolor* to estuarine sediments containing high concentrations of heavy metals. 1. General observation and adaptations to copper. J Mar Biol Assoc UK 51:207–217, 1971.

Bryan GW, Hummerstone LG: Adaptation of the polychaete *Nereis diversicolor* to estuarine sediments containing high concentrations of zinc and cadmium. J Mar Biol Assoc UK 53:839–859, 1973.

Burton DT, Jones AH, Cairns J, Jr: Acute zinc toxicity to rainbow trout (*Salmo gairdneri*): Confirmation of the hypothesis that death is related to tissue hypoxia. J Fish Res Bd Can 29:1463–1466, 1972.

Cairns J, Scheier A: The effects of periodic low oxygen upon the toxicity of various chemicals to aquatic organisms. Proc 12th Ind Waste Conf Purdue Univ Eng Ext Ser 94:165–176, 1958.

Cairns J, Scheier A: The effects of temperature and water hardness upon the toxicity of naphthenic acids to the common bluegill sunfish, *Lepomis macrochirus* Raf., and the pond snail, *Physa heterostropha* Say. Not Nat Acad Nat Sci Philadelphia No 353, 1962.

Cairns J, Jr, Scheier A: Environmental effects upon cyanide toxicity to fish. Not Nat Acad Nat Sci Philadelphia No 361, 1963.

Cairns J, Jr, Scheier A, Hess NE: The effects of alkyl benzene sulfonate on aquatic organisms. Ind Water Wastes 9:22–28, 1964.

Cairns J, Jr, Heath AG, Parker BC: Temperature influence on chemical toxicity to aquatic organisms. J Water Pollut Control Fed 47:267–280, 1975.

Carson WG, Carson WV: Avoidance of copper in the presence of humic acid by juvenile Atlantic salmon. Fish Res Bd Can Ms Rept Ser No 1237, 1973.

Chakoumakos C, Russo RC, Thurston RV: Toxicity of copper to cutthroat trout (*Salmo clarki*) under different conditions of alkalinity, pH, and hardness. Environ Sci Technol 13:213–219, 1979.

Chapman GA, McCrady JK: Copper toxicity: A question of form. In: Recent Advances in Fish Toxicology: A Symposium, edited by RA Tubb, pp. 132–151. U.S. EPA Rept EPA 660/3-77/085, 1977.

Chau YK, Lum-Shue-Chan K: Determination of labile and strongly bound metals in lake water. Water Res 8:383–388, 1974.

Cherry DS, Larrick SR, Dickson KL, Hoehn RC, Cairns J, Jr: Significance of hypochlorous acid in free residual chlorine to the avoidance response of spotted bass (*Micropterus punctulatus*) and rosyface shiner (*Notropis rubellus*). J Fish Res Bd Can 34:1365–1372, 1977.

Davies PH, Goettl JP, Jr, Sinley JR, Smith NF: Acute and chronic toxicity of lead to rainbow trout *Salmo gairdneri,* in hard and soft water. Water Res 10:199–206, 1976.

Davis JC: Minimal dissolved oxygen requirements of aquatic life with emphasis on Canadian species: A review. J Fish Res Bd Can 32:2295–2332, 1975.

Davis JS, Hoos RAW: Use of sodium pentachlorophenate and dehydroabietic acid as reference toxicants for salmonid bioassays. J Fish Res Bd Can 32:411–416, 1975.

Daye PG: Attempts to acclimate embryos and alevins of Atlantic salmon, *Salmo salar,* and rainbow trout, *S. gairdneri,* to low pH. Can J Fish Aquat Sci 37:1035–1038, 1980.

Dixon DG, Hilton JW: Influence of available dietary carbohydrate content on tolerance of waterborne copper by rainbow trout. J Fish Biol 19:509–517, 1981.

Dixon DG, Sprague JB: Acclimation-induced changes in toxicity of arsenic and cyanide to rainbow trout. J Fish Biol 18:579–589, 1981a.

Dixon DG, Sprague JB: Acclimation to copper by rainbow trout (*Salmo gairdneri*)—a modifying factor in toxicity. Can J Fish Aquat Sci 38:880–888, 1981b.

Dixon DG, Sprague JB: Copper bioaccumulation and hepatoprotein synthesis during acclimation to copper by juvenile rainbow trout. Aquat Toxicol 1:69–81, 1981c.

Doudoroff P, Shumway DL: Dissolved oxygen requirements of freshwater fishes. FAO Fish Tech Pap 86, 1970.

Doudoroff P, Leduc G, Schneider CR: Acute toxicity to fish of solutions containing complex metal cyanides, in relation to concentrations of molecular hydrocyanic acid. Trans Am Fish Soc 95:6–22, 1966.

Eedy W: Environmental cause/effect phenomena relating to technological development in the Canadian Arctic. Natl Res Counc Can Publ NRCC 13688, 1974.

EIFAC (European Inland Fisheries Advisory Commission): Water quality criteria for European freshwater fish. Report on monohydric phenols and inland fisheries. Water Res 7:929–941, 1973a.

EIFAC: Water quality criteria for European freshwater fish. Report on ammonia and inland fisheries. Water Res 7:1011–1022, 1973b.

EIFAC: Report on the effect of zinc and copper pollution on the salmonid fisheries in a river and lake system in central Norway. FAO Eur Inland Fish Adv Comm Tech Pap 29, 1977.

Eisler R: Some effects of a synthetic detergent on estuarine fishes. Trans Am Fish Soc 94:26–31, 1965.

Elson PF, Kerswill CJ: Impact on salmon of spraying insecticide over forests. In: Advances in Water Pollution Research, vol. 1, Proceedings of a Conference of International Associations on Water Pollution Research, Munich, pp. 55–74. Washington, D.C.: Water Pollution Control Federation, 1966.

Emerson K, Russo RC, Lund RE, Thurston RV: Aqueous ammonia equilibrium calculations: Effect of pH and temperature. J Fish Res Bd Can 32:2379–2383, 1975.

EPA: Quality criteria for water. U.S. Environmental Protection Agency, Washington, D.C., 256 p, 1976.

EPA: Water quality criteria. Fed Regist 43(97):21506–21518, 1978.

EPA: Interlaboratory comparisons of toxicity tests. U.S. EPA Environ Res Lab Duluth Q Rep, pp. 2–3, April–June 1979.

Ernst R, Allen HE, Mancy KH: Characterization of trace metal species and measurement of trace metal stability constants by electrochemical techniques. Water Res 9:969–979, 1975.

Ferguson DE, Ludke JL, Wood JP, and Prather JW: The effects of mud on the bioactivity of pesticides on fishes. J Miss Acad Sci 11:219–228, 1965.

Fogels A, Sprague JB: Comparative short-term tolerance of zebrafish, flagfish, and rainbow trout to five poisons including potential reference toxicants. Water Res 11:811–817, 1977.

Fry FEJ: Effects of the environment on animal activity. Univ Toronto Stud Biol Ser 55; Publ Ont Fish Res Lab 68, 1947.

Fry FEJ: Requirements for the aquatic habitat. Pulp Pap Mag Can 61:T61–T66, 1960.

Fry FEJ: The effect of environmental factors on the physiology of fish. In: Fish Physiology, vol. 6, Environmental Relations and Behavior, edited by WS Hoar, DJ Randall, pp. 1–98. New York: Academic, 1971.

Garside ET, Jordan CM: Upper lethal temperatures at various levels of salinity in the euryhaline cyprinodontids *Fundulus heteroclitus* and *F. diaphanus* after isosmotic acclimation. J Fish Res Bd Can 25:2717–2720, 1968.

Geckler JR, Horning WB, Nieheisel TM, Pickering QH, Robinson, EL, Stephan CE: Validity of laboratory tests for predicting copper toxicity in streams. U.S. EPA Ecol Res Ser EPA-600/3-76-116, 1976.

Giesy JP, Jr, Leversee GJ, Williams DR: Effects of naturally occurring aquatic organic fractions on cadmium toxicity to *Simocephalus serrulatus* (Daphnidae) and *Gambusia affinis* (Poeciliidae). Water Res 11:1013–1020, 1977.

Gudernatsch H: Verhalten von Nitrilotriessigsäure im Klärprozess und im Abwasser. Gas Wasserfach 111:511–516, 1970.

Guth DJ, Blankespoor HD, Cairns J, Jr: Potentiation of zinc stress caused by parasitic infection of snails. Hydrobiologia 55:225–229, 1977.

Henderson C, Pickering QH: Toxicity of organic phosphorus insecticides to fish. Trans Am Fish Soc 87:39–51, 1958.

Henderson C, Pickering QH, Cohen JM: The toxicity of synthetic detergents and soaps to fish. Sewage Ind Wastes 31:295–306, 1959a.

Henderson C, Pickering, QH, Tarzwell CM: Relative toxicity of ten chlorinated hydrocarbon insecticides to four species of fish. Trans Am Fish Soc 88:23–32, 1959b.

Herbert DWM, Shurben DS. A preliminary study of the effect of physical activity on the resistance of rainbow trout (*Salmo gairdneri* Richardson) to two poisons. Ann Appl Biol 52:321–326, 1963.

Herbert DWM, Shurben DS: The susceptibility of salmonid fish to poisons under estuarine conditions. II. Ammonium chloride. Int J Air Water Pollut 9:89–91, 1965.

Herbert DWM, Wakeford AC: The susceptibility of salmonid fish to poisons under estuarine conditions. I. Zinc sulphate. Int J Air Water Pollut 8:251–256, 1964.

Hicks DB, DeWitt JW: Effects of dissolved oxygen on kraft pulp mill effluent toxicity. Water Res 5:693–701, 1971.

Hodson PV: The effect of temperature on the toxicity of zinc to fish of the genus *Salmo*. PhD thesis, Univ of Guelph, Guelph, Ontario, Canada, 1974.

Hodson PV: Zinc uptake by Atlantic salmon (*Salmo salar*) exposed to a lethal concentration of zinc at 3, 11, and 19°C. J Fish Res Bd Can 32:2552–2556, 1975.

Hodson PV: Temperature effects on lactate-glycogen metabolism in zinc-intoxicated rainbow trout (*Salmo gairdneri*). J Fish Res Bd Can 33:1393–1397, 1976.

Hodson PV, Sprague JB: Temperature-induced changes in acute toxicity of zinc to Atlantic salmon (*Salmo salar*). J Fish Res Bd Can 32:1–10, 1975.

Hodson PV, Blunt BR, Spry DJ: pH-induced changes in blood lead of lead-exposed rainbow trout. J Fish Res Bd Can 35:437–445, 1978.

Hodson PV, Hilton JW, Blunt BR, Slinger SJ: Effects of dietary ascorbic acid on chronic lead toxicity to young rainbow trout (*Salmo gairdneri*). Can J Fish Aquat Sci 37:170–176, 1980.

Hokanson KEF, Smith LL, Jr: Some factors influencing toxicity of linear alkylate sulfonate (LAS) to the bluegill. Trans Am Fish Soc 100:1–12, 1971.

Holcombe GW, Fiandt JT, Phipps GL: Effects of pH increases and sodium chloride additions on the acute toxicity of 2,4-dichlorophenol to the fathead minnow. Water Res 14:1073–1077, 1980.

Houston AH: Osmoregulatory adaptation of steelhead trout (*Salmo gairdneri* Richardson) to sea water. Can J Zool 37:729–743, 1959.

Howarth RS, Sprague JB: Copper lethality to rainbow trout in waters of various hardness and pH. Water Res 12:455–462, 1978.

Inglis A, Davis EL: Effects of water hardness on the toxicity of several organic and inorganic herbicides to fish. U.S. Bur Sport Fish Wildl Tech Pap 67, 1972.

Irwin WH: Fifty-seven species of fish in oil-refinery waste bioassay. Trans 30th North Am Wildl Nat Resour Conf, pp. 89–99, 1965.

Johnson DW: Pesticides and fishes—A review of selected literature. Trans Am Fish Soc 97:398–424, 1968.

Johnson MW: The effectiveness of toxaphene at low temperatures. Minn Fish Game Invest Fish Ser 2:52–54, 1961.

Kinne O: Physiological aspects of animal life in estuaries with special reference to salinity. Neth J Sea Res 3:222–244, 1966.

Klapow LA, Lewis RH: Analysis of toxicity data for California marine water quality standards. J Water Pollut Control Fed 51:2054–2070, 1979.

Kleerekoper H, Waxman JB, Matis J: Interaction of temperature and copper ions as orienting stimuli in the locomotor behavior of the goldfish (*Carassius auratus*). J Fish Res Bd Can 30:725–728, 1973.

Koeppe R: The toxicology and toxicity of toxaphene with respect to fish and aquatic food animals. Z Fisch Deren Hilfswiss 9:771–794, 1961.

Kumaraguru AK, Beamish FWH: Lethal toxicity of Permethrin (NRDC-143) to rainbow trout, *Salmo gairdneri,* in relation to body weight and water temperature. Water Res 15:503–505, 1981.

Kwain W: Effects of temperature on development and survival of rainbow trout, *Salmo gairdneri,* in acid waters. J Fish Res Bd Can 32:493–497, 1975.

Lee DR, Buikema AR, Jr: Molt-related sensitivity of *Daphnia pulex* in toxicity testing. J Fish Res Bd Can 36:1129–1133, 1979.

Lett PF, Farmer GJ, Beamish FWH: Effect of copper on some aspects of the bioenergetics of rainbow trout (*Salmo gairdneri*). J Fish Res Bd Can 33:1335–1342, 1976.

Levitan WM, Taylor MH: Physiology of salinity-dependent naphthalene toxicity in *Fundulus heteroclitus.* J Fish Res Bd Can 36:615–620, 1979.

Lipschuetz M, Cooper AL: Toxicity of 2-secondary-butyl-4,6-dinitrophenol to blacknose dace and rainbow trout. NY Fish Game J 8:110–121, 1961.

Lloyd R: Effect of dissolved oxygen concentrations on the toxicity of several poisons to rainbow trout (*Salmo gairdnerii* Richardson). J Exp Biol 38:447–455, 1961a.

Lloyd R: The toxicity of ammonia to rainbow trout (*Salmo gairdnerii* Richardson). Water Waste Treatm J 8:278–279, 1961b.

Lloyd R: Factors that affect the tolerance of fish to heavy metal poisoning. Biological problems in water pollution, third seminar, 1962. U.S. Public Health Serv Publ 999-WP-25, pp. 181–187, 1965.

Lloyd R, Herbert DWM: The effect of the environment on the toxicity of poisons to fish. J Inst Public Health Eng 61:132–145, 1962.

Loch JS, MacLeod JC: Factors affecting acute toxicity bioassays with pulp mill effluent. Can Dept Environ Fish Mar Serv Tech Rept Ser No CEN/T-74-2, 1974.

Macek KJ: Growth and resistance to stress in brook trout fed sublethal levels of DDT. J Fish Res Bd Can 25:2443–2451, 1968.

Macek KJ, Hutchinson C, Cope OB: The effects of temperature on the susceptibility of bluegills and rainbow trout to selected pesticides. Bull Environ Contam Toxicol 4:174–183, 1969.

MacLeod JC, Pessah E: Temperature effects on mercury accumulation, toxicity, and metabolic rate in rainbow trout (*Salmo gairdneri*). J Fish Res Bd Can 30:485–492, 1973.

Mancy KH, Allen HE: A controlled bioassay system for measuring toxicity of heavy metals. U.S. EPA Rept EPA-600/3-77-037, 1977.

Marchetti R: Critical review of the effects of synthetic detergents on aquatic life. Stud Rev FAO Gen Fish Counc Mediterranean No. 26, 1965.

Marking LL: Effects of pH on toxicity of antimycin to fish. J Fish Res Bd Can 32:769–773, 1975.

Marking LL, Bills TD: Toxicity of rotenone to fish in standardized laboratory tests. U.S. Dept

Inter Fish Wildl Serv Invest Fish Control No. 72, 1976.

Mauck WL, Olson LE, Hogan JW: Effects of water quality on deactivation and toxicity of mexacarbate (Zectran) to fish. Arch Environ Contam Toxicol 6:385–393, 1977.

Mayer FL, Mehrle PM, Crutcher PL: Interactions of toxaphene and vitamin C in channel catfish. Trans Am Fish Soc 107:326–333, 1978.

McCrady JK, Chapman GA: Determination of copper complexing capacity of natural river water, well water and artificially reconstituted water. Water Res 13:143–150, 1979.

McKim JM: Evaluation of tests with early life stages of fish for predicting long-term toxicity. J Fish Res Bd Can 34:1148–1154, 1977.

McKim JM, Benoit DA: Effects of long-term exposures to copper on survival, growth, and reproduction of brook trout (*Salvelinus fontinalis*). J Fish Res Bd Can 28:655–662, 1971.

McLeay DJ, Gordon MR: Effect of seasonal photoperiod on acute toxic responses of juvenile rainbow trout (*Salmo gairdneri*) to pulp mill effluent. J Fish Res Bd Can 35:1388–1392, 1978.

McLeay DJ, Munro JR: Photoperiodic acclimation and circadian variations in tolerance of juvenile rainbow trout (*Salmo gairdneri*) to zinc. Bull Environ Contam Toxicol 23:552–557, 1979.

McLeay DJ, Walden CC, Munro JR: Influence of dilution water on the toxicity of kraft pulp and paper mill effluent, including mechanisms of effect. Water Res 13:151–158, 1979a.

McLeay DJ, Walden CC, Munro JR: Effect of pH on toxicity of kraft pulp and paper mill effluent to salmonid fish in fresh and seawater. Water Res 13:249–254, 1979b.

McLeese DW: Effects of temperature, salinity and oxygen on the survival of the American lobster. J Fish Res Bd Can 13:247–272, 1956.

McLeese DW: Toxicity of copper at two temperatures and three salinities to the American lobster (*Homarus americanus*). J Fish Res Bd Can 31:1949–1952, 1974.

Mehrle PM, Mayer FL, Johnson WW: Diet quality in fish toxicology: Effects on acute and chronic toxicity. In: Aquatic Toxicology and Hazard Evaluation, edited by FL Mayer and JL Hamelink, pp. 269–280. ASTM Spec Tech Rept 634, 1977.

Miller TG, Mackay WC: The effects of hardness, alkalinity and pH of test water on the toxicity of copper to rainbow trout (*Salmo gairdneri*). Water Res 14:129–133, 1980.

Mount DI: Chronic toxicity of copper to fathead minnows (*Pimephales promelas*, Rafinesque). Water Res 2:215–223, 1968.

Mount DI, Stephan CE: Chronic toxicity of copper to the fathead minnow (*Pimephales promelas*) in soft water. J Fish Res Bd Can 26: 2449–2457, 1969.

NAS/NAE (National Academy of Sciences, National Academy of Engineering): Water Quality Criteria 1972. U.S. EPA Ecol Res Ser EPA-R-73-033, p. 594, 1974.

Nriagu JO, Wong HKT, Coker RD: Particulate and dissolved trace metals in Lake Ontario. Water Res 15:91–96, 1981.

Olson R, Harrel RC: Effect of salinity on acute toxicity of mercury, copper, and chromium for *Rangia cuneata* (Pelecypoda, Mactridae). Contrib Mar Sci 17:9–13, 1973.

Opuszyński K: Temperature preference of fathead minnow *Pimephales promelas* (Rafinesque) and its changes induced by copper salt $CuSO_4$. Pol Arch Hydrobiol 18:401–408, 1971.

Oseid DM, Smith LL, Jr: Factors influencing acute toxicity estimates of hydrogen sulfide to freshwater invertebrates. Water Res 8:739–746, 1974.

Pagenkopf GK, Russo RC, Thurston RV: Effect of complexation on toxicity of copper to fishes. J Fish Res Bd Can 31:461–465, 1974.

Pascoe D, Cram P: The effect of parasitism on the toxicity of cadmium to the three-spined stickleback, *Gasterosteus aculeatus* L. J Fish Biol 10: 467–472, 1977.

Pesch CE, Morgan D: Influence of sediment in copper toxicity tests with the polychaeta *Neanthes arenaceodentata*. Water Res 12:747–751, 1978.

Phillips GR, Buhler DR: Influences of dieldrin on the growth and body composition of fingerling rainbow trout (*Salmo gairdneri*) fed Oregon moist pellets or tubificid worms (*Tubifex* sp.). J Fish Res Bd Can 36:77–80, 1979.

Pickering QH: Some effects of dissolved oxygen concentrations upon the toxicity of zinc to the bluegill, *Lepomis macrochirus*, Raf. Water Res 2:187–194, 1968.

Pickering QH, Henderson C: Acute toxicity of some important petrochemicals to fish. J Water Pollut Control Fed 38:1419–1429, 1966a.

Pickering QH, Henderson C: The acute toxicity of some heavy metals to different species of warmwater fishes. Int J Air Water Pollut 10:453–463, 1966b.

Pickering QH, Henderson C: The acute toxicity of some pesticides to fish. Ohio J Sci 66:508–513, 1966c.

Pickering QH, Henderson C, Lemke AE: The toxicity of organic phosphorus insecticides to different species of warmwater fishes. Trans Am Fish Soc 91:175–184, 1962.

Rehwoldt R, Menapace LW, Nerrie B, Alessandrello D: The effect of increased temperature upon the acute toxicity of some heavy metal ions. Bull Environ Contam Toxicol 8:91–96, 1972.

Reiff B, Lloyd R, How MJ, Brown D, Alabaster JS: The acute toxicity of eleven detergents to fish: Results of an interlaboratory exercise. Water Res 13:207–210, 1979.

Reinert RE, Stone LJ, Willford WA: Effect of temperature on accumulation of methylmercuric chloride and p,p'-DDT by rainbow trout (*Salmo gairdneri*). J Fish Res Bd Can 31:1649–1652, 1974.

Russo RC, Thurston RV, Emerson K: Acute toxicity of nitrite to rainbow trout (*Salmo gairdneri*): Effects of pH, nitrite species, and anion species. Can J Fish Aquat Sci 38:387–393, 1981.

Sanders HO, Cope OB: Toxicities of several pesticides to two species of cladocerans. Trans Am Fish Soc 95:165–169, 1966.

Sano H: The role of pH on the acute toxicity of sulfite in water. Water Res 10:139–142, 1976.

Schaefer ED, Pipes WO: Temperature and the toxicity of chromate and arsenate to the rotifer, *Philodina roseola*. Water Res 7:1781–1790, 1973.

Shepard MP: Resistance and tolerance of young speckled trout (*Salvelinus fontinalis*) to oxygen lack, with special reference to low oxygen acclimation. J Fish Res Bd Can 12:387–446, 1955.

Skidmore JF: Respiration and osmoregulation in rainbow trout with gills damaged by zinc sulphate. J Exp Biol 52:481–494, 1970.

Skidmore JF, Tovell PWA: Toxic effects of zinc sulphate on the gills of rainbow trout. Water Res 6:217–230, 1972.

Slonin AR: Acute toxicity of selected hydrazines to the common guppy. Water Res 11:889–895, 1977.

Smith LL, Oseid DM: Effects of hydrogen sulfide on fish eggs and fry. Water Res 6:711–720, 1972.

Smith MW: Copper sulphate and rotenone as fish poisons. Trans Am Fish Soc 69:141–157, 1939.

Sosnowski SL, Germond DJ, Gentile JH: The effect of nutrition on the response of field populations of the calanoid copepod *Acartia tonsa* to copper. Water Res 13:449–452, 1979.

Sparks RE, Walker WT, Cairns J, Jr: Effect of shelters on the resistance of dominant and submissive bluegills (*Lepomis macrochirus*) to a lethal concentration of zinc. J Fish Res Bd Can 29:1356–1358, 1972.

Spear PA, Pierce RC: Copper in the aquatic environment: Chemistry, distribution and toxicology. Natl Res Counc Can Environ Secretariat NRCC No. 16454, 1979.

Sprague JB: Promising anti-pollutant: Chelating agent NTA protects fish from copper and zinc. Nature (London) 220:1345–1346, 1968.

Sprague JB, Logan WJ: Separate and joint toxicity to rainbow trout of substances used in drilling fluids for oil exploration. Environ Pollut 19:269–281, 1979.

Sprague JB, Rowe DW, Westlake GF, Heming TA, Brown IT: Sublethal effects of treated liquid effluent from a petroleum refinery on freshwater organisms. Ottawa: Petroleum Association for Conservation of the Canadian Environment, and Fisheries and Environment Canada, Environmental Protection Service, 1978.

Steemann Nielsen E, Wium-Andersen S: Copper ions as poison in the sea and in freshwater. Mar Biol 6:93–97, 1970.

Stegeman JJ: Temperature influence on basal activity and induction of mixed function oxygenase activity in *Fundulus heteroclitus*. J Fish Res Bd Can 36:1400–1405, 1979.

Stiff MJ: Copper/bicarbonate equilibria in solutions of bicarbonate ion at concentrations similar to those found in natural water. Water Res 5:171–176, 1971a.

Stiff MJ: The chemical states of copper in polluted freshwater and a scheme to differentiate them. Water Res 5:585–599, 1971b.

Sunda WG, Guillard RR: Relationship between cupric ion activity and toxicity of copper to phytoplankton. J Mar Res 34:511–529, 1976.

Sylva RN: The environmental chemistry of copper (II) in aquatic systems. Water Res 10:789–792, 1976.

Teulin MP: An improved experimental medium for freshwater toxicity studies using *Daphnia magna*. Water Res 12:1027–1034, 1978.

Thurston RV, Phillips GR, Russo RC: Increased toxicity of ammonia to rainbow trout (*Salmo gairdneri*) resulting from reduced concentrations of dissolved oxygen. Can J Fish Aquat Sci 38:983–988, 1981.

Tovell PWA, Newsome C, Howes D: Effect of water hardness on the toxicity of a nonionic detergent to fish. Water Res 9:31–36, 1975.

Van den Berg CMG, Wong PTS, Chau YK: Measurement of complexing materials excreted from algae and their ability to ameliorate copper toxicity. J Fish Res Bd Can 36:901–905, 1979.

Vernberg WB, O'Hara J: Temperature-salinity stress and mercury uptake in the fiddler crab, *Uca pugilator*. J Fish Res Bd Can 29:1491–1494, 1972.

Voyer RA: Effect of dissolved oxygen concentrations on the acute toxicity of cadmium to the mummichog *Fundulus heteroclitus* (L.) at various salinities. Trans Am Fish Soc 104:129–134, 1975.

Waiwood KG, Beamish FWH: Effects of copper, pH and hardness on the critical swimming performance of rainbow trout (*Salmo gairdneri* Richardson). Water Res 12:611–619, 1978a.

Waiwood KG, Beamish FWH: The effect of copper, hardness and pH on the growth of rainbow trout *Salmo gairdneri*. J Fish Biol 13:591–598, 1978b.

Wilson RCH: Prediction of copper toxicity in receiving waters. J Fish Res Bd Can 29:1500–1502, 1972.

Woodward DF: Toxicity of the herbicides Dinoseb and Picloram to cutthroat (*Salmo clarkii*) and lake trout (*Salvelinus namaycush*). J Fish Res Bd Can 33:1671–1676, 1976.

Woodward DF, Mayer FL, Jr: Toxicity of three herbicides (butyl, isoocytl, and propylene glycol butyl ether esters of 2,4-D) to cutthroat trout and lake trout. U.S. Dept Inter Fish Wildl Serv Tech Pap 97, 1978.

Zitko V, Carson WG: A mechanism of the effects of water hardness on the lethality of heavy metals to fish. Chemosphere 5:299–303, 1976.

Zitko V, Carson WV, Carson WG: Prediction of incipient lethal levels of copper to juvenile Atlantic salmon in the presence of humic acid by cupric electrode. Bull Environ Contam Toxicol 10:265–271, 1973.

SUPPLEMENTAL READING

Alabaster JS, Lloyd R: Water quality criteria for freshwater fish. London: Butterworths, 1980.

Alderdice DF: Factor combinations. Responses of marine poikioltherms to environmental factors acting in concert. In: Marine Ecology, vol. 1, Environmental Factors, part 3, edited by O Kinne, pp. 1659–1722. London: Wiley-Interscience, 1972.

Brown VM: The calculation of the acute toxicity of mixtures of poisons to rainbow trout. Water Res 2:723–733, 1968.

Cairns J, Jr, Heath AG, Parker BC: Temperature influence on chemical toxicity to aquatic organisms. J Water Pollut Control Fed 47:267–280, 1975.

Fry FEJ: The effect of environmental factors on the physiology of fish. In: Fish Physiology, vol. 6, Environmental Relations and Behaviour, edited by WS Hoar, DJ Randall, pp. 1–98. New York: Academic, 1971.

Chapter 7

Toxicity of Chemical Mixtures

L. L. Marking

INTRODUCTION

Mixtures of chemicals have long been known to have advantages over chemicals applied singly. Historically, this knowledge was applied in the preparation of "magic potions" from roots and herbs. In the 20th century it has led to the evolution of the science of pharmacology and, more recently, to the development of chemical mixtures for use in agriculture and pest control. Reported advantages of mixtures include (1) increased effectiveness against target organisms, (2) increased safety of nontarget organisms, (3) applications of smaller quantities of material without a reduction in effectiveness, so that smaller residual quantities are left in the environment, and (4) reduced costs for material and application.

The concepts and terminology used in toxicology have been confusing because the methodologies used have not been standardized. Although each scientific discipline has addressed the problem somewhat differently, the literature suggests that procedures are similar enough to be standardized.

A frequent misconception is that the toxicity of chemical mixtures results from simple addition or summation of the activities of the components. Instead, additive toxicity covers the full range between the general terms antagonism and synergism, because at both extremes there is a summation of toxic action. The degree of antagonism or synergism must be defined and quantified before the advantages or disadvantages of chemical mixtures can be understood and assessed.

TERMINOLOGY AND DEFINITIONS

The terms synergism and antagonism are often used to describe a phenomenon in toxicology and pharmacology in which the effects resulting from exposure to mixtures of chemicals are greater than (synergism) or less than (antagonism) expected on the basis of the effects of exposure to each chemical individually. Because the terms are nonquantitative, they are often used ambiguously. A better system of terminology and quantitation is needed (Fingl and Woodbury, 1965). Sprague (1970) suggested that terms such as synergism and potentiation might well be avoided since they have been defined differently by different authors. Calamari and Alabaster (1980) reported that terminology on this subject is still confusing, and thought that the ideal model should describe the effects of mixtures of chemicals as simply additive, more than additive (synergistic), or less than additive (antagonistic) according to Sprague's (1970) interpretation.

Kobayashi (1978) compared methods for determining the toxicity of mixtures of chemicals and the terminology used to define the results. Many of the methods compared favorably in that they summed the toxic effects of chemical mixtures, but there was little consistency in the terminology. The literature on mixture toxicity reflects the inconsistent nomenclature, and more recent interpretations suggest that use of the terms "greater than additive," "additive," and "less than additive" would be helpful in quantitating the three categories of toxicity of mixtures. This additive toxicity concept is used here whenever appropriate, to promote the use of standard definitions and to enhance understanding of mixture toxicity. Among the terms that have been used to describe the three categories are the following:

Mixture toxicity studies are often referred to as interaction studies. The interactions are generally between the chemicals and physiological systems within the body rather than between the chemicals. Many interactions are so complex, obscure, or trivial that they remain undetected; however, the mechanisms of some of these interactions have been elucidated (Hayes, 1975; Frawley et al., 1957). Drug interactions may arise from alteration of the absorption, distribution, biotransformation, or excretion of one drug by another, or from a combination of their actions or effects (Fingl and Woodbury, 1965).

If two drugs have the same overt effect, they are termed homergic; if only one of a pair of drugs produces an effect, they are termed heterergic (Fingl and Woodbury, 1965). In either case, the combination of drugs can result in toxicity that is simply additive or greater than or less than additive.

Commercial synergists (e.g., methylenedioxyphenyl compounds) are often used to enhance the activity of insecticides. Piperonyl butoxide, sulfoxide, and Tropital are representative of such compounds and are used effectively in combination with insecticides (Parmer and Mukerjee, 1974) and fish toxicants (Marking, 1977). By definition, a synergist enhances or potentiates the activity of another compound. In the insecticide industry, the contribution of the synergist to toxicity is often discounted. However, the addition of a synergist to formulations of the piscicide rotenone produced a toxicity that was more than additive (synergistic) when calculated on the basis of the individual contributions of

Greater than additive	Additive	Less than additive
Synergism	Expected action	Antagonism
Supra-additive	Simple addition	Infra-additive
Synergistic action	Additive action	Antagonistic action
Potentiation	Addition	Competitive addition
Positive summation	Summation	Competitive antagonism
Joint action	Joint action	Joint action
Interaction	Interaction	Interaction

toxic effects of the synergists and rotenone (Marking, 1977).

HISTORY AND DEVELOPMENT OF MIXTURE TOXICITY CONCEPTS

Commercial use of drug and pesticide mixtures has become widespread only within the past few decades. In drug therapy and pest control, some mixtures have negative effects that may result in increased risk to a patient or to nontarget organisms in the environment. A better understanding of mixture toxicity is needed to help predict whether certain mixtures will have positive or negative effects.

Loewe and Muischnek (1926) devised a simple means of displaying results on chemical mixture toxicity that could be interpreted as greater than additive (synergism), additive, and less than additive (antagonism) (see Fig. 1). Their "isobole" concept was the basis for development of most of the procedures that eventually evolved for assessing toxicity of mixtures. The isobole [derived from isos (meaning equal) and bolos (blow or strike)] represents the results obtained with two com-

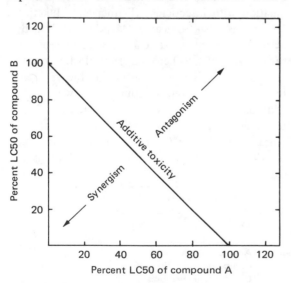

Figure 1 Isobole of LC50 values of compounds A and B; additive toxicity is represented by the diagonal line. *[Modified from Loewe and Muischnek (1926).]*

pounds administered in different ratios. The exception occurs at the 50% level, where components A and B contribute equal effects. The solid line in Fig. 1 is the isobole of exactly additive effects at all dosage ratios. For instance, the midpoint of the isobole indicates that 50% of the LC50 of compound A (LC50/2) plus 50% of the LC50 of compound B (LC50/2) will yield a mixture that produces one LC50. Likewise, 75% of the LC50 of compound A plus 25% of the LC50 of compound B will yield a mixture that produces one LC50. Additive action is the most common form of mixture toxicity, and greater than additive or less than additive actions are exceptions. The area to the right and above the isobole in Fig. 1 represents less than additive action (antagonism) and the area to the left and below it represents greater than additive action (synergism).

The basic concept of mixture toxicity (sometimes referred to as joint action) was described by Bliss (1939) and further defined by Finney (1942). Finney's concepts and formulas for additive joint toxicity provided a means of testing the hypothesis that the toxicity of chemical mixtures is simply additive on the basis of the harmonic means of the LC50s for mixture components. Finney's concepts were extremely detailed and complicated, and some investigators criticized the method because of its complexity (Sun and Johnson, 1960).

The toxic strength of an individual compound may be expressed as a "toxic unit"; the toxic strength of a mixture of compounds may be determined by summing the strengths of individual compounds. British researchers investigated methods of predicting the toxic effects of chemical mixtures in water by summing toxic units of individual toxic materials (Lloyd, 1961; Herbert and Shurben, 1964; Herbert and Vandyke, 1964; Brown, 1968; Brown et al., 1968, 1969; Brown and Dalton, 1970). Their original method was to sum fractions of threshold concentrations to obtain unity (1.0 toxic unit). The concept was basically similar to the isobole theory.

Sprague and Ramsey (1965) used the method

of summing toxic units to predict the toxicity of copper and zinc mixtures to Atlantic salmon (*Salmo salar*). They concluded that the exposure times required to produce mortality for the two metals were similar because the sum of the toxic units was 1.0. At higher concentrations of the metals, however, the summation of toxic units indicated more than additive effects, which supported previous reports in the literature. Later, Sprague and Logan (1979) demonstrated less than additive or additive toxicity of hydraulic drilling fluids to rainbow trout (*Salmo gairdneri*) by comparing results obtained with different ratios of fluids to isoboles for additive toxicity.

Calamari and Marchetti (1973) used the toxic unit concept to determine the toxicity of mixtures of metals and surfactants to rainbow trout in 14-d exposures. They concluded that metals and anionic detergents produced "more than additive" effects, but metals and nonionic detergents produced "less than additive" effects. However, their conclusions were based on toxic unit results rather than quantitative indices.

Other techniques for evaluating the toxicity of mixtures of chemicals to mammals were developed (Keplinger and Deichmann, 1967; Smyth et al., 1969), and most of them followed the mathematical model for additive toxicity (isobole theory) that yields the harmonic mean of the LC50s for the combined components. Smyth et al. (1969) normalized the values obtained from Finney's (1942) equation with a frequency distribution curve and adjusted the values to indicate additive toxicity with a zero. Smyth et al. (1970) derived joint toxicity values in terms of adjusted ratios for mixtures of industrial organic chemicals fed to rats.

RECENT DEVELOPMENTS IN MIXTURE TOXICITY ASSESSMENT

Marking and Dawson (1975) adapted existing methods, concepts, and terminology related to additive toxicity to derive a quantitative index for the toxicity of mixtures of chemicals in water.

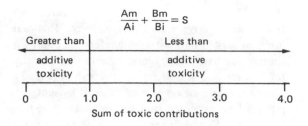

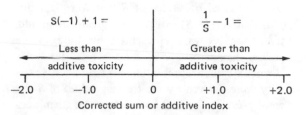

Figure 2 Sums S of toxic contributions for a chemical mixture, which are nonlinear for less than additive and greater than additive toxicity (top), are corrected for linearity and direction of plus and minus values (bottom). *[From Marking and Dawson (1975).]*

Their technique was based on the isobole theory and involved use of the toxic unit concept to sum the action of various components of a mixture according to the formula: $Am/Ai + Bm/Bi = S$, where A and B are chemicals, i and m are the toxicities (LC50s) of A and B individually and in a mixture, and S is the sum of activity.

Assuming that A and B are equitoxic and have similar modes of toxic action, any fractional combination of the two chemicals that equaled one toxicant would have the same effect as one toxic unit of either material. These values can be substituted into the formula; for instance, if each chemical contributes $\frac{1}{2}$ toxic unit, $Am/Ai + Bm/Bi = \frac{1}{2} + \frac{1}{2} = 1.0$ or S. This sum alone can be used as a quantitative indicator of additive toxicity, and some researchers have used the value S or a factor of S to define additive toxicity (Hayes, 1975; Carpenter et al., 1961). However, S values greater than 1.0 that indicate less than additive toxicity are not synchronous with values less than 1.0 that indicate greater than additive toxicity (Fig. 2).

Marking and Dawson (1975) devised a system in which additive, greater than additive, and less than additive effects are represented by zero, positive, and negative values, respectively. This was done by assigning zero as the reference point for simple additive toxicity and establishing linearity for greater and less than additive values (Fig. 2). The zero reference point was obtained by subtracting 1.0 (the expected sum for simple additive toxicity) from S, and linearity was achieved by using the reciprocal of values of S that were less than 1.0–that is, $[(1/S) - 1]$. Thus, greater than additive toxicity was represented by index values greater than zero.

Index values representing less than additive toxicity were derived by multiplying values of S that were greater than 1.0 by -1 to make them negative, and a zero reference point was established by adding 1.0 to this negative value $[S(-1) + 1]$. As a result, less than additive toxicity was represented by negative index values.

A sum S of 1.0 yields an index value of zero by either procedure and thus represents simple additive toxicity. A summary of the procedure follows:

$$\frac{Am}{Ai} + \frac{Bm}{Bi} = S, \text{ the sum toxic action}$$

$$\text{For } S \leqslant 1.0 \text{ the additive index} = \frac{1}{S} - 1.0$$

$$\text{For } S \geqslant 1.0 \text{ the additive index} = S(-1) + 1$$

For additional chemicals in the mixture, $Am/Ai + Bm/Bi + Cm/Ci + \ldots = S$.

The application of an additive toxicity index can be illustrated by selecting toxicity data from papers in which data were provided for components individually and in mixtures. Douderoff (1952), who studied the toxic activity of mixtures of zinc and copper, observed extraordinary toxic effects on fathead minnows (*Pimephales promelas*) in 8-h tests in which survival was recorded rather than LC50s. The additive index is $1.0/8.0 + 0.025/0.20 = 0.250$, which is less than 1.0; therefore $1/S - 1.0 = 1/0.250 - 1 = 3$, a value that strongly supports Douderoff's conclusions (Table 1). Lloyd (1961) and Sprague and Ramsay (1965) found no potentiation in zinc and copper mixtures, but they defined the toxicity with LC50s for longer exposures. However, they did report that lethal mixtures of those metal ions acted 2 to 3 times as fast as the metals did singly.

Cairns and Scheier (1968) reported "slight antagonistic interaction" of zinc and cyanide to fathead minnows, in contrast to the activity of combinations of zinc and copper. They attributed the effect to formation of chemical complexes. The additive index (-1.37) indicates less than additive toxicity. Chen and Selleck (1969) also found zinc and cyanide combinations to be very antagonistic, but they did not quantify the toxicity.

Howland (1969) reported additive effects for mixtures of two fish toxicants, antimycin and rotenone. The additive index calculated from his data was -0.39 (Table 1). Although the index value suggests less than additive toxicity, the significance of the value (discussed later) must be defined before the results can be interpreted.

The additive index method can be used to describe characteristics other than toxicity (Marking and Dawson, 1975). For instance, a mixture of two fish anesthetics that were known individually for rapid action (MS-222, tricaine methanesulfonate) and for sustained anesthetic effect [quinaldine sulfate (Qd SO$_4$)] had greater efficacy and a better safety factor than did either of the two compounds alone. An index value of 0.29 (Table 1) suggests greater than additive efficacy and agrees with Berger's (1969) interpretation that the action was synergistic, but no level of significance was assigned to the index value. Schoettger and Steucke (1970) discussed advantages of the anesthetic mixture, including a cost reduction of 60 to 80%. Dawson and Marking (1973) reported additive toxicity of mixtures of these anesthetics to six species of fish in laboratory tests. Mixtures of the therapeutants malachite green and formalin also had desirable effects in controlling fish diseases (Table 1).

Table 1   Toxicity or Efficacy of Chemicals Applied Individually and in Combination against Fishes and the Calculated Additive Index[a]

Chemical mixtures and toxic units	96-h LC50 or EC50 of chemicals		Additive index	Reference
	Individually	In combination		
Zinc[b] (mg/l) and	8.0	1.0	3.00	Doudoroff (1952)
Copper[b] (mg/l)	0.2	0.025		
Zinc (mg/l) and	4.2	3.90	−1.37	Cairns and Scheier (1968)
Cyanide (mg/l)	0.18	0.26		
Antimycin (μg/l) and	0.032	0.027	−0.39	Howland (1969)
Rotenone (μg/l)	57.0	31.0		
MS-222 (mg/l) and	80	30	0.29	Berger (1969)
QdSO$_4$ (mg/l)	25	10		
Malachite green (mg/l) and	0.2	0.05	0.83	Leteux and Meyer (1972)
Formalin[c] (mg/l)	50	15		

[a]From Marking and Dawson (1975).
[b]An 8-h time response, based on survival rather than LC50.
[c]Concentrations effective against parasites.

SIGNIFICANCE OF INDEX VALUES

Additive index values in Table 1 range from −1.37 to +3.00. The values near zero, such as +0.29 and −0.39, may not be significantly different from zero (additive toxicity). To deal with this, some investigators arbitrarily chose ranges of S to identify toxicity that was greater than or less than additive. For instance, on a nonlinear scale (where additive effects = 1.0), Kobayashi (1978) recommended that values of S between 0.5 and 2.0 be considered simple additive effects. In Kobayashi's review of literature on the subject, he also stated that a range of 0.67 to 1.5 and less than 1 degree (assume 1.0 unit) should be judged as additive toxicity. Because the assessments and ranges set for additive toxicity values are inconsistent, a more precise method is needed.

Marking and Dawson (1975) provided a system for judging whether additive index values were different from zero (additive toxicity). The significance of deviation from zero was determined by substituting the 95% confidence intervals for the LC50s into the additive index formula to establish a range for the additive indices. The range was derived by selecting values of the 95% confidence interval that yielded the greatest deviation from the additive index. The lower limits of the individual toxicants (Ai and Bi) and the upper limits of the mixtures (Am and Bm) were substituted for LC50s to determine the lower value of the index. Correspondingly, the upper limits of the individual toxicants (Ai and Bi) and the lower limits of the mixtures (Am and Bm) were substituted into the formula to determine the upper value of the index. Mixtures that resulted in ranges for the additive index that overlapped zero were judged to be only additive in toxicity; ranges that did not overlap zero were either greater or less than additive in toxicity.

Marking (1977) further enhanced the meaning of index values by defining magnification factors that describe the magnitude of additive toxicity. For instance, if the toxicity of a mixture increased twofold (magnification factor = 2) over the expected simple additive toxicity (that is, $Am = 1$, $Ai = 4$, $Bm = 1$, $Bi = 4$, and $Am/Ai + Bm/Bi = S$), then $\frac{1}{4} + \frac{1}{4} = \frac{1}{2}$ or 0.5. Since 0.5 is less than 1.0, the additive index is $1/S - 1 = 1/0.5 - 1 = 1.0$. Correspondingly, the magnification factors for mixtures are obtained with index values as follows:

Index value	Magnification factor
9	10×
1	2×
0	1×
−1	1/2×
−9	1/10×

Accordingly, the magnification factor can be obtained by adding 1.0 to the numerical index value. For less than additive values, the factor must be reciprocated.

Magnification of the toxicity of mixtures is difficult to judge by visual inspection of index values, especially if the ratios of chemicals are different from 1:1. According to Kobayashi (1978), Frawley et al. (1957) estimated that mixtures of EPN and malathion (two organophosphate insecticides) produced about a tenfold potentiation. When Kobayashi (1978) used the formula of Carpenter et al. (1961) to determine the degree of synergism, he obtained a value of 4.5. When the same values were introduced into the additive index formula, these values resulted: $Am/Ai + Bm/Bi = 6.6/65 + 167/1400 = 0.101 + 0.119 = 0.220$; additive index $= 1/S - 1.0 = 1/0.220 - 1 = 4.5 - 1 = 3.5$; magnification factor = additive index + 1.0 = 4.5. The magnification factor provided by Marking (1977) agrees with the degrees of synergism provided by Carpenter et al. (1961); only the terminology is different. The two calculated values were identical at 4.5, yet Frawley et al. (1957) estimated the potentiation to be about tenfold by visual inspection.

EXPERIMENTAL WORK WITH ADDITIVE INDEX CONCEPT

Marking (1977) gave examples of the use of mixtures of chemicals against rainbow trout to determine additive indices and ranges for the indices that were calculated from confidence limits. A mixture of the piscicide antimycin and the organic insecticide Dibrom was reported by Berger (1971) to be synergistically toxic to black bullheads (*Ictalurus melas*), largemouth bass (*Micropterus salmoides*), and yellow perch (*Perca flavescens*). However, the toxicity proved to be less than additive against rainbow trout because the range for the additive index of −0.574 did not overlap zero (Table 2).

The lampricides TFM and Bayer 73 are commonly applied in a 98:2 ratio and were reported to be synergistically toxic to sea lamprey (*Petromyzon marinus*) by Howell et al. (1964). However, Dawson et al. (1977) demonstrated in the laboratory that the same mixture was additive or less than additive in toxicity to sea lamprey. Bills and Marking (1976) concluded that the 98:2 ratio of lampricides was also additive in toxicity to rainbow trout (Table 2) as well as six other species of fish. However, Howell et al. (1964) based their judgment on the economic advantage of adding a chemical that was more toxic than TFM.

Mixtures of malathion and Delnav, two organophosphate insecticides, were reported to be synergistic against insects, and their combined toxicity to fish was definitely greater than additive (Table 2). The additive index value of 7.2 suggests that the combination is 8.2 (magnification factor) times more toxic than the individual chemicals.

Rotenone, a common insecticide, has been registered for use as a fish toxicant, and many formulations are available, including some that contain synergists. The toxicity of rotenone mixed with piperonyl butoxide or sulfoxide is more than additive; the additive indices were 2.36 and 2.13 when the chemicals were applied in a 1:1 ratio of their LC50s (Table 3). When the ratios of rotenone and sulfoxide were altered, the toxicity of the

Table 2 Toxicity and Additive Indices for Chemicals and Pairs of Chemicals against Rainbow Trout in Soft Water at 12°C[a]

Toxicant, unit, and ratio	LC50 and 95% confidence interval		Additive index and range
	Individually	In combination	
Antimycin (μg/l)	0.0312	0.0300	
	0.0266–0.0366	0.0272–0.0331	
and			−0.574
			−1.43 to −0.173
Dibrom (mg/l)	0.0490	0.0490	
(1:1 of LC50s)	0.0279–0.0633	0.0272–0.0331	
TFM lampricide (mg/l)	1.81	1.16	
	1.53–2.14	0.998–1.35	
and			−0.326
			−0.808 to 0.0295
Bayer 73 lampricide (mg/l)	0.0346	0.0237	
(98:2)	0.0297–0.0404	0.0204–0.0275	
Malathion (μg/l)	70.0	3.44	
	59.2–82.7	2.92–4.06	
and			7.20
			5.09 to 10.0
Delnav (μg/l)	47.2	3.44	
(1:1 of LC50s)	42.4–52.6	2.92–4.06	

[a]From Bills and Marking (1976) and Marking and Dawson (1975).

Table 3 Additive Toxicity of Paired Chemicals to Rainbow Trout in Soft Water at 12°C[a]

Mixture and ratio	Additive index	Range
Rotenone, piperonyl butoxide (1:1 of LC50s)	+2.36	
Rotenone, sulfoxide (1:1 of LC50s)	+2.13	
Rotenone, sulfoxide (1:2)	+1.81	
Rotenone, sulfoxide (1:1)	+1.39	
Rotenone, sulfoxide (2:1)	+0.416	

[a]From Marking (1977); copyright American Society for Testing and Materials, Philadelphia.

mixtures decreased from 1:2 to 1:1 and 2:1. The 1:1 ratio of rotenone to sulfoxide typifies Pro-Noxfish, a commercially available formulation containing 2.5% of each component. All ratios were synergistic, but the 1:2 ratio offers greater toxicity, may have economic advantages, and may be less contaminating. Also, the synergized rotenone in Pro-Noxfish (2.5%) was as effective as an equal amount of unsynergized formulation containing 5% rotenone (magnification factor >2). These data confirm the earlier observations of Hester (1959), who reported synergistic effects of sulfoxide and rotenone on fish.

The additive index concept has been recognized by many investigators as having advantages over previous procedures. Tucker and Leitzke (1979) described the quantitative advantages of the additive index concept. McLeese and Metcalfe (1979) used the additive index concept of Marking and Dawson (1975) and the toxic unit concept of Sprague and Ramsey (1965) to attempt to determine whether mixtures of phosphamidon and methidathion were additive or greater than additive in toxicity to lobsters (*Homarus americanus*). They found that both procedures identified the mixtures as additive or greater than additive in toxicity, and that the degree of toxicity was dependent on the ratio of the components. Gehrs et al. (1979) showed that the toxicities of effluent components to *Daphnia* were additive (index = 0.03 and 0.00). In studies with fathead minnows and rainbow trout, Broderius and Smith (1979) reported greater than additive toxicity for mixtures of zinc and hydrogen cyanide and mixtures of ammonia and hydrogen cyanide, but less than additive toxicity for chromium and hydrogen cyanide. Passino and Kramer (1980) demonstrated that mixtures of PCBs and arsenic were additive in toxicity to deepwater ciscoes (*Coregonus* sp.). Tsai and McKee (1978) used the procedure to define additive toxicity values for mixtures of chloramines, LAS, and copper to goldfish (*Carassius auratus*). Marking and Mauck (1975) also used it to study effects of mixtures of candidate forest insecticides on rainbow trout. Of the 20

mixtures used in their work, 9 produced less than additive, 9 additive, and 2 greater than additive toxicity.

DISCUSSION

Mixture toxicity studies have been reported for a wide variety of chemicals and organisms. Tests with organophosphate insecticides often indicate greater than additive toxicity. Kreitzer and Spann (1973) reported that malathion plus EPN and malathion plus trichlorofon were synergistically toxic to quail and pheasants, and 8 of 11 pairs of pesticides were synergistically toxic to rats, mice, dogs, and two species of insects. A mixture of malathion and Delnav produced an additive index of 7.2 (Marking, 1977) for rainbow trout, providing further evidence of broad-spectrum synergism of mixtures of organophosphate insecticides.

Most of the results referred to here were observed when pairs of chemicals were simultaneously added to test media. Inadvertent combinations of chemicals occur in the environment because some compounds persist for long periods or are applied repeatedly. More recently, combinations of chemicals have been applied to increase efficacy or reduce cost (Howell et al., 1964; Brown and Nishioka, 1967). Chemical combinations altered the tissue storage capacity for DDT in exposed rainbow trout (Mayer et al., 1970), and residues of the PCB Aroclor 1254 altered the sensitivity of rainbow trout to other chemicals (Bills et al., 1977). In houseflies, Plapp (1972) demonstrated that Aroclor 1254 was a powerful synergist for the carbamate insecticide carbaryl. In mice, dietary intake of polybrominated biphenyl (PBB) greatly enhanced the toxicity of carbon tetrachloride (Kluive and Hook, 1978). Statham and Lech (1975) reported that rainbow trout exposed to sublethal concentrations of carbaryl developed increased sensitivity to 2,4-D, dieldrin, rotenone, and pentachlorophenol. Chronic exposure of flagfish (*Jordanella floridae*) to cadmium and zinc mixtures resulted in additive toxicity, but uptake of one metal was not influenced by the presence of the other (Spehar et al., 1978).

Mechanisms of synergistic toxicity are not fully understood, but theories include increases in the rate of uptake, formation of toxic metabolites, reduction in excretion rates, alteration of distribution, and inhibition of detoxification mechanisms (Stolman, 1967; Wilkinson, 1968, 1974; Hodgson et al., 1973). Inhibition of detoxification appears to be the most popular theory, although several mechanisms may be responsible for some synergistic effects. There is evidence that methylenedioxyphenyl compounds used as synergists are metabolized by a mixed-function oxidase system, the primary system for oxidation of xenobiotics as well as normal substrates (Hodgson et al., 1973). Metabolism and biotransformation of foreign compounds are further discussed in Chapter 18.

The test for significance or range of the additive index is useful, especially when the index value is near zero. Some investigators have chosen an arbitrary value to detect or define greater than additive toxicity; selected values ranged from 0.35 to 1.0 unit beyond expected effects on the basis of nonlinear values of S (Bakuniak, 1973). In the tests for significance of additive indices presented here, values of 1.0 were greater than additive (the ranges did not overlap zero), but values of 0.3 were not. Values of 0.5 to 0.7 were greater than additive only when confidence intervals for LC50s were narrow, decreasing the range for additive indices. If ranges are not developed for additive indices, selected values for greater than additive toxicity should be 1.0 and greater, and selected values for less than additive toxicity should be −1.0 or less. Therefore, based on a linear relation, additive toxicity is involved for any index values > -1.0 and $< +1.0$. However, it is preferable to calculate the actual range for indices rather than select arbitrary values to differentiate the type of additive toxicity.

Interpretation of results of mixture toxicity data and application of the results to real situations are difficult and therefore easily misunderstood. Synergism appears spectacular because it is generally unexpected and seems to be an exception to additive toxicity. Also, it may be thought that antagonism is of little concern because the components of a mixture may actually interfere with each other so that their activity is not fully manifested. However, combinations of contaminants that have less than additive toxicity may become lethal to nontarget organisms. For this reason, all types of additive toxic action must be of concern to people and agencies that are attempting to protect the environment. Roales and Perlmutter (1974) reported that copper was antagonistic to the toxic action of methyl mercury, and Kim et al. (1977) reported that selenium dioxide was antagonistic to the toxic effects of mercuric chloride; however, both of these chemicals continue to increase the toxic burden of other sublethal or toxic substances in the environment.

In applying chemicals in aquatic environments one must consider the existing or potential toxic burden of the water. For instance, lampricides are applied to streams tributary to the Great Lakes. Although concentrations appropriate for treatment are chosen with caution, they are occasionally toxic to nontarget organisms; the result may be an unexpected fish kill. The increase in toxicity is most likely due to the combined effects of sublethal lampricide and sublethal contaminants present in the water. In this example, the toxicity of lampricides combined with contaminants could be less than additive, additive, or greater than additive. Chemical mixtures that result in more than additive toxicity present a greater hazard than an equal quantity of those producing less than additive toxicity, but both types of mixture toxicity can result in a hazard.

SUMMARY

Assessment of mixture toxicity began as an art, but it has developed into a science used in many disciplines: pharmacology, toxicology, physiology, human and veterinary medicine, agriculture, and especially pest control. Application of mixtures of chemicals has become popular because of their purported advantages over a single chemical. However, some chemical mixtures pose a greater hazard to nontarget organisms and to the environment. The advantages and disadvantages of using mixtures can be determined only by understanding the concepts of mixture toxicity and developing the ability to calculate quantitatively the additive toxicity of mixtures of chemicals. Investigators in various disciplines have attempted to describe synergism and antagonism; the result has been ambiguous terminology, even though the methodology has been fairly consistent. A number of additive toxicity procedures appear in the literature, but only a few are truly quantitative, and perhaps there is no one procedure that will accommodate all types of multiple exposures. Use of the additive toxicity index was developed from isobole theory and the summation of toxic units, as were many other methods. However, the index system has the advantages that (1) index values are linear for greater than and less than additive toxicity, (2) the significance of index values can be assessed to differentiate between the three categories of additive toxicity, and (3) magnification factors can be calculated to describe and express the expected activity or changes in unexpected activity. Furthermore, ranges for index values that overlap zero indicate additive toxicity, positive values indicate greater than additive toxicity, and negative values indicate less than additive toxicity. Synergism and antagonism are general terms and their use must be based on quantitative data. Both phenomena result from the summation of toxic units from multiple chemicals in the environment.

LITERATURE CITED

Bakuniak E: The synergism evaluating method of two-component insecticidal mixtures. Pol Pismo Entomol 43:395–414, 1973.

Berger BL: A synergic mixture of MS-222 and quinaldine sulfate as an anesthetic. 31st Midwest Fish Wildl Conf, 1969 (unpublished).

Berger BL: Fish toxicant compositions and method of using them. U.S. patent 3,608,072, 1971.

Bills TB, Marking LL: Toxicity of 3-trifluoromethyl-4-nitrophenol (TFM), 2',5-dichloro-4'-nitrosalicylanilide (Bayer 73), and a 98:2 mixture to fingerlings of seven fish species and to eggs and fry of coho salmon. U.S. Fish Wildl Serv Invest Fish Control 69, 1976.

Bills TD, Marking LL, Olson LE: Effects of residues of the polychlorinated biphenyl Aroclor 1254 on sensitivity of rainbow trout to selected environmental contaminants. Prog Fish Cult 39:150, 1977.

Bliss CI: The toxicity of poisons applied jointly. Ann Appl Biol 26:585–615, 1939.

Broderius SJ, Smith LL: Lethal and sublethal effects of binary mixtures of cyanide and hexavalent chromium, zinc, or ammonia to the fathead minnow (*Pimephales promelas*) and rainbow trout (*Salmo gairdneri*). J Fish Res Bd Can 36:164–172, 1979.

Brown E, Nishioka VA: Pesticides in water. Pestic Monit J 1:38–46, 1967.

Brown VM: The calculation of the acute toxicity of mixtures of poisons to rainbow trout. Water Res 2:723–733, 1968.

Brown VM, Dalton RA: The acute lethal toxicity to rainbow trout of mixtures of copper, phenol, zinc, and nickel. J Fish Biol 2:211–216, 1970.

Brown VM, Milrovic VV, Stark GTC: Effects of chronic exposure to zinc on toxicity of a mixture of a detergent and zinc. Water Res 2:255–263, 1968.

Brown VM, Jordon DHM, Tiller BA: The acute toxicity to rainbow trout of fluctuating concentrations and mixtures of ammonia, phenol, and zinc. J Fish Biol 1:1–9, 1969.

Cairns J, Scheier A: A comparison of toxicity of some common industrial waste components tested individually and combined. Prog Fish Cult 30:3–8, 1968.

Calamari D, Alabaster JS: An approach to theoretical models in evaluating the effects of mixtures of toxicants in the aquatic environment. Chemosphere 9:533–538, 1980.

Calamari D, Marchetti R: The toxicity of mixtures of metals and surfactants to rainbow trout (*Salmo gairdneri* Rich.). Water Res 7:1453–1464, 1973.

Carpenter CP, Weil CS, Palm PE, Woodside MW, Nair JH III, Smyth HF, Jr: Mammalian toxicity of 1-naphthyl-*N*-methyl-carbamate (Sevin insecticide). J Agric Food Chem 9:30–39, 1961.

Chen CW, Selleck RE: A kinetic model of fish toxicity threshold. J Water Pollut Control Fed 41:R294–R308, 1969.

Dawson VK, Marking LL: Toxicity of mixtures of quinaldine sulfate and MS-222 to fish. U.S. Fish Wildl Serv Invest Fish Control 53, 1973.

Dawson VK, Cumming KB, Gilderhus PA: Efficacy of 3-trifluoromethyl-4-nitrophenol (TFM), 2′,5-dichloro-4′-nitrosalicylanilide (Bayer 73), and a 98:2 mixture as lampricides in laboratory studies. U.S. Fish Wildl Serv Invest Fish Control 77, 1977.

Douderoff P: Some recent developments in study of toxic industrial wastes. Proc Annu Pac Northwest Ind Waste Conf 4:1–21, 1952.

Fingl E, Woodbury DM: General principles. In: Pharmacological Basis of Therapeutics, 3d ed., edited by LS Goodman, A Gilman, pp. 1–36. New York: MacMillan, 1965.

Finney DJ: The analysis of toxicity tests on mixtures of poisons. Ann Appl Biol 29:82–94, 1942.

Frawley JP, Fuyat HN, Hagan EC, Blake JR, Fitzhugh OG: Marked potentiation in mammalian toxicity from simultaneous administration of two anticholinesterase compounds. J Pharmacol Exp Ther 121:96–106, 1957.

Gehrs CW, Parkhurst BR, Shriner DS: Environmental testing. In: Application of Short-Term Bioassays in the Fractionation of Complex Environmental Mixtures, edited by MD Waters, S Nesnow, JL Huisingh, SS Sandher, L Clayton, pp. 319–330. New York: Plenum, 1979.

Hayes WJ: Toxicology of Pesticides. Baltimore: Williams & Wilkins, 1975.

Herbert DWM, Shurben DS: The toxicity to fish of mixtures of poisons. I. Salts of ammonia and zinc. Ann Appl Biol 53:33–41, 1964.

Herbert DWM, Vandyke JM: The toxicity to fish of mixtures of poisons. II. Copper-ammonia and zinc-phenol mixtures. Ann Appl Biol 53:415–421, 1964.

Hester FE: The tolerance of eight species of warm-water fishes to certain rotenone formulations. Proc Southeast Assoc Game Fish Comm 13:121–133, 1959.

Hodgson E, Philpot RM, Baker RC, Mailman RB: Effects of synergists on drug metabolism. Drug Metab Dispos 1:392–400, 1973.

Howell JH, King EL, Smith AJ, Hansen LH: Synergism of 5,2′-dichloro-4′-nitrosalicylanilide and 3-trifluormethyl-4-nitrophenol in a selective lampricide. Great Lakes Fish Comm Tech Rept 8, 1964.

Howland RM: Interaction of antimycin A and rotenone in fish bioassays. Prog Fish Cult 31:33–34, 1969.

Keplinger ML, Deichmann WB: Acute toxicity of combinations of pesticides. Toxicol Appl Pharmacol 10:586–595, 1967.

Kim JH, Birks E, Heisinger JF: Protective action of selenium against mercury in northern creek chubs. Bull Environ Contam Toxicol 17:132–136, 1977.

Kluive WM, Hook JB: Polybrominated biphenyl-induced potentiation of chloroform toxicity. Toxicol Appl Pharmacol 45:861–869, 1978.

Kobayashi S: Synergism in pesticide toxicity. J Med Soc Toho Univ 25:616–634, 1978.

Kreitzer JF, Spann JW: Tests of pesticidal synergism with young pheasants and Japanese quail. Bull Environ Contam Toxicol 9:250–256, 1973.

Leteux F, Meyer FP: Mixtures of malachite green and formalin for controlling *Icthyophthirius* and other protozoan parasites of fish. Prog Fish Cult 34:21–26, 1972.

Lloyd R: The toxicity of mixtures of zinc and copper sulfates to rainbow trout (*Salmo gairdneri* Richardson). Ann Appl Biol 49:535–538, 1961.

Loewe S, Muischnek H: Uber Kombinationswirkungen. Arch Exp Pathol Pharmakol 114:313–326, 1926.

Marking LL: Method for assessing additive toxicity of chemical mixtures. In: Aquatic Toxicology and Hazard Evaluation, edited by FL Mayer, JL Hamelink, pp. 99–108. Philadelphia: American Society for Testing and Materials, 1977.

Marking LL, Dawson VK: Method for assessment of toxicity or efficacy of mixtures of chemicals. U.S. Fish Wildl Serv Invest Fish Control 67:1–8, 1975.

Marking LL, Mauck WL: Toxicity of paired mixtures of candidate forest insecticides to rainbow trout. Bull Environ Contam Toxicol 13:518–523, 1975.

Mayer FL, Street JC, Neuhold JM: Organochlorine insecticide interactions affecting residue storage in rainbow trout. Bull Environ Contam Toxicol 5:300–310, 1970.

McLeese DW, Metcalfe CD: Toxicity of mixtures of phosphamidon and methidathion to lobsters (*Homarus americanus*). Chemosphere 2:59–62, 1979.

Parmer BS, Mukerjee SK: Synergism and antagonism in insecticides. Pesticides 8:54–56, 1974.

Passino DRM, Kramer JM: Toxicity of arsenic and PCBs to fry of deepwater ciscoes (*Coregonus*). Bull Environ Contam Toxicol 24:527–534, 1980.

Plapp FW: Polychlorinated biphenyl: An environmental contaminant acts as an insecticide synergist. Environ Entomol 1:580–582, 1972.

Roales RR, Perlmutter A: Toxicity of methylmercury on copper, applied singly and jointly, to the blue gourami, *Trichogaster trichopterus*. Bull Environ Contam Toxicol 12:633–639, 1974.

Schoettger RA, Steucke EW: Synergic mixtures of MS-222 and quinaldine as anesthetics for rainbow trout and northern pike. Prog Fish Cult 34:202–205, 1970.

Smyth HF, Weil CS, West JS, Carpenter CP: An exploration of joint toxic action: Twenty-seven industrial chemicals intubated in rats in all possible pairs. Toxicol Appl Pharmacol 14:340–347, 1969.

Smyth HF, Weil CS, West JS, Carpenter CP: An exploration of joint toxic action. II. Equitoxic versus equivolume mixtures. Toxicol Appl Pharmacol 17:498–503, 1970.

Spehar RL, Leonard EN, DeFoe DL: Chronic effects of cadmium and zinc mixtures on flagfish (*Jordanella floridae*). Trans Am Fish Soc 107:354–360, 1978.

Sprague JB: Measurement of pollutant toxicity to fish. II. Utilizing and applying bioassay results. Water Res 4:3–32, 1970.

Sprague JB, Logan WJ: Separate and joint toxicity to rainbow trout of substances used in drilling fluids for oil exploration. Environ Pollut 19:269–281, 1979.

Sprague JB, Ramsey BA: Lethal levels of mixed copper-zinc solutions for juvenile salmon. J Fish Res Bd Can 22:425–432, 1965.

Statham CP, Lech JL: Potentiation of the acute toxicity of several pesticides and herbicides in trout by carbaryl. Toxicol Appl Pharmacol 34:83–87, 1975.

Stolman A: Progress in Chemical Toxicology. New York: Academic, 1967.

Sun YP, Johnson ER: Synergistic and antagonistic actions of insecticide synergist combinations and their mode of action. J Agric Food Chem 8:261–266, 1960.

Tsai C, McKee JA: The toxicity to goldfish of mixtures of chloramines, LAS, and copper. No. 44, Water Resources Research Center, University of Maryland, 1978.

Tucker RK, Leitzke JS: Comparative toxicology of insecticides for vertebrate wildlife and fish. Pharmacol Ther 6:166–220, 1979.

Wilkinson CF: Detoxification of pesticides and the mechanism of synergism. In: Enzymatic Oxidations of Toxicants, edited by E Hodgson, pp. 113–142. Raleigh: North Carolina State University, 1968.

Wilkinson CF: Insecticide synergism. In: The Future for Insecticides: Needs and Prospects, edited by RL Metcalf, JJ McKelvey, Jr, pp. 195–218. New York: Wiley, 1974.

SUPPLEMENTAL READING

Banki L: Bioassay of Pesticides in the Laboratory, translated by G Gogyo. Budapest: Akadimiai Kiadom, 1978.

Brown VK: Acute Toxicity in Theory and Practice. New York: Wiley, 1980.

Filov VA, Golubev AA, Liublina EI, Tolokontsev NA: Quantitative Toxicology, translated by VE Tatorchenko. New York: Wiley, 1979.

Chapter 8
Microbial Toxicity Studies

P. H. Pritchard and A. W. Bourquin

INTRODUCTION

Toxicologists and microbiologists have been concerned with the effects of toxic materials on microbial growth and activities for many years. Studies of terrestrial microorganisms have been particularly plentiful, since the success of microbial geochemical events is very much a part of successful crop production. However, there have also been numerous studies of aquatic microorganisms because of the increasing incidence of toxicants in aquatic systems. Although the disruption of microbial activities could be catastrophic for an ecosystem, it has been found that in general bacteria are the most insensitive organisms to toxicants. In fact, there are very few reported cases of chemical toxicity to microorganisms at a concentration below that which adversely affects higher animals. One of the few cases is the compound N-Serve (Billen, 1975) developed specifically to inhibit denitrification in soil. This chemical is unique because it affects a very special bacterial process.

The relative insensitivity of bacteria to toxicants is due primarily to bacterial metabolic processes. Bacteria are small organisms whose metabolic processes have been reduced to a minimum so that they efficiently utilize carbon and energy sources and can reproduce rapidly. The simplicity of their metabolism and macromolecular organization is generally not characteristic of higher organisms, in which metabolic and structural complexity and specialization are commonplace. It is often because of this specialization that certain higher organisms are more sensitive to toxicants. In fact, many pesticides are designed to affect specific target organisms (Chapter 12) by disrupting one of these specialized processes or structures. A good example is the pesticide Dimilin, which specifically inhibits chitin synthesis. Although Dimilin is effective against insects, it also affects other organisms such as crustaceans, which synthesize chitin. As another example, organophosphate insecticides are designed to inhibit the enzyme acetylcholinesterase and nerve transmission, but bacteria, which have no enzyme system similar to that of insects, are relatively insensitive to organophosphates. Conversely, chemicals that are general inhibitors of metabolic processes common to all types of organisms are capable of adversely affecting bacteria.

Another important factor in the relative insensitivity of bacteria to toxic chemicals is the rather loose connection between disruption of cellular processes and cell death. Bacteria can become dormant and survive adverse conditions, whereas higher organisms generally lack this ability. In general, once the liver of a fish is adversely affected, the animal dies quite rapidly. Since bacteria have relatively few specialized organs or metabolic processes, death of the organism after impairment of a function may not occur for a considerable time. Likewise, if growth conditions are not ideal for a particular bacterium, it can slow down its growth and direct its energy to simply surviving. Frequently, the effect of chemical exposure on bacteria is biostatic (inhibiting cell growth but not killing cells) rather than biocidal (killing cells), and thus recovery of a normal population of bacteria following chemical exposure is quite high.

Finally, it appears that bacteria provide minimal access for a toxicant. Their transport mechanisms are very selective, and many toxicants are never transported into the cell. Bacteria lack gills, digestive tracts, livers, kidneys, mitochondria, and other typical organs and systems and consequently are far less likely to absorb a toxicant into the cell. Also, the complex bacterial cell wall and associated enveloping slime provide a more protective coating than, for example, the gut wall of an invertebrate.

Even if a toxicant is shown to have an adverse effect on a bacterium or a bacterial population, the environmental significance of such an effect is very difficult to assess for a number of reasons. First, bacteria grow relatively rapidly and can thus quickly regain their original density if only part of the population is killed. Second, in most cases bacterial specialization is in metabolic capabilities rather than structural aspects, and many bacteria of different genera carry out the same metabolic processes. If a prominent species in a population is eliminated, chances are good that a previously minor species will elaborate and adequately fill the temporary metabolic void. Therefore, since the same general metabolic processes are widespread among so many bacteria, it is unlikely that a toxicant will have a long-term effect. There are some unique metabolic processes that must be considered, however. For example, the types of bacteria associated with nitrification are very limited and are very slow growers. If these bacteria are specifically affected by a toxicant, functional recovery could be quite slow and the geochemical cycling of nitrogen could be impeded. Therefore, nitrifying bacteria constitute one group of microorganisms that should be considered first in toxicity assessments. Third, the ubiquity of bacteria and redundancy of metabolic processes within heterogeneous populations mean that localized effects of a toxicant can be compensated in a relatively short time. In aquatic environments, especially, there is great movement and mixing of bacterial populations, and it is quite easy for this exchange to compensate any damage to the population even from a chronic toxicity effect. If large numbers of bacteria were uniquely adapted for survival in a particular aquatic environment, this buffering effect would not be as great—for example, bacteria washed in from terrestrial environments could not replace the aquatic population. In general, this situation does not exist; terrestrial bacteria readily survive and reproduce in aquatic systems.

Despite the relative insensitivity and post-exposure recovery potential of bacterial populations, these organisms are useful for evaluating the toxicity of new chemicals in the aquatic environment, since this type of screening can lead to early identification of any new and potentially powerful bactericide before extensive environmental contamination has occurred. Certainly, if a chemical is found to be significantly toxic to bacteria, there is a substantial possibility that it may be even more toxic to higher plants and animals.

This chapter gives some examples of common methods used to determine the toxicity of chemicals to bacteria. Only the most common methods, particularly those that are easy to perform, are discussed. Numerous literature citations are included to help illustrate the use of each method and its advantages and disadvantages. The information presented is by no means a complete survey of the field. The supplemental reading list provides considerably more information on these methods.

TERMINOLOGY

Allochthonous. From without. Refers to organisms or organic material that is not produced or sustained within a particular environment.

Ammonification. A subset of mineralization in which organically bound nitrogen is released as ammonia.

Autochthonous. From within. Indigenous organisms or organic material.

Axenic culture. A pure culture, one free of other organisms.

Autotrophic. Obtaining carbon from the fixation of carbon dioxide and energy from the oxidation of specific inorganic compounds.

Bactericidal. Producing mortality; generally used in relation to toxic chemicals and disinfectants.

Bacteriostatic. Preventing growth and proliferation of bacterial cells without killing them.

Denitrification. The process of converting nitrogen compounds to molecular nitrogen (N_2).

Epifluorescence. The observation of fluorescence in certain chemicals by the use of high-energy light from hydrogen and halogen lamps.

Facultative anaerobes. Bacteria that can grow in the presence or absence of oxygen.

Gnotobiotic. Composition completely known, often referring to mixed populations of organisms.

Gram-negative or gram-positive. A general classification of bacteria used on the differential staining procedure developed by Hans Gram.

Heterotrophic. Requiring preformed organic substances for carbon and energy.

K_S. A constant referring to the concentration of substrate that will produce half the V_{max} (see below). Generally reflects the affinity of a catalytic unit (enzyme, cell, etc.) for a substrate.

Lipopolysaccharide. A chemical substance made of specific lipids and sugars that form the external surface of gram negative bacteria.

Methanogenic. Producing methane gas.

Mineralization. The biological process of transforming organic matter by complete oxidation into carbon dioxide, water, and other inorganic compounds.

Muramic acid. The chemical backbone of bacterial cell walls; unique to bacteria.

Nitrification. The process of converting ammonia to nitrite and nitrate.

Nitrogen fixation. The process of fixing molecular nitrogen into organic matter.

Obligate anaerobes. Bacteria that cannot grow in the presence of oxygen.

Plasmids. Extrachromosomal nonnuclear, self-replicating units of DNA that are not an essential part of the cell but can carry genetic information.

V_{max}. Maximum velocity (rate) of an enzyme-catalyzed reaction or biological process.

GENERAL BACKGROUND OF AQUATIC MICROBIOLOGY

Bacteria in aquatic environments can be found in very diverse habitats and communities. They are associated with all types of surfaces, including plants, rocks, animals, sediment, manufactured objects, and plankton, and they are found in environments that have extreme physical and chemical ranges: temperature −4 to +50°C, salinity 0 to 100 ppt, pressure 0 to 1000 atm, pH 5.5 to 8.5, and oxidation/reduction potential (Eh) +400 to −400 mV. The numbers, types, and activities of these bacteria are basically dictated by their environmental setting. Concentrations of organic and inorganic materials and temperature are probably the most restrictive factors controlling the growth of bacteria in aquatic habitats. Most bacteria are heterotrophs, deriving carbon and energy for growth from the dead remains of plant and animal material. Dissolved organic food material from these remains is often found in extremely low concentrations (μg/l) in aquatic habitats; thus, aquatic bacteria are efficient scavengers (Rheinheimer, 1971). Bacterial metabolism is geared to the utilization of small concentrations of nutrients that appear intermittently.

In the water column, bacteria are found free-swimming and attached. Those that attach often do so to themselves (aggregates), to inert organic and inorganic particulate matter, or to the surfaces of phytoplankton and zooplankton. In general, suspended particles have a favorable effect on microbial growth because they are focal points for adsorption and desorption processes that provide nutrients for attached bacteria and they neutralize toxic effects of other compounds.

Bacteria associated with sediment and with plant and animal surfaces are often found in greater numbers per unit area than those that are free-swimming. However, overall microbial activity may not reflect this mass difference because sediment and surface bacteria cells may be packed several cell layers thick. Those on the bottom layers are shielded from available nutrients and live essentially as dormant populations.

Aquatic environments typically have a distribution of bacterial populations in which cell numbers decrease with distance from shore and with depth. There are exceptions, of course. Surface slicks on lakes and bays are frequently rich in bacterial biomass and metabolic activities compared to the water immediately below. The same is true of the sediment-water interface, where a loose slurry of sediment (turbidity layer) may contain many of the mineralization activities associated with the aquatic environment. Thermoclines and euphotic zones of lakes and oceans can also have areas with greater bacterial numbers and sometimes greater bacterial activities.

The principal activity of bacteria is the transformation of organically bound carbon, nitrogen, phosphorus, magnesium, sulfur, and other elements into unbound oxidized states (nitrate, sulfate, phosphate). This process is called mineralization, and it is the key to nutrient cycling in aquatic systems. These nutrients provide plants with the essential factors needed for growth. Thus, toxicologists and microbiologists are concerned with the effects of toxic materials on bacteria and the processes they mediate. If mineralization and nutrient recycling become severely disturbed or curtailed, the functioning of the ecosystem will be dramatically affected since the two are so closely linked. Domestic sewage, for example, severely affects the microflora of waters. It changes the normal pattern of mineralization and has undesirable aesthetic and economic consequences. The massive increase in nutrients associated with sewage pollution causes algal blooms. The algae eventually die, leaving a large pool of readily degradable organic material which the bacteria attempt to eliminate through mineralization. Invariably, in heavily affected areas bacterial degradative activities become limited, and with oxygen depletion, large concentrations of sulfide accumulate, killing fish and other animals. Specific toxicants can have similar effects; thus it is important to routinely assess potential impacts on aquatic bacteria and the processes they catalyze.

Effects of Toxicants on Microbial Growth

Population growth is relatively easy to measure in the laboratory. It can be studied in natural mixed populations, synthetic gnotobiotic populations, or pure cultures. Some researchers consider that pure cultures are preferable for toxicity studies in certain situations; others think that mixed populations should be studied.

Growth studies with bacteria are generally simple and can employ a variety of experimental conditions related to specific physical and chemical characteristics of aquatic environments. Microbial populations spanning a range of physiological conditions and ecosystem types are easily accessible. Samples of sediments, soil, water, plants, and other material can be transported to the laboratory. With little additional effort, growth of microbial populations can be observed under laboratory conditions and the effect of a toxicant measured. Thus, initial estimates of toxicity invariably involve growth studies.

Enumeration of Bacteria in Aquatic Environments

To perform toxicity studies on bacteria it is necessary to be able to enumerate the bacteria in a specific population from a specific habitat and quantitatively measure metabolic activity. Many applicable techniques are discussed in subsequent sections. Because of their size, bacteria present unique problems that may make toxicity studies difficult to interpret.

For example, live bacterial cells are commonly enumerated by spreading a dilute water sample on an agar medium that will support growth. If individual cells are separated sufficiently from their neighbors, they will grow and divide, eventually producing a visible colony. The number of colonies equals the number of bacteria present in the diluted water sample. This is a mechanically simple exercise, but the interpretation can be confusing. First, there is no guarantee that a colony originated from a single cell. It may have aggregated during or prior to plating. If the toxicant provoked aggregation, the result would seem to be a reduction in cell numbers and an apparent toxicant-mediated mortality. Second, a toxicant may have a bacteriostatic effect, so that once it is washed away, the effect disappears. Enumeration techniques involving agar often ensure a constant concentration of toxicant, resulting in a misleading reduction in numbers not seen in nature. Third, the agar medium should

allow growth of all the bacteria in the water sample. In most situations, however, only a small percentage of the total bacteria in the sample will grow on a particular medium. With the diversity of metabolic types in natural bacterial populations, it is virtually impossible for all of the types to grow on a single type of medium. Thus, in a toxicity test, one never knows whether the bacteria that did not grow on a particular medium were more sensitive to the toxicant.

An alternative to counting viable cells on agar is counting bacteria directly with a microscope. This technique has been improved by the advent of epifluorescence counting (Daley and Hobbie, 1975). Cells are stained with acridine orange, a fluorescing dye that associates tightly with DNA and can be observed under a fluorescence microscope. The bacteria stand out vividly from the background, and all bacteria in the sample can easily be counted. However, many bacterial cells can remain intact even though functionally dead. Consequently, it is difficult to distinguish the live from the dead cells, which makes interpretation of a toxicity study difficult. Several variations on the epifluorescence technique have been used to differentiate live from dead bacteria. Nalidixic acid, for example, interferes with RNA synthesis in growing cells, causing them to enlarge and change shape, and this allows live bacteria to be distinguished morphologically from dead cells (Orndorff and Colwell, 1980). This technique may prove useful in toxicity tests with bacteria.

Direct counts invariably yield higher numbers of cells per unit volume than do plate counts, because dead cells and metabolically dormant cells are all counted together. However, direct counting has advantages, particularly in relation to microbial activity measurements, as will be shown in more detail below. Direct counts of bacteria are reasonable only if the numbers are generally higher than 10^3 or 10^4 cells per milliliter. At lower concentrations, the chance of detecting cells in a microscopic field is low. When cell concentrations are low, other counting techniques (such as plate counts) must be employed.

Several other methods for enumerating bacteria are also available, but their application to toxicity testing is limited. Bacterial growth in broth media causes increased turbidity, which can be quantitated with a spectrophotometer. The turbidometric method has been used extensively in microbiology, particularly with pure cultures. It is a very simple, reproducible technique. The classical multiphase growth response of bacterial cultures [lag phase (no growth), logarithmic growth phase (maximal growth), stationary phase (nutrient depletion), and death phase (cell lysis)] can be routinely assessed. This technique is also valuable when studying the phases of growth that are most sensitive to a toxicant. However, growth phases are essentially a laboratory artifact; caution is required in extrapolating the results of the field.

Several biochemical components of bacterial cells can be quantitated and related to cell numbers. Measurements of cellular ATP levels, cell wall components such as lipopolysaccharide or muramic acid, lipid phosphate and other lipid components, nuclear material such as DNA and RNA, and certain enzyme levels have been used with moderate success. In most cases, except for muramic acid and lipopolysaccharide, the measurements are not unique to bacteria; the presence of one algal cell or protozoan can greatly affect the concentration of these components and produce very misleading estimates of bacterial population densities. Muramic acid, which is found in the cell walls of cyanobacteria (blue-green algae), often gives misleading information, since many cyanobacterial cells are considerably larger than most bacteria.

In toxicity testing with microorganisms, it is important to be aware of the limitations of studies that concentrate on effects measurements related to changes in bacterial cell concentration or to mortality based on morphology rather than physiology. In other types of toxicity studies, a dead *Daphnia* or fish is obvious; the same clear-cut observation is not always possible with bacteria. In this chapter this limitation will be illustrated, and it will be shown how physiological indices, which represent a new and subtle approach to toxicity testing in higher organisms, are excellent effects-related parameters for bacterial populations.

Growth of Heterotrophic Microorganisms

The most common way to study the effects of toxic materials on microorganisms is to monitor growth inhibition on agar media by a viable plate count. Dilutions of natural water samples are plated on agar media that contain different concentrations of the toxicant, and the reductions in colony forming units (CFUs) relative to control plates containing no toxicant are then observed. The plate count technique is based on the principle that each viable organism will give rise to one colony. This method is simple, economical, suitable for statistical analysis, and amenable to the examination of large numbers of water samples. Numerous reports on this type of study are available (see Ware and Roan, 1970).

An example of this type of study is work on the toxicity of Kepone to estuarine microorganisms (Mahaffey et al., 1982; Bourquin et al., 1978). Kepone is an organochlorine pesticide that contaminated the James River estuary in Virginia. To determine its toxicity to microorganisms, samples of estuarine water from several sampling sites around Pensacola, Florida, were serially diluted and plated on Zobell's agar containing Kepone concentrations of 0.1–2.0 mg/l (ppm). A significant reduction ($\alpha = 0.05$) in CFUs relative to control plates was detected on plates containing 0.2 mg/l (Table 1). Twenty-three different colonies were selected from these plates and developed as pure microbial cultures. The physiological characteristics of these isolates are detailed in Table 2. These isolates, overall, were found to be sensitive to Kepone to varying degrees, but gram-negative isolates were generally least sensitive to this pesticide.

Since Kepone in the James River is primarily found in the sediments, it was important to determine whether the anaerobic organisms found primarily in estuarine sediments were also affected by Kepone. Kepone was not nearly as toxic to anaerobically grown microorganisms (Table 3).

Table 1 Effects of Kepone on Isolation of Aerobic Bacteria from Estuarine Water [a]

Sample source	Date[b]	Salinity (°/∞)	Temperature (°C)	CFUs × 10^2 per milliliter of water			
					Kepone[c] concentration (mg/l)		
				Control	0.02	0.20	2.00
Range Point	A	15	21	181.0	108.0 (41)[d]	73.0 (60)	35.0 (81)
	B	15	24	86.5	65.0 (25)	35.0 (60)	33.0 (61)
	C	20	23	17.7	12.0 (28)	13.0 (23)	13.0 (25)
Escambia Bay	A	11	22	267.0	81.0 (70)	233.0 (13)	130.0 (52)
	B	15	24	13.5	6.9 (50)	10.0 (26)	4.7 (66)
	C	18	22	11.6	11.0 (8)	9.0 (23)	8.9 (23)
Laboratory pond	A	20	20	479.0[e]	448.9 (7)[e]	409.0 (14)[e]	396.0 (18)[e]
	B	15	26	104.0	49.0 (53)	–	19.0 (82)
	C	20	27	544.0	501.0 (8)	437.0 (20)	309.0 (43)
Gulf of Mexico	A	33	18	270.0	62.0 (78)	32.0 (89)	46.0 (83)
	B	33	22	13.3	10.5 (21)	10.0 (25)	8.0 (40)
	D	33	24	15.0	6.1 (59)	1.2 (92)	0.7 (95)

[a] From Mahaffey et al. (1982).
[b] Sampling date (1977): A, April 1; B, April 17; C, April 29; D, May 7.
[c] Kepone added to Zobell's marine agar.
[d] Numbers in parentheses are percent reduction in CFUs normalized against growth on control plates of Zobell's marine agar containing no Kepone; all percent reductions are significant ($\alpha = 0.05$).
[e] CFUs × 10^3 per milliliter.

This difference is probably due to interference of Kepone with oxidation and respiration, similar to the mechanism described by Widdis et al. (1971) and Trudgill et al. (1971) for the toxicity of chlordane to *Bacillus* sp.

Orndorff and Colwell (1980) compared the viable plate counting technique with direct counting methods. The acridine orange epifluorescence method developed by Daley and Hobbie (1975) was used for direct counts of bacterial populations. In this method, acridine orange stains biological material and gives a distinct green color under the fluorescence microscope. To obtain an indication of the number of live bacteria comprising the total direct count, Orndorff treated the cells with nalidixic acid by the method of Kogure (1979). Nalidixic acid specifically inhibits RNA synthesis in live gram negative cells and causes a change in their shape, enabling them to be distinguished from dead cells. Since most aquatic micro-organisms are gram-negative, and Kepone is not toxic to gram-negatives, use of the Kogure technique is justified.

Results of Orndorff and Colwell (1980) in Table 4 indicate that viable direct counts (by fluorescence microscopy) comprised 2.5–56.7% of the total direct counts (mean $\bar{x} = 24.5\%$) and counts on the agar plates were 0.5–2 orders of magnitude less than the viable direct counts. It appears that the concentration-response curve is about the same, regardless of the counting method. The viable direct count is probably the most accurate method, yet the same relative toxicity can be established with the simpler viable plate counts.

In all these studies it is important to perform a statistical analysis on the data to determine whether effects resulting from a toxicant exposure are significant. Several statistical analyses can be used for this purpose. For example, in the work by

Table 2 Physiological Activities of Kepone-sensitive and Kepone-tolerant Microbes[a]

Culture number	Organism type	Gram stain	Alkane utilizer[b]	Aromatic utilizer[b]	Physiological function			Pesticide tolerance[c]
					Lipolytic	Amylolytic	Proteolytic	
Kepone-sensitive								
1	Rod	Positive	+	+	−	+	+	+
3	Rod	Positive	−	−	−	+	+	−
4	Cocc-bac	Negative	−	−	+	+	+	−
11	Cocc-bac	Positive	+	+	+	+	−	+
14	Rod	Positive	−	−	+	+	−	−
29	Rod	Positive	−	−	−	−	+	−
42	Coccus	Positive	−	−	+	−	−	−
54	Rod	Positive	−	+	−	+	+	−
8	Yeast	−	−	+	+	+	+	−
15	Fungus	−	+	+	ND[d]	ND	ND	−
Kepone-tolerant								
10	Rod	Negative	−	−	−	−	±	−
18	Pleo	Negative	+	−	+	−	−	−
20	Rod	Negative	+	−	ND	ND	ND	−
23	Rod	Positive	+	+	ND	ND	ND	+
40	Cocc-bac	Positive	+	−	+	−	+	+
45	Rod	Negative	−	−	+	−	+	−
46	Rod	Negative	−	−	+	−	−	+
56	Cocc-bac	Negative	−	−	+	+	−	+
59	Rod	Negative	−	−	−	−	−	−
2	Yeast	−	+	−	−	−	+	−
7	Yeast	−	−	−	+	+	+	−
27	Fungus	−	−	+	ND	ND	ND	+
44	Fungus	−	−	−	ND	ND	ND	+

[a]From Bourquin et al. (1978).

[b]Hydrocarbons tested were hexadecane, undecane, octadecane, benzene, naphthalene, biphenyl, xylene, and toluene.

[c]Pesticide tolerance test means growth in the presence of toxaphene, Aroclor 1242, methoxychlor, heptachlor, DDT, malathion, and pentachlorophenol.

[d]ND, not determined.

Table 3 Colony-forming Units in Sediments[a,b]

Date (1977)	Type	Kepone concentration (mg/l)			
		0	0.02	0.2	2.0
August 2	Aerobic	207.50 ± 22.00	197.50 ± 41.00	13.75 ± 13.00	33.20 ± 16.00
	Anaerobic	34.00 ± 4.30	30.60 ± 10.00	41.00 ± 10.00	36.25 ± 3.10
August 9	Aerobic	235.00 ± 75.00	74.00 ± 17.00	53.70 ± 18.00	26.25 ± 10.00
	Anaerobic	76.75 ± 12.70	68.25 ± 20.30	67.50 ± 25.00	59.50 ± 23.00
August 31	Aerobic	215.75 ± 51.30	243.50 ± 98.60	207.50 ± 99.50	62.25 ± 56.00
	Anaerobic	26.25 ± 7.00	24.50 ± 3.40	18.00 ± 8.00	13.25 ± 1.50

[a]From Mahaffey et al. (1982).

[b]Cells X 10^2 per milliliter, average of four replicates.

Table 4 Enumeration of Microbiological Populations from Colgate Creek, Maryland, in Water Samples with Different Concentrations of Kepone[a]

Sampling[b] date	TVC[c]	TC[d]	DVC[e] Kepone concentration (mg/l)			
			0	0.01	0.05	0.2
October	3.1×10^5	2.0×10^6	5.4×10^5	3.9×10^5	3.1×10^5	4.2×10^4
November	1.9×10^5	2.7×10^6	1.2×10^6	2.2×10^5	2.8×10^5	1.8×10^5
December	9.9×10^4	1.5×10^7	3.9×10^6	3.9×10^6	1.8×10^6	1.3×10^5
March	5.3×10^5	2.3×10^6	2.3×10^6	2.8×10^6	1.3×10^6	4.9×10^5

[a] From Orndorff and Colwell (1980).
[b] One sample was collected each month during 1978–1979.
[c] TVC, total viable heterotrophs per milliliter determined by plate count method.
[d] TC, total count per milliliter determined by acridine orange direct counting.
[e] DVC, direct viable counts per milliliter.

Mahaffey et al. (1982) the effect of Kepone on plate counts of bacteria was statistically analyzed by a three-factor model I analysis of variance (Zar, 1974). A comparison was made of 150 observations and 4 factors: Kepone concentration, aerobic versus anaerobic incubation, sampling date, and an air-treatment interaction component. A Student-Newman-Keuls (SNK) post hoc analysis was performed to evaluate the significant differences between population means. This test was used to constrast the Kepone-dependent reduction in CFUs under aerobic and anaerobic conditions. Figure 1 shows the mean number of CFUs for aerobic and anaerobic incubations plotted against

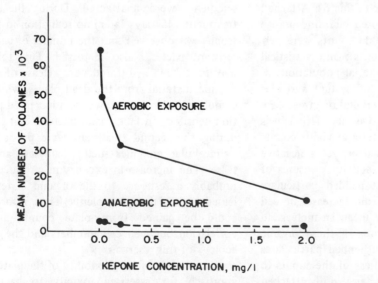

Figure 1 Effect of Kepone on the growth of natural marine microbial population under aerobic and anaerobic conditions. Control levels of colonies are shown at the zero concentration. *[From W. R. Mahaffey, P. H. Pritchard, and A. W. Bourquin (unpublished data).]*

Kepone concentration. The mean responses to aerobic and anaerobic treatments, on different sampling dates were significantly different at a confidence interval of $\alpha = 0.05$. The SNK post hoc analysis showed that populations grown under anaerobic conditions were not significantly affected by Kepone at any concentration tested. However, significant reductions in CFUs were observed under aerobic conditions. Significant differences ($\alpha = 0.005$) were observed between control populations and those grown aerobically in the presence of 0.2 and 2.0 mg/l Kepone. Differences were also observed between the 2.0 mg/l treatment and 0.02 and 0.2 mg/l treatments, indicating a minimum inhibitory concentration (MIC) of 0.2 mg/l Kepone.

Goulder et al. (1980) used bacterial growth studies to examine the relationships between heterotrophic bacterial populations and industrial pollution. This excellent paper can be used as a model for effect studies with bacteria. Many variables were assessed, including heavy-metal types and concentrations, bacterial activities and population densities, and environmental variables such as oxygen, salinity, organic content, and suspended particulate matter (Table 5). Attached and free bacteria were counted (acridine orange epifluorescence method); viable counts were performed (standard plate counts); and statistical correlations between the bacterial populations in the estuary and a number of system variables (Table 5) associated with the pollution stress were determined. A strong positive correlation was found between attached bacteria or viable counts and suspended particulate matter; yet a negative correlation existed between activity measures of bacterial populations and suspended particulate matter. This suggests that an increase in cell number does not necessarily mean an increase in activity, and degradation rates of these organic pollutants associated with suspended particulates may remain the same regardless of the inputs to the estuary. Numbers of bacteria, both attached and free, and bacterial activity were positively correlated with organic content. This can be interpreted as meaning that no widespread toxic effect existed because there was no correlation between these factors and the presence of toxic materials. The evidence also showed that heavy metals, particularly copper, may have inhibited bacterial growth at high concentrations. The inhibition was noted at an industrial outfall where copper concentrations were high.

The work described above demonstrates a useful methodology for determining the toxic effects of complex effluents. This method could readily be used to assess the potential dangers of an effluent to the microbial ecology of an estuarine environment. The number of determinations performed makes the method labor-intensive, but the measurements are simple and the results may be useful in long-term evaluations.

Fry et al. (1973) showed that monitoring of bacterial populations with viable plate counts was useful in developing a complete assessment of the effects of the herbicide paraquat. After the first application of paraquat to a large reservoir, all the macrophytes were killed. An immediate reduction in the number of heterotrophic bacteria in the water column was observed, but bacteria in the sediments were unaffected. During the second treatment (45 days later) no reduction in heterotrophs was observed, but the number of paraquat-resistant bacteria also increased. This tolerance may have been associated with release of soluble organic material from the dead plants, which also stimulated microbial growth and increased population densities. In fact, many bacteria that grew up during the second treatment were producers of extracellular enzymes such as amylase and protease. The increase in exoenzyme producers was probably a response to the organic material released by the decaying plants. Thus, information could be gained from plate counts and the correlation between cell numbers and the general ecology of this reservoir.

An example of the flexibility of the plate count approach for assessing toxicity to bacteria is presented by Guthrie et al. (1974), who described the natural bacterial population balance in a lake

Table 5 Significance Levels of Correlation Coefficients[a] between Bacterial and Environmental Variables in an Industrialized Estuary; Data from East Clough in Humber Estuary, England[b]

Bacterial measurements	Pollution-independent variable[c]				Indicator of organic pollution[c]						Heavy metals[c]								
	1	2	3	4	5	6	7	8	9	10	11	12	13	14	15	16	17	18	19
Attached bacteria	3	2	0	3	0	2	−1	0	0	−1	2	0	3	0	3	0	0	0	3
Free bacteria	0	1	0	0	0	0	0	0	0	0	0	0	0	0	0	−3	0	0	0
Viable bacteria	0	0	0	0	0	2	−1	3	0	0	0	−3	0	−2	0	0	−2	−2	0
V_{max}	0	0	0	1	0	0	0	1	−1	0	0	−2	0	0	0	0	−2	−2	0
Turnover time	0	0	0	0	0	0	0	0	1	0	0	2	0	0	0	0	2	2	0
Attached bacteria/suspended solids	0	0	1	0	0	0	0	0	0	1	0	0	0	0	0	0	0	0	0
V_{max}/bacterium	0	0	0	0	0	0	0	0	−1	0	−2	−3	0	0	0	0	−3	0	−1
Cu-tolerant bacteria	1	0	0	0	0	0	0	0	1	−1	3	0	1	0	2	0	2	0	3
Zn-tolerant bacteria	0	0	0	0	0	0	1	0	2	0	1	3	0	0	0	1	3	0	0

[a] 0 indicates no significant correlation ($p > 0.05$). Significant correlations are indicated by 1 ($p < 0.05$), 2 ($p < 0.01$), and 3 ($p < 0.001$). Minus signs indicate negative correlations.

[b] Reproduced with permission from Goulder et al. (1980); copyright, Pergamon Press, Ltd.

[c] 1, Suspended solids; 2, salinity; 3, oxygen; 4, suspended organic matter; 5, total permanganate O_2 demand; 6, particulate permanganate O_2 demand; 7, dissolved permanganate O_2 demand; 8, presumptive E. coli; 9, E. coli/viable bacteria; 10, organic matter as percent of suspended solids; 11, particulate Cu; 12, dissolved Cu; 13, particulate Pb; 14, dissolved Pb; 15, particulate Zn; 16, dissolved Zn; 17, Cu/suspended solids; 18, Pb/suspended solids; 19, Zn/suspended solids.

ecosystem. Samples of water from two different lake environments and from laboratory tank culture systems designed to simulate the lake environments were exposed to the herbicide diuron, and effects on bacterial populations were measured in three different ways. First, plate counts were performed and an overall net decrease in bacterial population was observed. An examination of colony morphology showed that the chromogenic (colored) colonies were significantly reduced. The apparent sensitivity of the chromogenic bacteria to this chemical is difficult to explain.

Second, disk sensitivity tests were performed. A pure culture of a bacterium isolated from the original plate counts was spread on an agar plate. Sterile filter paper disks saturated with different concentrations of toxicant (diuron) in aqueous solution were placed on the plate immediately after spreading. A zone of inhibition around the filter disks indicates toxicity (Fig. 2). The zone of inhibition crudely quantitates the degree of toxicity of the chemical to the bacteria. Surprisingly, many of the isolates, particularly the chromogenic types, were not affected by diuron in the disk sensitivity method. This suggests that a secondary, toxicant-related process affected the viability of the chromogenic forms.

Third, plate counts were performed on an agar medium supplemented with milk, Tween 80 (a surfactant), or starch. Many bacterial species secrete extracellular enzymes capable of hydrolyzing a number of these polymers. This activity

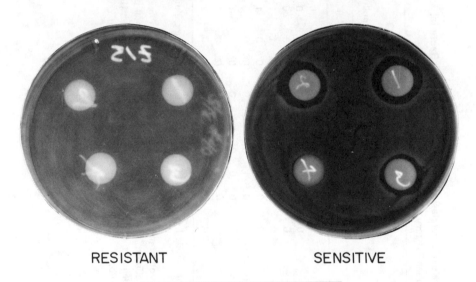

Figure 2 Example of the zone-of-inhibition method for determining toxicity of a chemical to growth of bacteria. Cloudiness on agar surface is microbial growth. White circles are filter paper disks saturated with the toxicant. Zones of clearing around disk indicate area where bacterial growth on agar was inhibited. *[From A. W. Bourquin (unpublished data).]*

results in a change in the consistency of the agar around each colony, and lipid hydrolyzers, starch hydrolyzers, and casein hydrolyzers can be readily detected. A toxicant that is more toxic to one physiological group than to the entire population can be easily observed; thus, a specific different toxic response can be assessed. In Guthrie's study, starch-, lipid-, and protein-hydrolyzing bacteria were present, but they did not show any differential sensitivity to the diuron (Table 6). In a similar study, Mahaffey et al. (1982) selected (on the basis of predominance) a total of 17 CFUs that grew in the presence of Kepone. Examination of the cell type and enzymatic activities of these purified isolates showed significant correlations with the amylolytic and lipolytic activities and the gram stain (see Table 2). Compared with 20 randomly selected isolates (no Kepone), 75% of the Kepone-tolerant isolates displayed amylolytic and lipolytic activities, whereas only 55% of the nontolerant isolates showed these activities. Ninety percent of the Kepone-tolerant isolates were gram-negative compared to 55% of the isolates from Zobell's marine agar (no Kepone). There was no significant difference between the two groups of isolates when compared with respect to the other characteristics tested.

After pure cultures of heterotrophic bacteria have been isolated, their individual growth responses can be scrutinized in relation to toxicant effects. These studies provide information on minimal toxicant concentration and on the range of sensitivity of various isolates. For example, to determine the toxicity of Kepone under different physiological conditions, growth studies were conducted with a rich, complex medium (yeast extract and proteins) and a defined medium (mineral salts and a single carbon source). The bacteria were isolated from estuarine environments in Pensacola, Florida. Isolate 32K, a gram-negative, rod-shaped bacterium, was not inhibited by Kepone at any concentration in complex media (Fig. 3). However, in a defined medium, the growth rate decreased as Kepone concentration increased.

Table 6 Effects of Diuron on the Population of Bacteria that Grow on Selective Culture Media[a]

Culture medium	Lake water[b] Keowee[d]	Lake water[b] Hartwell[d]	Laboratory diuron test[c] Keowee	Laboratory diuron test[c] Hartwell
Plate count	1×10^5	5×10^6	2×10^4	5×10^4
Protein	2×10^3	2×10^5	2×10^3	2×10^4
Starch	1×10^3	1×10^4	0	1×10^3
Lipid	0	3×10^4	0	2×10^4
Glucose salts	3×10^3	2×10^4	5×10^3	2×10^4

[a]From Guthrie et al. (1974).
[b]Counts shown are initial counts.
[c]Counts shown are final counts after test period.
[d]Lakes Keowee and Hartwell are located in South Carolina.

Similar growth studies performed on cultures of two gram-positive cocci (49K and 19K) which grew auxotrophically only in nutrient broth, involved different inoculum sizes (Fig. 4). A 4-fold reduction in growth was observed for the higher inoculum and a 20-fold one for the lower inoculum when they were exposed to 2.0 mg/l Kepone. Apparently, lysis or clumping of cells was responsible for the decline in optical density (growth) with the lower inoculum. In comparison, under the same conditions the growth of isolate 19K (Fig. 4) was depressed (28% optical density decrease) at a much smaller inoculum size, suggesting that 19K was more tolerant to Kepone. This is not surprising, considering that the organism was originally isolated from a toxic waste holding pond that receives a considerable loading of chlorinated hydrocarbons.

A unique autotrophic index was proposed by Matthews et al. (1980) as a possible test of toxic effects on microorganisms. Their approach involves analyzing the changes in the ratio of autotrophic to heterotrophic components of a stream microbial community. They measured microbial

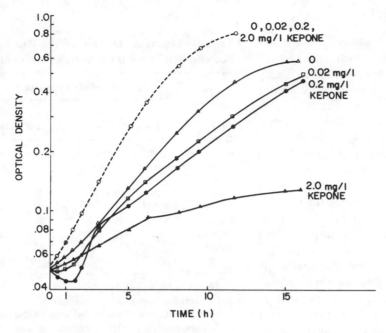

Figure 3 Growth response of isolate 32K on complex and defined media in the presence of Kepone. Controls contain amounts of acetone carrier equivalent to those used in treated cultures. (——) MSB/0.4% succinate medium (defined); (- - - -), Zobell's marine broth (complex) at 1.5% NaCl. *[From Mahaffey et al. (1982).]*

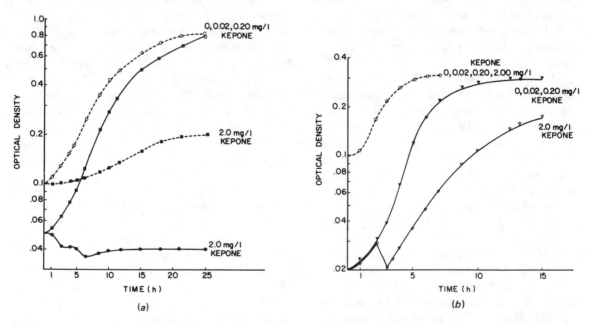

Figure 4 Effect of inoculum size on growth of isolates 49K and 19K in the presence of Kepone in marine broth. (*a*) Isolate 49K; initial optical densities were (——) 0.05 and (- - - -) 0.1. (*b*) Isolate 19K; initial optical densities were (——) 0.02 and (- - - -) 0.1. *[From Mahaffey et al. (1982).]*

190

biomass (ATP method) and chlorophyll *a* concentration under stressed conditions and then related these data to changes in the structure and function of the stream macroinvertebrate community. They hypothesized that any stress would promote a change in the heterotrophic/autotrophic balance as a result of the growth of tolerant species.

Data were collected from a small stream that received chlorinated sewage effluent near its headwaters and from a relatively unpolluted control stream. Polyurethane sponge substrates were suspended in the streams for 3, 7, and 10 d of colonization. At each sampling period, the microbial community was squeezed from the sponges, and the ATP and chlorophyll *a* content were determined. Microinvertebrates were sampled at the same time, using a box or Surber sampler, and classified into specific functional groups based on feeding habits.

The autotrophic index (AI)—the ratio of microorganism biomass (ATP) to chlorophyll concentration—was examined to determine whether the heterotrophic/autotrophic balance in the streams had been upset. Figure 5a is a plot of log AI versus percent of grazers (zooplankton that fed on bacteria and algae). As the AI value increased (i.e., the heterotrophic component increased relative to the autotrophic component) the change in invertebrate community structure was shown by a decreased grazer population. In another example

(Fig. 5b), the AI increased substantially and the invertebrate population diversity actually decreased. Thus, it appears that the balance between autotrophy and heterotrophy in the stream can be upset. Since both ATP and chlorophyll *a* are relatively simple measurements of standing biomass, and the data show definite relationships to traditional taxonomic responses to stress, this method of monitoring microbial communities could be useful in assessments of toxic effects on microorganisms.

Toward a Standard Bacterial Toxicity Test

Laboratory toxicity tests with fish, invertebrates, or algae are usually single-species tests in which the toxicity of a chemical is measured through mortality, decreased growth rate, and lowered reproductive capacity. These tests have been highly standardized and applied to a select group of organisms. Similar tests for bacteria have not been extensively developed. However, numerous studies have been performed with pure (axenic) cultures of bacteria, and certain types could be used for standard toxicity measurements. If a test organism is selected, there are several possible measurements of microbial activity and microbial growth that could be used in a standard test. Cell growth rates and oxygen uptake look promising for bacterial toxicity tests.

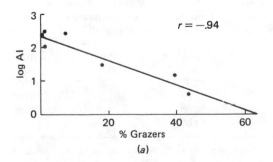 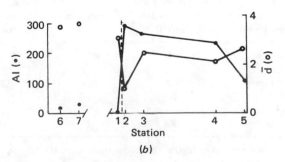

Figure 5 Use of the autotrophic index AI (ratio of microbial biomass to chlorophyll concentration) to assess pollution stress. (a) Linearity of the index with number of grazer organisms within a total invertebrate population. (b) Change in the index and in macroinvertebrate diversity $\bar{d}(0)$ at several river stations. *[From Matthews et al. (1980).]*

Growth rate constants of pure cultures of bacteria can be readily obtained. The organism can be inoculated into a compatible medium in a shake flask. Growth can be monitored by measuring optical density of the cell suspensions, and the values can be converted to dry weight for each organism tested. By plotting the natural logarithm (ln) of the cell weight against time and multiplying the slope by 7.303, a growth rate constant can be obtained. If the same experiment is performed in the presence of different concentrations of the toxicant, the investigator can determine inhibition or stimulation of the organism's growth.

Breazeale and Camper (1972) used pure cultures and changes in growth rate constants to measure the toxic effects of several selected herbicides (Table 7). The three test organisms were *Erwinia*, *Pseudomonas*, and *Bacillus*, all common inhabitants of terrestrial environments. Several of the chemicals tested inhibited growth (e.g., diquat completely inhibited growth of *Bacillus* sp.); others stimulated growth (nitralin versus *Pseudomonas*); and others had no effect (picloram versus *Erwinia*). Each organism showed a completely different spectrum of sensitivity to the toxicants. For particular chemicals, all of the organisms showed initial growth inhibition, but then apparently became acclimated and grew. This is a simple, straightforward pure culture toxicity test which can be considered as an acute toxicity test. Growth can easily be measured using increases in turbidity, in approximately 2–4 d. A test for the ability to adapt to better growth in the presence of the herbicide after a long incubation period could be considered a chronic test.

Trevors and Basaraba (1980) and Mahaffey et al. (1982) developed a pure culture toxicity test involving a respirometric or oxygen uptake method. In the former study, glucose was the principal carbon and energy source for a culture of *Pseudomonas fluorescens*. Cells grown in a compatible medium and washed three times in phosphate buffer provided a resting cell culture which was placed in a Warburg respirometer. Oxygen uptake measurements were made before and after the addition of glucose and in the presence and absence of a toxicant (Fig. 6). At relatively high concentrations (10 µg/ml) of benzoquinone and hydroquinone, oxygen uptake was significantly inhibited, even below endogenous levels.

Mahaffey et al. (1982) performed similar experiments to examine the effects of Kepone.

Table 7   Growth Responses[a] of *Erwinia carotovora*, *Pseudomonas fluorescens*, and *Bacillus* sp. to Selected Herbicides[b]

Herbicide	Erwinia carotovora		Pseudomonas fluorescens		Bacillus sp.	
	Minimal response concentration (µg/ml)	Response (%)	Minimal response concentration (µg/ml)	Response (%)	Minimal response concentration (µg/ml)	Response (%)
Diquat	25	40.8[c]	50	0	25	100[c]
Loxynil	25	71.0[c]	50	0	10	29.0[d]
Paraquat	50	25.5[c]	25	43.7[c]	5	100[c]
PCP	10	29.6[d]	25	65.8[d]	5	100[c]
Picloram	50	0	50	28.8[d]	50	0
Nitralin	50	0	25	22.0[d]	50	0

[a]All responses to the herbicides listed were inhibitory, except the response of *P. fluorescens* to nitralin, which was stimulatory.
[b]From Breazeal and Camper (1972).
[c]Significant at the 1% level.
[d]Significant at the 5% level.

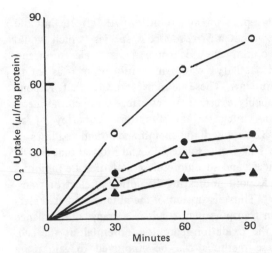

Figure 6 Inhibition of oxygen uptake by resting cells in the presence of (▲) benzoquinone and (△) hydroquinone at 10 μg/ml; (○) control and (●) endogenous condition. *[From Trevors and Basaraba (1980).]*

particulate fraction of cell extracts or the electron transport particle (ETP). To obtain the ETP preparation, cells grown for 18 h in succinate medium, harvested by centrifugation, washed, and resuspended in buffer were disrupted by sonication. Cell debris was removed by centrifugation and the supernatant centrifuged at 150,000 × g for 1 h at 2°C. The final pellet was completely homogenized in cold buffer. Succinooxidase activity in the ETP was assayed by measuring

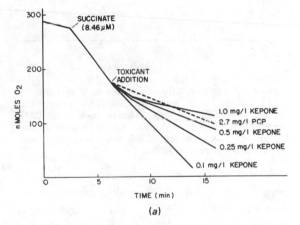

(a)

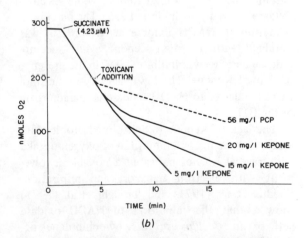

(b)

Cultures grown in a minimal salts medium were placed in a Gilford Oxygraph respirometer, and oxygen uptake rates were measured with an oxygen probe. At constant uptake, Kepone was added and its effect on the oxygen uptake was recorded continuously (Fig. 7). Respiration was reduced at about 20 mg/l Kepone. Kepone was considerably more toxic than pentachlorophenol. With one isolate, Kepone actually stimulated the production of oxygen (Fig. 8). The reason for this response is not yet known.

Respirometry provides data on metabolic processes that may not be observed in growth studies. The test is sensitive and short (about 1-2 h) and is easily standardized. It has been used for years to study intermediary metabolism in bacteria, and hence toxic effects can be related to the physiology of the organism. The procedure can be used to examine oxygen uptake by cell-free extracts of bacteria. Mahaffey et al. (1982) showed that Kepone toxicity may be related to the oxidative metabolism of microorganisms. The effects of Kepone on electron transport activity were studied by measuring the inhibition of NADH oxidase and succinooxidase activities in the

Figure 7 Oxygen uptake activity by whole cells. (a) Isolate 32 K (140 μg protein). (b) Isolate 28K (180 μg protein). Ten microliters of Kepone or PCP (reference toxicant), in dimethyl formamide carrier, was added to each reaction mixture after a constant rate of O_2 uptake was observed. *[From Mahaffey et al. (1982).]*

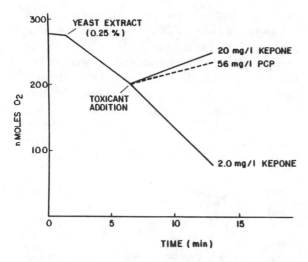

Figure 8 Oxygen evolution by whole cells of isolate 49 (200 μl protein) in the presence of high concentrations of Kepone and PCP. Ten microliters of toxicant in DMF carrier added to reaction mixture after a constant rate of O_2 uptake was observed. DMF alone had no effect. [From Mahaffey et al. (1982).]

oxygen uptake. A polarographic procedure was used similarly for NADH oxidase assays, and it was found that the NADH oxidase activity was inhibited 51% by 0.6 mg/l Kepone while succinooxidase activity was inhibited 25%. The maximum reduction in NADH oxidase activity (62%) was obtained with 1.2 mg/l Kepone, while succinooxidase activity was inhibited 50% in the presence of 6 mg/l Kepone. The lower activity of succinooxidase relative to NADH oxidase is characteristic of the ETP.

The lack of Kepone toxicity in anaerobic plate assays and the marked inhibition of oxygen uptake with several isolates indicated a possible involvement with electron transport and respiration. Widdus et al. (1971) and Trudgill et al. (1971) showed that the inhibition of NADH oxidase activity in *Bacillus subtilis* by chlordane occurred indirectly through apparent disruption of membrane-mediated electron transport. If similar mechanisms function during Kepone poisoning, a different effect would be expected from anaerobic and aerobic conditions. Trudgill et al. (1971) did

not report on anaerobic growth effects but did show that a *Streptococcus* species (which would have minimal cytochrome-mediated electron transport activity) was significantly more resistant to chlordane. These studies indicate that Kepone probably exerts a direct effect on bacterial membrane integrity and function. Mahaffey et al. (1982) studied the membrane-bound oxidases of the ETP from isolate 32K and showed that NADH oxidase and succinooxidase activities are inhibited by Kepone, indicating disruption of electron transport. Thus disruption of membrane-mediated electron transport may result in a transient imbalance in the oxidation-reduction potential of the cell. These methods can be employed to gain more information about the mechanism of toxicity to bacteria.

EFFECT OF TOXICANTS ON MICROBIAL ACTIVITIES

In toxicity studies with higher organisms, researchers have been examining mortality and growth as possible indicators of stress in pollution situations. Yet more subtle effects may be detectable if functional or physiological attributes are examined. Respiration (O_2 uptake or CO_2 production), gill ventilation rates, enzyme levels and activities in blood, avoidance, feeding rates, and assimilation could be more sensitive to a toxicant and could replace some of the tests involving growth and mortality.

A functional approach to the study of aquatic microbial toxicology has a number of appealing aspects. A large bank of physiological tests with bacteria can serve as alternative toxicity testing techniques. These physiological tests are considerably more developed and refined for microorganisms than they are for higher organisms. They include measures of general heterotrophic activity, geochemical cycling rates, and simple mineralization rates of organic materials. Geochemical cycling rates of sulfur, nitrogen, and phosphorus are particularly important because they are characteristic of a rather select group of microorganisms, and the disruption of these processes by a toxicant can have very obvious and dangerous environmental consequences. The oxidation of organic material under anaerobic conditions to methane and the decomposition of bulk organic matter (plant and animal litter) are good functional measures with which to gauge the harmful effects of a toxicant. The assessment consists of measuring substrate disappearance or the production of some product. The advantages and disadvantages of a variety of functional measures related to bacterial activities are discussed in the following sections.

Heterotrophic Activity

Numerous studies to characterize the metabolic activities of microorganisms in natural environments have concentrated on the rates at which bacteria transport solutes into the cell (Wright, 1978) and the rates at which bacteria mineralize a particular chemical to carbon dioxide (Harrison et al., 1971). The success of the kinetic approach for studying the natural activities of bacterial populations has led to a multifaceted application of the techniques to study aquatic microbial ecology. In heterotrophic activity studies, the metabolism of a radiolabeled organic substance (e.g., a sugar, amino acid, or organic acid) is measured with natural assemblages of microorganisms. It is assumed that if the concentration of the added substrate is kept low, it will be metabolized by the bacterial populations in a water sample at a rate similar to that actually occurring in the environment. The assay for metabolism is either uptake of the radioactive material into the cell or mineralization to carbon dioxide. The metabolic rates can be described by the Monod growth equation which relates bacterial growth to the concentration of a growth-limiting component, such as the carbon and energy source. This is an important relationship because it seems to apply to mixed microbial populations in which not all bacteria are active or active to the same extent. The Monod equation can be used to estimate rates at which certain

carbon compounds are metabolized by bacteria (turnover rates), the maximum growth rate of a microbial population, and the affinity of that population for the carbon source. Thus, it is a very useful method for measuring quantitatively the metabolic activities of natural heterotrophic populations. For further details of the technique and examples of the kinetic information derived in various types of studies, the reader is referred to Colwell and Morita (1974).

Hodson et al. (1977) illustrate the application of the technique to a specific toxicological problem: the potential effects of a crude oil spill on natural populations of marine bacteria. The experiments were part of the CEPEX program (Menzel and Case, 1977). Two large (68 m^3) polyethylene bags were used to enclose large water masses. Several crude oils were added to one bag to give a final hydrocarbon concentration of 10 $\mu g/l$ (ppb). The other bag served as the unexposed control. Seawater was removed from the control and oil-treated bags with 6-l Niskin bottles and the water samples were passed consecutively through 183- and 35-μm Nitex mesh filters and finally through 1-μm (pore diameter) Nucleopore filters. This effectively separated the photosynthetic organisms from the bacteria and thus permitted a specific study of the oil-induced changes in heterotrophic activity of natural bacterial populations.

To measure the effect of various concentrations of four types of crude oil on glucose assimilation into the cell, 25-ml filtered water samples (in triplicate) were placed in sterile bottles containing 0 to 3 ml oil-saturated aqueous solution. The bottles were capped and incubated in the dark at the temperature of the water sample at collection for 4 h, after which D-[^{14}C]glucose (about 10^5 cpm) was added to the bottles and incubation continued for 2 h. In many studies, serum bottles are used so that the radioactive glucose could be added with a syringe. (Glucose is one of several substrates that can be used; amino acids, hydrocarbons, glycolic acid, organic acids, and urea have all been successfully tested.) At the end of 2 h the water is filtered through a 0.22-μm membrane filter and washed in sterile seawater. The amount of radioactivity remaining on the filter gives the amount of glucose assimilated by the cells. It is assumed either that none of the substrate is lost by mineralization to CO_2 (due to the short incubation period) or that any loss is compensated by actual measurements (see below).

Two types of kinetic approaches (not described in the Hodson paper) have been used in assimilation experiments to ensure that the added substrate does not bias the assimilation rate (Wright, 1978). In one, a concentration of substrate below the *in situ* concentration (generally 50-100 $\mu g/l$ for aquatic environments) was used and therefore did not influence uptake rates by the bacteria. In the second, concentrations higher than natural levels were used, but several concentrations were tested. By plotting the rate of uptake (fraction assimilated per minute) against the reciprocal of the added substrate concentration, a straight line can usually be obtained. Extrapolation to zero added substrate gives the assimilation rate at natural substrate concentrations. Hodson et al. (1977) chose a concentration based on the workability of the radioactivity levels. The assumption is made that as long as the same concentration of substrate is used, sample-to-sample, the responses of bacterial populations to the substrate will be the same and relative effects of a toxicant can be easily observed.

Hodson et al. (1977) studied the effects of oil on mineralization (bacterial conversion of glucose to CO_2) in sealed (with rubber septa) culture tubes equipped with a hanging center-well to hold CO_2 trapping agent (Fig. 9). The trapping agent can be either a commercial preparation or a chemical such as phenylethylamine or ethanolamine. A small piece of fluted filter paper is usually placed in the cup to increase surface area and trapping efficiency. The tubes are inoculated and incubated as in the assimilation experiments, but at the end of the 2-h incubation, acid is added to the tube with a syringe by inserting a needle through the rubber septum to avoid opening the vessel. The acid stops the reaction and releases any dissolved radioactive CO_2 from the water. The trapping

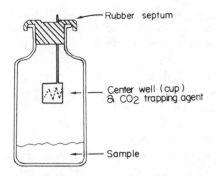

Figure 9 Reaction bottle used to study heterotrophic activity in natural microbial populations.

agent is added to the cup with a second syringe. After approximately one-half h all the CO_2 in the system is trapped. The bottles are opened, and the filter paper is placed directly into scintillation fluid for radioactivity counting. Since the radioactivity in the trapping agent is due entirely to radiolabeled CO_2, the extent of mineralization can be quantitated. This same procedure can be used to study mineralization of substrates in sediment-water slurries (Harrison et al., 1971).

An example of how the toxic effects of crude oils can be assessed in this way is shown in Fig. 10. The oils inhibited glucose assimilation, the effect increasing with increasing concentration of oil. Oil concentrations in excess of 300 $\mu g/l$ were required to produce inhibition, and the oils showed different degrees of toxicity. Bunker C fuel oil (80 $\mu g/l$) stimulated assimilation, probably as a result of the presence of growth-promoting substances. Similar results were observed with mineralization. The authors concluded that a 30-d exposure to crude oil in the enclosed water sample did not result in acclimation of the microbial population to the oil. This lack of acclimation could have been due to the exposure time, which was short compared to the time the bacteria were exposed in their natural substrate, or to the low oil concentration (~ 10 $\mu g/l$). Nevertheless, measurement of heterotrophic activity appears to be useful for measuring the toxic effects of chemicals to microbial populations.

Orndorff and Colwell (1980) used heterotrophic activity in toxic effects studies in a slightly different manner. Since two water samples with different heterotrophic activities may result from different concentrations of bacteria in the samples, measurements of heterotrophic activity were coupled with direct counting methods. By reporting a rate per cell, such as V_{max} (maximum growth rate) or uptake rate, a specific activity index is obtained. Wright (1978) counted bacteria by the acridine orange epifluorescence (ADOC) method and found habitat differences along a river and into an estuary. Orndorff and Colwell (1980) used the ADOC technique to determine the effects of Kepone on microbial populations in samples of

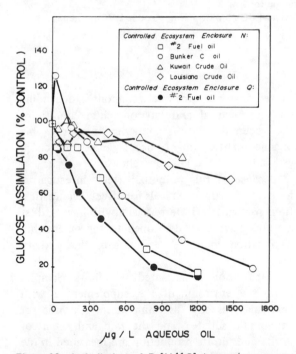

Figure 10 Assimilation of D-[U-^{14}C] glucose (as percent of control value) by 1-μm filterable population from "controlled ecosystem enclosure N" in the presence of increasing concentrations of No. 2 fuel oil, bunker C oil, Kuwait crude oil, and Louisiana crude oil and by 1-μm filtrate from "controlled ecosystem enclosure Q" in the presence of increasing concentrations of No. 2 fuel oil. Incubations were done in triplicate. In all cases, values for the replicates varied by less than 2% of the mean. *[From Hodson et al. (1977).]*

James River (Virginia) water. They modified the method according to the procedure of Kogure et al. (1979) to allow separation of live and dead cells (see section on Enumeration of Bacteria in Aquatic Environments). They based their specific activity measurement on the total uptake and mineralization of ^{14}C-labeled amino acids (MA) as a function of the viable ADOC number (DVC), taken as either Kepone-resistant or Kepone-sensitive bacteria.

The MA/DVC index based on Kepone-resistant bacteria (those able to grow in the presence of Kepone at $\geqslant 0.1$ mg/l) was not much different from that based on sensitive cells (Table 8). This means that bacteria resistant to Kepone have about the same metabolic activity as sensitive cells (at concentrations of Kepone below 0.1 mg/l), and it suggests that bacteria which predominate as a result of a toxicant stress will be able to carry on the same metabolic activity as those which were dominant before the stress. Thus microbial populations appear to be very adaptable to a range of perturbations caused by toxic chemicals. In similar studies, Goulder et al. (1980) (see section on Growth of Heterotrophic Microorganisms) used a specific activity index of V_{max} of glucose uptake per cell; the same relationship to toxicant stress was observed. In their studies V_{max} per cell was negatively correlated with copper concentration, whereas percent mineralization was not correlated. Thus specific activity indices appear to be an excellent measure of toxicity to actively metabolizing microbial populations in natural water samples. They are also useful as potential indicators of pollution stress.

Geochemical Cycling: Nitrogen

Cycling of inorganic nutrients involves the chemical and biological transformation of a variety of nitrogen, sulfur, and phosphorus compounds. Since the principles behind these transformations are similar, only nitrogen cycling will be discussed in relation to toxicity testing. Information on the other inorganic compounds can be found in the literature cited.

Mineralization of organic matter by bacteria

Table 8 Effect of Kepone on Respiration and Incorporation of ^{14}C-labeled L-Amino Acids and Metabolic Activity of Chesapeake Bay Microorganisms[a]

Kepone concentration (mg/l)	Eastern Bay				Colgate Creek			
	Respiration (%)[b]	Incorporation (%)[b]	MA Kepone DVC[c] ($\times 10^{-3}$)	DVC[c] ($\times 10$)	Respiration (%)	Incorporation (%)	MA Kepone DVC[c] ($\times 10^{-5}$)	DVC[c] ($\times 10$)
0.01	100	100	7.64[d]	5.93[e]	62.2	43.3	4.00[f]	2.09[g]
0.05	–	–	–	–	25.7	24.9	2.77	1.10
0.1	34.5	53.1	6.63	2.86	–	–	–	–
0.2	17.2	11.3	5.92	0.76	18.8	17.3	1.20	0.78
1.0	14.9	9.6	2.40	0.65	18.1	16.5	1.20	0.58
10.0	9.6	4.7	2.40	0.28	16.5	15.1	1.20	0.41

[a] From Orndorff and Colwell (1980).
[b] Percent of control, i.e., without added Kepone, after incubation for 2 h.
[c] Metabolic activity/cell = [(respiration + incorporation)/ml water]/[DVC/ml water or Kepone DVC/ml water].
[d] Eastern Bay control, MA/Kepone DVC = 8.50×10^{-1}.
[e] Eastern Bay control, MA/DVC = 6.06×10.
[f] Colgate Creek control, MA/Kepone DVC = 6.10×10^{-5}.
[g] Colgate Creek control, MA/DVC = 4.40×10^{-1}.

results in the production of ammonia (i.e., conversion of organically bound nitrogen to free nitrogen). Although ammonia is used by plants, nitrate is the principal inorganic nutrient used by rooted plants and algae since it is the form of nitrogen most readily assimilated. Much of the ammonia must therefore be converted to nitrate through nitrification. This conversion is mediated almost entirely by two groups of bacteria: *Nitrosomonas* sp., which oxidizes the ammonia to nitrite, and *Nitrobacter* sp., which oxidizes the nitrite to nitrate. The nitrifying bacteria are chemolithotrophs, which utilize the energy derived from nitrification to assimilate CO_2; consequently, they are slow growers. This is important in relation to toxicity studies. If these bacteria are killed or disturbed the population recovery could be quite slow; this could disrupt the nitrogen cycle significantly and have long-lasting effects on the productivity of an ecosystem. In contrast, organisms that release ammonia from organic materials (ammonification) quickly return to the soil and resume functioning rapidly after exposure to a toxicant. If the activity of the nitrifers is slowed or stopped for weeks to months, depending on the chemical and environmental conditions, the accumulation of ammonia from decaying organic matter might occur and this could generally foul the environment.

Because of this potential effect, investigators have tested many chemicals for effects on nitrification, particularly in terrestrial environments. Test methods have been developed to the extent that nitrification could be used as a routine toxicity test.

Nitrification is measured as follows. Samples from the environment are supplemented with ammonia (usually as ammonium chloride or ammonium sulfate), and the rate and extent of nitrite and nitrate production are measured in the presence and absence of a toxicant. For example, Jones and Hood (1980) examined the effects of seven thiophosphorus pesticides on ammonia oxidation. Ammonia-oxidizing bacterial populations were obtained by selective enrichment from sediment cores taken from an estuary. Subsamples of the sediment were removed from the cores and placed in a minimal salts medium containing ammonium chloride as the sole nitrogen source (selective for ammonia-oxidizing bacteria). Production of nitrite was determined by a standard colorimetric method in the presence and absence of the pesticides. The response of the natural populations of nitrifers to several pesticides at 10 mg/l is shown in Fig. 11. Control sediments produced nitrite in about 6 d of incubation and nitrite concentrations continued to rise until d 14. The pesticides all inhibited nitrification to some extent; fonofos and guthion (10 μg/l) were the most inhibitory of the pesticides tested, and methyl parathion and parathion were transiently inhibitory.

The principal degradation products were also examined for toxicity. Aminophenol, for example, was much more toxic (producing an effect at lower concentrations) than its parent compound, methyl parathion. Several pure cultures of bacteria capable of oxidizing ammonia were generally less sensitive to the pesticides than the mixed population from which they were originally isolated.

Studies of toxic effects of chemicals on nitrification rates can be difficult to interpret because of nitrate reduction, which commonly involves the conversion of nitrate to nitrogen gas (denitrification). Denitrification requires anaerobic conditions. In samples containing sediment, reducing conditions are likely to develop and stimulate denitrification. Such reducing conditions can also exist in microniches in apparently aerobic sediments, and denitrification can occur simultaneously with nitrification.

To separate these processes for a toxicological study, a test system for nitrification can be heavily aerated to diminish denitrification. The extent of denitrification can also be estimated by difference, using the chemical N-Serve to inhibit nitrification specifically (Billen, 1975). An alternative is to use the ^{15}N isotope dilution technique (Koike and Hattori, 1978). Sediment samples are placed in bottles and amended with sterile water, ^{15}N-labeled nitrate, and unlabeled ammonia. After complete mixing and incubation for various time periods, the contents are filtered through glass fiber filters, and the filtrate is saved for analysis. The analysis consists of converting all the nitrate in the sample to nitrite (by cadmium-copper reduction) and then converting the nitrite to nitrogen gas. The ratio of ^{29}N$_2$ (formed from the added ^{15}N nitrate) to ^{28}N$_2$ (from nitrification of unlabeled ammonia) is determined by mass spectrometry. Only nitrification and nitrate reduction are responsible for the nitrate change in sediments, and their rates can be calculated from the following equations:

$$N_2 - X_1 = Z - Y$$

$$N_2 X_2 - N_1 X_1 = Z\bar{x}Za - Y\bar{x}$$

where Y is the consumption of nitrate by bacterial nitrate reduction, Z is the production of nitrite by nitrification, N and X are the concentration of nitrate and its ^{15}N content, respectively, $\bar{x}$ and $\bar{x}Za$ are the average ^{15}N contents of nitrate and ammonia between times t_1 and t_2, respectively.

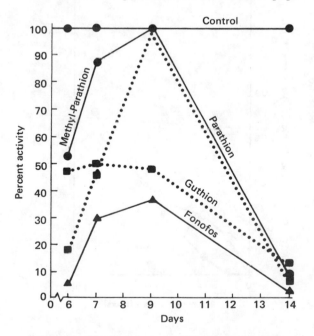

Figure 11 Effect of four thiophosphorus pesticides on ammonium oxidation by natural estuarine populations of nitrifiers. Activity is expressed as percent of control levels of nitrite released. [From Jones and Hood (1980).]

The type of data that can be developed by this technique (rates of nitrate reduction and nitrification) is shown in Fig. 12. The technique is reliable and can be easily applied to toxicological studies. Both nitrification and denitrification can be examined simultaneously, providing a much better indication of the toxicological effect of a chemical on the nitrogen cycle in natural systems.

A wealth of information exists on nitrogen fixation (the formation of nitrogen compounds from free N_2) in aquatic and terrestrial environments. This could provide another good criterion for the effect of a toxicant on a microbial system. Nitrogen fixation is carried out by several groups of microorganisms. In terrestrial environments, fixation of nitrogen by *Rhizobium* in symbiotic association with plant roots accounts for most of

the nitrogen converted into organic compounds. A number of free-living soil bacteria, such as *Azotobacter* and *Beijerinckia*, also fix nitrogen, but at a much lower rate. In aquatic environments, the major nitrogen fixers are the cyanobacteria *Nostoc* and *Anabaena*. These organisms are generally free-living and it is relatively easy to measure their nitrogen-fixing capability. Aquatic studies have shown that *in situ* measurements can be obtained with belljar-like systems (Bohool and Wiebe, 1978) or sealed cores (Herbert, 1975). A variety of methods are also available for studies with laboratory systems (Lee and Watanabe, 1977).

Studies of rates of nitrogen fixation have been facilitated by the development of the acetylene reduction method. This method is based on the fact that the enzyme nitrogenase, which is re-

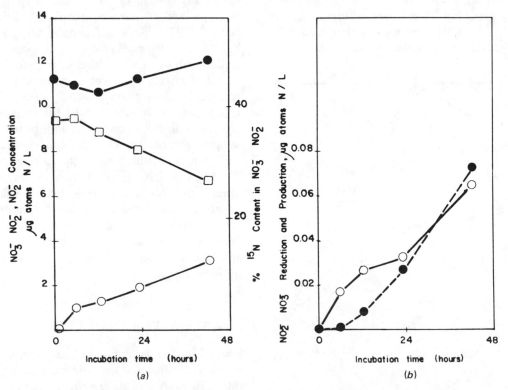

Figure 12 Nitrate reduction and nitrification in sandy sediments from Odawa Bay (November 20, 1976). (*a*) Changes with time in (○) nitrate and nitrite, (●) nitrite, and (□) ^{15}N content in nitrate and nitrite. (*b*) Nitrate (○) reduction and (●) production were calculated with equations in the text. *[From Koike and Hattori (1978).]*

sponsible for reducing N_2 to ammonia, also reduces acetylene. In this technique, vessels are purged of nitrogen and the atmosphere is replaced with helium and acetylene. Conversion of the acetylene (which acts as an N_2 analog) to ethylene is measured by flame ionization gas chromatography. The method works well in aquatic test systems. The results are often difficult to interpret in sediment-containing systems, where the measured rates may be more dependent on the diffusion of acetylene and ethylene to and from the active sediment sites (Lee and Wontanabel, 1977) than on N_2 fixation. Herbert (1975) found large differences between *in situ* and laboratory measurements, presumably due to gas diffusion limitations. Attempts to rectify this problem invariably result in disrupted sediment-water interfaces and uptake rates that cannot be unequivocally attributed to the natural system. However, the methods available for studying nitrogen fixation in aquatic environments are certainly adequate to provide information on relative toxicity. Although there have been numerous studies of nitrogen fixation in aquatic systems, few toxicological studies have been performed. To illustrate how nitrogen fixation can be studied in relation to toxicant input, some recent experiments have been made in soil systems whose results could be applied to aquatic systems.

Blue-green algae significantly influence the nitrogen economy of aquatic environments. DaSilva et al. (1975) used acetylene reduction to test six pesticides for their effect on nitrogen fixation by eight axenic cultures of a symbiotic blue-green alga. Mixed results were obtained; with some pesticides an initial depression in nitrogen-fixing activity of the algal species was followed by a dramatic increase in activity (Fig. 13). With others, such as monuron or MCPA (4-chloro-2-methyl-phenoxyacetic acid), significant inhibition was apparent throughout the exposure period. Some species were affected more than others (both stimulation and depression of activity), and in some cases acclimation to the presence of the pesticide occurred after extended incubation.

Charyulu et al. (1980) studied nitrogen fixation in a flooded rice paddy and effects of different concentrations of a benzimidazole pesticide. At the end of each incubation period, subsamples were spread on agar plates containing nitrogen-free medium to enumerate the symbiotic nitrogen-fixing organisms. Mannitol is usually used as the carbon source; great care must be taken to ensure that there is no combined nitrogen from other ingredients of the medium. Other subsamples were placed in tubes under an acetylene atmosphere, and nitrogen fixation was measured. The pesticide generally reduced cell numbers but did not substantially affect nitrogen fixation. This study indicates that an activity measure is better than a population measure because nitrogenase activity depends on the effectiveness of the individuals rather than their numbers. It also shows that this pesticide retarded the normal drop in oxidation-reduction potential for samples of flooded soil. Nitrogen fixation by microorganisms is very sensitive to Eh. The drop in Eh normally would favor the nitrogen-fixing organism *Azospirillum* (a common inhabitant of these soils); a stabilized Eh then would presumably inhibit the nitrogen-fixing potential of the soil.

Decomposition Processes

Bacteria and fungi are primarily responsible for the decomposition of bulk organic matter produced in aquatic environments. Most of this organic matter comes from plant debris. It is either transformed into soluble organic substances and eventually mineralized to carbon dioxide, or transformed into particulate organic carbon, which may become resistant to microbial breakdown. Accumulation of humic acids, pectins, lignins, and chitin (from animal sources) may be the result of the latter degradation processes. Microbial transformations require a wide range of enzymes, including cellulases for plant material, lipases for lipids, amylases for starch, proteases for proteins, amidases for chitin, and oxygenases for lignin. A single bacterial species probably will not have the genetic information for more than one or two of

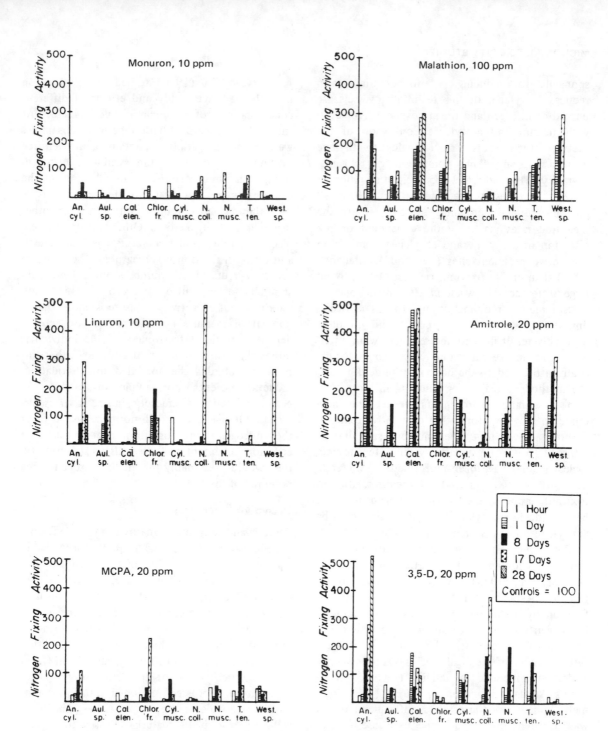

Figure 13 Effect of monuron, linuron, MCPA, malathion, amitrole, and 3,5-D on the nitrogen-fixing ability of *Anabaena cylindrica, Aulosira* sp., *Calothrix elenkenii, Chlorogloea fritschii, Cylindrospermum muscicola, Nostoc* sp. from *Collema, Nostoc muscorum, Tolypothrix tenuis,* and *Westiellopsis* sp. An initial inhibitory effect is more or less followed by gradual recovery. In some cases stimulation may occur. *[From DaSilva et al. (1975).]*

these enzymes. But these activities can be found in a typical interacting population of aquatic bacteria, where commensalistic and mutualistic coordination among bacteria themselves, between bacteria and fungi, and among bacteria and higher plants and animals can be found. A chemical that disrupts one of these enzymatic processes may ultimately alter the metabolic capability of the entire population.

Most streams and rivers have dense vegetation along their banks. When the vegetation dies, it commonly enters the water as leaf litter and serves as the dominant energy source, or an allochthonous input. Animal and microbial components of the stream are largely responsible for decomposing this litter material and releasing available energy. This decomposition process is a commensal relationship between animals and microbes. The animals shred the leaf litter into small chunks with large surface areas which can be colonized and decomposed by the bacteria and fungi. The microorganisms themselves are a nutrient source for grazing invertebrate animals. Thus, if the bacterial and fungal populations were disturbed or inhibited, a drastic change in community structure could occur and secondary productivity could be greatly reduced.

Giesy (1978) examined the toxic effects of cadmium by studying its impact on leaf litter decomposition. Fresh leaf material was placed in stainless steel screen envelopes and the package suspended 10 cm above the sediment surface in a model outdoor stream facility. The stream contained many of the assemblages of macrophytes, periphyton, micro- and macroinvertebrates, and fish typically found in a stream. Separate streams were treated continuously with $CdCl_2$ at 5 and 10 μgl, and changes in the leaf pack were noted. Both concentrations of cadmium reduced leaf litter decomposition, as indicated by changes in dry weight of the leaf pack. Visual observation showed that the exposed leaves (still green and intact after 28 d) were decaying more slowly than the control leaves (brown with only veins and petioles remaining). Pieces of the leaves were also fixed and observed under a scanning electron microscope. The exposed leaves showed much less colonization by bacteria and fungi than the control leaves (Fig. 14).

The apparent inhibition of leaf litter decomposition occurred at cadmium concentrations lower than those needed to inhibit other microorganisms (usually in pure culture) and their activities. It therefore appears that this decomposition process may be very sensitive to toxicants and an early indicator of pollutant stress. This example also shows that a complex mixed natural community may be a better system in which to carry out effects studies than its component parts (pure or axenic cultures).

Anaerobic environments occur in many ecosystems, and the activities of bacteria therein are crucial to the cycling of organic carbon. Methanogenic bacteria and many obligate anaerobic heterotrophic microorganisms have fermentative capacities. The persistence of a toxicant may increase under anaerobic conditions, because fewer organic structures are degraded under anaerobic than under aerobic conditions. A chemical that is also toxic to microbial communities could alter the microbial ecology of anaerobic environments.

There are two basic approaches to studying toxic effects in anaerobic systems. One is to study a specific microbiological process, such as methane production; the other is to study the integrated activities of a large number of organisms and chemical processes. Measurement of the respiratory electron transport system in aquatic sediments is an example of the latter approach.

Respiratory electron transport system (ETS) is a term used in connection with the respiration of organisms in sediments and is measured by the amount of oxygen taken up by a sediment sample. The oxygen demand is due largely to the activities of microorganisms in the sediment as they mineralize naturally occurring organic materials through biological oxidation. In this process different electron acceptors or sinks such as oxygen, nitrate, sulfate, and carbon dioxide are present. As these sinks are used up, they are reduced to H_2O, NO_2^-

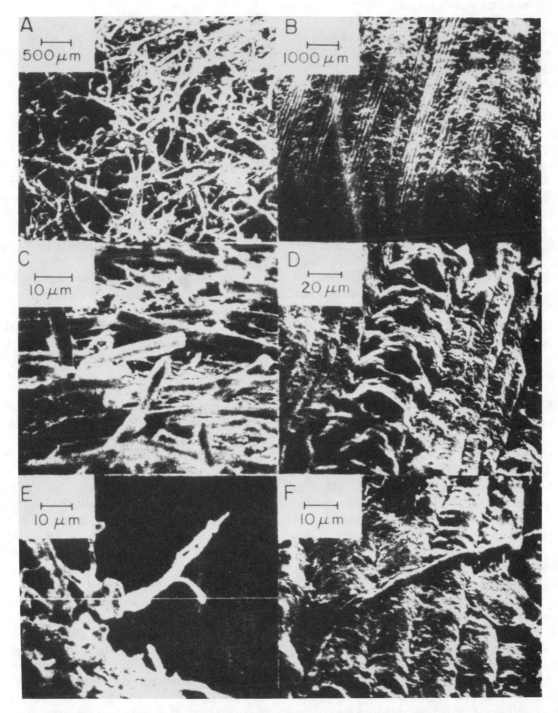

Figure 14 Effect of cadmium on microbial colonization of *Pseudomonas taoda*. (*a*) Control; (*b*) 10μg/l Cd; (*c*) control; (*d*) 10 μg/l Cd; (*e*) control; and (*f*) 5 μg/l Cd. *[Reproduced with permission from Giesy (1978); copyright 1978, Pergamon Press, Ltd.]*

or N_2, SO_2^{2-} or S^{2-}, and methane. As a result of these processes, electrons are transported actively among biological systems through specific chemical reactions of oxidation and reduction and are eventually passed to a final sink (i.e., oxygen, nitrate, sulfate, methane reduction). To measure these activities, researchers commonly add to natural sediments chemicals that are readily oxidized or reduced and whose oxidation-reduction reaction can be readily detected (e.g., by a spectrophotometric monitor). One example is the addition of NADH to sediments. By measuring its oxidation to NAD^+ spectrophotometrically, an indication of the respiratory activity of natural materials may be obtained. The method is known as the dehydrogenase assay since dehydrogenase mediates this process.

Another approach is to add a dye that is readily oxidized and reduced. Various tetrazolium salts, such as triphenyltetrazolium chloride (TTC), react with hydrogen and electrons under anaerobic conditions to form a red formazine compound, which can be measured colorimetrically. The method provides a relative measure of metabolic activity, usually expressed as dehydrogenase activity. Pamatmat and Bhagwat (1973) and Olanczuk and Vosjan (1977) thoroughly characterized the tetrazolium method and found it a quick and simple means of estimating natural rates of anaerobic metabolism by bacteria. It is an integrative method in which activities of all the bacteria growing under anaerobic conditions are considered. Unfortunately, this method has not been used extensively in toxic effects testing. It could be a relatively easy procedure for determining whether a toxic chemical inhibits anaerobic metabolism. Since the method can be used in the field (Pamatmat and Bhagwat, 1973), it is also possible that toxicant-induced stress to an environment can be observed through relative measurements of ETS activity.

Certain pesticides in natural environments may produce toxic residues that not only affect higher organisms but also inhibit the degradation of other pesticides which are not themselves particularly persistent. The use of two different pesticides on cropland may have an adverse effect not obvious with either one alone. Certain persistent xenobiotics (manufactured chemicals) are metabolized in nature only by the nonspecific enzymatic activities found in aquatic bacteria. Many bacteria may not be able to gain energy or carbon from a particular chemical but attack the chemical to some extent because it is similar to a substance readily utilized by the cell. This phenomenon has been referred to as cooxidation or cometabolism (Leadbetter and Foster, 1960). Agriculturally feasible combinations of chemicals may eventually interfere with each other's detoxification through cooxidation or some other more direct process. Engelhardt and Wallnofer (1975) found that a variety of carbamate and organophosphate insecticides inhibited phenylamide herbicide degradation by a pure culture (axenic) of Bacillus sphaericus. The effect was compound-specific and occurred at concentrations expected during normal pesticide application to crops. When the activity of crude cell-free preparations of the phenylamide-hydrolyzing acylamidase from cultures of the Bacillus species was tested in the presence of the carbamate insecticide, the inhibition was competitive. This means that the carbamate is capable of interfering with the active site of the enzyme or that the enzyme has low specificity. If this occurs in hydrolytic enzyme systems, then a variety of pesticides probably can nonspecifically inhibit degradative processes that require hydrolytic enzymes.

Anderson and Domsch (1980) observed the influence of several pesticides on the degradation of two thiocarbamate herbicides in soil. The degradation of radiolabeled triallate and diallate was followed by examining the parent compound, ^{14}C-labeled bound residues, and mineralization. Bound residues were defined as the radioactivity associated with soil particles that could not be extracted with solvents. Experiments were conducted with flasks containing a bed of soil and a system for trapping carbon dioxide. At the end of an incubation, the soil was extracted with solvent to recover any parent compound, then combusted to quantitate the radioactivity associated with the soil material (bound residue). After treatment with radioactive triallate and diallate herbicide, the soil samples were treated with several combinations of pesticide, fungicide, and herbicide formulations to simulate typical spray programs for crops (wheat and sugarbeets) in terms of both concentration and chronological application sequence. After 70 d of incubation, minimal influence of the pesticides on diallate degradation was observed (Table 9). Only the pesticide chlorpyrifos significantly inhibited diallate degradation. The effect was cumulative with incubation time. After 70 d, an average of 14% less $^{14}CO_2$ was produced than in the control, and 24% less bound residue was observed. The half-life of diallate (the period after which 50% of the applied concentration could no longer be extracted from the soil in the form of parent compound) was approximately 22 d in the control soils and 30 d in the chlorpyrifos-treated soil. Similar results were obtained with triallate. Chlorpyrifos was applied to the soils as the commercial formulation, and it was possible that one of the formulation components was the toxic agent. To test this, analytical grade chlorpyrifos was applied to soil in the flask and degradation of diallate was again determined. Inhibition was proportional to chlorpyrifos concentration; a concentration of 20 $\mu g/g$ (ppm) extended the half-life to 70 d. Thus, a formulation component was not the toxic ingredient. Bound residue formation and mineralization were affected to a similar extent. It can be concluded that these pesticides had relatively little effect on the degradation of diallate and triallate. Chlorpyrifos inhibition was not substantial and would probably translate to a minimal effect in the field. However, the experiments illustrate a potential sensitive test of toxicological hazard based on microbial activities.

Pritchard and Bourquin (unpublished information) studied toxic effects of pesticides in estuarine environments. Degradation of methyl parathion was studied in a special biodegradation test system known as an eco-core (Pritchard et al., 1978). This system (Fig. 15) permits the study of degradation while the sediment-water interface (one of the most microbially active areas in aquatic environments) is preserved. An intact sample of water and sediment was collected from a salt marsh with a sterile glass tube. The cores were brought into the laboratory, spiked with ^{14}C-labeled methyl parathion, and stoppered so that air could slowly be bubbled through the water column to maintain proper oxygen concentrations (bubbling does not disturb the sediment-water interface). At different time intervals, replicate cores were analyzed destructively for total parent compound concentration, bound residue formation, and mineralization to CO_2.

Kepone was tested in this system for its effect on the microbial degradation of methyl parathion. Kepone at 2 mg/l was found to significantly inhibit the microbially mediated conversion of methyl parathion to carbon dioxide (Fig. 16). The toxic effect was observed in sediment-water cores from two different estuaries: the Escambia (Range Point salt marsh) and James River estuaries. James River cores were considerably more active in biodegradation of methyl parathion. Although some studies have shown a Kepone concentration in sediments to be as high as 2 ppm, the concentration is variable and patchy. Since normal degradation of methyl parathion, or even other types of organics, occurs in many parts of the James River, it is unlikely that its persistence will be increased significantly. The experimental approach is another method of studying the toxic effects of certain organics to microorganisms and the processes they mediate.

UNIQUE ASPECTS OF THE EFFECTS OF TOXICANTS ON MICROORGANISMS

A variety of toxicology studies differ considerably from the norm, but their creativity and uniqueness merit special attention. These studies are not routine, but they offer new insights that may prove useful in the future development of toxicity

Table 9 Influence of Pesticide Mixtures on Microbial Degradation of [Carbonyl-^{14}C] Diallate in Soil[a,b]

Incubation time (d)	Distribution of ^{14}C-labeled compounds	[^{14}C] Diallate (0)	+ Pyrazon (0)	+ + Chlorpyrifos (0)	+ + + Dimethoate (14)	+ + + + Azinphosmethyl (28)	+ + + + + Thiophanate (35)
0	Soil[d]						
	Diallate	95.8	—	—	—	—	—
	Bound	3.0	—	—	—	—	—
14	Atmosphere						
	Diallate	4.2	3.8	4.6	—	—	—
	CO_2	22.5	22.6	17.9	—	—	—
	Soil						
	Diallate	56.3	58.6	62.1	—	—	—
	Bound	15.6	13.3	13.6	—	—	—
28	Atmosphere						
	Diallate	5.8	6.1	7.0	7.1	—	—
	CO_2	36.6	35.7	30.2	28.8	—	—
	Soil						
	Diallate	36.8	36.9	49.8	50.1	—	—
	Bound	19.2	19.3	11.2	12.1	—	—
35	Atmosphere						
	Diallate	6.6	6.6	8.1	7.7	8.4	—
	CO_2	37.7	40.4	37.9	30.5	33.9	—
	Soil						
	Diallate	36.3	32.3	41.1	47.6	45.8	—
	Bound	18.4	19.5	11.9	12.6	11.2	—
70	Atmosphere						
	Diallate	6.4	7.1	7.1	7.8	8.8	7.8
	CO_2	61.3	62.9	54.6	54.6	49.9	54.3
	Soil						
	Diallate	12.8	10.4	20.8	22.9	26.4	21.7
	Bound	18.5	18.7	15.3	12.9	13.3	15.1

[a]Results, which are averages from duplicate soil cultures and are in percent recovered radioactivity, show the distribution of ^{14}C residues between soil and the atmosphere above the soil. Radioactivity recovered (as percent of applied) was 98.3 ± 1.9 for a total of 38 extractions; lowest recovery was 96.0%.

[b]From Anderson and Domsch (1980).

[c]Diallate and thiophanate applied at 1 μg/g (active ingredient), all other compounds at 2 μg/g.

[d]All soil samples contained traces of water- and benzene-soluble radioactivity. These averaged 1.3–0.4 and 0.2–0.0% of the recovered radioactivity, respectively.

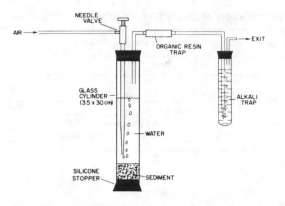

Figure 15 Diagram of eco-core test system. *[From Pritchard et al. (1978).]*

testing. They reflect some fascinating aspects of microbiology and may stimulate new thinking in the ecotoxicology of microbial processes.

Chemotaxis

Bacteria are capable of tactic responses to particular chemicals, including toxicants. Young and

Mitchell (1973) showed that toxicants can negatively affect chemotaxis in bacteria. Ordinarily, because bacteria are so small, this type of a response would be difficult to observe. Adler (1969), however, developed a method in which a capillary pipette is filled with a chemical or nutrient source and placed in a dilute culture of bacteria. After a short period of incubation, the mouth of the pipette is covered with bacterial cells (both in and around the pipette). This attraction to a chemical is called positive chemotaxis. When a toxic chemical is included in the nutrient broth in the capillary, the bacteria do not accumulate near the tip or inside; in fact, a distinct clearing zone is often noted around the tip. This is termed negative chemotaxis. Chemicals that neither stimulate nor inhibit chemotaxis are distinct because bacteria around the capillary tip are randomly distributed, and no bacteria are found inside the pipette. Young and Mitchell (1973) showed that bacteria can actively avoid unfavorable areas. Figure 17 shows the distribution of several marine bacterial

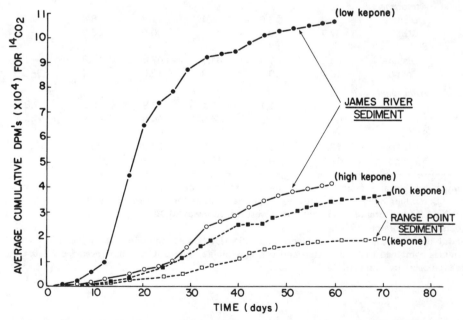

Figure 16 Effects of Kepone on methyl parathion mineralization in eco-cores: (○) 600 ppm and (●) 140 ppm Kepone in James River sediments; (□) 500 ppm Kepone and (■) control sediments from Florida salt marsh. *[From A. W. Bourquin and P. H. Pritchard (unpublished data.)]*

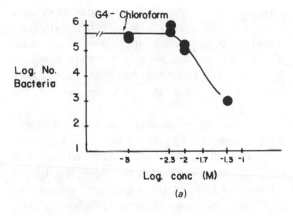

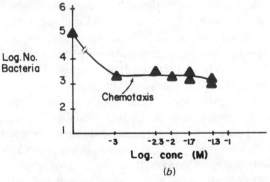

Figure 17 (a) Viability of bacterial isolate G4 in the presence of chloroform. (b) Number of bacteria entering capillary pipette in the presence of chloroform. [From Young and Mitchell (1973).]

isolates in nutrient broth in the presence of chloroform. As the concentration of chloroform is increased, fewer (two orders of magnitude) bacteria are found in the capillary pipette. Comparison of this curve with a survival curve (Fig. 17a) shows that chemotaxis occurs at a much lower concentration than that which causes cell death. Mitchell et al. (1972) reported on chemoreception, showing that seawater bacteria are attracted to a wide variety of organic materials, including sugars and amino acids. Isolates obtained from seawater in which the diatom *Skeletonema costatum* was the sole carbon source also showed chemotaxis toward this organism. In addition, they showed that phenol (0.6%), toluene (0.6%), and Kuwait crude oil (concentration unknown) inhibited the

chemotactic response to glucose by 80% compared to unexposed control. This tactic response measure has been minimally tested with toxicants, yet it has considerable potential as an effects method. It is quick, simple, easy to interpret, and could be used primarily as a screening tool. However, trying to find an ecological meaning for negative taxis is difficult.

Epiphytic Microorganisms

Almost any surface in any body of water has a layer of algae covering it. Invariably associated with the algae and adhering to them is a population of epiphytic bacteria. In this symbiotic relationship, the algae excrete organic materials for bacterial growth, and the bacterial metabolism supplies CO_2 and inorganic nutrients for algal growth. This symbiosis is important for the ecosystem, and it is desirable to know the extent to which a toxicant disturbs this community.

Fry and Ramsay (1977) examined the effect of the herbicide paraquat on the heterotrophic activity of bacteria associated with the leaf surfaces of *Elodea* spp. and *Chara* spp. A washed piece of plant leaf was suspended in a serum bottle containing ^{14}C-labeled glucose and was incubated in the presence of CO_2 trapping agent to measure mineralization (Harrison et al., 1971). Fry and Ramsey (1977) removed the epiphytes from the leaves by vigorously agitating the leaves (scraping the leaves was also successful) in sterile water for 5 min. The leaves were filtered out and the remaining cell suspension used to examine [^{14}C] glucose uptake and mineralization. After thoroughly scraping and cleaning the leaves, it was possible to run controls to determine how much glucose was taken up and mineralized by the plants. The epiphytes accounted for 60% of the glucose taken up by the plant system (Fig. 18). An autoradiographic technique with tritiated glucose showed that only bacteria were actively taking up the glucose, and that attributed to plants (40%) may have been due entirely to bacteria that were not removed.

The effect of paraquat was monitored by

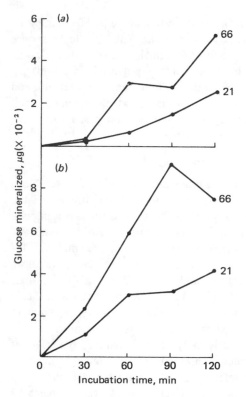

Figure 18 Effects of two concentrations (21 and 66 µg/l) of unlabeled glucose on mineralization of [^{14}C] glucose by epiphytic bacteria: (a) *Chara* and (b) *Elodea*. [From Fry and Ramsey (1977).]

determining the maximum velocity of uptake or mineralization by microorganisms (V_{max}), the glucose concentration that gives half the V_{max}, $K_s + S_n$, (where K_s is the concentration of substrate that gives half the maximal velocity and S_n is the natural glucose concentration), and the time taken for the natural substrate to be mineralized by natural populations (turnover time). Paraquat increased V_{max} and $K_s + S_n$ of bacteria associated with the *Elodea* (Fig. 19). Epiphytic bacteria on the surface of the *Chara* leaves remained unchanged. The herbicide may have stressed the *Elodea*, causing it to release soluble organic compounds which would stimulate growth of the epiphytic bacteria. *Chara* did not release organic materials, presumably because of its resistance to

paraquat. The bacterial activity may serve as a secondary indication of toxicity to plants. This technique of estimating kinetic constants is complicated by the variability in the data; however, there was little doubt that epiphytic bacteria were influenced by the release of nutrients from the host plant.

Using a slightly different approach, Bott and Rogenmuser (1978) assessed the toxic effects of the water-soluble fraction of crude oil and used crankcase oil on the attached algae of a typical woodland stream. Algal populations were developed on microscope slides by suspending the slides in a Plexiglas tank through which stream water flowed continually. Herbivores other than protozoans were removed from the slides daily. Once it appeared that the algal population was comparable on each slide, the water-soluble fraction of the oil was added to the tanks continuously.

Several different measurements were employed to determine how the algae responded. Species composition was determined by direct observation with a microscope. Algal biomass was measured by determining chlorophyll *a* and chlorophyll *c* (chlorophyll *c* is more often associated with diatoms). The cell concentration of cyanobacteria was followed through measurements of phycocyanin. Algal material accumulating on the slides was also checked for photosynthetic incorporation of radiolabeled CO_2 into cell material. The water-soluble fraction of these oils reduced algal biomass on the slides (lowered chlorophyll *a*) but caused an increase in cyanobacteria (Table 10). Some studies indicate that blue-green algae are a less desired food source for herbivores; thus their dominance may be an early indicator of adverse effects. Incorporation of radiolabeled CO_2 into cells during photosynthesis was both stimulated and inhibited by the oils. Number 2 fuel oil extracts at high concentrations depressed ^{14}C incorporation. Thus, following the activities of epiphytic algal and bacterial populations associated with surfaces in natural streams appears to offer an excellent approach to toxicity testing.

A variety of other methods can be used to

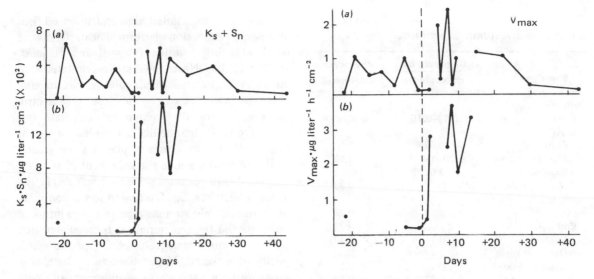

Figure 19 Changes in $K_s + S_n$ and V_{max} during mineralization of glucose by epiphytic bacteria of *Chara* and *Elodea* before and after treatment with paraquat. Only results having positive regressions are plotted. (a) *Chara* and (b) *Elodea*. Paraquat was applied on d 0. *[From Fry and Ramsey (1977).]*

monitor the effects of toxic chemicals on epiphytic microbial populations. Andrews and Kenerley (1978) plated out on agar medium the bacteria and fungi associated with apple leaf surfaces. Agar plates were inoculated with leaf washings, with spores that fell from the leaf surface, or by imprinting leaves on the agar. Light and electron microscopy were used to examine morphological and community structure changes on the leaf surfaces. Lactic acid-type bacteria and fluorescent pseudomonads were most depressed by a series of pesticides applied as in crop spraying. Although apple leaves were used, the same techniques could be applied to aquatic plants and vegetation.

Most toxicological studies on aquatic bacteria are performed with bacteria found in the water column, undoubtedly the easiest and most accessible populations to study. However, epiphytic microorganisms are an important part of the microbial community and should be considered for study whenever possible. In salt-marsh environments and wetland areas, epiphytic bacteria may be more important in the mineralization

of organic carbon from plants to CO_2 and inorganic nutrients than bacteria of the water column. Giesy (1978) showed that the epiphytes on rock surfaces are the major mineralizers in a stream ecosystem.

Incidence of Plasmid-containing Bacteria

The very low levels of organic and inorganic nutrients in marine environments may limit the growth and survival of many microorganisms. Consequently, marine bacterial populations maintain a delicate balance between genetic flexibility and metabolic capabilities. Maintenance of this balance may result in preferential loss of certain nonessential genetic elements, particularly extrachromosomal DNA or plasmids (Smith & Gardner, 1970). By studying the incidence of plasmids in marine bacterial populations, it may be possible to show that a pollutant is changing the nutrient conditions of the environment and consequently changing the genetic makeup of the indigenous bacteria.

Hada and Sizemore (1981) discussed effects of crude oil pollution on microorganisms which could

Table 10 Pigment Ratios of Algal Communities: Summer and Autumn Experiments[a]

Experiment	Chlorophyll c / chlorophyll a	Phycocyanin / chlorophyll a
Summer		
Start	0.11–0.15	0.03–0.05
End		
Control	0.08	0.06
Used crankcase	0.14	0.12
Nigerian crude	0.07	0.12
No. 2 fuel oil	0.15	0.33
Autumn		
Start	0.12	0.08
End		
Control	0.14	1.33
Used crankcase	0.17	0.96
Nigerian crude	0.13	0.93
No. 2 fuel oil	0.07	2.13

[14]C incorporation (dpm/μg of chlorophyll a) by algal communities exposed to water-soluble fractions of oils[b]

Extract exposure	July 19	August 13	August 24
Control	1869	1246	1890
Crankcase	1418	1542	1262
Nigerian crude	1369	1112	972
No. 2 fuel oil	1384	3691	927

[a]From Bott and Rogenmuser (1978).
[b]Corrected for dark fixation and excretion. Single determinations $\bar{x} \pm$ SD for 7/19 ($P°$) = 1510 ± 240 (16%).

be applicable in future assays for other toxic pollutants. They determined the incidence of DNA plasmids (extrachromosomal pieces of DNA found in the cytoplasm of bacterial cells) in marine *Vibrio* spp. in relation to the pollution history of the sampling area. The marine *Vibrio* spp. are gram-negative, facultatively anaerobic, rod-shaped bacteria common in many estuarine and marine environments. They are associated with diseases of humans and appear to be the "enteric bacteria" of the sea (Bauman and Bauman, 1977). Thus their survival could be coupled to pollution stress in the marine environment.

Hada and Sizemore (1981) isolated marine *Vibrio* spp. throughout the year from sampling stations in an unpolluted area and in an oil-field area near a production platform. The bacteria were lysed with Brij solution (Clewell and Helinski, 1969) and the DNA in the lysate precipitated with ethanol. The number of plasmids in this preparation was determined by agarose gel electrophoresis, where the components separate out according to their mobility and molecular weight (Table 11). The incidence of plasmids was greater at the oil-field stations than the control stations. The number of plasmids per isolate was also higher at the oil-field stations (compared to the controls). Since the oil-field stations receive a large influx of nutrients and toxic materials, it is speculated that these conditions were responsible for the multiplicity of plasmids. If this is correct, plasmids in microorganisms may serve as indicators of water

Table 11 Incidence of *Vibrio* spp. and Plasmid Containing *Vibrio* spp. for Gas and Oil-Field Stations and Control Site during Four Quarterly Cruises[a]

Season	Oil-field stations		Control stations	
	No. of Vibrio spp.	Percent Vibrio spp. with plasmids	No. of Vibrio spp.	Percent Vibrio spp. with plasmids
Fall	58	45	90	21
Winter	42	30	3	66
Spring	35	23	6	33
Summer	168	35	38	21

Plasmid multiplicity of plasmid-containing strains

Plasmid bands per strain	Percent of plasmid-containing strains	
	Oil-field isolates	Control station isolates
1	39.6	71
2	24.5	16
3	16.0	0
4	3.8	13
5	2.8	0
6	7.5	0
7	5.7	0

[a]From Hada and Sizemore (1981).

pollution. The results also suggest that the genetic and metabolic capabilities of these organisms may have changed, making it possible for some natural processes to be short-circuited or supplemented.

Bioaccumulation in Bacteria

Ko and Lockwood (1968) showed that chlorinated hydrocarbon pesticides (dieldrin, DDT, and the fungicide pentachloronitrobenzene) were readily accumulated by pure cultures of soil fungi and actinomycetes. Grimes and Morrison (1975) extended the observation to aquatic bacterial isolates. Pure cultures were grown in nutrient broth, washed by centrifugation, and resuspended in various pesticides (in acetone carrier) at a concentration of 0.1 μg/l. At specific time intervals, subsamples were removed and centrifuged; the concentration of the pesticide in the water was determined by gas chromatography. These pesticides were bioconcentrated (i.e., the ratio of pesticide in the cell to pesticide in the water increased) by factors ranging from 10 for lindane to as much as 59,000 for chlordane. Pesticides were ranked by bioconcentration potential: the more water-insoluble the pesticide, the higher the bioconcentration factor. Once inside the cells (equilibrium was reached within 15 min), the pesticides were difficult to extract. Extraction from the cells was also inversely related to water solubility. Because of the affinity of the insoluble pesticides for lipid-containing materials in the cell, pesticides would be expected to localize in cellular membranes. However, Grimes and Morrison (1975) found that the stalked bacterium *Caulobacter vibrioides,* which has the greatest cellular lipid content among bacteria, had the highest bioconcentration values.

Geller (1979) showed that bioaccumulation (at least for the herbicide atrazine) is a function of cell surface area. He observed that physiological and morphological groups of bacteria with different cellular volumes took up different amounts of atrazine. In contrast to the results of Grimes and Morrison (1975), Geller found that atrazine was readily taken up by the cells, but noted that cell

aggregates observed after extended incubation periods in liquid culture were less effective in absorbing atrazine. This might have resulted from a decreased surface area, or it might mean that actively growing cells (those not in aggregates) are the best bioconcentrators. In studies with the common aquatic myxobacterium *Cytophaga*, the high bioconcentration of atrazine was related to the extensive slime layer typically deposited on the surface of these cells. These studies indicate a general nonspecific mechanism of bioaccumulation which is more dependent on the biochemical composition of the cells than on a physiological or active transport mechanism. Since bacteria are the initial step in the food chain of aquatic systems, bioaccumulation may be a principal path by which toxic chemicals enter food chains, leading to damage and stress to ecosystems. Whether this is the case depends on how well the role of bacteria in the food chain can be described. It may also be possible that bacteria that accumulate pesticides can be used as biological sponges. Under controlled laboratory conditions, bacteria flocs could be used to remove pesticides from aquatic environments (Speidel et al., 1972).

ADVERSE EFFECTS OF MICROORGANISMS ON TOXIC SUBSTANCES

Toxicity of a chemical in an aquatic environment is tightly coupled to its chemical and biological fate. Some very toxic chemicals are innocuous in the environment because their degradation to nontoxic by-products is rapid. Biodegradation is one of the principal fates of these chemicals, and humans depend on the metabolic diversity of microbial populations to ensure that many synthetic organic materials do not accumulate in the environment. The biodegradation capabilities of bacteria have been overchallenged. Chemicals have been synthesized with structures that the enzymatic machinery of microorganisms cannot attack at significant rates, leading to major pollution problems with chemicals such as DDT, Kepone, and polychlorinated biphenyls (PCBs).

Biodegradation mechanisms and capabilities of aquatic organisms are discussed in Chapter 18. It is emphasized here, however, that biodegradation may generate a product more toxic than the parent compound. Although this is not well documented in nature, there are enough examples to concern microbiologists and to warrant studies of the toxicity of degradation products. Mercury is probably the most publicized example of a substance that was more toxic after microbial transformation. The anaerobic activities of microorganisms in sediments caused methylation of mercury (Bisogni and Lawrence, 1975; Olsen and Cooper, 1976). As a result, the mercury was made more water-soluble and was mobilized from the sediment and more thoroughly mixed with the water column. More toxic forms of the element (methyl and dimethyl mercury) resulted. Sayler et al. (1975) showed that bacteria, through bioaccumulation of mercury and consumption by higher organisms, can enhance the concentration of mercury in aquatic food chains. Methylation of other elements (cadmium, arsenic, tin) by microorganisms can also potentially produce a more toxic by-product.

The fate of the antimicrobial agent pentachlorobenzyl alcohol caused major concern in Japan. This chemical was applied to rice plants to control a common fungus. However, once the plants died and decayed in the soil, pentachlorobenzyl alcohol was converted to pentachlorobenzoic acid. This metabolic product was toxic to plants but no longer toxic to fungi. Pesticides such as DDT, mirex, heptachlor, and dieldrin can be slowly attacked by microorganisms and other degradative processes. The degradation products are usually resistant to further degradation and transformation, and their persistence and toxicity in the environment are of concern.

Crude oil contains many polynuclear aromatic hydrocarbons that are slowly degraded and could yield intermediate degradation products that are carcinogenic and mutagenic. Organophosphate insecticides have P=S bonds and could be oxidized by bacteria to corresponding P=O (oxone) deriva-

tives, which have considerably greater mammalian toxicity. Bacteria participate in N-alkylation and nitrosamination leading to the formation of nitrosamines from a variety of common precursors such as secondary amines and nitrites. Nitrosamines are powerful carcinogens and mutagens. Although many of these potential degradation products are not toxic to bacteria, bacterial activity leads to their formation.

SUMMARY

Microorganisms are an integral part of the nutrient cycling and energy flow processes of aquatic ecosystems. Their degradative and mineralization capabilities maintain the carbon balance of the ecosystem and also permit humans to dispose of synthetic wastes in aquatic environments. These environments have a certain assimilatory capacity for the wastes, and their biodegradation potential determines the magnitude of this capacity. Humans must not exceed this capacity. The generation of persistent or nonbiodegradable chemicals show how easily this capacity can be abused. The input of chlorinated hydrocarbons into the environment exceeded their biological detoxification, and major ecological damage resulted. Had the assimilatory capacity been properly assessed, environmental abuse might have been avoided.

The toxicity of chemicals to bacteria must be carefully observed and researched. If a new synthetic chemical is developed and allowed to pollute the environment, some microbial processes could be disturbed, and this could eventually have an indirect but catastrophic effect on the entire ecosystem. Severe inhibition of nitrification can affect plant communities. If photosynthetic production drops, the effect ripples throughout the ecosystem.

Bacteria and fungi and the processes they catalyze are fairly resistant to inhibition by synthetic chemicals. A small perturbation in one part of the environment can often be overcome because of the ubiquity of microorganisms and their great metabolic diversity. Nonetheless, toxicologists should incorporate microorganisms into testing schemes, since they may be potential indicators of environmental damage.

The importance of using a wide diversity of toxicity tests for microorganisms cannot be over-emphasized. Rapid methods for assessing chemical toxicity to microorganisms are needed for detecting chemicals that are potentially toxic to the ecosystem. Continued research in basic microbial ecology should help fill this need.

LITERATURE CITED

Adler J: Chemoreception in bacteria. Science 166:1588–1597, 1969.

Anderson JP, Domsch KH: Influence of selected pesticides on the microbial degradation of ^{14}C-triallate and ^{14}C-diallate in soil. Arch Environ Contam Toxicol 9:115–123, 1980.

Andrews JH, Kenerley CM: The effects of a pesticide program on non-target epiphytic microbial populations of apple leaves. Can J Microbiol 24:1058–1072, 1978.

Bauman P, Bauman L: Biology of the marine enterobacteria: *Beneckea* and *Photobacterium*. Annu Rev Microbiol 31:39–61, 1977.

Billen G: Evaluation of nitrifying activity in sediments by dark ^{14}C-bicarbonate incorporation. Water Res 9:51–57, 1975.

Bisogni JJ, Lawrence AW: Kinetics of mercury methylation in aerobic and anaerobic aquatic sediments. J Water Pollut Control Fed 47:135–152, 1975.

Bohool BB, Wiebe WJ: Nitrogen fixing communities in an intertidal ecosystem. Can J Microbiol 24:923–938, 1978.

Bott TL, Rogenmuser K: Effects of No. 2 fuel oil, Nigerian crude oil, and used crankcase oil on attached algal communities: Acute and chronic toxicity of water-soluble constituents. Appl Environ Microbiol 36:673–682, 1978.

Bourquin AW, Pritchard PH, Mahaffey WR: Effects of Kepone on estuarine microorganisms. Dev Ind Microbiol 19:489–497, 1978.

Breazeal FW, Camper ND: Effect of selected herbicides on bacterial growth rates. Appl Environ Microbiol 23:431–432, 1972.

Charyulu PBB, Ramakrishna C, Rao VR: Effect of 2-aminobenzimidazole on nitrogen fixers from flooded soil and their nitrogenase activity. Bull Environ Contam Toxicol 25:482–486, 1980.

Clewell DB, Helinski DR: Supercoiled circular DNA-protein complex in *Escherichia coli*: Purification and induced conversion to an open circular DNA form. Proc Natl Acad Sci USA 62:1159–1166, 1969.

Colwell RR, Morita RY: Effect of the ocean environment on microbial activities. In: Proceedings of the 2d U.S.-Japan Conference on Marine Microbiology. Baltimore: University Park Press, 1974.

DaSilva EJ, Henriksson LE, Henriksson E: Effect of pesticides on blue-green algae and nitrogen fixation. Arch Environ Contam Toxicol 3:193–204, 1975.

Daley RJ, Hobbie JE: Direct counts of aquatic bacteria by a modified epifluorescence technique. Limnol Oceanogr 20:875–882, 1975.

Englehardt G, Wallnofer, PR: Inhibition of phenylamide hydrolysis by *Bacillus sphaericus* with methyl carbamate and organophosphorous insecticides. Appl Environ Microbiol 29:717–721, 1975.

Fry JC, Brooker MP, Thomas PL: Changes in the microbial populations of a reservoir treated with the herbicide paraquat. Water Res 7:395–407, 1973.

Fry JC, Ramsey AJ: Changes in the activity of epiphytic bacteria of *Elodea canadensis* and *Chara vulgaris* following treatment with the herbicide paraquat. Limnol Oceanogr 22:556–561, 1977.

Geller A: Sorption and desorption of atrazine by three bacterial species isolated from aquatic systems. Arch Environ Contam Toxicol 8:713–720, 1979.

Giesy JP: Cadmium inhibition of leaf decomposition in an aquatic microcosm. Chemosphere 6:467–475, 1978.

Goulder R, Blanchard AS, Sanderson PL, Wright B: Relationships between heterotrophic bacteria and pollution in an industrial estuary. Water Res 14:591–601, 1980.

Grimes DJ, Morrison SM: Bacterial bioconcentration of chlorinated hydrocarbon insecticides from aqueous systems. Microb Ecol 2:43–59, 1975.

Guthrie RK, Cherry DS, Ferebee RN: The effects of diuron on bacterial populations in aquatic environments. Water Resour Bull 10:304–310, 1974.

Hada HS, Sizemore RK: Incidence of plasmids in marine *Vibrio* spp. isolated from an oil field in the northwestern Gulf of Mexico. Appl Environ Microbiol 41:199–202, 1981.

Harrison MJ, Wright RT, Morita RY: Method for measuring mineralization in lake sediments. Appl Microbiol 21:698–702, 1971.

Herbert RA: Heterotrophic nitrogen fixation in shallow estuarine sediments. J Exp Mar Biol Ecol 18:215–225, 1975.

Hodson RE, Azam F, Lee RF: Effects of four oils on marine bacterial populations: Controlled ecosystem pollution experiment. Bull Mar Sci 27:119–126, 1977.

Holm-Hansen O, Booth CR: The measurement of adenosine triphosphate in the ocean and its ecological significance. Limnol Oceanogr 11:510–519, 1966.

Jones RD, Hood NA: The effects of organophosphorous pesticides on estuarine ammonia oxidizers. Can J Microbiol 26:1296–1299, 1980.

Ko WH, Lockwood JL: Accumulation and concentration of chlorinated hydrocarbon pesticides by microorganisms in soil. Can J Microbiol 14:1075, 1968.

Kogure K, Simidu U, Taga N: A tentative direct microscopic method for counting living marine bacteria. Can J Microbiol 25:415–420, 1979.

Koike J, Hattori A: Simultaneous determinations of nitrification and nitrate reduction in coastal sediment by an ^{14}N dilution technique. Appl Environ Microbiol 35:853–857, 1978.

Leadbetter ER, Foster JW: Bacterial oxidation of gaseous alkanes. Arch Microbiol 35:92–194, 1960.

Lee KK, Watanabe J: Problems of the acetylene reduction technique applied to water-saturated paddy soils. Appl Environ Microbiol 34:654–660, 1977.

Mahaffey WR, Pritchard PH, Bourquin AW: Effect of Kepone on growth and respiration of several estuarine microorganisms. Appl Environ Microbiol 43:1419–1424, 1982.

Matthews RA, Kondratieff PF, Buikema AL: A field verification of the use of the autotrophic index in monitoring stress effects. Bull Environ Contam Toxicol 25:226–233, 1980.

Menzel DW, Case J: Concept and design: Controlled ecosystem pollution experiment. Bull Mar Sci 27:1–7, 1977.

Mitchell R, Fogel S, Chet I: Bacterial chemoreption: An important ecological phenomenon inhibited by hydrocarbons. Water Res 6:1137–1140, 1972.

Olanczuk-Neyman KM, Vosjan JH: Measuring respiratory electron-transport-system activity in marine sediments. Neth J Sea Res 11:1–13, 1977.

Olsen BH, Cooper RC: Comparison of aerobic and anaerobic methylation of mercuric chloride by San Francisco Bay sediments. Water Res 10:113–116, 1976.

Orndorff SA, Colwell RR: Effect of Kepone on estuarine microbial activity. Microb Ecol 6:357–368, 1980.

Pamatmat MM, Bhagwat AM: Anaerobic metabolism in Lake Washington sediments. Limnol Oceanogr 18:611–627, 1973.

Pritchard PH, Bourquin AW, Frederickson HL, Maziarz T: System design factors affecting environmental fate studies in microcosms. In: Proceedings of the Workshop: Microbial Degradation of Pollutants in Marine Environments, edited by AW Bourquin, PH Pritchard, pp. 251–272. EPA-600/9-79-012, U.S. Environmental Protection Agency, 1978.

Sayler GS, Nelson JD, Colwell RR: Role of bacteria in bioaccumulation of mercury in the oyster, *Crassostrea virginica*. Appl Microbiol 30:91–96, 1975.

Smith DH, Gardner P: The ecology of R factors. N Engl J Med 202:161–162, 1970.

Speidel HK, Bourquin AW, Mann JE, Fair JF, Bennett EO: Microbial removal of pesticides from aqueous environments. Dev Ind Microbiol 13:277–282, 1972.

Trevors JT, Basaraba J: Toxicity of benzoquinone and hydroquinone in short term bacterial bioassays. Bull Environ Contam Toxicol 25:672–675, 1980.

Trudgill PW, Widdus R, Ross JS: Effects of organochlorine insecticides on bacterial growth, respiration and viability. J Gen Microbiol 69:1–5, 1971.

Ware GW, Roan CC: Interaction of pesticides with aquatic microorganisms and plankton. Residue Rev 33:15–45, 1970.

Widdus R, Trudgill PW, Turnell DC: Effects of technical chlordane on growth and energy metabolism of *Streptococcus faecalis* and *Mycobacterium phlei*: A comparison with *Bacillus subtilis*. J Gen Microbiol 69:21–23, 1971.

Wright RJ: Measurement and significance of specific activity in the heterotrophic bacteria of natural waters. Appl Environ Microbiol 36:297–305, 1978.

Young CY, Mitchell R: Negative chemotaxis of marine bacteria to toxic chemicals. Appl Microbiol 25:972–975, 1973.

Zar JH: Biostatistical Analysis, pp. 151–162. Englewood Cliffs, N.J.: Prentice-Hall, 1974.

SUPPLEMENTAL READING

Anderson JR: Some method for assessing pesticide effects on non-target soil microorganisms and their activities. In: Pesticide Microbiology, edited by IR Hill, SJL Wright, pp. 247–533. New York: Academic, 1978.

Bourquin AW, Pritchard PH: Workshop: Microbial Degradation of Pollutants in Marine Environments, EPA-600 19/79-012; p. 545. U.S. Environmental Protection Agency, 1979.

Colwell RR, Morita RY: Effect of the ocean environment on microbial activities. In: Proceedings of the 2d U.S.-Japan Conference on Marine Microbiology. Baltimore: University Park, 1972.

Lynch JM, Poole NJ: Microbial Ecology: A Conceptual Approach. New York: Wiley, 1979.

Mitchell R: Water Pollution Microbiology, vol. 1. New York: Wiley-Interscience, 1972.

Pfister RM: Interactions of halogenated pesticides and microorganisms—a review. In: Microbial Ecology, edited by AI Laskin, H Lechevalier, pp. 1–33. Cleveland: CRC Press, 1972.

Rheinheimer G: Aquatic Microbiology. London: Wiley, 1971.

Tu, CM, Miles JRW: Interactions between insecticides and soil microbes. Residue Rev 64:17–65, 1976.

Ware GW, Roan CC: Interaction of pesticides with aquatic microorganisms and plankton. Residue Rev 33:15–45, 1970.

Sublethal Effects

Chapter 9
Behavior

G. M. Rand

INTRODUCTION

Behavior is "the whole complex of observable, recordable, or measurable activities of a living animal" (Verplanck, 1957). It is everything an animal does, including all of its integrated movements. Most animal behavioral patterns (responses) involve overt movements that are highly adaptive to environmental variables (or stimuli) of a physical, chemical, or biological nature. Through its normal adaptive behavior, an animal tends to mitigate or bring itself into favorable environmental conditions, thereby eliminating the effects of environmental perturbation. Ultimately, the most favorable relationships are those that promote the survival, growth, reproduction, and longevity of the population.

Genetic (hereditary or instinctive) and/or environmental (acquired learned information) influ-ences determine the development of animal behavioral patterns. Most behavioral responses are also based on the integration of underlying physiological and biochemical functions. Changes in these functions may be overlooked because they are often subtle and not readily observable, but they may be manifested in overt behavioral responses. The literature indicates that chemical agents may be "behaviorally toxic" in aquatic organisms, affecting both instinctive and learned behavior (Sprague, 1971).

Behavioral toxicity occurs when the introduction of a chemical or other stressful condition induces a behavioral change that exceeds the normal range of variability (Marcucella and Abramson, 1978). Many changes in behavior may indicate behavioral toxicity, but only chemically induced or physical changes that decrease an organism's ability to adapt and survive in the environment are

221

ecologically significant. For example, introduction of a chemical agent into the aquatic environment may affect (1) preference/avoidance responses to noxious stimuli (e.g., adverse temperature and salinity gradients and predators), (2) attraction to food and mates, (3) feeding behavior, (4) the ability to retain previously learned behavior and motivation, and (5) social behaviors (aggregation, territoriality, courtship, and parental care). Such effects may occur as a result of the impact of chemicals on sensory modalities (e.g., chemoreception, rheotaxis, phototaxis), motor activity (e.g., locomotor and swimming performance), or the central nervous system (CNS). Failure of any behavioral response system could eventually lead to reduced fitness and survival of individual organisms, resulting in adverse consequences at the population level.

Studies in behavioral toxicology require reliable measures and precise control over animal behavior under specified conditions. Experimental psychology has offered much to mammalian toxicology because of the extensive data base developed by researchers with rats, mice, pigeons, and primates. Because of this, behavior has received considerable attention as a sensitive end point for assessing the sublethal effects of chemical agents in mammalian toxicology. Although behavior has been shown to be a sensitive indicator of chemically induced stress in aquatic organisms, it has not been used to its fullest potential in aquatic toxicology.

At present there are no standardized aquatic behavioral toxicity tests that are widely used. However, the literature on fish and other aquatic organisms indicates that certain behavioral responses have been studied more extensively than others as indicators of sublethal chemical insult. In fact, similar techniques have been used by many different researchers, and thus show potential for standardization.

The purpose of the present chapter is to demonstrate the feasibility and importance of using aquatic organisms in behavioral toxicity studies with chemical agents. To accomplish this, some basic research prerequisites and considerations

of behavioral testing will first be integrated and presented. Then some state-of-the-art procedures and techniques that are currently available for monitoring the behavior of aquatic organisms will be discussed. Finally, a review of the literature, examining the effects of various chemical substances on behavioral responses, will be presented and the advantages, disadvantages, and implications of behavioral studies in aquatic toxicology will be evaluated.

GENERAL CONSIDERATIONS AND PREREQUISITES FOR BEHAVIORAL TOXICITY STUDIES WITH AQUATIC ORGANISMS

The objective of an aquatic behavioral toxicity test is to determine whether a chemical agent elicits an "abnormal" or "adverse" behavioral change outside the normal range of variability in aquatic organisms, during or after exposure to the chemical, which may seriously affect its fitness or decrease its chances for survival. Most organisms have evolved adaptive, defensive responses (e.g., shell valve closure of mollusks and burrowing of crabs) that enable them to tolerate, survive, and overcome temporary, transient stresses (e.g., introduction of a chemical or deleterious changes in temperature, pH, and dissolved oxygen) in their environment. However, at some level of stress or concentration of chemical these responses may be inadequate and the ability of the organism to respond normally may be impaired. Abnormal or aberrant behavioral responses may thus be observed. It is evident in measuring any behavior, just as with other end points (or effect criteria), that a threshold exists such that exposure to one concentration of a chemical elicits an adaptive defensive response and exposure to another, slightly higher chemical concentration may obliterate it and produce an aberrant behavioral response. The aberrant behavior indicates that the organism has been exposed to a concentration of a chemical that exceeds its tolerance limit and there may be physiological and/or biochemical damage to the sensory organs, the nervous system, or other parts of the body. Behavioral toxicity studies may be used to define the adaptive and aberrant behaviors produced as a result of exposure to chemicals and the conditions that must be present to elicit them.

Adaptive, defensive, and aberrant behavioral responses may be similar or different for different species of organisms exposed to concentrations of the same chemical. These responses may also be similar or different after exposure to different chemicals. Furthermore, changes in the chemical and physical properties of the environment in which the organisms live may have a direct impact on their behavioral responses because they may ultimately affect the general toxicity and behavioral toxicity of the chemical agents to which the organisms are exposed.

One of the first important things to consider in a toxicity testing program is whether a behavioral toxicity study is needed. Answers to some of the questions below may help in making this decision.

1 Is the compound behaviorally toxic or neurotoxic to mammalian organisms?

2 Does the compound structurally resemble other compounds that are behaviorally toxic or neurotoxic?

3 Are any of the transformation products or metabolites behaviorally toxic or neurotoxic?

It should be noted here that although a chemical may not elicit behavioral or neurotoxic properties in mammalian organisms, it may do so in aquatic organisms. The information above should serve only as a guide. Once it is decided that a behavioral toxicity test will be conducted, a variety of considerations and testing conditions have to be evaluated and planned. Some of these considerations and prerequisites may also be useful in eventually developing a standardized behavioral toxicity protocol. They are discussed below.

Selecting the Species

The type of species to use for testing is one of the most critical decisions. The organisms selected should be indigenous to or representative of the ecosystem that will be affected by the chemical. This should be determined on a site-by-site basis.

There are no "standard" test species for aquatic behavioral toxicity testing. However, several criteria listed in Chapter 1 may be helpful in selecting the appropriate species for behavioral tests. For instance, the organism should (1) be of sport, commercial, or economic value; (2) have a potential for interaction with and exposure to the test chemical; (3) have a considerable geographic distribution and abundance; (4) represent major trophic levels; (5) be easy to maintain and suitable for laboratory studies; (6) be a sensitive species whose susceptibility to chemical agents and consistency in response to these agents are known; and (7) be a species for which there is sufficient background information on "general" behavior or on some specific type of behavioral pattern (e.g., reproductive, feeding, or locomotor).

Probably the most significant criteria in selecting a species for behavioral toxicity tests are 5, 6, and 7 above. The ideal organisms for behavioral testing are species that are easy to maintain in the laboratory, for which a general toxicity data base on a large number of chemicals already exists, and for which background data are available on different behaviors. In this way, if a behavioral toxicity study is conducted along with other acute and longer term tests, the results can be used more effectively in assessing the safety of the chemicals under investigation.

Most aquatic tests species (e.g., fathead minnows, daphnids, mysids, sheepshead minnows) used for acute, early life stage, and chronic tests have been scarcely used in behavioral studies. Many of these species are ubiquitous, sensitive, and suitable for these kinds of laboratory toxicity tests, but there is little background data on their general behavior and biology so that their use in behavioral testing is limited.

A wealth of information is available from the pharmacology literature (Marcucella and Abramson, 1978) on the behavioral effects of drugs on aquarium fish such as Siamese fighting fish (*Betta splendens*), goldfish (*Carassius auratus*), mollies (*Mollienisia* sp.), Japanese carp (*Cyprinus carpio*), African mouthbreeders (*Tilapia macrocephala*), and paradise fish (*Macropodus opercularis*). However, these species have not been used extensively in behavioral toxicity studies with other types of chemicals because they are not widely distributed or indigenous to many areas, little information is available on their biology, and they may even be highly tolerant (e.g., goldfish) of chemical agents.

More than one species should be used in a behavioral testing program to determine variability in behavioral sensitivity. Depending on the part of the aquatic ecosystem that may be affected by the chemical, an invertebrate and a vertebrate species may be selected. Different stages of the life cycle of organisms may be behaviorally diverse because of differences in sensitivity. For example, the early larval stages of invertebrates (e.g., the fiddler crab, *Uca pugilator*) are more susceptible to chemical toxicants than the adults (DeCoursey and Vernberg, 1972). This is also generally true of fish (Chapter 3). Therefore different life stages should be examined separately.

Selection of a test species for a behavioral test should also depend on the objective of the test. For a comparison of avoidance of chemical agents, indigenous species may be appropriate for generating site-specific information. If the objective is to determine whether the chemical affects the "general" feeding behavior of aquatic organisms, then species may be used which are easily held in the laboratory and whose feeding behavior is well known.

Source of Test Species, Holding and Acclimation Conditions

Organisms may be collected directly from the study area outside the zone of influence or discharge site of the chemical or effluent being investigated. If species from the local area are not available, representative species from nearby areas may be used. Organisms may also be cultured and reared in the laboratory or purchased from a commercial grower. In any case, adequate documenta-

tion on nutrition, holding, and acclimation conditions should be kept and maintained.

Organisms held in the laboratory, either reared or obtained from a supplier, should be maintained in environmental conditions that resemble their normal requirements as closely as possible. Knowledge of the organisms' normal or typical environmental requirements from field observations are essential in determining such factors as size and shape of the holding tank, type of food and feeding schedule, optimum temperature, photoperiod (light-dark cycle), dissolved oxygen, pH, and salinity. For highly motile, fast-swimming organisms, elliptical aquaria should be used to prevent crowding in corners and damage to organisms striking the walls. Molluscan larvae tend to swim primarily along their vertical axis, so they require tall chambers. The type of food and time of feeding should be maintained for several weeks in the laboratory so that organisms are feeding normally before testing begins. Failure to eat is common in many organisms new to the laboratory. This period may be shortened by "social facilitation" (adding organisms that are already feeding). Organisms that are not eating or that stop eating for periods of time before testing should be eliminated from the experiment.

Optimum temperature, light intensity and photoperiod, dissolved oxygen concentration, pH, and salinity are important factors, because a variation in one may interact with the chemical being studied, making it more or less behaviorally toxic. Random fluctuations in these factors should be avoided. For example, the most desirable method of lighting is from above with a system that gradually increases and decreases light levels, simulating sunrise and sunset. With ichthyoplankton the source of illumination must be overhead, because they generally orient dorsally to light so that illumination from below or the side will lead to atypical body orientation. Other physical disturbances such as vibrations from pumps and refrigerators should also be avoided, since fish and invertebrates respond to sources of vibration and sound.

Loading requirements should be similar to those used for acute toxicity tests (see Chapter 2). Aggressive and cannibalistic organisms should be separated from the experimental organisms. Substrates should be suitable for burrowing by benthic organisms.

The acclimation period just before the experimental testing is very important. During this period the organisms must be maintained under environmental conditions that are within their adaptive range and the same as those to be used during the experiment. If fish and other aquatic organisms are not adequately acclimated, a major part of the variability or "noise" in a behavioral toxicity test may be a result of fluctuations in temperature, dissolved oxygen, pH, photoperiod, salinity, type of food and feeding schedule, and other abiotic factors and not of the chemical exposure.

Days, weeks, or months may be required for acclimation. This is dependent on the test species. For example, the blue crab (*Callinectus sapidus*) collected from the field may acclimate within 4 d before its ability to detect chemical stimuli is tested (Olla et al., 1980). Fish may be acclimated for several weeks to several months (Rand et al., 1975), and certain crabs (*Pachygrapsus crassipes*) may take a few hours (Kittredge et al., 1974). Standard procedures for routine toxicity tests suggest that test organisms such as fish may be acclimated for a week or longer. Since effect criteria differ in sensitivity, this acclimation period may not be sufficient for behavioral testing.

Because the purpose of behavioral toxicity tests is to define the potential effects of chemical agents on certain predefined behaviors, the fitness of the test organism is of utmost importance. The normal or typical behavior of the test organisms should be well understood so that diagnostic observations of subtle aberrant behaviors may be made before testing begins. Natural variability in behavior is so great that more subtle variations will not be apparent to the observer with only a superficial knowledge of the test species. Alterations in the following behaviors may be used in evaluating fitness:

feeding, photoactivity, sensitivity, excitability, motor activity, agonistic displays, loss of equilibrium, and opercular movements. These behaviors may be considered to reflect the relative health and state of the test organisms in order to determine whether they are acclimated and suitable as experimental subjects. This information should be accurately reported and documented with the physical and chemical data. It should be noted that the normal behavior of organisms in the laboratory may be different from that in the field. Evaluating changes in normal laboratory behavior is also important but may be difficult to extrapolate to the field.

Selection of a Response as an End Point or Criterion of Behavioral Effect

In selecting a behavioral response for a toxicity test, several criteria must be considered:

1 The behavioral pattern must be amenable to laboratory or controlled field investigations so that organisms can perform under controlled conditions and relevant behaviors can be isolated. That is, much of the background on the behavior being studied should be known.

2 The behavioral pattern must be sensitive to the chemical likely to occur at the locality of interest. The procedure or technique must also be sensitive to the change in behavior, especially if the change is subtle.

3 The behavioral pattern should be well studied so that the effects on it of major biotic and abiotic variables are known.

4 The response chosen should be ecologically relevant and understood in the context of the capabilities of the species for survival.

5 The behavioral test or technique must be practical to conduct in a routine manner, objective, and able to be used with a range of organisms and chemicals so that adequate comparisons can be made.

6 Behavioral patterns that integrate or depend on diverse sensory and/or motor mechanisms should be evaluated. For example, preference/avoidance behavior may depend on olfactory, visual, or acoustic detection followed by the appropriate locomotor response. However, depending on the nature (physical and chemical characteristics) of the chemical, it may disrupt chemoreception important for locating and detecting food, mates, and predators, but it may also affect turbidity and thus visually oriented behavior.

A particular behavior or behavioral pattern is best suited as an end point if the eventual behavioral alterations can be related to possible consequences in the field at the population and ecosystem levels. It is thus important that a behavioral toxicity test be selected on the basis of the natural behaviors or general behavioral repertoire of the organisms in the natural environment which, if significantly modified, may interfere with vital processes and lead to death. These processes include growth, reproduction, and development. Behavioral studies in the laboratory will have greater significance and relevance if they can be related to these processes.

Most aquatic invertebrates and vertebrates in their normal activities must meet a number of basic needs that are important for their survival, growth, reproduction, and development. Most significantly, they must:

1 Locate and remain in favorable environments,
2 Find and ingest appropriate food,
3 Avoid predation, and
4 Reproduce.

Locomotor Behavior

Movement of aquatic organisms may involve spontaneous, "undirected" (free-running) locomotor activity characterized by circadian and seasonal rhythmicity and not related to the direction of a stimulus. In this kind of behavior the direction of movement at any instant may be completely random. Movement may also involve orientation or "directed" locomotor responses to gradients of natural stimuli such as light, temperature, salinity, substratum, chemicals (pheromones, food odor),

and current and man-made stimuli such as chemical toxicants. Oriented movements under favorable conditions to the natural stimuli lead to species-specific distribution patterns that help keep the organisms at physiologically tolerable locations in these gradients. They enable the organisms to move adaptively and in a directed fashion in relation to physical, chemical, and biological stimuli. Environmental gradients may thus help guide feeding and migratory movements, favor discrimination between individuals, help in defense against predators, and aid reproductive behavior (e.g., finding mates and nesting sites). Sensory information is acquired, processed, and integrated in the nervous system and fed into control mechanisms which, on the basis of genetic and possibly ontogenetic acquired information, determine the nature of the orientated locomotion required by the environmental stimuli. Behavioral tests of undirected and directed locomotion will provide an indication of general nervous system function and motor and sensory capacity.

Feeding and Predatory Behavior

Feeding behavior or the acquisition of food involves searching, detection, capture (sometimes chase), and ingestion (Keenleyside, 1979). A hungry organism performs searching activities that increase the probability that it will find food. Once a potential food item is detected, a fish will orient toward it, approach it, and attempt to capture and ingest it. Feeding behavior of aquatic organisms involves many different strategies that require motor coordination and sensory modalities (Kleerekoper, 1969).

If aquatic organisms are to survive they must not only acquire food but avoid becoming food for other animals (Keenleyside, 1979). Fish have different mechanisms for countering their predators (Edmunds, 1974). These are termed primary and secondary defense mechanisms. Primary mechanisms include hiding and camouflage, which reduce the probability that a fish will be detected by hunting predators. Secondary mechanisms include those that reduce the chance of the fish being caught once an encounter between prey and predator begins. The fish may take action to avoid capture in three different ways: flee into a shelter, perform evasive action independently or as a member of a group, or show an aggressive defense posture to induce the predator to stop its attack. Fleeing by rapid movement away from an approaching predator is probably the most common escape tactic (Edmunds, 1974). In the absence of shelters, a single fish will often try to escape by swimming along an erratic, zigzag path. Predator avoidance by schooling fish often seems to be mediated by visual cues, both from attacking predators and from disturbed members of the school. One well-known escape response is initiated by chemical cues. This is the "alarm reaction," which was first described in the European minnow (*Phoxinus phoxinus*) by von Frisch (1938). Fish show an intense species-typical flight response to substances released from injured conspecifics. The effective material (Schreckstoff) is produced in specialized epidermal club cells and is released into the water when the cells are damaged. This alarm response has been documented for many fish species (Reed, 1969) and it occurs primarily but not exclusively among schooling fish (Pfeiffer, 1977).

Reproductive Behavior

Reproductive behavior has received considerable attention from behaviorists (Breder and Rosen, 1966). It includes selection and preparation of a site for spawning, courtship, mating, the spawning act, and parental care of the young. The study of any aspect of reproductive behavior is ecologically significant and relevant.

The behaviors listed above may be divided into those that require responses of individual organisms and those that involve responses of two or more individuals. They may require optimum functioning of different sensory modalities (chemoreception, which includes olfaction and gustation, vision, acoustic) and/or motor activity (locomotion). A number of specific behavioral responses have been used to evaluate the effects of sublethal concentrations of chemicals on aquatic organisms. These are listed in Table 1. Most behavioral studies in aquatic toxicology have concentrated on these basic responses, excluding reproductive behavior.

A behavioral response for testing may be selected from Table 1. The species selection and testing conditions should be carefully considered and the variables monitored. At present, there is no one species or behavioral response that is consid-

Table 1 Behavioral Responses Used to Monitor Sublethal Effects of Chemicals[a]

Individual response	Interindividual response
Locomotor	Predator-prey
Undirected locomotion	Social interactions:
Directed (orientative) locomotion to test stimuli:	Territoriality
Salinity gradients	Dominance
Temperature gradients	Aggregation (schooling)
Food odor or pheromone	
Light	
Chemical toxicant	
Current	
Feeding behavior/motivation	
Learning	

[a]Modified from Miller (1980).

ered better than another. If more than one behavioral test is planned, the simple tests should be conducted before the more complex ones.

Field and Laboratory Studies

Both direct and indirect methods have been used in the laboratory and field to study the behavioral effects of chemicals on aquatic organisms. In laboratory studies, variables such as dissolved oxygen, temperature, photoperiod, salinity, and general water quality can be adequately controlled. Thus cause and effect relationships between the chemical and the behavioral responses under investigation may be more definitively analyzed without interacting, masking, or modifying effects of environmental variables. The obvious limitation of laboratory studies is that the responses observed may not occur in nature. Field studies may be conducted in the natural aquatic ecosystem or in seminatural microcosms. Tests (e.g., cage tests) conducted in the natural ecosystem (e.g., pond or stream) are the most realistic and provide the best information. Systems are selected because they are examples of regions where chemical exposure is expected and because they have characteristics that satisfy the criteria for test systems. Subtle influences and behavioral interactions among individuals of the system that are not present in more simplified laboratory systems may be detected in field studies. Field studies may also be desirable for determining the predictability and realism of the laboratory data. In general, field studies of natural aquatic ecosystems are not easy to replicate and because of the complicating environmental variability, causal relationships are difficult to evaluate. In semimicrocosm studies, subsamples of the natural ecosystem are housed in enclosures and placed in the laboratory or in the natural environment. The most important advantage of microcosm test systems is that the behavioral effects and interactions of several different species can be identified. The limitation of microcosms is that they are oversimplifications of natural systems.

Most of the behavioral studies conducted to date have been done under controlled laboratory conditions. However, field studies should be conducted whenever possible in order to bridge the gap between responses in the laboratory and in the natural environment and to make more realistic predictions of behavioral effects.

Experimental Design

It is difficult to discuss a specific test design for a behavioral study because there are so many unanswered questions in the area of aquatic behavioral toxicology. A relatively simple approach should be considered, and some general comments about the design are listed below:

1 Organisms may be first exposed to the potential toxicant and then monitored in an experimental situation (e.g., response to odor, predator) to determine the behavioral effects of exposure. Organisms may also be exposed to the potential toxicant concurrently in the experimental situation (e.g., preference/avoidance, response to odor, predator) and monitored to determine the behavioral effects of exposure.

2 Behavioral effects of exposure to a range of 3–5 sublethal concentrations should be studied. Acute toxicity tests should first be conducted with the test organisms to determine the relative toxicity (LC50) of the chemical if it is unknown. Application factors (e.g., 0.1, 0.05) may then be applied to the acute LC50 value to estimate a safe concentration.. The range of test concentrations may include this estimated safe value and several others on either side of it. The method for determining these values may be similar to that used for the definitive acute test (see Chapter 2). Exposure concentrations for the behavioral test may also be based on those expected (estimated environmental concentration, EEC) in the aquatic environment likely to receive the chemical.

3 Concurrent control groups (untreated, positive, or solvent) should be used and tested in the same manner as the chemically exposed groups. Organisms may also serve as their own controls. For example, before exposure to the chemical the behavioral response (e.g., phototactic, locomotor, conditioned avoidance) of fish or invertebrates may be monitored. The organisms may then be exposed to the chemical for a period of time, after

which they are again monitored in the same experimental situation. The results before and after chemical exposure can be compared to determine the effects of the chemical.

4 Samples of organisms from the overall test population should be randomly selected for study. The number of organisms for each experimental group should be determined before the study begins. The size of each group must be large enough that statistical procedures can be applied to the data to determine their significance. The statistical procedures to be used (e.g., Analysis of Variance) should be considered before the study begins rather than after the data are collected.

5 Time is important in behavioral testing because various cyclic (daily, tidal, lunar) phenomena may predispose the reactions of animals to environmental stimuli, including chemicals, and make them more susceptible to exposure (Dicks, 1973). For example, the effects of crude oil on limpets (*Patella vulgata*) are greatly increased during active periods when they crawl over the oil. The rhythm of an animal's activity can substantially influence its susceptibility to chemicals, and this should be taken into consideration before behavioral testing.

6 Studies may be used to determine the behavioral effects of acute and/or chronic exposure to chemicals. The duration of exposure is dependent on the test organisms and the chemical. For example, if the effects are being studied with marine organisms from the shore (e.g., the acorn barnacle, *Balanus balanoides,* or the limpet, *P. vulgata* L.), exposure to the chemical should be of short duration because tidal cycles ensure considerable variation in exposure (e.g., a few hours) and chemical concentration. As another example, organophosphate insecticides have short half-lives in the environment compared to organochlorine insecticides, which may persist and produce chronic effects. Therefore, test organisms should be exposed to organophosphates for several hours or days, whereas with organochlorine compounds exposures may be much longer.

7 Recovery studies should be conducted whenever possible to determine whether there are persistent or delayed effects of exposure to the chemical.

8 Several types of tests with different behavioral end points (e.g., preference/avoidance, feeding, predator-prey interaction, learning) should be included. They should be conducted in a tier (stepwise) manner, with less complex behavioral responses (e.g., preference/avoidance) studied first and more complex ones (e.g., feeding and reproductive behavior, predator-prey interaction) studied later.

TECHNIQUES

Direct visual observations of behavior in the laboratory and field are tedious, time-consuming, sometimes too subjective, and often difficult to quantify and evaluate. Also, certain habitats in the field are inaccessible. Technological advances of the past 15 years have increased our ability to observe the behavior of aquatic organisms indirectly. Acoustic and radio telemetry, advanced photography, sonar, and closed-circuit television are examples of methods by which aquatic animals may be objectively observed in their natural habitat. Closed-circuit television, minicomputers, microprocessors, and other automated electronic tools greatly facilitate behavioral data collection and analysis in the laboratory.

Although many of these techniques that have been used to monitor behavioral responses can be used with both fish and invertebrates, most have been used to monitor fish behavior. The most commonly studied behavioral responses in aquatic toxicology are: locomotor (directed and undirected), feeding, predator-prey interaction, social behaviors, and learning.

Locomotor Behavior

Only motile species should be used to study locomotor behavior. Sedentary organisms should not be used, and organisms that move very fast or very slowly may be difficult to monitor. Territorial species may select areas of the monitoring tank as a home range and remain inactive. Thigmokinesis is a response to contact and a high intensity of contact stimulation which usually results in low activity (Fraenkel and Gunn, 1961). Species exhibiting positive thigmokinetic behavior would not swim throughout a tank. Territorial and thigmokinetic species should not be used in locomotor studies. Since activity can be affected by abiotic factors (e.g., temperature, dissolved oxygen), the health of the species and its reproductive status should also be considered when designing experiments on locomotor behavior.

Locomotor behavior has a high level of integration, yet it can be objectively described and quantified. Most aquatic behavioral toxicity studies deal with some type of locomotor response. Locomotor responses that have been studied are listed in Table 2. The techniques used to monitor the different responses are discussed separately.

Directed Orientation Responses

Locomotor responses are commonly but not always orientative and lead the animal to approach or avoid the source of the variable in question. Orientated locomotor behavior of this kind is widespread among animals and is of greatest significance in the localization of food and prey, conspecifics in general and mates in particular, and nesting and spawning sites; in the selection of an environment appropriate for normal physiological performance; and in the avoidance of inadequate conditions. Orientated locomotion is a very complex behavior involving many biological functions and requires at least three conditions. The variables in relation to which orientation is to occur must be perceived or "sensed" by the animal; there must be direction vectors in the environment relative to the locale of the source; and the

Table 2 Types of Locomotor Responses

Directed orientation responses (preference/avoidance)
  Orientation to chemical in the environment
  Effects of chemical exposure on orientation to stimuli:
    food odor, light, current, salinity, and temperature
    changes
Undirected locomotor responses (activity)
  Free
  Forced

---

animal must be physiologically capable of perceiving the vector and using it in its orientation.

Locomotor orientation of aquatic organisms may be affected by toxic substances in the environment. Several responses can occur. A motile naive fish—that is, a fish not previously exposed to the substance—may sense it as aversive and respond by orientating away from the source (avoidance), approach it (preference or attraction), or ignore it. A potentially toxic chemical responded to by avoidance will not have the harmful effect of one that elicits attraction or is responded to indifferently. Avoidance of toxic chemicals is usually beneficial. However, avoidance of nontoxic chemicals or sublethal levels of chemicals may not be beneficial, especially if it restricts the organism's normal feeding, mating, spawning, or migration. If the organism is attracted to or ignores a potentially toxic substance, orientation responses to sensory stimuli may be affected or death may occur. The affected responses may include those to light, current, odor (food, sex pheromones), salinity, and temperature. Monitoring locomotor orientation responses to these stimuli or avoidance of the chemical itself may indicate effects not only on neuromotor systems but also on sensory systems, because the chemical toxicant may interact with and damage chemoreceptors (or other sensory receptors) or mask the organism's ability to detect the source of stimulation.

There are significant differences in the interpretation of observations of locomotor orientation (preference/avoidance) to natural gradients (e.g., temperature or food odor) and to a potentially toxic chemical. If an organism avoids a chemical toxicant, the question is why. If the chemical is toxic and has been in the environment naturally, the avoidance behavior has adaptive significance. It has evolved because the organism has learned to avoid the stress or noxious stimuli it has been confronted with over time. However, if a chemical does not occur naturally in the environment and there is no history of prior exposure, no programmed response can be assumed. The organism may avoid a chemical that has a local inflammatory or irritant effect on exposed tissue, but many toxic chemicals are probably not detected or perceived. On the other hand, the preference for natural odors and the avoidance of natural predators can be understood. Therefore, the rationale for testing the preference/avoidance response to a potentially toxic chemical is to determine whether (1) the organism can generally detect or perceive it and (2) if it can, whether preference for the chemical poses a danger or avoidance provides a good escape. The latter two responses may be studied more completely with more sophisticated testing techniques.

Two types of preference/avoidance responses have been investigated: (1) alteration of a known preference/avoidance response to a natural abiotic factor or agent (e.g., food odor, light, temperature differential) by the chemical toxicant and (2) the direct preference/avoidance response to the chemical. Similar techniques have been used for both types of tests and for fish and invertebrates. The tank designs (rectangular or square, round, Y maze, or tube-shaped) used by different investigators to study locomotor behavior are illustrated in Fig. 1. Techniques used in this area are discussed.

Earlier preference/avoidance techniques were used to determine responses to gases and changes in water quality and temperature. The gradient tank method was introduced by Shelford and Allee (1913) to test reactions of fish to dissolved oxygen and CO_2. This method tested the reactions of fish to dissolved gases in 120 $\times$ 14 $\times$ 20 cm troughs (two parallel boxes, a reference and an experimental box) in which pure water (untreated) and a watery solution (treated) of the agent entered at opposite ends of the tank and drained from a common outlet in the middle. Although not well-defined, a "shallow" gradient was formed where the two fluids met. Three regions or zones were formed: the mixing zone (center) and untreated and treated zones at the ends. The fish were placed in the tank near the center and watched continuously for 20–90 min. Relative

positions of the fish were recorded as the residence time at each end, determined by the number of entries into the different zones. Wells (1915a) modified this technique slightly by inserting more outlets in the center drain to eliminate vertical stratification. The technique was used by many investigators (Wells, 1915b, 1918; Shelford and Powers, 1915; Shelford, 1917, 1918; Powers, 1921; Hall, 1925; Powers and Clark, 1943) in studies dealing with oxygen, CO_2, gradients of acidity and alkalinity, and the chloride, nitrate, and sulfate salts of ammonia, calcium, and magnesium. The work was extended to toxic pollutant substances including waste products associated with the manufacture of coal gas, such as ammonia and ammonium salts, aniline, hydrogen sulfide, sulfur dioxide, carbon bisulfide, acetone, phenol, cresols, naphthalene, carbon monoxide, and tar acids. Based on a similar principle, the steep gradient avoidance procedure was proposed by Jones (1947, 1948, 1951, 1952), who tested the reactions of small fish to different substances in a 58-cm horizontal glass tube (countercurrent system) in which fish were presented with a sharp differentiation between pure water and a known concentration of a test substance (e.g., mercuric chloride, zinc sulfate, chloroform, alcohol, Formalin) (Fig. 1). Untreated water was introduced into both ends of a Plexiglas tube and released at the center. Fish were introduced and allowed to acclimate for 10–15 min (control period) and then monitored for 10 min at $\frac{1}{2}$-min or 1-min intervals. Treated water was then released into one end and the movements of fish were recorded on graph paper for 7–120 min. Two parallel lines on graph paper represented the length of the "gradient tank," and minutes were marked on a vertical scale. The same approach was used by Olthof (1941) and Bishai (1962a, b) and was modified by Sprague (1964), who used four drains at the center to create a more defined separation of untreated and treated water. Sprague (1968) also improved the visual shielding, eliminated pump vibration, and increased water flow. A sharp vertical boundary was created at the middle of the hori-

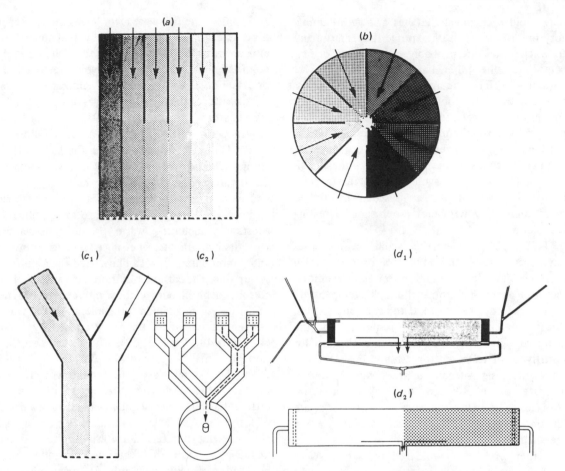

Figure 1 Basic tank designs used by different investigators to study locomotor behavior of aquatic organisms. Arrows indicate direction of water flow. (*a*) Gradients (Kleerekoper, 1969; Kleerekoper et al., 1972; Davy et al., 1972, 1973; Westlake and Lubinski, 1976; Hoglund, 1953). (*b*) Gradients (Kleerekoper, 1969; Rand, 1975, 1977a, 1977b). (*c₁*) Y maze (Hansen, 1969; Folmar, 1976, 1978). (*c₂*) Double Y maze (Hansen et al., 1972). (*d₁*) Countercurrent tube (Jones, 1947). (*d₂*) Rectangular countercurrent system (Sprague, 1964; Scherer and Nowak, 1973). *[From Scherer (1977) and Maciorowski et al. (1977b).]*

zontal Plexiglas tube (1.14 m long and 14.6 cm in diameter). Other investigators used this approach (Hill, 1968; Sprague et al., 1965; Sprague and Drury, 1969; Rehwoldt and Bida, 1970), and one group included a rectangular countercurrent tube with a recording device (Fig. 1) (Scherer and Nowak, 1973).

Jones et al. (1956) studied the reactions of juvenile salmonids to pulp mill wastes in a modified gradient tank (rectangular trough) with trans-verse baffles and also in a tank that was partitioned at one end into four parallel open channels having independent water supplies and drains. In the first apparatus, fish could select their preferred position in a gradient of stepwise-increasing concentration of the substance. In the second apparatus, the fish in unaltered water were confronted with an abrupt change of water quality at the openings of two of the four channels (the remaining two were control regions with untreated water), and they could choose between altered and unaltered water in the parallel channels. Fish movement was monitored by recording the number of entries into treated channels. A slight modification of this approach was developed by Whitmore et al. (1960) in a study of the reactions of salmonid and centrarchid fish to low oxygen concentrations. Collins (1952) conducted studies with similar troughs or avoidance tanks, but directly submerged them in streams to study reactions of fish in the "natural" environment.

A significant technique developed from the gradient tank is the fluvarium method (Fig. 1), which was first described by Hoglund (1953). It is based on the fact that a water mass flowing without disturbance should act like a stable system (i.e., a concentration gradient perpendicular to the direction of flow will vary little in a short time period). An angle gradient of any shape can be produced with this method and the reactions of unconditioned fish to different variables can be studied. Lindahl and Marcstrom (1958) introduced some technical improvements to stabilize the flow which were adopted and described by Hoglund (1961). Essentially, a fluvarium is a long trough; it consists of a test chamber in which fish swim freely and an apportionment box containing nine glass sheets which subdivide the middle part of the trough into 10 longitudinal sections (120 cm in length). Treated water was introduced into the apportionment box, forming a gradient of 10 concentration steps from pure water along one side to the highest concentration along the opposite side. Figure 2 illustrates a fluvarium that was used to produce a horizontal salinity gradient (12 concentrations) in a study of salinity preference. Fish

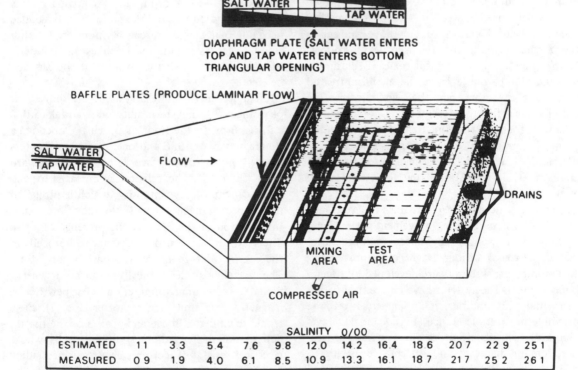

SALINITY 0/00											
ESTIMATED	1.1	3.3	5.4	7.6	9.8	12.0	14.2	16.4	18.6	20.7	22.9	25.1
MEASURED	0.9	1.9	4.0	6.1	8.5	10.9	13.3	16.1	18.7	21.7	25.2	26.1

Figure 2 Fluvarium used to produce a horizontal gradient of salinities. Estimated and actual salinities typical of the test area are tabulated. *[From Hansen (1972).]*

were first acclimated to fluvarium conditions and then the positions of the traversing fish were recorded per time period (e.g., 15 s).

Ishio (1965) refined earlier gradient tank approaches and designed a new horizontal gradient tank to prevent vertical stratification. The tank was divided into upper and lower paths by a horizontal sand layer. Untreated water was pumped into the lower path, ascended through the sandy layer, emerged into the upper path, and then moved directly toward a weir and out of the tank. The chemical solution was introduced into the upper path at the opposite end of the tank. The concentration decreased with distance toward the rear of the tank by mixing with newly supplied untreated tap water through the sandy layer. The water was aerated from a perforated tube buried in the sand to inhibit vertical gradients. Avoidance behavior was evaluated by the position of the fish in treated and untreated paths.

A widely used system for monitoring preference/avoidance behavior of aquatic organisms is the Y-maze test chamber (Hansen, 1969; Folmar, 1976) (Fig. 1). The chemical toxicant solution is introduced into one arm of the Y and untreated water into the other, and the two drain into the holding area for the fish. The responses (time, number of entries) to the treated and untreated (control) arms are observed and evaluated. A double Y maze (Fig. 1) has been used with fish (Hansen et al., 1972) and invertebrates (Hansen et al., 1973).

Basic tank designs have remained the same, but techniques for monitoring movement patterns and orientation responses have become more automated. Through various stages of improvement, two monitoring systems were developed by Kleerekoper (1969). The systems have different but complementary capabilities. One operates on the principle of multiple choice (Figs. 3 and 4). Movements of fish are monitored in a cylindrical tank (210 cm in diameter and 40 cm deep) with 16 hollow dividers, which are orientated radially from the periphery, leaving an open area in the center (100 cm in diameter). Alternate dividers contain a

light source, whose light is deflected by mirrors across the entrances of the neighboring compartments onto photoconductive cells in the adjacent dividers. The entrance to each of the 16 compartments is thus guarded by a photoelectric gate, which is triggered by the passage of a fish. The resulting electronic event and time of its occurrence are recorded by means of a logic interface by a paper tape punch located outside the chamber.

The tank has a peripheral channel from which water enters each compartment through a glass siphon. Water leaves the tank centrally through an overflow pipe. As the fish moves about, entries, exits, and times of these events are recorded for subsequent analysis of its orientation or preference or avoidance behavior. Physical and chemical conditions, single or in combination, can be controlled and varied in any of the compartments. For example, a chemical or food "odor" solution can be introduced into one or more of the compartments with solenoid pumps and the preference/avoidance behavior of a single fish can be monitored. Other stimuli, such as orientation to changes in temperature, light, sound, or the chemical itself, can also be tested.

In a second open-field system, the movement of a single fish may be monitored in a tank (5.0 $\times$ 5.0 $\times$ 0.6 m) in the floor of which is embedded a square matrix of 1936 photocells on 10-cm centers whose photosensitive faces are directed upward (Figs. 5 and 6). The cells are illuminated by collimated light of low intensity, which is projected uniformly overhead onto the surface of the water. Interception of the light by the presence of a fish affects the resistance of the shaded photocells in the matrix and generates the basic information. The system is electronically interfaced with a digital on-line minicomputer, a teletypewriter, a magnetic tape unit, and a plotter (Fig. 7). Electronic scanning of the x and y axes of the matrix determines the coordinates of photocells whose electrical resistance increases as a result of shading by the fish. This information (position) with the real time of the shading event is recorded on a magnetic tape and stored in a memory pack. These

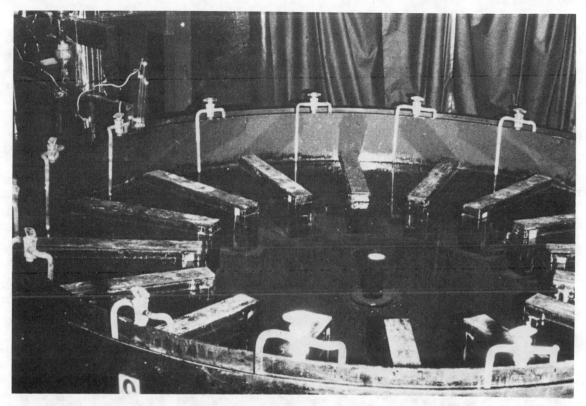

Figure 3 Photograph of cylindrical, multiple-choice monitoring tank. *[From H. Kleerekoper, Texas A&M University.]*

raw data and their sequence form the basis for computation of the position of the fish in the tank, its velocity, the magnitudes of turns, the lengths and orientation of steps between turns, the distances covered, and the frequency distributions of all these values over time.

Water can be admitted to any one of the four isolated channels, and it moves through the perforated baffles into the main body of the tank, from which it enters similar baffles in a channel located at the opposite end with an overflow. There is thus a close approximation of laminarity of water flow traversing the tank. Chemical gradients can be created in the tank by two means. The first method is to inject a solution of a chemical into the water supply of a whole channel or an isolated section of it, creating either a "polluted water mass" or a "slug" as it traverses the tank. The second method of introducing a localized chemical stimuli is through hypodermic needles embedded in the floor of the tank. Solutions of biological (e.g., food odor) or nonbiological (e.g., chemical toxicant) substances can be introduced through these needles at various rates and the locomotor responses of fish can be spatially and temporally evaluated.

Preference and avoidance responses can also be monitored with a minicomputer, which analyzes the signal from a video camera that scans a chamber into which fish (Gray et al., 1977; Lubinski et al., 1980; Westlake and Lubinski, 1976) or invertebrates (Greaves and Wilson, 1980; Miller et al., 1982) have been introduced. Gray et al. (1977) used a model raceway (rectangular trough 6 m

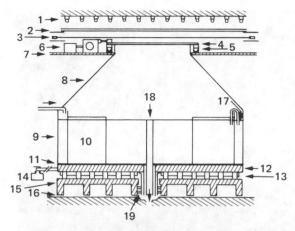

Figure 4 Schematic cross section of cylindrical monitoring tank: (1) Light source; (2 and 3) diffusers; (7) false ceiling; (8) light trap; (9) tank; (10) compartment dividers; (15 and 16) support; (17) water supply; (18) overflow. Components not identified are not relevant to experimentation. *[From H. Kleerekoper, Texas A&M University.]*

long) with a canopy overhead (to provide a uniform background) and two video cameras positioned under the canopy (Fig. 8). One camera was positioned upstream and one downstream of a simulated discharge to determine fish movement. A third camera was located directly above the discharge. Water entered through a slot in the bottom and the screen was raised by remote control to allow fish to swim or drift with the flow through the raceway. As the fish entered the discharge area, their reactions were recorded on videotape and a closed video switcher and playback system were used for analysis. This system can be used for preference/avoidance studies and also to determine swimming performance (see below) or the general ability of fish to maintain position in a current. Westlake and Lubinski (1976) used an open-field system similar to Kleerekoper's (1969), but in their approach the deep end

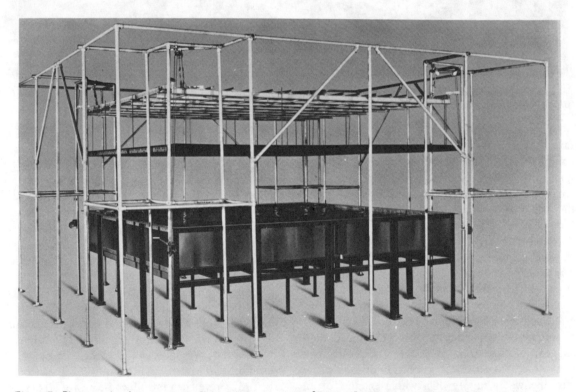

Figure 5 Photograph of square, open-field monitoring tank. *[From H. Kleerekoper, Texas A&M University.]*

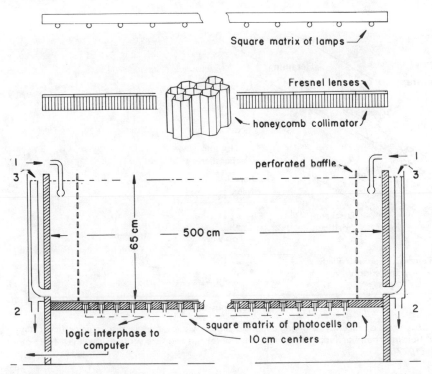

Figure 6 Schematic cross section of square monitoring tank: (1) Water inlet; (2) water outlet; (3) standing pipe for water level regulation. *[From Kleerekoper et al. (1972); reproduced by permission of the Minister of Supply and Services Canada.]*

of the monitoring tank received treated or untreated water that passed through a baffle to produce a laminar water flow, which then exited into a shallow area that contained a fish. Fish responses were monitored by a drop in voltage

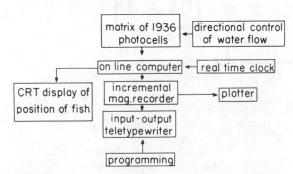

Figure 7 Block diagram of a data processing system. *[From Kleerekoper et al. (1972); reproduced by permission of the Minister of Supply and Services Canada.]*

from the fish movement recorded by an overhead TV camera interfaced with a computer. Locomotor patterns at different time intervals in relation to different chemicals could be analyzed. More recently, Lubinski et al. (1980) used a similar laminar-flow open-field tank enclosed in a protective housing (Fig. 9). Water from two sources (for treated and untreated water, respectively) was released into the deep end of the tank, which was separated by a divider, and then passed through a series of screens that created a laminar flow with a steep separation between treated and untreated water in the observation area.

The design produced an abrupt concentration gradient down the middle of the observation area when a chemical solution was slowly pumped into either compartment formed by the divider. A portable TV camera above the observation area was used to monitor the activity and position of

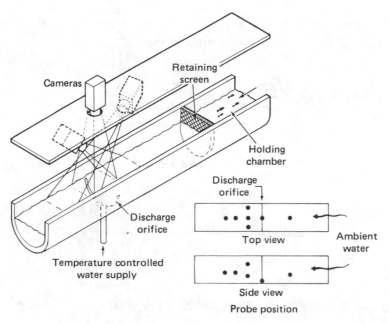

Figure 8 Schematic of raceway, showing overhead canopy video cameras, discharge orifice, retaining screen, holding chamber (upper left), and position of temperature probes (lower right). *[From Gray et al. (1977).]*

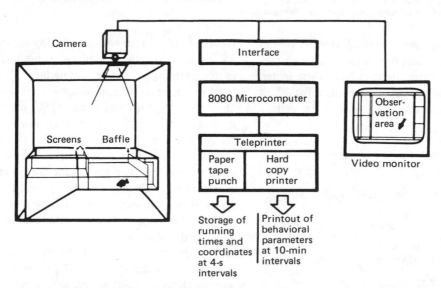

Figure 9 Diagram of behavior tank and television-computer monitor. A microcomputer was programmed to sample fish coordinates and experimental running times at 4-s intervals, and at 10-min intervals the behavioral parameters were calculated. *[From Lubinski et al. (1980); copyright, American Society for Testing and Materials, Philadelphia. Reprinted with permission.]*

the fish. The TV signal was directed to a video monitor for observation of movements and into a computer interface that recorded the position of a fish in an x-y coordinate grid system. A microcomputer could be programmed to sample coordinates and experimental running times at specific time intervals. The following locomotor parameters were calculated with this system: distance traveled, counts of movements, turns (left and right), straight paths and reversals, mean straight path lengths, accumulated left and right radians, and amount of time spent in each of four observation quadrants.

Miller et al. (1982) used a computerized video quantification system called the "bugsystem," which was developed by Greaves and Wilson (1980) to analyze directed (light) or undirected locomotor behavior of organisms ranging from bacteria to small fish. The main components of the system are shown in Fig. 10. Sequences of animal movement or spatial displacements are recorded on a videotape, which can play back the images of moving organisms into a video preprocessor ("bugwatcher"), which puts the image into x-y outline coordinates and then places them in the computer's memory access. The TV monitor is used for operator feedback.

Data input involves playing video information into the video-to-digital preprocessor (bugwatcher). This interface unit also conducts a

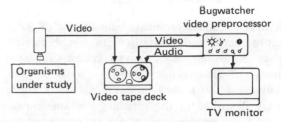

Figure 11 Apparatus used to collect behavioral data in the biological laboratory. *[From Greaves and Wilson (1980).]*

frame-by-frame analysis of the video record, per operator setting, permitting real-time input of the video signals to delineate the outline of moving organisms and reduce redundant information. The system is interactive and allows the user to follow the analysis sequence on the display in order to edit, manage, and transform data files to maximize the information obtained. Output may be on a line printer and plotter or cathode-ray tube (CRT) terminal display. The equipment used to collect the behavioral data is illustrated in Fig. 11. Organisms to be studied are placed in a dish or deep well slide and images of their movements are captured on videotape. The camera may be used with a microscope and the monitor is used to observe the experiment. The quality of the video image for computer input can be evaluated by playing the signal through the interface unit.

Undirected Locomotor Responses

Free

Freshwater as well as saltwater aquatic organisms show cyclic patterns in their daily activity (Schwassman, 1971). In fact, aquatic organisms may have an endogenously controlled diurnal rhythm of locomotor activity that persists in the absence of exogenous stimuli such as light and temperature (Reynolds and Casterlin, 1976).

Spontaneous, free-running locomotor activity and locomotor patterns are species-specific and highly variable over time, implying the need for prolonged observation. Therefore, precise assessment of locomotion, whether of "normal" (un-

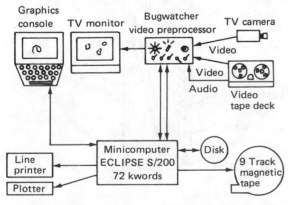

Figure 10 Block diagram of major components of the bug system. *[From Greaves and Wilson (1980).]*

treated or control) or of "exposed" (treated) animals, requires automated monitoring of locomotor activity or patterns with a sophisticated data acquisition and analysis system. The systems of Kleerekoper (1969), Westlake and Lubinski (1976), and Lubinski et al. (1980), which were described in the preceding section, can be used to monitor locomotor activity or patterns of freshwater or saltwater organisms, especially fish, in the absence of outside stimuli.

Spoor et al. (1971) developed an electrode chamber (33 X 8.5 X 15 cm) for recording respiratory and locomotor movements of free-swimming animals (Fig. 12). A fish is placed in a continuous-flow chamber, at opposite ends of which are stainless steel electrodes attached to a high-gain preamplifier and strip chart recorder. Movement (e.g., opercular, swimming) in the tank disturbs the electrochemical equilibrium at the electrode surface and changes its potential from a few to several hundred microvolts, depending on the velocity of water movement. One electrode is af-

fected more than another, and the potential difference is recorded as a wave on the strip chart recorder. By observing the activity and position of the animal in the chamber while the electrode potentials are being recorded, one can interpret the record to determine whether the movement is locomotor or opercular activity. The deflections are distinctive and sometimes their size will indicate the animal's location in the chamber, because the effectiveness of a movement is greater the nearer the electrode. Many investigators have used this technique to indicate the sublethal effects of chemicals (e.g., metals, pesticides) and effluents on fish "coughs" or "gill purges" [gill clearance actions that are interruptions of the normal ventilatory cycle of fish and serve to rid the gill surfaces of accumulated foreign material (Drummond and Carlson, 1977)].

The basic electrode technique was used in the development of a more open flow-through gradient tank (2 m X 30 cm X 12 cm) with multiple electrodes (Spoor and Drummond, 1972). The

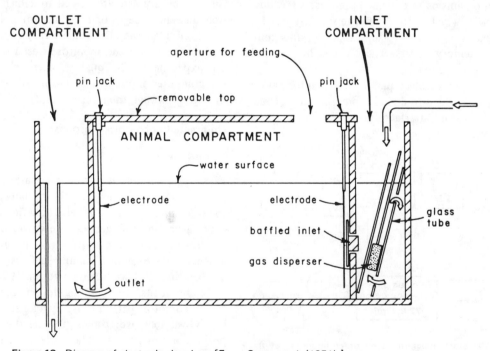

Figure 12   Diagram of electrode chamber. *[From Spoor et al. (1971).]*

tank was divided into four broadly connected compartments, each of which contained a pair of stainless steel electrodes. A fish's movement in each compartment, position, orientation, state of locomotor activity, and swimming speed could be determined continuously over long periods without disturbance by the observer. A similar system was used to monitor the movements of crayfish (Maciorowski et al., 1977a). After amplification, signals from crayfish were recorded by a microprocessor; the number of peaks in the electrical signal per time interval, corresponding to the total movement, was counted and recorded every 15 min. Several days of control data were recorded before exposure to the chemical in order to obtain the 95% confidence intervals of movement counts over the course of a day. Data taken during chemical exposure were compared with data on untreated controls. This statistical approach was similar to that of Cairns et al. (1973), who used a continuous monitoring system designed by Waller and Cairns (1972) to record fish movement patterns as a means of detecting exposure to pollutants. Test chambers were 5-gallon (41 X 21.5 X 26 cm) glass aquaria with a monitoring unit that consisted of light beams passing through red 650-nm filters, which traversed the tank at the bottom, middle, and just below the surface (Fig. 13). Photoresistors outside the tank at the opposite end were illuminated by the lamp sources. A fish swimming in front of light beam interrupted the light falling on the photoresistors, which operated relays via amplifiers, which in turn advanced a counter and deflected the pens of an event recorder. An automatic camera activated by a time switch took pictures of the counters every hour through a 24-h period. The fish activity data therefore consisted of cumulative light beam interruptions for each fish at three levels in the test tank during 1-h intervals. This activity monitoring system and a polygraph to record breathing signals from electrodes, along with an analog-to-digital converter, a minicomputer, and a teleprinter, were proposed for use in industrial plants or directly at an impact site to determine the effects of chemical

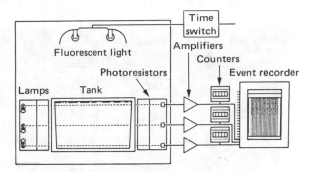

Figure 13 Monitoring apparatus, showing 5-gallon tank with lamp sources, photoresistors, two-transistor amplifiers, counters, and event recorder. *[Reprinted with permission from Waller and Cairns (1972); copyright 1972, Pergamon Press, Ltd.]*

exposure and to act as an early warning system (Cairns et al., 1973) (Fig. 14). It has been tested and found successful at an industrial site (Gruber et al., 1978).

Forced

Swimming performance or swimming ability is significant for survival of fish and is a good measure of sublethal chemical exposure (Cairns, 1966). Swimming performance tests monitor endurance and stamina, which permits an evaluation of processes such as respiratory metabolism, motor function, and swimming coordination. They are called "forced" activity tests because they are stress tests that measure sustained swimming speed or the ability of a fish to maintain its position in a current. Orientation and swimming are induced by creating a current. The response to water current is termed rheotaxis; swimming against the current is positive rheotaxis and swimming with the current negative rheotaxis (Keenleyside and Hoar, 1954). In fish, the response is dependent on visual, tactile, and labyrinth reflexes (Lyon, 1905; Gray, 1937). If a fish is exposed for a long time to current, positive rheotaxis may fail as a result of fatigue or adaptation of sensory mechanisms (Keenleyside and Hoar, 1954). Rheotaxis is to some extent a function of swimming ability. Critical swimming speed, defined by Brett (1964) as the maximum

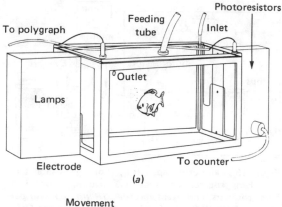

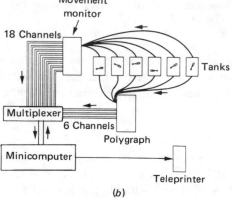

Figure 14 (*a*) Test chamber for monitoring fish activity and breathing. (*b*) Computerized monitoring system with fish as sensors. *[From Cairns et al. (1973); reprinted with permission from the American Water Resources Association.]*

velocity fish could maintain for a precise time period, is also used as a measure of swimming ability.

A number of devices have been suggested to measure swimming performance in fish (Blazka et al., 1960; Brett, 1964; Farmer and Beamish, 1969). They consist of a recirculating water tunnel with a swimming compartment (for fish) connected to a pump to create a current. Fish are "forced" (e.g., stimulated to maintain position by prodding with a glass rod or shocking when touched by an electric screen downstream) to swim against a current and subjected to a stepwise progression of velocity measurements until they

are fatigued (i.e., when, by repeated efforts, they can no longer hold themselves off the electric screen). Critical swimming speed is then calculated (Brett, 1964).

Several investigators have developed automated techniques for monitoring rheotaxis or the ability of the fish to maintain its position in moving water. Poels (1977) designed a swimming chamber (2 m × 62 cm × 25 cm) with a flow-through system for fish, employing photocells to determine loss of rheotaxis. The central part of the test basin consisted of three spatially separated chambers, each containing one fish and one monitoring system. When a fish in the chamber no longer displayed positive rheotaxis and moved to the downstream end of the swimming chamber, a series of photoelectric beams were interrupted and this caused a mild electric shock to be applied to the downstream part of the chamber. This electrical irritation persisted until fish moved back upstream away from the photocells. Another series of photoelectric cells indicated when the fish stayed in the downstream area regardless of the electrical stimulation. The behavior of each fish was registered on a printer. To reduce the chance that an alarm was triggered by random movements, the alarm switch operated only when at least two fish in the same measuring period (15 min) passed the photoelectric cells more than normally or when two fish remained in the extreme downstream part of the monitoring system for more than 5 min. Fish in the downstream part of the test chamber would be irritated twice electrically, and if this occurred it was classified as abnormal behavior. This monitoring system has been successfully applied on the Rhine River to monitor water quality. New fish are placed in the monitoring system every month to prevent adaptation.

Besch et al. (1977) developed a similar system in which loss of rheotaxis was measured by interruption of vertical light beams and the surfacing of fish was measured by horizontal light beams. A "kinetic screen" was present at the downstream end of the chamber. It produced electrical pulses which, when touched by the fish, provided a measure of the loss of swimming ability and of whether the fish swim closer to the bottom or to the surface when showing signs of fatigue during the stress periods. The basic assumption is that normal, healthy fish avoid contact of their caudal fins with the downstream limit of their confined area. Besch used alternating periods of resting (slow vertical current) and stress (strong longitudinal current) phases instead of continuous downstream flow of test water. Each interruption of light generated a signal, which was amplified and recorded. Swimming performance, schooling and surface behavior, incapacity to swim, and loss of equilibrium were automatically monitored.

In the rotatory-flow technique (Lindahl et al., 1977), a fish is placed in a horizontal tube that has water flowing through it and is rotated. At a certain rotational speed the fish is unable to compensate and will start to rotate. The critical number of revolutions at which the fish is just brought to rotate with the water is read and used as a measure of the ability of the fish to resist the torque of a rotating stream. An improved version of the rotatory-flow technique was developed to allow tests to be performed with fish of different sizes (Lindahl et al., 1977). This technique was used to compare cod from unpolluted and polluted areas.

Feeding and Reproductive Behavior

Feeding behavior is very complex because of the wide range of feeding strategies among aquatic organisms. Many aquatic organisms are herbivores, some are carnivores, and some vary their diet, so that omnivores are also prevalent. The primary feeding adaptation of herbivorous organisms is structural rather than behavioral. Since plants have no escape mechanisms, aquatic organisms do not require special capture strategies to eat them. To use plants for food, herbivores have specialized mouth parts and teeth. Most aquatic organisms, especially fish, are carnivores; they eat live prey at least during some part of their lives. This requires more elaborate capture techniques because the prey organisms use a wide range of behavioral and structural adaptations to avoid capture. Since

many aquatic organisms can serve as food, carnivorous organisms may utilize a number of behavioral strategies as well as structural adaptations to overcome their prey's defense mechanisms.

Different sensory modalities appear to be important in feeding behavior (search, detection, chase, capture, ingestion). For example, for many diurnally active fish visual and in some cases tactile cues play an important role in feeding, but chemical cues are more important in the feeding strategies of nocturnal organisms. In sharks, search behavior is initiated by chemical and acoustic cues; visual, chemical, and in some cases electrical cues are important in mediating approach and attack; and chemical and probably tactile cues are used to distinguish edible from inedible material in the mouth (Tester, 1963; Banner, 1972; Kalmijn, 1974). Locomotion is also important, especially during the search, detection, and capture (chase) phases.

Studies of feeding behavior in aquatic toxicology have mainly dealt with overt stereotypic feeding patterns of a few organisms. Observations are usually evaluated and quantified by a trained investigator after extensive study in the laboratory and, ideally, in the field. In most cases, automated techniques have not been used because they would not detect many subtle components of the behavioral pattern.

Observation periods are usually long; if the "normal" baseline behavior is not studied sufficiently, erroneous and misleading results may be obtained. Highly reproducible feeding patterns should be studied. For example, the mud snail (*Ilyanassa obsoleta*) and lobster (*Homarus americanus*) have stereotypic chemotactic feeding response sequences that consist of several discrete phases which can be easily studied (Hyland and Miller, 1979; Atema and Stein, 1974).

Chemoreception or food detection has also been studied in the Y maze (Evans et al., 1977) and in open-field and circular tanks (Kleerekoper, 1969); with the latter two types of tanks automation has been used. Feeding activity studies have also been automated (Spoor et al., 1971).

The methods described above are useful in demonstrating effects on feeding behavior, but it is possible that the altered behavior is secondary to such factors as respiratory stress or central nervous system (CNS) dysfunction and does not directly involve receptors. Electrophysiological studies might be useful in determining whether an organism can detect a chemical or whether the chemical damages chemoreceptors (Hara, 1971). Measurement of gross neural activity in chemoreceptor pathways (i.e., from receptors and second-order neurons) may be useful because they seem to be well correlated with relative behavioral thresholds for different compounds (Ottoson, 1971). A combination of behavioral, electrophysiological, and histological techniques may be most useful in determining the interaction between the chemical toxicant, the sensory tissue, and feeding behavior. This approach was successfully used by Bardach et al. (1965) in studying the effects of detergents on the yellow bullhead (*Ictalurus natalis*).

Although reproductive behavior has been studied extensively in aquatic organisms, it has scarcely been used in aquatic toxicology. It is also very complex because of the diversity of strategies used in spawning, courtship, and parental care. Reproductive behavioral studies rely predominantly on laboratory observations by trained investigators and are difficult to automate. These studies are not discussed here.

Predator-Prey Interaction

Predator-prey interaction has been studied with relatively simple and inexpensive test apparatus. Goodyear (1972) developed a test apparatus with two parts: a deep-water chamber for the predator (e.g., largemouth bass, *Micropterus salmoides*) and a shallow-water section for the prey (e.g., mosquitofish, *Gambusia affinis*). The shallow section is protected by a screen behind which the prey can hide. Kania and O'Hara (1974) used a similar apparatus with no screen but with a shallow shelf at one end for the prey and a deep end for the predators. Woltering et al. (1978) used large glass tanks with two Fiberglas screen shelves, one at each end

of the tank, to provide refuge for the prey but not the predators. Hatfield and Anderson (1972) used large outdoor circular concrete pools with gently sloping bottoms. Each pool contained a refuge which the prey (Atlantic salmon, *Salmo salar*) could pass through but the predator (brook trout, *Salvelinus fontinalis*) could not. Microcosm-type experimental tanks containing sand or gravel and vegetation have also been used in predator-prey studies (Sullivan et al., 1978; Tagatz, 1976). Field test plots and cages have also been used in the natural environment (Ward and Howes, 1974; Ward et al., 1976).

Predator-prey studies can include exposure of either prey or predator before initiating the experiment or exposure of both during the experiment. Exposure may be acute or long-term. Organisms are usually observed in the laboratory tank through a viewing window, and the number of swimming prey are counted and statistically analyzed at the end of the experiment.

Social Organization and Other Inter-Individual Relationships

Social organization of an animal population includes the sum of relationships among individuals of the population (Brown, 1975). Characteristics of these relationships can be understood only by observing the interactions of individual organisms. The different interactions are components of social behavior. The relationships between individuals are based on distance, home range, territory, and dominance (Keenleyside, 1979).

Territoriality (Symons, 1973) and dominance behavior (Henry and Atchison, 1979; Sparks et al., 1972) have received some attention in aquatic toxicology. Studies are conducted with the organisms observed in test tanks through viewing windows to identify behavioral patterns of individuals. Weeks to months of preliminary observations on the normal untreated test population are needed before the actual test periods begin in order to develop recording methodology and observation skills for reliability. Data are then statistically analyzed.

Learning

The ability to learn and retain a simple conditioned avoidance response has been used to measure chemically induced behavioral stress in aquatic organisms (Anderson and Peterson, 1969; Barthalmus, 1977; Jackson et al., 1970; Hatfield and Johansen, 1972; Warner et al., 1966; Weir and Hine, 1970). Fish can be classically conditioned to a stimulus (conditioned stimulus) presented at some time before the occurrence of a shock (unconditioned stimulus). The conditioned stimulus serves as a warning signal and is usually light or a sound. The time interval between the onset of the conditioned stimulus and the onset of the shock is set at a specified value; the stimulus usually remains on during the shock; and both shock and stimulus terminate at the same time. Avoidance is a response that postpones the occurrence of the shock (conditioned response to the unconditioned stimulus), while escape is a response that terminates the shock once it has been presented (unconditioned response). If the side of the conditioning tank on which the signal is to occur is not randomized or if the preshock interval is not variable, signaled avoidance is difficult to shape. The behavior that often develops is unsignaled avoidance, where the subject ignores the signal and uses temporal sensing to avoid or escape shock. Unsignaled avoidance conditioning without an external preshock signal has been studied in fish after exposure to a chemical agent (Rand and Barthalmus, 1980).

Conditioned avoidance training of organisms may be conducted in a shuttletank apparatus (Fig. 15). The tank measures 35 × 25 × 20 cm and is clear plastic. Stainless steel electrodes set into the long walls of the tank have small openings cut in them to permit the passage of light beams, which traverse the middle of the tank to reach the photocells. Only one of the two photocell circuits—the one on the opposite side of the fish—is functional at any time. When the beam is broken, the other circuit becomes functional; it remains so until its beam is broken, whereupon the first becomes functional again, and so forth. A response

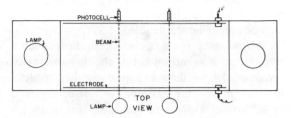
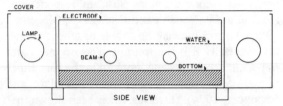

Figure 15 Shuttletank. *[From Rand and Barthalmus (1980); copyright American Society for Testing and Materials, Philadelphia; reprinted with permission.]*

is therefore defined as the breaking of the farthest photocell beam. The tank is enclosed in a darkened sound-attenuating chamber and is illuminated by 7.5-W lamps outside the tank.

One fish is conditioned at a time. Exposure to a chemical may occur before, after, or even during conditioning. A criterion of learning may be established after untreated fish are conditioned so that baseline values can be obtained and used for comparison. Conditioning of a simple tail reflex of fish can also be used to measure chemically induced stress (Anderson and Prins, 1970). Stimulation of the gular region of fish results in a weak propeller-like movement of the tail. This simple reflex can be elicited and learned with training.

BEHAVIORAL PATTERNS STUDIED IN THE LABORATORY

Behavioral response systems can be functionally affected by sublethal concentrations of toxic chemicals. A behavioral change may, in fact, be the first response of an organism to environmental perturbation (Slobodkin, 1968). If the behavioral response system reacts appropriately by eliminating contact with or exposure to the chemical, the probability of death and other sublethal effects may be reduced or negligible.

The presence of a noxious chemical may elicit a response such as movement of the organism away (avoidance) from the area containing the chemical, which will reduce exposure. For this or any type of behavioral response to occur, the chemical must be sensed, recognized as aversive, and responded to appropriately (Pearson and Olla, 1979; Olla et al., 1980). Organisms may be unable to sense a chemical, especially if it is novel to the environment and not similar to others encountered in the past either in substance or in occurrence (Slobodkin and Rapoport, 1974). However, it has been shown that blue crabs (Callinectus sapidus) can detect naphthalene at a threshold concentration of 10^{-7} mg/l (Pearson and Olla, 1980) and the water-soluble fraction of crude oil with similar sensitivity (Pearson et al., 1981). For the Dungeness crab (Cancer magister) the detection threshold for naphthalene was 10^{-2} mg/l (Pearson et al., 1980). Although the chemical is detected, the organism may not recognize it as aversive because of its novelty and therefore may not respond or may respond inappropriately. Mitigation of a perturbation is obviously dependent on the correct response.

Behavioral studies in aquatic toxicology may be divided into those that measure the ability of the organisms to mitigate the effects of chemicals (avoidance of chemicals) and those that measure abnormal behavior or departures from normal behavior (locomotor, feeding, predator-prey interaction) which may not lead to death but may have adverse biological effects (Olla et al., 1980). These studies are discussed below.

Preference/Avoidance of Chemicals

These studies monitor the ability of organisms to detect (sense) the presence of a chemical toxicant and to respond to it by moving toward the chemical (preference or attraction) or away from it (avoidance) into an untreated "clean" area. There are no typical preference/avoidance reactions of aquatic organisms to chemicals because organisms detect and avoid some chemicals but not others.

However, this response seems to be a good first step in the behavioral evaluation of chemical exposure. The literature on preference/avoidance responses is discussed below in terms of different chemical types.

Metals

Jones (1947) found that tenspine stickleback (Pygosteus pungitius) showed no special ability to detect or avoid mercuric chloride even at toxic concentrations. Zinc sulfate appeared to be detected and avoided. Copper sulfate was detected and avoided at high concentrations, but at low concentrations fish swam into the solution and became "stupified and ... motionless." Jones (1948) also found that threespine stickleback (Gasterosteus aculeatus) reacted positively (were attracted) to high concentrations of lead nitrate, but at low concentrations the response disappeared and was replaced by a negative reaction (avoidance). The minnow Phoxinus phoxinus L. also avoided dilute solutions of lead nitrate but was more sensitive than the stickleback because it detected and avoided these solutions at concentrations several orders of magnitude lower. Ishio (1965) showed that the minnow Zacco platypus avoided copper chloride solutions at high concentrations but then was attracted to them.

Some of the best documented work on preference/avoidance of metals is that with salmonids, which includes behavioral and physiological work that can be applied in the field. Sprague (1964) observed in the laboratory that Atlantic salmon (Salmo salar) avoided copper and zinc at 0.02 of the incipient lethal level. Rainbow trout tested with zinc sulfate showed a threshold avoidance level of 5.6 µg/l (0.01 of the lethal concentration); this was almost 0.1 of the threshold (53 µg/l) of Atlantic salmon under the same conditions (Sprague, 1968). Avoidance of zinc concentrations of 0.45 and 0.3 of the lethal concentration was reported by Ishio (1965) and Syazuki (1964), respectively. In contrast, Summerfelt and Lewis (1967) did not observe avoidance of lethal concentrations of copper and zinc by the green sunfish (*Lepomis megalotis*).

The effects of copper-zinc mining on the upstream spawning migration of Atlantic salmon was studied in the field (Saunders and Sprague, 1967). Counting of the fish at a fence below a copper-zinc mine effluent source showed that unusual downstream movements of adult salmon rose during periods when copper and zinc levels in the water were high (0.35–0.43 toxic unit). At about 0.8 toxic unit or higher, all upstream movement was blocked. Some 31% of the salmon returning downstream because of the pollution reascended during more favorable conditions; 62% were not seen again and about 7% were taken by anglers or commercial fisheries. There was no evidence that successive year classes were affected by the pollution.

The avoidance threshold for rainbow trout (*Salmo gairdneri*) to copper (4.4 μg/l) and nickel (23.4 μg/l) with a shallow gradient were within the 95% confidence interval of the results for the steep gradient (Giattina et al., 1982). Furthermore, rainbow trout avoided low copper concentrations and were attracted to higher ones (330–390 μg/l) during shallow-gradient tests, but under similar conditions they were attracted to low nickel concentrations (~6 μg/l) but avoided higher ones (>19 μg/l). Attraction to high concentrations of copper following avoidance to lower concentrations was also reported by Black and Birge (1980), who showed that rainbow trout avoided copper at 0.07 mg/l but were attracted to it at 0.46 and 0.76 mg/l. Maciorowski et al. (1977b) also found that the amphipod *Gammarus lacustris* showed a statistically significant avoidance of copper at 0.19 and 0.46 mg/l and a statistically significant preference for copper at 12.3 and 30.0 mg/l. In contrast, Costa (1966) found that *Gammarus pulex* avoided copper at 0.32, 31.8, and 318.0 mg/l.

Causes of preference/avoidance behavior have been related to narcotic effects (Jones, 1947, 1948) or to changes in the sensitivity of chemoreceptors (Hara et al., 1976; Sutterlin, 1974). For example, studies of water selection with adult salmon in laboratory tanks showed that low levels of copper alter the attractiveness of the home stream odor (Sutterlin and Gray, 1973). Hara (1972) showed that high copper levels caused a reduction in the electroencephalographic response from the olfactory bulb of salmon to a standard test odor. He postulated that this blocking effect was caused by interference of the copper ions with either receptor membranes or enzymatic components of the receptor membranes. Gardner and LaRoche (1973) found that 0.5 ppm copper damaged the olfactory mucosa in two species of estuarine fish. Hara et al. (1976) found that a threshold copper concentration of 8 μg/l was required to cause a minimal depression in the bulbar response of rainbow trout to the olfactory stimulant L-serine. The bulbar response was increasingly depressed at higher concentrations, and apparently irreversible damage to the olfactory receptor occurred at 50 μg/l.

Avoidance of metals, particularly copper and zinc, probably evolved as a mechanism for protecting fish from exposure to naturally occurring levels of these contaminants. Avoidance of these toxic solutions probably depends not only on the concentration, but also on the rate of change in concentration between two areas of water (Ishio, 1965). For copper, however, the direction of orientation appears to be relatively independent of the maximum concentration of the metal and dependent on the gradient of copper ions as the fish move into water containing copper (Kleerekoper et al., 1972; Timms et al., 1972; Westlake et al., 1974). A shallow gradient leading to the zones of maximum copper concentration (50 μg/l) attracted goldfish (*Carassius auratus*) and largemouth bass (*Micropterus salmoides*); a moderately steep gradient decreased that response somewhat; and a steep gradient resulted in significant avoidance. However, with a steep gradient, significant attraction was again observed when a temperature rise of 0.4°C was associated with the copper ions (0.01 ppm).

Phenol

Several investigators reported that fish do not avoid sublethal concentrations of phenol (Ishio,

1965; Jones, 1964; Sprague and Drury, 1969; Summerfelt and Lewis, 1967; Syazuki, 1964). Ishio (1965) and Syazuki (1964), in fact, reported avoidance thresholds at 1.1-2.5 times the lethal concentration. Skrapek (1963) reported escape reactions at 0.2-0.3 of the lethal level. In all the studies the concentrations used were above the olfactory threshold for the bluntnose minnow (*Hyborhynchus notatus*), which appeared to naturally dislike the odors of phenol and *p*-chlorophenol (Hasler and Wisby, 1950). Perhaps the phenol concentrations used in the avoidance studies were so high that they affected sensory perception by the fish. However, roaches (*Leuciscus rutilus*) display a preference for 2,4,6-trinitrophenol (3 × 10⁻⁶ *M*) (Lindahl and Marcstrom, 1958).

Pulp and Paper Mill Effluents

Young chinook salmon (*Oncorhynchus tshawytscha*) showed avoidance to 2.5-10% kraft mill effluent (KME) in seawater (Jones et al., 1956), and Columbia River smelt (*Thaleichthys pacificus*) avoided KME down to 0.5% in a field study (Smith and Saalfeld, 1955). Young coho salmon (*O. kisutch*), however, did not avoid KME at any concentrations up to 10% (Jones et al., 1956), nor did silver salmon avoid 3.5% KME (Holland et al., 1960). Atlantic salmon showed moderate avoidance of bleached KME at 10-100,000 ppm (Sprague and Drury, 1969); lower concentrations were not avoided. Experiments with unbleached KME gave similar results. In laboratory studies, lobsters (*Homarus americanus*) also did not avoid bleached KME at concentrations up to 20% (McLeese, 1970).

Hoglund (1961) observed avoidance by fish of a sublethal level (0.1-1.0 ppm) of sulfide waste liquor (SWL) and showed that the steepness of the gradient was important in the animals' ability to avoid toxic levels. Herring (*Clupea harengus*) avoided whole pulp mill effluent (PME) from a sulfite mill at a concentration threshold of 2.5-2.9 mg/l as sodium lignosulfonate (Wildish et al., 1976). Wildish et al. (1977) suggested that herring avoid long complex molecules such as lignosulfon-

ates and may avoid the lignin in PME rather than resin acids.

Pesticides

Green sunfish in the laboratory avoided chlordane (75% emulsifiable concentrate) at 20, 10, and 5 mg/l but were indifferent to 1.0 mg/l (Summerfelt and Lewis, 1967). Lindane [99% gamma isomer of benzene hexachloride (BHC or HCH)] was not avoided at 20 mg/l. Also, some fish in TVA (Tennessee Valley Authority) lakes moved out of areas treated with (2,4-dichlorophenoxyacetic acid (2,4-D) (Smith and Isom, 1967). Sheepshead minnows (*Cyprinodon variegatus*) avoided concentrations of DDT, endrin, Dursban, and 2,4-D, but a concentration-avoidance response curve was observed only with 2,4-D (Hansen, 1969). The fish did not avoid the test concentrations of malathion (up to 1.0 ppm) or Sevin (up to 10 ppm). Similarly, mosquitofish (*Gambusia affinis*) were able to avoid one or more concentrations of Dursban, DDT, malathion, Sevin, and 2,4-D but did not avoid endrin (Hansen et al., 1972). The concentration of each pesticide avoided was less than the 24-h LC50. Although mosquitofish were able to seek water free of pesticide, this behavior was not usually pronounced in all cases. Given a choice of two concentrations of the same pesticide, mosquitofish either did not discriminate between them or preferred or avoided the higher concentration.

Both susceptible and resistant populations of mosquitofish avoided endrin, toxaphene, and parathion (Kynard, 1974). DDT was avoided by susceptible fish but not by resistant fish. Scherer (1975) reported that goldfish (*Carassius auratus*) avoided fenitrothion with a threshold of about 10 µg/l. This is lower than some gustatory and olfactory thresholds determined for a number of test substances and species of fish.

Folmar (1976) found that rainbow trout avoided five herbicides (copper sulfate, dalapon, dimethylamine salt of 2,4-D, xylene, and acrolein) but did not avoid four others (glyphosate, aquathol K, diquat, trichloroacetic acid) at concentrations below the 24- or 96-h LC50. Mayflies (*Ephemerella walkeri*) avoided the highest test concentrations of copper sulfate, diquat, and Roundup but did not avoid the other herbicides (2,4-D DMA, acrolein, xylene, dalapon, and aquathol K) tested (Folmar, 1978). Except for diquat and aquathol K, the mayfly nymphs appeared to be less sensitive to the eight herbicides than the rainbow trout previously tested.

Petroleum and Related Hydrocarbons

Shelford (1917) reported that fish did not avoid sublethal levels of acetone, and Summerfelt and Lewis (1967) showed that green sunfish did not avoid lethal levels of benzene. However, the common shrimp (*Crangon crangon*) detected and avoided oil dispersants at a concentration 2 orders of magnitude below its 48-h TL50 (Portmann and Connor, 1968). The amphipod *Onisismus affinus* was repelled by lightly oiled sediments (0.05 ml oil per 15 g dry sediment) and rejected oiled food (Percy, 1977). The ability of this organism to discriminate between clean and oiled sediments disappeared when the oil concentration was 2.0 ml per 15 g dry sediment. This effect may have been due to temporary inactivation of chemosensory responses by the high concentrations of oil. Rice (1973) also reported avoidance of seawater extracts of Prudhoe Bay crude oil by pink salmon (*O. gorbuscha*) at oil concentrations as low as 1.6 mg/l, or approximately 0.1 of the 96-h TL50.

Organisms are not all repelled by oil. Percy (1977) found that the amphipod *Corophium clarense* and the isopods *Mesidotea entomon* and *M. siberica* were either oblivious to or neutral to oil. Lobsters may even be attracted by some kerosene products (Percy, 1977). Atema et al. (1973) observed that lobsters were attracted to and ingested kerosene-soaked objects; the attraction was probably to the water-soluble aromatic fraction and ingestion due to the saturated hydrocarbons.

Avoidance of Chemicals by Sessile Organisms

It is evident that fish and other highly motile, responsive organisms try to mitigate or avoid deleterious substances in their environment if they detect them and find them aversive. Species that are sessile and have limited motility must rely on other adaptive behavioral responses to mitigate or avoid exposure. Invertebrates such as barnacles, some annelids, and bivalves remain close to one place for most of their lives. These sessile organisms avoid exposure by closing themselves off from the rest of the environment. For example, Galtsoff (1960) found that oysters can effectively shut down by sealing their valves when exposed to crude oil; the period of valve closure was proportional to the concentration of the substance. The blue mussel (*Mytilus edulis*) also completely closed its valves when exposed to water-soluble extracts of Esso Extra or no. 2 home-heating oil for 60 min at concentrations of 24%, while at 12% the shells were open (Dunning and Major, 1974). Davenport and Manley (1978) showed that the blue mussel could detect low concentrations of copper sulfate. This was initially indicated by a sharp adduction of the valves, and was followed at higher concentrations by "testing" behavior—alternate opening and closing of the valves. Complete valve closure occurred at concentrations higher than the acute toxicity threshold. Although this response may not occur in the natural environment, the organisms do have the potential to close themselves off from the environment and thereby reduce their exposure.

Directed Locomotor Orientation Responses

Light

Normal photobehavior may be modified by sublethal exposure to chemicals. Parameters measured in photobehavior may include changes in the direction of orientation to a light stimulus (phototaxis), the intensity of the phototactic response, or the swimming rate (photokinesis) in response to the stimulus. Mercury (Vernberg et al., 1973), no. 2 fuel oil (Bigford, 1977), copper (Miller, 1980; Miller et al., 1982), and xanthene dyes (Bjornberg and Wilbur, 1968) altered phototaxis in fiddler crab larvae (*Uca pugilator*), rock crab larvae

(*Cancer irroratus*), barnacle nauplii (*Balanus improvisus*), and copepods, respectively. For example, Bigford (1977) found a reduction in the intensity of phototaxis in rock crab larvae exposed to 0.1 ppm no. 2 fuel oil (water-soluble fraction), but at 1.0 ppm this response was lost in three of five larval stages. Consequently, there are changes in the vertical distribution patterns of larvae in the water column which, in the field, could alter recruitment to adult populations.

Copper exposure was also shown to produce a shift from positive to negative phototaxis of barnacle nauplii (Miller, 1980; Miller et al., 1982). However, Vernberg et al. (1963) reported that mercury increased the intensity of positive phototaxis in fiddler crab larvae. These differences may be due to the use of different testing techniques.

Amiard (1976) measured the effects of metals (cobalt, strontium, silver) on photokinesis of the zoeal stage of two species of crustaceans. Hyperactivity was prevalent at low concentrations but was reduced at high concentrations. Copper and cadmium caused a significant initial increase of undirected (spontaneous) swimming activity of barnacle nauplii, followed by a reduction in speed below control levels as the exposure increased (Miller et al., 1982). Apparently, these metals produced a biphasic response, with exposure to low concentrations increasing locomotor activity while concentrations approaching acutely lethal levels suppressed it.

Photoresponses are important for vertical migration of plankton, for which the ambient level of illumination in the sea is the key stimulus (Forward, 1976). It is generally considered adaptive for zooplankton to move toward the surface at night to areas of high food density and to leave the euphotic zone during the day for protection against predators. The photoresponsiveness of vertically migrating species could be affected by chemical exposure.

Temperature

Temperature gradients were found to be important in directing the movements and distribution of fish in the laboratory (Sullivan and Fisher, 1954) and in nature (Smith and Saunders, 1958). Temperature selection is used by fish as a means of avoiding the deleterious effects of temperature extremes. When placed in a temperature gradient, fish select and move into a narrow range of temperatures. The temperature where the observed frequency of occurrence is greatest over a specific time period is called the "selected" or "preferred" temperature.

Pesticides have been found to alter the temperature selection responses of fish. Ogilvie and Anderson (1965) found that exposure of Atlantic salmon underyearlings for 24 h to sublethal concentrations of DDT (5–50 ppb) resulted in changes in the selected temperature. Low concentrations produced a downward shift of approximately $2°C$, whereas higher concentrations raised the selected temperature $6–10°C$ above control values. Warm-acclimated ($17°C$) fish appeared to be more affected by DDT than cold-acclimated ($8°C$) fish. Gardner (1973) investigated the effects of DDT and methoxychlor analogs (10–50 ppb) on temperature selection in brook trout fingerlings (*Salvelinus fontinalis*). All the compounds tested except DDE-type analogs altered temperature selection. When DDT- and methoxychlor-treated fish were placed in clean water, the lower selected temperature of the methoxychlor-treated fish returned to the control level in 5 d, whereas the lower selected temperature of the DDT-treated fish persisted for the duration of the study (9 d).

Peterson (1973) noted that DDT analogs and methoxychlor at low concentrations either did not affect or decreased the selected temperature of juvenile Atlantic salmon. Higher concentrations raised the selected temperature. The concentrations of the substances required to produce a given effect varied. However, the polychlorinated biphenyl Aroclor 1254 had no effect on temperature selection. Miller and Ogilvie (1975) also found that Aroclor 1254 had no effect on temperature selection of brook trout. However, they did find a typical biphasic concentration-response relationship for DDT and temperature. Low concentrations (10 ppb) depressed the mean temperature, while high concentrations (50 ppb) significantly increased the selected temperature by more than 4°C. Exposure to phenol produced a consistent downward shift in selected temperature.

Domanik and Zar (1978) found that the organophosphate pesticide malathion produced concentration-dependent decreases in the selected temperature (1.9–4.3°C below controls) of shiners (*Notropis cornutus*) acclimated at 17°C but not of those acclimated at 8°C. Two-yr-old fish at 1.0 μg/l showed the greatest lowering of selected temperature, followed by 2-yr-olds treated with 0.25 μg/l. One-yr-olds treated with 1.0 μg/l showed a slight lowering while young-of-the-year exhibited no downward shift.

The temperature selection response is probably mediated by the CNS. Since organochlorine and organophosphate pesticides affect neural transmission in the nervous system, it is not surprising that they may affect temperature selection. Such pesticide-induced temperature changes have the potential to produce changes not only in fish distribution but also in the timing of reproduction and growth.

Undirected Locomotor Activity: Free and Forced

Free

Effects of pesticides, metals, and petroleum hydrocarbons on fish and invertebrate locomotor behavior have been studied. Davy et al. (1972) found that the highly significant correlation between consecutive turns in the locomotor pattern of normal goldfish, which is attributed to a "memory" or retention process, was significantly reduced by exposing fish to water containing DDT (10 μg/l, prepared and renewed daily for 4 d). Keeping the fish in clean water for 130 and 139 d did not result in restoration of this correlation. Davy et al. (1973) also found that exposure to 10 ppb DDT for 4 d did not destroy the nonrandom exploratory pattern of goldfish. However, the frequency of shifts in position and the rate of activity showed different temporal oscillations

after DDT exposure. Also, the correlation between these two parameters changed significantly after DDT treatment.

Weiss and Weiss (1974) found that after 3 d of exposure to 1.0 ppb DDT, groups of goldfish swam faster, turned more often, and occupied a greater area. The increase in activity was associated with a decrease in schooling behavior. Seven days after the fish were returned to clean water there was no longer a significant difference in these categories. Fingerman et al. (1979) observed an increase in spontaneous activity of fiddler crabs (*Uca pugilator*) after 3 d exposure to 0.08 ppm DDT. However, the circadian nature of crab activity appears not to have been affected by the DDT. The latter finding agrees with the work on this species by Vernberg et al. (1974), who found that during a 2-wk exposure to 0.18 ppm mercury there was no change in the locomotor rhythm of adult crabs but there was suppressed activity. Mercury also induced changes in swimming patterns from linear paths to increasingly circular paths. Changes in the spatial pattern of swimming were also observed in barnacle nauplii exposed to copper (Miller, 1980).

Ellgaard et al. (1977) reported that exposure to sublethal concentrations of DDT elicited hyperactive locomotor responses in bluegill sunfish (*Lepomis macrochirus*) and the degree of the responses was concentration-dependent. Maximal effects were observed within 8 d after addition of DDT to the environment. Metals (cadmium, chromium, and zinc) also produced concentration-dependent hyperactive locomotor responses in the bluegill (Ellgaard et al., 1978).

Rand (1977a) demonstrated that exposure to sublethal concentrations of parathion for 24 h resulted in an overall decline in activity of goldfish. It is interesting to note that during the 24-h parathion exposure, fish remained listless on the bottom of the holding tank. When monitored in an automated system untreated fish displayed an orientation angle distribution characterized by a preponderance of small angles. After parathion exposure, in some fish, the distribution was modified and shifted to larger angles. A similar decline in activity was also observed in bluegill and large-mouth bass exposed to sublethal concentrations of parathion (Rand, 1977b).

Forced

Swimming performance has been cited as a sensitive indicator for cyanide (Neil, 1957), detergents (Cairns and Scheier, 1962), pulpwood food fiber (MacLeod and Smith, 1966), hydrogen sulfide (Oseid and Smith, 1972), sodium pentachlorophenate (Webb and Brett, 1973), fenitrothion (Bull and McInerney, 1974), copper (Waiwood and Beamish, 1978), and bleached pulp mill effluent (Howard, 1975). Swimming performance (or endurance) tests can be used to determine the effects of chemical exposure on active fish experiencing maximal exposure to chemicals.

Feeding Behavior

The search and feeding behavior of fish has been altered by sublethal concentrations of synthetic detergents (Bardach et al., 1965; Foster et al., 1966). Bardach et al. (1965) observed histological damage to the taste buds (on the barbels) of yellow bullhead catfish (*Ictalurus natalis*) after a 4-wk exposure to 0.5 ppm alkyl benzenesulfonate (ABS), but there were no such changes on the olfactory epithelium. Linear alkyl benzenesulfonates (LAS) produced similar degeneration of taste buds. Fish exposed to 1 ppm LAS or ABS for approximately 3 wk could not find food. After 6 wk in clean water, affected fish still could not sense or detect food. Foster et al. (1966) found that flagfish (*Jordanella floridae*) exposed to 10 ppm ABS for 4 wk detected and approached their food (tubificid worms) but then ejected it. Detergents at the higher concentrations may damage the olfactory epithelium, so that in one study the sense of smell was affected (Bardach et al., 1965) and in the other study the taste mechanism (Foster et al., 1966).

A 24-h exposure to a crude oil extract inhibited the feeding response of the shore crab (*Pachygrapsus crassipes*) to the amino acid taurine and the stereotypic responses of the male crab to the female sex pheromone (Takahashi and Kittredge, 1973; Kittredge et al., 1974). The monoaromatic hydrocarbons blocked chemoreception but the effects disappeared rapidly. The polynuclear aromatics produced chemosensory inhibition, which persisted for several weeks. Low concentrations of seawater extracts of the water-soluble kerosene (mostly benzenes and naphthalenes) also reduced the attraction of the mud snail (*Nassarius obsoletus*) to food extracts (Jacobson and Boylan, 1973). The reduced attraction to the food may have resulted from interference with chemoreception because an avoidance reaction to the kerosene extract alone did not appear. Chemically mediated feeding responses of the mud snail, such as the initial perception or arousal phase and the tasting phase, were inhibited by various fractions and concentrations of fuel oil. The arousal phase involves distance chemoreception, and tasting is a contact chemoresponse.

Atema and Stein (1974) found that lobsters exposed to whole crude oil took a longer time between detecting food and approaching it than either the control animals or those exposed to the water-soluble fraction. No morphological changes in odor receptors were detected by light or electron microscopy. The increased time was attributed not to chemoreceptor damage but to the noxious odor of oil, which reduced feeding motivation.

Most phases of feeding behavior in aquatic organisms involve some level of sensory perception, which include chemical, visual, and/or tactile sensing. Inhibition of food odor detection, lack of search behavior for food, and food rejection are all indications that there may be an alteration in chemoreceptors or some part of the CNS. To substantiate these findings, studies of the effects of chemicals on feeding behavior should be integrated with electrophysiological and histological studies.

Predator-Prey Interaction

Several laboratory studies have shown that chemicals affect the vulnerability of prey so that there is increased selectivity in predation by an unaffected or less affected predator, Hatfield and Anderson (1972) studied the effects of exposure to sublethal concentrations of DDT and Sumithion (fenitrothion) on the ability of Atlantic salmon parr to escape predation by large brook trout (*Salvelinus fontinalis*). After exposure for 24 h to 1.0 ppm Sumithion, Atlantic salmon parr were more vulnerable to predation than unexposed fish. Sumithion at 0.1 ppm and DDT at 0.07 ppm had no effect. Kania and O'Hara (1974) also observed that after 24 h exposure to sublethal concentrations of mercury (0.1, 0.05, and 0.01 ppm Hg^{2+}) there was selective predation, so that the ability of mosquitofish to avoid predation by bass was impaired. The effect was correlated with concentration.

Both acute (24-h) and subchronic (21-d) exposures of fathead minnows (*Pimephales promelas*) to cadmium (0.375 and 0.025 mg/l) increased their vulnerability to predation by largemouth bass when they were held in tanks with natural bottom materials and artificial vegetation for shelter (Sullivan et al., 1978). These levels were below the MATC for fathead minnows. On the other hand, fingerling rainbow trout (*Salmo gairdneri*) were more susceptible to predation by adults following exposure to phenol at 0.5 to 18.0 mg/l for 96 h (Schneider et al., 1980). At concentrations above 7.0 mg/l exposed prey were consumed more frequently than untreated fish. Acute mortality occurred at exposure concentrations greater than 10 mg/l, so that there was a narrow range between the sublethal effect (7.0 mg/l) and mortality (10.0 mg/l). This indicates that predator-prey interactions are not a sensitive indicator of sublethal exposure for phenol. The pesticide mirex also caused greater predation of grass shrimp (*Paleomonetes vulgaris*) by pinfish (*Lagodon rhomboides*) after 13 d exposure in an estuarine system (Tagatz, 1976).

The studies discussed above showed that prey are affected by chemicals, but the behavioral responses of predators may also be affected at sublethal concentrations. Woltering et al. (1978) exposed both the predator (largemouth bass) and the prey (mosquitofish) to sublethal concentrations of ammonia and found that NH_3 substantially decreased prey consumption and growth of bass. There were greater decreases in prey consumption and growth of bass at higher prey densities. The bass appeared to be more sensitive than the mosquitofish to ammonia. In contrast, Hedtke and Norris (1980) found that the prey (juvenile chinook salmon, *O. tshawytscha*) were more sensitive to the toxic effects of ammonium chloride than the predator (brook trout). The behavioral effect is clearly dependent not only on the particular chemical but also on the species of fish and the test technique.

Learning Behavior

Conditioned learning is a sensitive indicator of chemically induced stress in aquatic organisms. Since learning and conditioning have been extensively studied in fish by experimental psychologists, most of the studies on conditioned learning in aquatic toxicology have been with these organisms. One of the earliest investigations was conducted by Warner et al. (1966). They trained goldfish in a conditioned avoidance response apparatus and then showed that a 96-h exposure to 1.8 μg/l (0.04 TLM) toxaphene produced changes in conditioned avoidance responses reflecting behavioral pathology. Anderson and Peterson (1969) found that brook trout exposed to a sublethal concentration of DDT (20 ppb) failed to establish a visual conditioned avoidance response. Even after 7 d of exposure it appeared that the fish would never reach the training criterion. In addition, trout that learned the response and were then treated with DDT showed a decrease in performance success compared to controls. Anderson and Prins (1970) later stated that the latter effect may have been the result of sensory or motor impairment and not a direct effect on learning, which is a function of the CNS. They studied the sublethal effects of a 24-h exposure to DDT (20 ppb) on a conditioned response involving an extremely simple reflex (propeller-tail reflex), which is more likely to be a function of the CNS because of the reduced complexity of the sensory and motor apparatus required to elicit this response. More than half the brook trout could not be conditioned and the rest of the trout required more trials. The DDT effect disappeared 3–4 wk after testing. The CNS was implicated as the main target of DDT.

Jackson et al. (1970) reported that the work described by Anderson and Peterson (1969) was not as dramatic as previously suggested. They made certain modifications in the avoidance conditioning apparatus, such as lowering the water level in the shuttlebox, and found that both trout (*Salvelinus fontinalis*) and salmon (*Salmo salar*) pretreated with DDT (20 ppb) for 24 h were capable of acquiring the conditioned avoidance response.

Hatfield and Johansen (1972) studied the effects of four insecticides (DDT, methoxychlor, Sumithion, and Abate) at their 96-h LC50 and 0.1 of this concentration on the ability of Atlantic salmon parr to learn and retain a simple conditioned response. At the 96-h LC50 Sumithion completely inhibited learning, Abate retarded learning, DDT mildly enhanced learning, and methoxychlor had no observable effect. After 7 d of recovery, learning rates of Abate- and Sumithion-treated fish were the same as those of controls but the DDT-treated fish showed no improvement. Insecticides at 0.1 of the 96-h LC50 had no effect on learning ability.

Rand and Barthalmus (1980) studied the effects of 20 ppm 2,4-dichlorophenoxyacetic acid (2,4-D amine) on unsignaled conditioned avoidance learning in goldfish exposed at different times during conditioning. Fish treated for 24 h during conditioning showed no significant differences from controls. Those treated for 24 h on the first day of conditioning showed differences in the magnitude of avoidance responding. Fish exposed for 2 wk showed differences in the pattern, rate of acquisition, and maintenance of the avoidance baseline. Behavioral differences persisted during a postexposure period in the fish exposed for 2 wk.

Conditioned avoidance learning has also been used to study the effects of metals on aquatic organisms. Weir and Hine (1970) observed that sodium arsenate, mercuric chloride, lead nitrate, and selenium dioxide impaired conditioning performance in goldfish after 48 h exposure to sublethal concentrations of these metals. Furthermore, exposure of grass shrimp (*Palaemonetes pugio*) to sublethal concentrations of mercuric chloride (0.05 ppm) significantly impaired their conditioned avoidance responses by affecting initial acquisition and suppressing retention (Barthalmus, 1977).

Since learning is a critical element in many behavioral responses (e.g., territoriality, defense, migration), it has potential ecological significance for the overall behavioral activities of organisms in the natural environment.

EXTRAPOLATION OF LABORATORY RESULTS TO ECOSYSTEM EFFECTS IN THE NATURAL ENVIRONMENT

The literature review clearly indicates that different types of behaviors are altered by exposure to chemical agents in the laboratory. The question is whether these behavioral effects occur and are ecologically meaningful in the natural environment, with possible effects on species dynamics and animal populations. If the ecological function of the behavioral responses is well understood in the context of the overall behavioral repertoire of the organism, it may be possible to predict the effects on organisms in the field. However, the best way to support laboratory results is by conducting field validation studies.

One of the most complete studies, which includes both laboratory and field observations, is that of Krebs and Burns (1977). In 1969 a spill of no. 2 fuel oil provided an opportunity to study long-term (7 yr) effects of oil contamination of salt-marsh sediments on the population dynamics and behavior of the fiddler crab (*Uca pugnax*). The crabs were exposed to oil in both the sediment and the water. Behavioral observations were made in the field directly after the spill. Effects of the oil on the crabs were also studied in the laboratory by timing the escape responses from a standard stimulus.

Field observations after the oil spill showed dead and moribund *Uca*. Many migrated from the oiled creek areas and burrowed into the sandy sediments above the mean tide mark. Surviving crabs that remained in the oiled areas displayed aberrant locomotor and burrowing behavior. Adults also showed physiological disorders, such as increased molting and display of mating colors at the wrong time of the year. The normally rapid escape response was slow; crabs were lethargic and showed loss of equilibrium.

Laboratory experiments supported the field observations. The escape response times of crabs ingesting oil sediments more than doubled. Similar observations were obtained for decapod crustaceans exposed to oil emulsions and surfactants (Swedmark et al., 1971): impaired activity, loss of equilibrium, immobilization, and death were observed with exposure to increasing concentrations of toxicants. Slowed escape responses may also leave the crabs more vulnerable to predation (Ward et al., 1976).

Population data revealed that *Uca* densities were reduced for at least 7 yr. The reduction of fiddler crab populations by oil contamination is ecologically significant in that it affects the energy flow within salt marshes and between marshes and coastal waters. The impairment of locomotor ability and other behaviors accounted for the persistent reduction in fiddler crab populations.

Dicks (1973) also compared laboratory and field observations of the effects of crude oil on the limpet (*Patella vulgata* L.), which is important in the ecological balance of the rocky shore because its removal may upset the balance between algal and animal abundance. Crude oil caused detachment of the limpets from rocks, not by adhesion to the foot but by direct toxic effects on the foot muscles. Although the detached animals may not be killed, it was later shown that limpets on the shore might not have time to recover and reattach before becoming prey for gulls and other predators or might be washed into unsuitable environments by the incoming tide (Dicks, 1976). This organism is more susceptible to the effects of crude oil when

it is most active (at night) than when it is resting or least active (early morning).

Two important points can be emphasized here: (1) laboratory studies of behavioral toxicity with aquatic organisms may provide more meaningful results when field studies are also conducted, and (2) physical, chemical, or biological characteristics in the natural environment may mitigate or enhance the potential behavioral toxicity of chemicals, so that the results of field studies may not be similar to the results of laboratory studies.

ADVANTAGES, DISADVANTAGES, AND IMPLICATIONS OF BEHAVIORAL TOXICITY STUDIES

Studies of preference/avoidance of a potentially toxic chemical or its effects on a functional behavioral response have advantages in hazard assessment, especially if the environmental exposure concentrations are known and can be used in a behavioral testing program. These studies, however, should not be used alone for decision-making. They may be integrated with other acute and longer term tests to give a broader picture of what may be happening in the environment. In addition, it is clear that to be effective a testing program should be based on a multistage approach, with several different behavioral responses evaluated in different species.

Although there have been numerous studies in the area of aquatic behavioral toxicology, this area is still in the early stages of development. There are no standard test species or techniques and the overall amount of information available on the normal behavior of aquatic organisms is small, especially for the test species routinely used in acute, early life stage, and chronic tests. Furthermore, the behavioral results in aquatic toxicology are difficult to compare and evaluate for many chemicals because so many different techniques and test species have been used.

Exposure to sublethal concentrations of chemicals may be the most prevalent threat with which aquatic organisms are confronted in the environment. Behavioral modifications resulting from these exposures may not lead directly to death but may nonetheless cause disturbances of major ecological significance.

This area could benefit from adopting the techniques and procedures used successfully in experimental psychology and mammalian toxicology. In addition, some baseline behavioral information should be obtained on the test species used for standard toxicity tests so that behavioral toxicity studies can be conducted with these organisms.

SUMMARY

A behavioral response may be the initial reaction to chemical exposure in the natural environment. A chemical may be detected and avoided or may produce deleterious behavioral effects. Although there are currently no standard behavioral testing techniques in aquatic toxicology, several considerations for testing have been discussed and many of the monitoring techniques presented. The literature on several types of behavior (e.g., locomotor, feeding, predator-prey, learning) has been evaluated and the advantages and disadvantages of behavioral testing discussed. Several behaviors are promising indicators of sublethal stress of aquatic organisms exposed to chemical agents. However, in a behavioral testing program normal baseline behavioral data must first be obtained and then toxicity testing can be initiated. Several different types of behavioral tests should be conducted with different test species and may include different life stages.

LITERATURE CITED

Amiard JC: Les variations de la phototaxie des larves des crustaces sous l'action de divers pollutants metalliques: Mise au point d'un test de toxicite—sublethale. Mar Biol 34:239–245, 1976.

Anderson JM, Peterson MR: DDT: Sublethal effects on brook trout nervous system. Science 164:440–441, 1969.

Anderson JM, Prins HB: Effects of sublethal DDT on a simple reflex in brook trout. J Fish Res Bd Can 27:331–334, 1970.

Atema J, Stein LS: Effects of crude oil in the feeding behavior of the lobster, Homarus americanus. Environ Pollut 6:77–88, 1974.

Atema J, Jacobson S, Todd J, Boyland DB: The importance of chemical signals in stimulating behavior of marine organisms: Effects of altered environmental chemistry on animal communication. In: Bioassay Techniques and Environmental Chemistry, edited by GE Glass, pp. 177–197. Ann Arbor, Michigan: Ann Arbor Science, 1973.

Banner A: Use of sound in predation by young lemon sharks, Negaprion brevirostris (Poey). Bull Mar Sci 22:251–283, 1972.

Bardach JE, Fujiya M, Moll A: Detergents: Effects on chemical senses of the fish Ictalurus natalis. Science 148:1605–1607, 1965.

Barthalmus GT: Behavioral effects of mercury on grass shrimp. Mar Pollut Bull 8:87–90, 1977.

Besch WK, Kemball A, Meyer-Waarden K, Scharf B: A biological monitoring system employing rheotaxis of fish. In: Biological Monitoring of Water and Effluent Quality, edited by J Cairns, Jr, KL Dickson, GF Westlake, pp. 56–74. ASTM STP 607. Philadelphia: American Society for Testing and Materials, 1977.

Bigford TE: Effects of oil on behavioral responses to light, pressure and gravity in larvae of the rock crab. Cancer irroratus. Mar Biol 43:137–178, 1977.

Bishai HM: Reactions of larvae and young salmonids to water of low oxygen concentration. J Cons Cons Int Explor Mer 27:167–180, 1962a.

Bishai HM: Reactions of larvae and young salmonids to different hydrogen ion concentrations. J Cons Cons Int Explor Mer 27:187–191, 1962b.

Bjornberg TKS, Wilbur KM: Copepod phototaxis and vertical migration influenced by xanthene dyes. Biol Bull Woods Hole Mass 134:398–410, 1968.

Black JA, Birge WJ: An avoidance response bioassay for aquatic pollutants. Univ. Kentucky Water Resour Res Inst Res Rep 123, 1980.

Blazka P, Volt M, Cepella M: A new type of respirometer for the determination of the metabolism of fish in an active state. Physiol Bohemoslov 9:553–558, 1960.

Breder CM, Rosen DE: Modes of Reproduction in Fishes. New York: Natural History Press, 1966.

Brett JR: The respiratory metabolism and swimming performance of young sockeye salmon. J Fish Res Bd Can 21:1183–1226, 1964.

Brown JL: The Evaluation of Behavior. New York: Norton, 1975.

Bull CJ, McInerney JE: Behavior of juvenile coho salmon (*Oncorhynchus kisutch*) exposed to Sumithion (Fenitrothion), an organophosphate insecticide. J Fish Res Bd Can 31:1867–1872, 1974.

Cairns J: Don't be half-safe—The current revolution in bioassay techniques. Proc 21st Ind Waste Conf, Purdue Univ Eng Ext Ser 121:559–567, 1966.

Cairns J, Jr, Scheier A: The acute and chronic effects of standard alkylbenzene sulfonate upon the pumpkinseed sunfish, *Lepomis gibbosus* (Linn.) and the bluegill sunfish, *L. macrochirus* Raf. Proc 17th Ind Waste Conf, Purdue Univ Ser 112:14–28, 1962.

Cairns J, Jr, Lanza GR, Sparks RE, Waller WT: Developing biological information systems for water quality management. Water Resour Bull 9:81–99, 1973.

Collins GB: Factors influencing the orientation of migrating anadromous fishes. Fish Bull US Fish Wildl Serv 52:375–396, 1952.

Costa HH: Responses of *Gammarus pulex* L. to modified environment. I. Reactions to toxic solutions. Crustaceana (Leiden) 11:245–256, 1966.

Davenport J, Manley A: The detection of heightened sea-water copper concentrations by the mussel, *Mytilus edulis*. J Mar Biol Assoc UK 58:843–850, 1978.

Davy FB, Kleerekoper H, Gensler P: Effects of exposure to sublethal DDT on the locomotor behavior of the goldfish (*Carassius auratus*). J Fish Res Bd Can 29:1333–1336, 1972.

Davy FB, Kleerekoper H, Matis JH: Effects of exposure to sublethal DDT on the exploratory behavior of goldfish (*Carassius auratus*). Water Resour Res 9:900–905, 1973.

DeCoursey P, Vernberg WB: Effect of mercury on survival, metabolism and behavior of larval *Uca*

pugilator (Brachyura). Oikos 23:241–247, 1972.

Dicks B: Some effects of Kuwait crude oil on the limpet, *Patella vulgata*. Environ Pollut 5:219–229, 1973.

Dicks B: The importance of behavioural patterns in toxicity testing and ecological prediction. In: Marine Ecology and Oil Pollution, edited by JM Baker, pp. 303–319. New York: Wiley, 1976.

Domanik AM, Zar JH: The effect of malathion on the temperature selection response of the common shiner, *Notropis cornutus* (Mitchill). Arch Environ Contam Toxicol 7:193–206, 1978.

Drummond RA, Carlson RW: Procedures for measuring cough (gill purge) rates of fish. EPA-600/3-77-133. Duluth, Minn.: U.S. EPA Environmental Research Laboratory, 1977.

Dunning A, Major CW: The effects of cold sea-water extracts of oil fractions upon the blue mussel, *Mytilus edulis*. In: Pollution and Physiology of Marine Organisms, edited by FJ Vernberg, WB Vernberg, pp. 349–366. New York: Academic, 1974.

Edmunds M: Defense in animals: A survey of antipredator defenses. Harlow: Longman, 1974.

Ellgaard EG, Ochsner JC, Cox JK: Locomotor hyperactivity induced in the bluegill sunfish, *Lepomis macrochirus*, by sublethal concentrations of DDT. Can J Zool 55:1077–1081, 1977.

Ellgaard EG, Tusa JE, Malizia AA, Jr: Locomotor activity of the bluegill *Lepomis macrochirus*: Hyperactivity induced by sublethal concentrations of cadmium, chromium and zinc. J Fish Biol 1:19–23, 1978.

Evans GW, Lyes M, Lockwood APM: Some effects of oil dispersants on the feeding behavior of the brown shrimp, *Crangon crangon*. Mar Behav Physiol 4:171–181, 1977.

Farmer GJ, Beamish FWH: Oxygen consumption of *Tilapia nilotica* in relation to swimming speed and salinity. J Fish Res Bd Can 26:2807–2821, 1969.

Fingerman SW, VanMeter C, Jr, Fingerman M: Increased spontaneous locomotor activity in the fiddler crab, *Uca pugilator*, after exposure to a sublethal concentration of DDT. Bull Environ Contam Toxicol 21:11–16, 1979.

Folmar LC: Overt avoidance reaction of rainbow

trout fry to nine herbicides. Bull Environ Contam Toxicol 15:509–514, 1976.

Folmar LC: Avoidance chamber responses of mayfly nymphs exposed to eight herbicides. Bull Environ Contam Toxicol 19:312–318, 1978.

Forward RB, Jr: Light and diurnal vertical migration: Photophysiology and photobehavior of plankton. In: Photochemical and Photobiological Reviews, edited by KC Smith, pp. 157–209. New York: Plenum, 1976.

Foster NR, Scheier A, Cairns J, Jr: Effects of ABS on feeding behaviour of flagfish *Jordanella floridae*. Trans Am Fish Soc 95:109–110, 1966.

Fraenkel GS, Gunn DL: The orientation of animals. Dover Pub., New York.

Galtsoff PS: Environmental requirements of oysters in relation to pollution. In: Transactions, Second Seminar on Biological Problems in Water Pollution. April 1959. Tech Rep W60-3. Cincinnati, Ohio: U.S. Public Health Service, Robert A. Taft Sanitary Engineering Center, 1960.

Gardner DR: The effect of some DDT and methoxychlor analogs on temperature selection and lethality in brook trout fingerlings. Pest Biochem Physiol 2:437–446, 1973.

Gardner GR, La Roche G: Copper-induced lesions in estuarine teleosts. J Fish Res Bd Can 30:363–368, 1973.

Giattina JD, Garton RR, Stevens DG: The avoidance of copper and nickel by rainbow trout as monitored by a computer-based data acquisition system. Trans Am Fish Soc 111:491–504, 1982.

Goodyear CP: A simple technique for detecting effects of toxicants or other stresses on predator-prey interaction. Trans Am Fish Soc 101:367–370, 1972.

Gray J: Pseudo-rheotropism in fishes. J Exp Biol 14:95–103, 1937.

Gray RH, Genoway RG, Barraclough SA: Behavior of juvenile chinook salmon, *Oncorhynchus tshawytscha*, in relation to simulated thermal effluent. Trans Am Fis Soc 106:366–370, 1977.

Greaves JOB, Wilson RS: Development of an interactive system to study sublethal effects of pollutants on the behavior of organisms. EPA-600/3-80-10. Naragansett, R.I.: U.S. EPA Environmental Research Laboratory, 1980.

Gruber D, Cairns J, Jr, Dickson KL, Hendricks AC, Cavell MA, Landers JD, Jr, Miller WR, III, Showalter WJ: The Construction, Development and Operation of a Fish Biological Monitoring System. Springfield, Va.: National Technical Information Service, 1978.

Hall AR: Effects of oxygen and carbon dioxide on the development of the whitefish. Ecology 6:104–116, 1925.

Hansen DJ: Avoidance of pesticides by untrained sheepshead minnows. Trans Am Fish Soc 98:426–429, 1969.

Hansen DJ: DDT and malathion: Effect on salinity selection by mosquitofish. Trans Am Fish Soc 101:346–350, 1972.

Hansen DJ, Matthews E, Nall SL, Dumas DP: Avoidance of pesticides by untrained mosquitofish, *Gambusia affinis*. Bull Environ Contam Toxicol 8:46–51, 1972.

Hansen DJ, Schimmel SC, Keltner JM, Jr: Avoidance of pesticides by grass shrimp (*Palaemonetes pugio*). Bull Environ Contam Toxicol 9:129–133, 1973.

Hara TJ: Chemoreception. In: Fish Physiology, edited by WS Hoar, DJ Randall, pp. 79–120. New York: Academic, 1971.

Hara TJ: Electrical responses of the olfactory bulb of Pacific salmon *Oncorhynchus nerka* and *Oncorhynchus kisutch*. J Fish Res Bd Can 29:1351–1355, 1972.

Hara TJ, Law YMC, McDonald S: Effects of mercury and copper on the olfactory response in rainbow trout (*Salmo gairdneri*). J Fish Res Bd Can 33:1568–1573, 1976.

Hasler AD, Wisby WJ: Use of fish for olfactory assay of pollutants (phenols) in water. Trans Am Fish Soc 79:64–70, 1950.

Hatfield CT, Anderson JM: Effects of two insecticides on the vulnerability of Atlantic salmon (*Salmo salar*) parr to brook trout (*Salvelinus fontinalis*) predation. J Fish Res Bd Can 29:27–29, 1972.

Hatfield CT, Johansen PH: Effects of four insecticides on the ability of Atlantic salmon parr (*Salmo salar*) to learn and retain a simple conditioned response. J Fish Res Bd Can 29:315–321, 1972.

Hedtke JL, Norris LA: Effect of ammonium chloride on predatory consumption rates of brook trout (*Salvelinus fontinalis*) on juvenile chinook salmon (*Oncorhynchus tshawytscha*) in laboratory streams. Bull Environ Contam Toxicol 24: 81–89, 1980.

Henry MG, Atchison GJ: Influence of social rank on the behavior of bluegill, *Lepomis macrochirus* Rafinesque, exposed to sublethal concentrations of cadmium and zinc. J Fish Biol 15: 309–315, 1979.

Hill G: Oxygen preference in the spring cavefish, *Chologaster agassizi.* Trans Am Fish Soc 97: 448–454, 1968.

Hoglund LB: A new method of studying the reactions of fishes in gradients of chemical and other agents. Oikos 3:247–267, 1953.

Hoglund LB: The reactions of fish in concentration gradients. Fish Bd Swed Inst Freshw Res Drottingholm Rep 43:1–147, 1961.

Holland GA, Lasater JE, Neumann ED, Eldridge WE: Toxic effects of organic and inorganic pollutants on young salmon. Wash State Dep Fish Res Bull 5, 1960.

Howard TE: Swimming performance of juvenile coho salmon (*Oncorhynchus kisutch*) exposed to bleached kraft mill effluent. J Fish Res Bd Can 32:789–793, 1975.

Hyland JL, Miller DC: Effects of no. 2 fuel oil on chemically-evoked feeding behavior of the mud snail, *Ilyanassa obsoleta.* Am Petrol Inst Publ 4308, 1979.

Ishio S: Behavior of fish exposed to toxic substances. In: Advances in Water Pollution Research, pp. 19–33. Oxford: Pergamon, 1965.

Jackson DA, Anderson JM, Gardner DR: Further investigations of the effect of DDT on learning in fish. Can J Zool 48:577–580, 1970.

Jacobson SM, Boylan DB: Effect of seawater soluble fraction of kerosene on chemotaxis in a marine snail, *Nassarius obsoletus.* Nature (Lond) 241:213–215, 1973.

Jones JRE: The reactions of *Pygosteus pungitius* L. to toxic solutions. J Exp Biol 24:110–122, 1947.

Jones JRE: A further study of the reactions of fish to toxic solutions. J Exp Biol 25:22–34, 1948.

Jones JRE: The reactions of the minnows *Phoxinus phoxinus* to solutions of phenol, orthocresol and para-cresol. J Exp Biol 28:261–270, 1951.

Jones JRE: The reactions of fish to water of low oxygen concentration. J Exp Biol 29:403–415, 1952.

Jones BF, Warren CE, Bond CE, Doudoroff P: Avoidance reactions of salmonid fishes to pulp mill effluents. Sewage Ind Wastes 28:1403–1413, 1956.

Kalmijn AJ: The detection of electric fields from inanimate and animate sources other than electric organs. In: Handbook of Sensory Physiology, edited by A Fessard, vol. 3, pp. 147–200. Berlin: Springer, 1974.

Kania HJ, O'Hara J: Behavioral alterations in a simple predator-prey system due to sublethal exposure to mercury. Trans Am Fish Soc 103: 134–136, 1974.

Keenleyside MHA: Diversity and Adaptation in Fish Behavior. New York: Springer-Verlag, 1979.

Keenleyside MHA, Hoar WS: Effects of temperature on the responses of young salmon to water currents. Behavior 7:77–87, 1954.

Kittredge JS, Takahashi FT, Sarinara FO: Bioassays indicative of some sublethal effects of oil pollution. Proc Mar Technol Soc 10th Annu Meet Washington, D.C., pp. 871–897, 1974.

Kleerekoper H: Olfaction in Fishes. Bloomington: Indiana Univ Press, 1969.

Kleerekoper H, Westlake GF, Matis JH, Gensler PJ: Orientation of goldfish (*Carassius auratus*) in response to a shallow gradient of a sublethal concentration of copper in an open field. J Fish Res Bd Can 29:45–54, 1972.

Krebs CT, Burns KA: Long-term effects of an oil spill on populations of the salt-marsh crab *Uca pugnax.* Science 197:484–487, 1977.

Kynard B: Avoidance behavior of insecticide susceptible and resistant populations of mosquitofish to four insecticides. Trans Am Fish Soc 103:557–561, 1974.

Lindahl PE, Marcstrom A: On the preference of roaches (*Leuciscus rutilis*) for trinitrophenol, studied with the fluvarium technique. J Fish Res Bd Can 15:685–694, 1958.

Lindahl PE, Olofsson S, Schwanbom E: Rotatoryflow technique for testing fitness of fish. In: Biological Monitoring of Water and Effluent Quality, edited by J Cairns, Jr, KL Dickson, GF Westlake, pp. 75–84. ASTM STP 607. Philadelphia: ASTM, 1977.

Lubinski KS, Dickson KL, Cairns J, Jr: Effects of abrupt sublethal gradients of ammonium chloride on the activity level, turning, and preference—avoidance behavior of bluegills. In: Aquatic Toxicology, edited by JG Eaton, PR Parrish, AC Hendricks, pp. 328–340. ASTM STP 707. Philadelphia: ASTM, 1980.

Lyon EP: On Rheotropism. I. Rheotropism in fishes. Am J Physiol 12:149–161, 1905.

Maciorowski AF, Cairns J, Jr, Benfield EF: Laboratory simulation of an in-plant biomonitoring system using crayfish activity rhythms to detect cadmium induced toxic stress. Presented at the 25th Annual Meeting North American Benthological Society, Roanoke, Va., 1977a.

Maciorowski HD, Clarke RMcV, Scherer E: The use of avoidance-preference bioassays with aquatic invertebrates. In: Proceedings of the 3rd Aquatic Toxicity Workshop, pp. 49–58. EPS-5-AR-77-1. Environmental Protection Service, 1977b.

Macleod JC, Smith LL, Jr: Effect of pulpwood fiber on oxygen consumption and swimming endurance of the fathead minnow, *Pimephales promelas*. Trans Am Fish Soc 95:71–84, 1966.

Marcucella H, Abramson CI: Behavioral toxicology and teleost fish. In: The Behavior of Fish and Other Aquatic Animals, edited by DI Mostofsky, pp. 33–77. New York: Academic, 1978.

McLeese DW: Behavior of lobsters exposed to bleached kraft mill effluent. J Fish Res Bd Can 27:731–736, 1970.

Miller DC: Some applications of locomotor response in pollution effects monitoring. Rapp P V Reun Cons Int Explor Mer 179:154–160, 1980.

Miller DL, Ogilvie DM: Temperature selection in brook trout (*Salvelinus fontinalis*) following exposure to DDT, PCB or phenol. Bull Environ Contam Toxicol 14:545–551, 1975.

Miller DC, Lang WH, Greaves JOB, Wilson RS: Investigations in aquatic behavioral toxicology using a computerized video quantification system. In: Aquatic Toxicology and Hazard Assessment, edited by JG Pearson, R Foster, WE Bishop, pp. 206–220. ASTM STP 766. Philadelphia: ASTM, 1982.

Neil JH: Some effects of potassium cyanide on speckled trout (*Salvelinus fontinalis*). In: Proceedings of the 4th Ontario Industrial Waste Conference, pp. 74–96, Ontario Water Resource Committee, 1957.

Ogilvie DM, Anderson JM: Effect of DDT on temperature selection by young Atlantic salmon, *Salmo salar*. J Fish Res Bd Can 22:503–512, 1965.

Olla BL, Pearson WH, Studholme AL: Applicability of behavioral measures in environmental stress assessment. Rapp P V Reun Cons Int Explor Mer 179:162–173, 1980.

Olthof HJ: Die vergleichende Physiologie der Notatmung und verwandter Erscheinungen. Groningen-Batavia, Germany, 1941.

Oseid O, Smith LL, Jr: Swimming endurance and resistance to copper and malathion of bluegills treated by long-term exposure to sublethal levels of hydrogen sulfide. Trans Am Fish Soc 101:620–625, 1972.

Ottoson D: The electro-olfactogram. In: Handbook of Sensory Physiology, edited by LM Beidler, pp. 95–131. Berlin: Springer, 1971.

Pearson WH, Olla BL: Detection of naphthalene by the blue crab, *Callinectes sapidus*. Estuaries 2:64–65, 1979.

Pearson WH, Olla BL: Threshold for detection of naphthalene and other behavioral responses by the blue crab, *Callinectes sapidus*. Estuaries 3:224–229, 1980.

Pearson WH, Sugarman PC, Woodruff DL, Blaylock JW, Olla BL: Detection of petroleum hydrocarbons by the Dungeness crab, *Cancer magister*. US Fish Wildl Serv Fish Bull 73:821–826, 1980.

Pearson WH, Miller SE, Blaylock JW: Detection of the water-soluble fraction of crude oil by the blue crab, *Callinectus sapidus*. Mar Environ 5:3–11, 1981.

Percy JA: Responses of arctic marine benthic crustaceans to sediments contaminated with crude oil. Environ Pollut 13:1–10, 1977.

Peterson RH: Temperature selection of Atlantic salmon (*Salmo salar*) and brook trout (*Salvelinus fontinalis*) as influenced by various chlorinated hydrocarbons. J Fish Res Bd Can 30:1091–1097, 1973.

Pfeiffer W: The distribution of fright reaction and alarm substance cells in fishes. Copeia 1977:653–665, 1977.

Poels CLM: An automatic system for rapid detection of acute high concentrations of toxic substances in surface water using trout. In: Biological Monitoring of Water and Effluent Quality, edited by J Cairns, KL Dickson, GF Westlake, pp. 85–95. ASTM STP 607. Philadelphia: ASTM, 1977.

Portmann JE, Connor PM: The toxicity of several oil-spill removers to some species of fish and shellfish. Mar Biol 1:322–329, 1968.

Powers EB: Experiments and observations on the behavior of marine fishes toward the hydrogen-ion concentration of the seawater in relation to their migratory movements and habitat. Publ Puget Sound Biol Stn Univ Washington 3:1–22, 1921.

Powers EB, Clark RT: Further evidence of chemical factors affecting the migratory movements of fishes, especially the salmon. Ecology 24:109–113, 1943.

Rand G, Kleerekoper H, Matis J: Interaction of odour and flow perception and the effects of parathion in the locomotor orientation of the goldfish Carassius auratus L. J Fish Biol 7:497–504, 1975.

Rand GM: The effect of exposure to a subacute concentration of parathion on the general locomotor behavior of the goldfish. Bull Environ Contam Toxicol 18:259–266, 1977a.

Rand GM: The effect of subacute parathion exposure on the locomotor behavior of the bluegill sunfish and largemouth bass. In: Aquatic Toxicology and Hazard Evaluation, edited by FL Mayer, JL Hamelink, pp. 253–268. ASTM STP 634. Philadelphia: ASTM, 1977b.

Rand GM, Barthalmus GT: Use of an unsignalled avoidance technique to evaluate the effects of the herbicide 2,4-dichlorophenoxyacetic acid on goldfish. In: Aquatic Toxicology, edited by IG Eaton, PR Parrish, AC Hendricks, pp. 341–353. ASTM STP 707. Philadelphia: ASTM, 1980.

Reed JR: Alarm substances and fright reaction in some fishes from the southeastern United States. Trans Am Fish Soc 98:664–668, 1969.

Rehwoldt R, Bida G: Fish avoidance reactions. Bull Environ Contam Toxicol 5:205–206, 1970.

Reynolds WM, Casterlin ME: Locomotor activity rhythms in the bluegill sunfish, Lepomis macrochirus. Am Midl Natur 96:221–225, 1976.

Rice SD: Toxicity and avoidance tests with Prudhoe Bay oil and pink salmon fry. In: Proceedings of Joint Conference on Prevention and Control of Oil Spills, 1973. Published by American Petroleum Institute (API), Washington, DC. Sponsored by API, EPA, U.S. Coast Guard.

Saunders RL, Sprague JB: Effect of copper-zinc mining pollution on a spawning migration of Atlantic salmon. Water Res 1:419–432, 1967.

Scherer E: Avoidance of fenitrothion by goldfish (Carassius auratus). Bull Environ Contam Toxicol 13:492–496, 1975.

Scherer E: Behavioural assays—principles, results and problems. In: Proceedings of the 3rd Aquatic Toxicity Workshop, edited by WR Parker, E Pessah, PG Wells, GF Westlake, pp. 33–40. EPS-5AR-77-1. Environmental Protection Service, 1977.

Scherer E, Nowak S: Apparatus for recording avoidance movements of fish. J Fish Res Bd Can 30:1594–1596, 1973.

Schneider MJ, Barraclough SA, Genoway RG, Wolford ML: Effects of phenol on predation of juvenile rainbow trout Salmo gairdneri. Environ Pollut 23:121–130, 1980.

Schwassman HO: Biological rhythms. In: Fish Physiology, edited by WS Hoar, DJ Randall, vol. 6, pp. 371–421. New York: Academic, 1971.

Shelford VE: An experimental study of the effects of gas waste upon fishes with special reference to stream pollution. Bull Ill State Lab Nat Hist 11:381–412, 1917.

Shelford VE: The relation of marine fishes to acids with particular reference to the Miles acid process of sewage treatment. Publ Puget Sound Biol Stn Univ Washington 2:97–111, 1981.

Shelford VE, Allee WC: The reactions of fishes to gradients of dissolved atmospheric gases. J Exp Zool 14:207–266, 1913.

Shelford VE, Powers EB: An experimental study of the movements of herring and other marine fishes. Biol Bull Woods Hole Mass 28:315–334, 1915.

Skrapek K: Toxicity of phenols and their detection in fish. Ustav Ved Inform Min Zemed Lesn Vod Hospod Ziv Vyr 8:499–504, 1963.

Slobodkin LB: Toward a predictive theory of evolution. In: Population Biology and Evolution, edited by RC Lewontin, pp. 187–203. Syracuse, N.Y.: Syracuse Univ. Press, 1968.

Slobodkin LB, Rapoport A: An optimal strategy of evolution. Q Rev Biol 49:181–200, 1974.

Smith GE, Isom BG: Investigation of effects of large scale applications of 2,4-D on aquatic fauna and water quality. Pestic Monit J 1:16–21, 1967.

Smith MW, Saunders JW: Movement of brook trout, Salvelinus fontinalis (Mitchill) between and within fresh and salt water. J Fish Res Bd Can 15:1403–1449, 1958.

Smith W, Saalfeld RW: Studies on the Columbia River smelt, Thaleichthys pacificus (Richardson). Wash Dep Fish Fish Res Pap 1:3–26, 1955.

Sparks RE, Waller WT, Cairns J, Jr: Effect on the resistance of dominant and submissive bluegills (Lepomis macrochirus) to a lethal concentration of zinc. J Fish Res Bd Can 29:1356–1358, 1972.

Spoor WA, Drummond RA: An electrode for detecting movement in gradient tanks. Trans Am Fish Soc 101:714–715, 1972.

Spoor WA, Neiheisel TW, Drummond RA: An electrode chamber for recording respiratory and other movements of free-swimming animals. Trans Am Fish Soc 100:22–28, 1971.

Sprague JB: Avoidance of copper-zinc solutions by young salmon in the laboratory. J Water Pollut Control Fed 36:990–1004, 1964.

Sprague JB: Avoidance reactions of rainbow trout to zinc sulfate solutions. Water Res 2:367–372, 1968.

Sprague JB: Measurement of pollutant toxicity to fish. III. Sublethal effects and "safe" concentrations. Water Res 5:245–266, 1971.

Sprague JB, Drury DE: Avoidance reactions of salmonid fish to representative pollutants. In: Advances in Water Pollution Research, edited by SH Jenkins, pp. 169–179. London: Pergamon, 1969.

Sprague JB, Elson PF, Saunders RL: Sublethal copper-zinc pollution in a salmon river—a field and laboratory study. Int J Air Water Pollut 9:531–543, 1965.

Sullivan CM, Fisher KC: The effect of light on temperature selection of speckled trout, Salvelinus fontinalis (Mitchill). Biol Bull Woods Hole Mass 107:278–288, 1954.

Sullivan JF, Atchison GJ, Kolar DJ, McIntosh AW: Changes in the predator-prey behavior of fathead minnows (Pimephales promelas) and largemouth bass (Micropterus salmoides) caused by cadmium. J Fish Res Bd Can 35:446–451, 1978.

Summerfelt RC, Lewis W: Repulsion of green sunfish by certain chemicals. J Water Pollut Control Fed 39:2030–2038, 1967.

Sutterlin AM: Pollutants and the chemical senses of aquatic animals—perspective and review. Chem Senses Flavor 1:167–178, 1974.

Sutterlin AM, Gray R: Chemical basis for homing of Atlantic salmon (Salmo salar) to a hatchery. J Fish Res Bd Can 30:985–989, 1973.

Swedmark M, Braaten B, Emanuelsson E, Granmo A: Biological effects of surface active agents on marine animals. Mar Biol 9:183–201, 1971.

Syazuki K: Studies on the toxic effects of industrial waste on fish and shellfish. J Shimonoseki Coll Fish 13:157–211, 1964.

Symons PEK: Behavior of young Atlantic salmon (Salmo salar) exposed to or force-fed fenitrothion, an organophosphate insecticide. J Fish Res Bd Can 30:651–655, 1973.

Tagatz ME: Effect of mirex on predator-prey interaction in an experimental estuarine ecosystem. Trans Am Fish Soc 105:546–549, 1976.

Takahashi FT, Kittredge JS: Sublethal effects of the water soluble components of oil. In: Microbial degradation of oil pollutants, edited by DG Ahearn, SP Meyers, pp. 259–264. L.S.U. Press Public No. LSU-SG-73-01, 1973.

Tester AL: The role of olfaction in shark predation. Pac Sci 17:145–170, 1963.

Timms AM, Kleerekoper H, Matis J: Locomotor response of goldfish, channel catfish, and largemouth bass to a "copper-polluted" mass of water in an open field. Water Resour Res 8:1574–1580, 1972.

Vernberg WB, DeCoursey PJ, Padgett WJ: Synergistic effects of environmental variables on larvae of Uca pugilator. Mar Biol 22:307–312, 1973.

Vernberg WB, DeCoursey PJ, O'Hara J: Multiple environmental factor effects on physiology and behavior of the fiddler crab, *Uca pugilator*. In: Pollution and Physiology of Marine Organisms, edited by FJ Vernberg, WB Vernberg, pp. 381–425. New York: Academic, 1974.

Verplanck WS: A glossary of some terms used in the objective science of behavior. Psychol Rev 64:1–42, 1957.

von Frisch K: Zur psychologie des fischschwarmes. Naturwissenschaften 26:601–606, 1938.

Waiwood KG, Beamish FWH: Effects of copper, pH and hardness on the critical swimming performance of rainbow trout (*Salmo gairdneri* Richardson). Water Res 12:611–619, 1978.

Waller WT, Cairns J, Jr: The use of fish movement patterns to monitor zinc in water. Water Res 6:257–269, 1972.

Ward DV, Howes BL: The effects of abate, an organophosphorus insecticide, on marsh fiddler crab populations. Bull Environ Contam Toxicol 12:694–697, 1974.

Ward DV, Howes BL, Ludwig DF: Interactive effects of predation pressure and insecticide (Temefos) toxicity on populations of the marsh fiddler crab *Uca pugnax*. Mar Biol 35:119–126, 1976.

Warner RE, Peterson KK, Borgman L: Behavioural pathology in fish: A quantitative study of sublethal pesticide toxication. J Appl Ecol 3(Suppl):223–247, 1966.

Webb PW, Brett JR: The effects of sublethal concentrations of sodium pentachlorophenate on growth rate, food conversion efficiency, and swimming performance in underyearling sockeye salmon (*Oncorhynchus nerka*). J Fish Res Bd Can 30:499–507, 1973.

Weir PA, Hine CH: Effects of various metals on behavior of conditioned goldfish. Arch Environ Health 20:45–51, 1970.

Weis P, Weis JS: DDT causes changes in activity and schooling behavior in goldfish. Environ Res 7:68–74, 1974.

Wells MM: Reactions and resistance of fishes in their natural environment to acidity, alkalinity and neutrality. Biol Bull Woods Hole Mass 29:221–257, 1915a.

Wells MM: The reactions and resistance of fishes in their natural environment to salts. J Exp Zool 19:243–283, 1915b.

Wells MM: The reactions and resistance of fishes to carbon dioxide and carbon monoxide. Bull Ill State Lab Nat Hist 11:557–571, 1918.

Westlake GF, Lubinski KS: A chamber to monitor the locomotor behavior of free-swimming aquatic organisms exposed to simulated spills. In: Proceedings of the 1976 National Conference on Control of Hazardous Material Spills, pp. 64–69. Rockville, Md.: Information Transfer, Inc., 1976.

Westlake GF, Kleerekoper H, Matis J: The locomotor response of goldfish to a steep gradient of copper ions. Water Resour Res 10:103–105, 1974.

Whitmore CM, Warren CE, Doudoroff P: Avoidance reactions of salmonid and centrarchid fishes to low oxygen concentrations. Trans Am Fish Soc 89:17–26, 1960.

Wildish DJ, Akagi H, Poole NJ: Avoidance by herring of sulfite pulp mill effluents. International Council for the Exploration of the Sea Fisheries Improvement Comm. C.M. 1976/E:26. 8 pp.

Wildish DJ, Akagi H, Poole NJ: Avoidance by herring of dissolved components in pulp mill effluents. Bull Environ Contam Toxicol 18:521–525, 1977.

Woltering DM, Hedtke JL, Weber LJ: Predator-prey interactions of fishes under the influence of ammonia. Trans Am Fish Soc 107:500–504, 1978.

Chapter 10

Biochemistry/Physiology

P. M. Mehrle and F. L. Mayer

INTRODUCTION

Pollution of the aquatic environment by agricultural and industrial chemicals, spilled oil, mine effluents, and many other chemical contaminants has been recognized for years. Approaches used to evaluate the health and well-being of fish subjected to environmental insults have, in the past, focused primarily on short-term studies utilizing whole-animal responses such as gross abnormalities, behavioral changes, changes in growth rates, and mortality. In mammalian and veterinary toxicology, in contrast, physiological and biochemical techniques are used in conjunction with whole-animal responses to evaluate the health of animals exposed to toxic chemicals. Many of these techniques are routine clinical measurements that include blood chemistry profiles, blood cell analyses, and histopathological examinations of various

organs and tissues. The use of these clinical diagnoses in mammalian toxicology has been established by extensive research correlating physiological and biochemical responses with whole-animal responses. Such correlations enable the mammalian toxicologist to interpret the biological significance of physiological responses induced by toxic chemicals.

Similar diagnostic tests are not available to aquatic toxicologists because biochemical and physiological research has been less extensive in aquatic toxicology. The "state of the art" of physiological and biochemical measurements in aquatic toxicology was recently summarized in a workshop at Pellston, Michigan (Macek et al., 1978). Participants in the workshop rated the relative utility of 11 toxicity tests on the basis of several criteria: ecological significance of effects, scientific and legal defensibility, availability of acceptable methodology, utility of test results in predicting effects in aquatic environments, general applicability to all classes of chemicals, and simplicity and cost of the tests. In terms of utility in assessing hazards to aquatic environments, acute lethality tests were rated highest, followed by embryo-larval tests, chronic toxicity tests measuring reproductive effects, and residue accumulation studies. Histological tests ranked ninth, and physiological and biochemical tests ranked tenth in overall and present relative utility because it was not deemed possible to relate the results of these tests to adverse environmental impacts.

In this chapter the physiological and biochemical responses induced by chemical contaminants in fish are discussed. Chapter 18 concerns the metabolism and detoxification of chemicals by fish, whereas this chapter addresses the effects of chemicals on physiological and biochemical metabolic processes. In addition, this chapter includes considerations in designing physiological and biochemical investigations, and the relativity and utility of toxicant-induced responses in aquatic toxicology.

IMPORTANCE AND RELEVANCE OF TOXICANT-INDUCED PHYSIOLOGICAL AND BIOCHEMICAL RESPONSES

The aquatic toxicologist should consider three important factors in the design and interpretation of physiological and biochemical studies:

1 Understanding of the function and composition of organs primarily affected by toxic chemicals.
2 Knowledge of analytical procedures for measuring appropriate constituents, cellular morphology, and physiological responses.
3 Ability to interpret the significance of chemically induced biophysiological changes and relate them to the health and survival of the aquatic organism.

The first two of these factors have been addressed extensively in fishery research. A considerable number of biochemical, physiological, and histopathological investigations have been conducted with both freshwater and marine fish. Hunn (1967) showed that many techniques have been developed for determining organic and inorganic constituents of fish blood, and values for the constituents have been reported. Similarly, histopathological techniques have been used with various tissues and organs to describe lesions caused by diseases, chemical and physical agents, and nutritional factors (Ribelin and Migaki, 1975). The histological techniques used to evaluate the effects of potentially toxic chemicals are described in Chapter 11. The third factor, however, has been very difficult to address in fishery research and, more specifically, in aquatic toxicology. Although clinical techniques for measuring physiological and biochemical changes in mammalian toxicology have been successfully applied to various fluids and tissues of fish, chemically induced alterations have been of limited use in aquatic toxicology because they usually have not been related to impaired ability of fish to adapt or survive in natural habitats.

The problem of interpreting the toxicological significance of chemically induced changes in biochemical and physiological mechanisms in fish is twofold: (1) our understanding of physiological and biochemical regulatory mechanisms in fish is relatively limited, and (2) parallel changes in these factors have not been correlated with toxicant exposure and impaired ability of fish to survive. This lack of understanding encourages the extrapolation of mammalian clinical interpretations to responses observed in fish. However, the soundness of extrapolating mammalian clinical responses to poikilothermic animals is unproved and such extrapolation can lead to inaccurate interpretations of the status of fish health. Physiological and biochemical mechanisms in poikilothermic animals allows them to adapt to various environmental factors. These normal adaptive responses to environmental stresses due to toxic chemicals, diseases, water quality, and temperature fluctuations are reflected by changes in blood and tissue constituents, but deviations from physiological "norms" that fish and other aquatic animals can tolerate are not well understood (Grant and Schoettger, 1972). Since fluid and tissue constituents vary within species of fish, as well as among species and populations, it is difficult to establish the "normal" or baseline values that are needed to develop and apply diagnostic tests. Wedemeyer and Yasutake (1977) discussed this difficulty in their review on the use of clinical methods to assess the influence of environmental stress on fish health; they reported the expected concentration ranges and discussed the possible significance of changes in blood and tissue constituents of salmonids (Tables 1 and 2). However, many factors unrelated to environmental stresses and di-

Table 1 Outline Interpretation of Clinical Test Results Used to Assess Effects of Environmental Stress on Fish Health[a,b]

Clinical test	Possible significance if	
	Too low	Too high
Ammonia (in water, not ionized)	No recognized significance	Gill hyperplasia, predisposition to bacterial gill disease
Blood cell counts		
Erythrocytes	Anemias, hemodilution due to impaired osmoregulation, gill damage	Stress polycythemia, dehydration, hemoconcentration
Leukocytes	Leukopenia due to acute stress	Leukocytosis due to bacterial infection
Thrombocytes	Abnormal blood clotting time	Thrombocytosis due to acute or chronic stress
Chloride (plasma)	Gill chloride cell damage, compromised osmoregulation	Hemoconcentration, compromised osmoregulation
Cholesterol (plasma)	Impaired lipid metabolism	Fish under chronic stress, dietary lipid imbalance
Clotting time (blood)	Fish under acute stress, thrombocytopenia	Sulfonamides or antibiotic disease treatments affecting the intestinal microflora
Cortisol (plasma)	Interrenal exhaustion from severe stress	Fish under chronic or acute stress
Glucose (plasma)	Inanition	Acute or chronic stress
Glycogen (liver or muscle)	Chronic stress, inanition	Liver damage due to excessive vacuolation, diet too high in carbohydrate
Hematocrit (blood)	Anemias, hemodilution due to gill damage	Hemoconcentration, dehydration, stress polycythemia
Hemoglobin (blood)	Anemias, hemodilution due to gill damage, nutritional disease	Hemoconcentration, dehydration, stress polycythemia
Lactic acid (blood)	No recognized significance	Acute or chronic stress, swimming fatigue
Methemoglobin (blood)	No recognized significance	Excessive NO_2 in water or use of O_2 instead of air in fish-hauling trucks
Nitrite (water)	No recognized significance	Methemoglobinemia in fish population
Osmolality (plasma)	External parasite infection, heavy metal exposure, hemodilution	Dehydration, salinity increases in excess of osmoregulatory capacity, stress-induced diuresis, lactic acidosis
Total protein (plasma)	Infectious disease, kidney damage, nutritional imbalance, inanition	Hemoconcentration, impaired water balance

[a] Examples are based on salmonids but are applicable, with caution, to other fish.
[b] From Wedemeyer and Yasutake (1977).

Table 2 Mean Blood Chemistry Values (and Standard Deviations) for Selected Cold-, Cool-, and Warm-Water Fish of Interest in Environmental Monitoring[a,b]

Fish type and species	Hematological characteristic			
	Cl⁻ (meq/l)	Glucose (mg per 100 ml)	pH	Hematocrit (%)
Cold water				
Brown trout (*Salmo trutta*)	108.6 (6.9)	52.0 (6.5)	7.51 (0.08)	33.0 (4)
Brook trout (*Salvelinus fontinalis*)	108.6 (1.6)	59.2 (4.3)	7.71 (0.06)	31.0 (5)
Cool water				
Northern pike (*Esox lucius*)	104.8 (4.3)	53.4 (16.2)	7.64 (0.18)	30.0 (5)
Walleye (*Stizostedion vitreum*)	62.0 (10.5)	152.5 (78.3)	7.85 (0.08)	46.0 (4)
Warm water				
Channel catfish (*Ictalurus punctatus*)	114.0 (5.0)	29.1 (17.7)	7.55 (0.05)	32.1 (4.1)

[a]Normal ranges are not available but the mean values (±1.96 SD) can be used as a guide.
[b]Compiled by Wedemeyer and Yasutake (1977) from Hunn (1972) and Hunn and Schnick (unpublished results).

seases alter concentrations of blood constituents. Barnhart (1969) showed that diet, genetic strain, and age affected hematological characteristics of rainbow trout (*Salmo gairdneri*). Stress of handling, anesthesia, and various methods of capture also significantly altered blood characteristics in salmonids (Bouck and Ball, 1966; Housten et al., 1971; Miles et al., 1974). These studies showed that baseline concentrations of hematological and tissue constituents in fish are difficult to determine, and this is a major obstacle to the use of physiological and biochemical measurements in aquatic toxicology.

Equally important is the lack of unequivocal correlation of toxicant-induced physiological and biochemical responses with a whole-animal response critical to species or population survival (e.g., reproduction, growth, development, or adaptability). Studies conducted at the Columbia National Fisheries Research Laboratory illustrated this correlation very well. In rainbow trout exposed to sublethal concentrations of dietary endrin for 165 d, significant changes occurred in serum sodium, chloride, osmolality, total protein, cholesterol, cortisol, lactate, glucose, and liver glycogen (Grant and Mehrle, 1973). The major conclusions were that glycogenolysis and the cortisol stress-response mechanism were inhibited; this inhibition implied decreased survival because the ability of the trout to respond to environmental stresses had been reduced. Although the implication was correct, similar biochemical manifestations of the stress-response mechanisms can be induced by other nonspecific stresses such as fish handling and temperature shock (Selye, 1950; Wedemeyer, 1969). To adequately interpret the significance of the endrin-induced changes, aquatic toxicologists must have a better understanding of the extremes that trout can tolerate biochemically in stress-response mechanisms. This would better enable them to predict the eventual effects on fish of toxicants such as endrin.

In rainbow trout exposed to sublethal dietary concentrations of dieldrin for 300 d (Mehrle et al., 1972), liver phenylalanine hydroxylase activity was decreased and blood phenylalanine concentrations and urine concentrations of phenylpyruvic acid were increased. These responses were similar to the biochemical manifestations of phenylketo-nuria (PKU), an inherited metabolic disorder in humans. The disease is characterized by altered behavior and learning ability. However, since behavioral studies were not conducted with the trout, the significance of the biochemical manifestations of PKU in fish could not be assessed.

Christensen et al. (1977) reported altered hematological characteristics in brook trout (*Salvelinus fontinalis*) exposed to heavy metals: lead increased plasma chloride and lactate dehydrogenase activity and decreased plasma glucose, and methyl mercury increased plasma sodium and chloride and hemoglobin. These biochemical changes were used as an early sign of toxicity to derive no-effect exposure concentrations, although the changes could not be directly related to any adverse effect on the health of the fish. However, the authors discussed the need to better understand cause-effect relations at the molecular, tissue, and organ levels if biochemical changes are to be used in diagnostic tests for predicting threshold toxicity concentrations.

The studies mentioned above by no means represent a comprehensive review of the literature on the biochemical and physiological effects of toxic chemicals on fish. However, they show that if the aquatic toxicologist is to interpret toxicant-induced biochemical and physiological changes, it is essential that these changes be related to impairments of fish health or survival. Biochemical investigations and monitoring of effects for regulatory purposes and hazard assessment in aquatic toxicology cannot be based on unsupported assumptions or extrapolations from mammalian toxicology and human medicine. Such extrapolations can lead to erroneous conclusions concerning contaminant effects in aquatic animals whose biochemical adaptive capacities are not completely understood.

CONSIDERATIONS IN DESIGN OF STUDIES AND SELECTION OF RESPONSE MEASUREMENTS

The preceding discussion has shown that the state of the art of biochemical and physiological tests in aquatic toxicology is not well advanced. As previously indicated, the analytical techniques and instrumentation are well developed, and considerable research on physiological and biochemical responses to chemical toxicants has been conducted; however, in general, meaningful diagnostic tests have not been developed and are not part of the aquatic toxicologist's repertoire of measurements. The main reason for this lack of progress has been lack of a comprehensive, integrated approach in designing toxicological studies with fish. This disparity between the sublethal measurement and relevance to whole-animal response is the "design-gap syndrome" that most aquatic toxicologists exhibit when conducting physiological and biochemical studies. Typical signs of the syndrome are performing a battery of physiological or biochemical measurements and basing the interpretation on extrapolations from mammalian toxicology or human medicine. To overcome this problem, the aquatic toxicologist must design biochemical and physiological investigations in conjunction with toxicity studies that measure important and relevant whole-animal responses, and the measurements must be unequivocally related to whole-animal responses. Establishing this relation will help ensure the development of pertinent diagnostic tests that will be useful to the aquatic toxicologist. The choice of the whole-animal responses to be evaluated depends on the purpose of the toxicology program, but in most programs emphasis has been placed on toxicant effects on survival, growth and development, reproduction, and adaptability.

It was recently concluded (Macek et al., 1978) that the most meaningful information for hazard assessment with a wide variety of chemicals in aquatic environments is derived from laboratory toxicity tests such as those for acute lethality, partial chronic embryo or larval toxicity, chronic toxicity (including reproduction), and residue accumulation. Physiological and biochemical tests are generally not conducted for two reasons: (1) it is believed that they are mainly useful in evaluating the mode of action of chemicals

(Brungs and Mount, 1978) and (2) there is not enough basic information about fish physiology and biochemistry to ascertain the ultimate effects, because alterations in these processes do not necessarily indicate diminished survival and success of the organisms. To adequately assess the influence of contaminants on the aquatic environment and to overcome the avoidance of biochemical and physiological testing, investigators should develop techniques that can serve as diagnostic tests in the field, as well as in the laboratory, to estimate the "health" of a particular aquatic resource. However, biochemical and physiological changes must be viewed in light of the degree and duration of change to determine whether the organism can adapt or whether the changes lead to irreversible homeostatic disturbances and finally to the death or debilitation of the organism.

EXAMPLES OF PERTINENT PHYSIOLOGICAL AND BIOCHEMICAL STUDIES IN AQUATIC TOXICOLOGY

Several types of physiological and biochemical investigations in aquatic toxicology have received considerable attention and are relatively more advanced than others. Several of those that are being used or that show promise as diagnostic tools are reviewed here.

Toxicant Effects on Bone Development and Growth in Fish

For the past several years, we have studied the use of biochemical and physiological tests to predict and monitor effects of contaminants on growth and skeletal development in fish. The emphasis was on the unequivocal correlation of biochemical responses to the whole-animal response of growth. Growth of fish is usually evaluated by measuring weight or length. However, growth is the culmination of many biochemical phenomena that occur in a somewhat regulated pattern; therefore, contaminant intoxication should induce biochemical changes, especially in the skeletal system, before reductions in growth are observed. These subtle biochemical changes may be sensitive indicators of many readily observable manifestations that occur later.

Measurement of skeletal deformities in fish has been proposed for monitoring pollution in marine environments (Bengtsson, 1979). Likewise, measurements of vertebral composition and mechanical properties have been shown to be indicators of growth and development in fish exposed to organic contaminants (Mayer et al., 1977b). Skeletal and vertebral abnormalities have been reported in wild populations of marine fish (Orska, 1962; Gill and Fisk, 1966; Van de Kamp, 1977), and water pollution has often been suspected as the cause (Sneed, 1970; Wunder, 1975). In addition, vertebral anomalies in pond-cultured channel catfish were thought to be induced by either deficient nutrition or contaminants (Sneed, 1970).

Vertebral and skeletal abnormalities in fish have been attributed to heredity and abnormal embryonic development (Dahlberg, 1970), low dissolved oxygen concentration (Blaxter, 1969), water temperature variation during development (Brungs, 1971), parasitic infection (Hoffman et al., 1962), electric current (Spencer, 1967), vitamin C deficiency (Wilson and Poe, 1973), and chemical contaminants. Chemical contaminants have been reported to induce various degrees of vertebral lesions in fish; gross, observable lesions such as lordosis, scoliosis, and vertebral damage were induced by exposure to organophosphate pesticides (McCann and Jasper, 1972), metals such as zinc, cadmium, and lead (Bengtsson, 1975), Kepone (Couch et al., 1977), crude oil (Linden, 1976), and toxaphene (Mayer et al. 1977a; Mehrle and Mayer, 1975). Vertebral collagen, calcium, and phosphorus were altered in fish exposed to organic contaminants such as PCBs, toxaphene, di(2-ethylhexyl) phthalate, dimethylamine salt of 2,4-dichlorophenoxyacetic acid (Mayer et al., 1977b), triarylphosphate esters (Mayer et al., 1981), Kepone (Mehrle et al., 1981), and methoxychlor (P. Mehrle, unpublished data). Chronic effects of these toxicants on vertebral composition proved to be an early indication of reduced growth and altered bone development in fish (Mayer et al., 1977b). Furthermore, Hamilton (1980) reported that mechanical properties such as stress, strain, and elasticity of vertebrae in fish exposed to toxaphene were more sensitive than bone composition as indicators of bone structural integrity. In addition, the relation between bone composition and density was important in assessing the mechanical properties of vertebrae. Contaminant-induced vertebral lesions can be caused in at least two ways: by acute exposures that cause neurotoxic tetanic contractions of skeletal muscle, and by chronic exposures that alter bone composition and render the bone more fragile. Regardless of the etiology of the vertebral lesions, several possible adverse effects on essential biological functions have been described, including impaired swimming performance, decreased ability to escape predators, and altered feeding behavior (Kroger and Guthrie, 1971). Other adverse effects suggested by Hickey (1972) include decreased territorial defense, decreased ability to compete for sexual partners, and general physiological weakness.

A mode of action proposed for chronic effects of organic contaminants on vertebral quality in fish involved contaminant-induced competition for vitamin C between collagen metabolism in bone and microsomal mixed-function oxidases (see Chapter 18) that detoxify or metabolize a broad range of organic contaminants. The competition causes a decrease in bone vitamin C and reduction in collagen content, with a concomitant increase in bone minerals that renders the backbone more fragile (Mayer et al., 1978). This concept was expanded by Hamilton (1980), who showed that hydroxyproline concentration in vertebral collagen and vertebral density were also important factors in contaminant effects on mechanical properties and vertebral integrity. The mode of action of inorganic contaminants on vertebral structure has not been elucidated. Hodson et al. (1980) reported that lead-induced vertebral lesions were not directly related to vitamin C metabolism. However, Bhatanger and Hussain (1977) reported that cadmium, mercury, palladium, and platinum de-

creased collagen synthesis in mammalian lung tissue by binding essential sulfhydryl groups on prolyl hydroxylase. These investigations suggest that inorganic contaminants might decrease vertebral collagen concentration by binding active sites on prolyl hydroxylase, whereas organic contaminants decrease an essential cofactor for the enzyme.

Effects of organic and inorganic contaminants on collagen and vertebral integrity are similar, although they develop through different modes of action; this similarity makes vertebral collagen and mechanical property measurements useful for assessing the impact of an array of contaminants on vertebral integrity in fish. Such assessment is significant because of the large number of chemical contaminants from industrial, agricultural, and municipal sources (among others) that are potential toxicants. These chemicals are usually not measured in fish, but could still induce vertebral lesions. Thus bone development measurements represent an attractive diagnostic tool for the aquatic toxicologist in both laboratory and environmental studies.

Lead Inhibition of Aminolevulinic Acid Dehydratase Activity

The inhibition of δ-aminolevulinic acid dehydratase (ALAD) activity by lead is an example of a toxicant-induced response that is unique but that has limited application in aquatic toxicology. ALAD catalyzes the condensation of two moles of aminolevulinic acid to porphobilinogen and is involved in porphyrin and red blood cell metabolism (Gibson et al., 1955). ALAD activity in erythrocytes is inhibited by in vivo and in vitro exposures of fish, birds, and mammals to lead, and the enzyme inhibition appears to be relatively specific for lead. Although ALAD activity is inhibited in vitro by a number of substances such as EDTA, mercury, copper, silver, manganese (Hernberg and Nikkanen, 1972), and transiently by ethanol (Moore et al., 1971), the inhibitory effect of all these substances is less than that of lead. Although copper, cadmium, lead, mercury, silver, and zinc alter ALAD activity in fish, lead has the most significant effect (Jackin, 1973; Hodson et al., 1977). *In vivo* exposure to lead has been reported to decrease ALAD activity in the liver of mummichog (*Fundulus heteroclitus*) and winter flounder (*Pseudopleuronectes americanus*) (Jackin, 1973); in the blood of rainbow trout, brook trout, goldfish (*Carassius auratus*), and pumpkinseed (*Lepomis gibbosus*) (Hodson et al., 1977); and in the distal part of the kidney, the spleen, and the blood of rainbow trout (Johansson-Sjobeck and Larson, 1979). Measurement of ALAD activity is used clinically to detect lead intoxication in humans and as an index of lead shot ingestion in waterfowl. Similar responses have been observed in several freshwater species, and the inhibition of ALAD activity by lead has been proposed as a short-term indicator of long-term toxicity in fish (Hodson, 1976; Hodson et al., 1978, 1979). Hodson et al. (1977) reported significant inverse correlations between erythrocyte ALAD activity and lead concentration in the blood of brook trout and rainbow trout. Thus measurement of ALAD activity is a good indicator of lead accumulation in fish. In addition, Hodson et al. (1979) showed that ALAD activity can be used as a predictor of lead-induced lordosis and scoliosis in fish and an indicator of harmful lead concentrations in natural fish populations. This area of biochemical toxicology is the subject of both laboratory and field investigations.

Respiration and Oxygen Consumption

Studies of the effects of contaminants on oxygen consumption by fish are few; more data are available from experiments with mammals and terrestrial arthropods. The terminology used in respiration and oxygen consumption research with fish is not widely known and therefore several key terms are defined below.

Routine metabolism is the mean rate of oxygen consumption measured when precautions are taken against the fish being influenced by outside stimuli (Fry, 1967). External disturbances can introduce wide variability into this respiration measurement. Routine metabolism can be determined in any suitable container. A fish is placed in a respirometer and allowed to adjust for 1 h before oxygen measurements are made. Water should flow through the respirometer during the adjustment period and between measurements. The water flow is turned off for a specified period, before and after which a water sample is taken. Routine metabolism is best measured in a dark container to reduce activity of the fish and therefore variation; under these conditions, the end point is called the "low routine metabolic rate."

Standard metabolism is the minimum rate of oxygen consumption and should be determined by extrapolating the relations between oxygen consumption and spontaneous activity to zero activity (Fry, 1967). Standard metabolism can be measured with an apparatus described by Dickson and Kramer (1971). The chamber consists of a stainless steel pot fitted with a glass flowmeter. The flowmeter operates on a heat-loss principle. Fish movement results in loss of heat from the flowmeter and activation of a heater circuit. The time when the heater is on is an index of the spontaneous activity of the fish. Standard metabolism of each fish is estimated by plotting the logarithm of oxygen consumption against activity (five or six oxygen and activity measurements) and extrapolating to zero activity.

Active metabolism is the maximum steady rate of oxygen consumption under continuous forced activity (Fry, 1967). Measurements are made with an apparatus described by Dickson and Kramer (1971). The fish are forced to swim against a current produced by a propeller attached to a variable-speed electric motor. Each fish is allowed to adjust and orient itself in the chamber at a low water velocity. A water sample is then taken and the outlets and inlets are closed. The water velocity is slowly increased within a short period until the fish can just maintain its position. At the end of the forced-swimming period, the water velocity is greatly reduced and a water sample is collected.

Scope for activity is the difference between the

mean active (maximum) and mean standard (minimum) metabolic rates (Fry, 1947). It is an indication of the amount of respiration available for activity (Fry, 1957). The work of Dickson and Kramer (1971) should be consulted for details of the apparatus and references to literature on determining scope for activity.

Routine metabolism of bluntnose minnows (*Pimephales notatus*) increased when endrin was added to the water (Mount, 1962). Dowden (1966), who studied five insecticides, found either an increase or a decrease in routine metabolism depending on the water concentration of the insecticides. Pumpkinseeds subjected to dieldrin in water used more oxygen than controls when forced to swim against a current (Cairns and Scheier, 1964). Alterations of oxidative enzymatic activity may also alter oxygen consumption of affected organs and whole organisms. Bouck (1966) stated that sublethal levels of DDT halved the plasma lactate dehydrogenase activity in rock bass (*Ambloplites rupestris*). Colvin and Phillips (1968) found that succinate dehydrogenase and cytochrome oxidase were inhibited by endrin in *in vitro* studies of the liver of black bullhead (*Ictalurus melas*). Mayer (1970) also found *in vivo* inhibition of liver succinate dehydrogenase in rainbow trout exposed to dieldrin.

No significant effects of dietary dieldrin on standard or active metabolic rates were found in rainbow trout (Mayer, 1970), but standard metabolic rates were 15% less than those of the controls at the highest dieldrin dose. Dieldrin doses of 0, 0.04, 0.08, 0.12, 0.16, and 0.20 mg were given *per os* to fish averaging 172 g. The fish were dosed every other day for 2 wk with seven doses in all. Extensive liver damage was evident in fish given the higher doses and dieldrin reduced the swimming speed the trout could maintain. Such an effect could be of considerable importance in anadromous (salmon) and catadromous (eels) fish, many of which migrate great distances.

No other studies have been reported in which standard metabolic techniques were used to determine the effects of insecticides on fish metabolism. Riker et al. (1946) reported an increase of 23% in basal metabolic rates of rats, but this required feeding of a diet with a DDT level of 1000 mg/kg.

Mount (1962) found that endrin had no apparent effect on the ability of bluntnose minnows to swim against a current. Cairns and Scheier (1964) subjected pumpkinseeds to aqueous dieldrin concentrations of 0.75 and 1.7 μg/l for 12 wk and measured oxygen consumption and cruising speed weekly. Fish subjected to the higher dieldrin concentration consistently consumed more oxygen than the controls when forced to swim against a current and had a significantly reduced cruising speed.

Mayer and Kramer (1973), in a water reuse study (Larmoyeux and Piper, 1973) simulating hatchery conditions, found that active metabolism was reduced in rainbow trout after 300 d. Ammonia in the water of the affected fish ranged from 0.5–0.8 mg/l and oxygen from 3.3–4.9 mg/l. Oxygen concentrations of 5.6–7.7 mg/l and ammonia concentrations of 0.1–0.4 mg/l did not affect active metabolism. Standard metabolism was not affected by water reuse. Active metabolism was a more sensitive indicator of trout fitness than was growth or food conversion rate.

Mayer (1970) reported that scope for activity did not differ significantly among rainbow trout exposed to different concentrations of dieldrin (0.04–0.2 mg per dose), but was nominally greatest among those exposed to intermediate concentrations (0.08–0.12 mg per dose). Active metabolism was also highest at these concentrations. Scope for activity was lowest in the control fish. It is conceivable that the scope is higher in treated than in untreated animals. According to Beamish and Dickie (1967), "This index of scope might justifiably be considered as a measure of the scope for total energy expenditure, irrespective of the functions for which energy is used." Thus, the increased scope observed by Mayer (1970) may have been due to increased enzyme activity, repair of affected tissues, or both.

Routine metabolism and liver, kidney, and

brain metabolism were depressed in rainbow trout treated with low dieldrin concentrations (0.04–0.12 mg per dose), as was spontaneous activity (Mayer, 1970), but both were higher than those of controls at the highest dieldrin concentration (0.2 mg per dose). Mount (1962) found that routine metabolism of bluntnose minnows was slightly increased when endrin (0.3–0.5 μg/l) was added to the water. He attributed this to increased movement caused by tremors and convulsions. Dowden (1966) reported that chlordane increased or decreased routine metabolism in the bluegill (*Lepomis macrochirus*), depending on the water concentration; he described the response in terms of an "N-shaped curve." The N-shaped curve was characterized by a relative heightening of oxygen consumption at 0.1 μg/l and a second heightening at 5.0 μg/l. DDT elicited a response similar to that of chlordane in causing lower oxygen consumption at 1.0 μg/l than at the other two concentrations, but was different in depressing bluegill oxygen consumption at all three concentrations tested. Fish exposed to lindane exhibited a similar but less acute response than those exposed to DDT. Malathion and parathion had opposite effects on oxygen consumption by fish. Malathion, at the lowest (0.1 μg/l) and highest (5 μg/l) concentrations tested, depressed oxygen consumption to a greater extent than at the intermediate concentration (1 μg/l). In parathion, the fish exhibited increased oxygen consumption at the lowest and highest concentrations and depressed oxygen consumption at the intermediate concentration.

Spontaneous activity and oxygen consumption were increased in white suckers (*Catostomus commersoni*) exposed for 24 h to 0.04–0.1 mg/l methoxychlor, whereas no effects were noted at 0.01 mg/l (Waiwood and Johansen, 1974). The 96-96-h LC50 was 0.034 mg/l. Oxygen uptake rates of fish surviving methoxychlor exposure were similar to those of control fish.

In a study by Silbergeld (1973), both a decrease and an increase in oxygen consumption occurred in johnny darters (*Etheostoma nigrum*) exposed for 30 d to 2.3 μg/l dieldrin. Until d 15 the fish consumed less oxygen per gram of body weight than did the controls. After d 15 oxygen consumption increased, but the curve remained different in slope and intercept. Davis (1973) found a similar response: oxygen uptake increased in sockeye salmon (*Oncorhynchus nerka*) on initial exposure to 20% of the 96-h LC50 of bleached kraft pulp mill effluent. After overnight exposure to the effluent, oxygen consumption decreased and tended to approach preexposure levels. Changing effluent toxicity, acclimation phenomena, and physiological adjustment were discussed as possible explanations for the effects.

Doses of organochlorine insecticides required to cause appreciable alterations of whole-fish oxygen consumption are large enough to be extremely toxic to fish and to lead to death if exposure is prolonged. It would be more interesting to consider alterations of growth in long-term studies in which fish were exposed to low levels of insecticides, since a decrease in oxygen consumption and spontaneous activity might result in increased growth rates.

All the studies completed so far have been too short to show any differences in growth. However, Mount (1962) found that fish in 0.4 and 0.5 μg/l endrin were much more active than those in 0.1 μg/l or than controls. He also noted that mean daily increase in length was 48% greater in the 0.1 μg/l endrin treatment than in controls. Increases in growth at low levels of DDT exposure were observed by Allison et al. (1964) in cutthroat trout (*Salmo clarki*) fed 0.03–3.0 mg/kg per week and by Macek (1968) in brook trout fed 2–3 mg/kg per week.

Organochlorine insecticides at low concentrations may behave as "antithyroid" materials and reduce activity and oxygen consumption. Brown (1964) wrote that increased thyroid hormone would be expected to stimulate general activity in fish and deplete the energy available for growth. Growth rates of brown trout were reduced during periods of maximum thyroid activity (Swift, 1955). Decreases in oxygen consumption due to antithyroid materials such as thiourea have been reported in fish (Brown, 1964). The effect of organochlorine insecticides on the thyroid of fish is not understood, but some work has been done with higher vertebrates. Serum protein-bound iodine was lowered by *o,p'*-DDD in humans (Marshall and Tompkins, 1968). The compound was found to compete with thyroxine for thyroxine-binding globulin. Thyroxine in plasma is loosely bound to a globulin and enters tissue cells, where the thyroxine is dehalogenated and inorganic iodide is returned to the thyroid gland (Bell et al., 1965). Thyroxine regulates enzymes that control energy metabolism within the cell (Bell et al., 1965). It is possible that organochlorine insecticides reduce the amount of thyroglobulin that normally enters cells and that this reduction results in lower metabolic rates and higher growth rates.

Studies with other pesticides have given varied results. Respiration was not affected in bluegills exposed to 3 mg/l of the butoxyethanol esters of 2,4-D and 2,4,5-T for 30–60 min (Sigmon, 1979). However, exposure to dichlorvos, an organophosphate insecticide, decreased oxygen uptake in gill, brain, and muscle tissues of tilapia (*Tilapia mossambic*) after a 15-d exposure to 0.5 mg/l (Rath and Misra, 1980). The recovery of oxygen consumption in muscle after the fish were transferred to clean water was faster than that in the brain or gill.

Oxygen consumption should be a useful measure of sublethal effects because energy processes are indicators of overall physiological state. Brett (1958) proposed the use of scope for activity as a method of assessing the effect of pollutants on aquatic organisms. This may be justified for pollutants that greatly affect respiratory membranes or respiratory processes, but organochlorine insecticides do not appear to be in this category. No effect of dieldrin on the gill epithelium was observed by Mayer (1970) or Cairns and Scheier (1964). Furthermore, these and other studies indicated that quantities of organochlorine insecticides are required to induce a significant change in oxygen consumption by entire organisms.

Related research has dealt with respiratory activity and the cough response (Sparks et al., 1972; Morgan and Kuhn, 1974; Rice et al., 1977; Sloof, 1979), which appear to be better end points than oxygen uptake and show promise for use in monitoring effluents and predicting chronic fish toxicity (Maki, 1979). These techniques do not include the measurement of oxygen, but involve the nerve action potential associated with the opening and closing of the buccal cavity, branchial arches, and operculum.

Acetylcholinesterase

Acetylcholinesterase inhibition in aquatic organisms has been suggested as a measure of the impact of organophosphate and carbamate insecticides and related chemicals in the aquatic environment (Weiss, 1961, 1965; Weiss and Gakstatter, 1964; Williams and Sova, 1966; Holland et al., 1967; Morgan et al., 1973; Coppage and Braidech, 1976). Carbamates and organophosphates are usually less noxious than organochlorine chemicals because they break down rapidly in the environment and do not persist in animal tissues. Nevertheless, some of these insecticides are extremely toxic for short periods after application, during which they inhibit the neurotransmitter enzyme acetylcholinesterase in the central nervous system, usually causing death from paralysis. Acetylcholinesterase, which is normally present in all body tissues, is responsible for hydrolyzing acetylcholine into choline and acetic acid (O'Brien, 1967). This hydrolysis is an important biochemical process, especially for the transmission of nerve impulses across synapses and the operation of the sympathetic and autonomic nervous systems. Acetylcholinesterase is also inhibited or depressed in cases of severe infection, anemia, malnutrition, and liver disease.

Broad generalizations about the type of cholinesterase in a given tissue are usually not valid, and one cannot always predict the type, importance, or substrate specificity of cholinesterase by its location. There are two classical types—acetylcholinesterase and butyrylcholinesterase—which are found in mammalian erythrocytes and serum, respectively (O'Brien, 1967). In mammals, acetylcholinesterase preferentially hydrolyzes acetylcholine and butyrylcholinesterase preferentially hydrolyzes butyrylcholine. Some of these differences do not apply to insect cholinesterase. For example, fly head cholinesterase hydrolyzes butyrylcholine readily, but in other respects behaves like mammalian acetylcholinesterase. Butyrylcholinesterase in the sera of certain species, such as rats and ducks, is propionyl-specific rather than butyryl-specific. Rabbit serum contains both acetylcholinesterase and butyrylcholinesterase. Even nerve tissue contains both types of cholinesterase. The main enzyme in lake trout (*Salvelinus namaycush*) and crayfish (*Procambarus clarki*) was found to be acetylcholinesterase, while that in crab (*Uca pugnax*) was butyrylcholinesterase (Guilbault et al., 1972).

Acetylcholinesterase is vital for the neurological functioning of the sensory, integrative, and neuromuscular systems of fish. In salmonids, inhibition of this enzyme alters respiration (Klaverkamp et al., 1977), swimming (Matton and Lattam, 1969; Post and Leisure, 1974), feeding (Wildish and Lister, 1973; Bull and McInerny, 1974), and social interaction (Symons, 1973). Alterations in activity, an important factor in feeding and predator avoidance, were commonly observed.

The relation between brain acetylcholinesterase activity and organophosphate exposure appears to be close in birds regardless of species, age, and sex, but such relations are essentially unknown in aquatic invertebrates and fish. Inhibition of acetylcholinesterase in fish brains by organophosphate pesticides has been used to detect pollution of natural waters by these chemicals (Williams and Sova, 1966; Holland et al., 1967), but the interpretation of the relation of inhibition to exposure and death is controversial (Nicholson, 1967; Cox, 1968; Gibson et al., 1969). Death of fish after exposure to organophosphate pesticides in the laboratory was reported at brain activities ranging from 5.4 to 92% of normal (Weiss, 1958, 1961), but fish have survived at activities as low as 10-20% of normal (Weiss, 1961; Gibson et al., 1969).

If acetylcholinesterase measurements are to prove useful, further research is needed to better define the cholinesterases in aquatic organisms and to establish the biological significance of acetylcholinesterase inhibition in aquatic invertebrates and fish.

Osmoregulation and Gill Adenosinetriphosphatase

Salmonids and other euryhaline fish typically show increased gill $Na^+ + K^+$-adenosinetriphosphatase ($Na^+ + K^+$-ATPase) and ion pump activity before and after adaptation to seawater (Epstein et al., 1967; Kamiya and Utida, 1969; Kamiya, 1972). The fish maintain body fluid hypotonicity by drinking seawater, absorbing water and salts across the intestinal epithelium, and secreting NaCl across the gill epithelium while retaining the free water. The primary driving mechanism in both intestine and gill is the ion pump with which $Na^+ + K^+$-ATPase appears to be intimately involved (Janicki and Kinter, 1971a, 1971b). The increase in ATPase activity in the gill microsomal system begins in salmonids during smolting, prior to their entry into seawater, and peaks near the time when they show active migratory behavior (Zaugg and McLain, 1970; Zaugg and Wagner, 1973; McCartney, 1976).

ATPase activity in tissues other than gill has been inhibited by contaminants. ATPase systems were adversely affected in chronic *in vivo* studies with fathead minnows (*Pimephales promelas*) exposed to Aroclor 1242 and Aroclor 1254 (Koch et al., 1972) and *in vitro* studies with microsomal preparations of bluegill brain, liver, kidney, and muscle exposed to Aroclors 1221, 1242, 1254, and 1268 and a polychlorinated terphenyl, Aroclor 5460 (Yap et al., 1971; Cutkomp et al., 1972). Both *in vivo* and *in vitro*, the greatest effects were on Mg^{2+}-ATPase, with lesser effects on $Na^+ + K^+$-ATPase. The Aroclors in the intermediate range of chlorination, particularly Aroclor 1242, had the greatest inhibitory effect on ATPase.

Osmoregulation decreased in killifish (*Fundulus*

heteroclitus) acutely exposed to 0.25–0.75 mg/l DDT or 75 mg/l Aroclor 1221 (Kinter et al., 1972), and *in vitro* inhibition of ATPase activity by Kepone and its reduction product occurred in channel catfish brain (Desaiah and Koch, 1975). The $Na^+ + K^+$-ATPase in the microsomal fraction of gill homogenate of rainbow trout was inhibited by aldrin, chlordane, DDD, DDE, DDT, dicofol, dieldrin, heptachlor, lindane, methoxychlor, Perthane, Strobane, Thiodan, toxaphene, 2,4,5-T, and PCBs (Aroclors 1242 and 1254) but not by endrin, mirex, or 2,4-D (Davis and Wedemeyer, 1971; Davis et al., 1972).

Increased gill ATPase activity associated with the parr-smolt transformation in salmonids is being used to assess migration readiness, hypoosmoregulatory capability, and potential for ocean survival of anadromous fish (Wedemeyer et al., 1980). ATPase activity begins to increase in fresh water, and if the salmon enter salt water the gill ATPase activity continues to increase until it is three to four times that in fresh water, indicating that full osmoregulatory capability has been reached. There is also a substantial thyroid surge during smoltification, and thus it may be possible to monitor plasma thyroxine (T_4) as a method of following smoltification during rearing and of predicting ocean survival (Dickhoff et al., 1978). Smoltification and seawater adaptation in salmonids were reviewed by Folmar and Dickhoff (1980).

Exposure of salmonid smolts to environmental contaminants at levels commonly accepted as safe can affect the gill ATPase salt pump system and inhibit both migratory behavior and ability to adapt to seawater (Lorz and McPherson, 1976; Davis and Shand, 1978). This effect greatly reduces ocean survival and subsequent fishery success.

Effects of copper and zinc exposure on survival and growth of nonanadromous salmonids in fresh water are well documented (Lloyd, 1960; Sprague and Ramsay, 1965; McKim and Benoit, 1971; Chapman, 1973; Hodson and Sprague, 1975). However, much less information is available on smoltification and migration of anadromous fish exposed to traces of heavy metals (Wedemeyer et al., 1980). Exposure to trace levels was shown to affect numerous aspects of salmonid growth, development, and behavior. Studies by Sprague et al. (1965) and Saunders and Sprague (1967) indicated that pollution from copper and zinc mining interrupted the migratory behavior of returning Atlantic salmon (*Salmo salar*). Lorz and McPherson (1976) noted decreased gill ATPase activity and reduced migratory tendency and ability to cope with seawater in smolts of coho salmon (*Oncorhynchus kisutch*) exposed to sublethal concentrations of copper (20–30 µg/l). Davis and Shand (1978) obtained similar results with sockeye salmon and copper.

A study by Lorz et al. (1978b) is noteworthy because several heavy metals were shown to act in various ways. Exposure of coho salmon to nickel or chromium (5 mg/l) for 96 h in fresh water did not affect migratory behavior or capability for ocean survival, but sublethal mercury (50–300 µg/l) or cadmium (>4 µg/l) resulted in concentration-dependent mortalities in seawater. Exposure to cadmium or zinc during rearing did not adversely affect migratory behavior, but if copper (10 µg/l) was also present, downstream migration was reduced and gill ATPase activity was suppressed. Migratory success was reduced in coho salmon smolts exposed for 96 h to the herbicide Tordon 101 at 0.6–1.8 mg/l just before release (Lorz et al., 1978a).

Relatively little research has been done on contaminants and salmon; much more is warranted because this group of fish is one of the few that has been studied extensively in the field and because field techniques are available that greatly facilitate comparisons of laboratory results with field observations.

SUMMARY

Physiological and biochemical measurements have not been as integral a part of aquatic toxicology as they have been of mammalian toxicology. However, they are attracting more interest as aquatic toxicologists find a need for short-term tests that predict long-term toxicity, because the number of toxic chemicals and the cost of conducting chronic toxicity studies are increasing. Although they will not replace acute or chronic toxicity tests that determine effects on survival, growth, and reproduction in the laboratory, physiological and biochemical measurements will be useful in setting priorities for determining the chemicals for which more comprehensive hazard assessment is needed. They will also be useful in field investigations to determine the toxicological significance of contaminant residues in wild fish populations. Aquatic toxicologists need better diagnostic tools in order to better understand the impact of chemicals on fish and other aquatic organisms. The examples discussed here show that physiological and biochemical approaches will help to satisfy this need.

Underlying the efforts to develop diagnostic tools is the need to plan and execute the biochemical and physiological research within the framework of what exists in the real world. Unless the status of the environment we are attempting to preserve and improve is kept in proper perspective, much of our effort will be of little or no avail. Consequently, continued reassessment of aquatic toxicology in relation to the continued change in environmental needs is mandatory if the obvious objectives are to be reached. Yet the need for basic information must not be forgotten when research programs are designed, especially with aquatic organisms, for this information is ultimately the foundation for applied research.

LITERATURE CITED

Allison D, Kallman BJ, Cope OB, Van Valin CC: Some chronic effects of DDT on cutthroat trout. U.S. Bur Sport Fish Wildl Res Rept 64, 1964.

Barnhart RA: Effects of certain variables of hematological characteristics of rainbow trout. Trans Am Fish Soc 98:411–418, 1969.

Beamish FHW, Dickie LM: Metabolism and bio-logical production in fish. In: The Biological Basis of Freshwater Fish Production, edited by SD Gerking, pp. 215–242. New York: Wiley, 1967.

Bell GH, Davidson JN, Scarborough H: Textbook of Physiology and Biochemistry. Baltimore: Williams & Wilkins, 1965.

Bengtsson BE: Vertebral damage in fish induced by pollutants. In: Sublethal Effects of Toxic Chemicals on Aquatic Animals, edited by JH Koeman, JJTWA Strik, pp. 23–30. New York: Elsevier, 1975.

Bengtsson BE: Biological variables, especially skeletal deformities in our fish for monitoring marine pollution. Philos Trans R Soc London 286:457–464, 1979.

Bhatanger RS, Hussain MA: Interference with steps in collagen synthesis: A test for pulmonary toxicity of environmental agents. In: Proceedings of the Fourth Joint Conference on Sensing of Environmental Pollutants, pp. 527–531. Washington, D.C.: American Chemical Society, 1977.

Blaxter JHS: Development: Eggs and larvae. In: Fish Physiology, vol. 3, edited by WS Hoar, DJ Randall, pp. 177–252. New York: Academic, 1969.

Bouck GR: Changes in blood and muscle composition of rock bass (Ambloplites rupestris) as physiological criteria of stressful conditions. Thesis, Michigan State Univ., East Lansing, Mich., 1966.

Bouck GR, Ball RC: Influence of capture methods on blood characteristics and mortality in the rainbow trout (Salmo gairdneri). Trans Am Fish Soc 95:170–176, 1966.

Brett JR: Implications and assessments of environmental stress. In: The Investigation of Fish-Power Problems, edited by PA Larkin, pp. 69–83. H.R. MacMillan Lectures in Fisheries, Univ. of British Columbia, Vancouver, 1958.

Brown ME: The Physiology of Fishes, vol. 1, Metabolism. New York: Academic, 1964.

Brungs WA: Chronic effects of constant elevated temperature on the fathead minnow (Pimephales promelas Rafinesque). Trans Am Fish Soc 100:659–664, 1971.

Brungs WA, Mount DI: Introduction to a discussion of the use of aquatic toxicity tests for evaluation of the effects of toxic substances. In: Estimating the Hazard of Chemical Substances to Aquatic Life, edited by J Cairns, KL Dickson, AW Maki, ASTM STP 657, pp. 15–26. Philadelphia: American Society for Testing and Materials, 1978.

Bull CJ, McInerny JE: Behavior of juvenile coho salmon exposed to Sumithion, an organophosphate insecticide. J Fish Res Board Can 31:1867–1872, 1974.

Cairns J, Jr, Scheier A: The effect upon the pumpkinseed sunfish Lepomis gibbosus (Linn.) of chronic exposure to lethal and sublethal contrations of dieldrin. Not Nat Acad Nat Sci Philadelphia 370:1–10, 1964.

Chapman GA: Effect of heavy metals on fish. In: Heavy Metals in the Environment, pp. 141–162. Water Resources Research Inst., Oregon State Univ., Corvallis, 1973.

Christensen GM, Hunt E, Fiant J: The effect of methylmercury chloride, cadmium chloride and lead nitrate on six biochemical factors of the brook trout (Salvelinus fontinalis). Toxicol Appl Pharmacol 42:523–530, 1977.

Colvin HJ, Phillips AT: Inhibition of electron transport enzymes and cholinesterases by endrin. Bull Environ Contam Toxicol 3:106–115, 1968.

Coppage DL, Braidech T: River pollution by anticholinesterase agents. Water Res 10:19–24, 1976.

Couch JA, Winstead JT, Goodman LR: Keponeinduced scoliosis and its histological consequences in fish. Science 197:585–587, 1977.

Cox WS: Enforcing insecticide content water quality standards. Science 159:1123–1124, 1968.

Cutkomp LK, Yap HH, Desaiah D, Koch RB: The sensitivity of fish ATPases to polychlorinated biphenyls. Environ Health Perspect 1:165–168, 1972.

Dahlberg MD: Frequencies of abnormalities in Georgia estuarine fishes. Trans Am Fish Soc 99:95–97, 1970.

Davis JC: Sublethal effects of bleached kraft pulp mill effluent on respiration and circulation in sockeye salmon (Oncorhynchus nerka). J Fish Res Board Can 30:369–377, 1973.

Davis JC, Shand IG: Acute and sublethal copper sensitivity, growth and saltwater survival in young Babine Lake sockeye salmon. Fish Mar Serv Tech Rep 847, 1978.

Davis PW, Wedemeyer GA: Na^+, K^+-activated-ATPase inhibition in rainbow trout: A site for organochlorine pesticide toxicity? Comp Biochem Physiol 40:823–827, 1971.

Davis PW, Friedhoff JM, Wedemeyer GA: Organochlorine insecticide, herbicide and polychlorinated biphenyl (PCB) inhibition of NaK-ATPase in rainbow trout. Bull Environ Contam Toxicol 8:69–72, 1972.

Desaiah D, Koch RB: Inhibition of ATPase activity in channel catfish brain by Kepone[R] and its reduction product. Bull Environ Contam Toxicol 13:153–158, 1975.

Dickhoff W, Folmar L, Gorbman A: Changes in plasma thyroxine during smoltification of coho salmon Oncorhynchus kisutch. Gen Comp Endocrinol 36:229–232, 1978.

Dickson IW, Kramer RH: Factors influencing scope for activity and active standard metabolism of rainbow trout (Salmo gairdneri). J Fish Res Board Can 28:587–596, 1971.

Dowden BF: Effects of five insecticides on the oxygen consumption of the bluegill sunfish, Lepomis macrochirus. Ph.D. thesis, Louisiana State Univ., Baton Rouge, La., 1966.

Epstein FH, Katz AI, Pickford GE: Sodium and potassium-activated adenosine triphosphatase of gills: Role in adaptation of teleosts to salt water. Science 156:1245–1247, 1967.

Folmar LC, Dickhoff WW: The parr-smolt transformation (smoltification) and seawater adaptation in salmonids: A review of selected literature. Aquaculture 21:1–37, 1980.

Fry FEJ: Effects of environment on animal activity. Publ Ontario Fish Res Lab No 68, 1947.

Fry FEJ: The aquatic respiration of fish. In: Physiology of Fishes, vol. 1, edited by ME Brown, pp. 1–63. New York: Academic, 1957.

Fry FEJ: Responses of vertebrate poikilotherms to temperature. In: Thermobiology, edited by AH Rose, pp. 375–409. New York: Academic, 1967.

Gibson KD, Newberger A, Scottil JJ: Purification and properties of δ-aminolevulinic acid dehydrase. J Biochem 61:618–629, 1955.

Gibson RF, Ludke JL, Ferguson DE: Sources of error in the use of fish-brain acetylcholinesterase as a monitor for pollution. Bull Environ Contam Toxicol 4:17–23, 1969.

Gill DC, Fisk DM: Vertebral abnormalities in sockeye, pink, and chum salmon. Trans Am Fish Soc 95:177–182, 1966.

Grant BF, Mehrle PM: 1973. Endrin toxicosis in rainbow trout (Salmo gairdneri). J Fish Res Board Can 30:31–40, 1973.

Grant BF, Schoettger RA: The impact of organochlorine contaminants on physiologic functions in fish. Proc Tech Sessions Annu Meet Inst Environ Sci 18:245–250, 1972.

Guilbault GG, Lozes RL, Moore W, Kuan SS: Effect of pesticides on cholinesterase from aquatic species: Crayfish, trout and fiddler crab. Environ Lett 3:235–245, 1972.

Hamilton SJ: Mechanical properties of bone in fishes. M.S. thesis, Univ. of Missouri, Columbia, Mo., 1980.

Hernberg S, Nikkanen J: The effect of lead on σ-aminolevulinic acid dehydratase. Pracov Lek 24:77–83, 1972.

Hickey CR: Common abnormalities in fishes, their causes and effects. NY Ocean Sci Lab Tech Rep 0013, 1972.

Hodson PV: δ-Aminolevulinic acid dehydratase activity in fish blood as an indicator of a harmful exposure to lead. J Fish Res Board Can 33:268–271, 1976.

Hodson PV, Sprague JB: Temperature induced changes in acute toxicity of zinc to Atlantic salmon (Salmo salar). J Fish Res Board Can 32:1–10, 1975.

Hodson PV, Blunt BR, Spry DJ, Austen K: Evaluation of erythrocyte delta-aminolevulinic acid dehydratase activity as a short-term indicator in fish of a harmful exposure to lead. J Fish Res Board Can 34:501–508, 1977.

Hodson PV, Blunt BR, Spry DJ: Chronic toxicity of water-borne and dietary lead to a rainbow trout (Salmo gairdneri) in Lake Ontario water. Water Res 12:869–878, 1978.

Hodson PV, Blunt BR, Jensen D, Morgan S: Effect of fish age on predicted and observed chronic toxicity of lead to rainbow trout in Lake Ontario water. J Great Lakes Res 5:84–89, 1979.

Hodson PV Milton JW, Blunt BR, Slinger SR: Effects of dietary ascorbic acid on chronic lead

toxicity to young rainbow trout (Salmo gairdneri). Can J Fish Aquat Sci 37:170–176, 1980.

Hoffman GL, Dunbar EC, Bradford A: Whirling disease of trouts caused by Myxosoma cerebralis in the United States. U.S. Fish Wildl Serv Spec Sci Rept Fish No. 427, 1962.

Holland HT, Coppage DL, Butler PA: Use of fish brain acetylcholinesterase to monitor pollution by organophosphorus pesticides. Bull Environ Contam Toxicol 2:156–162, 1967.

Housten AH, Madden JA, Woods RJ, Miles HM: Variation in the blood and tissue chemistry of brook trout, Salvelinus fontinalis, subsequent to handling, anesthesia, and surgery. J Fish Res Board Can 28:635–642, 1971.

Hunn JB: Bibliography on the blood chemistry of fishes. U.S. Fish Wildl Serv Res Rept 72, 1967.

Hunn JB: Blood chemistry values for some fishes of the upper Mississippi River. J Minn Acad Sci 38:19–21, 1972.

Jackin E: Influence of lead and other metals on fish δ-aminolevulinate dehydrase activity. J Fish Res Board Can 30:560–562, 1973.

Janicki RH, Kinter WB: DDT inhibits Na$^+$, K$^+$, Mg^{++}-ATPase in the intestinal mucosae and gills of marine teleosts. Nature (Lond) 233:148–151, 1971a.

Janicki RH, Kinter WB: DDT: Disrupted osmoregulatory events in the intestine of the eel Anguilla rostrata adapted to sea water. Science 173:1146–1147, 1971b.

Johansson-Sjobeck ML, Larson A: Effects of inorganic lead on delta-aminolevulinic acid dehydratase activity and hematological variables in rainbow trout (Salmo gairdneri). Arch Environ Contam Toxicol 8:419–431, 1979.

Kamiya M: Hormonal effect on Na-K-ATPase activity in the gill of Japanese eel, Anguilla japonica, with special reference to seawater adaptation. Endocrinol Jpn 19:489–493, 1972.

Kamiya M, Utida S: Sodium-potassium-activated adenosinetriphosphatase activity in gills of freshwater, marine and euryhaline teleosts. Comp Biochem Physiol 31:671–674, 1969.

Kinter WB, Merkens LS, Janicki RH, Guarino AM: Studies on the mechanism of toxicity of DDT and polychlorinated biphenyls (PCBs): Disruption of osmoregulation in marine fish. Environ Health Perspect 1:169–173, 1972.

Klaverkamp JF, Duangsawadsi M, MacDonald WA: Majewski HS: An evaluation of fenitrothion toxicity in four life stages of rainbow trout, *Salmo gairdneri*. In: Aquatic Toxicology and Hazard Evaluation, edited by FL Mayer, JL Hamelink, ASTM STP 634, pp. 231–240. Philadelphia: ASTM, 1977.

Koch RB, Desaiah D, Yap HH, Cutkomp LK: Polychlorinated biphenyls: Effect of long-term exposure on ATPase activity in fish, *Pimephales promelas*. Bull Environ Contam Toxicol 2:87–92, 1972.

Kroger RL, Guthrie JF: Incidence of crooked vertebral columns in juvenile Atlantic menhaden, *Brevoortia tyrannus*. Chesapeake Sci 12(4): 276–278, 1971.

Larmoyeux JD, Piper RG: Some effects of water reuse on rainbow trout in hatcheries. Prog Fish Cult 35:2–8, 1973.

Linden O: The influence of crude oil and mixtures of crude oil dispersants on the ontogenic development of Baltic herring, *Clupea harengus membras* L. Ambio 5:136–140, 1976.

Lloyd R: Toxicity of zinc sulfate to rainbow trout. Ann Appl Biol 48:84–94, 1960.

Lorz HW, McPherson BP: Effects of copper or zinc in fish on the adaptation to sea water and ATPase activity and the effects of copper on migratory disposition of coho salmon (*Oncorhinchus kisutch*). J Fish Res Board Can 33: 2023–2030, 1976.

Lorz H, Glenn S, Williams R, Kunkel C, Norris L, Loper B: Effects of selected herbicides on smolting of coho salmon. EPA grant report R-804283. Corvallis, Ore.: U.S. EPA, 1978a.

Lorz HW, Williams RH, Fustish CA: Effects of several metals on smolting in coho salmon. Ecol Res Ser No EPA-600/3-78-090. Corvallis, Ore.: U.S. EPA, 1978b.

Macek KJ: Growth and resistance to stress in brook trout fed sublethal levels of DDT. J Fish Res Board Can 25:2443–2451, 1968.

Macek KJ, Birge W, Mayer FL, Buikema AL, Maki AW: Discussion session of synopsis of the use of aquatic toxicity tests for evaluation of the effects of toxic substances. In: Estimating the Hazard of Chemical Substances to Aquatic Life, edited by J Cairns, KL Dickson, AW Maki,

ASTM STP 657, pp. 27–32. Philadelphia, Pa.: ASTM, 1978.

Maki AW: Respiratory activity of fish as a predictor of chronic fish toxicity values for surfactants. In: Aquatic Toxicology, edited by LL Marking, RA Kimerle, ASTM STP 667, pp. 77–95. Philadelphia, Pa.: ASTM, 1979.

Marshall JS, Tompkins LS: Effect of *o,p'*-DDD and similar compounds on thyroxine binding globulin. J Clin Endocrinol 28:386–392, 1968.

Matton R, Lattam QN: Effect of the organophosphate Dylox on rainbow trout larvae. J Fish Res Board Can 26:2193–2200, 1969.

Mayer FL, Jr: Dynamics of dieldrin in rainbow trout and effects on oxygen consumption. Ph.D. thesis, Utah State Univ., Logan, Utah, 1970; University Microfilms, Ann Arbor, Mich.; Diss Abstr Int 32(1):527B, 1971.

Mayer FL, Jr, Kramer RH: Effects of hatchery water reuse on rainbow trout metabolism. Prog Fish Cult 35:9–10, 1973.

Mayer FL, Jr, Mehrle PM, Jr, Dwyer WP: Toxaphene: Chronic toxicity to fathead minnows and channel catfish. Ecol Res Ser No EPA-600/3-77-069. Duluth, Minn.: U.S. EPA, 1977a.

Mayer FL, Mehrle PM, Schoettger RA: Collagen metabolism in fish exposed to organic chemicals. In: Recent Advances in Fish Toxicology— A Symposium, edited by RA Tubb, pp. 31–54. Ecol Res Ser No EPA-600/3-77-085. Ore.: U.S. EPA, 1977b.

Mayer FL, Mehrle PM, Crutcher PL: Interaction of toxaphene and vitamin C in channel catfish. Trans Am Fish Soc 107:326–333, 1978.

Mayer FL, Adams WJ, Finley MT, Michael PR, Mehrle PM, Saeger VW: Phosphate ester hydraulic fluids: An aquatic environmental assessment of Pydraul 50E and 115E. In: Aquatic Toxicology and Hazard Assessment: Fourth Conference, edited by DR Branson, KL Dickson, ASTM STP 737. Philadelphia: ASTM, in press, 1981.

McCann JA, Jasper RL: Vertebral damage to bluegills exposed to acute levels of pesticides. Trans Am Fish Soc 101:317–322, 1972.

McCartney TH: Sodium-potassium dependent adenosine triphosphatase activity in gills and kidneys of Atlantic salmon (*Salmo salar*). Comp Biochem Physiol 53:351–353, 1976.

McKim JW, Benoit DA: Effects of longterm exposures to copper on survival, growth, and reproduction of brook trout (*Salvelinus fontinalis*). J Fish Res Board Can 28:655–662, 1971.

Mehrle PM, Mayer FL: Toxaphene effects on growth and bone composition of fathead minnows. *Pimephales promelas.* J Fish Res Board Can 32:593–598, 1975.

Mehrle PM, Jr, Mayer FL, Jr: Bone development and growth of fish as affected by toxaphene. In: Fate of Pollutants in Air and Water Environments, part 2, edited by JH Suffet, pp. 301–314, New York: Wiley Interscience, 1977.

Mehrle PM, Mayer FL, Buckler DR: Kepone and mirex: Effects on bone development and swim bladder composition in fathead minnows. Trans Am Fish Soc 110:636–641, 1981.

Mehrle PM, DeClue ME, Bloomfield RA: Phenylalanine metabolism altered by dietary dieldrin. Nature (Lond) 238:462–463, 1972.

Miles HM, Loehner SM, Michaud DT, Salviar SL: Physiological responses of hatchery reared muskellunge (*Esox masquinongy*) to handling. Trans Am Fish Soc 103:336, 1974.

Moore MR, Beattie AD, Thompson GG, Goldberg A: Depression of δ-aminolacvulinic acid dehydrase activity by ethanolamine in rat. Clin Sci 40:81–88, 1971.

Morgan RP, II, Fleming RF, Rasin VJ, Jr, Heinle DR: Sublethal effects of Baltimore harbor water on the white perch, *Morone americana,* and hogchoker, *Trinectes maculatus.* Chesapeake Sci 14:17–27, 1973.

Morgan WSG, Kuhn PC: A method to monitor the effects of toxicants upon breathing rate of largemouth bass (*Micropterus salmoides* Lacepede). Water Res 8:67–77, 1974.

Mount DI: Chronic effects of endrin on bluntnose minnows and guppies. U.S. Bur Sport Fish Wildl Res Rept 58, 1962.

Nicholson HP: Pesticide pollution control. Science 158:871–876, 1967.

O'Brien RD: Insecticides—Action and Metabolism. New York: Academic, 1967.

Orska J: Anomalies in the vertebral columns of the pike (*Esox lucius* L.). Acta Biol Cracov 5:327–345, 1962.

Post G, Leisure RA: Sublethal effect of malathion to three salmonid species. Bull Environ Contam Toxicol 12:312–319, 1974.

Rath S, Misra BN: Age-related changes in oxygen consumption by the gill, brain and muscle tissues of *Tilapia mossambica* Peters exposed to dichlorvos (DDVP). Environ Pollut (Ser A) 23:95–101, 1980.

Ribelin WE, Migaki G: The Pathology of Fishes. Madison: Univ. of Wisconsin Press, 1975.

Rice SD, Thomas RE, Short JW: Effect of petroleum hydrocarbons on breathing and coughing rates and hydrocarbon uptake-depuration in pink salmon fry. In: Physiological Responses of Marine Biota to Pollutants, edited by FJ Vernberg, A Calabrese, FP Thurberg, WB Vernberg, pp. 259–277. New York: Academic, 1977.

Riker WF, Jr, Huebner VR, Raska SB, Cattell M: Studies on DDT (2,2-bis[parachlorophenyl]-1,1-trichloroethane) effects on oxidative metabolism. J Pharmacol 88:327–332, 1946.

Saunders RL, Sprague JB: Effects of copper-zinc mining pollution on spawning migration of Atlantic salmon. Water Res 1:419–432, 1967.

Selye H: Stress and the general adaptive syndrome. Br Med J 1:1382–1392, 1950.

Sigmon C: Oxygen consumption in *Lepomis macrochirus* exposed to 2,4-D or 2,4,5-T. Bull Environ Contam Toxicol 21:826–830, 1979.

Silbergeld EK: Dieldrin effects of chronic sublethal exposure on adaptation to thermal stress in fresh water fish. Environ Sci Technol 7:846–849, 1973.

Sloof W: Detection limits of a biological monitoring system based on fish respiration. Bull Environ Contam Toxicol 23:517–523, 1979.

Sneed KE: Warmwater fish cultural laboratories. In: Progress in sport fisheries wildlife, U.S. Fish Wildl Serv Resour Publ 106, pp. 189–215, 1970.

Sparks RE, Cairns J, Jr, Heath AG: The use of bluegill breathing rates to detect zinc. Water Res 6:895–911, 1972.

Spencer SL: Internal injuries of largemouth bass and bluegills caused by electricity. Prog Fish Cult 29:168–169, 1967.

Sprague JB, Ramsay BA: Lethal levels of mixed copper-zinc solutions for juvenile salmon. J Fish Res Board Can 22:425–432, 1965.

Sprague JB, Elson PF, Saunders RL: Sublethal copper-zinc pollution in a salmon river. A field laboratory study. Proc 2nd Int Water Pollut Res Conf, Tokyo, pp. 61–82, 1965.

Swift DR: Seasonal variations in the growth rate, thyroid gland activity and food reserves of brown trout (Salmo trutta Linn.). J Exp Biol 32:751–764, 1955.

Symons PEK: Behavior of young Atlantic salmon exposed to or force-fed fenitrothion, an organophosphate insecticide. J Fish Res Board Can 30:651–655, 1973.

Van de Kamp G: Vertebral deformities of herring around the British Isles and their usefulness for a pollution monitoring programme. Int Counc Explor Sea 5, 1977.

Waiwood KG, Johansen PH: Oxygen consumption and activity of the white sucker (Catostomus commersoni) in lethal and nonlethal levels of the organochlorine insecticide, methoxychlor. Water Res 8:401–406, 1974.

Wedemeyer GA: Stress-induced ascorbic acid depletion and cortisol production in two salmonid fishes. Comp Biochem Physiol 29:1247–1251, 1969.

Wedemeyer GA, Yasutake WT: Clinical methods for the assessment of the effects of environmental stress of fish health. U.S. Fish Wildl Serv Tech Pap 89, 1977.

Wedemeyer G, Saunders RL, Clarke C: Environmental factors affecting smoltification and early marine survival of anadromous salmonids. Mar Fish Rev 42:1–14, 1980.

Weiss CM: The determination of cholinesterase in the brain tissue of three species of fresh water fish and its inactivation in vivo. Ecology 39:194–199, 1958.

Weiss CM: Physiological effect of organic phosphorus insecticides on several species of fish. Trans Am Fish Soc 90:143–152, 1961.

Weiss CM: Use of fish to detect organic insecticides in water. J Water Pollut Control Fed 37:647–658, 1965.

Weiss CM, Gakstatter JH: Detection of pesticides in water by biochemical assay. J Water Pollut Control Fed 37:647–658, 1964.

Wildish DJ, Lister NA: Biological effects of fenitrothion in the diet of brook trout. Bull Environ Contam Toxicol 10:333–339, 1973.

Williams AK, Sova RC: Acetylcholinesterase levels in brains of fishes from polluted waters. Bull Environ Contam Toxicol 1:198–204, 1966.

Wilson RT, Poe WE: Impaired collagen formation in the scorbutic channel catfish. J Nutr 103:1359–1364, 1973.

Wunder W: Ver Krüppelete Felchen uas der Biodensee. Zool Anz 194:279–292, 1975.

Yap HH, Desaiah D, Cutkomp LK, Koch RB: Sensitivity of fish ATPases to polychlorinated biphenyls. Nature (Lond) 233:61, 1971.

Zaugg WS, McLain LR: Adenosine triphosphatase activity in gills of salmonids: Seasonal variations and salt water influence in coho salmon, Oncorhynchus kisutch. Comp Biochem Physiol 35:587–596, 1970.

Zaugg WS, Wagner HH: Gill ATPase activity related to para-smolt transformation and migration in steelhead trout (Salmo gairdneri): Influence of photoperiod and temperature. Comp Biochem Physiol 45:955–965, 1973.

SUPPLEMENTAL READING

Baldwin E: An Introduction to Comparative Biochemistry. Cambridge, U.K.: Cambridge Univ Press, 1966.

Brown ME: The Physiology of Fishes, vol. 1, Metabolism, vol. 2, Behavior, New York: Academic, 1957.

Florey E: An Introduction to General and Comparative Animal Physiology. Philadelphia: Saunders, 1966.

Hoar WS, Randall DJ: Fish Physiology, vol. 1, Excretion, Ionic Regulation and Metabolism, vol. 2, Endocrine System, vol. 3, Reproduction and Growth, vol. 4, Nervous System, Circulation and Respiration, vol. 5, Sensory, vol. 6, Environmental Relations and Behavior, vol. 7, Locomotion, vol. 8, Bioenergetics and Growth. New York: Academic, 1969–1979.

Love MR: The Chemical Biology of Fishes. New York: Academic, 1970.

Singhal RL, Thomas JA: Lead Toxicity. Baltimore: Urban & Schwarzenberg, 1980.

Chapter 11

Histopathology

T. R. Meyers and J. D. Hendricks

INTRODUCTION

Overt signs of toxicity (loss of appetite, loss of equilibrium, discoloration, or death) are nearly always preceded by biochemical, physiological, and/or morphological changes in the organism. The ability to qualitatively or quantitatively measure these changes prior to death of the organism can often provide early indications of toxicity and valuable insights into the mechanisms of toxicity. This chapter concerns the field of

This work was supported in part by cooperative agreement CR809344-10 in the NCI/EPA Collaborative Program, Project 3, "Effects of Carcinogens, Mutagens and Teratogens in Nonhuman Species (Aquatic Animals)," administered by the Gulf Breeze Environmental Research Laboratory, and by Public Health Service grants ES01926 and ES00210 from the National Institute of Environmental Health Sciences. This is Technical Paper 5591 from the Oregon Agricultural Experiment Station, Oregon State University.

histopathology and its importance, use, and application in aquatic toxicology. Histopathology is the study of the structure of abnormal tissue. Examination of tissues from fish and other aquatic organisms after death may serve to identify the cause of death and possibly the causative agent. This information along with physiological and biochemical data may provide a more complete and accurate description of the activity of a chemical agent.

Although major advances have been made in recent years, the histology and histopathology of fish and aquatic invertebrates are still infant sciences compared with counterparts in mammals. There is probably no aquatic species whose normal histology is completely known. Only four atlases of normal histology exist: for the rainbow trout (Anderson and Mitchum, 1974), the channel catfish (Grizzle and Rogers, 1976), the American oyster (Galtsoff, 1964), and the blue crab (Johnson, 1980). These have been important contributions to the field, but represent only a fraction of the comprehensive literature that is available for mammals. The individual who desires to work in the area of aquatic animal histology or histopathology must draw heavily from basic mammalian histological and pathological concepts that are applicable to all living tissues and from the scattered literature on aquatic animal histology and pathology. Ultimately, such an individual may become the expert on a particular aquatic species, since it is possible that no one else has studied it.

The following sections present some routine diagnostic methods that may be used in aquatic histopathology to evaluate abnormal tissue changes resulting from exposure of the organism to a toxicant. Also included are definitions of commonly used terms and a review of the literature on toxic histopathology in aquatic organisms.

TERMINOLOGY

A glossary is presented below to define certain pathology terms mentioned within the text and literature review. Most definitions have been adapted from Stedman's Medical Dictionary (1976), Smith et al. (1972), and Schalm (1970). Another useful reference is the Glossary of Fish Health Terms (Post and Klontz, 1977).

Adenoma. Benign epithelial tumor in which cells form fairly well-differentiated glandular structures.

Adenomatous. Resembling an adenoma, sometimes referring to glandular hyperplasia.

Anemia. Reduction in the oxygen transport capabilities per unit volume of blood due to below-normal numbers of erythrocytes and/or a decreased hemoglobin concentration. Anemias are usually secondary diseases and are classified by cause and on the basis of morphological characteristics of erythrocytes.

Anisochromasia. Variability in staining characteristics of individual cell cytoplasms and/or nuclei within a population of cells; unequal cytoplasmic staining within a single cell as seen in

erythrocytes from certain anemias due to unequal distribution of hemoglobin.

Anisocytosis. Extreme differences in cell size within a normally uniform population, particularly seen in certain blood diseases.

Anophthalmia. Congenital defect where one or both eyes are absent.

Atrophy. Wasting of cells, organs, or entire body resulting from various causes including necrosis and reabsorption of cells, decreased cellular proliferation, malnutrition, decreased use, pressure, ischemia, or hormonal changes.

Ballooning degeneration. Separation of epithelial cells from one another classically seen in the deeper cell layers of the epidermis. Usually follows intracytoplasmic edema and vacuolation.

Catarrhal enteritis. Inflammation of any or all of the intestinal tract characterized by excessive mucus production accompanied by epithelial necrosis and desquamation. Necrosis may often predominate, in which case little or no mucus is evident from lack of a secreting membrane.

Centrilobular. Refers to the central area of hepatic parenchyma immediately surrounding the central vein of a liver lobule.

Ceroid. High molecular weight intracellular lipofuscin pigment resulting from autoxidation of phospholipids and unsaturated fats accompanied by polymerization. Thus, ceroid is insoluble in organic solvents, characteristically acid-fast, variably PAS-positive, sudanophilic in both frozen and paraffin sections, and negative with iron stains. Ceroid is found in cases of vitamin E deficiency, wasting diseases, and old age (Figs. 1 and 2).

Cirrhosis. Proliferative form of chronic hepatic inflammation characterized by replacement of parenchyma by new fibrous connective tissue generally beginning at the portal triads.

Cloudy swelling (acute cellular swelling). Earliest degenerative change within a cell, caused by influx of water, characterized by enlarged cell and homogeneous "ground glass" appearance of cytoplasm (Fig. 3).

Congestion. Excessive amount of blood within vessels producing a "pavementing" effect in the

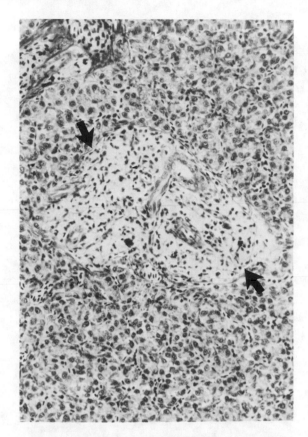

Figure 1 Portion of liver from a yearling rainbow trout after 1 yr on a diet containing 50 ppm sterculic acid, a cyclopropenoid fatty acid. Note the clear, lightly staining material in the cells of the expanded melanomacrophage center (arrows). H&E, ×440.

Edema. Excessive amounts of water collecting in intercellular spaces and/or body cavities.

Electron microscopy (EM). Use of a high-voltage electron beam with shorter wavelengths than visible light to observe fine structural detail not resolved with conventional light microscopy. Two-dimensional (transmission EM) and three-dimensional (scanning EM) viewing are routinely used.

Epithelioma. Benign neoplasm involving epithelial cells of the epidermis, including those of the adnexa.

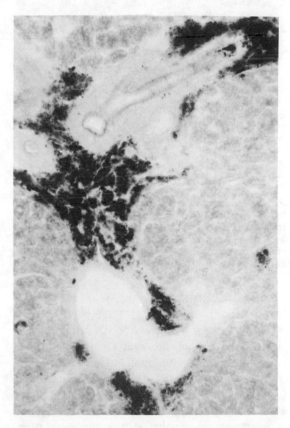

Figure 2 Frozen section of liver from the fish shown in Fig. 1, but stained with Sudan Black. Melanomacrophage centers are intensely sudanophilic, indicating the presence of a lipid material. In paraffin sections this material was also positive with periodic acid-Schiff reagent and was acid-fast, both characteristics of a ceroid pigment. ×440.

lumina. Cause is usually insufficient venous drainage of blood (passive).

Degenerative changes. Early abnormal pre-necrotic changes in cellular detail, many of which are reversible up to a certain point (i.e., fatty change, hydropic degeneration, cloudy swelling, etc.).

Desquamation. Sloughing of cells from an epithelial surface due to necrosis, some degenerative change, or from postmortem autolysis (Fig. 4).

Dysplasia. Abnormal alteration in size, shape and organization of adult cells or tissue (Figs. 5 and 6).

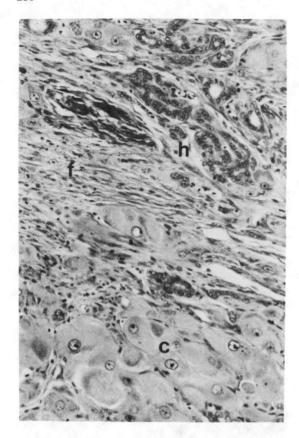

Figure 3 Section of liver from a 9-mo-old rainbow trout fed the control diet plus 100 ppm pyrrolizidine alkaloids for 6 mo. Replacement of degenerate hypertrophied hepatocytes with extensive fibrosis (f), cloudy swelling (c) of hepatocytes, and bile ductule hyperplasia (h) are illustrated. H&E, ×440. [From Hendricks et al. (1981).]

Erythema. Redness of the skin caused by inflammation.

Exophthalmos ("popeye"). Unilateral or bilateral extrusion of the eyes from their sockets commonly caused by accumulation of gas bubbles (nitrogen "gas bubble" disease) or edema fluids (osmoregulatory problems due to kidney lesions, etc.) beneath the eye globes.

Extravasation. Passing outside the vasculature, usually referring to blood or lymph. A large hemorrhage within a tissue.

Fatty change. Intracytoplasmic accumulation of neutral fat droplets. It is considered to be a

degenerative change independent of, but often occurring with, necrosis and is commonly found in the liver and kidney epithelium (Figs. 7 and 8). Fatty change results from inhibition of transport or metabolism of lipid. Because neutral fat is dissolved by organic solvents used in histological preparation, it appears as well demarcated unstained areas within the cell cytoplasm.

Fibrinoid degeneration. Degeneration occurring in fibrous connective tissue, probably resulting from a local antigen-antibody reaction. It appears to be either fibrin from an inflammatory exudate or degenerative collagen, which stains dirty pink

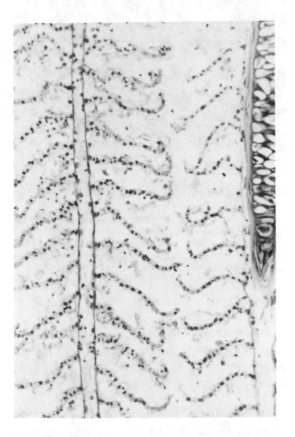

Figure 4 Portions of two gill filaments from a yearling coho salmon exposed to the herbicide dinoseb at 100 ppm in water for 114 h. Note the nearly complete necrosis and desquamation of the respiratory epithelium from the underlying pillar cells and blood sinuses. H&E, ×440.

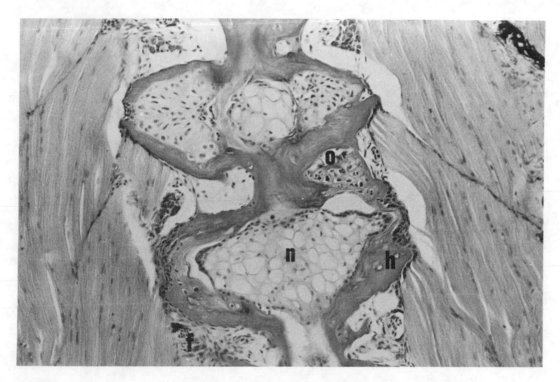

Figure 5 Vertebral dysplasia in *Cyprinodon variegatus* exposed for 30 d to 31 µg/l trifluralin in flowing seawater. Note the enlarged notochord (n), persistence and proliferation of osteoblasts (o) and/or fibroblasts (f), and semisymmetric hypertrophy (h) of the vertebral walls. H&E, ×258. *[Courtesy of Dr. John Couch, U.S. Environmental Protection Agency, Gulf Breeze, Florida.]*

and has fewer nuclei than surrounding normal tissues.

Fibroplasia or fibrosis. Adequate or excessive production of new fibrous connective tissue as a repair response to cell death following or concomitant with inflammation (Fig. 3).

Granuloma. Mass or focus of granulation tissue. There are two basic types: fibrous granuloma, which is composed of inflammatory cells, actively proliferating fibrous connective tissue, and numerous capillary buds, and reticuloendothelial granuloma, which contains proliferating macrophages or histiocytes, usually circumscribed by a collar of lymphocytes. A granuloma is a chronic host defense mechanism to wall off the site of infectious, toxic, or mechanical irritation.

Heinze bodies. Round, oval to serrated, cytoplasmic inclusion bodies observed within erythrocytes, usually indicative of hemolytic anemia following exposure to certain toxic compounds. Inclusions are refractile when unstained, blue when stained with new methylene blue. They are usually located adjacent to or protruding from the cell wall, but can be found free in the blood plasma.

Hemorrhage. Presence of blood outside the vasculature due to injury of the vessel walls.

Hemostasis. Stoppage of blood flow either by hemorrhage or in part of the vascular circulation.

Histochemistry. Qualitative identification of the normal and abnormal intracytoplasmic distribution of various cell products and assimilated chemicals (lipids, polysaccharides, nucleic acids, enzymes, etc.) and reaction sites by use of several methods including specific chemical stains, immunofluorescence, autoradiography, and electron microscopy.

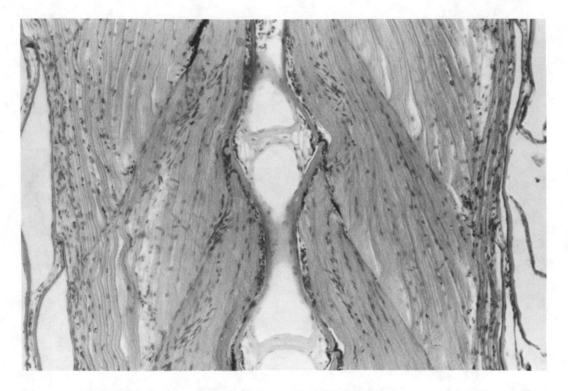

Figure 6 Normal vertebral structure from a control *Cyprinodon variegatus*, sectioned at the same level as the trifluralin-exposed specimen. Note vestigial notochord and thin-walled vertebrae. H&E, ×258. *[Courtesy of Dr. John Couch.]*

Histology. Study of normal microscopic and ultrastructural anatomy of animals or plants including the structure and function of cells, tissues, and organs. This is done by observing stained paraffin tissue sections with light microscopy and ultrathin sections with electron microscopy.

Howell-Jolly bodies. Round nuclear remnants eccentrically located in a young erythrocyte, usually one per cell. Can be indicative of a remissive anemia, but occur normally at low levels in the cat and the horse.

Hyalin degeneration. Cellular change characterized by glassy homogeneous eosinophilic material seen as droplets within cell cytoplasm or found replacing entire cells or cellular areas.

Hydropic degeneration. Accumulation of water within the cytoplasm of a swollen epithelial cell, appearing as a clear vacuole or vacuoles with an indistinct edge often adjacent to or surrounding the nucleus. This change may be a further sequence of cloudy swelling (Fig. 9).

Hyperchromic. More intensely staining.

Hyperemia. Excessive blood within the vasculature, distinguished from congestion by its "active" cause—dilated arteries delivering too much blood for proper venous drainage.

Hyperplasia. Increased proliferation of a cell population, usually in response to an irritant (toxic or infectious), endocrine imbalance, or nutritional deficiency. Normal tissue function and architecture may be impaired as observed in gill epithelium when hyperplasia causes overgrowth of cells ("clubbing") and cellular fusion of filaments and lamellae (Figs. 3, 10, and 11).

Hypertrophy. Increase in individual cell size and functional ability, sometimes resulting in a concomitant increase in tissue or organ size. Hypertrophy can occur from an increase in functional demand, which may be compensatory or hormonal in origin (Figs. 3, 5, 6, 7, 8, 10, 11).

Infarct. Localized area of tissue necrosis (usually coagulative) caused by insufficient blood supply due to vascular obstruction.

Inflammation. Dynamic process of events involving vascular and exudative stages occurring only in viable tissues that have been injured by an irritant. This response permits humoral and cellular elements of the immune system to interact with the causative agent at local sites of tissue damage in order that healing may occur. Inflam-

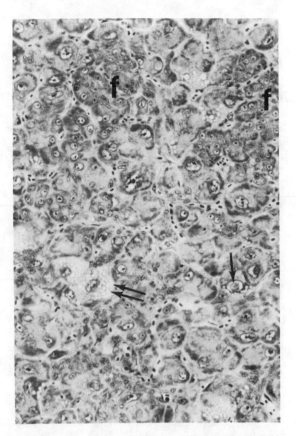

Figure 8 Portion of liver from a 9-mo-old rainbow trout fed the control diet plus 20 ppm mixed pyrrolizidine alkaloids from tansy ragwort plant for 6 mo. Note the great hypertrophy (megalocytosis) of the hepatocytes, the microdroplet fatty change (double arrow) in some of the cells, the abnormal cell shapes and staining characteristics, and intranuclear inclusion bodies (single arrow). Two foci (f) of small basophilic, regenerating hepatocytes are visible in the upper portion of the photomicrograph. H&E, ×440. *[From Hendricks et al. (1981).]*

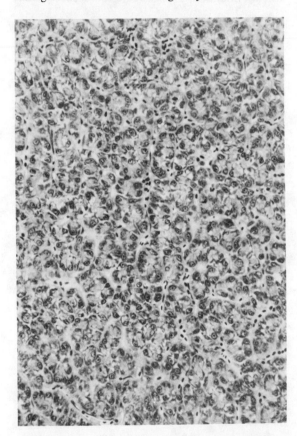

Figure 7 Portion of normal liver from 9-mo-old control rainbow trout. Note the small uniform size of the hepatic parenchymal cells and their nuclei. Hepatic tubulocords are two cells in width. H&E, ×440. *[From Hendricks et al. (1981).]*

mation is classified according to the morphological nature of the exudate, which varies with the type of tissue involved and the causative agent. Six forms of inflammation are recognized:

(*a*) *Serous inflammation,* characterized by a watery exudation of blood serum, often in peritoneal cavities or formed vesicles, with microscopic appearance of homogeneous pink staining precipitate mixed with a few leukocytes and slight amounts of fibrin.

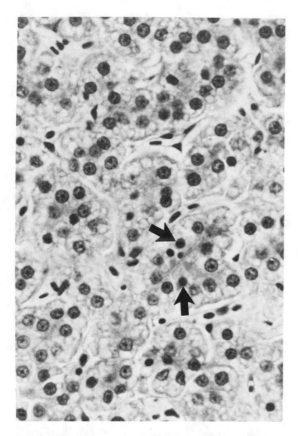

Figure 9 Portion of liver from a yearling coho salmon water exposed to 100 ppm of the herbicide amitrole for 144 h. Note the extreme hydropic degenerative changes in the hepatocytes, visualized as clear cytoplasmic vacuoles, some surrounding the nuclei. Several cells in each hepatic cord have undergone necrosis, as evidenced by pyknotic nuclei (arrows). H&E, ×1101.

(*b*) *Fibrinous inflammation*, with an exudate composed predominantly of clotted fibrin, usually occurring on mucous and serous membranes, particularly the pericardium. Microscopically, the exudate contains dirty pink staining fibrillar material adhering to a hyperemic parent surface usually accompanied by variable amounts of leukocytes, erythrocytes, and other precipitated serum proteins. A thick fibrin exudate that becomes firmly attached to its parent surface denotes a diphtheritic inflammation.

(*c*) *Purulent inflammation*, in which the exudate contains pus, which consists of variable numbers of necrotic and living neutrophils in or on the tissues accompanied by congestion and small amounts of fibrin, serum, and other leukocytes. If neutrophils predominate over other elements, the inflammation is said to be "suppurative." Although fish have neutrophils, purulent inflammation, particularly abscesses (circumscribed accumulations of pus), rarely occurs in teleosts.

(*d*) *Hemorrhagic inflammation*, consisting of an exudate that may contain many of the other exudative components above but also large accumulations of erythrocytes obviously outside vascular channels. This exudate can occur diffusely

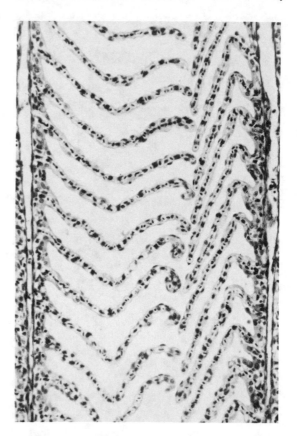

Figure 10 Normal gill structure from a yearling control coho salmon (*Oncorhynchus kisutch*). Note the single layer of squamous epithelial cells covering the lamellae and the basal interlamellar regions of the gill filament. H&E, ×440.

within tissues but more often involves mucous membranes.

(*e*) *Catarrhal or mucous inflammation*, which involves only mucous membranes since the principal component of the exudate is mucous secreted from host cells. Under the microscope, affected membranes may demonstrate hyperplasia of mucous goblet cells accompanied by attached overlying gray- or blue-staining strands of mucin. More often the membrane surface undergoes necrosis and desquamation, exposing an underlying hyperemic connective tissue infiltrated with varying amounts of lymphocytes.

(*f*) *Lymphocytic inflammation*, which results

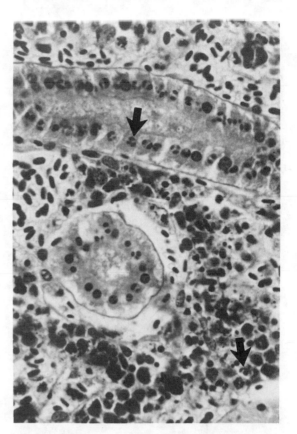

Figure 12 Portion of kidney tissue from a yearling coho salmon following water exposure to 100 ppm of the herbicide amitrole for 144 h. All the tubular cells and many of the surrounding hematopoietic cells have undergone necrosis; nuclear changes of pyknosis and karyorrhexis (arrows) are clearly visible. H&E, ×1101.

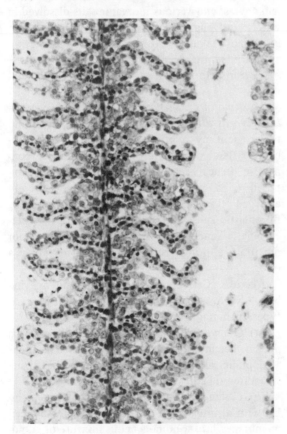

Figure 11 Gill filament from a yearling coho salmon following water exposure to 100 ppm paraquat for 120 h. Note both hypertrophy of individual epithelial cells and hyperplasia, particularly in the basal interlamellar region. H&E, ×440.

from infiltration of lymphocytes within affected tissues accompanied by some hyperemia. Histologically, tissues appear normal, except for slight vascular congestion and collections of lymphocytes, often surrounding the vessels (perivascular cuffing). Tissues in which this type of inflammation commonly occurs include nervous tissue, portal triads of the liver, and lamina propria of the gut. The latter two areas normally have resident populations of lymphocytes, which vary in number according to animal species.

Ischemia. Insufficient blood supply.

Karyolysis. Necrotic change characterized by

dissolution of a cell nucleus, recognized by incomplete stages where only nuclear outlines are visible.

Karyorrhexis. Necrotic change characterized by rupture of the nuclear membrane and fragmentation of the cell nucleus. These fragments may remain at the original site of the nucleus or may be scattered about with other necrotic debris (Fig. 12).

Lesion. Abnormal change within a cell, tissue, or organ.

Leukopenia. Abnormal reduction in circulating white blood cells per unit volume of blood.

Metaplasia. Change from one cell type to another within the limits of the original primary tissue, such as squamous cell metaplasia of cuboidal or columnar epithelium. Metaplasia has been seen only in epithelium and connective tissue. The cause is a change in demand of function.

Microphthalmia. Congenital defect in which one or both eyeballs are abnormally small.

Mucin. Mucopolysaccharide cellular secretion that stains gray to blue with hematoxylin and eosin.

Mucus. Viscid complex cellular secretion that functions as a cleansing agent, lubricant, and/or protective barrier at various membrane surfaces. Mucus is comprised of mucin, epithelial cells, leukocytes, and various inorganic salts dissolved in water, and may contain immunoglobulins and lysozymes, which provide localized protection against infectious agents.

Myositis. Inflammation of smooth or skeletal muscle.

Myxomatous degeneration (mucoid degeneration; serous atrophy of fat). Proliferation of and replacement by a primitive embryonal-type connective tissue where fibrous and/or adipose connective tissues occur. Myxomatous tissue is composed of a mucinous grayish to blue loosely arranged fibrillar ground substance containing fibroblastic cells with stellate to spherical hyperchromatic nuclei. The primary cause is poor nutrition, although certain toxemias may play a role.

Necrosis. Cell or tissue death within a living body. Necrosis is classified as several histological types, including:

(*a*) *Coagulative necrosis*, death of cells in which nuclei become pyknotic, cytoplasm becomes acidophilic, and cellular outlines and other tissue structures are still visible (Figs. 4, 9, 12).

(*b*) *Caseous necrosis*, loss of differential staining with disintegration of tissue structures and cell membranes into a homogeneous mixture of granular debris that is basophilic to purple with hematoxylin and eosin.

(*c*) *Liquefactive necrosis*, rapid and complete dissolution of cells and tissue structures leaving

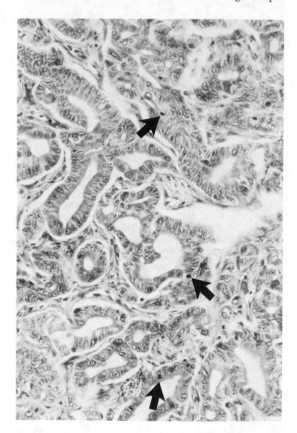

Figure 13 Portion of a cholangiocarcinoma induced in the liver of a rainbow trout by continuous feeding of 25 ppm *p,p'*-DDT for 21 mo. Note the irregular nature of the bile ducts and the frequent mitotic figures (arrows). H&E, ×440.

ragged-edged spaces filled with fluid, which may or may not have a residue of pink proteinaceous material when stained. An abscess produces a form of liquefactive necrosis in which fluid contains neutrophils, fibrin, and cellular debris.

(*d*) *Fat necrosis,* saponification of neutral fat into solvent-stable soap appearing solid and opaque within the dead fat cells. The soap may have small clefts from dissolved fatty acid crystals and should stain pink, purple, or blue, depending on which metallic ions (potassium, calcium, sodium, respectively) combined with the fatty acid radical during soap formation.

(*e*) *Zenker's necrosis,* which is similar to coagulative necrosis but occurs only in skeletal muscle, where changes are characterized by swelling of individual muscle fibers, marked homogeneous texture and acidophilia of the sarcoplasm, obscurity of myofibrils (striations), and pyknosis of nuclei.

Further descriptions of necroses may be based on distribution or location of the lesion—diffuse, focal, perivascular, and so on.

Neoplasia. Pathological transformation of a normal host cell resulting in uncontrolled proliferation into new cells without normal histological architecture or normal cellular functions. These cells usually bear some resemblance to the normal tissue of origin, although some malignant forms may appear so undifferentiated that cell identification of the growth or tumor is difficult (Fig. 13). For a discussion of tumor classification see the section on general types of tissue changes.

Nephrosis. Degenerative changes that may lead to necrosis in the nephrons of the kidney which do not involve an inflammatory process (called nephritis). Blood-borne toxic materials are common causes of nephrosis, particularly in renal tubular epithelium (Fig. 12).

Neutrophilia. Abnormally high percentage of neutrophil granulocytes in circulating blood, which may also cause an absolute increase in total number of peripheral white blood cells (leukocytosis).

Osteoblast. The cell responsible for the forma-

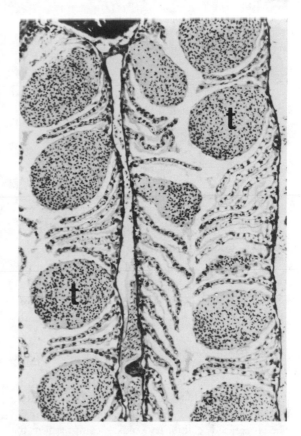

Figure 14 Portions of two gill filaments from a yearling coho salmon exposed to the herbicide atrazine at 15 ppm in water for 140 h. Note the severe telangiectasia (t) of the blood sinuses of the individual lamellae. H&E, X275.

tion of osteoid or bone matrix. An osteoblast is eventually surrounded by bone and then becomes an osteocyte (Fig. 5).

Pathology. The medical science concerned with the study of abnormal changes, and their causes, within the cells, tissues, and organs of an individual or a population.

Periportal. Referring to the area of tissue immediately surrounding a portal triad within the liver.

Petechiae. Small pinpoint hemorrhages.

Poikilocytosis. Distortion or abnormal variation in cell shape, usually referring to erythrocytes in certain blood diseases.

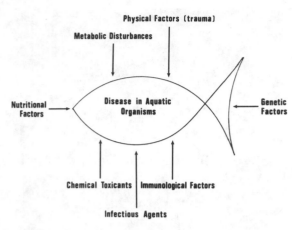

Figure 15 Etiologic factors of disease in aquatic organisms.

Polycythemia (erythrocytosis). Abnormal increase in the number of red blood cells per unit volume of blood.

Proliferative glomerulonephritis. Inflammation of the kidney glomeruli characterized by hypertrophy of glomerular tufts due to increased infiltration of leukocytes and proliferation of endothelial and visceral epithelial cells (podocytes). The increased cellularity causes compression of glomerular capillaries, leading to thrombosis and necrosis with subsequent hemorrhage into Bowman's space. Proliferating podocytes may cause adhesions with the parietal epithelium of Bowman's capsule, producing "epithelial crescents." There is no thickening of the glomerular basement membrane or alteration in foot processes of podocytes; these 2 anomalies help distinguish this condition from membranous glomerulonephritis.

Pyknosis. Necrotic change in cell nuclei characterized by a rounding up and condensation that causes hyperchromatic staining (Figs. 9 and 12).

Scoliosis. Lateral curvature of the spinal column. A combination of backward curvature with the lateral curvature is termed lordoscoliosis.

Telangiectasia. Marked dilation of terminal blood vessels within a part, usually capillaries (Fig. 14).

Thrombocytopenia. Abnormal reduction in thrombocyte or platelet cell numbers per unit volume of blood.

Thrombus. Blood clot, formed within a vessel or heart chamber of a living animal, which may obstruct blood flow or only partly so by attaching to the vessel wall.

Vasodilation. Enlargement of a vessel lumen.

POSSIBLE ETIOLOGIES OF HISTOPATHOLOGY IN AQUATIC ORGANISMS

In the science of pathology, the investigator must first know the normal variations of gross and microscopic anatomy in the necropsy (autopsy) subject. This is a challenge with fish and shellfish because there are many species that often differ somewhat in gross and histological appearance. For example, in lake trout the epithelium of the small distal portion of the convoluted tubule in the kidney often contains large cytoplasmic vacuoles (Walsh and Ribelin, 1975). In other fish species this might suggest a degenerative change, possibly resulting from toxic materials in the glomerular filtrate. In experimental situations, the use of normal unexposed control animals maintained under identical environmental conditions should eliminate confusion of normal features with those of true lesions. Although some field studies may require pathological interpretations without adequate control tissues for comparison, it cannot be overstressed that controls are indispensable for diagnosis of specific lesions and their etiologies.

The investigator must also be able to recognize postmortem pathology that begins immediately after death. This is due to the autolytic processes of extracellular and intracellular enzymes and to putrefaction by resident bacterial flora. Consequently, accurate interpretation of cellular and tissue morphology requires preservation and examination of tissues as soon after death as possible. For a useful discussion of invertebrate postmortem changes, the reader is referred to Sparks (1972).

Equally important is the distinction of toxicological lesions from those that may have resulted from other causes (Fig. 15). Collection, handling, and sampling procedures and design of animal maintenance facilities should be examined as possible sources of traumatic or self-inflicted injuries. Fin nipping by other fish and tank abrasions are quite common; they often result in white necrotic areas at fin tips or scraped and ulcerated regions on the body surface, particularly on the snout. These lesions may become secondarily infected with bacterial or fungal organisms and may ultimately lead to morbidity. In wild fish predator attacks can lead to stab, bite, or scrape lesions, which eventually heal via granulation tissue unless also infected by an opportunistic pathogen. Other physical factors in the environment can cause lesions in fish: particulate irritants including silt, ash, and dust can abrade delicate gill tissues, which usually respond by proliferation (hyperplasia) of epithelium; supersaturation of dissolved gases (nitrogen, oxygen) in the water can cause formation of gas bubbles in fish tissues (gas bubble disease). Lesions resulting from gas bubble disease may include external swellings, exophthalmia, gas emboli in vasculature, and edema of secondary gill lamellae and other tissues as well. Sunburn, probably caused by excessive exposure to ultraviolet radiation, can occur in cultured fish kept in uncovered shallow raceways, but it has also been reported in feral fish. The typical lesion is a focal necrosis on the crown of the head, which may become secondarily infected with bacteria or fungi. In young fish, necrosis and hemorrhage may involve the meninx primitiva and optic lobes of the brain, since they lie very close to the undersurface of the cranial capsule. Dietary photosensitization syndrome may be an alternative explanation for sunburn in fish (Roberts, 1978b).

Poor nutritional status, such as vitamin and amino acid deficiencies, can result in a wide variety of lesions, which could confuse identification of toxicological pathologies. For instance, proliferative gill lesions are often observed after exposure of fish to water-soluble toxicants. However, a deficiency in pantothenic acid, a necessary constituent of coenzyme A responsible for normal fat and carbohydrate metabolism, causes a similar gill pathology. Lesions of this "nutritional gill disease" consist of lamellar epithelial hyperplasia with eventual fusion of secondary lamellae near the tips of gill filaments (Cowey and Roberts, 1978). Since lesions may result from poor nutrition, fish used in toxicological studies must be fed a nutritionally adequate diet free of any contaminant that might bias the results. If a toxicant is administered orally with the food, its effect on the palatability of the diet is important. Refusal to feed if the diet is off-flavored results in malnutrition and no exposure to the toxicant.

Congenital anomalies, presumed to be gene-mediated disorders, can occur in fish offspring. These conditions include vertebral deformities, anomalous fin development, shortened operculae, foreshortened or overextended jaws, polycystic conditions in viscera of trout, hypoplastic swim bladder in certain cyprinodonts and Siamese twins (Roberts, 1978c). Genetically induced neoplasia was observed when two closely related species of aquarium fish were artificially hybridized: platy (*Xiphophorus maculatus*) and swordtail (*X. helleri*) crosses developed malignant melanomas (Gordon, 1959; Sobel et al., 1975).

Lesions in fish resulting directly from primary metabolic disturbances have been described only for sexually mature individuals that were ready to spawn. Vascular lesions, consisting of intimal hypertrophy, cartilaginous metaplasia, and fibrosis, occur in Pacific (*Oncorhynchus* sp.) and Atlantic (*Salmo salar*) salmon and steelhead trout concomitant with drastic changes in sexual hormone levels during spawning migration (Robertson et al., 1961; Van Citters and Watson, 1968; Maneche et al., 1972). Interestingly, these lesions regress in the steelhead that survive the spawning ordeal. In Pacific salmon increases in serum levels of 17-hydroxycorticosteroids cause an increase in cell numbers and intracellular products in the pituitary and adrenal glands. These changes are indicative of increased organ function; however, at full maturity cells of the pituitary undergo degenerative changes and the adrenal is hyperplastic (Robertson and Wexler, 1962a, 1962b). Hyperglycemia concurrent with hyperplasia of the endocrine pancreas (islets of Langerhans) may also occur (Love, 1970), as well as degeneration and atrophy of glomerular elements (Hay et al., 1976). Metabolic disturbances secondary to other primary causes are responsible for additional disease syndromes: sekoke disease of carp (*Cyprinus carpio*), initiated by silkworm pupae in the diet, is characterized by degranulation of B cells in the islets of the pancreas, causing diabetes mellitus accompanied by a retinopathy, thickening of the gill basement membranes, and telangiectasia of lamellar sinusoids (Yokote, 1974); goiter of the thyroid gland resulting from iodine deficiency (Cowey and Roberts, 1978).

Fish are immunologically competent, with cellular and humoral responses similar to those in higher vertebrates. Immediate type hypersensitivity reactions such as anaphylactic shock have been reported in various fish species (Dreyer and King, 1948), including goldfish (*Carassius auratus*) and channel catfish (*Ictalurus punctatus*) (Goven et al., 1980). It is likely that immune complex mediated or immunodeficiency diseases (and lesions) occur in fish; however, none have been reported as of this writing.

Infectious diseases are another major source of lesions, and close examination of tissues by use of histochemical techniques and microbiological procedures may be needed to eliminate bacteriological, viral, fungal, protozoal, or other parasitic etiologies. Because many of these pathogens are opportunistic, occurring as secondary invaders, the primary cause of a lesion may not be obvious despite the overwhelming presence of a particular infectious agent. Thus, caution must be exercised in interpreting lesions of this nature. An extremely helpful reference on necropsy and diagnostic procedures for infectious diseases of fish is provided by McDaniel (1979). Voluminous descriptive literature exists on infectious diseases of fish and resultant pathologies; the investigator is referred to Roberts (1978a) or Ribelin and Migaki

(1975) for further information. Overstreet (1978) is also a useful source for disease studies of marine fish and invertebrates.

It becomes apparent from the discussion above that, although various factors other than toxicants can be primary initiators of disease and tissue pathology, a histopathologic etiology may involve two or more of these factors acting in a synergistic manner; for instance, genetic inbreeding can produce immune-deficient offspring that are more susceptible to infectious disease. This type of relationship emphasizes the complexities that face the aquatic pathologist in interpreting lesions and diagnosing disease.

GENERAL TYPES OF TISSUE CHANGES

General Inflammatory Process

Regardless of cause, there are certain fundamental changes that can occur in tissues, and these changes form the basis of descriptive pathology. Many of these changes are part of or result from the inflammatory response in the living animal. Inflammation is a dynamic series of events that occur only in viable tissues in response to an irritant. The biological function of the inflammatory response is to destroy or "wall off" irritating substances so that damaged tissue may heal. Many entities can act as irritants, causing tissue damage and necrosis (necrotic tissue itself is an irritant) eliciting an inflammatory response; examples are infectious agents (bacteria, viruses, protozoans, fungi, metazoans) and their toxic metabolites, mechanical injuries, chemical toxicants, inanimate foreign bodies, antibody-antigen complexes, sequestered antigens, infarcts, and loss of nervous innervation. The events that comprise the inflammatory response are essentially the same in all vertebrates and have been described in great detail (Zweifach et al., 1965; Smith et al., 1972). Classic early inflammation involves vascular and exudative stages accompanied, in higher animals, by the four cardinal signs of redness, swelling, heat, and pain. In lower poikilothermic vertebrates heat is not likely to be one of the cardinal signs; however, the rate of the inflammatory process fluctuates directly with ambient temperature.

Inflammation begins following tissue damage, which initiates release of chemical mediators from resident mast cells and basophilic leukocytes. These mediators (histamine, serotonin, kinins, and so on) are vasoactive amines that affect vessels in the immediate area of injury by causing vasodilation and increased vascular permeability (enlargement of fenestrae in capillary walls). The vascular dilation allows an initial increase in blood flow (hyperemia causing redness and heat), while the more permeable vessel walls permit passage of serum proteins, erythrocytes, and migrating leukocytes (neutrophils, macrophages, lymphocytes) into nearby injured tissues (causing swelling). Fibrinogen, an important terminal component in the cascading clotting mechanism, is among the serum proteins that escape into the wound; it polymerizes (clots) to an insoluble protein, fibrin, which provides a fibrillar network for enhanced amoeboid migration of immunologically activated leukocytes. Continual loss of fluid from the blood and the adhesiveness of leukocytes finally cause a localized increase in blood viscosity with retardation of flow and eventual stasis. This passive congestion further enhances escape of humoral and cellular elements into the injured tissues. This exudative stage of inflammation is extremely important for tissue recovery because it is here that serum antibody and activated leukocytes of the immune system are liberated to attack the initial irritant (and its metabolites), necrotic host cells, and other deleterious products released by injured cells. These noxious substances and the exudative swelling irritate nerve endings, causing pain, the last of the cardinal signs.

Types of Inflammation

Inflammation is classified into various types according to the identity of the predominating elements in the exudate. Six types of inflammation have been recognized (see Terminology section for complete description of each): (1) serous inflammation, (2) fibrinous inflammation, (3) purulent inflammation, (4) hemorrhagic inflammation, (5) catarrhal or mucous inflammation, and (6) lymphocytic inflammation. Each type may be further classified according to duration and whether proliferation of new fibrous connective tissue has occurred. An acute inflammation is one that has a sudden clinical onset and progresses rapidly to recovery with no associated proliferation of connective tissue. A chronic inflammation is one that begins imperceptibly and continues for an indefinite period with resultant production of mature fibrous connective tissue. A subacute classification is intermediate, characterized by proliferation of new connective tissue that is not yet mature.

Results of Inflammation

The sequellae or outcome of inflammation in the host can be resolution, death, or continuation to chronicity. Resolution is characterized by complete restoration of tissues to their normal appearance and function by local proliferation of the necessary specific cell types (regeneration). In many acute inflammations, the host response is adequate in quickly removing the irritant, which is unable to cause extensive tissue injury. The degree of acute response is usually dependent on how well the host is able to recognize the irritant as nonself. This is also true for poikilotherms except, as mentioned before, the efficiency of foreign body recognition is dependent on optimum ambient temperatures, which vary among species.

In some cases acute inflammation is unable to destroy an injurious agent, and there is severe damage to vital tissues, followed by death. In extremely acute infectious diseases or toxicant exposures, death can occur so rapidly that tissue injuries appear insignificant and inflammatory changes have not yet had time to occur. Microscopic interpretation of such tissues may provide little information for diagnostic purposes.

Another possible outcome is that inflammation is unsuccessful in completely eliminating the initiating agent, which spreads and causes continuous and sometimes extensive tissue damage—a situation that allows little or no regeneration of parent tissue cells. This inadequate response often leads to a chronic inflammation with proliferation of new tissue, usually by fibrosis, as an attempt to wall off the irritant and replace lost cells. Since fibrous connective tissue can function only in a supportive manner, the specialized functions of replaced cells are lost. This process can continue indefinitely and may result in eventual death of the host due to replacement of vital tissues by the lesion.

The formation of fibrous granulomata is an example of a chronic proliferative inflammation that is quite common in fish and is usually caused by certain bacteria, fungi, or noninfectious foreign bodies. Early in development, these lesions are characterized by acute inflammation. This is followed by chronic multifocal proliferations, each of which appears as a central zone of necrotic cellular debris, often containing the causative agent, surrounded by a layer of epithelioid cells (macrophages resembling epithelial cells) interspersed with other leukocytes with encapsulation of the entire focus by new fibrous connective tissue. Another type of granuloma is formed principally by reticuloendothelial cells, which appear as small foci of proliferating macrophages or histiocytes, usually circumscribed by a collar of lymphocytes.

The inflammatory response can be excessive rather than adequate or inadequate. The inflammation may be able to eliminate or compromise the initiating irritant, but the severity or anatomic location of the response may threaten to kill the host before this can be accomplished. For example, exposure of fish to various infectious agents or toxic materials results in an exuberant proliferative inflammation of the gills. This is characterized by some infiltration of leukocytes and proliferation of connective tissue elements, but the outstanding feature is epithelial hyperplasia that causes fusion of secondary lamellae and clubbing of gill filaments. This loss of respiratory surface may result in death by anoxia before resolution of the initial insult.

Degenerative Changes in Cells

Cellular degeneration and death (necrosis) are not only fundamental to the inflammatory process but form the basis of many other descriptions in pathology. Most degenerative changes in cells are initiated by inability to maintain proper ionic balance. Cell injury causes an intracellular reduction in oxidative phosphorylation with a resultant drop in the level of adenosine triphosphate (ATP) and a concomitant shift toward acidosis (pH 6.0) due to glycolysis. The cation pump of the cell, which uses ATP as an energy source, breaks down, allowing an influx of sodium, chloride, calcium, and water. This causes cellular swelling and damages cell membranes, which leak intracellular ions (potassium), enzymes, and other proteins. Most degenerative changes in cells are reversible to a certain degree before cell death becomes inevitable. A condition known as acute cellular swelling, or cloudy swelling, is the earliest form of cellular degeneration and is often followed by a more advanced stage known as hydropic degeneration (vacuolar degeneration). Other types of degenerative changes in cells (see Terminology section) include fatty change, hyalin degeneration, fibrinoid degeneration, mucoid degeneration (i.e., serous atrophy of fat or myxomatous degeneration), and ballooning degeneration.

Necrosis

There is a point at which degenerative changes within a cell become irreversible, terminating in cell death or necrosis while the rest of the body still lives. This is especially true when intracellular membranes become damaged, allowing hydrolytic enzymes to leak out from ruptured lysosomes to further destroy cell integrity. Postmortem autolysis (necrosis after death of the body) is similar but is usually more generalized and lacks the vascular and cellular responses (inflammation) that occur around necrotic tissues during life. Necrotic changes in the nucleus determine whether cell death has occurred. These changes include pyknosis, karyorrhexis, karyolysis, or absence of the nucleus (except for the normally anucleate erythrocytes and thrombocytes of mammals). Less reliable features of necrosis include cytoplasmic changes such as increased acidophilia and cytoplasmolysis (dissolution of cytoplasm), which can also occur in living cells. Additional necrotic changes are characterized by loss of cell outlines and loss of differential staining between cytoplasm and nucleus or among different cell types. If a cell is detached or absent from its normal surface or location, it is assumed to have died. For example, desquamated epithelial cells in the gut lumen may stain normally, but by virtue of physical separation from parent tissues these liberated cells cannot survive and must be considered dead.

The specific causes (listed in the discussion of inflammation) of cellular injury and the kind of tissue in which it occurs determine the microscopic appearance of the necrotic process, thus forming a basis for classification. Five general types of necrosis (described in Terminology) are recognized: (1) coagulative necrosis; (2) caseous necrosis; (3) liquefactive necrosis; (4) fat necrosis; and (5) Zenker's necrosis.

Tumors/Neoplasia

Another tissue change that is fundamental in pathology is neoplasia, or tumor formation. Neoplasia is the pathological transformation of a normal host cell resulting in uncontrollable proliferation into new cells which resemble the original host tissue but lack normal histological architecture or normal cellular functions. The uncontrollable growth and the lack of contact inhibition make cancer an extremely destructive process. Proliferation of neoplastic cells can occur in two ways. A tumor can grow by expansion, causing compression atrophy of normal tissues outward from the enlarging focus of neoplastic cells. This is characteristic of a benign tumor, which generally is less destructive unless it occurs in a location where it compromises life functions (e.g., the brain). The other growth process is infiltration of neoplastic cells into and around normal tissue structures. This process, which is

characteristic of malignant tumors, is the most damaging one. By competitive exclusion of nutrients and oxygen, infiltrating malignant cells replace normal tissues, which are crowded out and disappear through necrosis. Eventually, malignant cells may invade a lymphatic channel or blood vessels, where clumps of the cells are likely to break off as emboli in the lymph or blood flow. These cells settle out in other organs and tissues and may proliferate into secondary malignant tumors. This proliferative dissemination of neoplastic cells from the primary site of growth is known as metastasis and is typical of most malignant tumors. Whether a tumor is benign or malignant is determined by histological examination. Cells of benign tumors are usually well differentiated and may be almost normal in architectural arrangement, closely resembling the tissues of origin. They usually show no tendency to infiltrate adjacent normal tissues, never metastasize, and are usually circumscribed or encapsulated with fibrous connective tissue. Invasive growth is rarely seen in certain types of tumors that are considered benign because they do not metastasize (e.g., lymphangioma of humans, equine sarcoid, basal cell carcinoma of humans and dogs). Besides erosive, infiltrative growth and metastasis, malignant tumors have other characteristics, which are used for classification if invasiveness is not apparent: (1) cells may be very anaplastic in that they appear undifferentiated and immature, having little or no recognizable arrangement to permit identification of the parent tissue; (2) in glandular tumors cells tend to "pile up," forming papillary projections in the lumina of acini; (3) tumors show increased cellularity, indicated by large numbers of closely spaced nuclei per unit area; (4) appearance of hyperchromatic, plump nuclei; and (5) a high mitotic index and/or the presence of abnormal mitotic divisions.

The prognosis or probable outcome of a neoplastic disease depends not only on whether the tumor is benign or malignant but also on its clinical behavior. Some malignancies do not grow rapidly, and metastasis occurs late, after tumor development is well advanced (e.g., hepato-carcinoma in rainbow trout). In these cases survival of the host is prolonged.

In vertebrates, nearly all living, dividing populations of cells comprising different types of tissues are capable of falling victim to the neoplastic process. This section is not intended to give detailed descriptions of tumor types, but rather to acquaint the investigator with the concept of neoplasia and the terminology used in its classification. For further information on neoplasia, the reader should consult Smith et al. (1972), Robbins (1974), and Moulton (1978). Tumors are classified according to the host cell(s) of origin belonging to one of the three basic categories of tissue: epithelium, supporting tissue (connective tissue, muscle, bone, cartilage, blood, and lymphoid tissue), and nervous tissue. Exceptions are mixed tumors and teratomas, which may consist of cell types from two or all three of the categories, respectively. Most epithelial tumors fall in three general classes: papillomas, adenomas, and carcinomas. Several other specialized tumor types exist but will not be mentioned here. A papilloma is a benign outgrowth of epithelium and is usually a complex arrangement of fingerlike projections with a fibrous connective tissue core. An adenoma is a benign epithelial tumor that forms acinar-like glandular structures, although tumors of nonacinar glands are also included. If the glandular epithelium of the adenoma, say of the pancreas, exhibits malignant characteristics, the tumor is reclassified as an adenocarcinoma of the pancreas. Therefore, the term "carcinoma" is used to denote malignancy in an epithelial tumor; another example is a squamous cell carcinoma.

Benign tumors of supporting tissues are classified similarly, with the suffix "oma" used after the tissue of origin: fibroma and chondroma refer to benign tumors of fibrous connective tissue and cartilage, respectively. The term "sarcoma" indicates a malignant tumor of supporting tissue origin and is used as a suffix, as in fibrosarcoma or chondrosarcoma.

Tumors of nervous tissue origin can occur in the central nervous system (brain or spinal cord) and the peripheral nervous system (all other nervous innervation of tissues and organs). Most notable are tumors of the brain and spinal cord, most of which are of neuroglial origin. These "gliomas" are of several types, conforming to the classes of neuroglial cells. Depending on the tumor type, gliomas have different rates of growth and locally invasive properties characterized by the terms benign and malignant. However, even a benign tumor of the brain or spinal cord can be destructive and life-threatening because of the fragile nature of nervous tissue and the specific location of the growth. Interestingly, malignant gliomas are not known to metastasize outside the cranial cavity or spinal canal (Smith et al., 1972; Robbins, 1974).

The suffix "blastoma" is often encountered in tumor terminology, as in neuroblastoma (tumor arising from nervous tissue during embryonal development), nephroblastoma (tumor of renal blastema from which kidney is formed), and ameloblastoma (tumor of the enamel organ, the embryologic predecessor of the tooth). As one might surmise from these definitions, blastoma refers to primary tumor formation in immature tissues encountered during embryonal development rather than in mature adult cells.

Causes of Neoplasia

Depending on the life span of the host species, tumor induction may have a latent period of months, years, or even decades. Unfortunately, the mechanisms and circumstances involved in transformation of a normal cell to one that is neoplastic are not well understood. Nonetheless, some factors have been identified as causing cancer. Overexposure to ultraviolet light from the sun or artificial sources is known to cause skin carcinomas in humans and certain bovine breeds. More destructive forms of cancer-causing irradiation are present in x-rays and in radioactive isotopes such as radium, thorium, and cobalt 60. Chemical carcinogens such as derivatives of 1:2-benzanthracene are perhaps the best known tumor-causing agents since many have been discovered through testing in a wide variety of laboratory animals, including fish. Hormones have also been implicated in cancer formation. For example, large doses of estrogenic hormones administered to certain laboratory animals have resulted in hyperplasia and neoplasia in organs normally under hormonal control. Infectious agents also play a role in tumor induction. Among metazoan parasites, the nematode *Spirocerca lupi* may cause malignant tumors in the esophagus of the dog. Oncogenic properties of some viruses have also been well documented with descriptions of papillomas, adenocarcinomas, fibromas, sarcomas, and lymphomas induced by viruses in avian and mammalian species.

The effects on an individual animal of each of the cancer-causing entities listed above are influenced by a unifying variable, heredity. That is, the relative susceptibility of an animal, or of an individual tissue in the animal, is genetically determined. For example, certain strains of mice may be highly resistant to induction of any tumor type, while other strains are susceptible to one or several kinds of tumors.

VARIABLES IN THE DEVELOPMENT OF TOXIC LESIONS

Many studies have shown that the lethality of a particular toxic compound varies depending on the age of the animal as well as the dose (or concentration) and time of exposure. Lesion development may be enhanced by larger doses, longer exposure periods, or use of juvenile experimental animals, which tend to be more susceptible to toxicant-induced insult than adults. The solubility of a toxic compound and its route of exposure may also influence the kinds of lesions observed. For example, compounds that are water-soluble or have water-soluble toxic components may be easily absorbed into the blood of fish or shellfish through direct contact with the respiratory epithelium of the gills or epidermal and sensory epithelium of the skin and buccal cavity. Therefore, it is not uncommon to find initial lesions involving the gills and epidermis, including the sensory epithelium of the olfactory and lateral line organs. However, water-soluble toxicants may not cause external epithelial lesions, but may be absorbed and produce systemic pathology elsewhere in the organism. Some of these compounds may become toxic only when altered by cellular metabolism. In saltwater fish, additional contact absorption of dissolved compounds and hence lesions can occur in the alimentary tract because these fish drink seawater to maintain osmotic equilibrium.

Chemical compounds that are not water-soluble or are only slightly soluble require other routes for cellular exposure. Many such compounds are soluble in lipids and are concentrated to toxic levels in the adipose tissues of prey animals. When such prey are eaten, fat digestion in the predator may release a lethal or, more likely, a sublethal dose of the toxicant that can produce chronic internal lesions during long periods of repeated low-level exposures. Experimentally, some water-insoluble toxic compounds can be dissolved in a carrier solvent and administered orally (directly into the mouth or in the diet) or parenterally (by injection). In either case, external lesions are uncommon. When interpreting lesions, the investigator should be aware that parenteral injections may also produce localized pathological changes due to trauma or a host–foreign body response (inflammation, fibrosis, and organ adhesions) to the carrier solvent. Examination of control animals given "sham" inoculations (injections without toxicant) prevents confusion of these artifacts with lesions resulting from the toxicant.

METHODOLOGY

Introduction

There are no standardized techniques for examining tissues in aquatic organisms. However, standard medical and veterinary techniques may be modified and used to diagnose tissue changes in fish and other aquatic organisms. Before beginning an experiment it is necessary to plan and coordinate the efforts involved, because histopathology is often only one of several types of information obtained from the experiment. The variables that should be considered in the experimental design include the most desirable animal species, numbers of animals, age of animals, diet, means of housing the animals, route of exposure, doses (or concentrations), length of exposure, effluent disposal, sampling schedule, tissues to be examined, tissue fixation (which is highly variable and depends on the techniques to be used), tissue processing, staining, and interpretation. The following are the general procedures followed in investigating toxicant-induced tissue changes or carcinogenesis in fish at the Food Toxicology and Nutrition Laboratory (FTNL) at Oregon State University.

Fish Methods

Species, Diet, Holding Conditions

The principal research animal used at FTNL is the Shasta strain of the rainbow trout, *Salmo gairdneri*. It has proved to be sensitive to many toxic compounds, is easy to rear in our laboratory, and, because of its large size, provides sufficient tissue (particularly liver) for *in vitro* metabolism studies. However, trout require large holding facilities and exacting criteria for water quality, and not all laboratories can conveniently rear them. Several other fish species are also used for toxicological research, including the channel catfish *Ictalurus punctatus*; goldfish *Carassius auratus*; carp, *Cyprinus carpio*; and bluegill, *Lepomis macrochirus*. More recently, several species of small aquarium fish have become popular in research. These include the Japanese medaka, *Oryzias latipes*; guppy, *Lebistes reticulatus*; zebrafish, *Brachydanio rerio*; fathead minnow, *Pimephales promelas*; mummichog, *Fundulus heteroclitus*; and sheepshead minnow, *Cyprinodon variegatus* (the latter two are estuarine species). These small species have the obvious advantages of low maintenance costs and smaller facility requirements. However, *in vitro* studies are limited by the smaller size of the species.

Rainbow trout at FTNL are fed a semipurified casein test diet (Sinnhuber et al., 1977), which supports adequate growth and permits reproducibility of experiments. Many commercial diets vary considerably from year to year, depending on availability and cost of the ingredients, which makes them undesirable for experimental work. The semipurified diet also facilitates incorporation of toxic materials since it is prepared as needed in the laboratory rather than premixed and pelleted like commercial rations.

The trout are reared in circular fiber glass tanks that receive an adequate flow of oxygenated, constant-temperature (12°C) well water. Groups of 100 fingerling trout may be held for up to 1 yr in a 4-ft-diameter (200-gal) tank, but for only 9 mo in a 3-ft (100-gal) tank, without overcrowding and stunting of growth. The standard procedure is to start a group of 100 fingerlings in a 3-ft tank, reduce the number through sampling to 60 at 9 mo, and terminate the experiment at 12 mo. If it is desirable to extend the experiment to 18 or 24 mo, a sample of 20 fish would be taken at 9 mo and the remaining 80 fish transferred to a 4-ft tank. Another 20-fish sample would be taken at 12 mo and the remaining 60 fish held in the 4-ft tank until 18 mo or more. Duplicate groups of fish for each experimental regime are routinely used to provide increased animal numbers and insurance against complete loss of data if water failure causes mortalities in one tank.

Exposure and Concentrations

Several routes of exposure to toxic chemicals are available when using rainbow trout or other fish species. These include diet, flow-through water, static water, and injection.

Many of the exposures to toxic chemicals at FTNL have been by the dietary route. This has proved convenient and effective since many of the compounds (aflatoxins, chlorinated hydrocarbons, and polyaromatic hydrocarbons) are highly lipid-soluble and easily added to the fish oil fraction of the diet. Depending on the experiment, a continuous low-concentration feeding exposure or sometimes a short-term, high-concentration, pulse-feeding exposure may be used. The main disadvantage of dietary exposure is that individual fish have unequal feeding rates and hence receive uneven concentrations of toxicant. A pecking order or dominance structure is established in each tank of fish, so that some fish eat more and some much less at each feeding.

Exposure of fish to low levels of toxicant dissolved in the water best represents their exposure in the environment. Thus, to determine the effects of environmental pollutants on fish, this route of exposure should be used. If fish are being used as a model system to test the toxicity or carcinogenicity of a compound in general, other routes of exposure, which require less elaborate facilities, are more desirable. The main disadvantages of flow-through exposure are that elaborate diluting and monitoring systems are required to deliver a constant concentration of toxicant, and a satisfactory waste treatment system is needed to dispose of the toxicant.

Static water exposures of fish to toxicants have been used extensively for short-term LC50 determinations. This method has advantages and disadvantages when compared to the flow-through method. Facility requirements are minimal and treatment and disposal of waste water are much easier, but length of exposure is limited. An adaptation of this method that is gaining popularity as a carcinogenicity test system is static exposure of fish embryos (eggs) to solutions of carcinogens (Hendricks et al., 1980d). It has proved effective with several mycotoxins and nitrosamines and the advantages over feeding exposures are that (1) it requires only a single handling of the carcinogen; (2) there is passive, uniform exposure of each egg to the carcinogen; (3) a small amount of carcinogen will expose large numbers of eggs; (4) detoxification and disposal of the carcinogen are convenient; and (5) in several cases, embryos have proved to be more sensitive to carcinogens than fingerlings (Wales et al., 1978). The main disadvantage is that it may be difficult or impossible to expose fish embryos to suffi-

ciently high concentrations of highly water-insoluble compounds.

Few long-term toxicity or carcinogenicity experiments use injection as the route of exposure; the main objection is to the continual stress and trauma placed on the fish by repeated handling. Injection can, however, be used effectively if care is taken and fish are of sufficient size to withstand the injection volume.

Regardless of the route of exposure, it is preferable to conduct short-term trials to determine the maximum tolerated concentration (MTC) of a compound before concentrations are selected for a long-term trial. Knowledge of the MTC and the nature of the compound will facilitate the selection of three to five concentrations, with the MTC as the high concentration, for a concentration-response study. If there are budget or space restrictions, a single concentration corresponding to the MTC may be used. In either case a negative control group is reared to ensure that the observed effect is due to the toxicant.

Sampling

The next variables to establish are the number of fish to sample and when to sample them to give the greatest amount of information. Depending on the objectives of the study, an experiment usually begins with duplicate groups of 100 trout for each concentration of a compound and controls. If the experiment is to run for 12 mo, random samples are taken of 20 fish at 6 mo, 20 fish at 9 mo, and 60 fish at 12 mo. If the experiment is to last 18 mo, the 20-fish samples will be taken at 6 or 9 mo and 12 mo and 60 fish at 18 mo.

Data Collected

The following data and tissue samples are routinely taken at each sampling date described above: individual body weight (growth), feed efficiency (diet consumption, recorded throughout the experiment), individual liver weight, ratio of liver weight to body weight, tissues for bioaccumulation analysis (three or more fish per group, killed and frozen whole), gross observations of external or internal lesions, and target tissues for fixation and later histopathologic examination.

The liver is often the target organ for many of the toxicants tested. However, if a toxicant is known to affect other organs, additional tissues may be fixed for observation; examples are mesonephric kidney, head kidney, alimentary tract, pancreas, spleen, thyroid, thymus, heart, gonads, swim bladder, gill, and brain. If a new compound is being tested for the first time, all tissues are fixed.

Tissue Fixation, Processing, and Staining

Light microscopy Toxicant-induced injuries in fish tissues are often difficult to discern grossly (except for large tumors); light microscopy is necessary to observe lesions at the cellular level. The following discussion concerns effective procedures for necropsy of fish specimens, tissue fixation, and histological preparations useful in light microscopy. Fish can be immobilized, a few at a time, by an overdose of tricaine methanesulfonate (MS 222) anesthetic or knocked unconscious by a sharp blow to the head. When all physical activity ceases, the fish are examined for external lesions, weighed individually, and one or more of the gill arches is cut to permit bleeding. The beating heart quickly pumps most of the blood from the body. This facilitates easy observation and subsequent removal of tissues. The body cavity is opened by a midlateral incision from the vent to the operculum and the liver is quickly removed by severing the anterior hepatic veins and the posterior portal vein and bile duct. Care must be taken to prevent spillage of bile from the gallbladder since bile causes necrosis of most tissues, especially liver. The liver is weighed and observed under a dissecting microscope for gross abnormalities before it is placed in a suitable fixative, usually Bouin's solution. Other organs are then removed, gross abnormalities noted, and portions fixed as above.

Before satisfactory histological sections can be produced from a tissue, attention must be given to its preparation. Proper fixation is fundamental.

The rapid autolysis of tissues after death means they must be handled rapidly to prevent degenerative changes in the specimen. This process is halted by fixation, which preserves the morphology of tissues in a condition as near as possible to that existing during life. Many simple and compound fixatives are used for light microscopy. The most common example of the former is neutral buffered formalin. Compound formaldehyde-containing fixatives include Bouin's solution, Helly's fixative, Orth's fixative, and Susa's fixative. Common fixatives that do not contain formaldehyde are Carnoy's and Zenker's fixatives. Liberal amounts of fixative, relative to the mass of tissue (at least 10:1), should be used to ensure rapid and complete fixation. Tissue specimens should be kept small ($\leqslant 1$ cm thick) to promote rapid penetration.

Depending on the preservative, tissue fixation requires 18–24 h; longer periods may be needed to make optimal preparations. After fixation is complete, the tissues are dissected and trimmed into acceptable sizes for processing and sectioning. They are put in small carriers and washed in running water before being placed in an automatic tissue processor for overnight dehydration, clearing, and paraffin infiltration. This machine, which operates on a timer, moves the tissues through a series of increasing concentrations of ethyl alcohol (70–100%), two or three changes of xylene (a clearing agent), and two changes of melted paraffin. In the morning, the tissues are embedded in molds containing clean melted paraffin and these are allowed to harden at room temperature. The hardened blocks are trimmed, mounted on tissue chucks, and sectioned on a microtome into ribbons at a thickness of 4–6 microns. Selected sections are floated and stretched on a hot-water bath, mounted on clean glass slides, and placed on a warming tray to dry and adhere.

At this point the tissues are ready for staining. For most routine histopathology, slides are stained with the nuclear cytoplasmic stain hematoxylin and eosin (H&E), which renders the nuclei blue and the cytoplasm pink. H&E is usually sufficient, but sometimes other stains are required to demonstrate or identify certain tissue or cellular components, abnormal structures, or inclusions. For further discussion of specific techniques the reader is referred to several excellent references (Luna, 1968; Humason, 1962; Putt, 1972; Lillie, 1965; Pearse, 1961; Thompson, 1966). Journals such as *Stain Technology* and the *Journal of Histochemistry and Cytochemistry* are good sources of specific techniques.

Histochemistry Histochemical techniques may be required to investigate the presence of certain chemicals (fat, carbohydrates, protein enzymes) in tissues. These techniques require different fixation procedures from routine light microscopy. For instance, to demonstrate glycogen with periodic acid–Schiff (PAS) stain, it is necessary to fix the tissue in an alcohol-based fixative (alcoholic formalin or Bouin's) to prevent dissolution of the water-soluble glycogen. For lipid stains such as Sudan IV and Sudan Black B, aqueous fixatives are used, preferably 10% formalin. If enzyme histochemical procedures are indicated, fresh frozen or formalin-fixed tissues are used for incubation procedures.

Transmission Electron Microscopy Histological examination of tissue sections from fish after acute or low-level chronic exposure to chemicals may not reveal any obvious lesions. However, examination of the ultrastructural features of the same tissue specimens may reveal significant pathological changes of cells or cellular organelles which could explain physiological or morphological irregularities not manifest at the light microscopic level.

For transmission electron microscopy (TEM), fixation in 2–5% glutaraldehyde in 0.1 M phosphate or cacodylate buffer (pH 7.4) is done overnight at 4°C, after which tissues are removed and postfixed to increase electron density in buffered 1–2% osmium tetroxide for 1–3 h at 4°C (cellular fixation is qualitatively enhanced and integrity of the dilute fixative is best preserved at low temperatures) (Pease, 1964). Postfixed tissues are rinsed in buffer and dehydrated through a series of ethanol baths (70–100%), with two or

three final changes of 100% ethanol for 5–10 min each to ensure complete dehydration. In this way there should be no problems later with infiltration and proper hardening of the resin blocks. If storage is desired, postfixed specimens rinsed in buffer may be kept indefinitely in 70% ethanol for later processing. Dehydrated tissues are placed in a mixture of 50% Spurr's low-viscosity resin (Spurr, 1969) and 50% absolute ethanol and allowed to infiltrate on a rotator overnight at room temperature. Complete resin infiltration is accomplished the next day by rotating the tissues in undiluted Spurr's resin for 4–6 h. Embedment is completed by adding tissues and fresh resin to BEEM capsules or other suitable plastic molds and placing them in an oven at 70°C. Spurr's resin cures in about 8 h, after which the molds may be peeled away to allow trimming and sizing of the block faces for sectioning. Trimmed blocks are placed in an ultramicrotome and thick sections (0.5–1.0 μm) are first cut for examination by light microscopy to determine if the desired field is present in the block for thin sectioning. Thick sections are floated on a water reservoir behind the cutting surface of the knife (glass or diamond) and placed on a clean glass slide with a small wire loop. The slide is heated over an alcohol flame for drying and adhesion of the sections to the glass surface. These sections are then deplasticized with a saturated solution of NaOH in absolute ethanol for 2–5 min (depending on thickness), rinsed in absolute ethanol and distilled water, and stained with toluidine blue (29% solution buffered with 2% sodium tetraborate) while heated on a slide warmer at 60°C. Staining time also varies with the thickness of the section and is usually 2–5 s. Stained slides are rinsed in distilled water and coverslipped with Permount. Cell nuclei stain purple-pink and cytoplasm is blue.

Thin sections (250–500 Å) are cut similarly, except that they are mounted on cleaned tiny copper meshed grids. This is done by gripping the grid with forceps and bringing it directly up under the floating section for proper seating. The grid and section are allowed to air-dry before staining with uranyl acetate (30 min) and counterstaining with lead citrate (2-5 min). Grids are then ready for viewing of cellular structure in the electron microscope.

The description above is a summary of a basic procedure applicable to many situations in TEM. However, there are several variations involving fixatives, buffers, stains and staining sequences, technique, embedding resins, and so on which may be more suitable for a specific need. More detailed descriptions of the procedures can be found in textbooks on TEM (Pease, 1964; Hayat, 1972, 1977) and in the literature (Hawkes, 1977, 1980).

Scanning Electron Microscopy Scanning electron microscopy (SEM) is useful for observing three-dimensional ultrastructural changes on the surfaces of tissues, cells, or other structures. Small tissue samples are preserved in a fixative, postfixed as above, and dehydrated through a series of acetone baths (25, 50, 75, and 90%). Dehydration is complete after two or three immersions in pure acetone for 5-10 min each. Dehydrated samples are dried in a special manner to prevent structural distortion due to pressure exerted by the surface tension of evaporating fluids, which normally occurs in air-drying. However, air-drying may be satisfactory for hard tissues such as chiton, shell, and bone. Soft tissues are dried in a critical-point dryer which, under pressure, replaces the acetone bath surrounding the specimens with liquid CO_2 or some other pressurized gas. The CO_2 is vaporized by increasing the pressure of the reaction vessel to the critical point (800–850 lb/in^2 or 1870 K/6.25 cm^2) by immersion in a hot-water bath. The gas is released slowly and the dried specimens are carefully removed for the next step. The specimens are mounted on an aluminum stub with double-sided tape or silver conducting paint. The stubs are placed in a vacuum evaporator which coats the surface detail of each specimen with a thin layer of metal dust by vaporizing a fine gold:palladium (60:40) wire. Stubs holding the coated specimens are removed from the evaporator and are ready for insertion into the scanning electron microscope. The metal dust coats the finest surface detail and conducts electrons from a focused electron beam, which produces an image of the specimen on a monitor screen. Again, this is a simplified version of a procedure that may vary depending on the results desired and the equipment available; critical-point dryers differ in the gases used and different metals may be employed to coat specimens. For further details on this protocol and others, see Hayat (1972, 1977) and Anderson (1969).

Invertebrate Methods

In most cases, many of the techniques used for fish tissues are applicable to invertebrates; however, these organisms are considerably more diverse in tissue, body structure, and physiology (Morton, 1971) than fish, so the investigator should regard this statement as a rule of thumb. For discussion, bivalve mollusks (oysters, scallops, mussels, clams) will be used as an example. Here the investigator must extract tissues for examination from between two opposing, often formidable, shells (valves). This is easily done by inserting a knife and severing the adductor muscles (one in oysters and scallops and two in mussels and clams), which hold the valves tightly closed. Histological procedures used for adult invertebrate tissues are similar to those outlined earlier for fish tissues. Many of the conventional histological and histochemical stains can be used effectively on paraffin-embedded invertebrate tissues, with H&E providing good routine microscopic detail (Buchanan, 1970; Meyers, 1981). Histological or histochemical procedures requiring frozen sections also work well in mollusks (Liddell, 1967; Meyers, 1979). Although the same general fixatives can be used, special attention should be given to the osmolarity if the animal was taken from salt water. Most invertebrates are conformers rather than regulators, which means that their cells are bathed in physiological fluids having a salt concentration approximating the salinity of ambient seawater. As with any tissues, this osmolarity should be maintained during fixation; adjustments can be made by adding NaCl or by preparing the fixative with salt water approximately equal in salinity to that from which the animals were taken. Difficult problems of fixation can result with larval mollusks that are too small (<2-3 mm) for tissues to be extracted with a scalpel. These animals must be fixed while in their valves, and all too often these are closed immediately or soon after addition of the fixative to the seawater. This results in poor penetration of the fixative and unsuitable preservation of cellular structure. Premature valve closure can be overcome by narcotizing the larvae with an anesthetic before addition of the fixative.

Because of the calcareous nature of the valves, decalcification of larvae is required before embedment. This can be accomplished in 10% formic acid adjusted to pH 4.5 with sodium citrate. Decalcified larvae should be embedded in Spurr's resin or other plastic media for routine light microscopy, since paraffin does not infiltrate the small larval samples as well. Although thick sections of plastic- or resin-embedded materials limit the use of various histological stains, easily stained frozen sections may be prepared in parallel from decalcified larvae embedded in cryosectioning medium (O.C.T. Compound, Lab Tek Products). An excellent treatise on fixation and decalcification problems in larvae as well as definitive descriptions of additional microtechniques and larval structures in invertebrate histology and TEM are presented by Elston (1980a, b).

Adult invertebrate tissues are prepared for TEM with procedures similar to those used for fish, except that osmolarity is again critical. A solution that works extremely well in providing proper ionic balance when mixed with glutaraldehyde is Millonig's phosphate buffer (pH 7.6). Larval samples that have been embedded in plastic resins for light microscopy are equally suitable for ultrasectioning and TEM, depending on the fixative and type of resin used. Additional information on procedures for TEM of adult mollusks is given in Perkins and Menzel (1967) and Perkins (1968, 1975). Procedures for SEM present no problems that are unique for invertebrates other than that

discussed for proper fixation in larvae. Further information regarding protocol is provided by Elston (1980a,b). For general references on invertebrate histology, ultrastructure, physiology, and biochemistry, see Malek and Cheng (1974), Galtsoff (1964), Sparks (1972), and Johnson (1980).

By using light microscopy, TEM, and SEM, the pathologist can observe, classify, and photographically document the lesions produced by a toxicant. In this chapter we have reviewed gross, histological, and ultrastructural lesions that have been described in aquatic animals exposed to toxic materials. These examples illustrate the types of lesions that can be expected.

LITERATURE REVIEW

The aquatic medium is a very efficient solvent for many chemical compounds or components thereof. Consequently, aquatic organisms are extremely vulnerable to toxic effects resulting from absorption or oral intake of these contaminants from the immediate environment. Various chemical compounds have been investigated to determine their potential toxicity to certain aquatic organisms, especially fish and to a lesser degree shellfish. However, many of these studies have been concerned with measuring lethality rather than the pathological effects of contaminants on the tissues. Table 1 lists several chemicals that have been examined for their potential to produce pathological changes in aquatic species. These aquatic species, along with specific toxicants and literature sources, are recorded in Table 2. Most of these studies employed an ambient water route of exposure, although some utilized per os (po) (through the mouth by incorporation into diet) or parenteral administration as well.

Nonspecific versus Diagnostic Lesions in Aquatic Toxicology

Unfortunately, toxicological studies of aquatic organisms have not revealed many tissue pathologies useful in diagnosing exposures to specific

Table 1 Organic and Inorganic Environmental Contaminants and Chemotherapeutic Agents Tested for Ability to Cause Pathological Changes in Tissues of Finfish and Shellfish

Organochlorines	Petroleum compounds	Organo-phosphates	Carbamates	Miscellaneous	Metals and nitrogenous compounds	Chemotherapeutic agents
Insecticides	Crude oil	Insecticides	Insecticides	Herbicides	Ammonia (NH_3)	Bradophen (disinfectant)
Chlordane	Whole	Abate	Carbaryl	Acrolein	Cadmium-109 ($^{109}Cd^{+2}$)	$CuSO_4$ (fungicide, algicide)
DDD	Saltwater-insoluble	Diazinon	(sevin)	Amitrole-T	Cadmium chloride ($CdCl_2$)	Dipterex
DDT	Saltwater-soluble	Dimethoate	Propoxur	Atrazine	Copper chloride ($CuCl_2$)	Emtrysidina
Dieldrin	Waste motor oil	Dursban		Dinoseb	Copper nitrate ($CuNO_3$)	Formalin (fungicide, ectoparasiticide)
Endosulfan	Oiled sediment	Dylox		Diquat	Copper sulfate ($CuSO_4$)	Hexa-ex (disinfectant)
Endrin	Oil slick	Fenthion		Hydrothol 191	Landfill leachates	Kanamycin
Heptachlor	Miscellaneous hydrocarbons	Malathion		Paraquat-CL	Lead acetate trihydrate ($C_4H_6O_4Pb$)	Malachite Green (fungicide, ectoparasiticide)
Kepone	Miscellaneous hydrocarbons and PCBs	Methyl parathion		Sodium trichloro-acetate ($NaTA_2$)	Lead nitrate ($PbNO_3$)	Methylene Blue (fungicide disinfectant)
Lindane	Naphthalene			Trifluralin	Mercuric chloride ($HgCl_2$)	Neguvon, Masoten
Methoxychlor	Phenol			Other	Methyl mercury chloride (CH_3HgCl_2)	Ozone (biocide)
Mirex				Bis(tri-n-butyltin) oxide (molluscicide)	Nitrite (NO_2)	Penicillin G Procain
Toxaphene				Dimethyl sulfoxide (DMSO)	Silver chloride (AgCl)	Dihydrostreptomycin sulfate
Herbicides				Sodium lauryl sulfate (SLS-detergent)	Sodium arsenate (Na_2HAsO_4)	Oxytetracycline
Dowpon				Triethylene phosphoramide (TEPA-insect chemosterilant)	Sodium arsenite ($NaAsO_2$)	Sulfamethazine
Dicamba				3-Trifluoromethyl 4-nitrophenol (TFM-lampreycide)	Zinc chloride ($ZnCl_2$)	Sulfonamides
Dichlobenil				Acid-alkaline pH (sulfuric acid; sodium hydroxide)	Zinc sulfate ($ZnSO_4$)	Thiabendazole
Diuron						Tobramycin
Dowicide G						Yomesan (anthelmintic)
Esteron						
2,4-D						
Kuron						
Kurosal						
Tordon 101						
Tordon 22k						
Industrial						
Chlorinated wastewater						
Polychlorinated biphenyls (PCBs)						
Aroclor 1248						
Aroclor 1254						
Miscellaneous						
PCBs						
Carbon tetra-chloride						

Table 2 Aquatic Species Examined for Pathological Changes in Tissues following Exposures to Organic and Inorganic Environmental Contaminants and Chemotherapeutic Agents

Common name	Scientific name	Literature source
		Trout
Brook trout	*Salvelinus fontinalis*	Daye and Garside, 1976 (alkaline-acid pH); Sangalang and O'Halloran, 1972 (CdCl$_2$).
Brown trout	*Salmo trutta*	King, 1962 (DDT).
Cutthroat trout	*Salmo clarki*	Allison et al., 1964 (DDT, malathion); Andrews et al., 1966 (heptachlor); Eller, 1971 (endrin); Van Valin et al., 1968 (mirex).
Lake trout	*Salvelinus namaycush*	Eller, L. L., unpublished, in Couch, 1975 (aroclor 1248, chlordane); Walsh and Ribelin, 1975 (DDT, dieldrin, endosulfan, 2,4-D, malathion, sevin, atrazine).
Rainbow trout	*Salmo gairdneri*	Abel and Skidmore, 1975 (SLS); Benville et al., 1968 (DMSO); Burkhalter and Kaya, 1977 (NH$_3$); Chliamovitch and Kuhn, 1977 [bis(tri-*n*-butyltin) oxide]; Christie and Battle, 1963 (TFM); Cope, 1966 (methoxychlor); Gingerich et al., 1978 (carbon tetrachloride); Halver et al., 1962 (DDT); Hawkes, 1977 (whole crude oil); Lowe, 1967 (sevin); Matton and LaHam, 1969 (dylox); McBride et al., 1975; 1979 (kanamycin, landfill leachates); Mitrovic et al., 1968 (phenol); Nestel and Budd, 1975 (aroclor 1254); Racicot et al., 1975 (carbon tetrachloride); Sivarajah et al., 1978 (Aroclor 1254); Smith and Piper, 1972, 1975 (formalin, NH$_3$); Wedemeyer et al., 1979 (ozone); Wobeser, 1975a,b (HgCl$_2$, CH$_3$HgCl$_2$); Wood, E. M., unpublished, in Couch, 1975 (endrin, heptachlor); Wood, E. M., unpublished, in Walsh and Ribelin, 1975 (DDT, lindane, methoxychlor, toxaphene, malathion, methyl parathion).
Steelhead trout	*Salmo gairdneri*	Wedemeyer and Yasutake, 1974, 1978 (formalin, NO$_2$).
Trout	Not specified	Reichenbach-Klinke, 1975 (bradophen, CuSO$_4$, malachite green, methylene blue, neguvon-masoten, sulfonamides).
		Salmon
Chinook salmon	*Oncorhynchus tshawytscha*	Benville et al., 1968 (DMSO); Buhler et al., 1969 (DDT); DeCew, 1972 (mixture penicillin, streptomycin and oxytetracycline); Hawkes et al., 1980 (miscellaneous PCBs and petroleum hydrocarbons); Wedemeyer and Yasutake, 1974 (formalin); Wood et al., 1957 (sulfamethazine).
Coho salmon	*Oncorhynchus kisutch*	Benville et al., 1968 (DMSO); Buckley et al., 1976 (chlorinated wastewater); Buckley, 1977 (chlorinated wastewater); Hawkes, 1977 (saltwater-soluble crude oil); Hendricks, 1979 (dicamba, esteron, tordon 101, tordon 22k, acrolein, amitrole-T, atrazine, dinoseb, diquat, paraquat-CL); Schneider et al., 1980 (tobramycin); Walsh and Ribelin, 1975 (DDT, dieldrin, endosulfan, 2,4-D, malathion, sevin, atrazine).
Sockeye salmon	*Oncorhynchus nerka*	Benville et al., 1968 (DMSO).

Table 2   Aquatic Species Examined for Pathological Changes in Tissues following Exposures to Organic and Inorganic Environmental Contaminants and Chemotherapeutic Agents (*Continued*)

Common name	Scientific name	Literature source
	Sunfish	
Bluegill	*Lepomis macrochirus*	Andrews et al., 1966 (heptachlor); Cope, 1963, 1966 (heptachlor, dichlobenil); Cope et al., 1969, 1970 (dichlobenil, 2,4-D); Eller, L. L., unpublished in Couch, 1975 (abate); Gilderhaus, 1966 (NaAsO$_2$); Kennedy et al., 1970 (methoxychlor); McCraren et al., 1969 (diuron); Van Valin et al., 1968 (mirex); Wood, E. M., unpublished, in Walsh and Ribeline, 1975 (kuron, kurosal).
Green sunfish	*Lepomis cyanellus*	Sorensen, 1976 (Na$_2$HAsO$_4$).
Redear sunfish	*Lepomis microlophus*	Eller, 1969 (hydrothol 191).
	Eels	
American eel	*Anguilla rostrata*	Ball and Baker, 1969–1970 (DDD); Janicki and Kinter, 1971 (DDT).
Lamprey eel	*Petromyzon marinus*	Christie and Battle, 1963 (TFM).
	Minnows and killifish	
Bream	*Abramis brama*	Waluga, 1966a,b (phenol).
Carp	*Cyprinus carpio*	Lakota et al., 1978 (methoxychlor, propoxur); Schulz, 1970, 1971 (NaTA$_2$, toxaphene); Sivarajah et al., 1978 (aroclor 1254); Reichenbach-Klinke, 1975 (CuSO$_4$, dipterex, emtrysidina, hexa-ex, malachite green, methylene blue, neguvon-masoten, sulfonamides, thiabendazole, yomesan).
Fathead minnow	*Pimephales promelas*	Mehrle and Mayer, 1975 (toxaphene).
Goldfish	*Carassius auratus*	Bromage and Fuchs, 1976 (SLS, ZnSO$_4$); Grant and Mehrle, 1970 (endrin); Tafanelli and Summerfelt, 1975 (CdCl$_2$); Van Valin et al., 1968 (mirex).
Mummichog	*Fundulus heteroclitus*	DiMichele and Taylor, 1978 (naphthalene); Eisler and Gardner, 1973 (CdCl$_2$ + CuCl$_2$ + ZnCl$_2$); Gardner and Yevich, 1970 (CdCl$_2$); Gardner and LaRoche, 1973 (CuCl$_2$); Gardner, 1975 (methoxychlor, CdCl$_2$, HgCl$_2$, AgCl); Wasserman and Koepp, 1977 (HgCl$_2$).
Sheepshead minnow	*Cyprinodon variegatus*	Couch et al., 1977 (Kepone); Couch et al., 1979 (trifluralin); Lowe, J. I., personal communication, in Couch, 1975 (dursban).
	Aquarium fish	
Cichlids	*Chichlasoma nigrofasciatum*	Ozoh, 1979b (C$_4$H$_6$O$_4$Pb).
	Herotilapia multispinosa	Jauch, 1979 (fenthion).
	Tilapia leucosticta	Jauch, 1979 (fenthion).
Guppy	*Poecilia reticulata*	Crandall and Goodnight, 1963 (dowicide G); King, 1962 (DDT); Mount, 1962 (endrin); Stock and Cope, 1969 (TEPA).
Medaka	*Oryzias latipes*	Aoki, 1978 (Cd 109).
Zebra fish	*Brachydanio rerio*	Ozoh, 1979a (CuNO$_3$, PbNO$_3$).

Table 2 Aquatic Species Examined for Pathological Changes in Tissues following Exposures to Organic and Inorganic Environmental Contaminants and Chemotherapeutic Agents (*Continued*)

Common name	Scientific name	Literature source
		Asian fish species
	Heteropneustes fossilis	Bhatnagar and Shrivastava, 1975 ($CuSO_4$).
	Ophiocephalus punctatus	Mathur, 1975 (dieldrin, lindane).
	Trichogaster fasciatus	Mathur, 1975 (dieldrin, lindane).
	Unspecified	Mathur, 1962 (DDT).
		Catfish
Asian catfish	*Channa punctatus*	Anees, 1976 (diazinon, dimethoate, methyl parathion); Sastry and Gupta, 1978a,b ($HgCl_2$, $PbNO_3$); Sastry and Sharma, 1978 (endrin).
Channel catfish	*Ictalurus punctatus*	Hinton et al., 1978 (miscellaneous PCBs); Kendall, 1977 ($CH_3 HgCl_2$); Klaunig et al., 1979 (miscellaneous PCBs); Mayer et al., 1978 (toxaphene).
		Marine flatfish
English sole	*Parophrys vetulus*	Hawkes, 1977 (saltwater-soluble crude oil).
Hogchoker	*Trinectes maculatus*	Trump et al., 1975 ($HgCl_2$).
Sand sole	*Psettichthys melanostictus*	Hawkes, 1980 (saltwater-soluble crude oil).
Starry flounder	*Platichthys stellatus*	Hawkes, 1977 (saltwater-soluble crude oil).
Winter flounder	*Pseudopleuronectes americanus*	Baker, 1969 ($CuSO_4$).
		Miscellaneous marine fish
Atlantic silverside	*Menidia menidia*	Gardner and LaRoche, 1973 ($CuCl_2$); Gardner, 1975, 1978 (whole, saltwater-insoluble, saltwater-soluble crude oil, waste motor oil).
Cunner	*Tautogolabrus adspersus*	Newman and MacLean, 1974 ($CdCl_2$); Payne et al., 1978 (oil slick).
Lisa	*Mugil auratus*	Establier et al., 1978a ($HgCl_2$, $CH_3 HgCl_2$).
Pacific herring	*Clupea pallasii*	Cameron and Smith, 1980 (whole crude oil).
Pinfish	*Lagodon rhomboides*	Lowe et al., 1971b (mirex).
Robalo	*Dicentrarchus labrax*	Establier et al., 1978c ($HgCl_2$).
Sapo	*Halobatrachus didactylus*	Gutierrez et al., 1978 ($CdCl_2$, $HgCl_2$).
Spot	*Leiostomus xanthurus*	Couch, 1975 (Aroclor 1254, sevin); Hawkins et al., 1980 ($CdCl_2$); Johnson, 1968 (endrin); Lowe, 1964, 1965 (toxaphene, endrin).
		Invertebrates
American oyster	*Crassostrea virginica*	Lowe et al., 1971a, 1972 (Aroclor 1254, DDT, toxaphene, parathion).
Bent-nosed clam	*Macoma nasuta*	Armstrong and Millemann, 1974 (sevin).
Hard clam	*Mercenaria mercenaria*	Fries and Tripp, 1976 (phenol).
Shrimp (langostino)	*Penaeus kerathurus*	Establier et al., 1978b ($CdCl_2$).

compounds. Most lesions have been extremely nonspecific and merely indicative of toxic insult. The nonspecific microscopic lesions reported in fish and shellfish species after exposures to different chemical compounds (see Table 1 for abbreviations of compounds) are summarized below. These lesions occurred either separately or in combination, depending on the compound used. The descriptions and interpretations provided are mostly in the words of the authors cited, which in some cases are vague or ambiguous. For further information on organ function or anatomic terminology not covered in the glossary, the reader should consult Hoar and Randall (1969) or Morton (1971).

Nonspecific Microscopic Lesions

Gills Epithelial hyperplasia with lamellar fusion, epithelial hypertrophy, telangiectasia, edema with epithelial separation from basement membranes, general necrosis, and/or epithelial desquamation have occurred following exposures to certain *organochlorines*: 2,4-D (Walsh and Ribelin, 1975); DDT (Walsh and Ribelin, 1975); dichlobenil (Cope, 1966); dieldrin (Walsh and Ribelin, 1975); diuron (McCraren et al., 1969); endosulfan (Walsh and Ribelin, 1975); endrin (Eller, 1971); esteron (Hendricks, 1979); heptachlor (Andrews et al., 1966; Wood, E.M., unpublished, in Couch, 1975); methoxychlor (Cope, 1966; Lakota et al., 1978); mirex (Van Valin et al., 1968); Tordon 22K (Hendricks, 1979); toxaphene (Lowe, 1964; Wood, E. M., unpublished, in Walsh and Ribelin, 1975); *petroleum compounds*: naphthalene (DiMichele and Taylor, 1978); phenol (Fries and Tripp, 1976; Mitrovic et al., 1968; Reichenbach-Klinke, 1965; Waluga, 1966b); saltwater-soluble crude oil (Hawkes, 1977); *organophosphates*: fenthion (Jauch, 1979); malathion (Walsh and Ribelin, 1975; Wood, E. M., unpublished, in Walsh and Ribelin, 1975); methyl parathion (Wood, E. M., unpublished, in Walsh and Ribelin, 1975); *carbamates*: propoxur (Lakota et al., 1978); sevin (Armstrong and Millemann, 1974; Walsh and Ribelin, 1975); *miscellaneous herbicides*:

acrolein (Hendricks, 1979); amitrole-T (Hendricks, 1979); atrazine (Hendricks, 1979; Walsh and Ribelin, 1975); dinoseb (Hendricks, 1979); diquat (Hendricks, 1979); hydrothol 191 (Eller, 1969); $NaTA_2$ (Schulz, 1970); paraquat-CL (Hendricks, 1979); *other miscellaneous compounds*: acid-alkaline pH (Day and Garside, 1976); bis(tri-n-butyltin)oxide (Chliamovitch and Kuhn, 1977); DMSO (Benville et al., 1968); SLS (Abel and Sidmore, 1975); TFM (Christie and Battle, 1963); *nitrogenous compounds*: NH_3 (Burkhalter and Kaya, 1977; Smith and Piper, 1975); NO_2 (Wedemeyer and Yasutake, 1978); *heavy metal salts*: $CdCl_2$ (Gardner and Yevich, 1970); $CuCl_2$ + $ZnCl_2$ + $CdCl_2$ (Eisler and Gardner, 1973); $CuSO_4$ (Baker, 1969; Bhatnagar and Shrivastava, 1975); $HgCl_2$ (Establier et al., 1978c; Wobeser, 1975a); CH_3HgCl_2 (Establier et al., 1978a; Wobeser, 1975a,b); $NaAsO_2$ (Gilderhaus, 1966); and *chemotherapeutic agents*: bradophen (Reichenbach-Klinke, 1975); formalin (Smith and Piper, 1972; Wedemeyer and Yasutake, 1974); malachite green (Reichenbach-Klinke, 1975); ozone (Wedemeyer et al., 1979).

Liver Hepatotoxic lesions of fatty infiltration, nuclear or general hypertrophy of hepatocytes, other degenerative changes in parenchyma (cytoplasmic vacuolation, cellular pleomorphism, deposition of bile or ceroid pigments, hydropic degeneration), loss of hepatic glycogen, coagulative hepatocyte necrosis, sinusoidal and vascular congestion, loss of normal muralial architecture, degeneration or necrosis of biliary epithelium, and perivascular or periportal fibrosis have been reported following exposures to several chemical compounds—for a review of pesticide pathology in fish liver up to 1972 see Couch (1975); *organochlorines*: Aroclor 1248 (Eller, L. L., unpublished, in Couch, 1975); Aroclor 1254 (Couch, 1975; Nestel and Budd, 1975; Sivarajah et al., 1978); carbon tetrachloride (Gingerich et al., 1978; Racicot et al., 1975); chlordane (Eller, L. L., unpublished, in Couch, 1975); 2,4,-D (Cope et al., 1970; Walsh and Ribelin, 1975); DDT (King, 1962; Mathur, 1962; Walsh and Ribelin; 1975);

dichlobenil (Cope et al., 1969); dieldrin (Mathur, 1965, 1975; Walsh and Ribelin, 1975); Dowicide G (Crandall and Goodnight, 1963); endosulfan (Walsh and Ribelin, 1975); endrin (Grant and Mehrle, 1970; Lowe, 1965; Mount, 1962; Sastry and Sharma, 1978; Wood, E. M., unpublished, in Couch, 1975); heptachlor (Andrews et al., 1966; Wood, E. M., unpublished, in Couch, 1975); kuron (Wood, E. M., unpublished, in Walsh and Ribelin, 1975); lindane (Mathur, 1975; Wood, E. M., unpublished, in Walsh and Ribelin, 1975); methoxychlor (Cope, 1966; Lakota et al., 1978; Wood, E. M., unpublished, in Walsh and Ribelin, 1975); tordon 101 and 22k (Hendricks, 1979); toxaphene (Wood, E. M., unpublished, in Walsh and Ribelin, 1975); *petroleum compounds*: crude oil (McCain et al., 1978); naphthalene (DiMichele and Taylor, 1978); *organophosphates*: abate (Eller, L. L., unpublished, in Couch, 1975); diazinon (Anees, 1976); dimethoate (Anees, 1976); dursban (Lowe, J. I. personal communication, in Couch, 1975); dylox (Matton and LaHam, 1969); malathion (Walsh and Ribelin, 1975; Wood, E. M., unpublished, in Walsh and Ribelin, 1975); methyl parathion (Anees, 1976; Wood, E. M., unpublished, in Walsh and Ribelin, 1975); *carbamates*: propoxur (Lakota et al., 1978); sevin (Couch, 1975; Walsh and Ribelin, 1975); *miscellaneous herbicides*: acrolein (Hendricks, 1979); amitrole-T (Hendricks, 1979); dinoseb (Hendricks, 1979); diquat (Hendricks, 1979); hydrothol 191 (Eller, 1969); paraquat-CL (Hendricks, 1979); *other miscellaneous compounds*: bis(tri-*n*-butyltin)oxide (Chliamovitch and Kuhn, 1977); DMSO (Benville et al., 1968); TFM (Christie and Battle, 1963); *nitrogenous compounds*: NH_3 (Smith and Piper, 1975); *heavy metal salts*: $CdCl_2$ (Gutierrez et al., 1978; Tafanelli and Summerfelt, 1975); $CuCl_2$ (Gardner and LaRoche, 1973); $CuSO_4$ (Baker, 1969); $PbNO_3$ (Sastry and Gupta, 1978b); $HgCl_2$ (Establier et al., 1978a,c; Gutierrez et al., 1978; Sastry and Gupta, 1978a); $CH_3 HgCl_2$ (Establier et al., 1978a; Kendall, 1977); $NaAsO_2$ (Gilderhaus, 1966); and *chemotherapeutic agents*: $CuSO_4$ (Reichenbach-Klinke, 1975); sulfametha-

zine (Wood et al., 1957); thiabendazole (Reichenbach-Klinke, 1975).

Liver neoplasia (hepatic cell carcinoma, cholangiocarcinoma) has been reported in rainbow trout following controlled exposures to various toxic compounds, most of which have not been potential contaminants in the aquatic environment (Sinnhuber et al., 1976; Grieco et al., 1978; Hendricks et al., 1980a,b,c; Hendricks et al., 1981). Moreover, certain industrial chemicals, such as PCBs, have been implicated as possible causes of liver neoplasia in populations of Atlantic hagfish (Falkmer et al., 1977), English sole (McCain et al., 1977), and Atlantic tomcod (Smith et al., 1979). At present, adequate experimental evidence on the carcinogenicity of PCBs in fish is not available. Nonetheless, investigations of certain other potential aquatic contaminants have shown that they can induce preneoplastic or neoplastic changes in the liver. Hendricks (unpublished data) found that dietary intake of the chlorinated hydrocarbon DDT produced hepatocellular and cholangiolar (Fig. 13) carcinomas in 21 and 69% of male and female rainbow trout, respectively. Hepatoma in DDT-fed rainbow trout was reported by Halver et al. (1962), while adenomatous changes were reported by Cope et al. (1969) in livers of centrarchid fish exposed to the herbicide dichlobenil and in cutthroat trout exposed to endrin (Eller, 1971).

Kidney Nephrotoxic lesions, including degenerative changes in tubular epithelium (cytoplasmic vacuolation, hydropic degeneration, hyperchromatic nuclei), dilation of tubular lumina, proteinaceous or cellular casts within tubular lumina, tubular necrosis and/or epithelial desquamation, necrosis of interstitial hematopoietic tissues, and excessive development of melanomacrophage centers, are some of the changes observed following exposure to: *organochlorines*: Aroclor 1254 (Nestel and Budd, 1975); DDT (King, 1962; Mathur, 1962); endrin (Mount and Putnicki, 1966; Wood, E. M., unpublished, in Couch, 1975); lindane (Wood, E. M., unpublished, in Walsh and Ribelin, 1975); *petroleum compounds*: naphthalene (DiMichele and Taylor, 1978); phenol (Waluga, 1966a); *organophosphates*: diazinon (Anees, 1976); dimethoate (Anees, 1976); methyl parathion (Anees, 1976; Wood, E. M., unpublished, in Walsh and Ribelin, 1975); *miscellaneous herbicides*: acrolein (Hendricks, 1979); amitrole-T (Hendricks, 1979); dinoseb (Hendricks, 1979); diquat (Hendricks, 1979); paraquat-CL (Hendricks, 1979); *other miscellaneous compounds*: DMSO (Benville et al., 1968); *heavy metal salts*: $CdCl_2$ (Gardner and Yevich, 1970; Gutierrez et al., 1978; Hawkins et al., 1980; Newman and MacLean, 1974; Tafanelli and Summerfelt, 1975); mixture of $CdCl_2$, $CuCl_2$, and $ZnCl_2$ (Eisler and Gardner, 1973); $CuCl_2$ (Gardner and LaRoche, 1973); $CuSO_4$ (Baker, 1969; Bhatnagar and Shrivastava, 1975); $HgCl_2$ (Establier et al., 1978c; Trump et al., 1975); CH_3HgCl_2 (Establier et al., 1978a; Wobeser, 1975b); *chemotherapeutic agents*: $CuSO_4$ (Reichenbach-Klinke, 1975); emtrysidina (Reichenbach-Klinke, 1975); formalin (Smith and Piper, 1975); kanamycin (McBride et al., 1975); malachite green (Reichenbach-Klinke, 1975); sulfamethazine (Wood et al., 1957); sulfonamides (Reichenbach-Klinke, 1975).

Intestine Toxic lesions most commonly reported in the intestine (and occasionally pyloric cecae) include hyperemia; degenerative changes in tips of villi; loss of structural integrity of mucosal folds; degeneration of mucosal epithelium (hypertrophy, vacuolation, hyperchromasia) and/or various smooth muscle layers; necrosis and/or desquamation of mucosal epithelium; cellular debris and excessive mucus in gut lumen; increased numbers of mucous goblet cells; vacuolation or necrosis of submucosa; degenerative changes or necrosis of submucosal vasculature; inflammatory infiltration of submucosa and/or lamina propria. These changes have occurred following exposures to *organochlorines*: miscellaneous PCBs (Hawkes et al., 1980); carbon tetrachloride (Gingerich et al., 1978); 2,4-D (Walsh and Ribelin, 1975); DDT (Janicki and Kinter, 1971; King, 1962; Mathur, 1962; Walsh and Ribelin, 1975); dieldrin (Walsh

and Ribelin, 1975); endosulfan (Walsh and Ribelin, 1975); *petroleum compounds*: miscellaneous hydrocarbons and PCBs (Hawkes et al., 1980); naphthalene (DiMichele and Taylor, 1978); phenol (Fries and Tripp, 1976); *organophosphates*: diazinon (Anees, 1976); dimethoate (Anees, 1976); malathion (Walsh and Ribelin, 1975); methyl parathion (Anees, 1976); *miscellaneous herbicides*: atrazine (Walsh and Ribelin, 1975); *nitrogenous compounds*: NH_3 (Smith and Piper, 1975); *heavy metal salts*: $CdCl_2$ (Gardner and Yevich, 1970; Gutierrez et al., 1978; Newman and MacLean, 1974); $HgCl_2$ (Establier et al., 1978a,c; Gutierrez et al., 1978; Sastry and Gupta, 1978a); CH_3HgCl_2 (Establier et al., 1978a); $PbNO_3$ (Sastry and Gupta, 1978b).

Spleen Atrophy, mottled or blanched in color, hypocellularity (reduction in red and white pulp), fibroplasia, and subcapsular necrosis of blood cells have been observed with *organochlorines*: Aroclor 1254 (Nestel and Budd, 1975); carbon tetrachloride (Gingerich et al., 1978); 2,4-D (Walsh and Ribelin, 1975); DDT (King, 1962; Walsh and Ribelin, 1975); dieldrin (Walsh and Ribelin, 1975); endosulfan (Walsh and Ribelin, 1975); *organophosphates*: malathion (Walsh and Ribelin, 1975); *carbamates*: sevin (Walsh and Ribelin, 1975); *miscellaneous herbicides*: atrazine (Walsh and Ribelin, 1975); *other miscellaneous compounds*: DMSO (Benville et al., 1968); *nitrogenous compounds*: NH_3 (Smith and Piper, 1975); and *chemotherapeutic agents*: formalin (Smith and Piper, 1972).

Pancreas Islet cell hyperplasia, subcapsular and acinar cell necrosis, vascular congestion, infarction, and edema have been reported following exposures to *organochlorines*: Dowpon (Schulz, 1971); endrin (Eller, 1971); *petroleum compounds*: naphthalene (DiMichele and Taylor, 1978); *organophosphates*: abate (Eller, L. L., unpublished, in Couch, 1975); *other miscellaneous compounds*: DMSO (Benville et al., 1968); and *chemotherapeutic agents*: sulfamethazine (Wood et al., 1957).

Adrenal Cortex Interrenal cell necrosis, cellular and nucleolar hyperplasia and hypertrophy, nuclear hypertrophy, hyperchromatic cytoplasm, cytoplasmic vacuolation, atrophy of cells with clumping of nucleoplasm, high mitotic index, and prominent sinusoids have been observed after exposures to *organochlorines*: DDT (King, 1962); dieldrin (Walsh and Ribelin, 1975); *petroleum compounds*: naphthalene (DiMichele and Taylor, 1978); *other miscellaneous compounds*: SLS (Bromage and Fuchs, 1976); *nitrogenous compounds*: landfill leachates (McBride et al., 1979); *heavy metal salts*: $ZnSO_4$ (Bromage and Fuchs, 1976); and *chemotherapeutic agents*: formalin (Smith and Piper, 1972).

Thyroid Gland Reduced follicular height and possible hyperplasia have been observed with *organochlorines*: endrin (Grant and Mehrle, 1970) and *heavy metal salts*: $CdCl_2$ (Gardner, 1975).

Hepatopancreas (digestive diverticula in some invertebrates) Atrophy, reduction in height of tubular epithelium, tubular dilation, necrosis, and desquamation of tubular epithelium have been noted after exposures to *organochlorines*: Aroclor 1254 (Lowe et al., 1972); DDT (Lowe et al., 1971a; toxaphene (Lowe et al., 1971a); *petroleum compounds*: phenol (Fries and Tripp, 1976); *organophosphates*: methyl parathion (Lowe et al., 1971a); and *heavy metal salts*: $CdCl_2$ (Establier et al., 1978b).

Testes Stimulation of spermatogenesis and exhaustion atrophy, development of ova-like cells within follicles, general atrophy and hypospermia (lower mean index of spermatogenic development), necrosis of tubular boundary cells with hemorrhage, vasodilation, and congestion, increased numbers of infiltrating macrophages with phagocytized debris, necrosis of primary germ cells with atrophy of seminiferous tubules, fibrosis, and infiltration of mononuclear inflammatory cells have been observed with *organochlorines*: kuron (Wood, E. M., unpublished, in Walsh and Ribelin, 1975); *miscellaneous herbicides*: hydrothol 191 (Eller, 1969); *other miscellaneous compounds*: TEPA (Stock and Cope, 1969); and *heavy metal salts*: $CdCl_2$ (Sangalang and O'Halloran, 1972; Tafanelli and Summerfelt, 1975).

Ovaries Hyperplasia of germinal epithelium and involution of some ova, decreased frequency of oocyte maturation, cytoplasmic clumping, and fragmentation and karyolysis of ova have been observed after exposure to *organochlorines*: Aroclor 1254 (Sivarajah et al., 1978) and endrin (Eller, 1971); and *heavy metal salts*: $CdCl_2$ (Tafanelli and Summerfelt, 1975) and $NaAsO_2$ (Gilderhaus, 1966).

Stomach Tunica muscularis with nuclear depolarization and cytoplasmic hyperchromasia, general edema, loss of pepsinogen granules from chief cells, disintegration of goblet cells, and degeneration and pyknosis of glandular epithelium with desquamation of gastric mucosa have occurred following exposures to *miscellaneous herbicides*: atrazine (Walsh and Ribelin, 1975); *heavy metal salts*: $CuSO_4$ (Bhatnagar and Shrivastava, 1975); $HgCl_2$ (Sastry and Gupta, 1978a); CH_3HgCl_2 (Establier et al., 1978a); and *chemotherapeutic agents*: sulfamethazine (Wood et al., 1957).

Esophagus Vacuolation and nuclear condensation (pyknosis) of mucosal epithelial cells and necrosis of all four tunics have been observed with *miscellaneous herbicides*: acrolein (Hendricks, 1979) and *other miscellaneous factors*: acid-alkaline pH (Daye and Garside, 1976).

Rectum Erosion of mucosa at tips of the villi have been reported after exposure to the *heavy metal salt*: $HgCl_2$ (Sastry and Gupta, 1978a).

Heart Degeneration of ventricular myocardium, hypotonicity with poor circulation, and hemostasis have been observed with *petroleum compounds*: whole crude oil (Gardner, 1975) and *heavy metal salts*: $C_4H_6O_4Pb$ (Ozoh, 1978b).

Blood Vessels Vascular anomalies, periodic acid-Schiff (PAS)-positive globular masses in lumina, endothelial separation from basement membrane, subendothelial myositis, and necrosis of arterial walls have been reported after exposures to *organochlorines*: 2,4-D (Cope et al., 1970); *petroleum compounds*: waste motor oil (Gardner, 1978); *miscellaneous herbicides*: hydrothol 191 (Eller, 1969); *heavy metal salts*: $NaAsO_2$ (Gilderhaus, 1966); and *chemotherapeutic agents*: sulfamethazine (Wood et al., 1957).

Peripheral Blood Microcytic, hypochromic, hemolytic anemia with high percentages of abnormal and immature erythrocytes; formation of Heinze and Howell-Jolly bodies; poikilocytosis, anisocytosis, hyperchromasia, anisochromasia, and presence of "smudge" cells among erythrocytes; polycythemia; morphological alterations of erythrocyte nuclei including karyorrhexis; neutrophilia; eosinophilia with deformed nuclei, cytoplasmic vacuolation, and reduction in granular mass; and irregularly shaped thrombocyte nuclei have been observed with *organochlorines*: heptachlor (Andrews et al., 1966); chlorinated wastewater (Buckley et al., 1976; Buckley, 1977); *heavy metal salts*: $CdCl_2$ (Gardner and Yevich, 1970; Gardner, 1975; Gutierrez et al., 1978; Newman and MacLean, 1974); and *chemotherapeutic agents*: formalin (Smith and Piper, 1972); methylene blue (Reichenbach-Klinke, 1975); ozone (Wedemeyer et al., 1979).

Skeletal Muscle Edema of myotomes, degenerative myotomal atrophy, and necrosis have been observed with *petroleum compounds*: naphthalene (DiMichele and Taylor, 1978); *miscellaneous herbicides*: atrazine (Walsh and Ribelin, 1975); $NaTA_2$ (Schulz, 1970); and *other miscellaneous compounds*: TFM (Christie and Battle, 1963).

Brain Hyperemia, hemorrhage, vascular congestion and dilation, infarction, cerebral edema, nuclear pyknosis, rupture and hemorrhage of meninx primitiva, and swelling of myelin sheaths around nerve fibers have occurred with exposures to *organochlorines*: 2,4-D (Cope et al., 1970; Walsh and Ribelin, 1975); DDT (Walsh and Ribelin, 1975); dieldrin (Walsh and Ribelin, 1975); endosulfan (Walsh and Ribelin, 1975); methoxychlor (Kennedy et al., 1970); *petroleum compounds*: naphthalene (DiMichele and Taylor, 1978); *organophosphates*: malathion (Walsh and Ribelin, 1975); *other miscellaneous compounds*: DMSO (Benville et al., 1968); *heavy metals*: $^{109}Cd^{+2}$ (Aoki, 1978); $CuCl_2$ (Gardner and LaRoche, 1973); and *chemotherapeutic agents*:

neguvon and masoten (Reichenbach-Klinke, 1975).

Spinal Cord Swelling of lipoid substance surrounding large nerve cells and "spirality" (twisting of the cord) have been observed with *heavy metal salts*: $CuNO_3$ (Ozoh, 1979a) and *chemotherapeutic agents*: dipterex (Reichenbach-Klinke, 1975).

Integument Reduction in mucous cell numbers and mucous secretion; increased thickness of epidermis; hypertrophy of squamous cells and mucous goblet cells; hyperplasia of mucous goblet cells; hypersecretion of mucus; abnormal melanogenesis of melanophores; generalized inflammation; hemorrhage, necrosis, and erosion of epithelium in pharynx, fins, and tail; epithelial vacuolation, and pyknosis with desquamation have been observed with *organochlorines*: toxaphene (Mayer et al., 1978); *petroleum compounds*: saltwater-soluble crude oil (Hawkes, 1977); phenol (Mitrovic et al., 1968; Reichenbach-Klinke, 1965; Waluga, 1966a); *organophosphates*: malathion (Walsh and Ribelin, 1975); *carbamates*: sevin (Armstrong and Millemann, 1974); *miscellaneous herbicides*; atrazine (Walsh and Ribelin, 1975); *other miscellaneous compounds*: bis(tri-*n*-butyltin) oxide (Chliamovitch and Kuhn, 1977); acid-alkaline pH (Daye and Garside, 1976); *heavy metal salts*: $CdCl_2$ (Newman and MacLean, 1974); $CuCl_2 + CdCl_2 + ZnCl_2$ (Eisler and Gardner, 1973); $C_4H_6O_4Pb$ (Ozoh, 1979b); $PbNO_3$ (Ozoh, 1979a); and *chemotherapeutic agents*: emtrysidina (Reichenbach-Klinke, 1975); hexa-ex (Reichenbach-Klinke, 1975); malachite green (Reichenbach-Klinke, 1975).

Lateral Line Organs Necrosis of sensory and sustentacular epithelium with pyknosis and karyorrhexis; necrosis of cuboidal cells lining canal; infiltration of granular leukocytes in canal lumina, walls, and peripheral connective tissues; reduction of goblet cell numbers lining canal; neuromast nuclei with enlarged nucleoli; and loss of nuclei in some cells have been reported following exposures to *organochlorines*: methoxychlor (Gardner, 1975); *petroleum compounds*: naphthalene (DiMichele and Taylor, 1978); and *heavy metal salts*: $CuCl_2$ (Gardner and LaRoche, 1973); $CuCl_2 + ZnCl_2 + CdCl_2$ (Eisler and Gardner, 1973); $HgCl_2$ (Gardner, 1975); CH_3HgCl_2 (Gardner, 1975); AgCl (Gardner, 1975).

Olfactory Organs Hyperplasia and cytoplasmic degeneration of neurosensory and sustentacular epithelium with cystlike formations containing cellular debris and remnants of sensory tissue; necrosis of mucosa with cellular debris in lumina, vasodilation, and congestion in submucosa, vacuolation and pyknosis in cells of lamina propria; epithelial metaplasia with replacement of neurosensory and sustentacular cells by a less differentiated epithelium and appearance of extracellular refractile rods in mucosa; and hypertrophy and hyperplasia of mucous goblet cells in mucosal lining have been observed with *petroleum compounds*: whole, saltwater-insoluble, and saltwater-soluble crude oil (Gardner, 1975); naphthalene (DiMichele and Taylor, 1978); *other miscellaneous factors*: acid-alkaline pH (Daye and Garside, 1976); and *heavy metal salts*: $CuCl_2$ (Gardner and LaRoche, 1973); $HgCl_2$ (Gardner, 1975); AgCl (Gardner, 1975).

Eye Enlarged abnormally soft lens; degeneration of lens fibers; other degenerative changes such that boundaries between capsule, lens epithelium, and fibers become indistinct; enlargement of lens capsule; corneal degeneration with necrosis of external squamous epithelium and vacuolation of basal epithelium; desquamation of corneal epithelium preceded by poor differentiation between epithelium and substantia propria; swelling of substantia propria after loss of corneal epithelium; hemorrhage in anterior chamber; hemorrhage in periorbital connective tissues; hemorrhage and leukocyte infiltration of limbus corneae; anophthalmia, microphthalmia, and exophthalmia have occurred after exposures to *petroleum compounds*: whole crude oil (Hawkes, 1977); oil slick (Payne et al., 1978); *carbamates*: sevin (Walsh and Ribelin, 1975); *miscellaneous herbicides*; atrazine (Walsh and Ribelin, 1975); *other miscellaneous compounds*: bis(tri-*n*-butyltin) oxide (Chliamovitch

and Kuhn, 1977); acid-alkaline pH (Daye and Garside, 1976); and *heavy metal salts*: $CuCl_2$ (Gardner and LaRoche, 1973); $C_4H_6O_4Pb$ (Ozoh, 1979b).

Pseudobranch Degeneration of secretory cells and hypertrophy of epithelial cells with nuclear swelling and occasional ballooning degeneration have been observed with *petroleum compounds*: whole crude oil (Gardner, 1975); *heavy metal salts*: CH_3HgCl_2 (Wobeser, 1975b); and *chemotherapeutic agents*: formalin (Smith and Piper, 1972).

Yolk Sac Developmental retardation with failure to absorb the yolk sac and occurrence of blue sac disease syndrome have been reported following exposures to *nitrogenous compounds*: NH_3 (Burkhalter and Kaya, 1977) and *heavy metal salts*: $PbNO_3$ (Ozoh, 1979a).

Swim Bladder Air distension in fry and edema have been reported after exposures to *organochlorines*: DDT (Burdick et al., 1964) and *miscellaneous herbicides*: atrazine (Walsh and Ribelin, 1975).

Pituitary Gland Degranulation of cells has been reported following exposure to the *organochlorine* DDD (Ball and Baker, 1969–1970).

Embryonic Tissues Teratomas have occurred in up to 15% of the progeny from parent fish exposed to a mixture of *chemotherapeutic agents*: penicillin G procain, dihydrostreptomycin sulfate, oxytetracycline (DeCew, 1972).

Microscopic Lesions of Diagnostic Significance

Some lesions that occur in fish appear to be useful in diagnosing exposures to certain toxic chemicals once nontoxic causes have been ruled out. Carbaryl (sevin) poisoning produces a syndrome characterized by hemorrhages within white skeletal muscle adjacent to the vertebral column, atrophy of the red skeletal muscle parallel to the lateral line, myxomatous degeneration of fat, and vacuoles in the molecular layer of the optic tectum and in the lateral geniculate body of the brain (Walsh and Ribelin, 1975).

Vertebral deformities are less specific but are suggestive of poisoning by several toxic compounds. For example, Kepone exposure of sheepshead minnows causes a neurologic dysfunction that is clinically observable as tetany or chronic rigor in skeletal muscle (Couch et al., 1977). This results in loss of control of caudal melanocyte patterns (blacktail), myotomal distortion, scoliosis, and fractures of vertebral centra in severe cases. These fractures undergo osteoblastic repair but, depending on severity, can cause further neurologic damage by compression of the lateral funiculi of the spinal cord. Toxaphene poisoning in fish appears similar to Kepone poisoning in that vertebral deformities occur; however, the mechanism of lesion production is different. Collagen metabolism is altered since toxaphene causes a functional vitamin C deficiency, resulting in reduced vertebral collagen and hence vertebral hyperfragility (Mehrle and Mayer, 1975; Mayer et al., 1978). Trifluralin exposure of sheepshead minnows produces a vertebral lesion that is unique in the literature of fish pathology (Couch et al., 1979). The resulting syndrome is one of hyperostosis (bone hypertrophy), characterized by vertebral dysplasia (Figs. 5 and 6, pages 287 and 288) seen as nearly symmetrical hypertrophy of vertebrae with foci of osteoblasts and fibroblasts actively producing bone and bone precursors. Hypertrophy of the notochord, compression of the spinal cord and mesonephric ducts of the kidney from vertebral outgrowths, and fusion of the vertebrae are accompanying lesions. Mechanisms proposed for trifluralin poisoning include alteration of calcium metabolism in the corpuscles of Stannius and the ultimobranchial glands, affecting bone deposition and/or direct or indirect stimulation of osteogenic cells. Additional compounds reported to produce vertebral deformities (scoliosis, lordoscoliosis) include malathion (Mount and Stephen, 1967; Weis and Weis, 1976), other organophosphates (akton, methyl parathion, trichlorfon, phosalone, demeton) (McCann and Jasper, 1972), carbamates (sevin) (Carter, 1971), and lead salts (Holcombe et al., 1976; Ozoh, 1979b).

In both humans (Robbins, 1974) and animals (Smith et al., 1972), bloodborne toxic chemicals do not usually cause glomerular lesions; instead, they produce tubular nephroses. As a rule, chemicals toxic to liver parenchyma often affect tubular epithelium to some degree (Smith et al., 1972). Soluble salts of mercury are noted for extreme nephrotoxicity and certain fish species are susceptible as well [hogchoker, *Trinectes maculatus* (Trump et al., 1975); mummichog (Wassermann and Koepp, 1977)]. Wobeser (1975b) and Establier et al. (1978a,c) noted that mercury and methyl mercury exposure of three fish species— rainbow trout, lisa (*Mugil auratus*), and robalo (*Dicentrarchus labrax*)—resulted in both tubular and glomerular lesions. This does not mean that toxic glomerular nephrosis in fish is a specific lesion for mercury poisoning, but neither is it common. Therefore, it may prove useful in narrowing the choice of a causative compound in a diagnostic situation. Other toxic chemicals that also produce some degree of glomerular change as well as other lesions in fish are cadmium (Hawkins et al., 1980), DMSO (Benville et al., 1968), erucic acid in rapeseed oil (Hendricks, J. D., unpublished data), pyrrolizidine alkaloids in tansy ragwort (Hendricks et al., 1981), amitrole-T (Fig. 12) (Hendricks, 1979), endrin (Mount and Putnicki, 1966), and methyl parathion (Wood, E. M., unpublished, in Walsh and Ribelin, 1975).

It should be noted in this section that the PAS-positive globules found within the vasculature of bluegills exposed to 2,4-D (Cope et al., 1970) are not considered a specific lesion. These globules have also been reported in bluegills exposed to methoxychlor (Kennedy et al., 1970) and in redear sunfish treated with hydrothol 191 (Eller, 1969). They are considered to be a nonspecific response to toxicants peculiar to centrarchid species (Walsh and Ribelin, 1975).

Ultrastructural Pathology in Aquatic Toxicology

Neoplasia is a pathological event which undoubtedly involves a series of complex ultrastructural preneoplastic changes, most of which cannot be recognized by light microscopy until overt cell transformation and tumor growth has occurred. Most of these changes and their chronology of occurrence are still to be defined by TEM and SEM. Since many of the pollutants in the aquatic environment are potential carcinogens, ultrastructural research should prove to be valuable for monitoring neoplasia in wild populations of aquatic species chronically exposed to low levels of various toxic compounds. Investigation of ultrastructural changes other than those of neoplasia is equally important for gaining insight into the environmental impact of various toxicants. The groups of compounds that have been studied most include organochlorines, petroleum compounds, and heavy metal salts. Following is a summary of ultrastructural lesions that have occurred in fish tissues after exposure to these and other groups of compounds. As with most toxicological lesions observed with light microscopy, the ultrastructural pathologies appear to be nonspecific with respect to the causative toxicant.

Gills

Chloride cell degeneration with hypertrophied perinuclear spaces and smooth endoplasmic reticulum; mitochondria having disorganized cristae and ruptured membranes; formation of autophagosomes, vacuoles, myelinlike bodies, and apical vesicles in epithelial cytoplasm; and reduction in thickness of apical homogeneous epithelial cytoplasm have been reported with *petroleum compounds*: saltwater-soluble crude oil (Hawkes, 1977); *other miscellaneous compounds*: bis(tri-*n*-butyltin) oxide (Chliamovitch and Kuhn, 1977); and *heavy metal salts*: $CuSO_4$ (Baker, 1969).

Liver

Distinct vacuolation of hepatocytes, enlargement and/or vesiculation of rough endoplasmic reticulum, presence of circular arrays of smooth-surfaced membranes and myelinlike bodies in hepatocyte cytoplasm, proliferation and "bizarre" whorls of smooth and rough endoplasmic retic-

ulum, loss of glycogen reserves in hepatocytes and presence of cochlear ribosomes, presence of intranuclear and intracytoplasmic electron-dense particles, increased size and numbers of lipofuscin granules, and abnormally enlarged mitochondria have been reported with *organochlorines*: Aroclor 1254 (Sivarajah et al., 1978); miscellaneous PCBs (Hawkes, 1980; Hinton et al., 1978; Klaunig et al., 1979); *petroleum compounds*: whole crude oil (Hawkes, 1977); and *heavy metal salts*: Na_2HAsO_4 (Sorensen, 1976).

Kidney

Focal degeneration of first and second proximal tubules with granular, vacuolated cytoplasm containing swollen or dense contracted mitochondria, some having a granular matrix and focal electron densities, epithelium of third proximal tubules having increased numbers of vacuoles, formation of autophagosomes, lipid droplets, nuclei with marginated chromatin, swollen nuclear envelopes and basal membranes contorted into myelinlike figures, distortion of tubular microvilli, and dilation of endoplasmic reticulum have been reported with *heavy metal salts*: $CdCl_2$ (Hawkins et al., 1980) and $HgCl_2$ (Trump et al., 1975; Wasserman and Koepp, 1977).

Intestine

Absence or reduction of brush border in mucosal epithelium, presence of abnormal inclusion bodies throughout cytoplasm or in apical cytoplasm of columnar epithelium, cytoplasmic vesiculation in columnar cells near luminal surface, abnormal reduction in cytoplasm density, increased amounts of rough endoplasmic reticulum in basal mucosal cells, and diffuse distribution of mitochondria have been reported with *organochlorines*: miscellaneous PCBs (Hawkes, 1980) and *petroleum compounds*: miscellaneous hydrocarbons (Hawkes, 1980).

Pancreas

Submicroscopic degeneration of acinar cells of exocrine pancreas has been reported following exposure to the *organochlorine* Dowpon (Schulz, 1971).

Testes

Damage to head region of spermatozoa and loss of serrations in outer membrane have been reported with the *organochlorine* Aroclor 1254 (Sivarajah et al., 1978).

Ovaries

Enlargement and proliferation of smooth endoplasmic reticulum have been observed with the *organochlorine* Aroclor 1254 (Sivarajah et al., 1978).

Skeletal Muscle

Numerous swollen mitochondria with some disruption of internal membranes and cristae and intercellular breakdown of membranes have been observed with *petroleum compounds*: whole crude oil (Cameron and Smith, 1980).

Brain

Enlarged and irregularly shaped non-membrane-bound perinuclear and intracellular spaces have been observed following exposure to *petroleum compounds*: whole crude oil (Cameron and Smith, 1980).

Integument

Increased numbers of mucus glands appearing dilated have been observed (with SEM) after exposure to *petroleum compounds*: saltwater-soluble crude oil (Hawkes, 1977).

Neurosensory Epithelium

Severe damage to receptor organelles in nares epithelium, including degeneration of chemosensory cilia and loss of microridges circumscribing epithelial cells surrounding olfactory organs, has been observed (with SEM) following exposure to *petroleum compounds*; saltwater-soluble crude oil (Hawkes, 1980).

BIOLOGICAL SIGNIFICANCE OF TOXIC PATHOLOGY

When an aquatic species encounters a toxic compound, the effect is direct, induced, or indirect. A direct effect is caused by direct action of the toxic substance on the aquatic organism. The most obvious direct effect is acute and consists of irreversible damage to vital organ function, resulting in rapid morbidity and death. Most commonly, this occurs as a toxic effect whereby the compound interferes with the integrity of tissue cells or cell processes, and is often manifested by overt gross, histological, and/or ultrastructural lesions. Acute toxic effects are often recognized in short exposure periods (hours or days), while longer periods of low-level exposure (weeks or months) may be required to elicit certain chronic effects. Acute direct effects are typical of experimental situations in the laboratory; if they occur in nature the resulting mass mortalities in aquatic animal populations are more likely to be observed than in the other examples discussed below.

A chronic direct effect differs from an acute one in that the toxicant causes a sublethal change in the host which may or may not be the eventual cause of death. Sublethal changes can occur from a single encounter or from continuous exposure to a toxicant over a long period of time. If a sublethal change is debilitative and predisposes the host to other environmental forces (infectious disease, predation), then the ensuing process (disease or predation) is said to be "induced." Of course, this can occur only if the environmental forces are present. Therefore, an induced effect is brought about by direct action of the toxicant on the aquatic organism but can occur only in the presence of another factor or agent. Chronic direct effects and induced effects of toxicant exposure are of particular importance to those concerned with the aquatic environment since they more closely represent natural situations: toxicants purposely or accidentally released into an aquatic environment are diluted rapidly by ambient waters to levels that are usually marginally lethal and very often sublethal. Exceptions do occur, with large volumes of toxic materials released in short periods of time, particularly at point sources of industrial effluents or ocean acid dump sites. In these cases, toxicant levels may be lethal and aquatic organisms in the immediate vicinity may suffer acute direct effects resulting in mortality. Actual animal losses occurring within a wild population due to chronic direct or induced effects have not been documented because it is nearly impossible to corroborate such data. This is because affected animals are eliminated randomly from the population by natural means which mask the real causative factors. For example, experimental and circumstantial evidence has shown that certain toxic compounds can disrupt sensory perceptions by affecting the lateral line and olfactory organs (Eisler and Gardner, 1973; Gardner and LaRoche, 1973; Gardner, 1975; Daye and Garside, 1976; DiMichele and Taylor, 1978; Hawkes, 1980) or the functioning of the eyes (Walsh and Ribelin, 1975; Daye and Garside, 1976; Chliamovitch and Kuhn, 1977; Hawkes, 1977; Payne et al., 1978; Ozoh, 1979b). These pathologies are chronic direct effects that would certainly adversely affect vital behavior patterns such as schooling, migration, prey selection or capture, and predator escapement, making survival unlikely.

That certain chemical compounds are carcinogenic to various fish species has been experimentally established. Neoplasia is a potentially life-threatening disease for most hosts and could be categorized as an acute direct effect, as discussed earlier. However, in the case of aquatic invertebrates and lower vertebrates, the chemically induced neoplasia reported in most studies may be more correctly classified as a chronic direct effect. Many such tumors are benign, involving nonvital tissues, and those that are malignant enlarge and metastasize so slowly that the life of the host is not immediately threatened. We have observed for nearly 16 mo a group of 100 rainbow trout exposed as embryos to the carcinogen N-methyl-N'-nitro-N-nitrosoguanidine. Nearly all of these fish developed nephroblastomas and hepatic cellular carcinomas, which were grossly visible as exaggerated bulges and swellings protruding from the abdominal area. Although a few mortalities (nine) have occurred, most of the affected fish are alive and feeding at this writing. Quite remarkably, this survival is despite severe debilitation of kidney and liver as well as other organ functions due to the massive displacement of normal tissues by the neoplastic growths. These tumors will eventually kill all of the fish in the tank. However, if the fish had been removed from the near-optimum conditions of the laboratory to a natural environment, they would have died early after tumor formation due to the selective processes of predation, secondary diseases, intra- and interspecific competition, and social hierarchy. Exceptions have been reported in which neoplasia appeared to be an acute direct effect causing mass mortalities: a captive population of feral kelp bass sustained mortalities from metastatic thyroid adenocarcinomas thought to have been caused by water quality factors (Blasiola et al., 1981); mortalities in certain bivalve mollusk populations exposed to possible pollutants have been associated with malignant neoplasms (Christensen et al., 1974; Mix et al., 1977b; Brown et al., 1977). For further information on neoplasia in lower vertebrates and invertebrates, the investigator is referred to the yearly activities report of the Registry of Tumors in Lower Animals, Smithsonian Institution (1979).

Physiological stress accompanies toxicant insult, and it has been shown to exert a chronic direct effect by adversely altering endocrine functions, as sometimes manifested by changes in endocrine histology and histochemistry. Abnormally high blood cortisol levels have been reported in goldfish exposed to sodium lauryl sulfate (Bromage and Fuchs, 1976), killifish exposed to naphthalene (DiMichele and Taylor, 1978), and steelhead trout exposed to therapeutic formalin (Wedemeyer and Yasutake, 1974). Cortisol, a glucocorticoid hormone, plays a major regulatory role in normal metabolism and thus influences the behavior of an individual (Prosser, 1973). In addition, production of androgenic hormones, which are essential for development of male accessory and secondary sexual characteristics and sexual behavior (Prosser, 1973), has been shown to be reduced in testes of brook trout exposed to cadmium chloride (Sangalang and O'Halloran, 1972). For survival of an individual or a population of organisms, normal behavior patterns are as essential as normal functioning of physiological processes and vital organs. Aberrant behavior invites predation or starvation and, when associated with the reproductive cycle, assures reduced population recruitment.

Toxicant-related physiological stress may also lead to induced effects. The physiological stress can directly enhance a host's susceptibility to infectious agents (latent viruses, bacteria, protozoans, etc.) endemic in a population of aquatic animals. The resulting induced effect is clinical disease that would not have surfaced in an otherwise healthy population of animals. Suppression of immunological competence and thus host resistance may be an important factor. The following are examples of the toxicant-infectious disease synergism: penaeid shrimp exposed to low levels of Aroclor 1254 showed a higher prevalance and intensity of infection by a shrimp-specific baculovirus (Couch and Courtney, 1977); rainbow trout exposed to copper showed greater susceptibility to infection with IHN virus (Hetrick et al., 1979); goldfish exposed to mirex developed clinical mycobacterial infections (Van Valin et al., 1968); mullet exposed to crude oils experienced outbreaks of bacterial fin rot disease (Giles et al., 1978); and American oysters exposed to a mixture of DDT, toxaphene, and parathion developed a secondary infection with a mycelial fungus (Lowe et al., 1971a). Surface lesions, resulting from contact with a toxicant, provide direct portals of entry for secondary bacterial or fungal infections, which can ultimately lead to death of the host. Pollutant-related infectious diseases are discussed by Brown et al. (1977).

Indirect effects represent another complex relationship, resulting from the action of a toxicant on something other than the aquatic organism which in turn has an effect on that organism. This can be illustrated by reviewing the use of the larvicide TFM to control the parasitic lamprey eel (*Petromyzon marinus*) in the Great Lakes commercial fishery during the early 1960s. TFM, applied in low doses, selectively killed lamprey larvae but left desirable fish species unharmed (Applegate and King, 1962). The indirect effect was a decline in fish losses due to lampreys and subsequent increase in commercial fish yield. However, as one might surmise, most toxicant-related indirect effects are deleterious rather than beneficial. A toxicant may selectively kill forage species of organisms, such as plankton, insects, or bait fish, which may be more susceptible to its lethal properties. Organisms that depend on those species as a food source are indirectly affected by having to find other forage or starve. Toxicants may exert additional indirect effects by adversely altering the physical properties of the aquatic environment, making survival for organisms difficult or impossible; for instance, the use of herbicidal compounds, such as copper sulfate, may result in anoxic (lack of dissolved oxygen) conditions caused by large quantities of dead and decaying aquatic vegetation (Surber and Everhart, 1950).

In addition to toxicants proved to be carcinogenic, there are many others that are suspected of being carcinogenic, perhaps because their residues have been detected in the tissues of neoplastic animals or at least within the ambient water or bottom sediments. As already noted, PCBs have been implicated in several examples of spontaneous neoplasia in feral finfish populations. Petroleum hydrocarbons have also been suspected as carcinogenic by those reporting neoplasia in bivalve mollusk species exposed to oil spills (Barry and Yevich, 1975; Brown et al., 1977; Yevich and Barszcz, 1977; Mix et al., 1977a,b, 1979; Lowe and Moore, 1978; Harshbarger et al., 1979). Unfortunately, there is little experimental evidence showing whether these two groups of compounds or certain others are indeed carcinogenic within a defined set of circumstances. To pursue these studies further, aquatic toxicologists will have to address the following problems: (1) difficulties in experimentally duplicating the environmental variables that exist in nature, particularly synergistic effects of behavioral, physical, and chemical parameters that may contribute to carcinogenesis; (2) technical inability to maintain certain aquatic fish and shellfish species in the laboratory; (3) lack of well-defined sensitive aquatic animal models for screening and investigation of the neoplastic process; and (4) inability or failure to maintain controlled sublethal toxicant exposures for periods of time long enough (12-24 mo) for carcinogenesis to occur.

SUMMARY

The far-reaching pathological effects of chemical pollution are often very difficult to define in populations of aquatic species. This is particularly true of subtle changes that occur over long periods of exposure to intermittent or continuous sublethal doses of one or several toxicants. It is these changes that aquatic toxicologists and pathologists will be most concerned with in years to come.

The many disciplines in the science of aquatic toxicology are joined in the task of identifying and comprehending each toxicant's mode of activity in organisms which is responsible for clinical signs of intoxication or death. This can be discerned to some degree through biochemical and physiological studies. However, effects are often due to physical changes in the tissues at the cellular or ultrastructural levels and can only be speculated upon unless they are visualized. Since these changes are not grossly apparent, histopathological studies with light microscopy, TEM, and SEM are necessary for the description and evaluation of potential lesions in aquatic animals exposed to various toxicants. Although many toxicant-induced tissue pathologies so far examined have been nonspecific, this is not surprising since aquatic toxopathology is in its infancy. As the science matures and more descriptive studies are made, lesions should emerge which will allow

greater specificity in diagnosing exposure to certain groups of compounds or perhaps to single toxicants. By combining histopathological results with results of biochemical and physiological studies, the complete reaction of an aquatic organism to a toxicant may be defined for future diagnostic purposes.

LITERATURE CITED

Abel PD, Skidmore JF: Toxic effects of an anionic detergent on the gills of rainbow trout. Water Res 9:759–765, 1975.

Allison DB, Kallman BJ, Cope OB, Van Valin CC: Some chronic effects of DDT on cutthroat trout. U.S. Fish Wild Serv Res Rep 64:1–30, 1964.

Anderson BG, Mitchum DL: Atlans of trout histology. Wyoming Game and Fish Dept Bull 13, 1974.

Anderson TF: Electron microscopy of microorganisms. In: Physical Techniques in Biological Research, vol. 3, part A, edited by G Oster and AW Pollister, 178–237. New York: Academic, 1969.

Andrews AK, Van Valin CC, Stebbings BE: Some effects of heptachlor on bluegills (*Lepomis macrochirus*). Trans Am Fish Soc 95:297, 1966.

Anees MA: Intestinal pathology in a freshwater teleost, *Channa punctatus* (Bloch) exposed to sublethal and chronic levels of three organophosphorus insecticides. Acta Physiol Latinoam 26:63–67, 1976.

Aoki K: Effects of cadmium on embryos and fry of the medaka, *Oryzias latipes*. Zool Mag 87:91–97, 1978.

Applegate VC, King EL: Comparative toxicity of 3-trifluoromethyl-4-nitrophenol (TFM) to larval lampreys and eleven species of fishes. Trans Am Fish Soc 91:342–345, 1962.

Armstrong DA, Millemann RE: Pathology of acute poisoning with the insecticide sevin in the bent-nosed clam, *Macoma nasuta*. J Invertebr Pathol 24:201–212, 1974.

Baker JTP: Histological and electron microscopical observations on copper poisoning in the winter flounder *(Pseudopleuronectes americanus)*. J Fish Res Board Can 26:2785–2793, 1969.

Ball JN, Baker BI: The pituitary gland: Anatomy and histophysiology. In: Fish Physiology, edited by WS Hoar, DJ Randall, vol. 2, p. 23. New York: Academic, 1969–1970.

Barry M, Yevich PP: The ecological, chemical and histopathological evaluation of an oil spill site. III. Mar Pollut Bull 6:171–173, 1975.

Benville PE, Jr., Smith CE, Shanks WE: Some toxic effects of dimethyl sulfoxide in salmon and trout. Toxicol Appl Pharmacol 12:156–178, 1968.

Bhatnagar SL, Shrivastava RS: Histopathological changes due to copper in *Heteropneustes fossilis*. (abstract). Indian Sci Congr Assoc Proc 62:173, 1975.

Blasiola GC, Jr., Turnier JC, Hurst EE: Metastatic thyroid adenocarcinomas in a captive population of kelp bass, *Paralabrax clathratus.* J Natl Cancer Inst 66:51–59, 1981.

Bromage NR, Fuchs A: A histological study of the response of the interrenal cells of the goldfish (*Carassius auratus*) to treatment with sodium lauryl sulphate. J Fish Biol 9:529–535, 1976.

Brown ER, Sinclair T, Keith L, Beamer P, Hazdra JJ, Nair V, Callaghan O: Chemical pollutants in relation to diseases in fish. Ann NY Acad Sci 298:535–546, 1977a.

Brown RS, Wolke RE, Saila SB, Brown CW: Prevalence of neoplasia in 10 New England populations of the soft-shell clam (*Mya arenaria*). Ann NY Acad Sci 298:522–534, 1977b.

Buchanan LR: Special invertebrate stain techniques. Annu Rept Am Malacol Union, pp. 56–58, 1970.

Buckley JA, Whitmore CM, Matsuda RI: Changes in blood chemistry and blood cell morphology in coho salmon (*Oncorhynchus kisutch*) following exposure to sublethal levels of total residual chlorine in municipal wastewater. J Fish Res Board Can 33:776–782, 1976.

Buckley JA: Heinze body hemolytic anemia in coho salmon (*Oncorhynchus kisutch*) exposed to chlorinated wastewater. J Fish Res Board Can 34:215–224, 1977.

Buhler DR, Rasmusson ME, Shanks WE: Chronic oral DDT toxicity in juvenile coho and chinook salmon. Toxicol Appl Pharmacol 14:535–555, 1969.

Burdick GE, Harris EJ, Dean HJ, Walker TM, Skea J, Colby D: The accumulation of DDT in lake trout and the effect on reproduction. Trans Am Fish Soc 93:127–136, 1964.

Burkhalter DE, Kaya CM: Effects of prolonged exposure to ammonia on fertilized eggs and sac fry of rainbow trout (*Salmo gairdneri*). Trans Am Fish Soc 106:470–475, 1977.

Cameron JA, Smith RL: Ultrastructural effects of crude oil on early life stages of Pacific herring. Trans Am Fish Soc 109:224–228, 1980.

Carter FL: *In vivo* studies of brain acetylcholinesterase inhibition of organophosphate and carbamate insecticides in fish. PhD thesis, Louisiana State Univ., Baton Rouge, La., 1971.

Chliamovitch YP, Kuhn C: Behavioural, haematological and histological studies on acute toxicity of bis-(tri-n-butyltin) oxide on *Salmo gairdneri* Richardson and *Tilapia rendalli* Boulenger. J Fish Biol 10:575–585, 1977.

Christensen DJ; Farley CA; Kern FG: Epizootic neoplasms in the clam *Macoma balthica* (L.) from Chesapeake Bay. J Natl Cancer Inst 52:1739–1749, 1974.

Christie RM, Battle HI: Histological effects of 3-trifluoromethyl-4-nitrophenol (TFM) on larval lamprey and trout. Can J Zool 41:51–61, 1963.

Cope OB: Sport fishery investigations in pesticide-wildlife studies. U.S. Fish Wildl Serv Circ 199:31, 1963.

Cope OB: Contamination of the freshwater ecosystem by pesticides. J Appl Ecol 3 (Suppl):33–44, 1966.

Cope OB, McCraren JP, Eller LL: Effects of dichlobenil on two fish pond environments. Weed Sci 17:158–165, 1969.

Cope OB, Wood EM, Wallen GH: Some chronic effects of 2,4,-D on the bluegill (*Lepomis macrochirus*). Trans Am Fish Soc 99:1–12, 1970.

Couch JA: Histopathological effects of pesticides and related chemicals on the livers of fishes. In: Pathology of Fishes, edited by WE Ribelin, G Migaki, pp. 559–584. Madison, Wis.: Univ. of Wisconsin Press, 1975.

Couch JA, Courtney L: Interactions of chemical pollutants and virus in a crustacean: A novel bioassay system. Ann NY Acad Sci 298:497–504, 1977.

Couch JA, Winstead JT, Goodman LR: Kepone-induced scoliosis and its histological consequences in fish. Science 197:585–587, 1977.

Couch JA, Winstead JT, Hansen DJ, Goodman LR: Vertebral dysplasia in young fish exposed to the herbicide trifluralin. J Fish Dis 2:35–42, 1979.

Cowey CB, Roberts RJ: Nutritional pathology of teleosts. In: Fish Pathology, edited by RJ Roberts, pp. 216–226, London: Bailliere Tindall, 1978.

Crandall CA, Goodnight CJ: The effects of sublethal concentrations of several toxicants to the common guppy. *Lebistes reticulatus*. Trans Am Microsc Soc 83:59, 1963.

Daye PG, Garside ET: Histopathologic changes in surficial tissues of brook trout, *Salvelinus fontinalis* (Mitchell), exposed to acute and chronic levels of pH. Can J Zool 54:2140–2155, 1976.

DeCew M: Antibiotic toxicity, efficacy and teratogenicity in adult spring chinook salmon (*Oncorhynchus tshawytscha*). J Fish Res Board Can 29:1513–1517, 1972.

DiMichele L, Taylor MH: Histopathological and physiological responses of *Fundulus heteroclitus* to naphthalene exposure. J Fish Res Board Can 35:1060–1066, 1978.

Dreyer NB, King JW: Anaphylaxis in fish. J Immunol 60:277, 1948.

Eisler RE, Gardner GR: Acute toxicology to an estuarine teleost of mixtures of cadmium, copper and zinc salts. J Fish Biol 5:131–142, 1973.

Eller LL: Pathology in redear sunfish exposed to hydrothol 191. Trans Am Fish Soc 98:52–59, 1969.

Eller LL: Histopathologic lesions in cutthroat trout (*Salmo clarki*) exposed chronically to the insecticide endrin. Am J Pathol 64:321, 1971.

Elston R: New ultrastructural aspects of a serious disease of hatchery reared larval oysters. J Fish Dis 3:1–10, 1980a.

Elston R: Functional anatomy, histology and ultrastructure of larval American oysters, *Crassostrea virginica.* Proc Natl Shellfish Assoc 70:65–93, 1980b.

Establier R, Gutierrez M, Arias A: Accumulation and histopathological effects of inorganic and organic mercury in the lisa (*Mugil auratus* Risso). Invest Pesq 42:65–80, 1978a.

Establier R, Gutierrez M, Rodriguez A: Accumulation of cadmium in the muscle and hepatopancreas of the shrimp (*Penaeus kerathurus*) and histopathological alterations produced. Invest Pesq 42:299–304, 1978b.

Establier R, Gutierrez M, Arias A: Accumulation of inorganic mercury from seawater by the robalo, *Dicentrarchus labrax* L., and the histopathological effects. Invest Pesq 42:471–483, 1978c.

Falkmer S, Marklund S, Mattsson PE, Rappe C: Hepatomas and other neoplasms in the Atlantic hagfish (*Myxine glutinosa*): A histopathologic and chemical study. Ann NY Acad Sci 298:342–355, 1977.

Fries C, Tripp MR: Effects of phenol on clams. Mar Fish Rev 38:10–11, 1976.

Galtsoff PS: The American oyster (*Crassostrea virginica*) Gmelin. U.S. Fish Wildl Serv Fish Bull 64:1–479, 1964.

Gardner GR: Chemically induced lesions in estuarine or marine teleosts. In: Pathology of Fishes, edited by WE Ribelin, G Migaki, pp. 657–693. Madison, Wis.: Univ. of Wisconsin Press, 1975.

Gardner GR: A review of histopathological effects of selected contaminants on some marine organisms. Mar Fish Rev 40:51–52, 1978.

Gardner GR, LaRoche G: Copper-induced lesions in estuarine teleosts. J Fish Res Board Can 30:363–368, 1973.

Gardner GR, Yevich PP: Histological and hematological responses of an estuarine teleost to cadmium. J Fish Res Board Can 27:2185–2196, 1970.

Gilderhaus PA: Some effects of sublethal concentrations of sodium arsenite on bluegills and the aquatic environment. Trans Am Fish Soc 95:289–296, 1966.

Giles RC, Brown LR, Minchew CD: Bacteriological aspects of fin erosion in mullet exposed to crude oil. J Fish Biol 13:113–117, 1978.

Gingerich WH, Weber LJ, Larson RE: Carbon tetrachloride-induced retention of sulfobromophthalein in the plasma of rainbow trout. Toxicol Appl Pharmacol 43:147–158, 1978.

Gordon M: The melanoma cell as an incompletely differentiated pigment cell. In: Pigment Cell Biology, edited by M Gordon, p. 215. New York: Academic, 1959.

Goven BA, Dawe DL, Gratzek JB: *In vivo* and *in vitro* anaphylactic type reactions in fish. Dev Comp Immunol 4:55–64, 1980.

Grant BF, Mehrle PM: Chronic endrin poisoning in goldfish, *Carassius auratus*. J Fish Res Board Can 27:2225–2232, 1970.

Grieco MP, Hendricks JD, Scanlan RA, Sinnhuber RO: Carcinogenicity and acute toxicity of dimethylnitrosamine in rainbow trout (*Salmo gairdneri*). J Natl Cancer Inst 60:1127–1131, 1978.

Grizzle JM, Rogers WA: Anatomy and histology of the channel catfish. Auburn Univ Agric Exp Stn, 1976.

Gutierrez M, Establier R, Arias A: Accumulation and histopathological effects of cadmium and mercury on the Sapo (*Halobatrachus didactylus*). Invest Pesq 42:141–154, 1978.

Halver JE, Johnson CL, Ashley LM: Dietary carcinogens induce fish hepatoma. Fed Proc 21:390, 1962.

Harshbarger JC, Otto SV, Chang SC: Proliferative disorders in *Crassostrea virginica* and *Mya arenaria* from the Chesapeake Bay and intranuclear virus-like inclusions in *Mya arenaria* with germinomas from a Maine oil spill site. Haliotis 8:243–248, 1979.

Hawkes JW: The effects of petroleum hydrocarbon exposure on the structure of fish tissues. In: Fate and Effects of Petroleum Hydrocarbons in Marine Ecosystems and Organisms, edited by DA Wolfe, pp. 115–128. New York: Pergamon, 1977.

Hawkes JW: The effects of xenobiotics on fish tissues: Morphological studies. Fed Proc 39:3230–3236, 1980.

Hawkes JW, Gruger EH, Jr., Olson OP: Effects of petroleum hydrocarbons and chlorinated biphenyls on the morphology of the intestine of chinook salmon (*Oncorhynchus tshawytscha*). Environ Res 23:149–161, 1980.

Hawkins WE, Tate LG, Sarphie TG: Acute effects of cadmium on the spot, *Leiostomus xanthurus* (Teleostei): Tissue distribution and renal ultrastructure. J Toxicol Environ Health 6:283–295, 1980.

Hay JB, Hodgins MB, Roberts RJ: Androgen metabolism in skin and skeletal muscle of the rainbow trout (*Salmo gairdneri*) and in accessory sexual organs of the spiny dogfish (*Squalus acanthias*). Gen Comp Endocrinol 29:402–413, 1976.

Hayat MA: Basic Electron Microscopy Techniques. New York: Van Nostrand Reinhold, 1972.

Hayat MA: Principles and Techniques of Electron Microscopy. Biological Applications, vols. 1–9. New York: Van Nostrand Reinhold, 1977.

Hendricks JD: Appendix II. Effect of various herbicides on histology of yearling coho salmon. In: Effects of Selected Herbicides on Smolting of Coho Salmon, edited by HW Lorz, SW Glenn, RH Williams, CM Kunkel, LA Norris, BR Loper, pp. 90–93. U.S. EPA 600/3-79-071, Corvallis Environmental Research Laboratory, 1979.

Hendricks JD, Sinnhuber RO, Loveland PM, Pawlowski NE, Nixon JE: Hepatocarcinogenicity of glandless cottonseeds and refined cottonseed oil to rainbow trout (*Salmo gairdneri*). Science 208:309–310, 1980a.

Hendricks JD, Sinnhuber RO, Wales JH, Stack ME, Hsieh DPH. The hepatocarcinogenicity of sterigmatocystin and versicolorin A to rainbow trout embryos. J Natl Cancer Inst 64:1503–1509, 1980b.

Hendricks JD, Scanlan RA, Williams JL, Sinnhuber RO, Grieco MP: The carcinogenicity of *N*-methyl-*N'*-nitro-*N*-nitrosoguanidine to the livers and kidneys of rainbow trout (*Salmo gairdneri*) exposed as embryos. J Natl Cancer Inst 64:1511–1519, 1980c.

Hendricks JD, Wales JH, Sinnhuber RO, Nixon JE, Loveland PM, Scanlan RA: Rainbow trout (*Salmo gairdneri*) embryos: A sensitive animal model for experimental carcinogenesis. Fed Proc 39:3222–3229, 1980d.

Hendricks JD, Sinnhuber RO, Henderson M, Buhler DR: Liver and kidney pathology in rainbow trout (*Salmo gairdneri*) exposed to dietary pyrrolizidine (*Senecio*) alkaloids. Exp Mol Pathol 35:170–183, 1981.

Hetrick FM, Knittel MD: Fryer JL: Increased susceptibility of rainbow trout to infectious hematopoietic necrosis virus after exposure to copper. Appl Environ Microbiol 37:198–201, 1979.

Hinton DE, Kendall MW, Silver BB: Use of histologic and histochemical assessments in the prognosis of the effects of aquatic pollutants. In: Biological Methods for the Assessment of Water Quality, edited by J Cairns, Jr., KL Dickson, pp. 194–208. ASTM STP528. Philadelphia: ASTM, 1973.

Hinton DE, Klaunig JE, Lipsky, MM: PCB-induced alterations in teleost liver: A model for environmental disease in fish. Mar Fish Rev 40:47–50, 1978.

Hoar WS, Randall DJ (eds.): Fish Physiology, vols. 1–9. New York: Academic, 1969.

Holcombe GW, Benoit DA, Leonard EN, McKim JM: Longterm effects of lead exposure on three generations of brook trout (Salvelinus fontinalis). J Fish Res Board Can 33:1731–1741, 1976.

Humason GL: Animal Tissue Techniques. San Francisco: Freeman, 1962.

Janicki RH, Kinter WB: DDT: Disrupted osmoregulatory events in the intestine of the eel. Science 173:1146–1148, 1971.

Jauch D: Gill lesions in cichlid fishes after intoxication with the insecticide fenthion. Experientia 35:371–372, 1979.

Johnson DW: Pesticides and fishes—a review of selected literature. Trans Am Fish Soc 97:398, 1968.

Johnson PT: Histology of the Blue Crab, Callinectes sapidus (Decapoda: Portunidae). A Model for the Decapoda. New York: Praeger, 1980.

Kendall MW: Acute effects of methylmercury toxicity in channel catfish (Ictalurus punctatus) liver. Bull Environ Contam Toxicol 18:143–151, 1977.

Kennedy HD, Eller LL, Walsh DF: Chronic effects of methoxychlor on bluegills and aquatic invertebrates. U.S. Bur Sport Fish Wildl Tech Pap 53, 1970.

King SF: Some effects of DDT on the guppy and the brown trout. U.S. Fish Wildl Serv Spec Sci Rep Fish 399:1–22, 1962.

Klaunig JE, Lipsky MM, Trump BF, Hinton DE: Biochemical and ultrastructural changes in teleost liver following subacute exposure to PCB. J Environ Pathol Toxicol 2:953–963, 1979.

Lakota S, Raszka A, Kupczak I, Hlond S, Stefan J, Roszkowski J: The effect of methoxychlor and propoxur on the health of carp fry (Cyprinus carpio L.). Acta Hydrobiol 20:197–205, 1978.

Liddell VA: Frozen section technique in shellfish research. J Invertebr Pathol 9:283–284, 1967.

Lillie RD: Histopathologic Technique and Practical Histochemistry. New York: McGraw-Hill, 1965.

Love RM: The Chemical Biology of Fishes. New York: Academic, 1970.

Lowe DM, Moore MN: Cytology and quantitative cytochemistry of a proliferative atypical hemocyte condition in Mytilus edulis (Bivalvia, Mollusca). J Natl Cancer Inst 60:1455–1459, 1978.

Lowe JI: Chronic exposure of spot, Leiostomus xanthurus, to sublethal concentrations of toxaphene in seawater. Trans Am Fish Soc 93:396, 1964.

Lowe JI: Some effects of endrin on estuarine fishes. Proc Annu Conf Southeast Assoc Game Fish Comm 19:271, 1965.

Lowe JI: Effects of prolonged exposure to sevin on an estuarine fish, Leiostomus xanthurus, Lacepede. Bull Environ Contam Toxicol 2:147–155, 1967.

Lowe JI, Wilson PD, Rick AJ, Wilson AJ, Jr.: Chronic exposure of oysters to DDT, toxaphene and parathion. 1970 Proc Natl Shellfish Assoc 61:71–79, 1971a.

Lowe JI, Parrish PR, Wilson AJ, Jr., Wilson PD, Duke TW: Effects of mirex on selected estuarine organisms. North Am Wildl Natur Resour Conf Trans 36, 1971b.

Lowe JI, Parrish PR, Patrick JM, Jr., Forester J: Effects of the polychlorinated biphenyl Aroclor 1254 on the American oyster Crassostrea virginica. Mar Biol 17:209–214, 1972.

Luna LG (ed.): Manual of Histologic Staining Methods of the Armed Forces Institute of Pathology. New York: McGraw-Hill, 1968.

Malek EA, Cheng TC: Medical and Economic Malacology. New York: Academic, 1974.

Maneche HC, Woodhouse SP, Elson PF, Klassen GA: Coronary artery lesions in Atlantic salmon (Salmo salar). Exp Mol Pathol 17:274–280, 1972.

Mathur DS: Studies on the histopathological changes induced by DDT in liver, kidney and intestine of certain fishes. Experientia 18:506–509, 1962.

Mathur DS: Histopathological changes in the liver of certain fishes induced by dieldrin. Sci Cult 31:258–259, 1965.

Mathur DS: Histopathological changes in the liver of fishes resulting from exposure to dieldrin and lindane. Toxicon 13:109–110, 1975.

Matton P, LaHam QN: Effect of the organophosphate dylox on rainbow trout larvae. J Fish Res Board Can 26:2193, 1969.

Mayer FL, Mehrle PM, Crutcher PL: Interactions of toxaphene and vitamin C in channel catfish. Trans Am Fish Soc 107:326–333, 1978.

McBride J, Strasdine G, Fagerlund UHM: Acute toxicity of kanamycin to steelhead trout (*Salmo gairdneri*). J Fish Res Board Can 32:5554–5558, 1975.

McBride JR, Donaldson EM, Derksen G: Toxicity of landfill leachates to underyearling rainbow trout (*Salmo gairdneri*). Bull Environ Contam Toxicol 23:806–813, 1979.

McCain BB, Pierce KV, Wellings SR, Miller BS: Hepatomas in marine fish from an urban estuary. Bull Environ Contam Toxicol 18:1–2, 1977.

McCain BB; Hodgins HO, Gronlund WD, Hawkes JW, Brown DW, Myers MS, Vandermeulen JH: Bioavailability of crude oil from experimentally oiled sediments to English sole (*Parophrys vetulus*) and pathological consequences. J Fish Res Board Can 35:657–664, 1978.

McCann JA, Jasper RL: Vertebral damage to bluegills exposed to acutely toxic levels of pesticides. Trans Am Fish Soc 101:317–322, 1972.

McCraren JP, Cope OB, Eller LL: Some chronic effects of diuron on bluegills. Weed Sci 17:497–504, 1969.

McDaniel D (ed.): Procedures for the Detection and Identification of Certain Fish Pathogens. Washington, D.C.: Fish Health Section, American Fisheries Society, 1979.

Mehrle PM, Mayer FL, Jr: Toxaphene effects on growth and bone composition of fathead minnows, *Pimephales promelas*. J Fish Res Board Can 32:593–598, 1975.

Meyers TR: Preliminary studies on a chlamydial agent in the digestive diverticular epithelium of hard clams, *Mercenaria mercenaria*, from Great South Bay, New York. J Fish Dis 2:179–189, 1979.

Meyers TR: Endemic diseases of cultured shellfish of Long Island, New York: Adult and juvenile American oysters (*Crassostrea virginica*) and hard clams (*Mercenaria mercenaria*). Aquaculture 22:305–330, 1981.

Mitrovic VV, Brown VM, Shurben DG, Berryman MH: Some pathological effects of subacute and acute poisoning of rainbow trout by phenol in hard water. Water Res 2:249–254, 1968.

Mix MC, Pribble HJ, Riley RT, Tomasovic SP: Neoplastic disease in bivalve mollusks from Oregon estuaries with emphasis on research on proliferative disorders in Yaquina Bay oysters. Ann NY Acad Sci 298:356–373, 1977a.

Mix MC, Riley RT, King KI, Trenholm SR, Schaffer RL: Chemical carcinogens in the marine environment. Benzo(a)pyrene in economically-important bivalve mollusks from Oregon estuaries. In: Fate and Effects of Petroleum Hydrocarbons in Marine Organisms and Ecosystems, edited by DA Wolfe, pp. 421–431. New York: Pergamon, 1977b.

Mix MC, Hawkes JW, Sparks AK: Observations on the ultrastructure of large cells associated with putative neoplastic disorders of mussels, *Mytilus edulis*, from Yaquina Bay, Oregon. J Invertebr Pathol 34:41–56, 1979.

Moulton JE: Tumors in Domestic Animals, 2d ed., edited by JE Moulton. Berkeley, Calif.: Univ. of California Press, 1978.

Mount DI: Chronic effects of endrin on bluntnose minnows and guppies. U.S. Fish Wildl Serv Res Rep 58, 1962.

Mount DI, Putnicki GJ: Summary report of the 1963 Mississippi River fishkill. North Am Wildl Natur Resour Conf Trans 31, 1966.

Mount DI, Stephan CE: A method for establishing acceptable toxicant limits for fish, of malathion and butoxyethanol ester of 2,4-D. Trans Am Fish Soc 96:185–193, 1967.

Morton JE: Molluscs. Essex, England: Anchor, 1971.

Nestel H, Budd J: Chronic oral exposure of rainbow trout (*Salmo gairdneri*) to a polychlorinated biphenyl (Aroclor 1254): Pathological effects. Can J Comp Med 39:208–215, 1975.

Newman MW, MacLean SA: Physiological response of the cunner, *Tautogolabrus adspersus*, to cadmium. VI. Histopathology. NOAA Tech Rep NMFS Spec Sci Rep Fish 681:27–33, 1974.

Overstreet RM: Marine Maladies? Worms, Germs, and Other Symbionts from the Northern Gulf of Mexico. Ocean Springs, Miss.: Mississippi-Alabama Sea Grant Consortium, 1978.

Ozoh PTE: Malformations and inhibitory tendencies induced to *Brachydanio rerio* (Hamilton-Buchanan) eggs and larvae due to exposures in low concentrations of lead and copper ions. Bull Environ Contam Toxicol 21:668–675, 1979a.

Ozoh PTE: Studies on intraperitoneal toxicity of lead to *Cichlasoma nigrofasciatum* (Guenther) development. Bull Environ Contam Toxicol 21:676–682, 1979b.

Payne JF, Kiceniuk JW, Squires WR, Fletcher GL: Pathological changes in a marine fish after a 6-mo exposure to petroleum. J Fish Res Board Can 35:665–667, 1978.

Pearse AGE: Histochemistry, Theoretical and Applied. Boston: Little, Brown, 1961.

Pease DC: Histological Techniques for Electron Microscopy. New York: Academic, 1964.

Perkins FO, Menzel RW: Ultrastructure of sporulation in the osyter pathogen, *Dermocystidium marinum*. J Invertebr Pathol 9:205–229, 1967.

Perkins FO: Fine structure of the oyster pathogen, *Minchinia nelsoni* (Haplosporida, Haplosporidiidae). J Invertebr Pathol 10:287–307, 1968.

Perkins FO: Fine structure of *Minchinia* sp. (Haplosporida) sporulation in the mud crab, *Panopeus herbstii.* Mar Fish Rev 37:46–60, 1975.

Post G, Klontz WG (eds): Glossary of Fish Health Terms. Washington, D.C.: Fish Health Section, American Fisheries Society, 1977.

Prosser CL (ed): Comparative Animal Physiology. Philadelphia: Saunders, 1973.

Putt FA: Manual of Histopathological Staining Methods. New York: Wiley, 1972.

Racicot JG, Gaudet M, Leray C: Blood and liver enzymes in rainbow trout (*Salmo gairdneri* Rich.) with emphasis on their diagnostic use: Study of CCl₄ toxicity and a case of *Aeromonas* infection. J Fish Biol 7:825–835, 1975.

Registry of Tumors in Lower Animals, 1979 Supplement: Activities Report. Washington, D.C.: National Museum of Natural History, Smithsonian Institution, 1979.

Reichenbach-Klinke H-H: Der phenolgehalt des wassers in seiner auswirkung auf den fish-organismus. Arch Fischereiwiss 16:176, 1965.

Reichenbach-Klinke H-H: Lesions due to drugs. In: Pathology of Fishes, edited by WE Ribelin, G Migaki, pp. 647–656. Madison, Wis.: Univ. of Wisconsin Press, 1975.

Ribelin WE, Migaki G (eds): Pathology of Fishes. Madison, Wis.: Univ. of Wisconsin Press, 1975.

Robbins SL: Pathologic Basis of Disease. Philadelphia: Saunders, 1974.

Roberts RJ (ed): Fish Pathology. London: Bailliere Tindall, 1978a.

Roberts RJ: The pathophysiology and systematic pathology of teleosts. In: Fish Pathology, edited by RJ Roberts, pp. 55–91. London: Bailliere Tindall, 1978b.

Roberts RJ: Miscellaneous non-infectious diseases. In: Fish Pathology, edited by RJ Roberts, pp. 227–234. London: Bailliere Tindall, 1978c.

Robertson OH, Wexler BC, Miller BF: Degenerative changes in the cardiovascular system of the spawning Pacific salmon (*Oncorhynchus tshawytscha*). Circ Res 9:826–834, 1961.

Robertson OH, Wexler BC: Histological changes in the pituitary gland of the rainbow trout (*Salmo gairdneri*) accompanying sexual maturation and spawning. J Morphol 110:157–169, 1962a.

Robertson OH, Wexler BC: Histological changes in the pituitary gland of the Pacific salmon (*Oncorhynchus*) accompanying sexual maturation and spawning. J Morphol 110:171–185, 1962b.

Sangalang GB, O'Halloran MJ: Cadmium-induced testicular injury and alterations of androgen synthesis in brook trout. Nature (Lond.) 240:470–471, 1972.

Sastry KV, Gupta PK: Effect of mercuric chloride on the digestive system of *Channa punctatus*: A histopathological study. Environ Res 16:270–278, 1978a.

Sastry KV, Gupta PK: Histopathological and enzymological studies on the effects of chronic lead nitrate intoxication in the digestive system of a freshwater teleost, *Channa punctatus.* Environ Res 17:472–479, 1978b.

Sastry KV, Sharma SK: The effect of endrin on the histopathological changes in the liver of *Channa punctatus.* Bull Environ Contam Toxicol 20:674–677, 1978.

Schalm OW: Veterinary Hematology. Philadelphia: Lea & Febiger, 1970.

Schneider SR, Hendricks JD, Constantine GH, Jr, Larson RE: Tobramycin nephrotoxicity and lethality in coho salmon. Toxicol Appl Pharmacol 54:399–404, 1980.

Schulz D: Research into the side effects of the herbicide NaTA$_2$ (sodium trichloroacetate) on the carp. Zentralbl Veterinaermed Reihe A 17:230–251, 1970.

Schulz D: Light microscopic, biochemical and electron microscopic changes on the exocrine pancreas of the carp caused by the herbicide Dowpon. Z Angew Zool 58:63–97, 1971.

Sinnhuber RO, Hendricks JD, Putnam GB, Wales JH, Pawlowski NE, Nixon JE, Lee DJ: Sterculic acid, a naturally occurring cyclopropene fatty acid, a liver carcinogen to rainbow trout (*Salmo gairdneri*). Fed Proc 35:505, 1976.

Sinnhuber RO, Hendricks JD, Wales JH, Putnam GB: Neoplasms in rainbow trout, a sensitive animal model for environmental carcinogenesis. Ann NY Acad Sci 298:389–408, 1977.

Sivarajah K, Franklin CS, Williams WP: Some histopathological effects of Aroclor 1254 on the liver and gonads of rainbow trout, *Salmo gairdneri*, and carp, *Cyprinus carpio*. J Fish Biol 13:411–414, 1978.

Smith CE, Piper RG: Pathological effects in formalin-treated rainbow trout (*Salmo gairdneri*). J Fish Res Board Can 29:328–329, 1972.

Smith, CE, Piper RG: Lesions associated with chronic exposure to ammonia. In: Pathology of Fishes, edited by WE Ribelin, G Migaki, pp. 497–514. Madison, Wis.: Univ. of Wisconsin Press, 1975.

Smith CE, Peck TH, Klauda RJ, McLaren JB: Hepatomas in Atlantic tomcod, *Microgadus tomcod* (Walbaum), collected in the Hudson River estuary in New York. J Fish Dis 2:313–319, 1979.

Smith HA, Jones TC, Hunt RD: Veterinary Pathology. Philadelphia: Lea & Febiger, 1972.

Sobel HJ, Marquet E, Kallman KD, Corley GJ: Melanomas in platy/swordtail hybrids. In: Pathology of Fishes, edited by WE Ribelin, G Migaki, pp. 945–981. Madison, Wis.: Univ. of Wisconsin Press, 1975.

Sorensen EMB: Ultrastructural changes in the hepatocytes of green sunfish, *Lepomis cyanellus* Rafinesque, exposed to solutions of sodium arsenate. J Fish Biol 8:229–240, 1976.

Sparks AK: Invertebrate Pathology. Noncommunicable Diseases. New York: Academic, 1972.

Spurr AR: A low viscosity epoxy resin embedding medium for electron microscopy. J Ultrastruct Res 26:31–43, 1969.

Stedman's Medical Dictionary. Baltimore: Williams & Wilkins, 1976.

Stock JN, Cope, OB: Some effects of TEPA, an insect chemosterilant, on the guppy, *Poecilia reticulata*. Trans Am Fish Soc 98:280–287, 1969.

Surber EW, Everhart MH: Biological effects of nigrosine used for control of weeds in hatchery ponds. Prog Fish Cult 12:135–140, 1950.

Tafanelli R, Summerfelt RC: Cadmium induced histopathological changes in goldfish. In: Pathology of Fishes, edited by WE Ribelin, G Migaki, pp. 613–645. Madison, Wis.: Univ. of Wisconsin Press, 1975.

Thompson SW: Selected Histochemical and Histopathological Methods. Springfield, Ill.: Thomas, 1966.

Trump BF, Jones RT, Sahaphong S: Cellular effects of mercury on fish kidney tubules. In: Pathology of Fishes, edited by WE Ribelin, G Migaki, pp. 585–612. Madison, Wis.: Univ. of Wisconsin Press, 1975.

Van Citters RL, Watson NW: Coronary disease in spawning steelhead trout (*Salmo gairdneri*). Science 159:105–107, 1968.

Van Valin CC, Andrews AK, Eller LL: Some effects of mirex on two warm-water fishes. Trans Am Fish Soc 97:185–196, 1968.

Wales JH, Sinnhuber RO, Hendricks JD, Nixon JE, Eisele TA: Aflatoxin B$_1$ induction of hepatocellular carcinomas in the embryos of rainbow trout (*Salmo gairdneri*). J Natl Cancer Inst 60:1133–1139, 1978.

Walsh AH, Ribelin WE: The pathology of pesticide poisoning. In: Pathology of Fishes, edited by WE Ribelin, G Migaki, pp. 515–557. Madison, Wis.: Univ. of Wisconsin Press, 1975.

Waluga D: Phenol effects on the anatomicohistopathological changes in bream (*Abramis brama* L.). Acta Hydrobiol 8:55–78, 1966a.

Waluga D: Phenol induced changes in the peripheral blood of the breams, *Abramis brama* (L.). Acta Hydrobiol 8:87–95, 1966b.

Wasserman J, Koepp SJ: An ultrastructural study

of mercury-induced injury in the intact proximal tubule of the common mummichog (*Fundulus heteroclitus*). NJ Acad Sci Bull 22:47, 1977 (abstract).

Wedemeyer GA, Yasutake WT: Stress of formalin treatment in juvenile spring chinook salmon (*Oncorhynchus tshawytscha*) and steelhead trout (*Salmo gairdneri*). J Fish Res Board Can 31:179–184, 1974.

Wedemeyer GA, Yasutake WT: Prevention and treatment of nitrite toxicity in juvenile steelhead trout (*Salmo gairdneri*). J Fish Res Board Can 35:822–827, 1978.

Wedemeyer GA, Nelson NC, Yasutake WT: Physiological and biochemical aspects of ozone toxicity to rainbow trout (*Salmo gairdneri*). J Fish Res Board Can 36:605–614, 1979.

Weis P, Weis JS: Abnormal locomotion associated with skeletal malformations in the sheepshead minnow, *Cyprinodon variegatus*, exposed to malathion. Environ Res 12:196–200, 1976.

Wobeser G: Acute toxicity of methyl mercury chloride and mercuric chloride for rainbow trout (*Salmo gairdneri*) fry and fingerlings. J Fish Res Board Can 32:2005–2013, 1975a.

Wobeser G: Prolonged oral administration of methyl mercury chloride to rainbow trout (*Salmo gairdneri*) fingerlings. J Fish Res Board Can 32:2015–2023, 1975b.

Wood EM, Yasutake WT, Johnson HE: Acute sulfamethazine toxicity in young salmon. Prog Fish Cult 19:64–67, 1957.

Yevich PP, Barszcz CA: Neoplasia in soft-shell clams (*Mya arenaria*) collected from oil-impacted sites. Ann NY Acad Sci 298:409–426, 1977.

Yokote M: Spontaneous diabetes in carp (*Cyprinus carpio*). Spec Publ Jpn Sea Fish Lab, pp. 67–74, 1974.

Zweifach BW, Grant L, McCluskey RI (eds): The Inflammatory Process. New York: Academic, 1965.

Editor's note: Two new atlases, on rainbow trout and striped bass, have been published since this chapter was written: Groman DB: Histology of the striped bass. Amer Fish Soc Monogr 3:1–116, 1982; Yasutake WT, Wales JH: Microscopic anatomy of salmonids: An atlas. U.S. Fish Wildl Serv Res Pub 150:1–190, 1983.

Specific Chemical Effects

Chapter 12

Pesticides

D. R. Nimmo

INTRODUCTION

The primary purpose of pesticides is to prevent, control, or eliminate pests. Pesticides have benefited humans by controlling insect and rodent disease vectors, noxious arthropods and plants, and crop and forest pests. Because they are designed to adversely affect certain organisms and to persist in the environment for a specific time, pesticides are considered a unique group of compounds.

Numerous chemical agents not usually considered by the public to be pesticides are actually classified as such. Examples are herbicides used as defoliants to remove leaves from agricultural crops prior to mechanical harvesting; chlorine used in power plant cooling systems to prevent fouling by periphyton or other sessile organisms; fumigants such as methyl bromide and *p*-dichlorobenzene; biocides in drilling fluids used in oil exploration; and such common wood preservatives as creosote and pentachlorophenol.

Pests are a major cause of crop losses in the field and in storage. Rudd (1964) estimated annual crop losses due to rodents in the United States to be $2 billion. Losses from insects were $4 billion. Even more surprising, losses due to weeds were $11 billion annually. If these estimates were reasonably accurate in 1964–1970, then the present-day losses, adjusted to current dollars, must be enormous.

In the past, chemical control of pests was accomplished with a relatively small number of inorganic copper and arsenic compounds or naturally occurring insecticides such as pyrethrum and rotenone. Development and effective use of organic chemicals for pest control were slow until World War II, when the discovery of a synthetic organic pesticide, DDT, initiated the development and expansion characteristic of the past 40 years. Until the discovery of DDT, the pesticide that had the greatest impact on natural aquatic ecosystems in many areas of the world was probably Paris green (copper acetoarsenite), which was applied to many mosquito breeding areas to control malaria.

DDT not only was highly toxic to a wide range of insect pests and had persistent properties that allowed it to remain active for months or years, it was also relatively inexpensive to manufacture. Its qualities stimulated the search for other synthetic organic chemicals for pest control. Initial research efforts concentrated on the particular group to which DDT belongs: the organochlorine or chlorinated hydrocarbon group. This expanded research produced a host of compounds—dieldrin, endrin, methoxychlor, and others.

Continued research has resulted in two other potentially effective groups, namely the organophosphate compounds (e.g., parathion and malathion) and the carbamates (e.g., Sevin). Examples will be discussed in detail in this chapter. In the past 5-10 yr new chemical groups of pesticides, such as pyrethroids or growth inhibitors have received much attention.

In the past three decades the use of synthetic pesticides in the United States has increased about 40-fold (weight basis) (Ridgway et al., 1978). The increase has probably been in existing types or classes of pesticides, since the number of new chemical compounds introduced annually has declined. Currently, only 70-100 new chemicals or biological control agents receive registration labels each year—a fraction of the thousands of industrial chemicals introduced each year for commercial use. World pesticide production in 1975 was estimated as 3.7 billion pounds, of which the United States produced half (Ridgway et al., 1978). On the basis of these estimates, about 70% of new chemicals produced in the United States are used in agriculture, and insecticides, herbicides, and fungicides comprise about 90% of all pesticides used in agriculture. According to Ridgway et al. (1978), about 70% of all pesticides are used on crops of cotton, corn, fruits, and vegetables; however, of all the pesticides used on farms, herbicide usage (Table 1) has increased far more than usage of fungicides, insecticides, fumigants, and other types.

In retrospect, it is difficult to understand how the discoveries of DDT and the other organochlorine compounds, which were so effective in controlling target pests and so resistant to degradation, did not include consideration of the possibility that their use on a large scale would have some deleterious and undesirable effects on nontarget species and the environment. Cautious and accurate forecasts of a few biologists prior to 1950 were ignored. For example, Ginsburg (1945) published on the toxicity of DDT to fish, and Sandholzer (1945) reported adverse effects of DDT on the Chesapeake Bay blue crab. It was almost 10 yr after the introduction and widespread use of DDT that the accumulation of evidence caused a reexamination of the question of whether pesticides should be considered environmental contaminants. Eventually, other materials became of equal concern in aquatic ecosystems.

Although this chapter concerns the impact of pesticides on aquatic life, references to polychlorinated biphenyls (PCBs) are made throughout.

Table 1 Quantities of Pesticides[a] by Type Used on U.S. Farms, 1964-1976[b]

Type of pesticide	Active ingredient (millions of pounds)			
	1964	1966	1971	1976
Fungicides	33	33	42	44
Herbicides	84	115	228	384
Insecticides	156	149	170	158
Fumigants, growth regulators, desiccants, and defoliants	44	46	52	57

[a]Does not include miticides, rodenticides, repellents, and others.
[b]Adapted from Ridgway et al. (1978).

PCBs are so closely related to many pesticides in their chemical, physical, and toxicological properties and widespread occurrence that they are almost inextricably associated with pesticides in discussions of chemical pollutants in the aquatic environment. The amount of scientific information on PCBs is so large that a separate chapter could be devoted to this single class of pollutants. Nevertheless, the next two paragraphs will briefly describe how PCBs are manufactured and used and why it is necessary to evaluate their movement in the environment and their toxicity to aquatic life. The reader should be aware of the environmental significance of PCBs and the reasons for inclusion (by association) in this chapter.

PCBs are chlorinated compounds formed by the direct chlorination of the biphenyl ring. They are very similar chemically to DDT, dieldrin, and aldrin. Mixtures of various isomers, often called chlorobiphenyls, were identified by U.S. manufacturers under the trade name "Aroclor" on the basis of percent of chlorine (e.g., 21, 42, 54, 60%). A common PCB was Aroclor 1254, a mixture of chlorinated biphenyl isomers with an average chlorine content of 54% by weight. Since the possible 209 individual components in the mixtures differ in physical, chemical, and biological properties, evaluation of the potential impact of the various Aroclor mixtures is complicated.

Unlike pesticides, PCBs were never intended to become part of the environment. Most uses were for "closed" systems such as electrical transformers and capacitors, and some applications were as lubricants, fluids in vacuum pumps and compressors, and heat transfer and hydraulic fluids. Of the approximately 1.25 billion pounds purchased by U.S. industry, it has been estimated in a report to the Office of Toxic Substances (Durfee et al., 1976) that about 750 million pounds are still in service, almost all in capacitors and transformers. Fifty-five million pounds have been destroyed by incineration or degraded in the environment, and about 44 million are still in the environment. About 290 million pounds are believed to be in landfills or dumps, and 150 million

are "free" in the environment and available to biota via air, water, soil, and sediments.

The first concern of the modern-day movement in ecology was with organic pesticides. The books *Silent Spring* (Carson, 1962), *Pesticides and the Living Landscape* (Rudd, 1964), and *Since Silent Spring* (Graham, 1970) have kept the problems, both real and imagined, before the public. *Pesticides—A New Factor in Coastal Environments* (Butler and Springer, 1963) alerted scientists and laymen to the fact that pesticides were so widely used that they must be considered a significant factor in the ecological relationships in coastal environments of fish and wildlife. Contamination with dioxin from Agent Orange (or Herbicide Orange, a defoliant), used extensively in Vietnam; the occurrence of Kepone in the James River, Virginia; buried wastes in the Love Canal at Niagara Falls, New York; 2,4,5-T spraying in the Northwest; and the ubiquity of PCBs keep the problems of synthetic organic chemicals, especially pesticides, under public scrutiny.

TARGET AND NONTARGET ORGANISMS

Pesticides may have dual actions. They are important in controlling injurious pests, but they may also present a hazard to species not considered to be pests in the environment. As a result, the concepts of "target" and "nontarget" organisms have arisen. For example, in many freshwater systems, control measures may be taken against undesirable target organisms such as mosquito larvae or unwanted algae. Nontarget organisms are those whose destruction is not intended and which are nevertheless affected. Furthermore, these nontarget organisms may play a key role in aquatic ecosystems. The distinction between target and nontarget species is not absolute, because the same group may be nontarget organisms in one area of the country but target organisms, under certain circumstances, in another area. For example, larvae of caddis flies (*Trichoptera* sp.) and naiads of mayflies (*Ephemeroptera* sp.) are important food sources for trout and other valuable freshwater fish. In certain areas, these species of insects occur in such large numbers that they are nuisance pests, and their immature stages are the target of planned control operations with pesticides. For example, Ali and Mulla (1977a,b) studied measures for control of nuisance midges at residential-recreational lakes in California.

The ideal situation in most control operations is to be able to destroy the undesirable species at pesticide concentrations that will have minimal adverse effects on the rest of the biota. However, some degree of contamination and hazard is assumed with nearly all pesticide use. The hazard to aquatic ecosystems depends on the chemical and physical properties of the pesticide, type of formulation, rate and method of application, and characteristics of the receiving water system.

TYPES OF PESTICIDES

Pesticides may be categorized according to their use or intended target (e.g., insecticide, herbicide, fungicide), chemical structure (organochlorine, organophosphate), or mode of action (chitin inhibitor, sex attractant). According to von Rumker et al. (1975b), there is no single authoritative categorization of pesticides, but use categories are presented (Table 2).

Pesticides were categorized by chemical structure in one review as follows (Lincer, 1975):

Insecticides
  Chlorinated hydrocarbons (organochlorines): DDT, aldrin, dieldrin, heptachlor, toxaphene, and chlordane.
  Organophosphates: malathion, parathion, diazinon, and Guthion.
  Carbamates: Sevin, Zectran, Baygon, and temik.
  Pyrethrins (house and garden sprays): allethrin and cyclethrin.
Fungicides
  Dithiocarbamates: ferbam, ziram, and maneb.
  Nitrogen-containing compounds: phenylmercuric acetate, triazines, quinones, heterocyclics, and some heavy metals.
  Hexachlorobenzene.

Table 2 Examples of Pesticide Use Categories[a]

Insecticides/miticides	
Aldrin	Methyl parathion
Carbaryl	Parathion
Carbofuran	Toxaphene
Chlordane	Disulfoton
Diazinon	Malathion
Herbicides/algicides	
Alachlor	Dichlobenil
Atrazine	Diuron
Bromacil	MSMA
2,4-D	Sodium chlorate
Neburon	Trifluralin
Fungicides and wood preservatives	
Captan	Maneb
Creosote	Pentachlorophenol
Fumigants	
Methyl bromide	p-Dichlorobenzene

[a]From von Rumker et al. (1975b).

Herbicides
  Phenoxy acids: 2,4-D and 2,4,5-T.
  Aquatic herbicides: endothal and diquat.

Some recent approaches to pest control emphasize novel ways to control insects. At a conference on this subject, Elliot (1976) reported on a class of compounds called pyrethroids. Pyrethroids, which are closely related to pyrethrum (natural extracts from the chrysanthemum family), are excellent insecticides and are relatively harmless to mammals. Unfortunately, natural pyrethrins are unstable and expensive to produce. As a result, in the synthesis of a pyrethroid, the photolabile portion of the pyrethrin molecule has been replaced with other groups, resulting in more stability (less susceptibility to degradation on exposure to air and light).

Insect growth regulators (IGRs) also represent new approaches. The best known is methroprene (trade name, Altosid IGR). An IGR is a substance that interferes with the normal physiological growth function. With some IGRs, death results when the adult fails to emerge. Another well-known IGR is diflubenzuron (trade name, Dimilin), whose specific action is interference in the formation of insect cuticle during the molting process.

Organotin compounds have extremely broad biological activity. According to Hunter (1976), triaryltins are active as antifoulants, bactericides, molluscides, algicides, anthelmintics, fungicides, insect antifeedants, acaracides, chemosterilants, and insecticides. The relatively low phytotoxicity of these compounds makes them excellent for plant protection. One of the best known organotins is the fungicide Duter. According to Kimbrough (1976), as early as the 1960s triphenyltin compounds were suggested as chemosterilants for insects.

Formamidines are a class of chemicals developed in the late 1950s and early 1960s which also appear to have a broad spectrum of useful activity. Some organisms sensitive to this class are the phytophagous and predaceous mites, ticks, Lepidoptera, and, more important, Homoptera (e.g., aphids, scales, leafhoppers, and psyllids) (Hollingworth, 1976). Common names for formamidines are Fundal, Galecron, and Amitraz.

Other insecticides besides pyrethrins are derived from plants. Soloway (1976) lists the following: nicotine alkaloid, nicotine sulfate, rotenone (cube), rotenone (derris), hellebore, ryania, and sabadilla. Soloway (1976) favored use of natural insecticides because of their generally low acute toxicity to mammals and their ease of metabolism. A disadvantage of natural insecticides is that they are complex mixtures, and determining the toxicological and metabolic properties of more than one component is difficult.

It must be recognized that most chemical pesticides are not applied to target areas as a pure material (i.e., active ingredients), but rather in a formulation. In conducting most aquatic toxicity studies necessary for the registration of a pesticide, it should be noted that the material used is pure or as pure as can be obtained by practical means. The various forms in which pesticides are applied are illustrated by the following definitions (Farm Chemicals Handbook, 1981):

Emulsifiable concentrate. Produced by dissolving the pesticide and an emulsifying agent in an organic solvent. A solvent substantially insoluble in water is usually selected, since water-miscible solvents have not, in general, proved feasible. The strength is usually stated in pounds of pesticide per gallon of concentrate.

Emulsifier. A surface-active substance that stabilizes (reduces the tendency to separate) a suspension of droplets of one liquid in another liquid, which otherwise would not mix.

Formulation. The prepared, or formulated, mixture concocted to give proper results. Few pesticidal substances are sold commercially without being mixed with other ingredients: carriers, diluents, solvents, wetting agents, emulsifiers, and so on. The chemicals are usually too concentrated and immiscible with water to be prepared directly for use by the purchaser. The process used by the manufacturer to prepare a pesticide for practical use is also termed *formulation.*

Surface-active agent. A substance that reduces the interfacial tension of two boundary layers. Most pesticide adjuvants can be considered surface-active agents. They are also known as surfactants.

Synergist. A material that exhibits synergism, the joint action of different agents such that the total effect is greater than the sum of the independent effects. The efficiency of one or more components of a mixture is greatly heightened or potentiated by a synergistic component. (Example: pesticide X kills 40% of an insect population; pesticide Y kills 20%; when applied together, X and Y kill 95%.) Newer developments in this field have stemmed from efforts to increase the activity or extend the supply of pyrethrum during World War II, when it was scarce.

Technical material. The pesticide chemical in pure form (usually 95–100% active ingredient) as manufactured by a chemical company prior to its formulation into wettable powders that are easily added to water to make a slurry, dust, emulsifiable concentrate, granule, or other form.

PHYSICAL AND CHEMICAL CHARACTERISTICS OF PESTICIDES

The physical and chemical characteristics of pesticides are significant for determining their activity and eventual effects on aquatic systems. Pesticides range from simple inorganic compounds to extremely complex organic molecules. They may have broad-spectrum activity or a single mode of action toward one particular species. The following characteristics help determine the relative hazard of a pesticide to the aquatic environment.

Aqueous Solubility

Pesticides have a wide range of solubilities (Table 3). For example, the solubility of DDT in water is 0.001 mg/l and that of dalapon (herbicide) is 80% (800,000 mg/l). In general, the solubility of most pesticides is in parts per million (ppm, mg/l). Determination of the water solubility of pesticides with values in the ppm range or more is relatively

Table 3 Solubility of Pesticides in Water

Pesticide	Solubility (mg/l)
Organochlorines	
DDT	0.0012
Aldrin	0.01
Heptachlor	0.056
Dieldrin	0.18
Lindane	7.0
Organophosphates	
Parathion	24
Diazinon	40
Malathion	145
Dimethoate	2500
Carbamates	
Carbaryl	40
Carbofuran	700
Herbicides	
Simazine	5.0
Atrazine	34
2,4,5-T	280
2,4-D	890
Diquat	(70%)
Dalapon	(80%)

simple; however, for strongly hydrophobic pesticides, such as DDT, whose solubility is in the parts per billion (ppb, μg/l) range, determination of water solubility is difficult because such chemicals form aggregates in aqueous solution. The presence of some pesticides in water can be detected by gas chromatography at the parts per trillion (ppt, μg/l) level, but the effects of such concentrations of pesticides on the organisms and systems in which they occur may not be perceived in many cases.

Pesticides that are insoluble in water are usually bound to suspended organic matter and bottom sediment of aquatic systems; otherwise, they may volatilize. Low water solubility may also indicate affinity of the compound to partitioning from water to lipid material, suggesting a potential for accumulation of the pesticide in the tissues of organisms. Highly water-soluble pesticides are more likely to be widely distributed in aquatic systems. These water-soluble substances tend not to adsorb to organics, are less likely to volatilize, are less persistent, and are more easily diluted and dispersed.

Stability and Persistence

The chemical structure of a pesticide determines its stability and persistence in aquatic systems. Pesticides range from very stable compounds that persist as residues for many years to unstable compounds that break down in a few hours. Malathion and carbaryl degrade in water in a few hours to a few days, while DDT, dieldrin, and endrin residues may persist for years under the same conditions. Persistent pesticides are a potential hazard to the aquatic ecosystem, since the organisms will be exposed to them for long periods of time after a single application. There is thus a potential for accumulation of the more persistent pesticides in fish and other aquatic organisms. For example, pesticide residues in fish may persist for days (organophosphates) or years (organochlorines). Persistence in the entire aquatic ecosystem is generally greatest for organochlorine insecticides, intermediate for organophosphate (organophosphorus) and carbamate insecticides, and least for biological control agents such as hormones and chitin inhibitors.

APPLICATION OF PESTICIDES

It might be useful to describe briefly a few methods of pesticide application to field crops, since household and garden uses of pesticides are more familiar. The best known method is aerial application, which is common in rural areas in this country. The formulation might be applied in dust (aircraft, venturi airblaster), liquid spray (tractor with a boom sprayer), or granular (aircraft with a venturi spreader or by a planter mounted on a tractor frame). Sometimes the ingredient is dispersed in a liquid carrier and applied in high volume (rather dilute), low volume, or ultra low volume, in which case no carrier or minimal carrier is used.

The best example of a granular material was mirex, the insecticide used to control fire ants (*Solenopsis saevissima richteri*) in the southeastern states. The granules, coarsely ground corncobs, were soaked in cottonseed oil in which mirex had been dissolved. After the granules were applied by aircraft, the ants were attracted to the oil, then carried the corncob granules into their burrows.

Applications of pesticides for various crops can be made by large tanker trucks (as large as a 1600-gal tank and 50-ft hydraulic wet booms). The pesticide may need to be directed toward a specific area of a row crop, in which case the tank may be mounted on a smaller row crop tractor with nozzles aimed at an angle. Often fertilizers and pesticides are applied concurrently by this method.

Applications of pesticides in liquid form on orchard crops or livestock may be less well known. The delivery of the liquid is similar to that above, except that the boom and nozzle are under direct control of the operator for thorough coverage.

For most pesticides the rates of application are usually expressed as pounds of active ingredient per acre. For instance, according to an EPA compendium (von Rümker et al., 1975a), Guthion may be used on apples at a rate of 6.0 lb active ingredient (12.0 lb, 50% wettable powder) per acre of application up to eight times per season. Each state pest management program may recommend a variation of this rate of usage.

PREPARATION OF SAMPLES FOR ANALYSIS OF PESTICIDES

The analysis of pesticides and PCBs in environmental samples varies with the type of sample: water, sediment (or soil), or biota. An extraction procedure almost always requires a specified amount of water to be extracted by one or more organic solvents in a separatory funnel, selectively concentrating the pesticide present in the original sample into a small volume of a solvent in which the pesticide is soluble. Next is a step to reduce the solvent volume, further concentrating the pesticide, before analysis by gas chromatography. For biota such as fish or oysters, or for sediment, the preparation is more involved. Samples are homogenized and extracted in a Soxhlet apparatus with an organic solvent such as hexane or methylene chloride. Next is a "cleanup" in which the samples are passed through a column of adsorbent material (Florisil is commonly used) to trap and remove debris and other materials that could interfere with the analysis. Further cleanup followed by a concentration step is necessary before analysis by electron capture (EC), flame ionization (FI), or multiple ion detection (MID) gas-liquid chromatography. In recent years, analysis by high-pressure liquid chromatography (HPLC) has become very popular. Often, after analysis, a further step is taken to verify the pesticide with mass spectrometry (MS). For a review of typical procedures used in the analysis of pesticides the reader is referred to Chapter 16 and to Goodman et al. (1979) and Veith et al. (1981).

TRANSPORT AND FATE OF PESTICIDES IN AQUATIC ENVIRONMENTS

Pesticides enter aquatic environments through intentional application, aerial drift, or runoff from applications or accidental release, and then become rapidly distributed through the action of wind and water. Some pesticides are applied directly to water to control aquatic weeds, algae, nongame fish, unwanted invertebrates, and noxious insects. Agricultural runoff from fields and grazing lands is considered the major route of pesticide movement into water (Li, 1975). For example, following a controlled flood to prevent frost damage in a cranberry bog, Miller et al. (1966) found that the runoff water transported diazinon and parathion, which had been used as insecticides on the crop. Vanderford and Hamelink (1977) found that bass contained high dieldrin residues from flood-control reservoirs that drain large areas of corn cropland in Indiana, but no dieldrin residues were found in smaller reservoirs in areas that had no corn cropland in their watersheds.

It has been estimated that industrial waste (effluents) from pesticide manufacturing is the second greatest source of pesticides in aquatic environments (Li, 1975). Examples are DDT, toxaphene, and Kepone. Waters of the Tombigbee-Mobile river system became contaminated to the extent of 1.9 ppb DDT from an industrial site (Mackenthun, 1965). River sediments contained 410 and 170 ppm DDT and the metabolite DDE, respectively, downstream from the outfall. Fish contained nearly 36 and 52 ppm DDT and DDE, respectively. Another release several years later, which gained much notoriety, was said to be the cause of the Mississippi fish kills of the early 1960s. These kills, described as "enormous" by Graham (1970), were due to a pesticide manufacturing plant near Memphis, Tennessee. Also reported by Graham (1970) was a release from a toxaphene plant into Terry Creek, Brunswick, Georgia. Sediments contained 2000 ppm and oysters had 6 ppm in their tissues.

Several investigators have studied pesticide contamination in marine waters off Southern California. Li (1975) concluded that the buildup of DDT in Southern California coastal marine organisms could be due to industrial waste discharge rather than to extensive agricultural usage.

Investigators in Southern California (Coastal Water Research Project, 1976–1980) have been studying various sources of pollutant inputs into coastal waters. The findings regarding pesticides and PCBs in water and sediments on a year-to-year basis were as follows:

1 1976—When municipal waste waters, industrial waste waters, river runoff, aerial fallout, and harbor discharges are compared, municipal wastes now contain only 5% of the DDT discharged in 1970. Aerial fallout has been the main source of DDT to the sea since 1974. Most PCBs enter the sea via outfalls, and the amount in 1975 was only one-tenth of that in 1972.

2 1977—The greatest decreases in monitored emissions were in DDT and PCBs. Amounts had fallen by 80–90% since 1972.

3 1978—Emissions of DDT were down 28% and PCBs down 34% from 1977 levels.

4 1979–1980—DDT concentrations in sediments off Palos Verdes decreased substantially in the upper 2 cm.

Perhaps the best known recent example of pesticide pollution from an individual source was Kepone in the James River and Chesapeake Bay estuary, Virginia. The extent of contamination is reviewed in a report by Lunsford (1981), who presents the results of monitoring Kepone in surface and bottom water samples. The toxicity to, and bioconcentration of, Kepone in aquatic species were studied by Bahner et al. (1977), Hansen et al. (1977a,b), Schimmel and Wilson (1977), and Walsh et al. (1977).

Significant atmospheric transport of pesticides to aquatic environments can also occur. This is due to three factors (Li, 1975): (1) aerial drift of pesticides, (2) volatilization from applications in terrestrial environments, and (3) wind erosion of treated soils. Nearly half of the DDT applied to the surface of a field may volatilize and thus contribute to the downwind distribution (Lloyd-Jones, 1971). Transport and input of DDT and PCB residues via particulate matter in the air and precipitation was found to be the most significant source in a Swedish lake ecosystem (Sodergren, 1973). Losses of pesticides Zinophos and Dyfonate occurred during applications to soil even though the distance between the spray nozzle and intended targets was short (Kiigemagi and Terriere, 1971). The authors concluded that the losses must be considerably higher when the pesticides are applied to plants, especially trees. It was recently shown that atmospheric deposition of organic pollutants in the Great Lakes represents a sizable, if not the major, source of pesticide contamination (Eisenreich et al., 1981).

Finally, another source of pesticides that is poorly understood and not well studied is that associated with hazardous waste disposal. In the late 1970s it was estimated that the weight of hazardous waste containing pesticides was more than 1800 metric tons per year in Florida (Carter et al., 1977). This did not include pentachlorophenol, creosote, and inorganic wastes produced by the wood processing industry.

Once in the water, pesticide residues may either become attached to suspended material, deposited on the bottom sediment, or absorbed by organisms, where they are detoxified or accumulated (Fig. 1). They may be transported through the aquatic system by diffusion in water currents or in the bodies of aquatic organisms. Some pesticides or their transformation products may also move back into the atmosphere by volatilization. There is a continuous interchange of pesticides between sediments and water, influenced by water movement, turbulence, and temperature.

Fish and invertebrates may accumulate pesticides at concentrations far in excess of that in the water in which they live because the chemicals

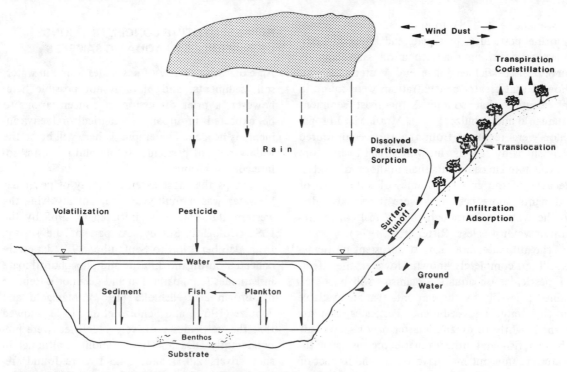

Figure 1 Movement of pesticides into and through aquatic ecosystems.

may be bound to suspended matter that is ingested. Baughman and Lassiter (1978) stated that sorption of compounds between water and biotic (e.g., microorganisms) and abiotic (e.g., sediments) components may be the single most important environmental process affecting the fate of pollutants. They reviewed five observations made by others regarding this process:

1 Sorption of highly insoluble organics by sediments and microorganisms is rapid (substantially complete in less than a few hours).
2 Sorption of highly insoluble organics by sediments and microorganisms is rapidly reversible.
3 Sediment sorption is strongest with the finer (smaller) particle size fractions in the case of both cations and hydrophobic organics.
4 Unless cation exchange is involved, the most insoluble compounds are usually the most strongly sorbed or most highly accumulated (by organisms).
5 Organic cations are likely to be strongly sorbed.

Wauchope (1978) found that many organochlorine pesticides, paraquat, and arsenical pesticides were strongly adsorbed on sediments. A survey of pesticides in several western streams showed that greater concentrations were found in the samples that contained the most sediment (Manigold and Schulze, 1969). Atrazine and propachlor were removed from the surface-contoured watersheds by storms and were found to be more concentrated in sediments than in the runoff water. Because of the greater volumes of water than of sediments, more pesticides were translocated due to the water even though their actual concentration in water was less (Ritter et al., 1974).

The ultimate fate of most persistent pesticides is still not completely known. However, the effects of pesticides on aquatic organisms will be determined primarily by the amounts that are available in the water and sediment. Pesticides that are sorbed tightly to organic matter may be less available to fish and other aquatic organisms in the water column but may have a profound impact on benthic organisms.

Several references may be mentioned that deal with the transport and fate of pesticides in aquatic environments by the use of various models. Baughman and Burns (1980) give an overview of the transport and transformation of chemicals in the environment, and Branson (1978) reviews several approaches to fate studies involving organic chemicals including pesticides. Leung (1978) uses a model to determine the fate of various substances in fish and gives excellent references pertaining to this aspect of fate and effects. Park et al. (1980) provide a very thorough effort in modeling the fate of organic substances in aquatic ecosystems. These efforts address the importance of various processes that affect the fate of chemicals in the environment and are designed eventually to extrapolate data from laboratory experiments and microcosms to natural environments. The ultimate goal is to understand the distribution, fate, and especially the concentrations of pesticides that can be expected to occur in aquatic systems.

REPRESENTATIVE CONCENTRATIONS OF PESTICIDES IN AQUATIC SAMPLES

An exhaustive review of pesticides found in water, soil, sediments, and biota is not possible here; however, a brief discussion of concentrations to be expected in urban and agricultural environments is needed. The emphasis here will be on the wide variety of pesticides found and not on absolute concentrations.

Perhaps the most extensive study of pesticides in water was a multiyear program involving the western states that was initiated in 1965 by the U.S. Geological Survey. As part of the survey, from October 1968 to September 1971 data were collected on organochlorine and phosphorothioate insecticides (e.g., parathion and diazinon). Reports by Brown and Nishioka (1967), Manigold and Schulze (1969), and Schulze et al. (1973) showed that the pesticides positively identified were preponderantly DDT and its metabolites, although in some rivers 2,4-D and 2,4,5-T were found frequently. Also found were 0.05 μg/l Diazinon in a

Missouri River sample at Nebraska City, Nebraska; 0.42 μg/l 2,4-D in the Yellowstone River near Billings, Montana, 0.02 μg/l DDD, 0.04 μg/l DDE, 0.01 μg/l DDT, 0.01 μg/l endrin, 0.02 μg/l lindane, and 0.02 μg/l endosulfan in a sample from the Gila River at Gillespie Dam, Arizona. Methyl parathion, parathion, Diazinon, and silvex were also found at Gillespie Dam. Interestingly, every station had several occurrences of herbicides, but the Green River, at Green River, Utah, had only one occurrence. The highest concentration of herbicide found was 0.99 μg/l 2,4-D from Feather River near Oroville, California, in December 1969.

Many factors influence the concentration or types of pesticides in water, one of the most obvious being land use. Samples of water, streambed material, fish, and soil were collected from four small drainage basins in Pennsylvania from 1969 to 1971 to determine the concentrations of insecticides and herbicides (Truhlar and Reed, 1976). Each basin represented a particular land use: forest, general farm, residential area, or orchard. DDT or a metabolite was the most frequently found pesticide and was in all media samples except forest soil. Median concentration in the orchard runoff was 0.12 μg/l and in the residential area was only 0.02 μg/l. However, the highest concentration of DDT and its metabolites (combined) in storm runoff samples was 11.4 μg/l in a sample from a stream in the residential area. Dieldrin was the next most frequently occurring pesticide, but others found were chlordane, heptachlor epoxide, and lindane. Aldrin was reported as a trace in one sample of fish. Each stream from each area contained at least one of the following: 2,4-D, silvex, and 2,4,5-T.

Wegman and Greve (1978) reported the results of a monitoring program, which took place from 1969 to 1975, on the organochlorines, cholinesterase inhibitors, and aromatic amines in the Rhine and Maas Rivers. Hexachlorobenzene (HCB) and α- and γ-benzene hexachloride (BHC) were almost always present in Rhine River samples, with HCB ranging from 0.6 to 0.14 μg/l, α-BHC from 0.06 to 0.22 μg/l, and γ-BHC from 0.04 to 0.13 μg/l.

Table 4 gives the concentrations of pesticides in the Rhine compared to those in the Maas. The authors noted that the concentrations of α-BHC in the Rhine and its tributaries are considered harmful to the reproduction of *Daphnia magna*.

Other researchers have found the following in fresh water: 0.2–7.7 μg/l 2,4,5-T in surface water samples during low stream discharge (Dudley and Karr, 1980); organochlorine residues of TDE, DDE, and PCBs as high as 1.96, 2.79, and 28.74 μg/kg, respectively, in sediments of American Falls Reservoir, Idaho (Kent and Johnson, 1979); and total DDT and metabolites below 0.01 μg/l in water samples from Indian River Lagoon, Florida, in the period 1977–1980 (Wang et al., 1980).

Some pesticides attach to particulates, and this phenomenon plays a major role in the disappearance of the pesticides from water. Other pesticides tend to stay in the water. Studies in major agricultural basins in California revealed that an average pesticide concentration of 0.1–0.2 μg/l in river water may mean that the bottom sediments contain 20–100 μg/kg (Li, 1975). Miles (1976) found that the proportion of TDE, a metabolite of DDT, to nonmetabolized DDT was <1 (μg/l) in water and >1 (μg/kg) in bottom sediments at Big Creek, Norfolk County, Ontario, Canada. Miles (1976) suggested that DDT was associated with eroded soil, then incorporated in the bottom mud, and

Table 4 Comparison of Highest Concentrations of Pesticides in the Rhine River Compared to Those in the Maas River[a]

	Residue (μg/l)	
Pesticide	Rhine	Maas
HBC	0.55	0.29
α-BHC	0.60	0.07
γ-BHC	0.42	0.18
Dieldrin	0.06	0.03
Endosulfan	0.81	0.09
Cholinesterase inhibitors	56	1.7
Aromatic amines	10	2.4

[a]From Wegman and Greve (1978).

gradually converted to TDE by microorganisms under anaerobic conditions. In contrast, he noted that Diazinon was present in all whole-water samples ($\leqslant$80 μg/l) but was not detected in any suspended sediment samples. He also found that the bed load (shifting mass of detritus and sediment collected with a Bogardi bed load sampler) had much greater DDT, dieldrin, and endosulfan concentrations than did bottom material (Table 5). Adsorption of insecticides on suspended material decreased in the order DDT > TDE > dieldrin > Diazinon, which is consistent with the increasing solubility of these compounds in water.

The following examples illustrate the extent of pesticides found in the tissues of fish. Organochlorine residues in fish from Lake Texoma, Texas and Oklahoma (Hunter et al., 1980), are shown in Table 6. PCBs (expressed as Aroclor 1254) were found in all species except largemouth bass and were present at all trophic levels of fish. DDT (as p,p'-DDT) was present in detritivores and carnivores at concentrations as high as 410 μg/g; p,p'-DDT as high as 127 μg/g; heptachlor as high as 37 μg/g; chlordane up to 24 μg/g; and dieldrin as high as 144 μg/g (expressed on a wet-weight basis).

Twenty-six composite samples of fish were collected during 1978 from watersheds near the Great Lakes and analyzed for PCBs. The PCBs and related organic chemicals (Veith et al., 1981) were found in 77% of the samples. Chemicals found were (in mg/kg, wet weight): total PCBs, 0.13–14.6; total DDT, <1.0–1.66; chlordane, <0.001–2.57; and hexachlorobenzene, <0.005–0.447.

Perhaps the most extensive sampling of pesticide concentrations in fish was that conducted by the U.S. Fish and Wildlife Service as part of the National Pesticide Monitoring Program (Schmitt et al., 1981). Organochlorine-type residues in fish were analyzed from about 100 stations in the western United States each year from 1970 to 1974. Overall conclusions of the study were: (1) DDT and metabolites showed a continued decline during the period of study; (2) PCB residues were virtually ubiquitous in fish, exceeding 0.5 μg/g (wet weight) in whole fish from all stations near urban or industrial areas, and (3) there was a trend toward increasing concentrations of toxaphene in freshwater fish. Residues of toxaphene commonly exceeded 1.0 μg/g; residues of approximately 1.0 μg/g have been associated with impaired growth and development of young fish (Schmitt et al., 1981).

Table 5   Insecticide Residues in Bed Load and Bottom Material of Big Creek, Norfolk County, Ontario, 1973[a,b]

Sampling date	Residues (μg/kg), dry weight)					
	DDT		Dieldrin		Endosulfan	
	Bed load	Bottom material	Bed load	Bottom material	Bed load	Bottom material
June 26	198	30	6	1.2	2	<0.1
July 10	45	26	4	1.3	<1	<0.1
August 14	21	27	1	1.7	3	0.7
September 25	100	35	8	1.3	3	1.2
October 2	30	18	2	1.1	1	0.6
October 16	62	18	2	0.7	1	0.2

[a]From Miles (1976).

[b]Bed load, shifting mass of detritus and sediment collected with the Bogardi bed load sampler; bottom material, more permanent bottom mud.

Table 6 Concentrations (ng/g) of Selected Organochlorine Residues in Fillets of Fish from Lake Texoma, October 1979[a]

Species	Number of samples	PCBs Med[b]	PCBs Max[c]	Chlordane Med	Chlordane Max	Mirex Med	Mirex Max	Dieldrin Med	Dieldrin Max	Endrin Med	Endrin Max	p,p'-DDE Med	p,p'-DDE Max	p,p'-TDE Med	p,p'-TDE Max	o,p'-DDT Med	o,p'-DDT Max	p,p'-DDT Med	p,p'-DDT Max	Heptachlor Med	Heptachlor Max	Heptachlor epoxide Med	Heptachlor epoxide Max
Herbivore																							
Gizzard shad	14	105	460	2	17	0	40	0	0	0	0	15	505	0	3	0	11	0	0	0	37	0	0
Total	14	105	460	2	17	0	40	0	0	0	0	14	505	0	3	0	11	0	0	0	37	0	0
Carnivores																							
Striped bass	8	50	100	0	8	0	0	0	0	0	0	4	37	0	0	0	0	0	0	0	0	0	0
White bass	14	75	110	0	0	0	0	0	144	0	0	4	12	0	0	0	0	0	410	0	0	0	34
White crappie	19	0	100	0	0	0	0	0	0	0	0	0	2	0	0	0	0	0	0	0	0	0	0
Largemouth bass	3	0	0	0	0	0	0	0	0	0	0	1	3	0	0	0	0	0	0	0	0	0	0
Blue catfish	2	50	100	0	0	0	0	0	0	0	0	12	20	0	0	0	0	0	0	0	0	0	0
Flathead catfish	1	120	120	5	5	0	0	0	0	0	0	34	34	0	0	0	0	0	0	0	0	0	0
Total	47	0	120	0	8	0	0	0	144	0	0	1	37	0	0	0	0	0	410	0	0	0	34
Detritivores																							
Smallmouth buffalo	13	185	1100	5	24	0	0	0	0	0	13	29	121	0	36	0	14	0	26	0	5	0	0
River carpsucker	11	100	300	1	14	0	0	0	0	0	10	35	27	0	9	0	11	0	10	0	0	0	0
Carp	7	50	100	0	6	0	0	0	0	0	0	8	54	0	0	0	0	0	0	0	0	0	0
Channel catfish	7	50	160	0	0	0	0	0	107	0	0	10	104	0	11	0	0	0	189	0	0	0	11
Total	38	100	1100	0	24	0	0	0	107	0	13	18	127	0	36	0	14	0	189	0	0	0	11

[a] From Hunter et al. (1980).
[b] Med, median value.
[c] Max, maximum value.

347

TRANSFORMATION OF PESTICIDES IN AQUATIC ENVIRONMENTS

In the aquatic environment pesticides may undergo transformation in the water through photochemical and chemical reactions (hydrolysis, oxidation, reduction). This subject has been extensively studied by Wolfe et al. (1976). Biological transformations may also occur in fish, invertebrates, and microorganisms. Whatever the mechanism of transformation, the original pesticide or parent compound will be changed. Transformation products may be more or less toxic than the original compound. The biological transformation (or metabolism) of pesticides is discussed below and the general principles of metabolism in aquatic organisms are discussed in Chapter 18.

ABSORPTION, METABOLISM, AND ELIMINATION OF PESTICIDES IN FISH

Fish can absorb pesticides directly from water as well as by ingesting contaminated food. The importance of each mechanism is discussed in the next section. The more lipophilic or fat-soluble the pesticide (or chemical), the more readily it will be taken up by aquatic organisms, especially if the concentration of the pesticide exceeds its water solubility. The size, age, and sex of the individual organism can affect the absorption rate. Furthermore, the same pesticide can be absorbed at different rates by different species.

The main uptake of pesticides by fish from water is direct but passive. The gills and the surrounding body are the primary sites of absorption. For example, Atlantic salmon (*Salmo salar*) exposed to 1.0 ppm DDT in solution (greater than its water solubility) absorbed the pesticide within 5 min through the gills and showed up to 31 ppm in the liver and spleen in 1 h (Premdas and Anderson, 1963).

Passive uptake of pesticides continues until an equilibrium level is attained. This level depends on the concentration of the pesticide in the surrounding water. The time required to achieve equilib-

rium depends on the nature of the pesticide, species of fish, physiological condition of individuals, and environmental factors. Equilibrium may be attained within a few hours or may require several weeks. Whether ingested or absorbed via the gills, pesticides appear in the blood and may be distributed to the tissues of all soft organs.

After absorption, pesticides (like other foreign organic chemicals or xenobiotics) are often modified by metabolism. Pesticide metabolism by organisms has been reviewed (Menzie, 1974; Matsumura, 1975). The important metabolic reactions that pesticides undergo are oxidation, hydrolysis, and reduction. These reactions may be followed by the excretion of metabolites either directly or after conjugation with endogenous molecules. These four reactions are discussed in Chapter 18.

Freshwater and marine organisms are capable of metabolizing a wide variety of pesticides. It has also been well documented that if pesticide exposure is discontinued—as when organisms are transferred to clean, pesticide-free water or fed uncontaminated food—they excrete the absorbed residues from their tissues usually in two phases: an initial rapid phase followed by a much slower gradual loss.

Elimination of the absorbed pesticide may occur simultaneously with its absorption (Chapter 17). This balance, or equilibrium, may be upset by high pesticide concentrations in the medium, but termination of exposure usually results in elimination of the stored pesticide. Elimination can involve the liver, kidneys, gills, and integument.

UPTAKE OF PESTICIDES FROM WATER AND FOOD: LABORATORY STUDIES

There are two main opinions about the importance of water versus food concentrations of pesticides in the aquatic environment. These perspectives are reviewed by Jarvinen et al. (1976) and Macek et al. (1979). For example, Jarvinen et al. (1976) noted that in fathead minnows DDT from the diet was concentrated about 1.2 times and DDT from the water about 100,000 times. They also noted, however, that the food used to feed the fish (clams) concentrated the DDT about 25,000 times. On the other hand, results of an investigation of cadmium, endrin, and Kepone indicated that the increased concentration of chemicals via food (sometimes called biomagnification) is relatively insignificant compared to direct uptake from water (Macek et al., 1979). The authors further concluded that DDT appeared to be the only chemical with a significant potential for accumulation through food chains.

With Aroclor 1254, a PCB, Nimmo et al. (1971) found that the substance was proportioned into specific tissues of penaeid shrimp by a variety of means, with high or low doses in water or high or low doses in the food. They noted that the PCB distribution in specific organs (hepatopancreas, heart, gills) of shrimp exposed in the laboratory to 0.2 μg/l PCB for 50 d was similar to that in shrimp from the field.

Extensive testing of Kepone showed that it is concentrated by estuarine animals when administered in food or water (Bahner and Oglesby, 1979). The uptake and retention of Kepone in blue crabs that received 0.25 μg/g of the pesticide in their food were not significantly different whether 0.03 or 0.3 μg/l Kepone was added to the water.

ACUTE EFFECTS OF PESTICIDES ON AQUATIC ORGANISMS AND FACTORS INFLUENCING TOXICITY

To obtain results quickly or to determine relative toxicity, an acute (48–96 h) LC50 or EC50 toxicity test can be conducted (see Chapters 1 and 2). The test species chosen should be indigenous to the area of potential exposure or at least representative of organisms likely to be exposed. Special precautions must be taken in conducting aquatic toxicity tests with pesticides because of their unusual characteristics. For example, some organochlorine pesticides adsorb to tank surfaces or are

easily lost from the water because of their volatility. Organophosphates form highly toxic metabolites. To avoid alterations in toxicity, exposure constancy in test conditions can be maintained in flow-through systems. Although this is the most appropriate type of test system for evaluating the acute effects of pesticides on aquatic organisms, most acute toxicity information has been obtained with static systems. This will be discussed in greater detail in the section on species sensitivity.

Literature on the acute toxicity of pesticides to aquatic species indicates that three laboratories have been major contributors. A recently published handbook includes 1587 acute tests on 271 substances (mostly pesticides) with 28 species of freshwater fish and 30 species of invertebrates (Johnson and Finley, 1980). These tests were conducted at the National Fisheries Research Laboratory in Columbia, Missouri, from 1965 to 1978. Portman and Wilson (1970) tested 140 substances on brown shrimp and several other marine species. Twenty-six of the chemicals tested were commonly used pesticides. Acute toxicity tests with pesticides were also conducted during the 1960s by J. I. Lowe and co-workers at the U.S. Environmental Protection Agency's Environmental Research Laboratory in Gulf Breeze, Florida. Results of many studies were summarized in several publications (Butler, 1962, 1963, 1964, 1965, 1966). The tests involved marine and estuarine species such as shrimps, crabs, oysters, and fish.

Effects of Pesticides on Plants and Protozoans in Acute Tests

Perhaps the most extensive studies of herbicides and aquatic plant species in terms of classes of herbicides, formulations, and numbers of species were those of Walsh (1972), Walsh et al. (1973), and Hollister et al. (1975). Important findings were that formulation materials enhanced oxygen evolution, and urea and triazine herbicides were the strongest inhibitors of oxygen evolution (Walsh, 1972). Diuron, neburon, and amytrene were the most toxic to algae. In a later paper, Walsh (1973) noted that the concentrations of herbicides required to kill mangroves appeared to be lower than those required to kill other species of tropical trees. Rates of picloram and 2,4-D combinations needed to kill seedlings of red mangrove, *Rhizophora mangle* L., were 4.4 and 1.6 kg/ha, respectively. Walsh theorized that the death of the seedlings was caused by the disruption of osmoregulatory ability of the roots.

Many organochlorine compounds are toxic to algae. For example, Sodergren (1968) reported that about 0.3 µg/l DDT reduced the growth (number of cells per unit volume) of the freshwater alga *Chlorella* sp. DDT reduced the rate of photosynthesis of five species of marine algae (Wurster, 1968), and about 1.0 mg/l mirex reduced photosynthesis in a freshwater species of *Chlamydomonas* (de la Cruz and Naqvi, 1973).

Mirex, the insecticide used against fire ants, and Aroclor 1254, a PCB, reduced growth rates and population densities of *Tetrahymena pyriformia,* a citiated protozoan, at 0.9 and 1.0 µg/l, respectively (Cooley et al., 1972). Aroclor 1248 and Aroclor 1260 reduced growth rates and populations at 1.0 mg/l (Cooley et al., 1973). In both studies, the authors noted the ability of the protozoans to concentrate the compounds, making them available to aquatic food chains.

Some Comparisons from Acute Tests with Invertebrates and Fish

Data summarized in the next few paragraphs for invertebrates and fish illustrate information obtained from acute tests that can be useful in making evaluations. The points discussed should not be taken as absolute, since they are based on a brief review of the toxicological literature. As data bases for various chemicals are enlarged, some of the generalizations and conclusions will require modification.

Data in Table 7 lead to some general conclusions regarding organophosphate insecticides. For instance, acute effects on populations of aquatic insects, crustaceans, and mollusks would likely be of immediate concern with these chemicals since they are apparently substantially more

Table 7 Comparison of LC50s: Invertebrates and Fishes Exposed to Organophosphate Pesticides[a]

	LC50 (96-h, µg/l)		
Pesticide	Invertebrates	Non-game fish	Fish
Malathion	49 (15)[b]	3099 (5)	162 (1)
Ethyl parathion	24 (12)		1391 (13)
Methyl parathion	11 (5)		5411 (14)
Diazinon	7 (4)		640 (4)
Chlorpyrifos	4 (3)		81 (5)

[a]From Johnson and Finley (1980).
[b]Number of species is given in parentheses.

toxic to aquatic invertebrates than to fish. The difference in sensitivity to methyl parathion is easily observed in Table 8, which shows that fish are two to six orders of magnitude more tolerant than invertebrates.

By contrast, in a similar comparison with the herbicide trifluralin, fish were generally more sensitive than invertebrates (Table 9). A study by Eisler (1970) showed that with some marine fish chlorinated insecticides were considerably more toxic than a group of organophosphates (Table 10).

Species Sensitivity

Perhaps the best data illustrating differences in species sensitivity and also tolerance to different pesticides are those in a report from the U.S. EPA (1981) (Tables 11 and 12). These data were chosen because they are all from tests conducted in flowing seawater by similar methods, and with one exception, all represent measured concentrations. Calculated LC50s, in some cases, show wide differences in sensitivity to the same chemicals; for example, the LC50 of EPN in the sheepshead minnow is 190 µg/l and in the pink shrimp is 0.29 µg/l—a difference of 655 times (Table 12). LC50s in some closely related taxonomic groups (e.g., crustaceans) differ by no more than a factor of 2 or 3 for several chemicals. The range of differences in sensitivity of fish to the same pesticide is notable. Examples are carbophenothion in spot and sheepshead minnow (Table 11) and EPN and Ethoprop (Table 12), which differ by a factor of 10 in sheepshead minnow and pinfish.

It is difficult to make generalizations about species sensitivity because of the differences in reporting values in the literature and in test methodologies. It is also difficult to generalize about the toxicity of a group of compounds because of lack of data for a group of organisms (e.g., mol-

lusks). When variables have not been controlled or at least specified, they may be the source of differences incorrectly regarded as due to species sensitivity. When all experimental variables are controlled or corrected for, striking differences can be attributed to species sensitivity.

Size and Age

There is evidence that larger, or older, fish are less susceptible than smaller, or younger, fish. For ex-

Table 8 Comparison of Acute Toxicity of Methyl Parathion to Invertebrates and Fish[a]

Invertebrates			Fish		
Test organism	Temperature (°C)	96-h LC50 95% CI (µg/l)	Test organism	Temperature (°C)	96-h LC50 95% CI (µg/l)
Simocephalus sp.	15	0.37[b] 0.23–0.57	Bluegill	17	4380 3480–5510
Daphnia magna	21	0.14[b] 0.09–0.20	Largemouth bass	18	5220 4320–6310
Gammarus fasciatus	15	3.8 2.6–5.5	Yellow perch	18	3060 2530–3700
Orconectes sp.	15	15[c]	Coho salmon	12	5300 4900–5600
Ischnura sp.	15	33[c]	Cutthroat trout	12	1850[c] 1390–2470
			Rainbow trout	12	3700 3130–4380
			Brown trout	12	4700 3130–4380
			Lake trout	12	3780 3900–5090
			Goldfish	18	9000 8100–9900
			Carp	18	7130 6440–7870
			Fathead minnow	18	8900 7780–10,200
			Black bullhead	18	6640 4970–8880
			Channel catfish	18	5240 4270–6440
			Green sunfish	18	6860 5590–8420

[a]From Johnson and Finley (1980).
[b]48-h EC50.
[c]Tested in hard water, 162–272 ppm $CaCO_3$.

Table 9   Comparison of Acute Toxicity of Trifluralin to Invertebrates and Fish[a]

Invertebrates			Fish		
Test organism	Temperature (°C)	96-h LC50 95% CI (μg/l)	Test organism	Temperature (°C)	96-h LC50 95% CI (μg/l)
Simocephalus sp.	15	900[b] 651–1245	Bluegill	22	58 47–70
Daphnia magna	21	560[b,c] 320–1000	Largemouth bass	18	75[c] 65–87
Daphnia pulex	15	625[b] 446–876			
Gammarus fasciatus	21	2200 1400–3400	Rainbow trout	12	41 26–62
Pteronarcys sp.	15	2800 2100–3700	Fathead minnow	18	105 83–134
			Goldfish	18	145 108–195
			Channel catfish	22	2200 1420–3410

[a]From Johnson and Finley (1980).
[b]48-h EC50.
[c]Tested in hard water, 272 ppm $CaCO_3$.

ample, Mount (1962) reported 96-h LC50s for endrin of 0.27 μg/l in 30-mm-long fish and 0.47 μg/l in 60-mm-long fish (for both guppies and bluntnose minnows, *Pimephales notatus*). Pickering et al. (1962) conducted a variety of acute toxicity tests with 13 organophosphate pesticides and concluded that bluegills averaging 10 g were slightly more tolerant than 2-g bluegills to dioxathion, parathion, and malathion. Fathead minnow fry 2 to 30 d old were 10 times more sensitive to dioxathion than were adults, but age had little effect on sensitivity to TEPP in this fish. The eggs and sac fry were the most tolerant, followed by the sensitive fry stages (7 to 14 d old). Increased

Table 10   Ranges of LC50s for Six Species of Estuarine Fish[a] Exposed to Chlorinated Hydrocarbon and Organophosphate Insecticides

Chlorinated hydrocarbon	LC50 (μg/l)	Organophosphate	LC50 (μg/l)
Endrin	0.05–3.1	Dioxathion	6.0–75
DDT	0.4–89	Malathion	27–3,250
Heptachlor	3.0–188	Phosdrin	65–800
Dieldrin	5.0–34	DDVP	1,250–2,680
Lindane	9.0–60	Methyl parathion	5,700–75,800
Aldrin	13–36		
Methoxychlor	12–150		

[a]Atlantic silversides, bluehead, striped killifish, American eel, mummichog, and northern puffer.
[b]From Eisler (1970).

Table 11 Acute Toxicity of Acephate, Aldicarb, Carbophenothion, and DEF to Estuarine Organisms in Flowing Seawater Tests[a,b]

Species	Acephate	Aldicarb	Carbophenothion	DEF
Mysidopsis bahia, mysid shrimp	7,300 (300–190,000)	16 (13–20)	3.0 (2.4–3.7)	4.6 (4.2–4.9)
Penaeus duorarum, pink shrimp	3,800 (2,000–7,300)	12 (7.5–18)	0.47 (0.36–0.66)	14 (10–18)
Palaemonetes pugio, grass shrimp	—	—	4.6 (3.8–6.2)	22 (19–23)
Wildstock larvae, 1–7-d	—	—	2.0 (1.8–2.6)	—
Laboratory-reared, 49-d	—	—	2.9 (2.5–3.3)	—
Cyprinodon variegatus, sheepshead minnow	910,000[c]	41	2.8 (0.85–9.6)	<440
Menidia menidia, Atlantic silversides	—	—	7.7 (5.7–12.0)	—
Lagodon rhomboides, pinfish	85,000 (7,800–933,000)	80 (43–150)	7.7 (4.6–12)	290 (240–379)
Leiostomus xanthurus, spot	—	—	>206	130 (100–170)

[a]From U.S. EPA (1981).
[b]Values are 96-h LC50s, except where indicated. Measured concentrations are in µg/l and 95% confidence intervals are in parentheses.
[c]96-h EC50 (nominal concentrations) based on loss of equilibrium.

Table 12 Acute Toxicity of EPN, Ethoprop, Methyl Parathion, and Phorate to Estuarine Organisms in Flowing Seawater Tests[a,b]

Species	EPN	Ethoprop	Methyl parathion	Phorate
Mysidopsis bahia, mysid shrimp	3.4 (2.5–5.8)	7.5 (6.4–9.2)	0.77 (0.65–0.98)	0.33 (0.27–0.43)
Penaeus duorarum, pink shrimp	0.29 (0.1–1.1)	13 (4.7–37)	1.2 (0.91–1.4)	0.11 (0.08–0.16)
Cyprinodon variegatus, sheepshead minnow	190 (150–260)	180 (85–390)	—	1.3 (0.97–1.7)
Lagodon rhomboides, pinfish	18 (15–24)	6.3 (4.78–8.4)	—	—
Leiostomus xanthurus, spot	26 (19–24)	—	59 (45–74)	3.9 (3.1–5.6)

[a]From U.S. EPA (1981).
[b]Values are 96-h LC50s; measured concentrations are in µg/l and 95% confidence intervals are in parentheses.

tolerance was observed in 60- to 90-d fry and particularly in adults. Schimmel et al. (1974) found a similar age sensitivity pattern with sheepshead minnow (*Cyprinodon variegatus*) eggs, embryos, fry, juveniles, and adults treated with Aroclor 1254. Hughes (1970) concluded that striped bass larvae were more tolerant than fingerlings to parathion, methyl parathion, copper sulfate, and trichlorfon. In contrast, larvae were less tolerant than fingerlings to diuron, potassium dichromate, potassium permanganate, and 2,4-D.

The effects of age and size on toxicity may be a result of the following factors:

1 Small individuals of a species have a greater body surface area for absorption of pesticide per amount of body mass.

2 Small or young animals have higher respiration rates (or gill movements) than larger animals.

3 Young have incompletely developed organ systems for detoxification or excretion of xenobiotics.

Temperature

The effect of temperature on toxicity of pesticides to aquatic organisms is well documented. It is important to note, however, that differences or changes in temperature can themselves affect the general activity, metabolism, and behavior of fish and other aquatic organisms, and this can influence the effect of the pesticide. Temperature can also affect the chemical and the physical state of the pesticide, the time it remains in solution or suspension, its persistence, and the rate of pesticide uptake by aquatic organisms.

In most acute aquatic toxicity studies on a wide range of pesticides, it is reported that most compounds are increasingly toxic at higher temperatures. Iyatomi et al. (1958) found that endrin was several hundred times as toxic to carp (*Cyprinus carpio*) at 27°C than at 7°C. Bridges (1965) reported that heptachlor was five times as toxic to redear sunfish (*Lepomis microlophus*) at 24°C than at 7°C. Cope (1965) substantiated the positive effects of increased temperature on the tox-

icity of pesticides (e.g., endrin, lindane, dieldrin, and aldrin) to bluegills. Fish pretreated with 2.3 μg/l dieldrin for 30 d and then exposed to increasing temperatures, had higher mortality than fish not pretreated with dieldrin (Silbergeld, 1973).

Conversely, the toxicity of some pesticides has been found to increase with decreasing temperature. This negative temperature correlation was characteristic of the acute toxicity of DDT. The 96-h LC50 of DDT for bluegills (Cope, 1964) and rainbow trout (Cope, 1965) was less at lower temperatures. Methoxychlor was more toxic to bluegills at low than at high temperatures (Cope, 1968). A negative temperature coefficient for methoxychlor was reported earlier by Crosby et al. (1966) in a *Daphnia* toxicity test.

Macek et al. (1969) reported 24-h and 96-h LC50s for a number of pesticides at three temperatures for rainbow trout (*Salmo gairdneri*) and bluegills (*Lepomis macrochirus*) in static tests. Toxicity generally increased with increasing temperature during the first 24 h of exposure but with methoxychlor the susceptibility of both species decreased with increasing temperature. Bluegills showed no change in reaction over the temperature range tested with lindane and azinphosmethyl (Guthion). After 96 h, the effect of temperature on susceptibility of both test species was less than in 24-h tests, except with trifluralin (a herbicide) in rainbow trout. Respiration, and thus pesticide intake, could be greater at higher than at lower temperatures; the oxygen demand of the fish is also greater. In static tests the amount of pesticide available is limited so that the effect of temperature is more marked before 24 h has elapsed than after (Macek et al., 1969). Furthermore, increased metabolism and oxygen uptake lead to a decrease in dissolved oxygen in water and in high concentrations of waste, which increase susceptibility. This lends further support to the use of flow-through test systems with pesticides.

Hardness and pH

The effect of pesticides and other substances on aquatic organisms may be influenced by water characteristics such as hardness, alkalinity, and pH. Since natural waters usually differ widely in these characteristics, routine toxicity tests or screening studies for potential pesticides should be conducted with dilution water of uniform water characteristics (see Chapter 2) or in duplicate with hard and soft waters.

An interesting example of the effects of water hardness and alkalinity on pesticide toxicity are field and laboratory studies on the molluscicide Bayluscide. A study of the impact of Bayluscide on aquatic snails and other fauna was carried out in South Africa in two different types of streams, one soft and the other moderately hard (Harrison, 1966). In soft-water streams treated at 0.10 ppm, fish died within minutes of Bayluscide spraying. Fish kill was much slower in hard water; mortality was not observed until 2 h after spraying with 0.20 ppm Bayluscide. This was confirmed in laboratory studies by Marking and Hogan (1967). At all exposure periods, Bayluscide was found to be more toxic to rainbow trout and other fish in soft water than in hard water.

TFM (3-trifluoromethyl-4-nitrophenol) toxicity to larval lampreys is markedly affected by water hardness and pH. The compound is most effective in soft, acid waters. As the pH and alkalinity increase, the effective concentrations needed to kill larval lampreys increase. In soft, acid waters the minimum lethal concentration in 0.5 ppm, while in the hardest alkaline waters the minimum lethal concentration for the larvae was 8.0 ppm. Therefore, the amount of TFM required for effective treatment of a stream may be greater in hard, alkaline waters than in soft, acid waters (Applegate et al., 1961). This effect of hardness on TFM toxicity was confirmed by Howell et al. (1964).

The relationship between pH, alkalinity, and hardness is also well documented for the piscicide antimycin (Walker et al., 1964). Basic studies were conducted in the laboratory, followed by semi-natural field studies in large wading pools and natural hatching ponds. Antimycin at 10 ppb was effective in killing fish in the hatching ponds but not in the wading pools. Massive plant growth in the wading pools converted the relatively hard water that was used to fill the pools to soft water because of a decrease in calcium. There was a shift from bicarbonate to free hydroxide with a consequent increase in pH from 7.5 to more than 10. Calcium ions were removed and magnesium ions predominated, similar to the shift observed in softer waters. In contrast, the effectiveness in the hatching ponds was a result of the high buffering capacity of the water and low hydroxide concentration. Even when the pools and the hatching ponds had the same pH and total alkalinity, there was more free hydroxide in the pools. These chemical changes accelerated the degradation of toxicant in the pools, where 20–40 ppb antimycin was needed to kill the fish.

An activity half-life for antimycin was determined by evaluating the toxicity of antimycin solutions of pH ranging from 6 to 10 (Marking and Dawson, 1972). The half-life decreased from 310 at pH 6 to 1.5 at pH 10. This indicates that pH can influence the rate of degradation and therefore the toxicity of a chemical. Calcium and magnesium ions do not themselves affect the toxicity of pesticides unless accompanied by pH and alkalinity changes (Amend, 1974; Inglis and Davis, 1972).

Acute toxicity of both organochlorine and organophosphate pesticides to fathead minnows was found to be small and not significant in water of varying hardness (20 and 400 mg/l as calcium carbonate) (Henderson et al., 1960). The only 96-h LC50s that differed between hard and soft water were those for trichlorphon (an organophosphate), for which the LC50 in hard water was less than one-third of that in soft water. This was due to a rapid breakdown of the pesticide to more toxic products at the higher pH.

It appears that changes in hardness may not affect the toxicity of pesticides to aquatic organisms unless changes in pH are produced at the same time. Changes in pH, alkalinity, and hardness should be continually monitored in routine acute toxicity tests with aquatic organisms.

Flow

Static acute toxicity tests have been the primary tool for evaluating short-term effects of pesticides and other foreign compounds on aquatic organisms. With certain pesticides, however, losses due to volatilization or to adsorption on glass, tubing, or particulates occurred with time and highly toxic metabolic products were produced, seriously altering the LC50 values. To avoid such alterations in toxicity, static tests have been supplemented and in some cases replaced by tests with continuous flow-through systems to evaluate acute toxicity.

A comparative study of static and flow-through systems was conducted with endrin and DDT in fathead minnows over a 48-h period (Lincer et al., 1970). The flow-through 48-h LC50 of endrin was 74% of the static value. After 96 h the value was 51%. For DDT, the situation was reversed: the 48-h LC50 for the flow-through system was more than 5.4 times that for the static system. It was concluded that a drop in oxygen from 70% to 16% saturation and high ammonia concentrations in the static tanks caused increased respiration rates in the fish, resulting in greater uptake of DDT via the gills. It was suggested that ammonia may also have acted synergistically with DDT.

Results of flow-through and static tests with eight pesticides are presented in Table 13. In general, the LC50s from the static tests are greater than those from the flow-through tests; exceptions are sheepshead minnows with EPN and mysid shrimp with Aldicarb. In most cases the differences are a factor of 2 or 3. Flow-through test methods give a more accurate measurement of the LC50 because they provide a superior simulation of field exposure. However, well-designed static tests can be useful in determining acute toxicities for comparative studies or as indicators for further acute or chronic tests.

Formulations and Carriers

Few pesticides are directly soluble in water. Most pesticides are of very low water solubility or almost completely insoluble. These compounds are, however, soluble in different oils (solvents) in which they can be formulated, so that when added to water they produce very fine emulsions. The formulations can be oil solutions, wettable powders, emulsifiable concentrates, water-miscible formulations, or granular formulations. These formulations are designed to ensure maximum dispersion of the pesticide.

In view of the important role of solvents in formulations, it has become apparent that some of these components may contribute to the toxic effects and absorption of pesticides. This could be important in evaluating results and comparing different pesticide treatments in the field. Emulsifiable concentrates of organophosphates were found to be more toxic to fathead minnows and bluegills than technical grade materials (Pickering et al., 1962). Hiltibran (1967) observed that granular formulations of some herbicides were less toxic to fish than liquid formulations, possibly due to slow release of the herbicides from the granules.

Commercial formulations should be tested because it is impossible to determine the LC50 from the concentration of the active ingredients or technical material (Alabaster, 1969). In addition, the other components themselves may be toxic. Table 14 gives examples of variations in toxicity for several DDT formulations. A DDT formulation in oil (naphtha) was more toxic than an aqueous suspension.

Several formulations of the phenoxy herbicides 2,4-D and 2,4,5-T showed wide variations in LC50s for bluegills depending on whether an amine or an ester group was attached (Table 15) (Hughes and Davis, 1963). The esters were, in most cases, more toxic than the amines, and there were some wide differences within the esters, probably associated with the different manufacturers.

Routine acute toxicity tests with insoluble pesticides usually require solvents (or carriers) to dissolve and disperse the substances in water (see Chapter 2). If a solvent is used, its concentration should be minimal and a solvent control should be included in the test design.

Table 13 Comparison of Acute Toxicity of Eight Pesticides to Estuarine Organisms in Flowing Seawater Tests (Top Line in Each Data Pair) and Static Tests (Bottom Line in Each Data Pair)[a,b]

Species	EPN	Ethoprop	Methyl parathion	Phorate	Acephate	Aldicarb	Carbophenothion	DEF
Mysidopsis bahia,[c] mysid shrimp	3.4 (2.5–5.8)	7.5 (6.4–9.2)	0.77 (0.65–0.98)	0.33 (0.27–0.43)	7,300 (300–190,000)	16 (13–20)	3.0 (2.4–3.7)	4.3 (4.2–4.9)
Mysidopsis bahia,[d] mysid shrimp, 24 h old	13 (10–18)	23 (19–27)	0.98 (0.81–1.2)	1.9 (1.0–3.2)	–	13 (10–15)	13 (10–17)	5.3 (4.4–6.8)
Cyprinodon variegatus,[c] sheepshead minnow	190 (150–260)	180 (85–390)	–	1.3 (0.97–1.7)	910,000	41 (55–72)	2.8 (0.85–9.6)	>440
Cyprinodon variegatus,[d] sheepshead minnow	140 (59–500)	740 (585–1,070)	12,000 (10,000–14,000)	4.0 (3.5–4.5)	>3,200,000	168 (102–320)	17 (14–21)	440 (410–473)
Leiostomus xanthurus,[c] spot, 28 d old	26 (19–24)	–	59 (45–74)	3.9 (3.1–5.6)	>100,000	–	>206	130 (100–170)
Leiostomus xanthurus,[d] spot	37 (33–40)	33 (0–48)	93 (56–320)	5.0 (4.2–5.6)	–	202 (116–293)	500 (390–630)	158 (135–220)

[a] From U.S. EPA (1981).
[b] Values are 96-h LC50s as measured concentrations in flowing seawater tests and nominal concentrations in the static tests. The 95% confidence intervals are in parentheses.
[c] Flowing seawater tests.
[d] Static tests.

Table 14 Toxicity of Different Pesticide Formulations[a,b]

Pesticide	Composition (%)	24-h LC50 (μg/l)
p,p'-DDT	100	13
o,p'-DDT	100	30
Commercial DDT	75 p,p'-DDT, 20 o,p'-DDT)	1.4
Shell "Arkotine" DDT	18 DDT	200
Murphy "De De Tane 25"	(25 DDT, 3 emulsifier, 48 naphtha, 24 water)	140
Murphy "De De Tane Paste"	(50 DDT, 24 suspending agent, 26 water)	10,700
2,4-D (BEE)	100	1,000
2,4,5-T (BEE)	100	1,000
Econal 13086	(50 2,4-D, 25 2,4,5-T)	230

[a]From Alabaster (1969).
[b]Test species, *Rasbora heteromorpha.*

(fish)

Other Variables

A number of other factors are known to affect the LC50 in acute toxicity tests. These are the physiological condition of the fish, food quantity and type, light intensity and periodicity, oxygen and carbon dioxide content of the test water, length of the acclimation period, randomization and selection of test organisms, and purity of toxicants. Many of these factors can be adequately controlled in toxicity tests (Chapter 2).

Acute Effects of Pesticides on Aquatic Organisms—Sublethal

Studies of sublethal effects of pesticides following acute exposure are listed in Table 16. Reduced shell growth of oysters, hatching success of eggs, and effects on feeding activity are important observations. Not all the changes observed are necessarily adverse—especially under actual field conditions, where the organism can avoid the stressing agent. Many sublethal effects do not persist as exposure continues; there is commonly a return to normal conditions (Brungs and Mount, 1978). It is vital, however, that the investigator recognize the effects and further test whether the effects are real and important ecologically.

For additional information on the acute effects of pesticides, the reader is referred to studies with invertebrates (Muncy and Oliver, 1963; Gaufin et

Table 15 Toxicity of Various Phenoxy Herbicides (LC50 Values as mg/l Acid Equivalent)[a,b]

Form	24-h LC50
2,4-D	
Alkanolamine	450–900
Dimethylamine	166–542
Di-N,N-dimethylcocoamine	1.5
Acid + emulsifiers	8.0
Iso-octyl ester	8.8–66.3
Propylene glycol butyl ether ester	2.1
Butoxyethanol ester	2.1
Butyl ester	1.3
Isopropyl ester	0.9
Ethyl ester	1.4
2,4,5-T	
Dimethylamine	144
Iso-octyl ester	10.4–31
Propylene glycol butyl ether ester	17
Butoxyethanol ester	1.4
Fenoprop	
Potassium salt	83
Iso-octyl ester	1.4–15.5
Propylene glycol butyl ether ester	19.9
Butoxyethanol ester	1.2

[a]From Hughes and Davis (1963); reproduced with permission of the Weed Science Society of America.
[b]Test species, *Lepomis macrochirus.*

Table 16 Some Acute Effects of Pesticides on Aquatic Organisms for Criteria other than Death

Test species	Test material	Criterion/observed effect	Effective concentration	Reference
Crassostrea virginica, American oyster	Chlordane	Reduced shell growth	6.2 µg/l	Parrish et al. (1976)
Four marine algae	Kepone	Effect on growth of cultures	350–600 µg/l	Hansen et al. (1977a)
Pimephales promelas, fathead minnow	Kelthane Dursban Disulfoton Pydrin Permethrin	Alteration in normal schooling behavior after 24 h	218 µg/l 44 µg/l 413 µg/l 3.6 µg/l 7.2 µg/l	Holcombe et al. (1982)
Perca flavescens, yellow perch	Methoxychlor	Effect on respiration	5.0 µg/l	Merna and Eisele (1973)
Arenicola cristata, lug worm	Sodium pentachlorophenate	Effect on feeding activity	80 µg/l	Rubenstein (1978)
Callinectes sapidus, juvenile blue crabs	Mirex	Paralysis	Mirex bait	Lowe et al. (1971)
Culex pipiens quinque fasciatus, southern home mosquito	FLIT MLO	Extension of the larval period	Rate of 0.75 to 2.5 gal/acre	Mickes (1970)
Lagodon rhomboides, pinfish	Naled (Dibrom)	Brain acetylcholinesterase inhibition	84–99% inhibition at lethal concentrations	Coppage and Matthews (1975)
Tresus capax, gaper clam *Macoma nasuta,* bent-nosed clam	Sevin	Reduction in population field exposure	2.3–4.6 kg/acre	Armstrong and Milleman (1974
Cyprinodon variegatus, sheeps-head minnow	Dursban, DDT, endrin, endrin, malathion, Sevin, 2,4-D	Avoidance	Avoided DDT, endrin, Dursban, 2,4-D; no avoidance of malathion or Sevin	Hansen (1969)
Salvelinus fontinalis, brook trout	DDT	Prevents the establishment of a visual conditioned avoidance response	20–60 µg/l	Anderson and Peterson (1969)
Lepomis macrochirus, bluegill sunfish *Micropterus salmoides,* large-mouth bass	Parathion	Effect on locomotor orientation	10–25 µg/l	Rand (1977)
Palaemonetes pugio, grass shrimp	Methyl or ethyl parathion	Impairment of antipredation behavior	0.1 µg/l	Farr (1977)
Cyprinodon variegatus, sheeps-head minnow	Kepone	Scoliosis	0.8 µg/l	Couch et al. (1977)
Leptodius floridanus, Panopeus herbstii (crab larvae)	Dieldrin	Impaired development, mortality during the first zoeal stage	1.0 µg/l	Epifanio (1971)

al., 1965; Eisler, 1969; Saunders and Cope, 1966; Cardwell et al., 1977), freshwater fish (Pickering et al., 1962), and marine fish (Eisler, 1970).

CHRONIC TOXICITY OF PESTICIDES TO AQUATIC ORGANISMS

For some time aquatic toxicologists have known that acute tests (~96-h duration) conducted in the laboratory are usually inadequate for predicting long-term effects of substances on populations of organisms in the field. As early as the late 1950s, Henderson and Pickering (1957) suggested that an adjustment could be applied to concentrations used in acute studies to provide for "a safe concentration for the test fish." They further suggested, on the basis of their tests with organophosphate insecticides, that to protect the test fish the adjustment might be half of the acute value, whereas to protect all aquatic life the adjustment may be as much as one-tenth the acute TLM or LC50. It is sometimes difficult to arrive at appropriate adjustments of values from acute and chronic tests for application to the situation in the environment; reasons for this were summarized by Stern and Walker (1978).

1 The test population may not be representative of the same species in the environment because of different environmental histories.

2 Acute tests rely on a single life stage tested for an extremely short time.

3 The 96-h LC50, representing a theoretical concentration lethal to 50% of the organisms, is an unrealistic environmental concentration; at best it provides an understanding of the threshold of acute toxicity.

4 Data from a laboratory test cannot be easily extrapolated to an environmental situation because of difficulty in predicting concentrations of the substance in the field and understanding the physical-chemical fluctuations that affect behavior of the chemical in the aquatic environment.

If chronic tests are contemplated, the obvious questions that arise are: (1) How long should an organism be exposed to a substance to determine sublethal effects (assuming that they will occur)? (2) What criteria of effect should be considered significant biologically or ecologically? and (3) How does one standardize for assessing the differences between acute and chronic tests since organisms vary so greatly in their life histories? The ultimate goal is to develop a methodology for establishing acceptable toxicant limits for various aquatic species.

The concept of "application factor" (AF), introduced in the early 1960s, eventually led to the concept of the maximum acceptable toxicant concentration (MATC) (see Chapters 1, 3, and 4). After observing that the pesticide Delnav had a cumulative toxic effect on fish, Pickering et al. (1962) believed that an application factor would be necessary when using short-term static toxicity test results to estimate safe concentrations in the field. A method for establishing acceptable toxicant limitations for fish was designed by Mount and Stephan (1967). This method involves determining acceptable concentrations of toxic materials from laboratory studies by selecting a measurable effect or criterion to indicate that the test fish are in an unacceptable environment. Mount and Stephan (1967) suggested that the "laboratory fish production index" (LFPI) be used as the measure of effect and that the MATC be established as a basis of chronic exposures. The LFPI requires data on such criteria as growth, reproduction, spawning behavior, and viability of eggs over at least one generation. It was also suggested that when MATCs could not be calculated from data developed in laboratory studies, AFs be used to estimate "safe" or acceptable concentrations for species that were not or could not be tested (Mount and Stephan, 1967). Later studies showed that AFs, computed by dividing the MATCs by the 96-h LC50s, were similar and therefore useful in estimating long-term safe concentrations from the results of short-term tests (Eaton, 1970).

By use of the MATC/AF, data have been generated that are useful in making comparisons or predictions. MATCs have been used for diverse groups of organisms (e.g., marine and freshwater species across phylogenetic groups) and have become widely accepted for developing new testing procedures and deriving water quality criteria that eventually result in limitations or standards for various constituents.

Table 17 gives examples of pesticide studies in which the AFs calculated from acute and chronic tests were similar. For example, the limits on the AFs for *Daphnia magna* and *Pimephales promelas,* tested with the same pesticides (e.g., acrolein, heptachlor, trifluralin, and atrazine), are almost identical. Similar AFs for saltwater species (*Mysidopsis bahia* and *Cyprinodon variegatus*) are calculated for Kepone. Other AF ranges are available for the following pesticides and are also similar:

	Limits of AF (µg/l)
Toxaphene:	
D. magna	0.007–0.01
M. bahia	0.03–0.05
Malathion:	
P. promelas	0.02–0.06
C. variegatus	0.08–0.18
Heptachlor:	
D. magna	0.16–0.32
C. variegatus	0.09–0.18
Trifluralin:	
D. magna	0.012–0.037
P. promelas	0.017–0.044
C. variegatus	0.007–0.25

There are AFs for the same pesticides, however, that are quite different. The AFs computed from tests with endosulfan in *D. magna* and *P. promelas,* and also with lindane in *D. magna* or *P. promelas,* differ by a factor of 10. Interestingly, the AFs for trifluralin are similar in all tests species shown except for *M. bahia,* a species not affected by acute or chronic exposures even at a concentration greater than the solubility limit of the chemical (Nimmo et al., 1981).

Aquatic species respond differently when chronically exposed to the same pesticide, as shown by exposure of a variety of fish and invertebrates to the insecticide chlordane (Cardwell et al., 1977). In entire life cycle or as partial chronic

tests, the lowest aqueous concentration of technical chlordane to have deleterious effects was 0.32 µg/l, at which brook trout embryo viability was reduced. Chronic effects for bluegills and chironomids occurred at about 2 µg/l. Apparently, chronic sensitivities to chlordane were lower for fathead minnows, daphnids, and amphipods, which were unaffected by the pesticide at 5–10 µg/l. The authors cautioned that the experiments with brook trout and bluegills were begun with yearling fish and not fry or embryos; greater effects might have been observed had entire life cycle studies been conducted.

A variety of effects have been documented in fish after chronic exposure to pesticides. Some have been valuable for determining MATCs and, eventually, developing data for water quality criteria. It is not our intention here to review the vast literature on the subject, but there are some excellent examples. Endrin incorporated in diets of male goldfish for 3–4 mo affected growth, gonad development, thyroid activity, serum characteristics, total and differential body fat, behavior, and mortality (Grant and Merhle, 1970). Maturing yearling brook trout fed DDT for 156 d (Macek, 1968) and fish fed the higher dosage produced fewer mature ova than untreated fish. There was a marked increase in mortality of cutthroat trout following a 20-mo exposure to DDT in the diet and water through one spawning cycle (Allison et al., 1964).

One of the most significant advances in determining chronic physiological effects of pesticide poisoning in fish resulted with toxaphene. Tests with this pesticide led to the recommendation that collagen and hydroxyproline in the vertebral column be considered early biochemical indicators of growth and developmental changes in fish (Mayer et al., 1975). These studies showed that effects on growth of brook trout were correlated with biochemical parameters. In similar studies on growth, reproduction, mortality, and bone development, the MATC of toxaphene in water was 25–54 µg/l for fathead minnows and 49–72 µg/l for channel catfish (Mayer et al., 1977). A 50%

Table 17 Some Comparisons of 96-h LC50s and Maximum Acceptable Toxicant Concentrations of Various Pesticides to Freshwater and Saltwater Species

Species and chemical	96-h LC50 (μg/l)	MATC limits (μg/l)		Limits of application factors (μg/l)	Reference
Daphnia magna[a]					
Acrolein	57	>16.9	<33.6	0.30–0.59	Macek et al. (1976a)
Atrazine	(6.9 mg/l)	>0.14	<0.25	0.02–0.04	Macek et al. (1976b)
Endosulfan	166	>2.7	<7.0	0.016–0.042	Macek et al. (1976a)
Heptachlor	78	>12.5	<25.0	0.16–0.23	Macek et al. (1976a)
Lindane	485	>11.0	<19.0	0.02–0.03	Macek et al. (1976c)
Toxaphene	10	>0.07	<0.12	0.007–0.01	Sanders (1980)
Trifluralin	193	>2.4	<7.2	0.012–0.037	Macek et al. (1976a)
Pimephales promelas					
Acrolein	84	>11.4	<41.7	0.14–0.05	Macek et al. (1976a)
Atrazine	15	>0.21	<0.52	0.01–0.03	Macek et al. (1976b)
Endosulfan	0.86	>0.20	<0.40	0.23–0.47	Macek et al. (1976a)
Heptachlor	7.02	>0.86	<1.84	0.12–0.26	Macek et al. (1976a)
Lindane	69	>9.1	<23.5	0.13–0.34	Macek et al. (1976c)
Malathion	9000	>200	<580	0.02–0.06	Mount and Stephan (1967)
Trifluralin	115	>1.9	<5.1	0.017–0.044	Macek et al. (1976a)
Mysidopsis bahia					
DEF	4.55	<0.34		<0.08	Nimmo et al. (1981)
Diazinon	4.82	>1.16	<3.27	0.23–0.68	Nimmo et al. (1981)
Dimilin	1.97	>0.075[b]		0.04	Nimmo et al. (1981)
EPN	3.01	>0.44	<4.13	0.15–1.37	Nimmo et al. (1981)
Kepone	10.29	>0.26	<0.34	0.002–0.03	Nimmo et al. (1981)
Leptophos	3.31	>0.64	<1.77	0.19–0.53	Nimmo et al. (1981)
Methyl parathion	0.77	>0.11	<0.16	0.14–0.20	Nimmo et al. (1981)
Phorate	0.33	>0.09	<0.14	0.27–0.42	Nimmo et al. (1981)
Sevin	7.7	—		—	Nimmo et al. (1981)
Toxaphene	2.67	>0.07	<0.14	0.03–0.05	Nimmo et al. (1981)
Trifluralin	>136.0	—		—	Nimmo et al. (1981)
Cyprinodon variegatus					
Carbofuran	386.0	>15.0	<23.0	0.04–0.06	Parrish et al. (1977)
Chlordane	12.6	>0.5	<0.8	0.04–0.06	Parrish et al. (1978)
Diazinon	1470.0	>0.47		<0.0003	Goodman et al. (1979)
Endrin	0.34	>0.12	<0.31	0.35–0.91	Hansen et al. (1977)
Heptachlor	10.5	>0.97	<1.9	0.09–0.18	Hansen and Parrish (1977)
		or <0.71		or <0.07	
Kepone	69.5	>0.074	<0.12	0.001–0.002	Goodman et al. (1982)
Malathion	51.0	>4.0	<9.0	0.08–0.18	Parrish et al. (1977)
Methoxychlor	49.0	>12.0	<23.0	0.024–0.47	Parrish et al. (1977)
Pentachlorophenol	442.0	>47.0	<88.0	0.11–0.20	Parrish et al. (1978)
Trifluralin	190.0	>1.3	<4.8	0.007–0.025	Parrish et al. (1978)

[a]*Daphnia magna* tests were 48 h in duration.
[b]Estimated concentration.

reduction in brain acetylcholinesterase activity of bluegill sunfish exposed to malathion for several months was accompanied by evidence of spinal deformity (Eaton, 1970). Sheepshead minnows exposed to malathion for 26 wk had reduced acetylcholinesterase levels in brain tissue (Holland and Lowe, 1966). In a similar study, acetylcholinesterase activity varied inversely with exposure concentration of Diazinon during a partial life cycle test (Goodman et al., 1979). Fish maintained in the highest concentration (6.5 μg/l) averaged 71% inhibition.

Similar studies have been conducted with marine invertebrates. Oysters, *Crassostrea virginica,* reared from juveniles to sexual maturity in flowing seawater with DDT, toxaphene, and parathion added in combination (1.0 μg/l each) were smaller than controls (Lowe et al., 1971). Weights and lengths of oysters in seawater containing about 1.0 μg/l of each pesticide were not significantly different from those of controls. For nine pesticides, the zoeal stages of the Dungeness crab, *Cancer magister,* were 5–10 times more sensitive (mortality) and 10–100 times more sensitive than juveniles and adult crabs, respectively (Caldwell, 1977). *Cancer magister* and *Hemigrapsus nudus* exposed to methoxychlor were less resistant to periods of low salinity than control crabs (Caldwell, 1974). Results of several acute and life cycle tests with the mysid shrimp, *Mysidopsis bahia,* showed that criteria used to establish MATC limits varied (Nimmo et al., 1981). Effects were observed on growth, reproduction, and mortality; with two pesticides, however, effects on reproduction and mortality were observed at the same concentrations. Perhaps the two issues implicit in this section are (1) the importance of long-term or chronic studies and (2) discoveries of useful criteria for determining effects of pesticides on test species. Limiting the duration of testing or narrowing the design of the study to a single criterion can result in important effects being overlooked. For example, in some acute tests Kepone was found to be toxic to sheepshead minnows, *Cyprinodon variegatus,* with a 96-h LC50 of 69.5 μg/l (Schim-

mel and Wilson, 1977). Couch et al. (1977) described pathological anomalies (scoliosis) in sheepshead minnows exposed to 4 μg/l for 10–17 d. Hansen et al. (1977a) reported a 28-d LC50 of 1.3 μg/l for adult fish and also found that the average standard lengths of juvenile progeny were significantly less after an exposure to $\geqslant$0.08 μg/l. An entire life cycle of 141 d led to external signs of Kepone poisoning such as darkening of the posterior third of the body in fish exposed to $\geqslant$0.07 μg/l (Goodman et al., 1982). In these studies short test regimes and effects based solely on mortality would have resulted in a serious under-estimation of toxicity. However, the biological significance of the effect observed (such as limited change in pigmentation) should also be considered when using that effect as a criterion of toxic response.

COMPOUNDING FACTORS: INSECTICIDE RESISTANCE AND PESTICIDE INTERACTIONS

Two intriguing discoveries were made in studies of the toxic effects of pesticides. These are (1) the development of resistance of aquatic species to pesticides and (2) the unexpected effects of various substances and pesticides combined.

Perhaps the most notable report on pesticide-resistant populations was that of Vinson et al. (1963) on the resistance to DDT of the mosquito fish, *Gambusia affinis.* Several years later, Ferguson (1968) showed that many populations of fish from a pesticide-contaminated area in the Mississippi Delta exhibited higher tolerance to many pesticides than did fish from an uncontaminated site. Although most of the earlier studies showed resistance to the cyclodiene derivatives (e.g., dieldrin, endrin), cross resistance as a result of past exposure to toxaphene was suggested. Some fish were 300 times as resistant as animals from uncontaminated areas. Later, as organophosphate pesticides were used, fish were found to be tolerant to parathion, methyl parathion, and Dursban. In 24-h toxicity tests, freshwater shrimp, *Palaemonetes kadiakensis,* from three areas in the Mississippi Delta were 1–25 times more resistant to seven organochlorine, three organophosphorous, and one carbamate insecticide than those from an uncontaminated area (Naqvi and Ferguson, 1970).

Toxicity of mixtures of two or more chemicals is commonly referred to as synergistic, additive, or antagonistic, depending on its relation to the toxicity of the individual components (Marking, 1977). This is discussed in Chapter 7, and only some examples involving pesticides will be discussed here. In studies by Marking (1977), mixtures of malathion and Delnav were found to be highly synergistic in toxicity to rainbow trout, with an index of 7.20. Mixtures of commercial synergizers (sulfoxide and piperonyl butoxide) plus rotenone produced greater than additive effects on rainbow trout, with indices of 2.13 and 2.36. Further, Marking found that antimycin was detoxified by potassium permanganate ($KMnO_4$), and a mixture produced an additive index of −91.8. Toxicities of cadmium, methoxychlor, and a PCB to pink shrimp, *Penaeus duorarum,* appeared to be additive and independent regardless of the length of exposure (96 h or 30 d) (Bahner and Nimmo, 1975; Nimmo and Bahner, 1976). Mixtures of phosphamidon and methidathion tested in adult lobsters, *Homarus americanus,* were much more toxic than expected from the results with the individual chemicals in 48-h tests (McLeese and Metcalfe, 1979).

EFFECTS OF PESTICIDES ON POPULATIONS AND COMMUNITIES OF AQUATIC ORGANISMS

Although there is ample evidence that pesticides can adversely affect aquatic species in the environment, some studies have not shown such effects. Field tests with Dibrom 14 concentrate, applied by thermal fogging or aerially, showed little or no observable effect on estuarine test animals held in cages in their natural environments (Bearden, 1967). Similar findings were reported after application of malathion 95 on salt marsh areas near Pensacola, Florida (Tagatz et al., 1974). Deaths

due to the pesticide were not observed among crabs, shrimps, or fish. No dramatic mortalities of aquatic species in a freshwater marsh were recorded after DDT was applied at a rate of 0.2 lb per acre (Meeks and Peterle, 1967). These examples provide evidence for mitigation of expected adverse effects in the environment, possibly due to factors such as method of application, and inavailability to biota because of adsorption or degradation.

Some novel techniques have been used to determine the effects of pesticides on communities in the laboratory. Perhaps one of the best designs was that of Hansen (1976), who showed that Aroclor 1254 and toxaphene altered the composition of estuarine communities. The communities developed from planktonic larvae in salt water that flowed through small aquaria with and without the respective toxicants. Similar results were reported with pentachlorophenol (Tagatz et al., 1977) and Dowicide G-ST (79% sodium pentachlorophenate) (Tagatz et al., 1978). Several examples can be given of studies on experimental pesticide exposures in streams or field plots. Effects of acute exposure to Abate, Dursban, and methoxychlor on blackfly larvae and on "nontarget" stream invertebrates were studied by means of cone, rock, Surber, and drift samples (Wallace et al., 1973). Posttreatment drift of nontarget invertebrates indicated considerable disturbance of the aquatic community. Blackfly larvae were either greatly reduced or eradicated in the treated streams. A similar study, conducted over 1 yr with methoxychlor, showed that most invertebrate populations were reduced (Eisele and Hartung, 1976). The riffle invertebrate community (colonizing artificial substrates) showed a temporary decrease in diversity by both richness and evenness. The chitin inhibitor diflubenzuron, applied to three farm ponds at rates of 10, 5, and 2.5 μg/l and to a lake at 5 μg/l, inhibited emergence of adult *Chaoborus asticopus* (Apperson et al., 1978). Suppression of zooplankton crustaceans also occurred at all treatment concentrations. Bluegill sunfish, which fed predominantly on cladocerans and copepods, switched to chironomid midges and terrestrial insects after the treatment. In a saltwater study, the insecticide Sevin significantly reduced numbers of juvenile clams in plots treated with 2.3 and 4.6 kg per acre (Armstrong and Milleman, 1974).

Pesticides can adversely affect populations of organisms by being directly toxic to aquatic species or by contaminating organisms such as fish, which are then eaten by other wildlife or humans (Table 18). As far as can be determined, the pesticides listed are from normal use sources and, in the case of Kepone, from an accidental source. Documented effects range from the development of pesticide-tolerant species to physiological consequences such as reduced acetylcholinesterase activity. Some of the cases serve as unfortunate models of pesticide misuse and provide a basis for future approaches to testing needs for registration. They reinforce the need to address not only acute and chronic toxicity but also the fate and translocation of chemical contaminants, metabolism, and impacts on different trophic levels of biotic communities.

SUMMARY, CONCLUSIONS, AND FUTURE RESEARCH

Synthetic organic compounds are likely to continue to be used against a variety of pests, and recent trends indicate that widespread use of organochlorine-type chemicals will diminish. A variety of newer chemical types with different and unique modes of action will probably become available. Current pest control methods tend to involve use of several different chemicals mixed in varying proportions. Infestations of pests (e.g., the Mediterranean fruit fly) that threaten an entire region or a major crop will probably still be controlled with well-known chemicals, but wide application of a single pesticide will probably diminish.

Methods of assessing impacts of chemicals are evolving from single toxicity tests to the integration of many factors discussed in this chapter (such as the physical-chemical behavior of the compound). Toxicity tests will continue to be a vital part of the evaluation process, as for routine screening, but the checklist of factors necessary for substantiation of the impact continues to grow. Temperature, pH, photosensitivity, method of application, rates of metabolism, and many other factors will become increasingly important in the consideration of "hazard" or "impact." In toxicity testing of pesticides, there appears to be a trend toward longer-term tests and toward investigation of sublethal effects. Emphasis is also being placed on problems associated with extrapolation of laboratory results to conditions in the field (validation) and use of microcosms to evaluate new chemicals before production.

If biological control methods become more

Table 18 Some Effects on, or Contamination of, Biota after Exposures to Pesticides in Field Populations

Observed effects and organisms	Pesticide	Reference
Documenting the presence of pesticide-tolerant fish	Strobane and Chlordane	Ferguson (1968)
Failure to reestablish populations of bass	Several	Bingham (1970)
Failure of sea trout egg development	DDT	Butler et al. (1970)
Depressed acetylcholinesterase activity in brain tissue of fish	Malathion	Coppage and Duke (1971)
Reduced growth and spinal deformities in fish	Toxaphene	Mayer et al. (1975)
Eggshell thinning of brown pelican eggs	DDE	Blus et al. (1972)
Toxicity to fish and aquatic invertebrates in ponds	Dursban	Macek et al. (1972)
Contamination of James River and Chesapeake Bay biota	Kepone	Hansen et al. (1977b)
Reductions in some nontarget insects and significant increases in other nontarget insects	Methoprene (Altosid)	Steelman et al. (1975)

widely used, the evolution of hazard assessment and testing will probably change direction. Increasing use of such biological controls such as sporulating agents, pheromones, and sterilants will necessitate entirely new testing procedures for determining hazards to aquatic organisms.

Perhaps one of the greatest needs today is to understand the potential of effects and translocation of complex wastes containing pesticides. For example, a biological sludge dumped by a chemical company in the Gulf of Mexico contained more than 100 organic materials plus metals (Atlas et al., 1980). Potentially hazardous wastes generated by firms surveyed in Florida totaled about 580,000 metric tons per year (including pesticides) (Carter et al., 1977).

LITERATURE CITED

Alabaster JS: Survival of fish in 164 herbicides, insecticides, fungicides, wetting agents and miscellaneous substances. Int Pest Control 11:29–35, 1969.

Ali A, Mulla MS: Chemical control of nuisance midges in the Santa Ana River basin, Southern California. J Econ Entomol 70:191–195, 1977a.

Ali A, Mulla MS: The IGR diflubenzuron and organophosphorus insecticides against nuisance midges in man-made residential-recreational lakes. J Econ Entomol 70:571–577, 1977b.

Allison D, Hallman BJ, Cope OB, Valin CV: Some chronic effects of DDT on cutthroat trout. U.S. Dept Inter Fish Wildl Serv Res Rep 64, 1964.

Amend DF: Comparative toxicity of two iodophors to rainbow trout eggs. Trans Am Fish Soc 103:73–78, 1974.

Anderson JM, Peterson MR: DDT: Sublethal effects on brook trout nervous system. Science 164:440–441, 1969.

Appelgate VC, Howell JH, Moffet JW, Johnson BGH, Smith MA: Use of 3-trifluoromethyl-4-nitrophenol as a selective sea lamprey larvicide. Tech Rep Great Lakes Fish Comm No 1, 1961.

Apperson CS, Schaefer CH, Colwell AE, Werner GH, Anderson NL, Dupnas EF, Jr, Lorganecker DR: Effects of diflubenzuron on *Chaoborus*

astictopus and nontarget organisms and persistence of diflubenzuron in lentic habitics. J Econ Entomol 71:521–527, 1978.

Armstrong DA, Milleman RE: Effects of the insecticide carbaryl on clams and some other intertidal weed flat animals. J Fish Res Board Can 31:466–470, 1974.

Atlas E, Brooks J, Trefry J, Sauer T, Schwab C, Bernard B, Schofield J, Giam CS, Meyer ER: Environmental aspects of ocean dumping in the western Gulf of Mexico. J Water Pollut Contr Fed 52:329–350, 1980.

Bahner LH, Nimmo DR: Methods to assess effects of combinations of toxicants, salinity and temperature on estuarine animals. In: Trace Substances in Environmental Health IX. A Symposium, edited by DD Hemphill, pp. 169–177. Columbia: Univ. of Missouri, 1975.

Bahner LH, Oglesby JL: Test of a model for predicting Kepone accumulation in selected estuarine species. In: Aquatic Toxicology, edited by LL Marking, RA Kimerle, pp. 221–231. STP 667. Philadelphia: ASTM, 1979.

Bahner LH, Wilson AJ, Jr, Sheppard JM, Patrick JM, Jr, Goodman LR, Walsh GE: Kepone bioconcentration, accumulation, loss and transfer through estuarine food chains. Chesapeake Sci 18:299–308, 1977.

Baughman GL, Burns LA: Transport and transformation of chemicals in the environment: A perspective. In: Handbook of Environmental Chemistry (vol. 2), pp. 1–17, edited by O Hutzinger. New York: Springer, 1980.

Baughman GL, Lassiter RR: Prediction of environmental pollutant concentration. In: Estimating the Hazard of Chemical Substances to Aquatic Life, edited by J Cairns, Jr, KL Dickson, AW Maki, pp. 35–54. ASTM STP 657. Philadelphia: ASTM, 1978.

Bearden CM: Field tests concerning the effects of "Dibrom 14 concentrate" (Naled) on estuarine organisms. Contrib Bears Bluff Lab No 45, Wadmalaw Island, S.C., 1967.

Bingham CR: Comparison of insecticide residues from two Mississippi oxbow lakes. Proc 23rd Annu Conf Southeast Assoc Game Fish Comm, Mobile, Ala., pp. 275–280, 1970.

Blus LJ, Gish CD, Belisle AA, Prouty RM: Logarithmic relationship of DDE residues to eggshell thinning. Nature (Lond) 235:376–377, 1972.

Branson DR: Predicting the fate of chemicals in the aquatic environment from laboratory data. In: Estimating the Hazard of Chemical Substances to Aquatic Life, edited by J Cairns, Jr, KL Dickson, AW Maki, pp. 55–70. ASTM STP 657. Philadelphia: ASTM, 1978.

Bridges WR: Effects of time and temperature on the effects of heptachlor and Kepone to redear sunfish. In: Biological Problems in Water Pollution, 3d Seminar 1962 Transactions. Cincinnati, Ohio: U.S. Dep Health Educ Welfare, Public Health Serv, Division of Water Supply and Pollution Control, 1965.

Brown E, Nishioka YA: Pesticides in selected western streams—A contribution to the national program. Pestic Monit J 1:38–46, 1967.

Brungs WA, Mount DI: Introduction to a discussion of the use of aquatic toxicity tests for evaluation of the effects of toxic substances. In: Estimating the Hazard of Chemical Substances to Aquatic Life, edited by J Cairns, Jr, KL Dickson, AW Maki, pp. 15–26. ASTM STP 657. Philadelphia: ASTM, 1978.

Butler PA: Effects on commercial fisheries. U.S. Dep Inter Fish Wildl Serv Circ 143, pp. 21–24, 1962.

Butler PA: Commercial fisheries investigations. U.S. Dep Inter Fish Wildl Serv Circ 167, pp. 11–25, 1963.

Butler PA: Commercial fishery investigations. U.S. Dep Inter Fish Wildl Serv Circ 199, pp. 5–28, 1964.

Butler PA: Effects of pesticides on fish and wildlife. Fish Wildl Serv Circ 226, pp. 65–77, 1965.

Butler PA: The problem of pesticides in estuaries. Trans Am Fish Soc Spec Publ No 3, pp. 110–115, 1966.

Butler PA, Childress R, Wilson AJ, Jr: The association of DDT residues with losses in marine productivity. In: FAO Technical Conference on Marine Pollution and Its Effects on Living Resources and Fishing, pp. 1–13. FIR:MP/70/E-76. ROme: FAO, 1970.

Butler PA, Springer PF: Pesticides—A new factor in coastal environments. Trans 28th North Am Wildl Natl Res Conf, pp. 378–390, 1963.

Caldwell RS: Osmotic and ionic regulation in deca-

pod crustacea exposed to methoxychlor. In: Pollution and Physiology of Marine Organisms, edited by FJ Vernberg, WB Vernberg, pp. 197–223. New York: Academic, 1974.

Caldwell RS: Biological effects of pesticides on the dungeness crab. Ecol Res Ser EPA-600/3-77-131, 1977.

Cardwell RD, Foreman DG, Payne TR, Wilbur DJ: Acute and chronic toxicity of chlordane to fish and invertebrates. EPA 600/3-77-019. Duluth, Minn.: U.S. Environmental Research Laboratory, 1977.

Carson RL: Silent Spring. Boston: Houghton Mifflin, 1962.

Carter CE, Fink LL, Teaf CM, Herndon RC: Hazardous waste survey for the state of Florida. Final report, EPA grants L-004161-01 and L-004224-01-0. Tallahassee: Department of Environmental Regulation, 1977.

Coastal Water Research Project: Annual Reports 1976, 1977, 1978, 1979–80, Summary of Findings. El Segundo: Southern California Coastal Water Research Project, 1976–1980.

Cooley NR, Keltner JM, Jr, Forester J: Mirex and Aroclor 1254: Effect on and accumulation by *Tetrahymena pyriformis* strain W. J Protozool 19:636–138, 1972.

Cooley NR, Keltner JM, Jr, Forester J: The Polychlorinated biphenyls, Aroclor 1248 and 1260: Effect on and accumulation by *Tetrahymena pyriformis*. J Protozool 20:443–445, 1973.

Cope OB: Sport fishery investigations. Circ Fish Wildl Serv Wash No 199, 29:29–43, 1964.

Cope OB: Sport fishery investigations. Circ Fish Wildl Serv Wash No 226, 51:51–63, 1965.

Cope OB: U.S. Bur Sport Fish Wildl Resource Publ 64:125–132, 1968.

Coppage DL, Duke TW: Effects of pesticides in estuarines along the Gulf and southeast Atlantic coasts. In: Proceedings of the Second Gulf Coast Conference on Mosquito Suppression and Wildlife Management, in conjunction with Annual Meetings of the Louisiana Mosquito Control Association and the Gulf States Council of Wildlife, Fisheries and Mosquito Control, New Orleans, La., pp. 24–31, 1971.

Coppage DL, Matthews E: Brain acetylcholinesterase inhibition in a marine teleost during lethal and sublethal exposures to 1,2-dibromo-2,2-

dichloroethyl dimethyl phosphate (Naled) in seawater. Toxicol Appl Pharmacol 31:128–133, 1975.

Couch JA, Winstead JT, Goodman LR: Kepone-induced scoliosis and its histological consequences in fish. Science 197:585–587, 1977.

Crosby DG, Tucker RK, Aharonson N: The detection of acute toxicity with *Daphnia magna*. Food Cosmet Toxicol 4:503–514, 1966.

de la Cruz AA, Naqvi SM: Mirex incorporation in the environment. Uptake in aquatic organisms and effects on the rates of photosynthesis and respiration. Arch Environ Contam Toxicol 1: 255–264, 1973.

Dudley DR, Karr JR: Pesticides and PCB residues in the Black Creek watershed, Allen County, Indiana 1977–78. Pestic Monit J 13:155–157, 1980.

Durfee RL, Contos G, Whitmore FC, Borden JD, Hackman EE, III, Westin RA: PCBs in the United States, Industrial Use and Environmental Distributions. Washington, D.C.: U.S. EPA, Office of Toxic Substances, 1976.

Eaton JG: Chronic malathion toxicity to the bluegill (*Lepomis macrochirus* Rafinesque). Water Res 4:673–684, 1970.

Eisele PJ, Hartung R: The effects of methoxychlor on riffle invertebrate populations and communities. Trans Am Fish Soc 105:628–633, 1976.

Eisenreich SJ, Looney BB, Thornton JD: Airborne organic contaminants in the Great Lakes ecosystem. Environ Sci Technol 15:30–38, 1981.

Eisler R: Acute toxicities of insecticides to marine decapod crustaceans. Crustaceana 16:302–310, 1969.

Eisler R; Acute toxicities of organochlorine and organophosphorus insecticides to estuarine fishes. U.S. Dep Inter Bur Sport Fish Wildl Tech Pap 46, pp. 3–12, 1970.

Elliott M: Properties and applications of pyrethroids. Environ Health Perspect 14:3–14, 1976.

Epifanio CE: Effects of dieldrin in seawater on the development of two species of crab larvae *Leptodius floridanus* and *Panopeus herbstii*. Mar Biol 11:356–362, 1971.

Farm Chemicals Handbook. 67th ed. Willoughby, Ohio: Meister, 1981.

Farr JA: Impairment of antipredator behavior in

Palaemonetes pugio by exposure to sublethal doses of parathion. Trans Am Fish Soc 106: 287–290, 1977.

Ferguson DE: Characteristics and significance of resistance to insecticides in fishes. Reservoir Fishery Resources Symposium, Athens, Ga., April 5–7, 1967, pp. 531–536, 1968.

Gaufin AR, Jensen LD, Nebeker AV, Nelson T, Teel RW: The toxicity of ten organic insecticides to various aquatic invertebrates. Water Sewage Works 112:276–279, 1965.

Ginsburg JM: Toxicity of DDT to fish. J Econ Entomol 38:274–275, 1945.

Goodman LR, Hansen DJ, Coppage DL, Moore JC, Matthews E: Diazinon: Chronic toxicity to, and brain acetylcholinesterase inhibition in, the sheepshead minnow, *Cyprinodon variegatus*. Trans Am Fish Soc 108:479–488, 1979.

Goodman LR, Hansen DJ, Manning CS, Faas LF: Effects of Kepone on the sheepshead minnow (*Cyprinodon variegatus*) in an entire life-cycle toxicity test, Arch Environ Contam Toxicol 11:335–342, 1982.

Graham F, Jr: Since Silent Spring. Boston: Houghton Mifflin, 1970.

Grant BF, Mehrle PM: Chronic endrin poisoning in goldfish, *Carassius auratus*. J Fish Res Board Can 27:2225–2232, 1970.

Hansen DJ: Avoidance of pesticides by untrained sheepshead minnows. Trans Am Fish Soc 98: 426–429, 1969.

Hansen DJ: Techniques to assess the effects of toxic organics on marine organisms. In: Water Quality Research of the U.S. Environmental Protection Agency, Proceedings of an EPA-sponsored Symposium, pp. 63–76. EPA-600/3-76-079. Washington, D.C.: U.S. EPA, 1976.

Hansen DJ, Goodman LR, Wilson AJ, Jr: Kepone: Chronic effects on embryo, fry, juvenile, and adult sheepshead minnows (*Cyprinodon variegatus*). Chesapeake Sci 18:227–232, 1977a.

Hansen DJ, Nimmo DR, Schimmel SC, Walsh GE, Wilson AJ, Jr: Effects of Kepone on estuarine organisms. In: Recent Advances in Fish Toxicology, a Symposium, pp. 20–30. Ecological Research Series, EPA-600-3-77-085. Washington, D.C.: U.S. EPA, 1977b.

Hansen DJ, Schimmel SC, Forester J: Endrin: Effects on the entire life cycle of a saltwater fish, *Cyprinodon variegatus*. J Toxicol Environ Health 3:721–733, 1977c.

Harrison AD: The effects of Bayluscide on gastropod snails and other aquatic fauna. Hydrobiologia 28:371–384, 1966.

Henderson C, Pickering QH: Toxicity of organic phosphorus insecticides to fish. Trans Am Fish Soc 87:39–51, 1957.

Henderson C, Pickering QH, Tarzwell CM: The toxicity of organic phosphorus and chlorinated hydrocarbon insecticides to fish. In: Biological Problems in Water Pollution, Transactions, 2d Seminar, pp. 76–88. Cincinnati, Ohio: U.S. Dep Health Educ Welfare, Public Health Serv, Division of Water Supply & Pollution Control, 1960.

Hiltibran RC: Effects of some herbicides on fertilized fish eggs and fry. Trans Am Fish Soc 96:414–416, 1967.

Holcombe GW, Phipps GL, Tanner DK: The acute toxicity of kelthane, Dursban, disulfoton, pydrin, and permethrin to fathead minnows (*Pimephales promelas*) and rainbow trout (*Salmo gairdneri*), Environ Pollution Series A 29:167–178, 1982.

Holland HT, Lowe JI: Malathion: Chronic effects on estuarine fish. Mosquito News 26:383–385, 1966.

Hollingworth RM: Chemistry, biological activity, and uses of formamidine pesticides. Environ Health Perspect 14:57–69, 1976.

Hollister TA, Walsh GE, Forester J: Mirex and marine unicellular algae: Accumulation, population growth and oxygen evolution. Bull Environ Contam Toxicol 14:753–759, 1975.

Howell JH, King EL, Smith AJ, Hanson LH: Synergism of 5,2'-dichloro-4'-nitro-salicylamide and 3-trifluoromethyl-4-nitrophenol in a selective lamprey larvicide. Tech Rep Great Lakes Fish Comm No 8, 1964.

Hughes JS: Tolerance of striped bass, *Morone saxatilis* (Walbaum), larvae and fingerlings to nine chemicals used in pond culture. Proc Conf Southeast Assoc Game Fish Comm 24:431–438, 1970.

Hughes JS, Davis JT: Variations in toxicity to bluegill sunfish of phenoxy herbicides. Weeds 11:50–53, 1963.

Hunter RC: Organotin compounds and their use for insect and mite control. Environ Health Perspect 14:47–50, 1976.

Hunter RC, Carroll JH, Randolph JC: Organochlorine residues in fish of Lake Texoma, October 1979. Pestic Monit J 14:102–107, 1980.

Inglis A, Davis EL: Effects of water hardness on the toxicity of several organic and inorganic herbicides to fish. Tech Pap Fish Wildl Serv 67, 1972.

Iyatomi K, Tamura T, Itazawa Y, Hanyu I, Sugiura S: Toxicity of endrin to fish. Prog Fish Cult 20:155–162, 1958.

Jarvinen AW, Hoffman MJ, Thorslund TW: Toxicity of DDT in food and water exposure to fathead minnows. EPA-600/3-76-114. Duluth, Minn.: Environmental Research Laboratory, 1976.

Johnson DW, Finley MT: Handbook of acute toxicity of chemicals to fish and aquatic invertebrates. U.S. Dep Inter Fish Wildl Sect Resource Publ 137, 1980.

Kent JC, Johnson DW: Organochlorine residues in fish, water, and sediment of American Falls Reservoir, Idaho, 1974. Pestic Monit J 13:28–34, 1979.

Kiigemagi U, Terriere LC: Losses of organophosphorus insecticides during application to the soil. Bull Environ Contam Toxicol 6:336–342, 1971.

Kimbrough RD: Toxicity and health effects of selected organotin compounds: A review. Environ Health Perspect 14:51–56, 1976.

Leung DK: Modeling the bioaccumulation of pesticides in fish. CEM Rep 5. Troy, N.Y.: Center for Ecological Modeling, Rensselaer Polytechnic Institute, 1978.

Li M: Pollution in nation's estuaries originating from the agricultural use of pesticides. In: Estuarine Pollution Control and Assessment, Proceedings of a Conference, pp. 451–466. Washington, D.C.: U.S. EPA, Office of Water Planning and Standards, 1975.

Lincer JL: The impact of synthetic organic compounds on estuarine ecosystems. In: Estuarine Pollution Control, Proceedings of a Conference, pp. 425–443. U.S. EPA, Office of Water Planning and Standards, 1975.

Lincer JL, Solon JM, Nair JH: DDT and endrin fish toxicity under static versus dynamic bioassay conditions. Trans Am Fish Soc 99:13–19, 1970.

Lloyd-Jones CP: Evaporation of DDT. Nature (Lond) 229:65–66, 1971.

Lowe JI, Parrish PR, Wilson AJ, Jr, Wilson PD, Duke TW: Effects of mirex on selected estuarine organisms. Trans 36th North Am Wildl Nat Res Conf pp. 171–186, 1971.

Lowe JI, Wilson PD, Rick AJ, Wilson AJ, Jr: Chronic exposure of oysters to DDT, toxaphene and parathion. Natl Shellfish Assoc 61:71–79, 1971.

Lunsford CA: Kepone distribution in the water column of the James River Estuary—1976–78. Pestic Monit J 14:119–124, 1981.

Macek KJ: Reproduction in brook trout (*Salvelinus fontinalis*) fed sublethal concentrations of DDT. J Fish Res Board Can 25:1787–1796, 1968.

Macek KJ, Hutchinson C, Cope OB: The effects of temperature on the susceptibility of bluegills and rainbow trout to selected pesticides. Bull Environ Contam Toxicol 4:174–183, 1969.

Macek KJ, Lindberg MA, Sauter S, Buxton KS, Costa PA: Toxicity of four pesticides to water fleas and fathead minnows. EPA-600/3-76-099. Duluth, Minn.: U.S. Environmental Research Laboratory, 1976a.

Macek KJ, Buxton KS, Sauter S, Gnilka S, Dean JW: Chronic toxicity of atrazine to selected aquatic invertebrates and fishes. EPA-600/3-76-047. Washington, D.C.: U.S. EPA, 1976b.

Macek KJ, Buxton KS, Derr SK, Dean JW, Sauter S: Chronic toxicity of lindane to selected aquatic invertebrates and fishes. EPA-600/3-76-046. Washington, D.C.: U.S. EPA, 1976c.

Macek KJ, Petrocelli SR, Sleight BH, III: Considerations in assessing the potential for, and significance of, biomagnification of chemical residues in aquatic food chains. In: Aquatic Toxicology, edited by LL Marking, RA Kimerle, pp. 251–268. ASTM STP 667. Philadelphia: ASTM, 1979.

Macek KJ, Walsh DF, Hogan JW, Holz DD: Toxicity of the insecticide Dursban to fish and aquatic invertebrates in ponds. Trans Am Fish Soc 101:420–427, 1972.

Mackenthun KM: Report on pollution of inter-state waters of the Tombigbee-Mobile River System, Florida. U.S. Dep Health Educ Welfare, Public Health Serv, 1965.

Manigold DB, Schulze JA: Pesticides in water (Pesticides in selected western streams—A progress report). Pestic Monit J 2:124–135, 1969.

Marking LL: Method for assessing additive toxicity of chemical mixtures. In: Aquatic Toxicology and Hazard Evaluation, edited by FL Mayer, JL Hamelink, pp. 98–108. ASTM STP 634. Philadelphia: ASTM, 1977.

Marking LL, Dawson VK: The half-life of biological activity of antimycin determined by fish bioassay. Trans Am Fish Soc 101:100–105, 1972.

Marking LL, Hogan JW: Toxicity of Bayer 73 to fish. Invest Fish Cont No 19. LaCrosse, Wis: Bur Sport Fish & Wildlife, 1967.

Matsumura F: Toxicology of Insecticides. New York: Plenum, 1975.

Mayer FL, Jr, Mehrle PM, Jr, Dwyer WP: Toxaphene effects on reproduction, growth, and mortality of brook trout. EPA-600/3-75-013. Fish-Pesticide Research Laboratory, Columbia, Missouri, for U.S. EPA, Duluth, Minn., 1975. 42 pp.

Mayer FL, Jr, Mehrle PM, Jr, Dwyer WP: Toxaphene: Chronic toxicity to fathead minnows and channel catfish. EPA-600/3-77-069. Fish-Pesticide Research Laboratory, Columbia, Missouri, for U.S. EPA, Duluth, Minn., 1977. 33 pp.

McLeese DW, Metcalfe CD: Toxicity of mixtures of phosphamidon and methidathion to lobsters (*Homarus americanus*). Chemosphere 8:59–62, 1979.

Meeks RL, Peterle TJ: The cycling of Cl^{36} labeled DDT in a marsh ecosystem. Rep C00-1358-3, RF Project 1794. The Ohio State University Research Foundation, Columbus, 1967.

Menzie CM: Metabolism of pesticides—An update. U.S. Dep Inter Fish Wildl Serv Spec Sci Rep Wildl No 184, 1974.

Merna JW, Eisele PJ: The effects of methoxychlor on aquatic biota. EPA-R3-73-046. Duluth, Minn.: U.S. EPA, National Water Quality Laboratory, 1973.

Micks DW: Mosquito control agents derived from petroleum hydrocarbons. IV. Further larval abnormalities produced by FLIT MLO. J Econ Entomol 63:1118–1121, 1970.

Miles JRW: Insecticide residues on stream sediments in Ontario, Canada. Pestic Monit J 10: 87–91, 1976.

Miller CW, Zuckerman BM, Charig AJ: Water translocation of diazinon-C^{14} and parathion-S^{35} off a model cranberry bog and subsequent occurrence in fish and mussels. Trans Am Fish Soc 95:345–349, 1966.

Mount DI: Chronic effects of endrin on bluntnose minnows and guppies. U.S. Bur Sport Fish Wildl Res Rep 58, 1962.

Mount DI, Stephan CE: A method for establishing acceptable toxicant limits for fish—malathion and butoxyethanol ester of 2,4-D. Trans Am Fish Soc 96:185–193, 1967.

Muncy RJ, Oliver AD, Jr: Toxicity of ten insecticides to the red crawfish, *Procambarus larki* (Girard). Trans Am Fish Soc 92:428–431, 1963.

Naqvi SM, Ferguson DE: Levels of insecticide resistance in fresh-water shrimp, *Palaemonetes kadiakensis*. Trans Am Fish Soc 99:696–699, 1970.

Nimmo DR, Bahner LH: Metals, pesticides and PCBs: Toxicities to shrimp singly and in combination. In: Estuarine Processes, vol. 1, Uses, Stresses, and Adaptation to the Estuary, edited by M Wiley, pp. 523–532. New York: Academic, 1976.

Nimmo DR, Blackman RR, Wilson AJ, Jr, Forester J: Toxicity and distribution of Aroclor 1254 in the pink shrimp *Penaeus duorarum*. Mar Biol 11:191–197, 1971.

Nimmo DR, Hamaker TL, Matthews E, Moore JC: An overview of the acute and chronic effects of first and second generation pesticides on an estuarine mysid. In: Biological Monitoring of Marine Pollutants, edited by FJ Vernberg, A Calabrese, FP Thurberg, WB Vernberg, pp. 3–20. New York: Academic, 1981.

Park RA, Connoly CI, Albanese JR, Clesceri LS, Heitzman GW, Herbrandson HH, Indyke BH, Loehe JR, Ross S, Sharma DD, Shuster WW: Modeling transport and behavior of pesticides and other toxic organic materials in aquatic environments. CEM Rep 7. Troy, N.Y.: Center for Ecological Modeling, Rensselaer Polytechnic Institute, 1980.

Parrish PR, Dyar EE, Enos JM, Wilson WG: Chronic toxicity of chlordane, trifluralin, and pentachlorophenol to sheepshead minnow (*Cyprinodon variegatus*). EPA-600/3-78-010. Gulf Breeze, Fla.: U.S. EPA, 1978.

Parrish PR, Dyar EE, Lindberg MA, Shanika CM, Enos JM: Chronic toxicity of methoxychlor, malathion, and carbofuran to sheepshead minnows (*Cyprinodon variegatus*). EPA-600/3-77-059. Gulf Breeze, Fla.: U.S. EPA, 1977.

Parrish PR, Schimmel SC, Hansen DJ, Partick Jm, Jr, Forester J: Chlordane: Effect on several estuarine organisms. J Toxicol Environ Health 1: 485–494, 1976.

Pickering QH, Henderson C, Lemke AE: The toxicity of organic phosphorus insecticides to different species of warm water fishes. Trans Am Fish Soc 91:175–184, 1962.

Portmann JE, Wilson KW: The toxicity of 140 substances to the brown shrimp and other marine animals. Minist Agric Fish Food Shellfish Inf Leaflet 22, 1971.

Premdas F, Anderson JM: The uptake and detoxification of C^{14} labelled DDT in Atlantic salmon. J Fish Res Board Can 20:827–837, 1963.

Rand GM: The effect of subacute parathion exposure on the locomotor behavior of the bluegill sunfish and large mouth bass. In: Aquatic Toxicology and Hazard Evaluation, edited by FL Mayer, JL Hamelink, pp. 253–268. ASTM STP 634. Philadelphia: ASTM, 1977.

Ridgway RL, Finney JC, MacGregor JT, Starler NJ: Pesticide use in agriculture. Environ Health Perspect 27:103–112, 1978.

Ritter WF, Johnson HP, Lovely WG, Molnan M: Atrazine, propachlor, and diazinon residues on small agricultural watersheds: Runoff losses, persistence and movement. Environ Sci Technol 8:38–42, 1974.

Rubenstein NI: Effect of sodium pentachlorophenate on the feeding activity of the lugworm, *Arenicola cristata* Stimpson. In: Pentachlorophenol: Chemistry, Pharmacology and Environmental Toxicology, edited by K Ranga Rao, pp. 175–179. New York: Plenum, 1978.

Rudd RL: Pesticides and the Living Landscape. Madison, Wis.: Univ. of Wisconsin Press, 1964.

Sanders HO, Cope OB: Toxicities of several pesticides to two species of cladocerans. Trans Am Fish Soc 95:165–169, 1966.

Sanders HO: Sublethal effects of toxaphene on daphnids, scuds, and midges. EPA-600/3-80-006. Duluth, Minn.: U.S. EPA, 1980.

Sandholzer LA: The effect of DDT upon the Chesapeake Bay blue crab (*Callinectes sapidus*). Fish Mark News 7:2–4, 1945.

Schimmel SC, Hansen DJ, Forester J: Effects of Aroclor 1254 on laboratory-reared embryos and fry of sheepshead minnows (*Cyprinodon variegatus*). Trans Am Fish Soc 103:582–586, 1974.

Schimmel SC, Wilson AJ, Jr: Acute toxicity of Kepone to four estuarine animals. Chesapeake Sci 18:224–227, 1977.

Schmitt CJ, Ludke JL, Walsh DF: Organochlorine residues in fish: National pesticide monitoring program, 1970–74. Pestic Monit J 14:136–206, 1981.

Schulze JA, Manigold DB, Andrews FL: Pesticides in selected western streams—1968–71. Pestic Monit J 7:73–85, 1973.

Silbergeld EK: Dieldrin. Effects of chronic sublethal exposure on adaptation to thermal stress in freshwater fish. Environ Sci Technol 7:846–849, 1973.

Sodergren A: Uptake and accumulation of C^{14}-DDT by *Chlorella* sp. (Chlorophyceae). Oikos 19:126–138, 1968.

Sodergren A: Transport, distribution, and degradation of DDT and PCB in a South Swedish lake ecosystem. Vatten 2:90–108, 1973.

Soloway SB: Naturally occurring insecticides. Environ Health Perspect 14:109–117, 1976.

Steelman CD, Farlow JE, Breaud TP, Schilling PE: Effects of growth regulators on *Psorophora columbiae* (Dyar and Knab) and non-target aquatic insect species in rice fields. Mosquito News 35:67–76, 1975.

Stern AM, Walker CR: Hazard assessment of toxic substances: environmental fate testing of organic chemicals and ecological effects testing. In: Estimating the Hazard of Chemical Substances to Aquatic Life, edited by J Cairns, Jr, KL Dickson, AW Maki, pp. 81–131. ASTM STP 657. Philadelphia: ASTM, 1978.

Tagatz ME, Bosthwick PW, Cook GH, Coppage DL: Effects of ground applications of mala-

thion on salt-marsh environments in northwestern Florida. Mosquito News 34:309–315, 1974.

Tagatz ME, Ivey JM, Moore JC, Tobia M: Effects of pentachlorophenol on the development of estuarine communities. J Toxicol Environ Health 3:501–506, 1977.

Tagatz ME, Ivey JM, Tobia M: Effects of Dowicide G–ST on development of experimental estuarine macrobenthic communities. In: Pentachlorophenol, edited by K Ranga Rao, pp. 157–163. New York: Plenum, 1978.

Truhlar JF, Reed LA: Occurrence of pesticide residues in four streams draining different land-use areas in Pennsylvania, 1967–71. Pestic Monit J 10:101–110, 1976.

U.S. EPA: Acephate, aldicarb, carbophenothion, DEF, EPN, ethoprop, methyl parathion, and phorate: Their acute and chronic toxicity, bioconcentration potential, and persistence as related to marine environments. EPA-600/4-81-023. Washington, D.C.: 1981.

Vanderford MJ, Hamelink JL: Influence of environmental factors on pesticide levels in sport fish. Pestic Monit J 11:138–145, 1977.

Veith GD, Kuehl DW, Leonard EN, Welch K, Pratt G: Polychlorinated biphenyls and other organic chemical residues in fish from major United States watersheds near the Great Lakes, 1978. Pestic Monit J 15:1–8, 1981.

Vinson SB, Boyd CE, Ferguson DE: Resistance to DDT in the mosquito fish, *Gambusia affinis*. Science 139:217–218, 1963.

von Rumker R, Kelso GL, Horay F, Lawrence KA: A study of the efficiency of the use of pesticides in agriculture. EPA 540/1-74-001. Washington, D.C.: U.S. EPA, 1975a.

von Rumker R, Lawless EW, Meiners AG, Lawrence KA, Kelso GL, Horay F: Production, distribution, use and environmental impact potential of selected pesticides. EPA 540/1-74-001. Washington, D.C.: U.S. EPA, 1975b.

Walker CR, Lennon RE, Berger BL: Preliminary observations on the toxicity of antimycin A to fish and other aquatic animals. Invest Fish Control Circ Bur Sport Fish Wildl No 186:1–18, 1964.

Wallace RR, West AS, Downe AER, Hynes HBN: The effects of experimental blackfly (Diptera: Simuliidae) larviciding with Abate, Dursban, and methoxychlor on stream invertebrates. Can Entomol 105:817–831, 1973.

Walsh GE: Effects of herbicides on photosynthesis and growth of marine unicellular algae. Hyacinth Control J 10:45–48, 1972.

Walsh GE, Ainsworth K, Wilson AJ: Toxicity and uptake of Kepone in marine unicellular algae. Chesapeake Sci 18:222–223, 1977.

Walsh GE, Barrett R, Cook GH, Hollister TA: Effects of herbicides on seedlings of the red mangrove, *Rhizophora mangle* L. Bio-Science 23: 361–364, 1973.

Wang TC, Johnson RS, Bricker JL: Residues of polychlorinated biphenyls and DDT in water and sediment of the Indian River Lagoon, Florida—1977–78. Pestic Monit J 13:141–144, 1980.

Wauchope RD: The pesticide content of surface water draining from agriculture fields—A review. J Environ Qual 7:459–472, 1978.

Wegman RCC, Greve PA: Organochlorines, cholinesterase inhibitors, and aromatic amines in Dutch water samples, September 1969–December 1975. Pestic Monit J 12:149–162, 1978.

Wolfe NL, Zepp RG, Baughman GL, Fincher RC, Gordon JA: Chemical and photochemical transformation of selected pesticides in aquatic systems. EPA-600/3-76-067. Washington, D.C.: U.S. EPA, 1976.

Wurster CF, Jr: DDT reduces photosynthesis by marine phytoplankton. Science 159:1474–1475, 1968.

SUPPLEMENTAL READING

Corbett JR: The Biochemical Mode of Action of Pesticides. New York: Academic, 1974.

Edwards CA: Environmental Pollution by Pesticides. New York: Plenum, 1973.

Johnson DW: Pesticides and fishes—A review of selected literature. Trans Am Fish Soc 97:398–424, 1968.

Khan MAQ: Pesticides in Aquatic Environments. New York: Plenum, 1977.

Moriarty F (ed): Organochlorine insecticides: Persistent organic pollutants. New York: Academic, 1975.

Muirhead-Thompson RC: Pesticides and Freshwater Fauna. New York: Academic, 1971.

O'Brien RD: Insecticides: Action and Metabolism. New York: Academic, 1967.

Pimentel D: Ecological Effects of Pesticides on Non-target Species. Washington, D.C.: Government Printing Office, 1971.

Tucker RK, Leitzke JS: Comparative toxicology of insecticides for vertebrate wildlife and fish. Pharmacol Ther 6:167–220, 1979.

Wilkinson CF (ed): Insecticide Biochemistry and Physiology. New York: Plenum, 1976.

Chapter 13
Trace Metals

H. V. Leland and J. S. Kuwabara

INTRODUCTION

Many trace metals are important in plant and animal nutrition, where, as micronutrients, they play an essential role in tissue metabolism and growth. The essential trace metals include cobalt, copper, chromium, iron, manganese, nickel, molybdenum, selenium, tin, and zinc. Requirements of different plant and animal species vary substantially, but optimal concentration ranges for micronutrients are frequently narrow. Severe imbalances can cause death, whereas marginal imbalances contribute to poor health and retarded growth. Some nonessential trace metals, such as lead, cadmium, and mercury, also can be toxic at concentrations commonly observed in soils and natural waters.

Adverse environmental effects associated with redistribution of trace metals, such as by mining and fossil fuel combustion, have long been recog-

nized. Information about the polluted state of rivers of the lead-mining districts of the British Isles can be found in the fifth report of the River Pollution Commission of 1874 (reviewed in Jones, 1964). Research on the effects of trace metals in natural waters during the first half of this century focused on lead, zinc, and copper pollution from mining and industrial effluents (reviewed in Doudoroff and Katz, 1953; Jones, 1964). During this era, much was learned about trace metal requirements of plants and animals and their limits of tolerance. However, the recent expansion of environmental research on trace metals was triggered not so much by interest in the essential trace metals as by revelations about the widespread occurrence and potential health hazards of nonessential trace elements, particularly cadmium, lead, and mercury.

Public and private support provided during the

past decade to document and control the distribution of these and other potentially hazardous trace metals has led to a large body of literature on their environmental effects. Reviews have appeared that consider the toxicity to aquatic organisms of copper (Hodson et al., 1979; U.S. EPA, 1980a), zinc (Whitton, 1980; Pagenkopf, 1980; U.S. EPA, 1980b), lead (U.S. EPA, 1980c), and mercury (U.S. EPA, 1980d). These reviews give references to data on trace metal concentrations that are lethal to different aquatic species. The aim of this chapter is to summarize recent toxicological and ecological research findings that characterize the effects of trace metal contamination of aquatic environments. Information on toxicological and homeostatic responses of organisms is emphasized. As much pertinent research on biochemical processes and metabolism of trace metals has been conducted only on mammalian and higher plant tissues, and homologies exist between aquatic and terrestrial organisms, results of some investigations of nonaquatic organisms are included. Elements considered in detail are copper, lead, mercury, and zinc.

ENVIRONMENTAL CONCENTRATIONS

Anthropogenic enrichment of trace metals in aquatic environments has been frequently observed (Table 1). Vertical distributions of most trace metals, including copper, lead, mercury, and zinc, exhibit characteristic profiles in open ocean waters removed from direct anthropogenic influence. Total concentrations of copper, zinc, and cadmium in surface waters have been positively correlated with macronutrient concentrations, suggesting a role in biogeochemical cycling (Bruland et al., 1978; Boyle et al., 1976; 1977; Boyle and Edmond, 1975). Spencer and Brewer (1969), however, calculated that copper uptake by plankton in the Sargasso Sea and the Gulf of Maine cannot account for variations in surface water copper concentrations. Total concentrations of copper, zinc, and cadmium generally increase with depth, presumably due to mineralization during particle sinking (Boyle et al., 1977).

Schaule and Patterson (1978) observed lead enrichment in surface waters of the North Pacific between California and Hawaii, and attributed this

Table 1 Concentration Ranges of Selected Trace Metals, Reflecting Localized Anthropogenic Inputs, in Water and Sediments of Freshwater and Marine Environments[a]

Element	Seawater (µg/l)	Marine sediments (mg/kg)	Fresh water (µg/l)	Freshwater sediments (mg/kg)	Anthropogenic sources cited
Copper[b]	0.2–500	2–700	0.3–9000	<5–2000	Copper mining and smelting, steel production, fossil fuel combustion
Mercury[c]	0.001–0.7	0.01–800	0.01–30	0.02–10	Coal combustion, acetaldehyde and chlor-alkali production, fungicide application
Lead[d]	0.005–0.4	10–200	0.2–900	3–20,000	Lead smelting, lead alkyl production
Zinc[e]	0.01–20	5–100,000	0.1–50,000	<10–10,000	Municipal sewage discharge, mining

[a]Lower values in the concentration ranges are typical baseline concentrations; higher values are concentrations reported at sites affected by human activities.

[b]From Boyle (1979); Hodson et al. (1980); Merlini (1971); Thornton (1980); Ward et al. (1976); Nordstrom et al. (1977).

[c]From Koch (1980); Pillay et al. (1973); Holden (1972); Fitzgerald (1979).

[d]From Koch (1980); Collinson and Shimp (1972); Patterson (1973); Forstner and Wittmen (1979).

[e]From Koch (1980); Forstner and Wittmen (1979); Young et al.(1980); Martin et al. (1980); Nordstrom et al. (1977).

enrichment to atmospheric inputs from automobile and smelter emissions. Windom et al. (1975) noted seasonal variations of soluble mercury concentration in surface waters of the southeastern Atlantic continental shelf and, like Schaule and Patterson (1978), linked these variations to atmospheric inputs from the continental United States. Mercury is enriched in deep seawaters by hot springs discharge (Bostrom and Fisher, 1969; Carr et al., 1975). Copper introduction into Pacific deep seawater from surficial sediments was hypothesized by Boyle et al. (1977). Notable exceptions to the depth dependence of concentrations in open ocean waters are concentrations of strontium, cesium, rubidium, uranium, and molybdenum (Bolter et al., 1964; Forstner and Wittman, 1979), which remain fairly constant with depth.

In contrast to characteristic vertical distributions in open ocean waters, copper, lead, mercury, and zinc concentrations of fresh water and coastal seawater display great spatial and temporal variability, generally as a result of localized anthropogenic inputs. Low and high values of metal concentrations in Table 1 represent typical baseline levels and high concentrations reported for areas receiving anthropogenic effluents, respectively. Higher metal concentrations have been reported

for polluted fresh water than for polluted seawater, whereas high coastal marine sediment concentrations generally exceed high freshwater sediment concentrations. This observation, supported by examples presented in Table 1, suggests that oceans serve as the final sink for these pollutants.

ACUTE TOXICITY

Trace metal toxicity to aquatic organisms is manifested in a wide range of effects, from slight reduction in growth rate to death. Comparison of concentration ranges of trace metals in surface waters (Table 1) with acute toxicity data for these metals (Tables 2 and 3) shows that concentrations determined to be lethal (96-h LC50) in laboratory tests occur commonly in nature. For example, concentration ranges for copper, lead, mercury, and zinc in fresh water (Table 1) consistently overlap acute toxicity ranges for freshwater crustaceans (Table 3). Mollusks and fish generally survive higher trace metal concentrations than do other phyla tested (Tables 2 and 3). This trend shows the importance of examining toxic responses of several test organisms representative of the aquatic community in question when water quality standards are to be set. The U.S. Environmental Protection Agency

Table 2 Acute Toxicity (48- 96-h LC50 or EC50) Data for Certain Phyla Commonly Used as Marine Test Organisms[a,b]

Test organism	Copper	Mercury	Lead	Zinc
Arthropoda (crustaceans)	50–100,000	4–400	700–3000	200–5000
Annelida	100–500	10–90	–	800–50,000
Mollusca	200–8000	4–30,000	800–30,000	100–40,000
Vertebrata (Salmonidae)	30–500	–	–	20,000–70,000
Algae				
Chlorophyta	–	<5–400	–	50–7000
Chrysophyta (diatoms)	5–50	0.1–10	–	200–500

[a]From Hodson et al. (1979) and U.S. EPA (1980a-d).

[b]Total concentration ranges (μg/l) given for the four trace elements reflect variations in experimental design (i.e., chemical, physical, and biological characteristics) as well as inherent randomness in organism response. Concentration ranges for algae represent concentrations causing significant growth inhibition. Dashes indicate that sufficient data were not obtained to determine an LC50 or EC50 range, generally because tests in this category had emphasized sublethal toxicity and bioaccumulation.

Table 3 Acute Toxicity (48- 96-h LC50 or EC50) Data for Certain Phyla Commonly Used as Freshwater Test Organisms[a,b]   .3-9000

Test organism	Copper	Mercury	Lead	Zinc
Arthropoda (crustaceans)	5–3000	0.02–40	–	30–9000
Annelida	6–900		–	–
Mollusca	40–9000	90–2000	–	500–20,000
Vertebrata (fish)				
Salmonidae	10–900	3–20,000	1000–500,000	50–7000
Centrachidae	700–10,000	3000–10,000	20,000–400,000	1000–20,000
Cyprinidae	20–2000	–	2000–500,000	400–50,000
Algae				
Chlorophyta	1–8000	<0.8–2000	500–1000	30–8000
Chrysophyta (diatoms)	5–800	–	–	–

[a]From Hodson et al. (1979) and U.S. EPA (1980a–d).
[b]Total concentration ranges (μg/l) given for the four trace elements reflect variations in experimental design (i.e., chemical, physical, and biological characteristics) as well as inherent randomness in organism response. Concentration ranges for algae represent concentrations causing significant growth inhibition. Dashes indicate that sufficient data were not obtained to determine an LC50 or EC50 range, generally because assays in this category had emphasized sublethal toxicity and bioaccumulation.

computes water quality criteria based on available acute toxicity data from all tested phyla (U.S. EPA, 1980b).

It is interesting to note (Tables 2 and 3) that major differences in 96-h LC50 concentrations are not evident between freshwater and marine organisms of the same phylum. Hodson et al. (1979) also noted, from their compilation of copper toxicity data, a lack of striking differences between acutely lethal concentrations for freshwater and marine organisms. This apparent lack of difference in sensitivity may be due to the diversity of experimental conditions used to obtain the mortality data (LC50) and to variations in sensitivity of test species within a phylum.

The utility of laboratory-derived data in predicting responses of natural populations is dependent on understanding the limitations of laboratory toxicity tests and the effects of physicochemical variables at the field site. Numerous physiological, chemical, and physical processes control toxicant availability as well as an organism's response to metals. A few generalizations can be made about the laboratory tests used to generate the toxicity data summarized in Tables 2 and 3.

1 Data are for total metal concentrations added to test media. Anions of metals added were not identical in all tests (Saliba and Krzyz, 1976).
2 Experiments were usually carried out in batch (static) cultures instead of continuous-flow cultures to facilitate replicability at lower cost and lower labor intensity. Testing of fish was an exception, with approximately half the data based on flow-through experiments (U.S. EPA, 1980a). Chemical characteristics such as pH, dissolved oxygen (DO), and dissolved organic carbon (DOC) may have varied during the toxicity test period as a result of metabolic activities.
3 Results are provided for tests in single species of various physiological states, for example, size, stage of development, extent of acclimation, sex, and nutritional status (refer to Chapter 6).

Toxicity test characteristics described above pose serious limitations on the direct application of test results. Consideration of total metal concentration alone can be misleading because chemical speciation of trace metals significantly affects availability to aquatic organisms and hence toxicity. Uncomplexed metal ions (Cd^{2+}, Cu^{2+}, Pb^{2+}, and Zn^{2+}) are apparently more readily assimilated by organisms than are complexed forms (Eichhorn, 1975; Sunda and Guillard, 1976; Anderson et al., 1978; Sunda et al., 1978; Dodge and Theis, 1979; Allen et al., 1980; Hart, 1981). It is therefore evident that the effects of chemical processes that control chemical speciation (e.g., inorganic complexation, chelation, precipitation, and adsorption) should be monitored or, if possible, controlled. Techniques for measuring free metal ion concentrations in aqueous media are at present restricted in their applications. Ion-selective electrodes, which measure free ion activity directly, typically yield a less than optimal (i.e., non-Nernstian) response below submicromolar total concentrations (McKnight, 1979). In addition, chloride ion interference restricts the use of certain ion-selective electrodes to solutions of low ionic strength. Anodic stripping voltammetry measures concentrations of labile copper species, including free copper ions and weakly bound copper complexes. Knowledge of the complexing capacities of various organic and inorganic ligands in the sample is therefore necessary to make distinctions between concentrations of each species.

An alternative to analytical estimation of trace metal speciation is the use of chemically defined media (e.g., Morel et al., 1979), whereby metal speciation can be estimated by using chemical equilibrium computer programs (e.g., Truesdell and Jones, 1974; McDuff and Morel, 1973; Westall et al., 1976). An example of such a computation with REDEQL2 (Table 4) demonstrates the effects on trace metal speciation of the addition of copper (total concentration, 50 $\mu g/l$) to a chemically defined freshwater growth medium, SANM(E) (Kuwabara, 1981). The basal formulation and preparation of SANM(E) is identical to that of Synthetic Algal Nutrient Medium (Miller et al., 1978), except that nutrient stock solutions other than trace metal stocks are passed through columns of Chelex-100 resin to remove divalent metal contaminants prior to trace metal stock additions (Davey et al., 1970). Trace element speciation in SANM(E) is dominated by complexation with ethylenediaminetetraacetic acid (EDTA). Note that copper addition not only increased the computed copper free ion concentration, but competition for a fixed concentration of ligand (EDTA) sites also resulted in slight increases in free ion concentrations of the other metals. To attribute differences observed in organism response as a result of exposure to these media solely to an increase in total copper concentration may therefore

Table 4   Change in SANM(E) Trace Nutrient Speciation due to Copper Addition[a]

Nutrient	Basal SANM(E)		50 $\mu g/l$ Cu added	
	Concentration (nM)	Major species (%)	Concentration (nM)	Major species (%)
Metals				
Fe^{3+}	$(5.9 \times 10^2, 1 \times 10^{-10})$	Fe-EDTA (100)	$(5.9 \times 10^2, 4 \times 10^{-10})$	Fe-EDTA (97)
Mn^{2+}	$(2.1 \times 10^3, 7 \times 10^2)$	Mn-EDTA (66) Uncomplexed (34)	$(2.1 \times 10^3, 1 \times 10^3)$	Uncomplexed (62) Mn-EDTA (37)
Cu^{2+}	$(<2, <3 \times 10^{-5})$	Cu-EDTA (100)	$(7.9 \times 10^2, 2 \times 10^{-2})$	Cu-EDTA (100)
Zn^{2+}	$(2.4 \times 10^1, 4 \times 10^{-2})$	Zn-EDTA (100)	$(2.4 \times 10^1, 0.1)$	Zn-EDTA (99)
Co^{2+}	$(6.0, 2 \times 10^{-2})$	Co-EDTA (100)	$(6.0, 6 \times 10^{-2})$	Co-EDTA (99)
Ligands				
$B(OH)_4^-$	$(3.0 \times 10^3, 8 \times 10^1)$	$HB(OH)_4$ (98)	$(3.0 \times 10^3, 8 \times 10^1)$	$HB(OH)_4$ (98)
MoO_4^{2-}	$(3.0 \times 10^5, 3 \times 10^5)$	Uncomplexed (100)	$(3.0 \times 10^1, 3 \times 10^1)$	Uncomplexed (100)

[a]Concentrations are given in the following format: (total concentration, computed free-ion concentration) (Kuwabara, 1981).

be an oversimplification. Computed estimates of this type are obviously only as precise as the thermodynamic data used in the computations and the techniques by which concentrations of media constituents are defined or controlled.

Adaptation of acutely lethal concentration data according to measured water hardness has been proposed, using the mathematical expression

$$C = \exp \{a [\ln (\text{hardness})] + b\}$$

or

$$\ln C = a \ln (\text{hardness}) + b$$

where a and b are constants determined by linear regression of ln (hardness) against the natural logarithm of the median acutely lethal concentration C (U.S. EPA, 1980c). Water hardness was selected as the dependent variable in the expression above because "while there are many such [physical-chemical] factors which may alter [zinc] toxicity, the only factor for which the effect is well documented is hardness." Although this qualifying statement was made with regard to zinc toxicity, serious limitations to this approach also exist for other trace metals.

Toxicity tests involving batch (static) cultures are widely used in toxicological research because they have the following advantages (Oswald and Gaonkar, 1969; Miller et al., 1978):

1 Smaller laboratory space requirements relative to continuous-flow systems. Each experimental replicate merely requires space for a culturing flask.
2 Fewer equipment requirements relative to continuous-flow systems reduce maintenance time and costs.
3 Lower volume requirements for growth media. This is a labor-intensive phase of trace element research when chemically defined media are employed (Morel et al., 1979; Kuwabara and North, 1980; Anderson et al., 1978).

Continuous-flow (flow-through) toxicity tests, however, provide chemical parameter consistency not achievable in static cultures (Fencl, 1966). A continuous-flow system (chemostat) not subject to buildup of metabolites and depletion of toxicants clearly represents a more appropriate model of an open system in nature than does a static culture (Porcella, 1969; Davis, 1978). Flow-through cultures are especially important for larger test organisms, e.g., fish (Lorz and McPherson, 1976; Solbe, 1974; Sprague, 1964).

Isolating a single species for study greatly simplifies the test method because necessary measurements (e.g., survival percentages) usually increase markedly with the number of species under observation. However, species interactions are important and limit predictability when an attempt is made to directly apply results of single-species tests to the analysis of natural communities. Attempts (Medine et al., 1977; Tagatz et al., 1979; Cantelmo et al., 1979; Bowling et al., 1980; Leland and Carter, 1984a) have been made to quantify these interactions by using multispecies laboratory and field tests. Model streams (Harris, 1980; McIntire, 1966) have been used to examine toxic effects on benthic community structure while maintaining a higher degree of control over environmental parameters than is possible in the field. Leland and Carter (1984a; 1984b) examined community responses to continuous, long-term (months) copper exposure in natural stream channels. Menzel and Case (1977) investigated mercury effects on marine and estuarine plankton dynamics, using a 1700-m^3 polyethylene enclosure.

Water temperature and light intensity are factors that can limit the predictability of toxic responses by natural populations (Pirson et al., 1959; Heit and Fingermann, 1977; Trainor, 1978). The reader is directed to the earlier discussion of abiotic factors (see Chapter 6).

Finally, interpretation of toxicity data may be dependent on the manner in which experimental results are numerically analyzed. Various statistical algorithms have been created to estimate LC50 values from percent survival data (Finney, 1971; Hamilton et al., 1977). Statistical biases, if any, in the selected algorithm should certainly be understood. Statistical methods applied in aquatic toxicology are discussed in Gelber et al. (Chapter 5).

There is a need for further research to quantify effects of factors discussed above on results of acute toxicity assays. Water quality criteria for trace metals can be most judiciously set if environmental factors that can alter the toxic response in the field are identified and it is possible to estimate quantitatively how these factors in combination affect responses of aquatic organisms.

CHRONIC TOXICITY

Fish

The embryonic and larval stages of aquatic animals are generally the most sensitive stages of the life cycle to heavy metals and other toxicants. Consequently, toxicity tests with early life stages have been recommended for estimating maximum acceptable toxicant concentrations (MATCs) and obtaining data for the establishment of water quality criteria (see Chapter 3). In 56 life cycle toxicity tests performed with 34 organic and inorganic chemicals and four fish species, embryo-larval and early juvenile stages were the most, or among the most, sensitive life stages (McKim, 1977). Sac fry and early juveniles of eight freshwater fish were more sensitive than embryos to continuous exposures to copper (McKim et al., 1978) or cadmium (Eaton et al., 1978). In a study of the effects of zinc on developmental stages of the minnow (*Phoxinus phoxinus*), mortality of newly hatched fry was a more sensitive test than measures such as number of deposited eggs, hatching percentage, and mortality of under-yearlings, yearlings, and mature minnows (Bengtsson, 1974). Spehar (1976) examined toxicity and accumulation of cadmium and zinc in the flagfish, *Jordanella floridae*. In chronic tests, spawning and hatching success were the most sensitive indicators of cadmium toxicity, being inhibited at 8.1 μg/l Cd; survival of fry and growth of adults were the most sensitive indicators of zinc toxicity, being reduced

at 85 and 51 μg/l Zn, respectively. Ward and Parrish (1980) examined hatching success, juvenile mortality, and juvenile growth of the saltwater sheepshead minnow, *Cyprinodon variegatus,* to estimate specific application factors (the ratio of chronic to acute toxicity) for 18 organic chemicals. Comparisons of effect concentrations showed that juvenile mortality is a more sensitive indicator of toxicity than is hatching success of embryos. Growth of sheepshead minnows during early life stages was not a statistically sensitive indicator of toxicant effect for 16 of 18 compounds tested. These results all indicate the value of toxicity tests on tolerances of embryos, larvae, or early juveniles of sensitive resident species in estimating maximum acceptable concentrations for fish.

Developing fish embryos are particularly sensitive to heavy metals during early embryogenesis (Weis and Weis, 1977; Sabodash, 1977). Permeability of the egg decreases and the chorion hardens during the first few hours after release, allowing the egg to become more resistant with time (Lee and Gerking, 1980). Onset of mortality of embryos continuously exposed from the time of fertilization is therefore frequently observed to precede egg hardening. When *Fundulus heteroclitus* embryos were exposed to 0.03 mg/l Hg at the early blastula stage, the percentage of successful axis formation was reduced and a significant proportion of the embryos developed cyclopia (Weis and Weis, 1977). The severity of these effects was less if embryos were exposed at the late blastula stage. Embryos that developed in 1 mg/l Pb were normal in appearance until hatching, but then were unable to uncurl from the position they had in the chorion. Growth of surviving embryos may also be adversely affected. Pacific herring, *Clupea harengus pallisi,* exposed to copper before hardening grew significantly more slowly than larvae hatched from eggs exposed during later developmental stages (Rice and Harrison, 1978).

Comparison of the sensitivities to a given toxicant of early life cycle stages is complicated by several factors. (1) Embryonic impairments may contribute to the high sensitivity of postembryonic stages; this is supported by high incidences of teratogenesis in embryos exposed to copper (Birge and Black, 1979) and mercury (McKim et al., 1976). (2) Because egg yolk accumulates significant concentrations of test toxicants (McKim et al., 1976; Holcombe et al., 1976), individuals exposed during embryonic development may receive increased exposure during final resorption and assimilation of the principal yolk mass. McKim et al. (1976) found that mercury was transferred to embryos from brook trout, *Salvelinus fontinalis,* exposed during maturation to methyl mercury. Eggs of brook trout exposed during maturation to lead also contained elevated lead residues (Holcombe et al., 1976). Newly hatched alevins had negligible lead residues, however, indicating that most of the lead was contained in the egg membrane and not in the embryo. (3) The quality of the test water may also differentially affect metal toxicity to different developmental stages (Birge et al., 1979).

Hodson et al. (1979) summarized published data on effects of prolonged exposure to copper on fish growth and reproduction, the primary determinants of production. Spawning, growth, and long-term survival of the freshwater species tested were apparently affected at total copper concentrations between 5 and 40 µg/l in waters low in organic complexing matter. Lett et al. (1976) studied the effects of copper on appetite, growth, and proximate body composition of the rainbow trout, *Salmo gairdneri.* The initial copper effect was a cessation of feeding, with a gradual return to control levels. The higher the copper concentration, the slower the return of appetite. Growth rates were depressed by copper but recovered with appetite to approach those of control fish after 40 d. Assimilation efficiency was unchanged, indicating that depressed growth represented a response to appetite suppression rather than a decreased ability to digest. Waiwood and Beamish (1978) also found growth to be suppressed by copper when appetite was normal, because of a lower gross conversion efficiency of copper-exposed fish. The reduced growth rate of

copper-exposed rainbow trout may be attributed to an increased maintenance energy requirement and decreased efficiency of energy utilization.

A cessation of feeding, with a gradual return (within 10–20 d) to control levels, was also observed for juvenile salmon, *Salmo salar,* exposed to zinc (Farmer et al., 1979). After 45 d of exposure, food intake was greater than that of controls. Growth rates of salmon exposed to zinc (maximum concentrations ≤21-d LC50) and offered rations of 2.0–3.5% of the body weight per day were not reduced during a 3-mo period. The response of salmon was to increase food intake and decrease caloric content.

Invertebrates

In general, each successive developmental stage of bivalve mollusks is more resistant than the former stage to trace metals (Cunningham, 1972; Thurberg et al., 1975). The period of larval settlement is a critical point in the life cycle, however, since retardation in larval growth can prolong the pelagic stage, thereby increasing the chance of larval loss through predation, disease, and dispersion (Calabrese and Nelson, 1974).

Interspecific comparisons of the 48-h EC50 (estimated concentration resulting in failure of 50% of the test population to develop normally to the straight-hinge larval stage) responses of embryos of *Crassostrea virginica* and *Mercenaria mercenaria* showed that embryos of *C. virginica* were more sensitive to silver and lead, equally sensitive to mercury, and less sensitive to zinc and nickel than embryos of *M. mercenaria* (Calabrese et al., 1973; Calabrese and Nelson, 1974). Embryos of both species exhibited sensitivity to trace metals in the order Hg > Ag > Zn > Ni > Pb. Calabrese et al. (1977) measured growth of larvae of the same species exposed to EC50 concentrations of trace metals. For *M. mercenaria,* EC50 concentrations of mercury (0.015 mg/l), silver (0.032 mg/l), copper (0.016 mg/l), nickel (5.7 mg/l), and zinc (0.195 mg/l) retarded shell growth to 69, 66, 52, 0, and 62% of control growth, respectively. Nickel was the least toxic metal tested, yet at EC50 concentrations it had the greatest inhibitory effect on growth. Each of these metals also retarded shell growth of *C. virginica*. Growth rates of 48-h veligers of *Crassostrea gigas* were reduced at 0.05 mg/l Zn in an estuary contaminated with metal-rich mine water, although development was normal (Brereton et al., 1973). Practically no umbo development occurred at 0.15 mg/l Zn and veligers were abnormal. Boyden et al. (1975) reported increased larval mortality of *C. gigas* with increasing zinc concentrations and a decline in the percentage of larvae that settle as spat after a 5-d exposure.

Although EC50s (Nelson et al., 1976) and oxygen consumption (Thurberg et al., 1975) are common criteria for determining toxicity of metals to spat and juveniles of bivalve mollusks, shell growth rate is more frequently used (Cunningham, 1976). Retardation of *C. gigas* spat shell growth to 78 and 51% of controls at 0.25 and 0.50 mg/l Zn, respectively, was reported by Boyden et al. (1975). Shell growth of juvenile *C. virginica* exposed to 0.01 and 0.10 mg/l Hg for 47 d was reduced to 67 and 23% of controls (Cunningham, 1976). The inhibitory effect of zinc and mercury on shell growth was found to be reversible after juveniles were returned to ambient seawater.

Stage of development is also a critical factor to consider in the sensitivity of crustaceans to trace metals. Vernberg et al. (1974) examined the effects of inorganic mercury over a range of temperature and salinity conditions with larval and adult fiddler crabs, *Uca pugilator*. Zoeal stages I, III, and V and megalopal stages were tested; characteristics measured were survival, oxygen consumption, and swimming activity. Larval crabs were several orders of magnitude more sensitive to mercury than were postlarval stages. Respiratory rates of larvae reared to the first zoeal stage in 1.8 μg/l Hg (optimal salinity and temperature) were significantly depressed (Vernberg et al., 1973), but this concentration did not depress oxygen consumption of crabs reared to the third zoeal stage.

Sensitivities of estuarine crustaceans to trace metals can be substantially altered by salinity or temperature interactions. McKenney and Neff (1979) found the rate of larval development of the grass shrimp, *Palaemonetes pugio*, to be progressively reduced by increasing zinc concentrations from 0.25 to 1.0 mg/l. The salinity-temperature conditions allowing for maximal developmental rates were greatly restricted by exposure to sublethal concentrations of zinc. Similarly, at salinities and temperatures outside the optimal range for maximal development, exposure to zinc further prolonged the period for successful completion of metamorphosis above that observed for nonoptimal salinities and temperatures. Both zoeal and megalopal developmental rates of *Rhithropanopeus harrisii* were retarded by mercury at low temperatures, whereas only megalopal rates were reduced by mercury at high salinities (McKenney and Costlow, 1977). Epifanio (1971) suggested that a delay in metamorphosis may represent a generalized response of decapod crustaceans to environmental stress.

Depressed scope-for-growth measurements appear to be particularly useful indicators of toxicant stress in crustaceans and bivalve mollusks (Bayne et al., 1976, 1978; Gilfillan, 1980). Scope for growth is an experimentally derived estimate of the instantaneous growth rate in animals for which ingestion, assimilation, and respiration rates can be experimentally determined. The product of ingestion rate and assimilation ratio is the rate of assimilation of food. When respiration rate is subtracted (in appropriate units) from assimilation rate, the scope for growth is obtained. When scope-for-growth values are positive, the animal has energy available for growth and reproduction; when they are negative, the animal is losing energy. Gilfillan (1980) observed quantitative dose-response relationships between tissue burdens of aromatic hydrocarbons and scope for growth in *Mya arenaria*. Periodic measurements of scope for growth for two or more populations of the clam allowed prediction of the relative growth rates of the populations. Bayne et al. (1976; 1978) found that scope for growth was correlated with other measures of stress and with fecundity and survival of eggs and larvae of *Mytilus edulis*. Few studies appear to have been conducted on the effects of toxicants on scope for growth in invertebrates other than crustaceans and bivalve mollusks (Bayne et al., 1980).

SUBLETHAL EFFECTS

General Effects of Specific Metals

Zinc

Zinc is a ubiquitous trace metal essential for normal cell differentiation and growth in both plants and animals. It is essential because it is an integral part of a number of metalloenzymes and a cofactor for regulating the activity of specific zinc-dependent enzymes. The concentration of zinc in cells can govern many metabolic processes—specifically carbohydrate, fat, and protein metabolism and nucleic acid synthesis or degradation—through initiation and/or regulation of the activity of these enzymes. The decrease in activity of a particular enzyme in response to deficient zinc nutrition depends on the tightness of binding of zinc to the protein or the speed of its exchange with ligands.

Some zinc-dependent enzymes contain metal-binding sites that are essential for structural stability; examples are alkaline phosphatase and carbonic anhydrase. Under controlled experimental conditions, the activity of alkaline phosphatase is a good indicator of zinc supply. Under field conditions, however, the activity of alkaline phosphatase is subject to large individual variation (Kirchgessner and Roth, 1980; Wolfe, 1970) so that it has limited value as a measure of zinc supply in nature. Zinc is an essential constituent of the DNA-dependent DNA and RNA polymerases. These transcription enzymes have a key position in nucleic acid metabolism and hence also in protein biosynthesis.

Anemia is a common symptom of sublethal zinc intoxication in mammals and results from induced copper and, in some cases, iron deficiencies brought about by interference with absorption and utilization of these elements (Underwood, 1977). The levels of dietary zinc at which toxic effects are evident depend markedly on the concentration ratio of zinc to copper. Exposure to aqueous zinc at 0.5 to 1.2 mg/l for 24 h significantly depressed mean white blood cell-thrombocyte counts in salmon (McLeay, 1975). Decreases were proportional to zinc concentration. However, erythrocyte counts remained unchanged. Prolonged exposure of rainbow trout fry to sublethal concentrations of zinc caused extensive edema and necrosis of liver tissue (Leland, 1983).

Zinc is a metabolic antagonist of cadmium, so that high zinc intakes in animals afford some protection against the potentially toxic effects of cadmium exposure (Underwood, 1977).

Copper

Copper is an essential component of many enzymes. However, not all of these enzyme activities are so decreased in copper deficiency that they are metabolically limiting. Poor growth and loss of weight due to copper deficiency in terrestrial animals are most often related to loss of cytochrome oxidase activity, as evidenced by a depression of succinooxidase activity. The succinooxidase system has a higher oxygen consumption rate than any other mitochondrial dehydrogenase system and thus requires more cytochrome oxidase (Gallagher, 1979).

Animals have some ability to cope with stresses on trace metal (including copper) balance. Nyberg (1974) isolated wild stock of *Paramecium aurelia* that were resistant to copper due to a mutational adaptation in this inbreeding species. In general, more outbreeding ciliate species have greater resistance to stress (Nyberg, 1974). Many higher organisms have specific cellular mechanisms that conserve copper when it is deficient and excrete it if an excess amount enters the body (Gallagher, 1979; Bryan, 1976). If periods of deficiency or excess are not long-lasting, mechanisms that regulate copper balance may successfully prevent the occurrence of severe abnormalities. In all animals studied, continued ingestion of copper in excess of nutritional requirements led to some accumulation in tissues, especially liver. The capacity for hepatic copper storage varies greatly among species, and differences among species in tolerance to high copper intakes are also great.

Chronic administration of copper to mammals forces deposition of the metal in the liver, kidney, and other organs. Copper accumulates when the excretory capacity of liver cells is exceeded (Luckey and Venugopal, 1977). Fractionation of liver homogenates and morphological studies of copper-exposed animals showed (1) an increase in hepatic copper concentration; (2) a change in the subcellular distribution of copper with an increase in the proportion in mitochondria and lysosomes and a marked decrease in the proportion in cytosol of hepatocytes; and (3) increased numbers and prominence of copper-

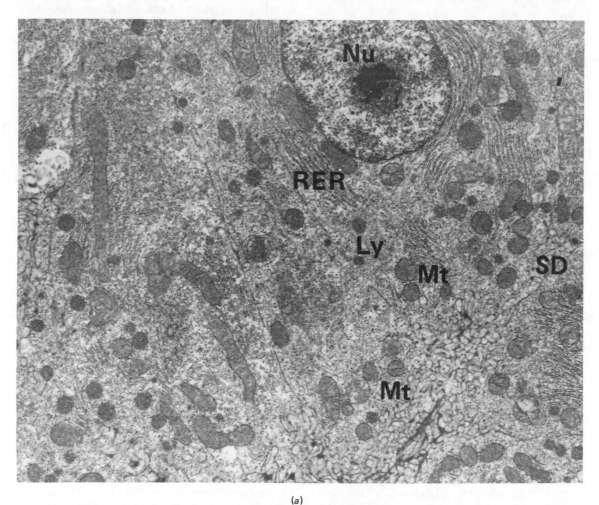

(a)

Figure 1 (a) Electron micrograph of typical juvenile rainbow trout hepatocytes adjacent to a sinusoid. Mitochondria (Mt) basally in the hepatocytes tend to "ring" the space of Disse (SD). One cell displays a nucleolus (Nu). Mitochondria are round to oval or rod-shaped. Few lysosomes (Ly) are present. Rough endoplasmic reticulum (RER) is present in moderate amounts and divided between random and parallel arrays. Smooth endoplasmic reticulum is rare. ×7,200.

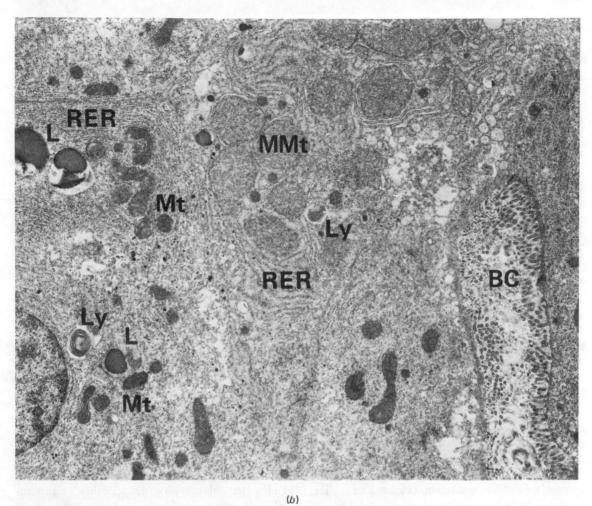

(b)

Figure 1 (*Continued*) (*b*) Electron micrograph of hepatocytes of juvenile rainbow trout exposed to 17 µg/l Cu from hatch to approximately 1 mo after initiation of feeding. Many hepatocytes contain membrane-bound lipid droplets (*L*). Lysosomes are more abundant and complex than in controls. Mitochondria are generally dense. A few cells contain megamitochondria (*MMt*), which are less electron-dense, rounded, and have angular and irregular cristae. Rough endoplasmic reticulum shows increased vesiculation. BC, bile canaliculi. X7,200.

containing lysosomes (Luckey and Venugopal, 1977; Bremner, 1979).

Ultrastructural studies of the liver of juvenile rainbow trout, *Salmo gairdneri,* during development of copper toxicosis provided information on changes that occur as copper accumulates in liver (Leland, 1983). There were increases in the num-

ber of lysosomes and increased vesiculation of the endoplasmic reticulum in hepatocytes (Fig. 1). Also observed were swelling and contraction of mitochondria and increased numbers of multilaminar and globular inclusions, intranuclear granules, and number of lipid droplets. At advanced stages of copper toxicosis, interruptions of the plasma membrane and degeneration of mitochondria occurred and an increasing number of necrotic cells appeared around the portal tracts.

Lead

Sublethal lead poisoning in vertebrates is characterized by neurological defects, kidney dysfunction, and anemia. Nervous system and renal effects are usually recognizable only during the phase of overt lead toxicity. Lead blocks both impulse transmission and acetylcholine release (Kostial and Voak, 1957). Anemia results from two basic defects: shortened erythrocyte life span and impairment of heme synthesis. Cells of the proximal renal tubule are the most severely affected renal tissue in mammals (Goyer et al., 1968). Dysfunction of these cells was manifested by impaired reabsorption of glucose, amino acids, and phosphate. Mitochondria in proximal renal tubular lining of experimental animals with lead poisoning showed swelling and dilation of matrical granules, probably secondary to increased membrane permeability. Such changes are similar to the nonspecific swelling that occurs in early stages in other forms of cellular injury.

Several enzymes are sensitive to lead at very low concentrations. Lead strongly inhibits several ATPases and lipoamide dehydrogenase, an enzyme crucial to cellular oxidation (Ulmer and Vallee, 1969). Lead appears to be a specific inhibitor of aminolevulinic acid dehydratase, which is involved in the biosynthesis of heme.

Significant increases in tissue lead storage can occur when diets contain less than the animal's physiological requirement for calcium. Six and Goyer (1970) showed that decreased dietary calcium intake in mammals produced a redistribution of lead from storage in bone to tissues such as kidney. This may be due to a smaller total binding capacity of bone for lead in animals fed a low-calcium diet.

Mercury

The primary effect of mercury on cells appears to be binding with sulfhydryl groups on surface membrane proteins (Luckey and Venugopal, 1977). Mercury has an extremely high affinity for sulfhydryl groups. As virtually all proteins have sulfhydryl groups and their conformations are dependent on these functional groups, at some concentration mercury can inhibit the function of virtually any enzyme. The important lesion for mercury toxicity in plants and animals appears to involve cell membranes and affect membrane permeability. One important effect is that sodium leaks in and potassium leaks out, with subsequent volume shifts in the cell.

Early subacute mercury poisoning in mammals generally has a neurological manifestation. Toxicity to methyl mercury is first evident through its action on the peripheral nervous system (Chang and Hartmann, 1972). Ingestion of inorganic mercury salts affected liver and kidney tissues of all animals studied and may also have caused proteinuria and necrosis of the intestinal tract (Underwood, 1977). Trump et al. (1975) observed selective necrosis of the nephron of hogchokers, *Trimectes maculatus,* injected with 16 mg/kg $HgCl_2$. The second segment, and perhaps the first, of the proximal tubules was affected, but the collecting tubules were unaltered. These results imply selective concentration of mercury in certain segments of the nephron.

Physicochemical properties—for example, lipid and water solubility or dissociability of mercurials—are important factors in tissue distributions of mercury. However, these properties may be modified during metabolism. In mammals, mercurials appear to be metabolized primarily in a manner that decreases lipid solubility and increases water solubility ($Hg^{\circ} \rightarrow Hg^{2+}$; $RHg^{+} \rightarrow R + Hg^{2+}$, where R is an alkyl or aryl moiety). The subcellular distribution is also related to the physicochemical properties of mercurials. In rat liver, after inorganic mercury injection, mercury is found principally in lysosomes. After methyl mercury injection, methyl mercury is principally associated with microsomes, and the lysosomal content of mercury is mainly inorganic (Norseth, 1969; Magos, 1973). Comparable studies have not been conducted on physicochemical factors influencing tissue distributions of mercury in aquatic organisms.

Respiration, Osmoregulation, Neurotransmission

Toxic agents damage respiratory membranes of aquatic animals in superficially similar ways, but future studies should demonstrate reactions diagnostic of some toxicants, possibly related to their specific modes of action. Investigations by Carpenter (1927, 1930) and Ellis (1937) of the toxicity of trace metal salts to fish led to the "coagulation film anoxia" hypothesis, in which acute toxicity was attributed to asphyxiations brought on by metal ions reacting with some constituent of the mucus secreted by gills. Before death, fish were covered with a film much like coagulated mucus; within the operculum, gills were covered by a thicker film of an apparently similar nature. Ellis (1937) described acute toxicity as a three-step process: (1) the spaces between the gill filaments fill with precipitate, so that water flowing through the branchial chambers cannot reach the gill epithelial cells; (2) the spaces between the gill lamellae become filled, so that movement of the gill filaments is impossible and blood circulation in the gill capillaries is inhibited; and (3) this stasis affecting blood circulation in the gills leads to heart block, with heart beat dropping to about half the normal rate. This hypothesis was subsequently supported by other investigators (Westfall, 1945; Schweiger, 1957). Lloyd (1960), however, observed no precipitation on the gills of rainbow trout that succumbed to zinc sulfate exposure and postulated that acute metal toxicity may be attributable instead to necrosis of gill tissues. Subsequent histological studies of fish exposed to trace metals have supported this conclusion.

Skidmore and Tovell (1972) reported that gill tissue deterioration caused by exposure of rainbow trout to zinc sulfate included swelling of epithelial cells, adhesion of secondary lamellae, detachment of epithelium from the pillar cell system, discharge of mucous cells, and hematomas (Fig. 2). Similar responses were observed in gill tissues of rainbow trout exposed to the anionic detergent sodium lauryl sulfate (Abel and Skidmore, 1975). The reaction to zinc sulfate is primarily an inflammatory response, with chloride cells becoming detached in a characteristic manner and pillar cells becoming vacuolated. The latter traits are not evident in trout exposed to sodium lauryl sulfate. Inflammation has not been reported in all studies of gill damage, possibly because it does not occur at all acutely toxic concentrations of toxicants.

With both zinc sulfate and detergent poisoning of rainbow trout, the size of cells in subepithelial spaces remains unchanged, indicating that an osmotically normal internal environment is maintained. Patterns of lamellar hematomas after exposure to these toxicants indicate that the integrity of the outer epithelial layers is upheld even in the final stages of poisoning and that the resistance of the pillar cell system relative to that of the epithelium may not be great. Morgan and Tovell (1973) suggested that epithelial lifting between the secondary lamellae may exert a protective effect, hindering toxicant uptake by increasing diffusion distance. Clearly, this response would occur at the expense of respiratory efficiency and would be a handicap in later stages of acute poisoning, especially when asphyxia is the immediate cause of death. Barton et al. (1972) demonstrated that lactic acid, a product of anaerobic glycolysis, is increased in zinc-poisoned fish just before death. Lactic acid production and glycogen utilization in white muscle of rainbow trout increase with time of exposure to a lethal concentration of zinc (Hodson, 1976a).

At near-lethal copper concentrations, rainbow trout show increased coughing frequency, ventilation frequency, and amplitude of opercular and buccal respiratory pressure changes (Sellers et al., 1975). These changes are accompanied by little variation in arterial oxygen tension and indicate less of a respiratory response to copper than to zinc. Whereas zinc causes death through gill destruction and hypoxia, osmoregulatory failure is the more likely basis of acute copper toxicity (Lewis and Lewis, 1971; Lorz and McPherson, 1976). Exposure of fish to other trace metals also results in some loss of osmoregulatory capacity.

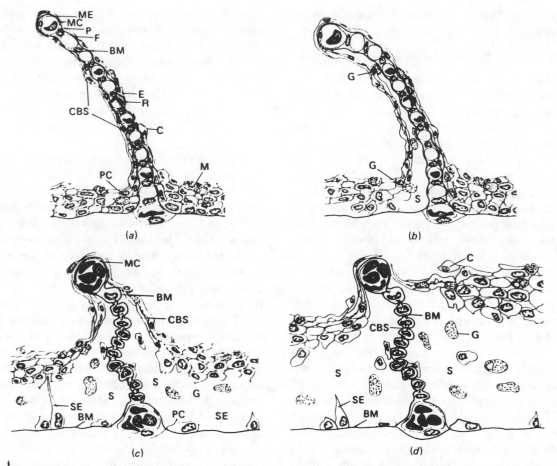

Figure 2 Diagrams of a secondary lamella in transverse section, showing four stages in the pathogenesis of zinc-induced cell damage. *[from Skidmore and Tovell (1972).]* (*a*) Control tissue before exposure to zinc. (*b*) After 60% of the estimated survival time. Shows separation of the epithelium on the concave side of the lamella, the maximum distance of the lamellar margin from the filament surface being reduced by 20%. (*c*) At overturn of the fish. Shows partial occlusion of central blood spaces, but proximal and marginal channels enlarged. Further separation of epithelium and enlargement of subepithelial space, which has now formed on both surfaces of the lamella. Lamellar height reduced by 50%, with gross curling of the pillar cell system. Epithelium still normally attached along marginal channels. (*d*) At immobilization of the opercula. Epithelium is elevated further following considerable enlargement of the subepithelial space. Central blood spaces completely occluded. Abbreviations: basement membrane, *BM*; chloride cell, *C*; central blood space, *CBS*; epithelial cell, *E*; pillar cell flange, *F*; granulocyte, *G*; mucous cell, *M*; marginal channel, *MC*; marginal endothelial cell, *ME*; pillar cell, *P*; proximal channel, *PC*; red blood cell, *R*; subepithelial space, *S*; stretched epithelial cell, *SE*.

Both inorganic mercury and methyl mercury inhibit branchial sodium uptake and renal sodium transport in the marine teleost *Fundulus heteroclitus* (Schmidt-Nielson, 1974), promoting a net increase in sodium efflux.

Abnormal values for several blood chemistry parameters, including transient declines in plasma chloride concentration, are characteristically observed in freshwater fish exposed to sublethal levels of copper (McKim et al., 1970; Christensen et al., 1972). Golden shiners, *Notemigonus cryso-leucas,* challenged by exposures to copper or zinc, exhibit transient but significant decreases in serum osmolarity (Lewis and Lewis, 1971); this effect can be eliminated by the addition of sodium chloride to test solutions. Decreases in plasma electrolyte levels of goldfish, *Carassius auratus,* exposed to cadmium tend to be coupled with increases in concentrations of tissue electrolytes, particularly sodium and chloride, the major extracellular electrolytes (McCarty and Houston, 1976). Increased water loads of freshwater fish exposed to trace metals may therefore be largely localized in extracellular phases.

Fish are capable of some degree of compensating for the initial effects of sublethal metal exposure. Transient increases in hematocrit, hemoglobin, and numbers of erythrocytes of brook trout (McKim et al., 1970) and brown bullheads (Christensen et al., 1972) disappear after approximately 3 wk during continuing exposure to copper, as do decreases in plasma chloride and osmolarity. The increased hematocrit, hemoglobin, and erythrocyte counts might be offset by hemodilution, as shown by reduced osmolarity.

A failure in osmoregulation, resulting from disruption of the transporting surface epithelium, may also be the primary lethal effect of copper in mollusks. Sullivan and Cheng (1975) found that epithelial cells of the rectal ridge of the freshwater snail *Biomphalaria glabrata* become greatly distended when exposed to lethal doses of copper. Cytopathologic features include a modified appearance of the epithelial surface, loss of digitiform projections from the bases of cells, disintegration of the underlying basal lamina and distended appearance of loose vascular connective tissue of the rectal ridge (Cheng, 1979). Gill epithelial cells of oysters, *Crassostrea virginica,* exposed to copper are swollen and rounded compared to controls, and mitochondria with rarified matrices occur (Engel and Fowler, 1979). The tissue is also edematous.

Lead-induced acute toxicity in fish may derive more from lead effects on central nervous system coordination of activity and metabolism than from direct effects of lead on the enzymes of intermediary metabolism (Somero et al., 1977). Oxygen consumption by isolated gill tissues of the marine teleost *Gillichthys mirabilis* (longjaw mudsucker) that contain extremely high concentrations of lead is not different between control and lead-exposed individuals, whereas whole-organism oxygen consumption is higher in lead-exposed individuals. Hyperactivity, erratic swimming, muscular spasms, and loss of equilibrium are all characteristic of fish poisoned by lead, indicating involvement of the nervous system (Holcombe et al., 1976). While the mode of action by which lead produces neurotoxicity remains unknown, it has been hypothesized that it involves interactions between lead and calcium at sites important in neurotransmission. Some recent mammalian studies support this hypothesis. Studies of the *in vitro* effects of lead on neuromuscular and ganglionic function show that lead-induced defects are reversible by added calcium and are potentiated by decreased calcium (Kostial and Voak, 1957). *In vitro* studies have also been done on the accumulation of tyrosine and choline, precursors of the neurotransmitters norepinephrine and acetylcholine. Increased lead and decreased calcium concentrations have similar effects on transport of these precursors into synaptosomal preparations (Silbergeld et al., 1975).

In summary, few investigators have considered modes of action of lethal concentrations of trace metals or attempted to correlate physiological and biochemical responses with whole-animal responses. Studies designed specifically to examine mechanisms of toxicity of copper and zinc to fish indicate that zinc causes death through gill necrosis and hypoxia but that osmoregulatory failure is the more likely basis of acute copper toxicity. Lead and mercury affect nervous system coordination of activity in fish and mercury contributes to some loss of osmoregulatory capacity, but the primary mechanisms of acute toxicity of these metals are unknown.

Sensory Membranes

Sensory membranes of aquatic animals are not shielded by external barriers or the internal complexing and detoxifying systems that protect internal tissues. As shown by electrophysiological experiments, sublethal concentrations of trace metals can block the function of chemoreceptors within a few seconds after exposure begins (Hidaka and Yokata, 1967; Hidaka, 1970). Surprisingly, information on cytopathological effects of trace metals on sensory tissue is quite limited. Gardner and LaRoche (1973) found that brief exposures (several hours) of the marine teleost *Fundulus heteroclitus* to 0.5 mg/l copper produced severe degenerative and hyperplastic changes in olfactory and lateral line tissues. Similar results were obtained for mercury and lead (Gardner, 1975). Cytopathological effects in sensory tissue were not observed in *F. heteroclitus* exposed to sublethal concentrations of zinc. Rates of accumulation of trace metals into olfactory epithelium of the goldfish, *Carassius auratus,* and resulting histological changes were determined by Vigayamadhavan and Iwai (1975). Rates of accumulation of trace metals into olfactory epithelium were found to decrease in the order Hg > Cu > Zn > Pb. Mercury damaged not only taste buds, but entire epithelial layers within 30 min. Lead affected mucous cells more than it did taste buds. The extent of degenerative changes in olfactory tissue varied with the metal concentration and duration of exposure.

The sensitivity of sensory receptors to trace metals has been exploited in the development of laboratory avoidance tests. Avoidance thresholds of 2 µg/l Cu and 54 µg/l Zn were reported for Atlantic salmon (Sprague et al., 1965). These concentrations are less than one-tenth of the incipient lethal concentrations. Avoidance of sublethal levels of zinc by fish in laboratory studies was also reported by Ishio (1965), Sprague (1968), and Syazuki (1964). Avoidance thresholds ranged from 0.01 to 0.45 toxic unit (fraction of the incipient lethal concentration) in these studies. Depending on the steepness of the gradient and the availabil-

ity of other sensory cues, goldfish either avoided or were attracted to sublethal levels of copper (Kleerekoper et al., 1972; Westlake et al., 1974). Sutterlin (1974) has reviewed the literature on the possible types of interactions between pollutants and chemosensory organs. Responses to several major classes of pollutants were considered and caution was recommended in extending information from laboratory avoidance tests to field conditions, where there are other variables such as gradient steepness as well as other motivational factors.

Hematology

Pathological effects are frequently evident in hematopoietic tissues of animals after prolonged trace metal exposure. Anemia is an early manifestation of acute or chronic lead intoxication in vertebrates and is nearly always present when other symptoms of lead toxicity occur. The anemia results from two basic defects: shortened erythrocyte life span and impairment of heme synthesis. The activity of δ-aminolevulinic acid dehydratase (ALAD), an enzyme involved in the biosynthesis of heme, appears to be specifically inhibited by lead; hence, measurement of ALAD activity can serve as an indicator of the toxic effects of lead absorption. Total aqueous lead concentrations as low as 13 µg/l caused a significant inhibition of ALAD activity in rainbow trout blood (Hodson, 1976b), and it was proposed that assay of this enzyme's activity be used to diagnose lead intoxication in fish. Fish exposed to 300 µg/l Pb also showed an anemic response and basophilic stippling of erythrocytes (Johansson-Sjöbeck and Larsson, 1979). This lead exposure does not alter significantly the composition or number of white blood cells. Absence of erythrocyte ALAD inhibition in fish exposed to cadmium, copper, mercury, and zinc indicates that this enzyme is quite specific for lead (Johansson-Sjöbeck and Larsson, 1979; Hodson et al., 1977). Lead poisoning also results in accumulation of excess protoporphyrin. Spectrofluorometric determination of zinc protoporphyrin in blood is now widely used clinically to detect lead poisoning in humans (Joselow and Flores, 1977). Its applicability in aquatic toxicology has not been tested.

Lead exposure results in rapid loss of potassium from erythrocytes, leaving a shrunken cell with a decreased capacity for survival. The integrity of the cell membrane is related to the cationic transport system of membrane $Na^+ + K^+$-ATPase. Unlike δ-aminolevulinic acid dehydratase, which has no residual function in the mature erythrocyte, $Na^+ + K^+$-ATPase is considered a critical determinant of cation permeability of the cell and of erythrocyte survival. Angle et al. (1975) found a linear depression of erythrocyte membrane $Na^+ + K^+$-ATPase with increasing blood lead level in children. Inhibition of $Na^+ + K^+$-ATPase activity in hematopoietic tissue of fish following *in vivo* exposure has also been observed for cadmium and mercury (Kuhnert et al., 1976; Natochin et al., 1975).

Development of hemolytic anemia in copper poisoning in mammals is preceded by a reduction in blood glutathione concentration to nearly zero and by an increase in methemoglobin concentration (Bremner, 1979), indicating that marked oxidative changes occur in the erythrocyte. Concentrations of these constituents have apparently not been measured in fish exposed to copper, but many other hematological responses have been observed. After 6 d of exposure to 50 μg/l Cu, blood glucose concentrations of brown bullheads, *Ictalurus nebulosus*, were 2–8 times control levels and the elevated concentrations persisted for at least 30 d (Christensen et al., 1972). No change was seen at 600 d, indicating long-term adaptation to copper. Hematocrit and hemoglobin values were also elevated at 6 and 30 d, but the total red blood cell count was constant; this indicated an increase in average cell size due to either cellular swelling or mortality of small immature cells and replacement by larger cells from the spleen.

The underlying mechanism of copper-induced hemolysis is not clearly established. Metz and Sagone (1972) postulated that the injury to red blood cells stems primarily from accelerated oxidation of glutathione, with resulting oxidative injury to hemoglobin and the cell membrane. When copper accumulates in mammalian tissue, a significant rise in serum transaminases and lactic dehydrogenase (LDH) occurs. Determination of serum glutamic-oxaloacetic transaminase (GOT) levels has therefore been proposed as an aid in detection of chronic copper poisoning. Christensen et al. (1972) observed that plasma LDH levels in brown bullheads were unaffected by copper exposure, whereas plasma GOT was reduced at copper concentrations above 27 μg/l after a 600-d exposure. Increased levels of plasma GOT usually indicate liver damage and release of the enzyme into the blood. Therefore, the observed decreased activity of GOT may represent direct inhibition of the enzyme by copper in fish. Hemolytic crises in mammals are also accompanied by extensive focal necrosis of liver tissue, neutrophilia, and high blood urea levels.

Significant changes in plasma protein levels, plasma osmolality, hematocrit, hemoglobin, and mean corpuscular hemoglobin were detected in the blood of winter flounder, *Pseudopleuronectes americanus*, exposed to mercuric chloride (10 μg/l Hg) for 60 d (Calabrese et al., 1975). Mercury concentrations in the blood of exposed flounder were also much higher than in control fish (mean of 3.8 versus <0.04 μg/g Hg). Factors regulating partitioning of mercurial compounds between blood cells and plasma appear to be the permeability of erythrocytes to the compound and the number of binding sites in intracellular and extracellular components of blood. Rothstein (1973) showed that the permeability of erythrocytes is inversely related to the degree of mercurial dissociation. Short-chain alkyl mercury compounds rapidly penetrate the red cell membranes and bind to hemoglobin. Binding of methyl mercury to intracellular hemoglobin is reversible by extracellular sulfhydryl groups (Giblin and Massaro, 1973). Gel filtration chromatography of soluble liver proteins of rainbow trout yielded identical elution profiles for methyl mercury administered as the free salt and bound in erythrocytes (Massaro, 1974).

There have been few studies of the effects of elevated trace metal concentrations on circulatory fluids of invertebrates. Ruddell and Rains (1975) related environmental copper and zinc concentrations to basophil levels of oyster, *Crassostrea gigas* and *C. virginica,* and some limited monitoring has been undertaken on serum ion composition of ocean scallops, *Placopecten magellanicus* (Thurberg et al., 1978). Considerable additional research is needed before generalizations about effects of trace metals on invertebrate circulatory fluids can be made.

Accumulation

The mechanisms of accumulation and storage of trace metals in aquatic animals are diverse, varying with chemical form of the metal, mode of uptake, and animal species (Luoma, 1983). Concentrations of the uncomplexed metal ion are closely correlated with toxicity, and thus uptake, of solutions of cadmium, copper, and zinc in crustaceans (Andrew et al., 1977; Sunda et al., 1978) and fish (Pagenkopf et al., 1974; Zitko et al., 1973). Penetration of epithelial membranes by uncomplexed metal ions appears to involve special transport associated with a carrier molecule. Such a mechanism is necessary for toxicants that lack sufficient lipid solubility to move rapidly through cell membranes.

Certain metal complexes may also be directly available. Over the range of pH and alkalinity conditions expected in natural waters, copper toxicity to animals has been related to Cu^{2+} and $CuOH^+$, but not $Cu(CO_3)^{\circ}$ or $Cu(OH)_2^{\circ}$ (Andrew et al., 1977; Howarth and Sprague, 1978). Complexing ligands, such as hydroxyl and carbonate ions, play a dominant role in regulating speciation, and separation of the effects of different copper species is difficult (Magnuson et al., 1979). Correlations between observed toxicity to fish and concentrations of Zn^{2+} and $ZnOH^+$ are not as strong as those observed for Cu^{2+} and $CuOH^+$ (Pagenkopf, 1980). Complexation of trace metals with natural humic and fulvic substances generally effects a reduction in toxicity. However, in some circumstances, complexation with natural organic compounds may enhance uptake rates (Giesy et al., 1977).

Ingested food may also be a significant source of metals assimilated by aquatic organisms. Pentreath (1976a,b) compared tissue distributions of mercury in plaice, *Pseudopleuronectes platessa,* exposed to inorganic mercury and methyl mercury in food and in solution. Only individuals exposed to methyl mercury in food had tissue distributions similar to those observed in nature. Bryan and Uysal (1978) concluded from tissue distribution data that food is the primary source of cadmium, cobalt, lead, and zinc, but possibly not silver and copper, in the burrowing clam, *Scrobicularia plana.*

Absorption of dietary copper and zinc in higher animals appears to be regulated in part by metal thioneins, low molecular weight proteins containing high levels of cysteine. These metal-binding proteins may regulate the form of metal that passes from mucosal cells into the circulatory fluid. Fluctuations in the zinc content of intestinal cells of vertebrates (Cousins and Failla, 1980) and mussels (Talbot and Magee, 1978) can be largely accounted for by metallothionein. Synthesis of metallothionein apparently provides the intestinal cell with an additional pool of binding sites with which to alter the net flux of zinc ions. Depending on the physiological status of the animals, zinc may equilibrate with metalloproteins and metallothionein, be absorbed into the plasma, or be secreted (Evans and Johnson, 1978). All of these transitions ensure an adequate supply of zinc to the plasma carrier for transport to the tissues.

Several ligands are involved in the metabolism and transport of copper (Evans, 1973). Within hepatic cells of vertebrates, copper initially bound to a copper-binding protein eventually appears in ceruloplasmin, copper-dependent enzymes, and bile (Terao and Owen, 1973). Ceruloplasmin has several important functions. It mobilizes iron into the plasma from iron storage cells in the liver, and it is a vehicle for copper transport, comparable to transferrin. Copper initially secreted into the bile is apparently bound to amino acids and/or bile acids.

Metal concentrations of selected tissues of brook trout, *Salvelinus fontinalis,* exposed to high but sublethal solutions of lead and methyl mercury (Fig. 3) illustrate the variability in tissue distribution of metals that occurs when animals are exposed to toxicants of substantially different polarities and lipid solubilities. Metal concentrations in gill, liver, kidney, muscle, spleen, gonads, and erythrocytes were sampled periodically during 38-wk exposures. Residues of lead in gill, liver, and kidney tissues reached a steady-state concentration after 20-wk exposure to 235 µg/l Pb, but did not reach a steady state at lower exposure concentrations (34 and 119 µg/l Pb) (Holcombe et al., 1976). Muscle tissue did not accumulate lead to

any substantial degree at these exposure concentrations. Erythrocytes accumulated lead in direct proportion to the solution concentration of lead during the first 9 wk of exposure. Dissipation of lead from tissues of exposed brook trout transferred to uncontaminated water showed that lead excretion occurred. After 2 wk, residues were lower in gill and kidney but higher in liver. After 12 wk, lead levels were significantly lower in all three tissues.

Blood, spleen, and kidney of brook trout accumulated methyl mercury more rapidly than did other tissues and contained the highest mercury concentrations (Fig. 3). Other tissues, in order of decreasing mercury residues, were liver, gill, brain,

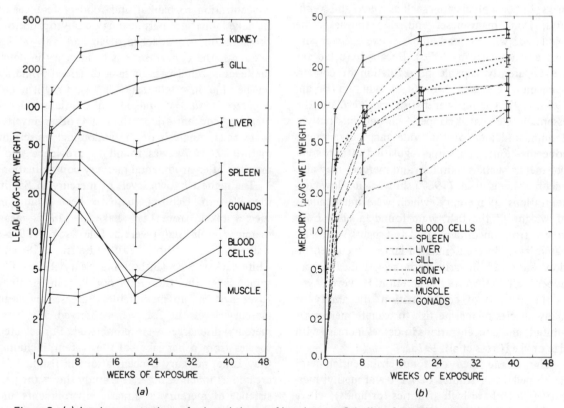

Figure 3 (*a*) Lead concentrations of selected tissues of brook trout, *Salvelinus fontinalis,* exposed to a near-lethal concentration of lead chloride (235 µg/l Pb). Error bars indicate the standard error of 10 samples. *[From Holcombe et al., (1976).]* (*b*) Mercury concentrations of selected tissues of brook trout exposed to a near-lethal concentration of methyl mercuric chloride (0.93 µg/l CH₃Hg). Error bars indicate the standard deviation of 4–10 samples. *[Modified from McKim et al. (1976).]*

gonad, and muscle. Steady-state concentrations of mercury were reached in all tissues after 20–28 wk of continuous exposure to methyl mercury in water (McKim et al., 1976). The rate of mercury excretion from rainbow trout is slow and biphasic, with an estimated half-retention time of 200 d for the first 100-d phase (Massaro and Giblin, 1972). Subsequent excretion is apparently governed by the rate of release of methyl mercury from skeletal muscle.

Many aquatic animals are able to excrete a higher than normal proportion of their metal intake under contaminated conditions and thus maintain trace metal concentrations in the body at a normal level. Regulation of trace metals is generally poor in bivalve and perhaps gastropod mollusks, but in polychaetes such as *Nereis* and *Nephthys,* iron, manganese, and zinc appear to be regulated, whereas cadmium, copper, silver, and lead are not (Bryan, 1976). Decapod crustaceans are apparently capable of regulation of copper, manganese, and zinc, but not of cadmium (Bryan, 1968, 1976). Freshwater fish can regulate the essential elements copper, chromium, molybdenum, and zinc over a wide range of ambient concentrations, and some regulation of nonessential metals such as cadmium and mercury may also occur. Johnels et al. (1967) showed that low concentrations of mercury, which were independent of weight of the fish, were found in pike, *Esox lucius,* from uncontaminated and slightly contaminated lakes. In contaminated lakes, the concentration increased linearly with size, indicating an upper limit to the rate of excretion. However, even in the absence of contamination, the ability of many species of marine fish to excrete mercury is limited, and concentrations in tissues increase with size or age (Cross et al., 1973).

The classic idea of food chain enrichment, developed from studies of DDT and methyl mercury (which have high affinities for lipids), where the highest trophic levels contain the highest toxicant concentrations, does not hold for most heavy metals. The more typical distribution was demonstrated by Leland and McNurney (1974) for lead,

a metal with a low distribution coefficient in natural waters (Fig. 4). Sediments generally contain higher concentrations of heavy metals than are present in aquatic organisms; consequently, if significant accumulation through food ingestion occurs, sediment-feeding organisms contain higher metal concentrations than do other consumers.

The Wabigoon-English-Winnipeg River system of northwestern Ontario was one of the waterways in Canada most heavily contaminated with mercury before early 1970, when mercury discharges in effluents from chloralkali plants were first regulated. Armstrong and Hamilton (1973) determined mercury concentrations in invertebrates and small vertebrates of Clay Lake, a part of the river system, in an attempt to relate differences in mercury concentration to habitat and food preferences of the lake fauna. Animals feeding on phytoplankton, zooplankton, or attached algae had only about one-tenth the concentrations of mercury in detritus feeders, omnivores or taxa that feed primarily on benthic invertebrates (Fig. 4). Crayfish, *Orconectes virilis,* contained substantially higher mercury concentrations than did other invertebrate taxa. Analysis of the abdominal muscle of mature *O. virilis* was found to provide a good monitor of environmental mercury contamination.

The highest known levels of mercury in fish in the Western Hemisphere have been found in species taken from Clay Lake. In 1970, mean mercury levels (μg/g) were as follows: pike, 9.24; walleye, 12.1; burbot, 22.0; whitefish, 3.58; and white sucker, 3.83 (Bishop and Neary, 1976). For some lakes in the Wabigoon-English-Winnipeg River system, no measurable decreases in mean mercury levels in fish were observed 5 y after mercury discharges were eliminated. For selected species from other lakes of the system, including Clay Lake, mercury concentrations in fish had decreased as much as 50%. This study shows the persistence of mercury in aquatic environments and the significance of its cycling in food chains. Until natural scouring and sedimentation processes remove the recent additions of mercury from circulation through transport out of the river system or

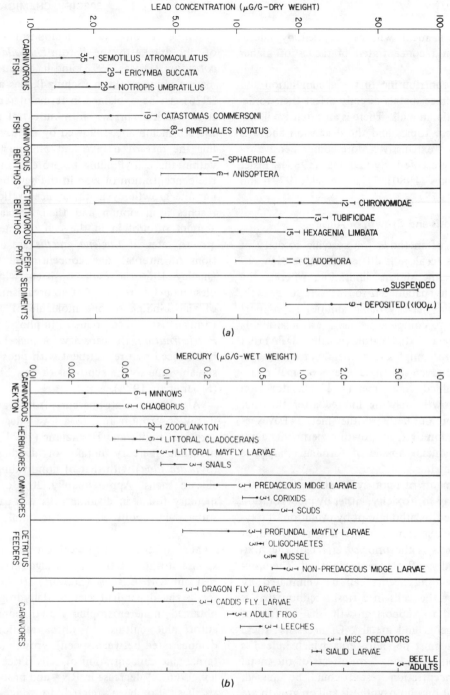

Figure 4 (a) Relationship between whole-body lead concentration and food selection for organisms in a small river (Vermilion River, Illinois) of a rural area. Numbers indicate sample size; lines and points refer to the standard deviation and arithmetic mean, respectively. *[Modified from Leland and McNurney (1974).]* (b) Relationship between whole-body mercury concentration and food selection for organisms in Clay Lake, Ontario, June 1970. Numbers indicate sample size; lines and points refer to the range and geometric mean, respectively. *[Modified from Armstrong and Hamilton (1973).]*

burial, the element will be recycled by micro-organisms and concentrated in tissues of higher organisms.

Factors contributing to the accumulation and storage of trace metals directly affect their toxicity to aquatic animals. There is an extensive literature on these topics and the discussion above is by no means exhaustive. More comprehensive reviews are presented by Luoma (1983), Eisler (1980), Stokes (1980), Leland et al. (1979), and Miettinen (1975).

Photosynthesis and Growth of Algae

The choice of methods for assaying toxicity of trace metals to algae is difficult because each suffers from some serious limitation. Whereas the most obvious parameter to measure is growth, natural waters have variable abilities to support growth and to complex metals. If artificial media are used, the added chelators (usually EDTA) that are needed to complex trace metal nutrients, especially iron, reduce the toxic effects of small quantities of added trace metals. If chelators are omitted, growth may be limited after the first week by iron and perhaps other metals (Davey et al., 1973). Moreover, in growth experiments algae liberate products capable of forming complexes with heavy metals.

Measurements of photosynthesis are frequently made to assay for toxicity, either by incorporation of ^{14}C-labeled bicarbonate or by evolution of oxygen. The assumption is made that reduction of photosynthesis is the primary effect of the toxicant or rapidly reflects the toxic effect. The problem of chelating agents can be eliminated by resuspending the cells in a fresh medium that is not required to support growth (that is, free of chelating agents and metals). Of necessity, these experiments must be short-term, which indeed is an attraction. Any long-term effects of the metal at the concentration tested could be missed. Assays based on photosynthesis and on growth are essentially complementary.

Uptake of trace metals by algae appears to be primarily a passive process, although one that can

be influenced directly by metabolism. The kinetics of zinc uptake by the diatom *Phaeodactylum tricornutum* (Davies, 1973) and lead uptake by two marine phytoplankton (Schulz-Baldes and Lewin, 1976) can be explained in terms of rapid absorption (which occurs within minutes) of metal onto the cell membrane, followed by diffusion controlling the rate of uptake and binding to proteins within the cell. Binding to proteins may control the concentration of zinc in the cell, because during the growth cycle the concentration of zinc reaches a maximum and then decreases as the amount of protein in the cell declines. Specific growth rates of *Euglena gracilis* are linear functions of internal zinc concentration (Price and Quigley, 1966), a result consistent with the simplest model of response of an organism: one atom of zinc binding to one molecule of a ligand to form an essential component. In phosphate-starved *P. tricornutum,* the capacity for nickel absorption is enhanced by pretreatment with phosphate, presumably due to the synthesis of new binding sites (Skaar et al., 1974).

Algae accumulate mercury from water primarily by absorption and, to a lesser degree, by adsorption. Fujita and Hashizume (1974) compared inorganic mercury uptake of dividing diatoms (*Synedra ulna*) with that of nondividing cells and silicate shells. Approximately 20% of the total mercury found in dividing cells was passively adsorbed and about 50% was accumulated within cells.

Most of the detailed work on physiological responses to zinc deficiency in algae has been carried out with *Euglena* (Stewart, 1974). Evidence for a zinc-dependent lactate dehydrogenase was obtained in heterotrophic growth conditions. In autotrophic cultures, a linear relationship was demonstrated between specific growth rate and internal zinc concentration of cells (Price and Quigley, 1966). A decrease in RNA and protein synthesis has also been related to zinc deficiency (Wacker, 1962).

The importance of copper as a trace nutrient in plant metabolism is well recognized. It is necessary for plastocyanin synthesis and functions in photosynthetic electron transport. Copper is also involved in the enzymatic oxidation of ascorbate and polyphenolic compounds (Bidwell, 1974).

The optimal concentration range for essential trace elements in aquatic environments may be very narrow. Copper inhibits photosynthesis and growth of sensitive algal species at concentrations (as low as 1-2 µg/l total Cu) often found in pristine waters (Steemann Nielsen and Wium-Andersen, 1970). Organic and inorganic cupric complexes, which constitute the major copper species in natural waters, are apparently relatively nontoxic to algae. Culture experiments with the diatom *Thalassiosira pseudonana* showed that growth rate inhibition and copper content of cells are related to cupric ion activity and not to total copper concentration (Sunda and Guillard, 1976). Cupric ion activity was altered independently of total copper concentration by varying the chelator concentration and the pH. Copper inhibited the growth rate of *T. pseudonana* at cupric ion activities above 2 ng/l and growth ceased at activities above 300 ng/l. Anderson et al. (1978) demonstrated that zinc ion activity (in contrast to total zinc concentration) can limit the growth rate of *Thalassiosira weissflogii* and that the limitation occurs at zinc ion activities naturally present in unpolluted seawater. Toxicity of zinc ion activity to *T. weissflogii* was observed in the range 65-650 ng/l Zn. The range over which *T. weissflogii* grows at its maximum rate spans only two orders of magnitude (0.65-65 ng/l Zn). The natural zinc ion activity of marine waters is approximately 3 ng/l.

Wagemann and Barica (1979) determined rates of disappearance of total dissolved copper in six hard-water lakes treated with copper as an algicide. Less than 0.5% of total dissolved copper was calculated to be present at any time as free cupric ion. The total dissolved concentration of added copper declined with time through precipitation of the copper as tenorite, CuO (in some cases malachite, $Cu_2(OH)_2CO_3$), and through adsorption on solids.

The mechanisms of toxicity of trace metals to aquatic plants are not fully known. Several trace metals, including copper, lead, mercury, and zinc, retard the flow of electrons in electron transfer reactions of plant mitochondria (Koeppe and Miller, 1970; Bittell et al., 1974) and thus can be expected to have a detrimental effect on respiration. Each of these elements also inhibits photosynthetic rate of algae. Gaechter (1976) observed that rates of inhibition of photosynthesis of natural freshwater phytoplankton assemblages decreased in the order $Hg \geqslant Cu > Cd > Zn > Pb$. Berland et al. (1976) determined concentrations of cadmium, copper, mercury, and lead that inhibit growth of marine unicellular algae. Mercury was the most toxic metal, and lead retarded growth less than did the other elements.

Copper inhibits both photosynthesis and respiration of algae (Steemann Nielsen et al., 1969; Steemann Nielsen and Wium-Andersen, 1970). Photosynthesis is generally the more sensitive measure. The most sensitive site of the green alga *Chlorella* sp. to cupric ion is the oxidizing side of photosystem II (Cedeno-Maldonado, 1973). Copper concentrations that inhibit photosynthesis and respiration in *Chlorella* have no immediate effect on the ultrastructure of cells. Overnell (1975) compared the relative sensitivities of photosynthetic inhibition and potassium loss from cells as measures of response of unicellular marine algae to trace metals. With cadmium, lead, thallium, and zinc, inhibition of photosynthesis is either more sensitive or equally affected. With copper, release of potassium occurs at a lower concentration than does inhibition of photosynthesis.

Population growth rate and pigment composition of the marine green alga *Dunaliella salina* exposed to copper and lead were determined by Pace et al. (1977). Copper (0.5-2.5 mg/l) delayed the onset of the logarithmic phase of growth and increased the extractable pigment concentrations of cells; lead (0.3-15 mg/l) reduced extractable chlorophyll and carotenoid concentrations, but population growth rate was not affected during the logarithmic phase. Saifullah (1978) determined inhibitory effects of copper on three species of marine dinoflagellates in batch and continuous cultures. Chlorophyll concentration, rate of [^{14}C] bicarbonate uptake, and population growth rate were equally sensitive response parameters. The inhibitory effect of copper was most pronounced at the end of the logarithmic phase of growth.

Lead retarded the flow of electrons in electron transfer reactions of plant mitochondria (Koeppe and Miller, 1970) and chloroplasts (Bazzaz and Govindjee, 1974) and thus can be expected to have a detrimental effect on both respiration and photosynthesis. In studies of isolated corn mitochondria, lead concentrations as low as 1 μg/g reduced oxidation of succinate and modified general membrane integrity (Koeppe and Miller, 1970). Photosynthesis was completely suppressed by 7.5 mg/l Pb in cells of the marine diatom *Phaeodactylum* in short-term (24-h) tests, whereas respiration was reduced to 25% at this concentration (Woolery and Lewin, 1977). Vital activities of cells treated for 48 or 72 h were progressively more inhibited; total lead concentrations as low as 75 μg/l reduced photosynthesis and respiration rates by 25–50%. The severity of effects of lead on reproduction, viability, and motility of the marine flagellate *Platymonas subcordiformis* also depended primarily on metal concentration and duration of exposure (Hessler, 1974). Log phase cells of *P. subcordiformis* are more sensitive than stationary phase cells. Sublethal concentrations of lead (2.5 and 10 mg/l) retard population growth by delaying cell division and daughter cell separation. Lethal concentrations cause inhibition of growth and cell death. Motility varies with lead concentration of the medium and length of exposure.

Whitton (1970) measured growth inhibition of freshwater green algae by lead (and copper and zinc) under standard test conditions. All species tested were considerably more tolerant of lead than of zinc or copper, with inhibition occurring at 3–60 mg/l Pb. *Cladophora* is a relatively sensitive genus and may be a useful indicator of metal toxicity in streams.

Lead is adsorbed strongly by biological membranes, and its binding significantly influences the effects observed. There is a high passive affinity of lead for mitochondrial membranes (Bittell et al., 1974). The number of binding sites for lead on mitochondrial membranes is greater than for calcium, but generally comparable to that for other trace elements such as manganese, nickel, cadmium, and zinc. Very high lead concentrations (>70,000 μg/g) can occur in benthic algae in streams receiving effluents from lead mines and mills (Gale et al., 1973, 1976). The ability of algae to grow under these conditions is attributable to the fact that virtually all lead assimilated by the cells is bound to cell walls and membranes.

Sick and Windom (1974) determined rates of uptake of inorganic mercury and cadmium by selected unicellular marine algae and effects of the metals on population growth and cell physiology. Inorganic mercury concentrations of 0.03 to 0.350 μg/l significantly depressed algal growth. Lowered cell-division rates were accompanied by decreases in total cellular nitrogen and lipid and increases in cellular carbon and mercury concentrations. Freeberg (1977) measured maximum specific growth rates, chlorophyll *a* per cell, and [^{14}C] bicarbonate uptake of two marine phytoplankton exposed to inorganic mercury in continuous culture. Maximum specific growth rates were generally enhanced at low metal concentrations and markedly reduced as metal concentrations increased above a threshold value. Chlorophyll *a* per cell and [^{14}C] bicarbonate uptake were not affected by inorganic mercury at less than near-lethal concentrations. Semiconservative DNA synthesis in *Chlorella* and *Chlamydomonas* was inhibited by inorganic mercury (Wihlidal et al., 1976), and repair capacity was inhibited depending on mercury concentration.

Organomercurials generally inhibit the growth and availability of algae even more effectively than inorganic mercury (Matida et al., 1971). As little as 0.1 μg/l of some alkyl mercurial fungicides decreased growth and photosynthesis of sensitive marine and freshwater phytoplankton (Harriss et al., 1970; Nuzzi, 1972). Algae may be highly susceptible to alkyl mercurials because of the high lipid content of their cell membranes (Boney and Corner, 1959).

Ecological interactions between phytoplankton species and biochemical interactions affecting trace metal uptake and toxicity compound the problem of predicting toxicity of trace metals in natural environments. Mixed cultures of marine phytoplankton respond more adversely and at lower concentrations to copper than do the same species in unialgal cultures, suggesting that information on effects of competition should be included in interpretations of effects of trace metals on phytoplankton growth (Fielding and Russell, 1978). Breaek et al. (1976) showed that joint effects of copper and zinc on marine phytoplankton cannot be predicted on the basis of toxicity of the individual metals. Responses of the dinoflagellate *Amphidinium carteri* and the diatom *Thalassiosira pseudonana* clearly indicated synergism, whereas the same metals acted as antagonists toward the diatom *Phaeodactylum tricornutum*. Zinc toxicity to *P. tricornutum* increased at low concentrations of magnesium.

TOLERANCE MECHANISMS

Considering the importance of toxicant-resistant populations of aquatic species in animal and plant toxicology, relatively few field studies of metal tolerance have been conducted. Populations of phytoplankton, *Scenedesmus acutiformis* and *Chlorella fusca,* from metal-contaminated lakes near Sudbury, Ontario, were found to be more resistant to the toxic effects of copper and nickel than populations of these species from uncontaminated areas (Stokes et al., 1973; Stokes and Hutchinson, 1976). Populations of the polychaete *Nereis diversicolor* from estuaries contaminated with copper, cadmium, lead, and zinc were able to accumulate more copper than nontolerant *N. diversicolor* from less contaminated areas (Bryan and Hummerstone, 1971, 1973; Bryan, 1974). *Nereis diversicolor* from some, but not all, of the contaminated estuaries were also resistant to zinc.

No resistance to cadmium or lead was detectable in *N. diversicolor,* despite high concentrations of these metals in the sediments. Populations of the isopod *Asellus meridianus* from sites receiving mine drainage were shown by toxicity tests and growth rate experiments to be tolerant to copper and lead (Brown, 1976, 1977). Copper tolerance confers tolerance to lead in *A. meridianus,* but lead tolerance is not accompanied by increased resistance to copper.

Luoma (1977) proposed the study of resistant populations to detect trace contaminant effects in aquatic ecosystems. If one population of a species is more resistant to a toxicant than other populations in an ecosystem, it may be direct evidence that the toxicant is present in a high enough concentration to exert an effect on that species. Use of toxicant resistance to detect contaminant effects has the advantage over extrapolation of laboratory toxicity data to natural environments that it eliminates the need to correlate toxicity and contaminant concentrations.

Tolerance in organisms suggests the presence of a mechanism to prevent toxic substances from affecting metabolism or damaging sensitive structures within cells. Tolerance mechanisms fall into two broad categories, namely exclusion from cells and intracellular changes. Exclusion is brought about in several ways: (1) Algae may release organic material, which can then chelate free metal ions in solution (Davey et al., 1973; Swallow et al., 1978; Jackson and Morgan, 1978). Extracellular material produced by an associated organism also can effect a reduction in toxicity. (2) Cell wall alginates can sequester metal ions. Silverberg (1975) found that metal tolerance exhibited by the green alga *Stigeoclonium tenue* resulted from partial exclusion of metal ions by the cell wall. (3) Changes in cell membrane permeability can alter the dynamics of metal uptake and excretion. Hall et al. (1979) demonstrated such changes in copper-tolerant strains of the alga *Ectocarpus siliculosus.*

In the absence of an exclusion mechanism, tolerance can occur only if there are changes within the cell. These changes involve one or more of the following detoxification mechanisms: (1) biological oxidation, reduction, or hydrolysis of metals into more water-soluble and more acidic products, which enhances excretion; (2) incorporation of the metal into macromolecules, such as metallothionein, that are harmless; and (3) sequestering of the toxicants in less mobile tissues, or organelles, thus limiting access to the more sensitive tissues and organelles. Investigations of detoxication of trace metals in aquatic organisms have largely been limited to the latter two mechanisms.

Silverberg et al. (1976) showed that copper-tolerant *Scenedesmus* sp. deposit copper within nuclear inclusions. Fine-structural examination of tolerant *Scenedesmus* cells exposed to copper revealed the presence of nuclear inclusions in the form of central dense-core complexes and the occasional presence of cytoplasmic structures resembling the intranuclear inclusions (Silverberg et al., 1976). X-ray microanalysis of the structures provided evidence that the inclusions contained copper. These results suggest that the formation of inclusions may be an important cellular detoxifying mechanism in which copper is complexed by protein ligands, and that by this mechanism cytoplasmic organelles are, to some extent, protected from the toxic effects of copper. Formation of insoluble intracellular metal-protein complexes is apparently also characteristic of some types of trace metal, particularly lead, intoxication (Goyer, 1973) in animals, and has been reported in a variety of plant and animal tissues (Choie and Richter, 1972; Moore and Goyer, 1974).

The tolerance of crustaceans to high concentrations of trace metals in the environment may be partially attributed to the formation of granules within cells of the alimentary canal. Production of granules in cells of the gut of several species of amphipods, isopods, and decapods is restricted to the hepatopancreatic caeca (Icely and Nott, 1980). Most intracellular granules in tissues of crustaceans can be separated into two distinct types on the basis of structure and composition: (1) homogeneous electron-dense material, which always contains copper and sulfur, and (2) a dense material having

concentric layers, which usually contain calcium, magnesium, and phosphorus. Other metals that occur in the second type include zinc, potassium, iron, and lead. Production of the homogeneous type of granule in some species has been correlated directly with the concentration of copper in the environment (Icely and Nott, 1980).

High concentrations of zinc and other trace metals occurred in membrane-lined vesicles of kidney tissues of *Mytilus edulis* (George and Pirie, 1980) and the scallop *Pecten maximus* (George et al., 1980). The granules appeared to be predominantly insoluble phosphates of calcium, manganese, and zinc. Over an extended range of seawater zinc concentrations (10–1000 µg/l), zinc uptake by *M. edulis* was proportional to the concentration in seawater. Immobilization of zinc in tissues is evidenced by the presence of insoluble zinc granules in membrane-lined vesicles, in the kidney cells, and in circulating amoebocytes. The amoebocytes probably make a significant contribution to the zinc concentrations in tissues such as muscle and mantle. In contrast, neither cadmium nor mercury could be identified in amoebocytes of *M. edulis,* but were present in hemolymph (Janssen and Scholz, 1979). Transport via hemolymph and selective discrimination at the basement lamina of the midgut gland tubuli appear to be primary factors affecting accumulation of cadmium and mercury. In the tubuli, both metals are immobilized in membrane-bound vesicles, which are finally defecated.

A common characteristic of herbaceous plants growing in zinc-contaminated habitats is the evolution of zinc-tolerant ecotypes (Antonovics et al., 1971). Tolerant ecotypes are distinguished from sensitive ones not only by their degree of tolerance but by production rates, requirements for nutrients, and the development of self-fertility (Mathys, 1977). Gene flow between tolerant and nontolerant populations is very low, and therefore tolerant species are often isolated from their sensitive ecotypes. This tolerance is highly specific, so cotolerance for both zinc and copper is not induced by zinc exposure. Mathys (1980) proposed a mechanism of zinc tolerance for herbaceous plants based on the formation of zinc-malate complexes. Malate is thought to function as a transport vehicle for zinc between cytoplasm and vacuoles. Strong complexing agents in the vacuoles effect a constant concentration gradient for unidirectional transport of zinc from plasma to vacuoles. Restricted uptake or translocation of zinc may also occur.

Acquired tolerance to trace metals in animals can result from increased synthesis of metallothionein. In higher organisms, this protein is usually stored as a soluble constituent of liver and kidney cytoplasm. Metallothionein produced in response to cadmium, copper, or mercury contains zinc in approximately half of its binding sites (Leber, 1974; Bremner and Davies, 1975). Zinc has a much lower affinity than cadmium or mercury for metallothionein binding sites. On a second exposure to cadmium or mercury, these elements replace zinc on metallothionein, and thus zinc, rather than one of the more toxic metals, is released into the cytoplasm. Cadmium or mercury also displace copper from metallothionen.

Pathological effects result if there are not enough zinc- or copper-containing binding sites on metallothionein to detoxify all the mercury or cadmium, or if synthesis of metallothionein is slower than uptake of the toxic metal. Brown and Parsons (1978) reported that pathological effects occur in chum salmon, *Oncorhynchus keta,* and zooplankton when synthesis of metallothionein is slower than metal influx. In salmon liver, as mercury increases in metallothionein, there is a concomitant decrease of copper and zinc in metallothionein. In zooplankton, copper and zinc are not displaced by increasing levels of mercury in metallothionein. The difference between fish and zooplankton may be due to different tissue types or lower cytoplasmic mercury levels in zooplankton at corresponding environmental mercury concentrations.

Metallothionein in vertebrates can be induced by a number of trace metals and is especially important in the binding of cadmium, zinc, copper, and mercury. Another low molecular weight protein, specific for copper, also exists. The predominant protein depends on whether induction initially occurs as a result of exposure to copper or another trace element, such as cadmium (Winge et al., 1975). Two low molecular weight copper-binding proteins also occur in the clam *Protothaeca staminea* (Roesijadi, 1980) and the crab *Carcinus maenus* (Rainbow and Scott, 1979). The estimated molecular weight of the smaller protein and its ability to bind copper, zinc, and cadmium are similar to properties described for metallothionein. Copper was found to occur on "copper-binding protein" in gills and muscle of the clam and on metallothionein-like protein in kidneys and viscera. The midgut gland is probably central to the metabolism of copper, cadmium, and zinc in *C. maenus.*

Many trace metals, including cobalt, lead, manganese, and nickel, do not induce synthesis of metallothionein following repeated exposure (Mogilnicka et al., 1975). However, such ions may increase the hepatic zinc pool and thus indirectly induce synthesis of metallothionein.

COMMUNITY EFFECTS

In contrast to the wealth of data in the literature on concentrations of trace metals in various marine and freshwater species, field studies examining impacts of trace metals on population dynamics, species abundances and diversity, and community function are rare. One of the more informative fisheries investigations dealt with the impact of base metal mining on the ecology of northwest Miramichi Atlantic salmon, *Salmo salar* (Sprague and Ramsey, 1965; Saunders and Sprague, 1967). A strong relationship between downstream migration of adult salmon and the occurrence of high copper and zinc concentrations in the Miramichi River (New Brunswick, Canada) was observed. When mining in the upper watershed was active, metal levels were high and a high percentage of adults returned downstream before spawning. Only about one-third reascended. During years of no mining, more fish ascended the river, fewer returned before spawning, and overall spawning was more successful. Effects attributed to mining operations were a 25% reduction of adult stock from the spawning grounds, removal of about 25% of the rearing ground from production of salmon, and a reduction of late-run populations to a level such that several generations were needed for recovery (Elson, 1974).

Beamish (1974) examined the gradual disappearance of fish populations from unexploited remote lakes in Ontario, Canada, which resulted from atmospheric fallout of acid. Losses of fish populations were attributed both to long-term lethal effects and to an absence of recruitment of young into the populations due to a failure in reproduction. Losses of fish populations were attributed to acidity and not the relatively high concentrations of several trace metals observed in the lakes.

An experimental investigation of responses of stream macroinvertebrates (Winner et al., 1975) and fish (Geckler et al., 1976) to copper was conducted in Shayler Run, Claremont County, Ohio. Copper sulfate was added continuously to this stream for 33 mo at a concentration (120 μg/l Cu) at the point of discharge which was expected, on the basis of laboratory toxicity test data, to adversely affect some, but not all resident fish species. The stream also received a domestic waste water effluent and thus contained variable but unknown concentrations of copper-complexing species. Most of the common fish and macroinvertebrate species resident in the stream were adversely affected by the addition of copper, with effects including death, avoidance, and restricted spawning (Geckler et al., 1976). Except for a failure to display avoidance, responses of the resident fish to copper could have been reliably predicted from laboratory toxicity test data. Winner et al. (1975) found the index "number of species" to be more sensitive to changes in benthic invertebrate community structure than either Margalef's or Shannon's diversity index.

Changes in function and structure of the Aufwuchs (i.e., periphyton) community of an oligotrophic stream during continuous, low-level exposure to copper were determined by Leland and Carter (1984a, 1984b). The study site, Convict

Creek, is located on the eastern escarpment of the Sierra Nevada in California. Total copper concentrations maintained in stream water of the four study sections for 1 yr were ≤ 1 (control), 2.5, 5, and 10 μg/l. Inhibition of photosynthetic carbon fixation and sulfate assimilation was observed within the first 48 h at 5 and 10 μg/l Cu, but not at 2.5 μg/l Cu. Additional effects observed during long-term, continuous exposure to the two higher copper concentrations were reductions in rate of colonization (chlorophyll a and ash-free dry weight), rate of nitrogen fixation, rate of microbial decomposition of leaf litter, and algal species diversity. An inhibitory effect of copper on community function at 2.5 μg/l Cu during long-term continuous exposure was evidenced by reduced rates of photosynthetic carbon fixation and sulfate assimilation relative to the control, and by lower rates of colonization of artificial substrates and microbial decomposition of leaf litter. The threshold of tolerance of most epiphytic rotifers and ciliated protozoans was found to be greater than 2.5 μg/l but less than 7 μg/l Cu (Leland and Kent, 1981). These results indicate the extreme toxicity of copper in waters containing little organic complexing matter. Convict Creek waters are moderately hard (60 mg/l as $CaCO_3$) and alkaline (pH 8), but the complexing capacity of the stream water for copper is low.

Thomas et al. (1977) examined effects of low concentrations of copper on standing crop and productivity of marine phytoplankton in large (65 m^3) plastic enclosures at Saanich Inlet, British Columbia. At 10–50 μg/l, copper initially inhibited standing crops, photosynthesis, and growth rates; however, at the end of the experiment (27 d), these values did not differ from controls. Copper was added only once, at the beginning of the test period. There was a significant change in species composition in the copper-treated enclosures, with the dominant diatom (*Chaetoceros* sp.) replaced by copper-insensitive algae (microflagellates, *Nitzschia delicatissima,* and *Navicula distans*) (Thomas and Seiberg, 1977). Marked increases in relative numbers and activity of bacterial heterotrophs were observed in the copper-treated enclosures, presumably due to release of available organic carbon from copper-sensitive plankton (Vaccaro et al., 1977). Stable isotope tracer techniques were used to examine the effects of copper on silica uptake by phytoplankton (Goering et al., 1977). At 25 μg/l Cu, mean silica uptake was only 61% (range, 49–98) of the control. Harrison et al. (1977) reported that sublethal concentrations of copper also inhibited uptake of nitrate, synthesis of nitrate reductase, and photosynthetic carbon assimilation. Fluctuations in zooplankton abundance, species composition, and secondary production were also determined following additions of copper (5, 10, and 50 μg/l) to the enclosures. Abundances of ctenophores and medusae were reduced at all three concentrations (Gibson and Brice, 1977). Major ciliate groups were eliminated at 50 μg/l; ciliate species composition was significantly altered at the two lower copper concentrations (Beers et al., 1977). Among the important micrometazoan taxa, naupliar copepod abundances were lower relative to controls at 50 and 10 μg/l, but not at 5 μg/l. Laboratory experiments on ingestion, filtration, and fecal pellet production rates of copepods from the enclosures showed reduced activity at all three concentrations (Reeve et al., 1977).

SUMMARY AND RECOMMENDED RESEARCH

Recent efforts to document and control the environmental distribution of potentially hazardous trace metals have led to a large body of literature on biological effects of metals in aquatic environments. Much of this literature considers lethal solution concentrations for individual species, or trace metal bioavailability and body burdens of common or commercially important species. Recent reviews of these topics are referenced in the text. This chapter focuses on the toxicology of trace metals and the responses of aquatic organisms to metal exposure.

Established criteria for metal toxicity to aquatic organisms are acute mortality, growth retardation, and impaired reproduction with mortality of offspring. Although many clinical techniques for measuring cytopathological, physiological, and biochemical changes in mammalian and higher plant tissues have been successfully adapted for the detection of trace metal stress in aquatic organisms, few useful diagnostic tests are available. Measurement of the activity of plasma δ-aminolevulinic acid as an indicator of the toxic effects of lead absorption in fish is a notable exception. Little is known about normal adaptive responses of aquatic organisms, thus making it difficult to establish baseline values for diagnostic tests or to extrapolate laboratory toxicity data to field conditions. It is not clear, for example, whether many hematological changes during sublethal exposures represent deleterious effects of trace metals or merely the normal adaptive mechanisms of the organism. Equally difficult is the lack of unequivocal correlation of metal-induced physiological or cytopathological responses with impaired, whole-animal responses critical to population survival. Comprehensive studies are sorely needed in which whole-animal responses critical to population survival, cellular morphological changes, and biochemical reaction rates are linked.

Pathological effects occur in tissues when the rate of influx of a toxicant exceeds rates of detoxification and excretion. For example, if synthesis of metallothionein in animals is slower than influx of cadmium or mercury, toxic symptoms result. Further study is needed on the mechanisms of uptake, metabolism, and depuration of trace metals in aquatic organisms, particularly the kinetics of these processes as they affect the tissue distribution of trace metals and the development of toxic symptoms.

Field studies critically examining impacts of trace metals on population dynamics, species abundances and diversity, and community function are rare. There is a need to develop biological indices appropriate to field investigations that are a function of the stress acting on the individual or population and that are sensitive over the range of trace metal concentrations typically encountered.

Measurement of the energy available to individuals for growth and production of gametes after the demands of respiratory metabolism are met is a potentially suitable index. Measurement of changes in tolerance to evaluate stress could also be applied to field conditions, although this could include genetic as well as physiological adaptation. Numerical classification (similarity) is a common and, if properly employed, sensitive index of community-level responses. Trace metal concentrations that reduce the number of species of an aquatic community may also be expected to affect sensitive indices of community function, such as nutrient cycling and rates of primary and secondary production.

LITERATURE CITED

Abel PD, Skidmore JF: Toxic effects of an anionic detergent on the gills of rainbow trout. Water Res 9:759–765, 1975.

Allen HE, Hall RH, Brisbin TD: Metal speciation; effects on toxicity. J Am Chem Soc 14:441–446, 1980.

Anderson MA, Morel FMM, Guillard RRL: Growth limitation of a coastal diatom by low zinc ion activity. Nature (Lond) 276:70–71, 1978.

Andrew RW, Biesinger KE, Glass GL: Effects of inorganic complexing on the toxicity of copper to *Daphnia magna*. Water Res 11:309–315, 1977.

Angle CR, McIntire MS, Stelmak KL: High urban lead and decreased red blood cell survival. Proc Int Conf Heavy Metals Environ, pp. 87–104, Toronto, Ontario, 1975.

Antonovics J, Bradshaw AD, Turner RG: Heavy metal tolerance in plants. Adv Ecol Res 7:1–85, 1971.

Armstrong FAJ, Hamilton AL: Pathways of mercury in a polluted northwestern Ontario lake. In: Trace Metals and Metal-Organic Interactions in Natural Waters, edited by PC Singer, pp. 131–156. Ann Arbor, Mich.: Ann Arbor Science, 1973.

Barton DT, Jones AH, Cairns J: Acute zinc toxicity to rainbow trout (*Salmo gairdneri*); confirmation of the hypothesis that death is related to tissue hypoxia. J Fish Res Board Can 29: 1463–1466, 1972.

Bayne BL, Livingstone DR, Moore MN, Widdows J: A cytochemical and a biochemical index of stress in *Mytilus edulis* L. Mar Pollut Bull 7: 221–224, 1976.

Bayne BL, Holland DL, Moore MN, Lowe DM, Widdows J: Further studies on the effects of stress in the adult on the eggs of *Mytilus edulis*. J Mar Biol Assoc UK 58:825–841, 1978.

Bayne BL, Anderson J, Engel D, Gilfillan E, Hoss D, Lloyd R, Thurberg FP: Physiological techniques for measuring the biological effects of pollution in the sea. Rapp PV Reun Cons Int Explor Mer 179:88–99, 1980.

Bazzaz MB, Govindjee: Effects of lead chloride on chloroplast reactions. Environ Lett 6:175–191, 1974.

Beamish RJ: Loss of fish populations from unexploited remote lakes in Ontario, Canada, as a consequence of atmospheric fallout of acid. Water Res 8:85–95, 1974.

Beers JR, Stewart GL, Hoskins KD: Dynamics of micro-zooplankton populations treated with copper; controlled ecosystem pollution experiment. Bull Mar Sci 27:66–79, 1977.

Bengtsson BE: The effects of zinc on the mortality and reproduction of the minnow, *Phoxinus phoxinus* (L.). Arch Environ Contam Toxicol 2:342–355, 1974.

Berland BR, Bonin DJ, Kapkov VI, Maestrini SY, Arlhac DP: Toxic effects of four heavy metals on the growth of unicellular marine algae. CR Hebd Seances Acad Sci Ser D Sci Natur 282: 633–636, 1976.

Bidwell RGS: Plant Physiology. New York: Macmillan, 1974.

Birge WJ, Black JA: Effects of copper on embryonic and juvenile stages of aquatic animals. In: Copper in the Environment, part 2, Health Effects, edited by JO Nriagu, pp. 373–399. New York: Wiley-Interscience, 1979.

Birge WJ, Black JA, Hudson JE, Bruser DM: Embryo-larval toxicity tests with organic compounds. In: Aquatic Toxicology, edited by LL Marking, RA Kimerle, pp. 131–147. Spec Tech Publ 657. Philadelphia: ASTM, 1979.

Bishop JN, Neary BP: Mercury levels in fish from northwestern Ontario, 1970–1975. Inorganic Trace Contaminants Section, Ministry of the

Environment, Rexdale, Ontario: Laboratory Services Branch, 1976.

Bittell J, Miller RJ, Koeppe DE: Sorption of heavy metal cations by corn mitochondria and the effects on electron and energy transfer reactions. Physiol Plant 30:226–230, 1974.

Bolter E, Turekian KK, Schutz DF: The distribution of rubidium, cesium and barium in the oceans. Geochim Cosmochim Acta 28:1459–1466, 1964.

Boney AD, Corner EDS: Application of toxic agents in the study of the ecological resistance of intertidal red algae. J Mar Biol Assoc UK 38:267–275, 1959.

Bostrom K, Fischer DE: Distribution of mercury in East Pacific sediments. Geochim Cosmochim Acta 33:743–745, 1969.

Bowling JW, Giesy JP, Kania HJ, Knight RL: Large-scale microcosms for assessing fates and effects of trace contaminants. In: Microcosms in Ecological Research, edited by JP Giesy, pp. 224–247. Washington, D.C.: Technical Information Center, Department of Energy, 1980.

Boyden CR, Watling H, Thornton I: Effect of zinc on the settlement of the oyster Crassostrea gigas. Mar Biol 31:227–234, 1975.

Boyle EA: Copper in natural waters. In: Copper in the Environment, part 1, edited by JO Nriagu, pp. 77–88. New York: Wiley-Interscience, 1979.

Boyle EA, Edmond JM: Copper in surface water south of New Zealand. Nature (Lond) 253:107–109, 1975.

Boyle EA, Sclater FR, Edmond JM: On the marine geochemistry of cadmium. Nature (Lond) 263:42–44, 1976.

Boyle EA, Sclater FR, Edmond JM: The distribution of dissolved copper in the Pacific. Earth Planet Sci Lett 37:38–54, 1977.

Breaek GS, Jensen A, Mohus A: Heavy metal tolerance of marine phytoplankton. III. Combined effects of copper and zinc ions on cultures of four common species. J Exp Mar Biol Ecol 25:37–50, 1976.

Bremner I: Copper toxicity studies using domestic and laboratory animals. In: Copper in the Environment, part II, Health Effects, pp. 285–306. New York: Wiley-Interscience, 1979.

Bremner I, Davies NT: The induction of metallothionein in rat liver by Zn injection and restric-

tion of food intake. Biochem J 149:733–738, 1975.

Brereton A, Lord H, Webb JS: Effect of zinc on growth and development of larvae of the Pacific oyster Crassostrea gigas. Mar Biol 19:96–101, 1973.

Brown BE: Observations on the tolerance of the isopod Asellus meridianus Rac. to copper and lead. Water Res 10:555–559, 1976.

Brown BE: Uptake of copper and lead by a metal-tolerant isopod Asellus meridianus Rac. Freshwater Biol 7:235–244, 1977.

Brown DA, Parsons TR: Relationship between cytoplasmic distribution of mercury and toxic effects to zooplankton and chum salmon (Oncorhynchus keta) exposed to mercury in a controlled ecosystem. J Fish Res Board Can 35:880–884, 1978.

Bruland KW, Knauer GA, Martin JH: Zinc in north-east Pacific water. Nature (Lond) 271:741–743, 1978.

Bryan GW: Concentrations of zinc and copper in the tissues of decapod crustaceans. J Mar Biol Assoc UK 48:303–321, 1968.

Bryan GW: Adaptation of an estuarine polychaete to sediments containing high concentrations of heavy metals. In: Pollution and Physiology of Marine Organisms, edited by FJ Vernberg, WB Vernberg, pp. 123–135. New York: Academic, 1974.

Bryan GW: Some aspects of heavy metal tolerance in aquatic organisms. In: Effects of Pollution on Aquatic Organisms, edited by APM Lockwood, pp. 7–34. London: Cambridge Univ. Press, 1976.

Bryan GW, Hummerstone LG: Adaptation of the polychaete Nereis diversicolor to estuarine sediments containing high concentrations of heavy metals. I. General observations and adaptation to copper. J Mar Biol Assoc UK 51:845–863, 1971.

Bryan GW, Hummerstone LG: Adaptation of the polychaete Nereis diversicolor to estuarine sediments containing high concentrations of zinc and cadmium. J Mar Biol Assoc UK 53:839–857, 1973.

Bryan GW, Uysal H: Heavy metals in the burrowing bivalve Scrobicularia plana from the Tamar estuary in relation to environmental levels. J Mar Biol Assoc UK 58:89–108, 1978.

Calabrese A, Nelson DA: Inhibition of embryonic development of the hard clam, *Mercenaria mercenaria* by heavy metals. Bull Environ Contam Toxicol 11:92–97, 1974.

Calabrese A, Collier RS, Nelson DA, MacInnes JA: The toxicity of heavy metals to embryos of the American oyster, *Crassostrea virginica*. Mar Biol 18:162–166, 1973.

Calabrese A, Thurberg FP, Dawson MA, Wenzloff DR: Sublethal physiological stress induced by cadmium and mercury in winter flounder, *Pseudopleuronectes americanus*. In: Sublethal Effects of Toxic Chemicals on Aquatic Animals, edited by JH Koeman, JJTWA Strik, pp. 15–21. Amsterdam: Elsevier, 1975.

Calabrese A, MacInnes JR, Nelson DA, Miller JE: Survival and growth of bivalve larvae under heavy metal stress. Mar Biol 41:179–184, 1977.

Cantelmo FR, Tagatz ME, Ranga K: Effect of barite on meiofauna in a flow-through experimental system. Mar Environ Res 2:301–310, 1979.

Carpenter KE: The lethal action of soluble metallic salts on fishes. Br J Exp Biol 4:378–390, 1927.

Carpenter KE: Further researches on the action of metallic salts on fishes. J Exp Zool 56:407–422, 1930.

Carr RA, Jones MM, Warner TB, Cheek CH, Russ ER: Variations in time of mercury anomalies at the Mid-Atlantic Ridge. Nature (Lond) 258:588–589, 1975.

Cedeno-Maldonado A: Studies on the Mechanism of Copper Toxicity in *Chlorella*. Ph.D. thesis, Dept. of Biology, Univ. of California, Riverside, 1973.

Chang LW, Hartmann HA: Ultrastructural studies of the nervous system after mercury intoxication. II. Pathological changes in the nerve fibers. Acta Neuropathol 20:316–334, 1972.

Cheng TC: Use of copper as a molluscicide. In: Copper in the Environment. Part II. Health Effects, edited by JO Nriagu, pp. 401–432. New York: Wiley-Interscience, 1979.

Choie DD, Richter GW: Lead poisoning: Rapid formation of intranuclear inclusions. Science 177:1194–1195, 1972.

Christensen GM, McKim JM, Brungs WA, Hunt EP: Changes in the blood of the brown bull-head (*Ictalurus nebulosus* (Lesuer)) following short and long term exposure to copper (II). Toxicol Appl Pharmacol 23:417–427, 1972.

Collinson C, Shimp NF: Trace Elements in Bottom Sediments from Upper Peoria Lake, Middle Illinois River, pp. 1–22. Urbana, Ill.: Illinois State Geological Survey, 1972.

Cousins RJ, Failla ML: Cellular and molecular aspects of mammalian zinc metabolism and homeostasis. In: Zinc in the Environment, Part II. Health Effects, pp. 121–135. New York: Wiley-Interscience, 1980.

Cross FA, Hardy LH, Jones NY, Barber R: Relations between total body weight and concentration of manganese, iron, copper, zinc and mercury in white muscle of bluefish (*Pomatomus saltatrix*) and a bathyl-demersal fish *Antimora rostrata*. J Fish Res Board Can 30:1287–1291, 1973.

Cunningham PA: The effects of mercuric acetate on the adults, juveniles, and larvae of the American oyster, *Crassostrea virginica*. M.S. thesis, pp. 1–77, Univ. of Delaware, Newark, Del., 1972.

Cunningham PA: Inhibition of shell growth in the presence of mercury and subsequent recovery of juvenile oysters. Proc Natl Shellfish Assoc 66:1–5. 1976.

Davey EW, Gentile JH, Stanton JE, Setzer P: Removal of trace metals from marine culture media. Limnol Oceanogr 15:486–488, 1970.

Davey EW, Morgan MJ, Erickson SJ: A biological measurement of the copper complexation capacity of seawater. Limnol Oceanogr 18:993–997, 1973.

Davies AG: Kinetics of and a preliminary model for the uptake of radiozinc by *Phaeodactylum tricornutum* in culture. In: Radioactive Contamination of the Marine Environment, pp. 403–420. Vienna: International Atomic Energy Agency, 1973.

Davis CO, Breitner NF, Harrison PJ: Continuous culture of marine diatoms under silicon limitation. III. A model of Si-limited diatom growth. Limnol Oceanogr 23:41–51, 1978.

Dodge EA, Theis TL: Effect of chemical speciation on the uptake of copper by *Chironomous tentans*. Environ Sci Technol 13:1287–1288, 1979.

Doudoroff P, Katz M: Critical review of literature on the toxicity of industrial wastes and their components to fish, II. Metals as salts. Sewage Ind Wastes 25:802–839, 1953.

Eaton JG, McKim JM, Holcombe GW: Metal toxicity to embryos and larvae of seven freshwater fish species–I. cadmium. Bull Environ Contam Toxicol 13:95–103, 1978.

Eichhorn G: Active sites of biological macromolecules and their interaction with heavy metals. In: Ecological Toxicology Research, edited by AD McIntyre, CF Mills, pp. 123–142. New York: Plenum, 1975.

Eisler R: Accumulation of zinc by marine biota. In: Zinc in the Environment, Part II, Health Effects, edited by JO Nriagu, pp. 259–351. New York: Wiley-Interscience, 1980.

Ellis MM: Detection and measurement of stream pollution. Bull U.S. Bur Fish 48:365–437, 1937.

Elson PF: Impact of recent economic growth and industrial development on the ecology of northwest Miramichi Atlantic salmon (Salmo salar). J Fish Res Board Can 31:521–544, 1974.

Engel DW, Fowler BA: Copper and cadmium induced changes in the metabolism and structure of molluscan gill tissue. In: Marine Pollution: Functional Responses, edited by WB Vernberg, FP Thurberg, A Calabrese, FJ Vernberg, pp. 239–256. New York: Academic, 1979.

Epifanio CE: Effects of dieldrin in seawater on the development of two species of crab larvae, Leptodius floridanus and Panopeus herbstii. Mar Biol 11:356–362, 1971.

Evans GW: Copper homeostasis in the mammalian system. Physiol Rev 53:535–570, 1973.

Evans GW, Johnson PE: Copper and zinc binding ligands in the intestinal mucosa. In: Trace Element Metabolism in Animals, edited by M Kirchgessner, vol. 3, p. 98. Friesing-Weihenstephan, West Germany: Institüt für Ernährungsphysiologie, 1978.

Farmer GJ, Ashfield D, Samant HS: Effects of zinc on juvenile Atlantic salmon Salmo salar: Acute toxicity, food intake, growth and bioaccumulation. Environ Pollut 19:103–117, 1979.

Fencl Z: Theoretical analysis of continuous culture systems. In: Theoretical and Methodological Basis of Continuous Culture of Microorganisms, edited by I Malek, Z Fencl (translated by J Liebster). New York: Academic, 1966.

Fielding AH, Russell G: The effect of copper on competition between marine algae. J Appl Ecol 13:871–876, 1978.

Finney DJ: Probit Analysis. London: Cambridge Univ. Press, 1971.

Fitzgerald WF: Distribution of mercury in natural waters. In: The Biogeochemistry of Mercury in the Environment, edited by JO Nriagu, pp. 161–173. Amsterdam: Elsevier/North-Holland Biomedical, 1979.

Forstner U, Wittman GTW: Metal Pollution in the Aquatic Environment. Berlin: Springer-Verlag, 1979.

Freeberg LR: The effects of light intensity, temperature, cell density and heavy metals (mercury and chromium) on two marine phytoplankters in continuous culture. Diss Abstr Int B 37:5920, 1977.

Fujita M, Hashizume K: Status of uptake of mercury by the freshwater diatom, Synedra ulna. Water Res 9:889–894, 1974.

Gaechter R: Heavy metal toxicity and synergism to natural phytoplankton in the eutrophic Lake Alpnach and the mesotrophic Horw Bay. Schweiz Z Hydrol 38:97–119, 1976.

Gale NL, Wixson BG, Hardie MB, Jennett JC: Aquatic organisms and heavy metals in Missouri's "new lead belt." Water Res Bull 9:673–688, 1973.

Gale NL, Bolter E, Wixson BG: Investigation of Clearwater Lake as a potential sink for heavy metals from lead mining in southeast Missouri. Trace Subst Environ Health 10:187–196, 1976.

Gallagher CH: Biochemical and pathological effects of copper deficiency. In: Copper in the Environment, Part II, Health Effects, edited by JO Nriagu, pp. 57–82. New York: Wiley-Interscience, 1979.

Gardner GR: Chemically induced lesions in estuarine or marine teleosts. In: The Pathology of Fishes, edited by WE Ribelin, G Migaki, pp. 657–694. Madison: Univ. of Wisconsin Press, 1975.

Gardner GR, LaRoche G: Copper induced lesions in estuarine teleosts. J Fish Res Board Can 30:363–368, 1973.

Geckler JR, Horning WB, Neiheisel TM, Pickering QH, Robinson EL, Stephan CE: Validity of laboratory tests for predicting copper toxicity in streams, pp. 1–192. EPA 600/3-76-116. Duluth, Minn.: U.S. EPA, 1976.

George SG, Pirie BJS: Metabolism of zinc in the mussel, *Mytilus edulis* (L.): A combined ultrastructural and biochemical study. J Mar Biol Assoc UK 60:575–590, 1980.

George SG, Pirie BJS, Coombs TL: Isolation and elemental analysis of metal-rich granules from the kidney of the scallop, *Pecten maximus* (L.). J Exp Mar Biol Ecol 42:143–156, 1980.

Giblin FJ, Massaro EJ: Pharmacodynamics of methylmercury in the rainbow trout (*Salmo gairdneri*): Tissue uptake, distribution and excretion. Toxicol Appl Pharmacol 24:81–91, 1973.

Gibson VR, Grice GD: Response of macro-zooplankton populations to copper: Controlled ecosystem pollution experiment. Bull Mar Sci 27:85–91, 1977.

Giesy JP, Leversee GJ, Williams DA: Effects of naturally-occurring aquatic organic fractions on cadmium toxicity to *Simocephalus serrulatus* (Daphnidae) and *Gambusia affinis* (Poeciliidae). Water Res 11:1013–1020, 1977.

Gilfillan ES: The use of scope-for-growth measurements in monitoring petroleum pollution. Rapp PV Reun Cons Int Explor Mer 179:71–75, 1980.

Goering JJ, Boisseau D, Hattori A: Effects of copper on silicic acid uptake by a marine phytoplankton population: Controlled ecosystem pollution experiment. Bull Mar Sci 27:58–65, 1977.

Goyer RA: The renal tubule in lead poisoning. I. Mitochondrial swelling and aminoaciduria. Lab Invest 19:71–77, 1968.

Goyer RA: Formation of intracellular inclusion bodies in heavy metal poisoning (lead, bismuth, and gold). Environ Health Perspect 4:97–98, 1973.

Hall A, Fielding AH, Butler M: Mechanisms of copper tolerance in the marine fouling alga *Ectocarpus siliculosus*—evidence for an exclusion mechanism. Mar Biol 54:195–199, 1979.

Hamilton MA, Russo RC, Thurston RV: Trimmed Spearman-Karber method for estimating median lethal concentrations in toxicity bioassays. Environ Sci Technol 11:714–719, 1977.

Harris WF: Microcosms as potential screening tools for evaluating transport and effects of toxic substances. Oak Ridge Natl Lab Environ Sci Div Publ 1506, EPA-600/3-80-042, 1980.

Harrison WG, Eppley RW, Renger EH: Phytoplankton nitrogen metabolism, nitrogen budgets, and observations on copper toxicity; controlled ecosystem pollution experiment. Bull Mar Sci 27:44–57, 1977.

Harriss RC, White DB, Macfarlane RB: Mercury compounds reduce photosynthesis by plankton. Science 170:736–737, 1970.

Hart BT: Trace metal complexing capacity of natural waters; a review. Environ Technol Lett 2:95–110, 1981.

Heit M, Fingerman M: The influence of size, sex and temperature on the toxicity of mercury to two species of crayfishes. Bull Environ Contam Toxicol 18:572–580, 1977.

Hessler A: The effects of lead on algae. I. Effects of Pb on viability and motility of *Platymonas subcordiformis* (Chlorophyta: Volvocales). Water Air Soil Pollut 3:371–385, 1974.

Hidaka I: The effects of transition metals on the palatal chemoreceptors of the carp. Jpn J Physiol 20:599–609, 1970.

Hidaka I, Yokota S: Taste receptor stimulation by sweet-tasting substances in the carp. Jpn J Physiol 17:652–666, 1967.

Hodson PV: Temperature effects on lactate-glycogen metabolism in zinc-intoxicated rainbow trout (*Salmo gairdneri*). J Fish Res Board Can 33:1393–1397, 1976a.

Hodson PV: δ-Aminolevulinic acid dehydratase activity of fish blood as an indicator of a harmful exposure to lead. J Fish Res Board Can 33:268–271, 1976b.

Hodson PV, Blunt BR, Spry DJ, Austin K: Evaluation of erythrocyte δ-amino levulinic acid dehydratase activity as a short-term indicator in fish of a harmful exposure to lead. J Fish Res Board Can 34:501–508, 1977.

Hodson PV, Borgmann U, Shear H: Toxicity of copper to aquatic biota. In: Copper in the Environment, Part II. Health Effects, edited by JO Nriagu, pp. 307–372. New York: Wiley-Interscience, 1979.

Hodson PV, Hilton JW, Blunt BR, Slinger SJ: Effects of dietary ascorbic acid on chronic lead toxicity to young rainbow trout (*Salmo gairdneri*). Can J Fish Aquat Sci 37:170–176, 1980.

Holcombe GW, Benoit DA, Leonard EN, McKim JM: Long-term effects of lead exposure on three generations of brook trout (*Salvelinus fontinalis*). J Fish Res Board Can 33:1731–1741, 1976.

Holden AV: Present levels of mercury in man and his environment. In: Mercury Contamination in Man and His Environment, Tech Rep 137, pp. 143–168. Vienna: International Atomic Energy Agency, 1972.

Howarth RS, Sprague JB: Copper lethality to rainbow trout in waters of various hardness and pH. Water Res 12:455–462, 1978.

Icely JD, Nott JA: Accumulation of copper within the "hepatopancreatic" caeca of *Corophium volutator* (Crustacea: Amphipoda). Mar Biol 57:193–199, 1980.

Ishio S: Behavior of fish exposed to toxic substances. In: Advances in Water Pollution Research, edited by O Jang, pp. 19–33. New York: Pergamon, 1965.

Jackson GA, Morgan JJ: Trace metal-chelator interactions and phytoplankton growth in seawater media; theoretical analysis and comparison with other reported observations. Limnol Oceanogr 23:268–282, 1978.

Janssen HH, Scholz N: Uptake and cellular distribution of cadmium in *Mytilus edulis*. Mar Biol 55:133–141, 1979.

Johansson-Sjobeck ML, Larsson A: Effects of inorganic lead on delta-aminolevulinic acid dehydratase activity and hematological variables in the rainbow trout, *Salmo gairdneri*. Arch Environ Contam Toxicol 8:419–431, 1979.

Johnels AG, Westermark T, Berg W, Persson PI, Sjostrand B: Pike (*Esox lucius* L.) and some other aquatic organisms in Sweden as indicators of mercury contamination in the environment. Oikos 18:323–333, 1967.

Jones JRE: Fish and River Pollution. London: Butterworth, 1964.

Joselow MM, Flores J: Application of the zinc protoporphyrin (ZP) test as a monitor of occupational exposure to lead. Am Ind Hyg Assoc J 38:63–66, 1977.

Kirchgessner M, Roth HP: Biochemical changes of hormones and metalloenzymes in zinc deficiency. In: Zinc in the Environment, Part II. Health Effects, pp. 77–103. New York: Wiley-Interscience, 1980.

Kleerekoper H, Westlake GF, Matis JH, Gensler PJ: Orientation of goldfish (*Carassius auratus*) in response to a shallow gradient of a sublethal concentration of copper in an open field. J Fish Res Board Can 29:45–54, 1972.

Koch RD, Elliot RL, O'Leary RM, Risoli DA: Trace element data for stream-sediment heavy-mineral concentrate samples for Bradfield Canal Quadrangle, Southeastern Alaska, U.S. Geol Surv Open File Rep 80-910C, pp. 1–68, 1980.

Koeppe DE, Miller RJ: Lead effects on corn mitochondrial respiration. Science 167:1376–1377, 1970.

Kostial K, Voak VB: Lead ions and synaptic transmission in the superior cervical ganglion of the cat. Br J Pharmacol 12:219–222, 1957.

Kuhnert PM, Kuhnert BB, Stokes RM: The effect of *in vivo* chromium exposure on Na/K- and Mg-ATPase activity in several tissues of the rainbow trout (*Salmo gairdneri*). Bull Environ Contam Toxicol 15:383–397, 1976.

Kuwabara JS: Toxicity to *Selenastrum capricornutum* (Chlorophyceae) relative to copper introduction rate. Paper presented at the Annual Phycological Society Meeting, Univ. of Indiana, Bloomington, 1981.

Kuwabara JS, North WJ: Culturing microscopic stages of *Macrocystis pyrifera* (Phaeophyta) in Aquil, a chemically defined medium. J Phycol 16:546–549, 1980.

Leber AP: A mechanism for cadmium- and zinc-induced tolerance to cadmium toxicity; involvement of metallothionein. PhD. thesis, Purdue Univ., West Lafayette, Ind., 1974.

Lee RM, Gerking SD: Sensitivity of fish eggs to acid stress. Water Res 14:1679–1681, 1980.

Leland IIV: Ultrastructural changes in the hepatocytes of juvenile rainbow trout and mature brown trout exposed to copper or zinc. Environ Toxicol Chem, 2:353–368, 1983.

Leland HV, Carter JL: Effects of copper on species composition of periphyton in a Sierra Nevada, California, stream. Freshwater Biol (in press), 1984a.

Leland HV, Carter JL: Effects of copper on production of periphyton, nitrogen fixation and processing of leaf litter in a Sierra Nevada, California, stream. Freshwater Biol (in press), 1984b.

Leland HV, Kent E: Effects of copper on microfaunal species composition in a Sierra Nevada, California stream. Verh Int Ver Limnol 21: 819–829, 1981.

Leland HV, McNurney JM: Lead transport in a river ecosystem. In: Proceedings of the International Conference on Transport of Persistent Chemicals in Aquatic Ecosystems, pp. 17–23. Ottawa, Canada, 1974.

Leland HV, Luoma SN, Fielden, JM: Bioaccumulation and toxicity of heavy metals and related trace elements. J Water Pollut Control Fed 51: 1592–1616, 1979.

Lett PF, Farmer GJ, Beamish FWH: Effect of copper on some aspects of the bioenergetics of rainbow trout (Salmo gairdneri). J Fish Res Board Can 33:1335–1342, 1976.

Lewis SD, Lewis WM: The effect of zinc and copper on the osmolarity of blood serum of the channel catfish, Ictalurus punctatus Rafinesque, and golden shiner, Notemigonus crysoleucas Mitchill. Trans Am Fish Soc 100:639–643, 1971.

Lloyd R: The toxicity of zinc sulphate to rainbow trout. Ann Appl Biol 48:84–94, 1960.

Lorz HW, McPherson BP: Effects of copper or zinc in freshwater on the adaptation to seawater and ATPase activity, and migratory disposition of coho salmon (Oncorhynchus kisutch). J Fish Res Board Can 33:2023–2030, 1976.

Luckey TD, Venugopal B: Metal Toxicity in Mammals. New York: Plenum, 1977.

Luoma SN: Detection of trace contaminant effects in aquatic ecosystems. J Fish Res Board Can 34:436–439, 1977.

Luoma SN: Bioavailability of trace elements to aquatic organisms. Sci Total Environ 28:1–22, 1983.

Magnusson VR, Harriss DK, Sun MS, Taylor DK, Glass GE: Relationships of activities of metalligand species to aquatic toxicity. In: Chemical Modeling in Aqueous Systems, edited by EA Jenne, pp. 657–680. Washington, D.C.: American Chemical Society, 1979.

Magos L: Factors affecting the uptake and retention of mercury by kidneys in rats. In: Mercury, Mercurials and Mercaptans, edited by MW Miller, TW Clarkson, pp. 167–186. Springfield, Ill.: Thomas, 1973.

Martin JH, Knauer GA, Flegal AR: Distribution of zinc in natural waters. In: Zinc in the Environment, Part I. Ecological Cycling, edited by JO Nriagu, pp. 193–197. New York: Wiley-Interscience, 1980.

Massaro EJ: Pharmacokinetics of toxic elements in rainbow trout. EPA-660/3-74-027, pp. 1–30. Buffalo: State Univ. of New York, 1974.

Massaro EJ, Giblin FJ: Uptake, distribution and concentration of methylmercury by rainbow trout (Salmo gairdneri) tissues. In: Trace Substances in Environmental Health, edited by DD Hemphill, pp. 107–112. Columbia, Mo.: Univ. of Missouri Press, 1972.

Mathys W: The role of malate, oxalate, and mustard oil glucosides in the evolution of zinc-resistance in herbage plants. Physiol Plant 40: 130–136, 1977.

Mathys W: Zinc tolerance by plants. In: Zinc in the Environment, Part II. Health Effects, edited by JO Nriagu, pp. 415–437. New York: Wiley-Interscience, 1980.

Matida Y, Kumada H, Kimura S, Nose T, Yokota M, Kawatsun H: Toxicity of mercury compounds to aquatic organisms and accumulation of the compound by the organisms. Bull Freshwater Fish Res Lab Tokyo 21:197–227, 1971.

McCarty LS, Houston AH: Effects of exposure to sublethal levels of cadmium upon water-electrolyte status in the goldfish (Carassius auratus). J Fish Biol 9:11–19, 1976.

McDuff RE, Morel FMM: Description and use of the chemical equilibrium program REDEQL2. Tech Rep EQ7302, WM Keck Engineering Laboratories, California Inst. of Technology, Pasadena, Calif., 1973.

McIntire CD: Some effects of current velocity on periphyton communities in laboratory streams. Hydrobiologia 27:559–570, 1966.

McKenney CL, Costlow JD: Interaction of temperature, salinity, and mercury on larval development of the xanthid crab, Rhithropanopeus harrisii (Gould). Ann Zool 17:922, 1977.

McKenney CL, Neff JM: Individual effects and

interactions of salinity, temperature, and zinc on larval development of the grass shrimp *Palaemonetes pugio*. I. Survival and developmental duration through metamorphosis. Mar Biol 52:177–188, 1979.

McKim JM: Evaluation of tests with early life stages of fish for predicting long-term toxicity. J Fish Res Board Can 34:1148–1154, 1977.

McKim JM, Christensen GM, Hunt EP: Changes in the blood of brook trout (*Salvelinus fontinalis*) after short-term and long-term exposure to copper. J Fish Res Board Can 27:1883–1889, 1970.

McKim JM, Olson GF, Holcombe GW, Hunt EP: Long-term effects of methylmercuric chloride on three generations of brook trout (*Salvelinus fontinalis*): Toxicity, accumulation, distribution, and elimination. J Fish Res Board Can 33:2726–2739, 1976.

McKim JM, Eaton JG, Holcombe GW: Metal toxicity to embryos and larvae of eight species of freshwater fish. II. Copper. Bull Environ Contam Toxicol 19:608–616, 1978.

McKnight DM: Interactions between freshwater plankton and copper speciation. PhD. thesis, Massachusetts Inst. of Technology, Cambridge, Mass., 1979.

McLeay DJ: Sensitivity of blood cell counts in juvenile coho salmon (*Oncorhynchus kisutch*) to stressors including sublethal concentrations of pulpmill effluent and zinc. J Fish Res Board Can 32:2357–2364, 1975.

Medine AJ, Porcella DB, Cowen PA: Microcosm Dynamics and Response to a Heavy Metal Loading in a Lake Powell Sediment-Water-Gas Ecosystem, pp. 1–131. Logan, Utah: Utah State Univ. and Utah State Foundation, 1977.

Menzel DW, Case J: Concept and design: Controlled ecosystem pollution experiment. Bull Mar Sci 27:1–7, 1977.

Merlini M: Heavy metal contamination. In: Impingement of Man on the Oceans, edited by DW Hood, pp. 461–486. New York: Wiley, 1971.

Metz EN, Sagone AL: Effect of copper on the erythrocyte hexose manophosphate. J Lab Clin Med 80:405, 1972.

Miettinen JK: The accumulation and excretion of heavy metals in organisms. In: Ecological Toxicology Research, edited by AD McIntyre, CF Mills, pp. 215–229. New York: Plenum, 1975.

Miller WE, Greene JC, Shiroyama T: The *Selenastrum capricornutum* Printz Algal Assay Bottle Test: Experimental Design, Application, and Data Interpretation Protocol, pp. 1–126. EPA-600/9-78-018. Corvallis, Ore.: U.S. EPA, 1978.

Mogilnicka EM, Piotrowski JK, Trojanowska B: Effect of certain metals (cadmium, mercury, zinc, copper, lead, manganese, vanadium) on the metallothionein level in rat liver and kidneys. Med Pr 26:147–155, 1975.

Moore JF, Goyer RA: Lead-induced inclusion bodies: Composition and probable role in lead metabolism. Environ Health Perspect 7:121–127, 1974.

Morel FMM, Rueter JG, Anderson DM, Guillard RRL: Aquil: A chemically defined phytoplankton culturing medium for trace metal studies. J Phycol 15:135–141, 1979.

Morgan M, Tovell PWA: The structure of the gill of the trout, *Salmo gairdneri* (Richardson). Z Zellforsch Mikrosk Anat 142:147–162, 1973.

Natochin YV, Krayushkina LS, Maslova MN, Sokolova MM, Bakhteeva VT, Lavrova EA: Enzyme activity in gills and kidneys and endocrine factors in the regulation of ion exchange in down-stream migrating and spawning sockeye salmon, *Oncorhynchus nerka*. J Ichthyol 15:131–140, 1975.

Nelson DA, Calabrese A, Nelson BA, MacInnes JR, Wenzloff DR: Biological effects of heavy metals on juvenile bay scallops *Argopecten irradians* in short term exposures. Bull Environ Contam Toxicol 16:275–282, 1976.

Nordstrom DK, Jenne EA, Averett RC: Heavy metal discharges into Shasta Lake and Keswick reservoirs on the upper Sacramento River, California; a reconnaissance during low flow, pp. 1–25, Rep 76-49, U.S. Geological Survey, Menlo Park, Calif., 1977.

Norseth T: Studies of intracellular distribution of mercury. In: Chemical Fallout, edited by MW Miller, GG Berg, pp. 408–419. Springfield, Ill.: Thomas, 1969.

Nuzzi R: Toxicity of mercury to phytoplankton. Nature (Lond) 237:38–40, 1972.

Nyberg D: Breeding systems and resistance to environmental stress in ciliates. Evolution 28: 367–380, 1974.

Oswald WJ, Gaonkar SA: Batch assays for determination of algal growth potential. In: Proceedings Eutrophication and Biostimulation Assessment Workshop, edited by EJ Middlebrook, TE Maloney, CF Powers, LM Kaack, pp. 23–39. Berkeley: Univ. of California, 1969.

Overnell J: The effects of heavy metals in photosynthesis and loss of cell potassium in two species of marine algae, *Dunaliella tertiolecta* and *Phaeodactylum tricornutum.* Mar Biol 29:99–103, 1975.

Pace F, Ferrara R, DelCarratore G: Effects of sublethal doses of copper sulphate and lead nitrate on growth and pigment composition of *Dunaliella salina.* Teod. Bull Environ Contam Toxicol 17:679–685, 1977.

Pagenkopf GK: Zinc speciation and toxicity to fish. In: Zinc in the Environment, Part II. Health Effects, edited by JO Nriagu, pp. 353–361. New York: Wiley-Interscience, 1980.

Pagenkopf GK, Russo RC, Thurston PV: Effect of complexation on toxicity of copper to fishes. J Fish Res Board Can 31:462–465, 1974.

Patterson CC: Lead in the environment. In: Lead Poisoning in Man and the Environment, pp. 71–87. New York: MSS Information Corp., 1973.

Pentreath RJ: The accumulation of organic mercury from seawater by the plaice, *Pleuronectes platessa* (L.) J Exp Mar Biol Ecol 24:121–132, 1976a.

Pentreath RJ: The accumulation of mercury from food by the plaice *Pleuronectes platessa* (L.). J Exp Mar Biol Ecol 25:51–65, 1976b.

Pillay KKS, Thomas CC, Sondel JA, Hyche CM: Mercury pollution of Lake Erie ecosphere. In: Mercury Poisoning, Part I, edited by E Mayz, pp. 88–97. New York: MMS Information Corp., 1973.

Pirson A, Lorenzen H, Koepper A: A sensitive stage in synchronous cultures of *Chlorella.* Plant Physiol 34:353–355, 1959.

Porcella DB: Continuous-flow (chemostat) assays. In: Proceedings Eutrophication and Biostimulation Assessment Workshop, edited by EJ Middlebrook, TE Malone, CF Powers, LM Kaack, pp. 7–22. Berkeley: Univ. of California, 1969.

Price CA, Quigley JW: A method for determining quantitative zinc requirements for growth. Soil Sci 101:11–16, 1966.

Rainbow PS, Scott AG: Two heavy metal-binding proteins in the midgut gland of the crab *Carcinus maenas.* Mar Biol 55:143–150, 1979.

Reeve MR, Gamble JC, Walter MA: Experimental observations on the effects of copper on copepods and other zooplankton; controlled ecosystem pollution experiment. Bull Mar Sci 27:92–104, 1977.

Rice DW, Harrison FL: Copper sensitivity of Pacific herring, *Clupea harengus pallasi,* during its early life history. Fish Bull 76:347–356, 1978.

Roesijadi G: Influence of copper on the clam *Protothaca staminea:* Effects on gills and occurrence of copper-binding proteins. Biol Bull 158: 233–247, 1980.

Rothstein A: Mercaptans, the biological targets for mercurials. In: Mercury, Mercurials and Mercaptans, edited by MW Miller, TW Clarkson, pp. 68–95. Springfield, Ill.: Thomas, 1973.

Ruddell CL, Rains DW: The relationship between zinc and copper and the basophils of two crassostreid oysters, *Crassostrea gigas* and *Crassostrea virginica.* Comp Biochem Physiol 51A: 585–591, 1975.

Sabodash VM: Size of eggs and larvae from carps of different ages under normal conditions and under the effect of elevated levels of zinc sulfate. Biol Nauka 20:62, 1977.

Saifullah SM: Inhibitory effects of copper on marine dinoflagellates. Mar Biol 44:299–308, 1978.

Saliba LJ, Krzyz RM: Acclimation and tolerance of *Artemia salina* to copper salts. Mar Biol 38: 231–238, 1976.

Saunders RL, Sprague JB: Effects of copper-zinc mining pollution on a spawning migration of Atlantic salmon. Water Res 1:419–432, 1967.

Schaule B, Patterson C: The occurrence of lead in the northeast Pacific and the effects of anthropogenic inputs. In: Proceedings of an International Experts Discussion on Lead: Occurrence, Fate and Pollution in the Marine Environment, edited by M Branica, pp. 31–43. Oxford: Pergamon, 1978.

Schmidt-Nielsen B: Osmoregulation: Effect of

salinity and heavy metals. Fed Am Soc Exp Biol 33:2137–2146, 1974.

Schulz-Baldes M, Lewin RA: Lead uptake in two marine phytoplankton organisms. Biol Bull 150:118–127, 1976.

Schweiger G: Die toxicologische Einwirkung von Schwermetallsalzen auf Fische und Fischnährtiere. Arch Fischereiwiss 8:54–78, 1957.

Sellers CM, Heath AG, Bass ML: The effect of sublethal concentrations of copper and zinc on ventilatory activity. Blood oxygen and pH in rainbow trout (*Salmo gairdneri*). Water Res 9: 401–408, 1975.

Sick LV, Windom HL: Effects of environmental levels of mercury and cadmium on rates of metal uptake and growth physiology of selected genera of marine phytoplankton. In: Proceedings of a Symposium on Mineral Cycling in Southeastern Ecosystems, Augusta, Ga., pp. 239–249. Energy Research and Development Administration, 1974.

Silbergeld EK, Carroll PT, Goldberg AM: Neurotoxicity of lead: A review of experimental studies. In: Proceedings of an International Conference on Heavy Metals in the Environment, edited by TC Hutchinson, University of Toronto, pp. 213–228, 1975.

Silverberg BA: Ultrastructural localization of lead in *Stigeoclonium tenue* (Chlorophyceae, Ulothrichales) as demonstrated by cytochemical and X-ray microanalysis. Phycologia 14:265–274, 1975.

Silverberg BA, Stokes PM, Ferstenberg LB: Intranuclear complexes in a copper-tolerant green alga. J Cell Biol 69:210–214, 1976.

Six KM, Goyer RA: Experimental enhancement of lead toxicity by low dietary calcium. J Lab Clin Med 76:933–942, 1970.

Skaar H, Rystad B, Jensen A: The uptake of [63]Ni by the diatom *Phaeodactylum tricornutum*. Physiol Plant 32:353–358, 1974.

Skidmore JF, Tovell PWA: Toxic effects of zinc sulphate on the gills of rainbow trout. Water Res 6:217–230, 1972.

Solbe JF de LG: The toxicity of zinc sulfate to rainbow trout in very hard water. Water Res 8: 389–391, 1974.

Somero GN, Yancey PH, Chow TJ, Snyder CB: Lead effects on tissue and whole organism respiration of the estuarine teleost fish, *Gillichtys mirabilis*. Arch Environ Contam Toxicol 6: 349–354, 1977.

Spehar RL: Cadmium and zinc toxicity to flagfish, *Jordanella floridae*. J Fish Res Board Can 33: 1939–1945, 1976.

Spencer DW, Brewer PG: The distribution of copper, zinc and nickel in seawater of the Gulf of Maine and the Sargasso Sea. Geochim Cosmochim Acta 33:325–339, 1969.

Sprague JB: Lethal concentrations of copper and zinc for young Atlantic salmon. J Fish Res Board Can 21:17, 1964.

Sprague JB: Avoidance reactions of rainbow trout in zinc sulphate solution. Water Res 2:367–372, 1968.

Sprague JB, Ramsay B: Lethal levels of mixed copper-zinc solutions for juvenile salmon. J Fish Res Board Can 22:425–432, 1965.

Sprague JB, Elson PF, Saunders RL: Sublethal copper-zinc pollution in a salmon river: A field and laboratory study. Int J Air Water Pollut 9: 531–543, 1965.

Steemann Nielsen E, Kamp-Nielsen L, Wium-Andersen S: The effect of deleterious concentrations of copper on the photosynthesis of *Chlorella pyrenoidosa*. Physiol Plant 22:1121–1133, 1969.

Steemann Nielsen E, Wium-Andersen S: Copper ions as poison to the sea and freshwater. Mar Biol 6:93–97, 1970.

Stewart WDP: Algal Physiology and Biochemistry. Los Angeles: Univ. of California Press, 1974.

Stokes PM: Copper accumulation in freshwater biota. In: Copper in the Environment, Part I, Ecological Cycling, edited by JO Nriagu, pp. 357–381. New York: Wiley-Interscience, 1980.

Stokes PM, Hutchinson TC: Copper toxicity to phytoplankton as affected by organic ligands, other cations and inherent tolerance of algae to copper. In: Toxicity to Biota of Metals Forms in Natural Water, edited by RW Andrew, PV Hodson, DE Konasewich, pp. 159–185. Windsor, Ont.: International Joint Commission. Great Lakes Research Advisory Board, 1976.

Stokes PM, Hutchinson TC, Krauter K: Heavy metal tolerance in algae isolated from contaminated lakes near Sudbury, Ontario. Can J Bot 51:2155–2168, 1973.

Sullivan JT, Cheng TC: Heavy metal toxicity to *Biomphalaria glabrata* (Mollusca: Pulmonata). Ann NY Acad Sci 266:437–444, 1975.

Sunda W, Guillard RRL; The relationship between cupric ion and the toxicity of copper to phytoplankton. J Mar Res 34:511–529, 1976.

Sunda WG, Engel DW, Thuotte RM: Effect of chemical speciation on the toxicity of cadmium to grass shrimp *Paleomanetes pugio:* Importance of free cadmium ion. Environ Sci Technol 12:409–413, 1978.

Sutterlin AM: Pollutants and the chemical senses of aquatic animals; perspective and review. Chem Senses Flavor 1:167–178, 1974.

Swallow KC, Westall JC, McKnight DM, Morel NML, Morel FMM: Potentiometric determination of copper complexation by phytoplankton exudates. Limnol Oceanogr 23:538–542, 1978.

Syazuki K: Studies on the toxic effects of industrial waste on fish and shell-fishes. Suisan Daigakko Kenkyu Hokoku 13:158–211, 1964.

Tagatz ME, Ivey JM, Lehman HK, Ogelsky JL: Effects of Sevin on the development of experimental estuarine communities. J Toxicol Environ Health 5:643–652, 1979.

Talbot V, Magee RJ: Naturally occurring heavy metal binding proteins in invertebrates. Arch Environ Contam Toxicol 7:73–81, 1978.

Terao T, Owen CA, Jr: Nature of copper compounds in liver supernate and bile of rats; studies with [67]Cu. Am J Physiol 224:682–686, 1973.

Thomas WH, Seiberg DLR: Effects of copper on the dominance and the diversity of algae; controlled ecosystem pollution experiment. Bull Mar Sci 27:23–33, 1977.

Thomas WH, Holm-Hansen O, Seibert DLR, Azam F, Hodson R, Takahashi M: Effects of copper on phytoplankton standing crop and productivity; controlled ecosystem pollution experiment. Bull Mar Sci 27:34–43, 1977.

Thorton I: Copper in soils and sediments. In: Copper in the Environment, Part I, Ecological Cycling, edited by JO Nriagu, pp. 171–216. New York: Wiley-Interscience, 1980.

Thurberg FP, Cable WD, Dawson MA, MacInnes DR, Wenzloff DR: Respiratory response of larval, juvenile and adult surf clams, *Spisula solidissima,* to silver. In: Respiration of Marine Organisms, edited by JJ Cech, DW Bridges, DB Horton, pp. 41–52. Portland, Maine: TRIGOM, 1975.

Thurberg FP, Gould E, Dawson MA: Some physiological effects of the "Argo Merchant" oil spill on several marine teleosts and bivalve molluscs. In: In the Wake of the "Argo Merchant," pp. 103–108. Kingston, R.I.: Univ. of Rhode Island, 1978.

Trainor FR: Introductory Phycology. New York: Wiley, 1978.

Truesdell AH, Jones BF: WATEQ, a computer program for calculating chemical equilibria of natural waters. J Res U.S. Geol Surv 2:233–248, 1974.

Trump BF, Jones RT, Sahaphong S: Cellular effects of mercury on fish tubules. In: Pathology of Fishes, edited by WE Ribelin, G Migaki, pp. 585–612. Madison, Wis.: Univ. of Wisconsin Press, 1975.

Ulmer DD, Vallee BL: Effects of lead on biochemical systems. Trace Subst Environ Health 2, Proc Univ Mo Annu Conf 1968, pp. 7–27, 1969.

Underwood EJ: Trace Elements in Human and Animal Nutrition. New York: Academic, 1977.

U.S. Environmental Protection Agency: Guidelines for deriving water quality criteria for the protection of aquatic life. Fed Regist 42:21506, 1978; Fed Regist 43:29028, 1978.

U.S. Environmental Protection Agency: Ambient Water Quality Criteria for Copper. EPA 440/5-80-036. Washington, D.C.: U.S. EPA, 1980a.

U.S. Environmental Protection Agency: Ambient Water Quality Criteria for Zinc. EPA 440/5-80-079. Washington, D.C.: U.S. EPA, 1980b.

U.S. Environmental Protection Agency: Ambient Water Quality Criteria for Lead. EPA 440/5-80-057. Washington, D.C.: U.S. EPA, 1980c.

U.S. Environmental Protection Agency: Ambient Water Quality Criteria for Mercury. EPA 440/5-80-058. Washington, D.C.: U.S. EPA, 1980d.

Vaccaro RF, Azam F, Hodson RE: Response of natural marine bacterial populations to copper; controlled ecosystem pollution experiment. Bull Mar Sci 27:17–22, 1977.

Vernberg WB, DeCoursey PJ, Padgett WJ: Synergistic effects of environmental variables on larvae of *Uca pugilator.* Mar Biol 22:307–312, 1973.

Vernberg WB, DeCoursey PJ, O'Hara J: Multiple environmental factor effects on physiology and behavior of the fiddler crab *Uca pugilator*. In: Pollution and Physiology of Marine Organisms, edited by FJ Vernberg, WB Vernberg, pp. 381–425. New York: Academic, 1974.

Vijayamadhavan KT, Iwai I: Histochemical observations on the permeation of heavy metals into taste buds of goldfish. Bull Jpn Soc Sci Fish 41: 631–639, 1975.

Wacker WE: Nucleic acids and metals, III. Changes in nucleic acid, protein, and metal content as a consequence of zinc deficiency in *Euglena gracilis*. Biochemistry 1:859–865, 1962.

Wagemann R, Barica J: Speciation and rate of loss of copper from lakewater with implications for toxicity. Water Res 13:515–523, 1979.

Waiwood KG, Beamish FWH: The effect of copper, hardness and pH on growth of rainbow trout (*Salmo gairdneri*). J Fish Biol 13:591–598, 1978.

Ward GS, Parrish PR: Evaluation of early life-stage toxicity tests with embryos and juveniles of sheepshead minnows (*Cyprinodon variegatus*). In: Aquatic Toxicology, edited by JG Eaton, Parrish PR, AC Hendrichs, pp. 243–247. STP 707. Philadelphia: ASTM, 1980.

Ward WE, Brooks RR, Reeves RD: Copper, cadmium, lead and zinc in soils, streams, waters and natural vegetation around the Tui Mine, Te Aroha, New Zealand. NZ J Sci 19:81–89, 1976.

Weis JS, Weis P: Effects of heavy metals on development of the killifish, *Fundulus heteroclitus*. J Fish Biol 11:39–44, 1977.

Westall JC, Zachary JL, Morel FM: MINEQL; a computer program for the calculation of chemical equilibrium composition of aqueous systems, Ralph M. Parsons Water Quality Lab Tech Note 18, pp. 1–91, Cambridge: Massachusetts Institute of Technology, 1976.

Westfall BA: Coagulation film anoxia in fishes. Ecology 26:283–287, 1945.

Westlake GF, Kleerekoper H, Matis J: The locomotor response of goldfish to a steep gradient of copper ions. Water Resour Res 8:103–106, 1974.

Whitton BA: Toxicity of zinc, copper and lead to Chlorophyta from flowing waters. Arch Microbiol 72:353–360, 1970.

Whitton BA: Zinc and plants in rivers and streams. In: Zinc in the Environment, Part II. Health Effects, edited by JO Nriagu, pp. 363–400. New York: Wiley-Interscience, 1980.

Wihlidal H, Stehlik G, Elsenreich W, Biebl R: Effect of mercury ions on the DNA synthesis and DNA repair in *Chlorella fusca* and *Chlamydomonas reinhardi*. Bodenkultur 27:221–228, 1976.

Windom HL, Taylor FE, Waiters EM: Possible influence of atmospheric transport on the total mercury content of southeastern Atlantic continental shelf surface water. Deep Sea Res 22: 629–633, 1975.

Winge DR, Premakumar R, Rajagopalan KV: Metal-induced formation of metallothionein in rat liver. Arch Biochem Biophys 170:242–252, 1975.

Winner RW, VanDyke JS, Caris N, Farrell MP: Response of the macroinvertebrate fauna to a copper gradient in an experimentally-polluted stream. Verh Int Ver Limnol 19:2121–2127, 1975.

Wolfe DA: Zinc enzymes in *Crassostrea virginica*. J Fish Res Board Can 27:59–69, 1970.

Woolery ML, Lewin RA: The effects of lead on algae. IV. Effects of lead on respiration and photosynthesis of *Phaeodactylum tricornutum* (Bacillariophyceae). Water Air Soil Pollut 6:25–31, 1977.

Young DR, Jan T, Hershelman GP: Cycling of zinc in the nearshore marine environment. In: Zinc in the Environment, Part I, Ecological Cycling, edited by JO Nriagu, pp. 297–335. New York: Wiley-Interscience, 1980.

Zitko V, Carson WV, Carson WG: Prediction of incipient lethal levels of copper to juvenile Atlantic salmon in the presence of humic acid by cupric electrodes. Bull Environ Contam Toxicol 10:265–271, 1973.

Chapter 14

Polycyclic Aromatic Hydrocarbons

J. M. Neff

INTRODUCTION

Polycyclic aromatic hydrocarbons (PAH) constitute one of several classes of organic pollutants that are released into the environment in large quantities due in large part to human activities. PAH are components of crude and refined petroleum and of coal. Oil spills are a major source of PAH in freshwater and marine environments. Combustion of organic materials in fires or in internal combustion engines produces PAH which are released to the environment in exhaust particulates and in solid residues (ash).

Concern about PAH in the environment arises from the fact that many of them are quite persistent and some are known to be potent carcinogens in mammals. The environmental effects of most of the PAH that are not carcinogenic are poorly understood. The purpose of this review is

to summarize and synthesize what is known about the impact of PAH on aquatic organisms and ecosystems.

TERMINOLOGY

PAH are composed of carbon and hydrogen arranged in the form of two or more fused aromatic (benzene) rings. Two aromatic rings are said to be fused when a pair of carbon atoms is shared. The resulting structure is a molecule with all the carbon and hydrogen atoms lying in a single plane. Naphthalene ($C_{10}H_8$), which consists of two fused aromatic rings, is the PAH with the lowest molecular weight. The largest fused-ring aromatic system is graphite, an allotropic form of elemental carbon. Of primary environmental concern are mobile hydrocarbons ranging in molecular weight (MW) from naphthalene ($C_{10}H_8$, MW 128.16) to coronene ($C_{24}H_{12}$, MW 300.36). PAH of higher molecular weight are relatively immobile because of their large molecular volumes and extremely low volatility and solubility. Among the mobile forms are thousands of compounds that differ in the number and position of aromatic rings and in the number, chemistry, and position of substituents on the basic ring system.

Several systems of nomenclature have been used to describe PAH ring structures. Nomenclature used in this review is that adopted by the International Union of Pure and Applied Chemistry (IUPAC) and described in detail in The Ring Index (Patterson et al., 1960). Carbon atoms are numbered clockwise, and carbons common to two or more rings are not numbered. Ring faces, except those shared by two aromatic rings, are lettered; side "a" is the ring face between carbons 1 and 2, and the letters proceed around the molecule in a clockwise direction. Structural formulas of some typical PAH, with examples of the numbering and lettering system, are shown in Fig. 1.

PAH undergo three types of chemical reactions characteristic of aromatic hydrocarbons: electrophilic substitution, oxidation, and reduction. Oxidation and reduction reactions destroy the aromatic character of the affected benzene ring, but electrophilic substitution does not.

SOURCES OF AQUATIC POLYCYCLIC AROMATIC HYDROCARBONS

Until recently, it was generally considered that PAH are formed only during high-temperature (e.g., 700°C) pyrolysis of organic materials. The discovery in fossil fuels of complex mixtures of PAH spanning a wide molecular weight range has led to the conclusion that, given sufficient time (e.g., millions of years), pyrolysis of organic materials at temperatures as low as 100–150°C can lead to production of PAH (Blumer, 1976). In addition, there has been considerable speculation during the past 20 yr, and some experimental evidence, that PAH are synthesized by bacteria, fungi, and plants. Thus, PAH may be formed in

three ways: high-temperature pyrolysis of organic materials, low- to moderate-temperature diagenesis of sedimentary organic material to form fossil fuels, and direct biosynthesis by microbes and plants.

Biosynthesis

A wide variety of organic molecules containing fused-ring polyaromatic systems are synthesized by organisms, particularly bacteria, fungi, and higher plants (Gerarde and Gerarde, 1962). Many of these compounds are not true PAH since they contain oxygen, nitrogen, or sulfur substituents. Microorganisms, higher plants, and even a few animals synthesize a wide variety of polycyclic quinone pigments (Thompson, 1971). Structures of two polyaromatic quinone pigments are shown in Fig. 2. Naphthoquinones are common in flowering plants. Vitamin K_2 is a naphthoquinone. The largest group of naturally occurring polycyclic quinones is the anthraquinones.

Polycyclic quinones are readily reduced to the corresponding hydroquinones and to the parent PAH with further reduction. Conditions suitable for the reductive synthesis of PAH from biogenic polycyclic quinones may occur in highly anaerobic water basin sediments and waterlogged soils. Perylene, presumably derived from reduction of biogenic perylene quinones (Fig. 2), has frequently been reported at high concentrations in anaerobic freshwater and marine sediments (Orr and Grady, 1967; Aizenshtat, 1973; Rose, 1977; Wakeham, 1977). PAH assemblages produced by reduction of biological quinones are expected to be compositionally quite simple.

Since the early 1960s, several attempts have been made to demonstrate the de novo biosynthesis of PAH by bacteria, algae, and higher plants. Several investigators have provided circumstantial evidence that such biosynthesis does take place (Graf and Diel, 1966; Borneff et al., 1968; Mallet, 1972). More recent investigations have shown that, in most cases, increasing concentrations of PAH in experimental bacteria or plants could be attributed to accumulation by the organisms of PAH from

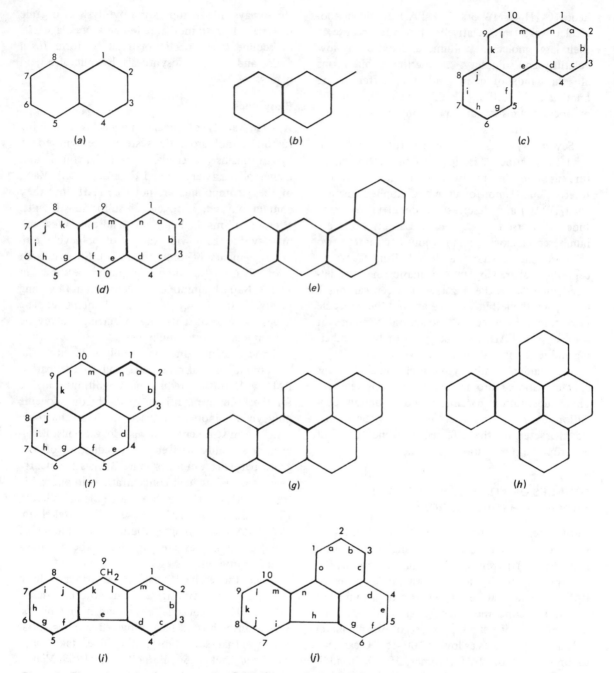

Figure 1 Ring structures of representative PAH. The numbering and lettering system for several PAH is also given. Compounds are: (a) naphthalene, (b) 2-methylnaphthalene, (c) phenanthrene, (d) anthracene, (e) benz[a]anthracene, (f) pyrene, (g) benzo[a]pyrene, (h) benzo[e]pyrene, (i) fluorene, and (j) fluoranthene.

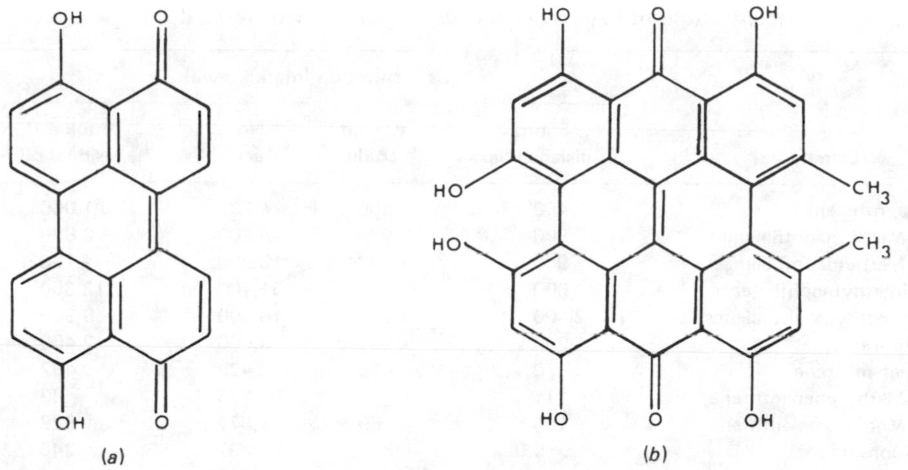

Figure 2 Examples of natural products with a PAH-like structure: (a) 4,9-Dihydroxyperylene-3,10-quinone from the fungus *Daldinia concentrica*. Closely related pigments are found in the insect family Aphididae. (b) Hypericin from St. John's wort, *Hypericum perforatum*.

the ambient medium (Grimmer and Duval, 1970; Payer et al., 1975; Hase and Hites, 1976). Therefore, evidence for direct biosynthesis of PAH remains equivocal.

Fossil Fuels

Coal is generally considered an aromatic material. As much as 75% of the carbon present in bituminous coal may be in aromatic form (Wiser, 1973). Six-membered rings are dominant, but five-membered rings are also present. Most of the aromatic units in coal are covalently linked to form a high molecular weight polymeric material. Therefore PAH are not extracted easily from coal. Several PAH have been identified in coal by special techniques (Hayatsu et al., 1975; Woo et al., 1976). They include naphthalene, phenanthrene, fluorene, fluoranthene, benz[a]anthracene, benzo[a]pyrene, benzo[e]pyrene, dibenzo[cd,m]-pyrene, and perylene.

Crude petroleum and most refined petroleum products are extremely complex mixtures of many thousands of organic compounds. Hydrocarbons are most abundant, usually representing more than 75% of the weight of the oil. The remainder is made up primarily of various sulfur-, oxygen-, and nitrogen-containing organic compounds (Speers and Whitehead, 1969). Petroleums from different sources vary tremendously in relative concentrations of the different hydrocarbon types present. Typical crude petroleums may contain from 0.2 to more than 7% PAH. Kerosene, gasolene, and diesel oil have relatively low concentrations of tricyclic and larger PAH, while heavy oil products such as bunker c oil (residual oil) and asphalt may contain several percent PAH (Guerin et al., 1978). Shale oil and coal-derived synthetic crude oils may contain as much as 15% PAH. Thus, crude and refined oils contain significant quantities of PAH. Shale oil and coal-derived synthetic crudes tend to have the highest concentrations.

The chemical complexity of petroleum has hampered attempts to identify and quantify specific PAH in oil samples. The four API (American Petroleum Institute) reference oils have been used extensively in biological effects studies and considerable information is available about their chemical composition (Anderson et al., 1974; Pancirov, 1974; Pancirov and Brown, 1975; Youngblood and Blumer, 1975). Concentrations of several PAH in these oils are listed in Table 1. Most oils contain the same hydrocarbons, but the relative propor-

Table 1 Concentrations of PAH in Two Crude Oils and Two Refined Oils[a]

Compound	Concentration (mg/kg, ppm)			
	South Louisiana crude	Kuwait crude	No. 2 fuel oil	Bunker C residual oil
Naphthalene	400	400	4,000	1,000
1-Methylnaphthalene	800	500	8,200	2,800
2-Methylnaphthalene	900	700	18,900	4,700
Dimethylnaphthalenes	3,600	2,000	31,100	12,300
Trimethylnaphthalenes	2,400	1,900	18,400	8,800
Fluorenes	200	<100	3,600	2,400
Phenanthrene	70	26	429	482
1-Methylphenanthrene	111	—	173	43
2-Methylphenanthrene	144	89	7,677	828
Fluoranthene	5.0	2.9	37	240
Pyrene	3.5	4.5	41	23
Benz[a]anthracene	1.7	2.3	1.2	90
Chrysene	17.56	6.9	2.2	196
Triphenylene	10	2.8	1.4	31
Benzo[ghi]fluoranthene	1	<1		
Benzo[b]fluoranthene	<0.5	<1		
Benzo[j]fluoranthene	<0.9	<1		
Benzo[k]fluoranthene	<1.3	<1		
Benzo[a]pyrene	0.75	2.8	0.6	44
Benzo[e]pyrene	2.5	0.5	0.1	10
Perylene	34.8	<0.1	—	22
Benzo[ghi]perylene	1.6	<1		

[a]The oils are API reference oils. Naphthalene-fluorenes from Anderson et al. (1974b) and phenanthrene-benzo[ghi]perylene from Pancirov and Brown (1975).

tions of different hydrocarbons vary widely from one oil to another. Nearly always, alkyl homologs are present at higher concentrations in crude and refined oils than are the parent PAH (Pancirov and Brown, 1975; Youngblood and Blumer, 1975; Blumer, 1976). This is reflected in the relative concentrations of naphthalene and C_1–C_3 naphthalenes in the four API oils. PAH in crude and shale oils are usually more highly alkylated than those in refined oils. C_2–C_4 homologs are usually most abundant and there is a decreasing frequency of PAH with seven or more alkyl carbons. A similar predominance of alkyl PAH is seen in several petroleum by-products such as creosote, tar, and asphalt (Wallcave et al., 1971).

Pyrolysis

Most PAH in the environment are formed during incomplete combustion of organic matter at high temperatures (Suess, 1976). Several mechanisms have been proposed for the formation of PAH by pyrolysis. Complex organic molecules are partially cracked to lower molecular weight free radicals. Pyrosynthesis of PAH then proceeds by rapid combination of free radicals containing one, two, or many carbons (Badger et al., 1960). Although almost any type of organic compound can be a precursor of PAH under the right pyrolytic conditions, cyclic compounds, both saturated and unsaturated, are particularly good precursors. Optimal conditions for PAH pyrosynthesis include a fuel-rich flame (high fuel-to-air ratio) and a flame temperature above about 500°C. Nearly all of the airborne PAH produced by flame pyrolysis are associated with the particulate fraction produced during combustion (soots and carbon blacks).

A great many domestic and industrial activities involve pyrosynthesis of PAH. The resulting PAH may be released to the environment in airborne particulates or in solid or liquid by-products of the pyrolytic process. Domestic activities that produce significant quantities of PAH include cigarette smoking, home heating with wood or fossil fuels, waste incineration, broiling and smoking of foods, and use of internal combustion engines. Industrial activities that produce large quantities include coal coking; production of carbon blacks, creosote, coal tar, and related materials from fossil fuels; petroleum refining; synfuel production from coal; and use of Soderberg electrodes in aluminum smelters, ferrosilicium and iron works, and so on.

RATES AND ROUTES OF ENTRY INTO THE AQUATIC ENVIRONMENT

Polycyclic aromatic hydrocarbons formed by the processes discussed above may reach the aquatic environment by a variety of routes. Major routes of entry of PAH into marine and fresh waters include biosynthesis, spillage and seepage of fossil fuels, discharge of domestic and industrial wastes, fallout or rainout from air, and runoff from land.

Andelman and Snodgrass (1972) suggested that most of the PAH in the marine environment are derived from endogenous sources (e.g., biosynthesis). However, as indicated above, direct PAH biosynthesis has not been demonstrated conclusively. The compositional complexity of PAH assemblages in marine and freshwater sediments is much greater than would be expected if these assemblages were produced by biosynthesis (Youngblood and Blumer, 1975; Hites, 1976; Hites et al., 1980). If PAH biosynthesis does occur, it would be restricted to anoxic sediments, and the PAH

assemblages formed would be compositionally simple and probably immobile (Suess, 1976).

Spillage and seepage of petroleum into marine and fresh waters is an important source of PAH. World oil production in 1971 is estimated as 2478.4 million metric tons (NAS, 1975). Annual world oil production rose sharply during the 1970s and only now is beginning to level off as demand decreases (Flower, 1978). Approximately 6 million metric tons of oil (about 0.25% of production) enters the oceans each year from natural and anthropogenic sources (NAS, 1975). Since crude and refined oils may contain up to several percent total PAH, this accidental spillage and natural seepage represents a quantitatively important input of PAH to the aquatic environment.

Industrial and domestic sewage often contains high concentrations of particulate and soluble PAH. Several of the industrial sources of these PAH were discussed above. Storm sewage (runoff from roadways) contains PAH from wear and leaching of asphalt road surfaces, wear of vehicle tires that contain carbon black, condensation from vehicular exhaust, and from the all too common practice of oiling roadsides and unpaved roadways with used crankcase oil, which is high in PAH. MacKenzie and Hunter (1979) identified used crankcase oil as the main source of PAH and related sulfur heterocyclics in stormwater runoff from Philadelphia, Pennsylvania.

Treated and sometimes untreated liquid sewage is nearly always discharged to any available water body (e.g., river, lake, estuary). Solid residues from activated sludge treatment of wastes may be disposed of in the ocean or in landfills. Liquid domestic sewage usually contains less than 1 μg/l total PAH, industrial sewage 5–15 μg/l (Borneff and Kunte, 1965), and sewage sludge 1–30 mg/kg (Grimmer et al., 1978; Nicholls et al., 1979).

Most of the PAH emitted to the atmosphere during pyrolysis of organic matter are adsorbed on microscopic particles (NAS, 1972; Suess, 1976). However, lower molecular weight PAH (naphthalene and pyrene) have sufficiently high vapor pressures that they can exist at significant concentrations in the vapor phase (Pupp et al., 1974). Atmospheric processes that result in deposition of airborne PAH on land and water include rainout, dry fallout, and vapor phase deposition onto surfaces. The first two processes are the primary mechanisms for deposition of airborne particulate PAH. Residence time of particulate PAH in the atmosphere depends on rates of chemical degradation and photodegradation and on settling rate. Suess (1976) estimated that, in the absence of rainfall, submicrometer particles remain in the atmosphere from a few days to several weeks, whereas particles in the range 1–10 μm are deposited in a few days or less. Rainfall can be expected to reduce residence time of airborne particulates.

Long-range transport of airborne particulate PAH has been demonstrated (Lund and Bjorseth, 1977; Bjorseth et al., 1979b). Concentrations of PAH in air samples collected in southern Norway and western Sweden varied depending on season and wind direction. High PAH loads (20–30 ng/m^3) occurred in air masses that had passed over Great Britain or Europe. Stationary air or air masses moving south from northern Scandinavia contained little PAH. Thus PAH can persist at relatively high concentrations in aerosols transported through long distances.

The estimated total annual input of PAH to the aquatic enivironment from the sources discussed above is approximately 230,000 metric tons (Neff, 1979). Surface runoff from land and fallout from the air appear to be the main sources of high molecular weight PAH in the aquatic environment, while petroleum spillage is the main source of total PAH. This reflects the relatively high PAH content (mainly bi- and tricyclic PAH) of petroleum in comparison to other major PAH sources.

DISTRIBUTION IN THE AQUATIC ENVIRONMENT

The estimated amounts of benzo[a]pyrene (BaP) and total PAH entering the aquatic environment from all sources are significantly lower than estimated inputs to the atmosphere and to land. If these aquatic PAH were evenly distributed through the world's oceans and freshwater bodies, their concentrations would be undetectable and inconsequential. However, they are not evenly distributed. Most of the environmental PAH burden remains relatively near the point sources of PAH, and concentrations decrease approximately logarithmically with distance from the source. Thus most of the PAH entering the aquatic environment are localized in rivers, estuaries, and coastal marine waters.

PAH are less sensitive to photooxidation and therefore are more persistent in water than in air. When incorporated into anoxic sediments, they may persist for long (even geologic) times. The cycle of PAH in the aquatic environment appears to be relatively simple. PAH entering water from various sources quickly become adsorbed on organic and inorganic particulate matter and large amounts are deposited in bottom sediments. Leaching or biological activity in the sediments may return a small fraction of these PAH to the water column. PAH are readily accumulated by aquatic biota, reaching levels higher than those in the ambient medium. Relative concentrations of PAH in aquatic ecosystems are generally highest in the sediments, intermediate in aquatic biota, and lowest in the water column. Routes of removal of PAH from the aquatic environment include volatilization from the water surface (mainly low molecular weight PAH), photooxidation, chemical oxidation, microbial metabolism, and metabolism by higher metazoans.

PAH in Water

Aqueous solubilities of PAH are quite low, reflecting their nonpolar, hydrophobic nature (Table 2). Solubility tends to decrease as number of aromatic rings or molecular weight increases. Naphthalene has a solubility of about 30 ppm, while five-ring PAH have solubilities in the range 0.5–5.0 ppb. Alkyl PAH usually have lower solubilities than unalkylated parent compounds. Linear mole-

Table 2 Recent Values for the Solubility of PAH in Distilled Water at 25–27°C

Compound	No. of aromatic rings	Molecular weight	Solubility (μg/kg, ppb)
Naphthalene	2	128.2	22,000[a], 31,300[b], 31,690[c], 31,700[d]
1-Methylnaphthalene	2	142.2	25,800[b], 28,500[d]
1,5-Dimethylnaphthalene	2	156.2	27,740[b], 3,380[d]
1-Ethylnaphthalene	2	156.2	8,000[b], 10,700[d]
Fluorene	2	166.2	1,685[c], 1,980[d]
Anthracene	3	178.2	30[a], 44.6[c], 73[d]
Phenanthrene	3	178.2	1,002[c], 1,070[b], 1,290[d]
2-Methylanthracene	3	192.3	21.3[c], 261[d]
Fluoranthene	3	202.3	206[c], 236[a], 260[d]
Pyrene	4	202.3	132[c], 135[d], 171[a]
Benz[a]anthracene	4	228.3	9.4[c], 14[d]
Chrysene	4	228.3	1.8[c], 2[d]
Benzo[a]pyrene	5	252.3	3.8[d]
Perylene	5	252.3	0.4[d]
3-Methylcholanthrene	5	268.4	2.9[d]
Benzo[ghi]perylene	6	276.3	0.26[d]

[a]Schwarz and Wasik (1976).
[b]Eganhouse and Calder (1976).
[c]May (1980).
[d]Mackay et al. (1980).

cules are usually less soluble than more condensed isomers (e.g., anthracene and phenanthrene).

The limited data available indicate that PAH are slightly less soluble in seawater than in fresh water due to salting out. Differences are not large. For instance, Eganhouse and Calder (1976) reported solubility values at 25°C of 31.3 and 22.0 ppm, for naphthalene in fresh water and seawater, respectively. Temperature has a much greater effect on aqueous solubility of PAH. The solubility of phenanthrene in distilled water increases from 423 to 1277 ppb between 8.5 and 29.9°C (May et al., 1978).

Because of their low aqueous solubility and hydrophobic character, PAH are readily adsorbed on particulate materials and solid surfaces in water. Adsorption and concentration occur on such substrates as activated carbon, calcareous material, silica, glass, clay, soil, and organic particles (Andelman and Suess, 1970; Herbes, 1977; May et al., 1978). Organic particles tend to adsorb PAH more readily than clay particles (Meyers and Quinn, 1977; Herbes, 1977). It appears that in natural waters there is an equilibrium between adsorbed and particulate PAH. While this equilibrium favors the particulate form, a significant fraction of the total PAH is present in solution or collodial suspension except in heavily PAH-contaminated waters.

Concentrations of PAH in fresh waters are quite variable, reflecting the variety of sources of these waters and uses to which they have been put. River water often contains significant quantities of PAH. In most cases, there is a direct relationship between PAH concentrations in river water and degree of industrialization and other human activity along the banks and adjacent floodplain. Rivers flowing through heavily industrialized areas may contain 1–5 μg/l (ppb) total PAH. Unpolluted rivers, ground water, drinking water, and seawater usually contain less than 0.1 μg/l total PAH (Neff, 1979).

PAH in Sediments

Most of the PAH in fresh and marine waters are adsorbed on suspended organic and inorganic particles. They tend to settle with these particles and accumulate in the bottom sediments. Once deposited on the bottom, the PAH are much less subject to photochemical, chemical, or biological degradation than they were in the water column. Concentrations of PAH in sediments are nearly always greater by a factor of 1000 or more than those in the water column. Sediment PAH assemblages have frequently been used as indices of the rate of PAH input to aquatic environments. Sediments have a substantial integrating effect on temporal patterns of PAH input and offer good geographic resolution, especially when current patterns, sediment origins, and settling rates are known (Dunn and Stich, 1976). However, the composition and relative concentrations of the PAH assemblage in the sediment may be different from those in the PAH source because of differential partitioning of PAH between sediment and aqueous phases (Hase and Hites, 1977).

Concentrations of BaP and total PAH in freshwater and marine sediments vary widely. Sediments from water bodies receiving drainage from industrial areas may have total PAH concentrations of 100 mg/kg (ppm) or more (Bjorseth et al., 1979; Greist, 1980). Sediments in areas remote from human activity usually have PAH concentrations in the low ppb range. It is generally thought that PAH in sediments from remote sites are derived from long-range aerosols, forest fire particulates, or oil seeps (Shaw et al., 1979; Platt and Mackie, 1979; Hites et al., 1980; Stich and Dunn, 1980).

There have been many reports on the presence of PAH, and particularly BaP, in tissues of aquatic organisms (Neff, 1979). BaP concentrations in tissues of freshwater and marine animals are generally in the low ppb range, except near point sources of PAH pollution. Several surveys of BaP in marine bivalve mollusks (mainly mussels, *Mytilus* spp.) along the Pacific coast of Canada and

the United States have shown a high degree of correlation with industrial, urban, and recreational uses of the coastal water (Dunn and Stich, 1975, 1976; Dunn and Young, 1976; Mix et al., 1977; Mix and Schaffer, 1979). Creosoted wooden structures were found to be an important source of PAH contamination of mussels and other marine invertebrates (Zitko, 1975; Dunn and Stich, 1976; Dunn and Fee, 1979). Other sources are industrial effluents, domestic sewage, and spilled oil.

TRANSFORMATION IN THE AQUATIC ENVIRONMENT

PAH in the aquatic environment are subject to chemical transformation and degradation through a variety of processes. The most important of these are photooxidation, chemical oxidation, and biological transformation by bacteria, fungi, and animals. Since most natural mechanisms of oxidative transformation of PAH require molecular oxygen, sunlight, or both, PAH are generally quite stable and persistent once incorporated into oxygen-poor bottom sediments of water bodies.

Photodegradation

Chemical reactions of photoinduced oxidation of PAH in the aqueous phase by singlet oxygen, ozone, OH radicals, and other oxidizing agents are similar to those involved in photooxidation of airborne PAH; until recently, they were thought to be the primary pathways of photoinduced transmation of PAH in solution or adsorbed on waterborne particles (NAS, 1972). In most studies of photoreactions of PAH in water, solubilizers such as acetone were used to increase the aqueous solubility of the PAH. Under these conditions and in the presence of high oxygen concentrations, direct and indirect photooxygenations predominate. Zepp and Schlotzhauer (1979) showed that when PAH are present in true solution in "pure" fresh water or seawater, direct photolysis reactions are quantitatively much more important than photooxygenation reactions involving singlet oxygen. These direct photochemical transformations can take place in the absence of molecular oxygen or in the presence of mercuric chloride, a quencher of triplet-state reactions. There is a strong tendency for sensitivity to direct photolysis in the aqueous phase to increase with increasing PAH molecular weight. Thus naphthalene is quite insensitive to photolysis and BaP is quite sensitive. Linear PAH such as anthracene and naphthalene are much more sensitive than angular or condensed PAH such as phenanthrene and chrysene. Because light intensity decreases rapidly with depth in the water column, the rate of PAH photolysis also decreases with depth. Sorption on bottom sediments decreases photolysis rate further, particularly for higher molecular weight PAH.

The situation apparently is quite different in an oil slick on the surface of the water. Here the primary mechanism of photodegradation of PAH is photooxygenation involving singlet oxygen (Larson et al., 1976, 1977).

Chemical Oxidation

Chlorination and ozonation are often used to destroy pathogens in drinking water and sometimes to oxidize organic compounds in industrial waste water effluents. Investigations of the efficiency of these methods for destroying aqueous PAH have yielded variable results, due in part to lack of control of factors such as chlorine or ozone concentration, pH, and temperature (Harrison et al., 1975). Under the conditions that exist in a water treatment plant, sodium hypochlorite is effective in oxidizing most PAH (Harrison et al., 1976a,b). Temperature, free chlorine concentration, and water pH (by affecting hypochlorous ion concentration) all have a profound effect on the rate and extent of chlorine-mediated PAH degradation.

PAH tend to undergo electrophilic substitution reactions with chlorine ions to produce chlorinated aromatic compounds. Since polychlorinated naphthalenes (Green and Neff, 1977) and probably other polychlorinated PAH are highly toxic and persistent in aquatic organisms, consideration should be given to using alternative methods for purifying waste water or drinking water containing high concentrations of PAH.

Ozonation is one such alternative method for water purification. Ozone reacts readily with aqueous PAH (NAS, 1972; Radding et al., 1976). Reaction products may include quinones, aromatic aldehydes, and carboxylic acids (Meineke and Klamberg, 1978). Ozonation is more efficient than chlorination in removing PAH from water. However, ozone is removed from water so rapidly by volatilization and reaction with organics that it is difficult to maintain a high enough ozone concentration in a water purification system to effect complete removal of PAH.

Bacteria and Fungi

Bacteria and fungi show tremendous diversity and adaptability in utilization of different organic molecules as a carbon source. Some microorganisms are able to oxidize some aromatic hydrocarbons completely to carbon dioxide and water and use them as a source of energy and as a source of carbon for biomass accretion. Others are not able to carry out this complete oxidation of aromatics, but if an alternative growth substrate is available, they are able to metabolize them partially to various oxygenated metabolites. The latter process is called cooxidation (Gibson, 1977).

PAH are oxidized by bacteria to dihydrodiols (Jerina et al., 1971; Gibson, 1977). These may be oxidized further in a series of reactions to catechols and eventually to carbon dioxide and water. An extremely important feature of the bacterial pathway is that a *cis*-dihydrodiol apparently is produced through a dioxetane intermediate, whereas in the mammalian microsomal system a *trans*-dihydrodiol is produced through an arene oxide intermediate. The arene oxides, or their immediate oxidation products, appear to be responsible for the carcinogenicity or mutagenicity of PAH with these properties (Jerina and Daily, 1974; Lehr et al., 1980).

Many studies have been performed on the ability of marine water column and sediment bacteria to degrade petroleum hydrocarbons,

including PAH. Aliphatic and aromatic hydrocarbons are degraded much more rapidly under
aerobic than under anaerobic conditions (Lee et
al., 1978; Delaune et al., 1980; Ward et al., 1980).
Rate of PAH degradation tends to decrease with
increasing PAH molecular weight (Herbes and
Schwall, 1978). Bacterial populations from oil-
contaminated areas metabolize PAH more readily
than populations from clean areas.

Fungi (yeasts and molds), unlike bacteria, metabolize PAH by a cytochrome P-450–dependent
mixed-function oxygenase system somewhat similar to that found in mammalian liver microsomes
(Ferris et al., 1973, 1976). As in the mammalian
microsomal system, the initial product of fungal
attack on PAH is a *trans*-dihydrodiol produced
through an arene oxide intermediate (Cerniglia et
al., 1978, 1980).

Aquatic Animals

In mammals, the enzyme system variously known
as the cytochrome P-450–dependent mixed-
function oxidase, mixed-function oxygenase
(MFO), aryl hydrocarbon hydroxylase, or drug-
metabolizing system is responsible for initiating
the metabolism of various lipophilic organic compounds, including xenobiotics (foreign organic
compounds such as alkanes, PAH, pesticides, and
drugs) and endogenous compounds such as steroid
hormones and bile salts. Although this system effectively detoxifies certain xenobiotics, others,
such as certain PAH and alkenes, may be transformed to intermediates that are highly toxic,
mutagenic, or carcinogenic to the host. Oxidative
metabolism of PAH in this system proceeds
through highly electrophilic intermediate arene
oxides, some of which bind covalently to cellular
macromolecules such as DNA, RNA, and protein.
It is now generally agreed that metabolic activation by the MFO system is a prerequisite for PAH-
induced carcinogenesis and mutagenesis (Jerina
and Daly, 1974; Huberman et al., 1976; Jerina et
al., 1978). For instance, the carcinogenicity of BaP
is though to be due primarily to 7,8-dihydroxy-
9,10-epoxy-7,8,9,10   tetrahydrobenzo[a]pyrene

(Sims et al., 1974; Lehr and Jerina, 1977; Yang et
al., 1977).

Considerable progress has been made in identifying and quantifying the MFO system and
its components in aquatic invertebrates and
vertebrates. This is discussed in detail in Chapter 18.

Among the invertebrates, MFO activity seems
to be restricted primarily to some members of the
phyla Arthropoda and Annelida (Neff, 1979; Lee,
1981). Of course, most invertebrate phyla have
not been investigated. Coelenterates and ctenophores apparently lack MFO activity (Lee, 1975).
Among the Echinodermata, sea urchins, *Strongylo-
centrotus* sp., and starfish, *Asterias* sp., have low
levels of MFO (Payne and May, 1979). Five species
of marine polychaete worms have been examined,
and all but one species (*Arenicola* sp.) have at least
a limited ability to transform PAH (Rossi, 1977;
Lee et al., 1979; Lee, 1981; Payne and May,
1979). The situation among the Mollusca is more
complicated. Several investigators have been unable to detect MFO activity in several species of
bivalve mollusks including *Mytilus edulis, Mya
arenaria, Ostrea edulis,* and *Anodonta* sp. (Lee et
al., 1972a; Vandermeulen and Penrose, 1978;
Payne and May, 1979). However, Anderson (1978)
measured a low level of MFO activity in oysters,
Crassostrea virginica, that had been exposed to
BaP for long periods of time. Stegeman (1980)
reported low levels of MFO activity in the hepatopancreas of the mussels *Mytilus edulis* and *Modiolus modiolus.* Moore et al. (1980) were able to
detect aldrin epoxidase, NADPH-neotetrazoleum
reductase, and glucose-6-phosphate dehydrogenase
(enzymes thought to be associated with the MFO
system) in tissues of *M. edulis.* Enzyme activity
was highest in blood cells and mantle tissue. Khan
et al. (1974) also detected aldrin epoxidase activity in several species of freshwater bivalve mollusks. It is possible that epoxidation of aldrin to
dieldrin takes place by a pathway other than the
MFO system in bivalve mollusks. Little information is available on other molluscan classes. Low
levels of MFO activity have been reported in snails,

Littorina sp., and squid, *Illex illecebrosus* (Payne, 1977; Payne and May, 1979).

MFO activity has been detected in more than a dozen species of marine and freshwater crustaceans (Neff, 1979). Levels of *in vitro* MFO activity in crustacean hepatopancreatic preparations are usually low and variable. However, *in vitro* activity may not accurately reflect true PAH-metabolizing capability in the intact animal. The crustacean hepatopancreas is a digestive gland containing high concentrations of powerful hydrolytic enzymes. Homogenization releases these enzymes and inhibits *in vitro* MFO activity (Pohl et al., 1974). In addition, nonhepatic tissues of crustaceans such as the green gland, gonads, and stomach may have MFO activity as high as or higher than the hepatopancreas (Singer and Lee, 1977; Singer et al., 1980). Metabolite identification experiments with several marine crustaceans have shown that the intact animal can produce PAH metabolites very rapidly (Corner et al., 1973; Lee, 1975; Lee et al., 1976; Sanborn and Malins, 1977).

Other enzymes involved in PAH transformation—epoxide hydratase and glutathione *S*-transferase—are also present in tissues of many species of aquatic animals (James et al., 1979). Epoxide hydratase is associated with the microsomal fraction, while glutathione *S*-epoxidetransferase is present primarily in the cytoplasmic fraction in invertebrates and fish. Both enzymes are present at significant levels in hepatic and several extrahepatic tissues of marine bivalve mollusks, crustaceans, elasmobranchs, and teleosts. There is a general trend among the species tested to date for hepatic microsomal epoxide hydratase activity (with BaP-4,5-oxide as substrate) to be higher in crustaceans than in fish or mollusks, and for glutathione *S*-epoxidetransferase activity to be higher in fish than in crustaceans and mollusks. The significance of these differences is uncertain. However, relative activities of these two enzymes will in large part determine the ultimate metabolic fate of PAH. Thus it may be predicted that fish will preferentially tend to produce glutathione conjugates, while crustaceans will preferentially tend to produce dihydrodiols and phenols.

The types of PAH metabolites produced by marine and freshwater animals are similar to those produced by mammals. They include PAH dihydrodiols, phenols, and quinones as well as PAH conjugates with sulfate, glucuronic acid, and glutathione. The major metabolite produced from phenanthrene by the Norway lobster, *Nephrops norvegicus,* is 9,10-dihydroxy-9,10-dihydrophenanthrene, the same as the major metabolite in mammals (Palmork and Solbakken, 1979). Blue crab (*Callinectes sapidus*) microsomes metabolize phenanthrene, benz[*a*]anthracene, and chrysene primarily to diols (Singer et al., 1980). Dimethylbenz[*a*]anthracene and benzo[*a*]pyrene are converted primarily to phenols. Naphthalene is converted primarily to naphthoquinone, naphthalene-1,2-dihydrodiol, and α-naphthol by larval spot shrimp, *Pandalus platyceros* (Sanborn and Malins, 1980). Trout, *salmo trutta lacustris,* starry flounder, *Platychthys stellatus,* and coho salmon, *Oncorhynchus kisutch,* liver microsomes metabolize BaP to a number of metabolites similar to those produced by rat liver microsomes (Ahokas et al., 1979; Varanasi and Gmur, 1980) (Table 3). The major identified metabolites produced by the fish microsomes are the 7,8- and 9,10-dihydrodiols, which are precursors of the major carcinogenic BaP metabolite.

In fish, as in mammals, most MFO activity is localized in the liver (Lindstrom-Seppa et al., 1981). Gills and kidney also contain significant MFO activity. Activity in other tissues is low (less than 10% of the activity in liver microsomes).

Distribution of other PAH-metabolizing enzymes is somewhat different. Uridine diphosphate-glucuronic acid transferase activity is higher in gills than in liver of vendace, *Coregonus albula* (Lindstrom-Seppa et al., 1981). Intestine, heart, and kidney have activities of about half that in the liver. Distribution of glutathione *S*-epoxide transferase and epoxide hydratase activity seems roughly parallel to that of MFO activity in the teleosts studied to date (James et al., 1979). With

Table 3 Metabolism of [³H] Benzo[a]pyrene Catalyzed by the 10,000× g Liver Supernatant Fractions (Microsomes plus Cytosol) from Starry Flounder, *Platichthys stellatus*, Coho Salmon, *Oncorhynchus kisutch*, and Sprague-Dawley Rats[a,b]

Compound	Starry flounder			Coho salmon			Rat	
	Control	3-MC[d]-treated	BaP[d]-treated	Control	3-MC-treated	BaP-treated	Control	3-MC-treated
Percent of total radioactivity								
Unreacted BaP	40	13	8	59	5	5	62	35
Ethyl acetate-soluble metabolites	39	52	59	20	40	51	6	38
Aqueous phase metabolites	21	35	33	21	55	44	32	27
Ethyl acetate-extractable metabolites (percent of ethyl acetate radioactivity)								
Quinones	6.8	4.2	4.9	7.8	8.9	10.5	23.9	26.7
Phenols	15.3	7.6	3.8	30.6	13.8	10.7	24.6	30.8
4,5-Dihydrodiol	0.6	2.2	1.6	2.7	6.6	2.9	3.2	5.1
7,8-Dihydrodiol	47.3	38.3	34.9	31.8	24.9	37.4	14.4	13.8
9,10-Dihydrodiol	24.3	25.9	36.4	16.5	22.0	17.0	13.1	14.0
Unclassified[c]	3.8	17.1	15.0	5.9	15.0	16.1	13.3	8.0
At origin	1.8	4.7	3.4	4.7	8.8	5.5	7.6	1.6

[a]Microsomal preparations were incubated with 5 nmol [³H] BaP (500 mCi/mmol) for 15 min at 15°C (fish) or 37°C (rats).

[b]From Varanasi and Gmur (1980); reprinted with permission of Pergamon Press Ltd.

[c]Primarily "prediol" metabolites having lower R_f values than BaP-9,10-dihydrodiol on thin-layer chromatographic plates; may include conjugates.

[d]3-MC = 3-methylcholanthrene; BaP = Benzo[a] pyrene.

BaP-4,5-oxide or styrene-7,8-oxide as the substrate, activity is highest in liver, intermediate in kidney and intestine, and low in gill.

The pattern among aquatic invertebrates is quite different. In the blue crab, *Callinectes sapidus*, highest BaP hydroxylase activity occurs in the green gland (analogous to the teleost kidney) and the pyloric stomach (Singer and Lee, 1977). The hepatopancreas (roughly analogous to the teleost liver) has low activity. Other crab tissues with significant MFO activity include gill and testes. The distribution of MFO activity is quite different in another crustacean, the barnacle *Balanus eburneus* (Stegeman and Kaplan, 1981). Digestive gland (hepatopancreas) and intestine have about equal concentrations of cytochrome P-450, but the digestive gland contains about twice as much BaP hydroxylase activity as the intestine. Other tissues in barnacles which have BaP hydroxylase activity include ovaries, testes, and cirri. Nearly all the MFO activity in the marine worm *Nereis virens* is associated with the tissues of the lower intestine (Lee et al., 1979). In aquatic caddisfly larvae *Limnophilus* sp., activity of aldrin epoxidase (an MFO enzyme) occurs only in the gut and fat body (Krieger and Lee, 1973). Thus levels of hepatopancreatic MFO and related enzyme activities do not, in most cases, reflect the true metabolic capabilities of aquatic invertebrates.

A great many endogenous and exogenous factors may influence the activity of the MFO system in tissues of aquatic animals. For a complete discussion of these, see Chapter 18. Only factors that affect PAH activity will be discussed here. Chambers and Yarbrough (1979) reported seasonal cycles of the hepatic microsomal cytochrome P-450 and b_5 concentration and activity of several microsomal cytochrome reductases in natural populations of mosquito fish, *Gambusia affinis*. Highest values for most parameters were in the late fall and winter. Levels of NADPH–cytochrome *c* reductase and BaP hydroxylase activity were greater in liver microsomes of killifish, *Fundulus heteroclitus*, acclimated in the laboratory to 6.5°C than in those acclimated to 16.5°C (Stegeman,

1979). This suggests that seasonal effects are at least partly mediated by temperature change.

Sexual differences in levels and activities of MFO components have been observed in fish and crustaceans. BaP hydroxylase activity was nearly two orders of magnitude higher in green gland of mature female blue crabs, *Callinectes sapidus*, than in green gland of mature males of the same species (Singer and Lee, 1977). Cytochrome P-450 concentration was significantly higher in hepatic microsomes of gonadally mature male brook trout, *Salvelinus fontinalis*, and rainbow trout, *Salmo gairdneri*, than in hepatic microsomes of gonadally mature females of the same species (Stegeman and Chevion, 1980). However, BaP hydroxylase activity, when normalized to cytochrome P-450 concentration, was higher in liver and kidney microsomes of gonadally mature females than in gonadally mature males. Immature male and female brook trout had similar levels of hepatic BaP hydroxylase activity, and these were significantly lower than levels of enzyme activity in gonadally mature males and females.

Embryos and larvae of fish (Binder and Stegeman, 1980) and aquatic amphibians (Doherty and Khan, 1981) have low but detectable levels of MFO activity. Activity increases during juvenile development.

Singer and Lee (1977) observed large changes in BaP hydroxylase activity in the green gland of female blue crabs during the molting cycle. MFO activity is high during late intermolt and falls to very low levels just before and during the molt (ecdysis). It rises to its highest levels about 48 h after the molt. These dramatic changes in MFO activity during the normal molting cycle of a crustacean strongly suggest that green gland MFO activity functions to control the concentration of steroid molting hormones (crustecdysones) in the hemolymph of the crab (steroids are normal substrates for MFO). High levels of MFO activity during the intermolt and postmolt periods would ensure low ecdysteroid titers, preventing untimely initiation of the molting process. Reduction in MFO activity during proecdysis would allow ecdysteroid titers to rise to levels high enough to initiate molting.

Induction of MFO Activity

Enzyme induction is the process whereby the concentration or activity of an enzyme is increased in response to exposure of the organism to the normal substrate of the enzyme. This is discussed in Chapter 18. Several investigators have shown that exposure to PAH or complex mixtures of hydrocarbons such as petroleum results in rapid (within 1 to 10 d) induction of elevated levels of MFO activity in some aquatic species. MFO activity in liver microsomes of several species of fish is increased severalfold within a few days after intraperitoneal (ip) injection of single or multiple doses of PAH (Pedersen et al., 1976; Gerhart and Carlson, 1978; James and Bend, 1980). The degree and time course of induction are highly species- and PAH-specific. Pedersen et al. (1976) induced elevations in BaP hydroxylase activity in five strains of rainbow trout, *Salmo gairdneri,* by ip injection of 3-methylcholanthrene. The degree of induction varied from 2.3- to 47.7-fold. Greatest induction occurred in the strain that had the lowest control (uninduced) activity. This may indicate, as Bend et al. (1978) suggested, that some control fish are already partially induced, presumably by exposure to inducers in their environment. One way to distinguish between induced and uninduced MFO activity in fish hepatic microsomes is to assay for *in vitro* activity in the presence of α-naphthoflavone, which selectively inhibits the induced component of total hepatic microsomal MFO activity and stimulates activity in the uninduced fraction.

Increases in MFO activity resulting from induction are not always accompanied by significant increases in the concentration of microsomal cytochrome P-450. Usually, a small increase in cytochrome P-450 concentration accompanies a large increase in MFO activity (James and Bend, 1980; Willis et al., 1980). This may be due to the fact that six or more distinct cytochrome P-450s may be present, and only one will be induced by a particular inducer (Yang et al., 1978). Epoxide

hydratase and glutathione S-epoxidetransferase usually have not been induced in the fish species examined to date (James and Bend, 1980).

Since different components of the PAH-metabolizing system are induced to different degrees, it is not surprising that the relative proportion of different types of PAH metabolites produced by uninduced and induced hepatic microsomes are different (Table 3). Relative proportions of BaP phenols produced by PAH-induced hepatic microsomes decreased about threefold compared to those in uninduced controls in starry flounder, *Platychthys stellatus,* and coho salmon, *Oncorhynchus kisutch* (Varanasi and Gmur, 1980). Relative proportions of BaP dihydrodiols, some of which are precursors of carcinogens, increased. Such changes could be important in relation to PAH-induced cancer in aquatic animals.

PAH show some variability in ability to induce hepatic microsomal MFO activity in fish. Gerhart and Carlson (1978) reported that ip injection of chrysene and BaP induced elevations in MFO activity in rainbow trout (*Salmo gairdneri*) hepatic microsomes, but naphthalene, phenanthrene, pyrene, and fluoranthanthene were ineffective. In addition, exposure of the fish to pyrene and fluoranthene in solution in the ambient medium did not induce MFO activity, but exposure to BaP in solution did. MFO induction could also be effected by providing the fish with food containing 3-methylcholanthrene (Addison et al., 1978; Willis et al., 1980).

The time course of 3-methylcholanthrene-mediated induction of MFO activity in sheepshead (*Argosargus probatocephalus*) is season- (temperature-) dependent (James and Bend, 1980). In summer, at 26°C, BaP hydroxylase activity reached a maximum at 3 d and returned to the control level after 14 d. In winter, at 14°C, maximum activity was reached 8 d after dosing, but elevated activity persisted for more than 28 d. Intraperitoneal injection of BaP in killifish (*Fundulus heteroclitus*) acclimated to 16.5°C resulted in a significant induction of hepatic microsomal BaP hydroxylase activity, NADPH–cytochrome *c* reductase activity, and cytochrome P-450 concentration in 2–4 d (Stegeman, 1979). The same treatment of another group of fish that had been acclimated to 6.5°C was without effect on these MFO parameters at 4 d. It is possible that some induction would have been observed in the cold-acclimated fish after a longer time, as James and Bend (1980) showed.

Much less research has been performed on induction of MFO activity in aquatic invertebrates. Several attempts to induce MFO activity in species of algae, mollusks, crustaceans, annelids, and echinoderms by exposure to PAH or petroleum have failed (Payne, 1977; Vandermeulen and Penrose, 1978; Payne and May, 1979; Singer et al., 1980). However, Anderson (1978) apparently was able to induce a very low level of BaP hydroxylase activity in oysters (*Crassostrea virginica*) by exposure for 5–9 mo to 1 μg/l BaP or methylcholanthrene in the ambient medium. Lee et al. (1979) induced MFO activity in the polychaete worm (*Capitella capitata*) by exposing the worm to benz[a]anthracene or crude oil in its sand substrate for 3–10 wk. Exposure of copepods (*Calanus helgolandicus*) for 7 d to seawater solutions of naphthalene, 2-methylnaphthalene, 3-methylcholanthrene, or BaP (50–200 μg/l) resulted in a significant elevation of BaP hydroxylase activity in whole-animal homogenates (Walters et al., 1979).

Several investigators observed induction of MFO activity in fish as a result of exposure in the laboratory or the field to petroleum. Hepatic microsomal MFO activity was induced in coho salmon (*Oncorhynchus kisutch*) by exposure of fish in the laboratory to low concentrations of crude oil in the water or food (Gruger et al., 1977a,b). Similar results were obtained with cunner (*Tautogolabrus adspersus*) (Walton et al., 1978; Payne and May, 1979). Exposure of the fish to 1-2 ppm crude oil in water or 500 ppm crude oil in food resulted in a two- to sixfold increase in MFO activity above uninduced levels. Activity was induced in all tissues examined except brain (Table 4). Extent of induction varied from about 4 to 10 times the control level.

Other components of the MFO system are subject to petroleum-mediated induction. In mullet (*Mugil cephalus*) exposed to Empire Mix or Saudi Arabian crude oil, hepatic cytochrome P-450 and b_5, and NADPH–cytochrome c and NADPH–dichlorophenolindophenol reductases were induced, but NADH–cytochrome c and NADH–cytochrome b_5 reductases were not (Chambers, 1979). Moore et al. (1980) reported induction in mussel (*Mytilus edulis*) blood cell microsomes of NADPH-neotetrazoleum reductase (thought to be associated with MFO) and the NADPH-generating

Table 4 Induction of Mixed-Function Oxygenase Activity in Several Tissues of Cunners, *Tautogolabrus adsperus,* Exposed to a Surface Slick of Venezuelan Crude Oil for 3 d[a,b]

Tissue	MFO specific activity (units per mg protein per 10 min)		
	Control	Oil-exposed	Induced/control
Liver	9.9 ± 4.4	61.59 ± 10.26	6.2
Heart	0.48 ± 0.35	4.98 ± 1.83	10.4
Kidney	1.29 ± 1.22	8.47 ± 2.31	6.6
Gills	0.54 ± 0.19	2.10 ± 0.20	3.9
Spleen	0	0.52 ± 0.36	—
Brain	0	0	—

[a]Activity was measured as rate of hydroxylation of 2,5-diphenyloxazole.
[b]From Payne and May (1979); with permission from the American Chemical Society.

enzyme glucose-6-phosphate dehydrogenase following exposure of the mollusks to North Sea crude oil.

Payne (1976) reported significantly higher levels of MFO activity in cunners (*Tautogolabrus adspersus*) from oil-polluted stations than in those from unpolluted stations along the coast of the Avalon Peninsula, Newfoundland. Based on these and other results, he recommended use of fish hepatic microsomal MFO activity as a monitor for oil pollution. Kurelec et al. (1977) reported that hepatic MFO activity in a natural population of blennies (*Blennius pavo*) was increased dramatically within 7 d after an oil spill near Rovinj, Yugoslavia. BaP hydroxylase activity in the fish reached a maximum within 3 wk after the spill (about eight times the basal level) and subsequently dropped to about three times the prespill level 3 wk later. It remained relatively constant at this elevated level for at least 5 mo. Stegeman (1978) reported elevated levels of BaP hydroxylase activity and cytochrome P-450 concentration in killifish (*Fundulus heteroclitus*) collected from Wild Harbor Marsh, Massachusetts, the site of a spill of fuel oil 8 yr earlier.

It is apparent that a great many endogenous and exogenous factors can influence levels of PAH and related enzyme activity and concentrations of MFO components in the tissues of aquatic animals. Each species seems to respond somewhat differently to these factors and there are even significant intraspecific (probably genetic) differences. Endogenous factors may include age, sex, nutritional status, and period of the molt cycle (in arthropods). Primary exogenous factors influencing rate of PAH metabolism include temperature, season, possibly salinity (though this has not been studied), current, and previous history of exposure to potential inducers or inhibitors of different components of the microsomal PAH-metabolizing system.

ACCUMULATION AND RELEASE BY AQUATIC ORGANISMS

The presence of PAH in tissues of a wide variety of freshwater and marine organisms indicates that these organisms are able to accumulate PAH present at low concentrations in the ambient medium, food, or sediments. This is not surprising, since PAH are highly hydrophobic and lipophilic. Intrinsic lipid-water partition coefficients strongly favor rapid transfer of PAH from the aqueous phase into lipophilic compartments such as biological membranes, macromolecules, and depot lipid stores in organisms (Leo et al., 1971; Neely et al., 1974). Release of PAH from tissues of contaminated organisms may be passive, reflecting an equilibrium distribution between the aqueous phase and lipophilic compartments in contact with it, or it may be active and involve metabolic transformation of PAH to polar water-soluble metabolites, which are more readily excreted. A great deal of research has been done on accumulation and release by aquatic organisms of PAH from solution, food, sediments, and particularly petroleum.

Accumulation from Water

Freshwater and marine microalgae rapidly accumulate PAH to high concentrations during exposure to low concentrations in the ambient medium (Soto et al., 1975; Dobroski and Epifanio, 1980). Much of this apparent uptake may be merely adsorption of PAH on cell surfaces (Herbes, 1977). However, the PAH are not readily released back to the water.

Marine polychaete worms *Neanthes arenaceodentata* and *Arenicola marina* also accumulated [14C]naphthalene rapidly from the water (Rossi, 1977; Lyes, 1979). Both species released [14C]-naphthalene from their tissues rapidly when returned to isotope-free seawater. Nearly two-thirds of the radioactivity released is in the form of polar metabolites.

Bivalve mollusks, which lack or have very low PAH-metabolizing ability, tend to accumulate PAH from water more readily and retain them in their tissues longer than other aquatic animals. Relative rates of accumulation and release of different PAH vary (Neff et al., 1976b; Hansen et al., 1978). Lee et al. (1978) showed that rates of accumulation of several PAH from very low concentrations in solution by oysters (*Crassostrea virginica*) were approximately inversely related to PAH molecular weight. Rates of release of PAH from oyster tissues were also inversely related to molecular weight. Despite the very limited ability of mollusks to metabolize PAH, all species so far studied are able to release most of the accumulated PAH from their tissues in periods varying from a few days to several weeks.

Patterns of accumulation and release of PAH in solution by aquatic crustaceans are somewhat different, probably reflecting their greater activity and greater PAH-metabolizing ability. A freshwater zooplankton species, the water flea *Daphnia pulex,* accumulated and released PAH rapidly (Herbes and Risi, 1978; Southworth et al., 1978). Most PAH reached equilibrium concentrations in *Daphnia* tissues within 24 h. Bioconcentration factors (concentration in tissues divided by concentration in water) increase with PAH molecular weight (Table 5) from 131 for naphthalene to 10,109 for benz[*a*]anthracene. Thus, in *Daphnia,* the bioaccumulation potential of PAH increased by nearly a factor of 10 with each additional ring in the PAH structure. As shown for many other hydrophobic pollutant chemicals (Hamelink and Spacie, 1977), the *n*-octanol-water partition coefficient of a PAH is a good predictor of its bioaccumulation potential by *Daphnia*. Elimination was rapid for all PAH, with half-lives ranging from 0.4

to 5 h. Only 6% of the anthracene released by *Daphnia* after exposure to this PAH was in the form of polar metabolites, indicating that metabolism plays a minor role in PAH kinetics in this small freshwater crustacean.

Most fish can metabolize and excrete PAH even more rapidly than crustaceans. Equilibrium concentrations of PAH were often reached in fish tissues in 24 h or less (Lee et al., 1972b; Anderson et al., 1974b). As in macrocrustaceans, PAH equilibrium concentration increased and PAH release rate tended to decrease in fish tissues as the PAH molecular weight and octanol-water partition coefficient increased. Most of the PAH were excreted as polar metabolites or conjugates via the gallbladder (in bile) or the urine. PAH and their metabolites tended to accumulate selectively in gallbladder, liver, brain, visceral depot fat, and spleen (Lee et al., 1972b; Statham et al., 1976; DiMichele and Taylor, 1978). Fish skin is also an important site of PAH accumulation and elimination (Varanasi et al., 1978).

Accumulation from Food

Accumulation by aquatic animals of PAH from contaminated food appears in most cases to be less efficient and more variable than PAH uptake from solution. Information about bioavailability of PAH from food is essential for assessing the

Table 5 Accumulation of PAH from Solution (0.3–1000 µg/l Exposure Concentrations) by the Freshwater Water Flea, *Daphnia pulex*[a,b]

Compound	Molecular weight	Number of rings	Partition coefficient[c]	Bioaccumulation factor ± SE
Naphthalene	128	2	2.00×10^3	131 ± 10
Phenanthrene	178	3	2.82×10^4	325 ± 56
Anthracene	178	3	2.82×10^4	917 ± 48
9-Methylanthracene	192	3	1.32×10^5	4,583 ± 1,004
Pyrene	202	4	7.94×10^4	2,702 ± 245
Benz[*a*]anthracene	228	4	3.98×10^5	10,109 ± 507
Perylene	252	5	1.15×10^6	7,191 ± 804

[a]Bioconcentration factors, calculated after 24-h exposure, are concentration in tissues divided by concentration in water.
[b]From Southworth et al. (1978); with permission from Pergamon Press.
[c]*n*-Octanol–water partition coefficient calculated from Leo (1975).

potential for biomagnification of PAH in aquatic food webs.

The marine polychaete worm *Neanthes arenaceodentata* did not assimilate significant amounts of radioactivity in its tissues when it was fed for 16 d food containing 10–15 ppm 2-[^{14}C] methylnaphthalene (Rossi, 1977). Larvae of the hardshell clam *Mercenaria mercenaria* accumulated BaP to a concentration of 18.6 µg/g larvae after 9 d of feeding diatoms, *Thalassiosira pseudodana,* contaminated with BaP at 42.2 µg/g (Dobroski and Epifanio, 1980). It was calculated that BaP accumulation from food (trophic transfer) was several times less efficient than direct uptake from solution. However, in a contaminated environment, both routes of uptake would contribute significantly to body burdens of PAH in mollusks.

The situation is quite different in marine crustaceans and fish. Marine copepods *Calanus helogolandicus* accumulated [^{14}C] naphthalene more efficiently from food (algae and dead copepod larvae) than from water (Corner et al., 1976a; Harris et al., 1977). Approximately 60% of naphthalene ingested with food was assimilated. Almost half of the assimilated naphthalene was retained in copepod tissues; the other half was released as naphthalene or its metabolites.

Fish show considerable variability in absorption of PAH from food, but there are some general trends. In most species, more than half the administered dose remains associated with the digestive tract or its contents, part of it apparently strongly adsorbed or bound to the stomach wall (Corner et al., 1976b; Whittle et al., 1977). The assimilated fraction, which varied from about 4% (starry flounder, *Platychthys stellatus*) (Varanasi et al., 1979) to more than 90% (spiny dogfish, *Squalus acanthius*) (Solbakken and Palmork, 1980) of the administered dose, usually accumulates first in liver. PAH and PAH metabolites produced in the liver are then carried by the blood to other organs and tend to accumulate in depot fat and muscle (Solbakken and Palmork, 1980), brain (Collier et al., 1978), and skin (Varanasi et al., 1978). Main routes of excretion of PAH and metabolites are directly from liver into the gastrointestinal tract via the bile; from the kidney in the urine; and through the skin, bound to mucus (Palmork et al., 1978; Varanasi et al., 1978). Conjugated metabolites predominate in bile, while in urine and skin unconjugated metabolites are more abundant (Solbakken et al., 1980). A portion of the metabolite fraction is retained in certain tissues, particularly muscle, long after the parent PAH has been completely metabolized and/or excreted (Palmork et al., 1978). Retention of dietary PAH and metabolites in liver, brain, kidney, and blood increased at low temperatures (Collier et al., 1978).

From the limited data available, there appear to be large interspecific differences in ability to absorb and assimilate PAH from food. Polychaete worms have a very limited ability to do so, while in fish absorption of PAH from the gut is extremely variable, depending on species and possibly also on the PAH and the food in which it is administered. Crustaceans, on the other hand, apparently readily assimilate PAH from contaminated food. In all cases where assimilation of dietary PAH was observed, metabolism and excretion of PAH were rapid. Thus, the potential for food-web biomagnification of PAH seems to be limited. For such biomagnification to occur, the material must be readily absorbed from food and, once assimilated, relatively resistant to metabolism or excretion.

Accumulation from Petroleum

Crude and refined petroleums may contain several percent PAH by weight. When oil is spilled in water, PAH in the oil may enter the water column in solution, in dispersed form (micro and macro oil droplets), or adsorbed on organic and inorganic particles. The physical behavior of oil in natural waters is extremely complex and poorly understood. Dispersed oil droplets are similar in composition, at least initially, to the spilled oil. The degree to which different hydrocarbons leave oil droplets or surface slicks and dissolve in the water column depends on their concentration in the oil, aqueous solubility, and oil-water partition coefficient. Apparent solubility and oil-water partition coefficients may be influenced by surfactants in the oil and cosolutes and solubilizing agents in the water.

The physical form in which oil-derived PAH occur in the water and bottom sediments may significantly affect their bioavailability and rate of accumulation by aquatic organisms. There is a large literature dealing with accumulation by aquatic organisms of petroleum-derived PAH from water and sediments (Varanasi and Malins, 1977; Neff and Anderson, 1981). In general, petroleum-derived PAH in solution or very fine dispersion in water behave biologically very much like the pure PAH in solution. Cosolutes in the water, including other petroleum hydrocarbons and natural dissolved organic matter, seem to have little effect on bioavailability of PAH in solution (Boehm and Quinn, 1976; Eganhouse and Calder, 1976). However, PAH associated with suspended oil droplets or adsorbed on organic and inorganic particles (including sediments) appear to be substantially less available to aquatic organisms than PAH in solution (Neff et al., 1976; Lyes, 1979).

Accumulation from Sediment

Much of the PAH entering lakes, rivers, and coastal marine waters ultimately becomes adsorbed on particulate matter and is deposited in bottom sediments. Large populations of microorganisms, plants, and animals live on the surface of or buried in bottom sediments, particularly in estuarine and coastal marine environments. Many benthic animals ingest sediment and remove organic materials from it as a source of nutrition (deposit feeders). The extent to which these organisms accumulate sediment-adsorbed PAH has received relatively little attention, although it would be a mechanism by which PAH could be mobilized from sediments into the aquatic food chain. Bioaccumulation of PAH by benthic organisms might also pose a health hazard to predators (including humans) of benthic organisms.

The available evidence indicates that sediment-adsorbed PAH have very limited bioavailability to

marine animals. In the deposit-feeding worm *Arenicola marina,* bioaccumulation factors for uptake of naphthalene by different tissues from sediment varied from 0.12 for blood to 4.1 for stomach wall (Lyes, 1979). The high value for stomach wall may have been due to contamination with sediment particles.

Clams (*Macoma inquinata*) were exposed in the laboratory to sediment containing detritus contaminated with Prudhoe Bay crude oil and spiked with four different ^{14}C-labeled PAH (Roesijadi et al., 1978). One group of clams was exposed directly to the sediment, while another group was suspended in the overlying water column. This permitted estimation of the relative efficiency and magnitude of PAH uptake from detritus and water. After 7 d the sediment, water, and clams were analyzed for ^{14}C activity. Efficiency of PAH uptake from sediments was much lower than from water. Bioaccumulation factors for uptake of the four PAH from contaminated sediments were 0.2 or less, indicating no significant bioaccumulation of PAH by this route. Accumulation of PAH from sediment, when it occurs at all, may be attributed in large part to uptake of PAH desorbed from sediment particles into the interstitial water.

Effects of Endogenous and Exogenous Factors

Endogenous biological factors such as size, nutritional status, body composition, age, and sex, as well as exogenous physical factors such as salinity and temperature, may affect patterns of uptake and release of PAH by aquatic organisms. Relatively few investigations have been performed in these areas.

Harris et al. (1977) studied accumulation of ^{14}C naphthalene from solution by nine species of marine and estuarine copepods. Retention of ^{14}C naphthalene following 24 h varied nearly 16-fold among the different species. Strong positive correlations were drawn between total lipid content of copepods and naphthalene retention.

Mature male and gravid female polychaete worms, *Neanthes arenaceodentata,* accumulated naphthalenes at a similar rate from the water-soluble fraction of no. 2 fuel oil (Rossi and Anderson, 1977). However, males rapidly released naphthalenes when returned to oil-free seawater, while gravid females retained them until spawning occurred about 300–500 h after the beginning of the depuration period. Newly released zygotes contained high concentrations of naphthalenes and retained them during early developmental stages to the trochophore stage several days later. Trochophore and later juvenile stages released naphthalenes rapidly. Gravid female *Neanthes* have high concentrations of lipids, primarily associated with the ovaries and developing eggs. Naphthalenes apparently accumulated in these gonadal lipid stores and were released in eggs at spawning. Yolk lipid stores are not utilized in this species until larvae reach the trochopore stage. When the lipids were mobilized, naphthalenes were released rapidly. Thus, aromatic hydrocarbons that become associated with stable lipid pools such as depot lipids and gonadal lipid stores may be retained until the animals mobilize the lipids for nutritional purposes, while aromatic hydrocarbons that become associated with more labile hydrophobic compartments such as membrane lipids and cellular macromolecules may be released rapidly when ambient hydrocarbon levels decrease. Such a two-compartment model may partly explain the observation that release of chronically accumulated aromatic hydrocarbons is a two-phase process, characterized by initial rapid release followed by gradual release of remaining aromatic hydrocarbons (Lake and Hershner, 1977).

Temperature and salinity of the ambient medium have a profound effect on many physiological functions in marine organisms. They also affect solubility, adsorption-desorption kinetics, octanol-water partition coefficients, and other properties of PAH in water. One would therefore, expect salinity and temperature to have a significant effect on accumulation and release of PAH by marine organisms; however, little research has been done in this area.

Temperature had a slightly significant effect on rate of uptake of naphthalenes from south Louisiana crude oil by the clams *Rangia cuneata* and *Protothaca staminea* (Fucik and Neff, 1977). Rate of uptake was highest at the lowest temperature used and decreased with increasing temperature.

Harris et al. (1977) also found an inverse relationship between temperature and amount of [^{14}C] naphthalene accumulated by the copepod *Calanus helgolandicus* during exposure to 1 μg/l for 24 h. Accumulation of [^{14}C] naphthalene decreased by about 39 pg, or 3.23 pg/μg copepod lipid, per 10° rise in temperature. Herbes (1977) measured the effect of temperature on the adsorption of anthracene from solution (0.02 μg/l) on nonliving yeast cells. The fraction adsorbed by the yeast cells decreased significantly with increasing temperature. Calculated heat of adsorption for this process was 5.2 kcal/mol, which is characteristic of simple physical (van der Waals) adsorption. As the temperature rose, the strength of this weak chemical bond decreased, favoring desorption of PAH from the particles. Because partitioning of PAH between soluble and adsorbed phases is determined by relative rates of adsorption and desorption reactions, adsorption will be favored over desorption as temperature decreases. Therefore, temperature affects PAH uptake primarily at the initial step of the process—adsorption from water onto the surface of a biological membrane.

BIOLOGICAL EFFECTS IN THE AQUATIC ENVIRONMENT

PAH do not readily undergo chemical reactions with cellular biochemicals (e.g., covalent bonding to protein or DNA), except for certain specific enzyme reactions discussed earlier. However, they may interact physically with hydrophobic sites in the cell, causing molecular deformation and perturbation. Alternatively, PAH metabolites, being more hydrophilic, reactive, and electrophilic, may undergo a variety of spontaneous or enzyme-mediated chemical reactions. The most important of these are reactions leading to covalent bonding of PAH to cellular macromolecules such as proteins and DNA, leading to cell damage, mutagenesis, teratogenesis, and cancer.

Aromatic hydrocarbons appear to bind selectively to the surface of plasma membranes (Roubal, 1974; Roubal and Collier, 1975). A charge-transfer mechanism may direct them away from the hydrophobic interior of the membrane to the more polar surface, where they are held by weak bonds. This binding of aromatic hydrocarbons to the membrane surface causes perturbations in surface organization, increasing membrane permeability (Van Overbeek and Blondeau, 1954; Goldacre, 1968). By disrupting membrane organization, aromatic hydrocarbons might also affect the activity of the many enzymes bound to plasma membranes and essential for cell function.

Acute Toxicity

It may be predicted that the degree of membrane perturbation, and thus the toxicity of an aromatic hydrocarbon, will be proportional to the concentration of the hydrocarbon associated with the membrane surface. This, in turn, will be proportional to activity (product of mole fraction and activity coefficient) of the aromatic hydrocarbon in the aqueous phase (Hutchinson et al., 1980). Since the activity coefficient is inversely proportional to solubility, less soluble aromatics should have a greater effect at a given concentration than more soluble ones.

Although acute toxicity of aromatic hydrocarbons to aquatic organisms increases as molecular weight increases (and aqueous solubility decreases), the relationship is not absolute and there is much variability in response to PAH with similar molecular weights (Tables 6 and 7). Only PAH in the molecular weight range from naphthalene (MW 128) to fluoranthene and pyrene (MW 202) are acutely toxic to aquatic organisms. Higher molecular weight PAH are not acutely toxic to aquatic organisms, apparently because solubility falls below the aqueous concentration required to cause a response (Gehrs, 1978).

It should be recognized that the acute toxicity data do not adequately reflect the potential impact of chronic low-level PAH contamination on aquatic organisms and ecosystems. Chronic exposure to low concentrations of PAH in water, sediment, or food may produce sublethal responses in aquatic organisms. These sublethal effects may be detrimental to the long-term survival of an organism in its normal environment. In addition, chronic exposure to certain PAH may induce mutation and cancer in sensitive species.

Sublethal Effects: Bacteria and Plants

Depending on their type and concentration, PAH may either stimulate or inhibit growth and cell division in aquatic bacteria and plants. At low concentrations (10^{-5}–10^{-7} M), PAH known to be carcinogenic to mammals, such as BaP, benz[a]-anthracene, and dibenz[ah]anthracene, stimulated growth of the bacterium Escherichia coli (Hass and Applegate, 1975). Other PAH such as anthracene, phenanthrene, and chrysene inhibited growth at similar concentrations. Growth of two species of marine bacteria was inhibited by several PAH (Calder and Lader, 1976). Only pyrene increased the growth rate. Toxicity and degree of growth inhibition increased with increasing PAH molecular weight. Low concentrations (~µg/l) of several PAH, particularly those known to be carcinogenic in mammals, stimulated growth in freshwater microalgae (Graf and Nowak, 1966) and marine red macroalgae (Boney and Corner, 1962; Boney, 1974). The most effective growth stimulators for the red alga Antithamnion plumula were 6-methylbenz[a]anthracene and 9,10-dimethylbenz[a]-anthracene, both known mammalian carcinogens. Several PAH stimulated growth at low concentrations and inhibited it at higher concentrations. Boney (1974) found that the growth-stimulating effect of some PAH in red algae sporlings was increased rate of cell production by the apical cell cavity. This was accompanied by some reduction of cell size. The molecular mechanism of PAH-induced growth stimulation is unknown.

At higher concentrations (~mg/l), most PAH are acutely toxic to aquatic plants. They reduce the rate of cell division, inhibit photosynthesis,

Table 6 Acute Toxicity, Measured as LC50 (Concentration Causing Mortality of 50% of the Test Population in the Time Indicated), to Selected Species of Marine Animals

Compound	Species	Concentration (ppm)	Effect[a]	Reference
Naphthalene	*Neanthes arenaceodentata* (marine polychaete)	3.8	96-h LC50	Rossi and Neff (1978)
	Cancer magister (stage I zoeae, dungeness crab)	2.0	96-h LC50	Caldwell et al. (1977)
	Elasmopus pectenicrus (marine amphipod)	2.7	96-h LC50	Lee and Nicol (1978)
	Eurytemora affinis (marine copepod)	3.8	24-h LC50	Ott et al. (1978)
	Palaemonetes pugio (grass shrimp)	2.4	96-h LC50	Neff et al. (1976)
	Cyprinodon variegatus (sheepshead minnow)	2.4	24-h LC50	Anderson et al. (1974b)
	Oncorhynchus kisutch (coho salmon fry)	3.2	96-h LC50	Moles (1980)
1-Methylnaphthalene	*Cancer magister*	1.9	96-h LC50	Caldwell et al. (1977)
	Cyprinodon variegatus	3.4	44-h LC50	Anderson et al. (1974b)
2-Methylnaphthalene	*Cancer magister*	1.3	96-h LC50	Caldwell et al. (1977)
	Palaemonetes pugio	1.1	96-h LC50	Neff et al. (1976)
	Eurytemora affinis	1.5	24-h LC50	Ott et al. (1978)
	Cyprinodon variegatus	2.0	24-h LC50	Anderson et al. (1974b)
2,6-Dimethylnaphthalene	*Neanthes arenaceodentata*	2.6	96-h LC50	Rossi and Neff (1978)
	Palaemonetes pugio	0.7	96-h LC50	Neff et al. (1976)
	Eurytemora affinis	0.9	24-h LC50	Ott et al. (1978)
2,3,6-Trimethylnaphthalene	*Neanthes arenaceodentata*	2.0	96-h LC50	Rossi and Neff (1978)
2,3,5-Trimethylnaphthalene	*Eurytemora affinis*	0.3	24-h LC50	Ott et al. (1978)
Fluorene	*Neanthes arenaceodentata*	1.0	96-h LC50	Rossi and Neff (1978)
	Palaemonetes pugio	0.3	96-h LC50	Wofford and Neff (unpublished)
	Cyprinodon variegatus	1.7	96-h LC50	Wofford and Neff (unpublished)
Phenanthrene	*Neanthes arenaceodentata*	0.6	96-h LC50	Rossi and Neff (1978)
	Palaemonetes pugio	0.3	96-h LC50	Young (1977)
1-Methylphenanthrene	*Neanthes arenaceodentata*	0.3	96-h LC50	Rossi and Neff (1978)
Fluoranthene	*Neanthes arenaceodentata*	0.5	96-h LC50	Rossi and Neff (1978)
Chrysene	*Neanthes arenaceodentata*	1.0	NAT	Rossi and Neff (1978)
Benzo[a]pyrene	*Neanthes arenaceodentata*	1.0	NAT	Rossi and Neff (1978)
Dibenz[ah]anthracene	*Neanthes arenaceodentata*	1.0	NAT	Rossi and Neff (1978)

[a]LC50, median lethal concentration in the time specified; NAT, not acutely toxic in 96 h.

or kill cells outright. Toxicity of PAH to algae, measured as the concentration required to reduce the rate of photosynthetic carbon fixation by 50%, tends to increase with increasing PAH molecular weight, as is the case in animals (Table 7) (Hutchinson et al., 1980). Estimated toxicity of pyrene was nearly 50 times that of naphthalene in

two species of freshwater algae. *Chlamydomonas angutosa* was more sensitive than *Chlorella vulgaris* to all PAH tested. The difference in relative sensitivity of the two species decreased with increasing PAH molecular weight. Photosynthetic carbon fixation by three species of green macroalgae of the genus *Acrosiphonia* was inhibited by 44, 37, and 11% during exposure for 2 h to 5 ppm naphthalene (Kusk, 1980). Thus, there is considerable interspecies difference in relative sensitivity of aquatic algae to PAH.

Sublethal Effects: Animals

When unfertilized eggs of the sea urchin *Paracentrotus lividus* were exposed to 5 µg/ml BaP bound to horse serum proteins for 3 h and then fertilized, cleavage was abnormal and stopped at the morula stage (Ceas, 1974). If exposure to BaP was delayed until after fertilization, development progressed normally (Bresch et al., 1972). However, if newly fertilized eggs were exposed to 7,12-dimethylbenz[*a*]anthracene before the first cleavage, mesenchyme cells in the blastula were abnormal and the embryonic skeleton of the pluteus larvae was reduced in size and often abnormal in form (DeAngelis and Giordano, 1974).

Early larval stages of mud crabs, *Rhithropanopeus harrisii,* were more sensitive to phenanthrene and naphthalene than were later larval stages (Laughlin and Neff, 1979). Phenanthrene was much more toxic than naphthalene. Toxic effects of phenanthrene and naphthalene were increased

Table 7 Comparative Acute Toxicity of Several PAH to the Freshwater Microalgae
Chlamydomonas angulosa and *Chlorella vulgaris*[a,b]

Compound	*Chlamydomonas angulosa*	*Chlorella vulgaris*
Naphthalene	9.6	19.2
1-Methylnaphthalene	1.7	5.1
2-Methylnaphthalene	4.5	9.0
Phenanthrene	0.9	1.2
Anthracene	0.2	0.5
Pyrene	0.2	0.3

[a]Values are concentration (mg/l) of PAH required to reduce rate of photosynthetic $^{14}CO_2$ fixation by 50% during a 3-h incubation. Values for anthracene and pyrene are above the solubility of these PAH and are extrapolated.
[b]From Hutchinson et al. (1980); with permission from Plenum Press.

by lower than optimal salinity and temperature. Duration of larval development to the megalops stage was increased by exposure to sublethal concentrations of phenanthrene and decreased by exposure to sublethal concentrations of naphthalene. Megalops stage larvae that had been exposed continuously during larval development to phenanthrene or naphthalene had significantly lower weights than controls (Laughlin and Neff, 1980). This effect was greatest at low salinity (5 ppt). Exposure to sublethal concentrations of phenanthrene usually resulted in an increase in respiration rate of the larvae. Magnitude of the respiratory response was dependent on the stage of larval development and on the salinity or temperature regime. The most dramatic respiratory responses were observed in early larval stages exposed to phenanthrene at low salinity. The authors hypothesized that phenanthrene and, to a lesser extent, naphthalene increased the metabolic cost of osmoregulation in the larvae, possibly by increasing membrane permeability. As a result, less energy was available for growth, and growth rate decreased.

When marine copepods, *Eurytemora affinis,* were exposed for the complete life cycle (up to 29 d) to 10 µg/l naphthalene or methyl-, dimethyl-, or trimethylnaphthalene, there was a statistically significant reduction in life span, brood size, and total number of nauplii produced (Ott et al., 1978). Rate of egg production and total number of eggs produced per female were both reduced by approximately 50%. Trimethylnaphthalene had a greater effect than the other naphthalenes on these reproductive parameters.

Blue crabs, *Callinectes sapidus,* detected extremely low concentrations of naphthalene in solution and responded by increased antennular flicking rate (Pearson and Olla, 1979, 1980). The lowest concentration detected was 10^{-7} mg/l (10 pptr). Oriented locomotor activity and defensive displaying began at 2 mg/l (ppm). Several PAH abolished positive phototaxis in nauplii of barnacles, *Balanus amphitrite niveus,* at concentrations ranging from about 0.14 ppm dimethylnaphthalene to 0.42 ppm phenanthrene (Donahue et al., 1977). It is not known whether this was a behavioral or an anesthetic response.

Several histopathologic effects of exposure to PAH have been reported in mollusks and fish. Some of these will be discussed below; for a complete description, see Chapter 11.

Injected anthracene caused destabilization of lysosomal membranes in epithelial cells of the digestive tubules and pericardial glands of the mussel *Mytilus edulis* (Moore et al., 1978, 1980). Destabilization was accompanied by release of hexoseaminidase (an enzyme involved in catabolism of mucopolysaccharides) and evidence of cytolysis. Recovery was complete within 168 h after injection.

In oysters, *Crassostrea virginica,* exposed intermittently for 51 d to 3-methylcholanthrene in water, Couch et al. (1979) described a lesion consisting of incipient perivascular inflammatory foci in the mantle. Blood cells making up the lesion had pleomorphic nuclei and increased mitotic activity, and were larger than normal oyster leukocytes. The lesions had some characteristics of sarcomoid neoplasms but could not be identified unequivocally as cancerous.

A variety of histological changes occurred in the liver of mullet, *Mugil cephalus,* 4–11 d after they received a single injection of 30 mg/kg 3-methylcholanthrene (Schoor and Couch, 1979). At d 4 there was evidence of depletion of hepatic glycogen reserves. By d 7 there was substantial proliferation of the smooth and rough endoplasmic reticulum of hepatocytes. This change was undoubtedly correlated with induction of the hepatic microsomal (endoplasmic reticulum) mixed-function oxygenase system. Some degenerative changes were also observed after 11 d, including mitochondrial swelling, pigment deposition, and nuclear degeneration, suggestive of early necrosis.

Consumption for up to 28 d of a diet containing 5 ppm of a mixture of several hydrocarbons had little effect on the normal histology of the digestive tract of Chinook salmon, *Oncorhynchus tshawytscha* (Hawkes et al., 1980). Histopatholo-

gic changes included appearance of unusual cellular inclusions, vesiculation of the apical cytoplasm of columnar cells of the intestinal mucosa, and a decrease in cytoplasmic density and increase in rough endoplasmic reticulum in basal cells of the mucosa.

A wide variety of histopathologic and physiological responses to naphthalene exposure was described in the mummichog *Fundulus heteroclitus* (DiMichele and Taylor, 1978; Levitan and Taylor, 1979). Gill hyperplasia was the most consistent pathological condition noted and occurred even in fish exposed to as little as 2 μg/l naphthalene for 15 d. Hemorrhages of gill filaments were also noted in fish exposed to naphthalene at $\geqslant$2 mg/l. Fish were more sensitive to naphthalene when exposure occurred at high ambient seawater salinity (33 ppt) than when it occurred at intermediate or low salinity. At high ambient salinity, exposure to 4 mg/l naphthalene caused a large increase in respiration rate, an elevation in blood cortisol and glucose concentration, and osmoregulatory imbalance. It appears that naphthalene-mediated damage to gill lamellae interfered with the ability of *Fundulus* to osmoregulate at ambient salinities hyperosmotic to the body fluids.

At all but the lowest naphthalene concentration, there were signs of necrosis of neurosensory cells in epithelia of the lips, mouth, and pharynx and in the olfactory organ and lateral line system. In fish exposed to 2–30 ppm naphthalene, focal necrosis, hyperplasia, and ischemia were observed in several organs including the pancreas, liver, and brain. These histopathologies were attributed to blood stasis, probably caused by an increase in rigidity of erythrocyte membranes which prevented free passage of erythrocytes through finer blood vessels and capillaries.

The results of these investigations support the conclusion that a major mode of PAH toxicity, particularly with the lower molecular weight compounds, is through interference with cellular membrane function and membrane-associated enzyme systems.

PAH-Induced Cancer in Aquatic Animals

The main reason for concern about PAH in the environment is the observation that some of them can cause cancer in mammals, including humans (IARC, 1973; Zedeck, 1980). Carcinogenicity varies widely among the known PAH carcinogens. Four-, five-, and six-ring PAH tend to be more carcinogenic than those with smaller or larger ring systems. Highly angular configurations tend to be more carcinogenic than either linear or highly condensed ring systems.

PAH themselves are not carcinogenic; metabolic activation to reactive electrophilic metabolites is required (DePierre and Ernster, 1978). Thus, the degree of carcinogenicity is related to the structure and reactivity of the major metabolites produced by the cytochrome P-450 MFO and epoxide hydratase systems.

Different species of organisms vary substantially in sensitivity to PAH-induced carcinogenesis. This may result from interspecific differences in the levels of MFO–cytochrome P-450 activity, stereochemistry of the reactions catalyzed by enzymes from different species, activity of epoxide hydratase, and rate at which conjugating enzymes convert activated metabolites or their precursors to less active products. Many aquatic animals have the enzyme systems needed for metabolic activation of PAH. Evidence is growing that these enzyme systems are able to produce metabolites that behave like the known carcinogenic PAH metabolites. Hepatic microsomal enzyme preparations from several species of marine and freshwater teleost fish converted BaP to metabolites that were active in the Ames bacterial mutagenicity test (Ahokas et al., 1977; Stegeman, 1977; Payne et al., 1978; Kurelec et al., 1979). The Ames Salmonella/mammalian microsome test is widely used as a preliminary screening test for chemical carcinogens, based on the hypothesis that molecular mechanisms of mutagenesis and carcinogenesis are similar (i.e., that most mutagens are carcinogens) and that substances mutagenic to bacteria will be mutagenic to eukaryotes (Ames et al., 1975).

A critical step in PAH carcinogenesis in mammals appears to be the covalent binding of metabolically activated PAH to nucleophilic residues in cellular macromolecules, especially DNA (Heidelberger, 1976; Pelkonen et al., 1978). Metabolites of BaP produced by liver microsomal preparations from lake trout, Salmo trutta lacustris, readily bound to nucleosides of deproteinized DNA in vitro (Ahokas et al., 1979). Liver microsomes of the roach (a fish) Rutilus rutilus were relatively inactive in producing DNA-binding BaP metabolites. The DNA-binding metabolites produced by trout microsomes included BaP diol-epoxides and phenols. In similar experiments, Varanasi and Gmur (1980) demonstrated covalent bonding in vitro to salmon sperm DNA of BaP metabolites produced by liver preparations of PAH-induced starry flounder, Platichthys stellatus, and coho salmon, Oncorhynchus kisutch. The flounder liver was more active than the salmon liver in producing DNA-binding metabolites. BaP-9,10-dihydrodiol and BaP-7,8-dehydrodiol were the major BaP metabolites produced by both species. The 7,8,9,10-diol-epoxide is considered to be the most carcinogenic metabolite of BaP in mammals. Thus, fish can activate BaP and presumably other carcinogenic PAH to highly reactive electrophilic metabolites, similar to those produced by mammalian microsomes, which covalently bind to DNA and cause mutations in Salmonella.

Despite the ability of teleost fish to produce mutagenic, and by inference carcinogenic, metabolites from PAH, they appear to be quite resistant to PAH-induced cancer. Embryos of zebrafish, Brachydanio rerio, developed tail necrosis, tumor-like growths, enlarged pericardium, and shortened body when exposed during development to 0.56 ppm 7,12-dimethylbenz[a]anthracene (Jones and Huffman, 1957). Epithelial cells and nuclei of PAH-exposed embryos were enlarged and granular, suggestive of a precancerous condition. Ermer (1970) was able to produce skin lesions which he identified as epitheliomas in two short-lived fish—the three-spined stickleback, *Gasterosteus aculeatus,* and the bitterling, *Rhodeus amurus*—but not in a long-lived fish, the carp, *Cyprinus carpio,* by painting the skin twice a week for 3–6 mo with 0.5 mg 3-methylcholanthrene or BaP. In another experiment, he injected *G. aculeatus* with 0.1 ml 1% BaP in glycerol 10 times (10 mg BaP) and observed the fish for 4 mo. This treatment produced injection site necrosis but no neoplasms. Exposure to 7,12-dimethylbenz[a]anthracene inhibited mitosis and induced an increase in the number of multinucleate cells in cultures of cells derived from trout (*Salmo gairdneri*) gonadal fibroblasts and fathead minnow (*Pimephales promelas*) epithelium (Bourne and Jones, 1973). In fathead minnow epithelial cell cultures exposed to the carcinogen, many cells were extremely abnormal, with reduced cytoplasm, clumped chromatin, and basophilic cytoplasm. These cellular changes are all highly suggestive of an interaction between the carcinogen or its metabolites and nuclear DNA to produce precancerous changes in cellular function.

Several investigators have induced formation of cancerous lesions in aquatic amphibians by injecting PAH or implanting PAH crystals in the tissues (Seilern-Aspang and Kratochwil, 1962, 1963; deLustig and Matos, 1971; Neukomn, 1974). If a regenerative field is induced near the site of PAH injection by amputation of a limb, formation of a tumor may be inhibited or stimulated, indicating an interaction between the cellular processes underlying tissue regeneration and carcinogenesis.

There have been no reports of induction of cancer in aquatic animals by exposure to environmentally realistic levels of carcinogenic PAH in the water, food, or sediments. In addition, carcinogenic PAH have not been identified unequivocally as the causative agent for an increased incidence of cancer in any natural population of aquatic organisms.

There have been several reports of an increased incidence of cancerlike lesions in marine animals from the vicinity of an oil spill (Hodgins et al., 1977). Yevich and Barszcz (1977) reported a high incidence of gonadal neoplasms in soft-shell clams, *Mya arenaria,* from Long Cove, Searsport, Maine, and of hematopoietic neoplasms in the same species from Harpswell Neck, Maine. Although both sites had been contaminated with refined oil products high in aromatics, the authors could not say that the oil was a causative factor in inducing the neoplasms.

Black et al. (1980) reported a high incidence of tumors in bottom fish from the Buffalo River near its confluence with the Niagara River in Buffalo, New York. Extracts of sediments from the river were highly mutagenic in the Ames bacterial mutagenesis assay. More than 40 PAH were identified by gas chromatography-mass spectrometry in the sediment samples, including the mammalian carcinogens benz[a]anthracene and benzo[a]pyrene. Fish and invertebrates from the site were contaminated with the types of PAH found in the sediments. These findings provide strong circumstantial evidence of a link between mutagenic PAH in sediments and a high incidence of proliferative tissue lesions in bottom-living fish in the area.

SUMMARY AND CONCLUSIONS

Polycyclic aromatic hydrocarbons are formed by a variety of processes, including indirect and direct biosynthesis, diagenesis of organic material to produce fossil fuels, and incomplete combustion of organic matter. Ability of organisms to synthesize PAH is questionable. If PAH biosynthesis does occur, it is likely to be of little quantitative importance to the cycle of PAH in the environment. Fossil fuels, including peat, coal, and petroleum, are relatively rich in PAH. Assemblages of PAH in crude and refined petroleum are extremely complex. Pyrolysis of organic matter at temperatures between 400 and 2000°C results in generation of a wide variety of PAH. Reducing conditions in the pyrolytic environment favor PAH production.

There are many routes by which PAH from diverse sources enter the aquatic environment. PAH indigenous to fossil fuels may enter in coal dust, in leachate of peat bogs, or in petroleum spillage into water bodies. The latter is the most important quantitatively. Pyrosynthesized PAH are released into the atmosphere adsorbed to soot. Residence time of particulate PAH in the atmosphere is long enough to allow dispersal over long distances. Airborne PAH enter the aquatic environment through dry fallout, rainfall, and deposition from the vapor phase onto water surfaces. PAH deposited on land may reach the aquatic environment in surface run-off. Industrial and domestic waste waters are often rich in PAH. Sewage treatment processes remove some PAH, but the remainder are released to the aquatic environment.

It is estimated that nearly 230,000 metric tons of total PAH enter the aquatic environment each year from various sources. Main routes of entry are petroleum spillage and fallout or rainfall. Most of the PAH entering the aquatic environment remain close to sites of deposition, so that lakes, rivers, estuaries, and coastal marine environments near centers of human population are primary repositories of aquatic PAH.

Because of their low aqueous solubilities, PAH in the aquatic environment rapidly become adsorbed to organic and inorganic particulate materials and are deposited in bottom sediments or accumulated in the tissues of aquatic organisms. Aquatic organisms often have tissue PAH concentrations orders of magnitude higher than aqueous PAH concentrations, but equal to or less than those in bottom sediments.

Several processes reduce concentrations of PAH in water and sediments. These include evaporation, photooxidation, and metabolic degradation by aquatic bacteria, fungi, and animals.

Aquatic organisms are able to accumulate PAH from water, food, and sediment. In most cases, accumulation from water is more efficient than accumulation from food or sediment. Sediment-adsorbed PAH have very limited bioavailability to aquatic organisms. Benthic infaunal animals rarely have higher concentrations of PAH than the sediments in which they live.

Most aquatic animals can degrade PAH to more polar metabolites and excrete them rapidly. Even species lacking PAH-metabolizing ability can release accumulated PAH rapidly when they are returned to a PAH-free environment. Thus, food chain biomagnification of PAH occurs to a very limited extent, if at all.

PAH are acutely toxic to aquatic organisms at concentrations of about 0.2–10 ppm. Deleterious sublethal responses in aquatic organisms are sometimes observed at concentrations in the range 5–100 ppb PAH. Many of these PAH-induced responses involve interference of PAH with key membrane-mediated physiological and biochemical processes.

Metabolic intermediates of some PAH are highly carcinogenic, mutagenic, and/or teratogenic. PAH-induced cancerlike growths or developmental anomalies have been described in several aquatic animals and plants. Attempts to identify PAH as causative agents of cancer in natural populations of aquatic organisms have met with limited success. The role of PAH in carcinogenesis in aquatic organisms or humans is unknown.

LITERATURE CITED

Addison RF, Zinck ME, Willis DE: Induction of hepatic mixed-function oxidase (MFO) enzymes in trout (*Salvelinus fontinalis*) by feeding Aroclor 1254 or 3-methylcholanthrene. Comp Biochem Physiol 61C:323–325, 1978.

Ahokas JT, Paakkonen R, Raunio V, Karki N, Pelkonen O: Oxidative metabolism of carcinogens by trout liver resulting in protein binding and mutagenicity. In: Microsomes and Drug Oxidations, edited by V Ullrich, I Roots, A Hildebrandt, RW Estabrook, AH Conney, pp. 435–441. Oxford: Pergamon, 1977.

Ahokas JT, Saarni H, Nebert DW, Pelkonen O: The *in vitro* metabolism and covalent binding of benzo[*a*]pyrene to DNA catalyzed by trout liver microsomes. Chem Biol Interact 25:103–111, 1979.

Aizenshtat Z: Perylene and its geochemical significance. Geochim Cosmochim Acta 37:559–567, 1973.

Ames BN, McCann J, Yamasaki E: Methods for

detecting carcinogens and mutagens with *Salmonella*/mammalian-microsome mutagenicity test. Mutat Res 31:347–364, 1975.

Andelman JB, Snodgrass JE: Incidence and significance of polynuclear aromatic hydrocarbons in the water environment. CRC Crit Rev Environ Control 4(1):59–83, 1972.

Andelman JB, Suess MJ: Polynuclear aromatic hydrocarbons in the water environment. Bull WHO 43:479–508, 1970.

Anderson JW, Neff JM, Cox BA, Tatem HE, Hightower GM: Effects of oil on estuarine animals: Toxicity, uptake and depuration, respiration. In: Pollution and Physiology of Marine Organisms, edited by FJ Vernberg, WB Vernberg, pp. 285–310. New York: Academic, 1974.

Anderson RS: Benzo[a]pyrene metabolism in the American oyster *Crassostrea virginica.* EPA Ecol Res Ser EPA-600/3-78-009, 1978.

Badger GM: Mode of formation of carcinogens in the human environment. Natl Cancer Inst Monogr 9:1–16, 1962.

Badger GM, Kimber RWL, Spotswood TM: Mode of formation of BP in human environment. Nature (Lond) 187:663–665, 1960.

Bend JR, Foureman GL, James MO: Partially induced hepatic mixed-function oxidase systems in individual members of certain marine species from coastal Maine and Florida. In: Aquatic Pollutants. Transformation and Biological Effects, edited by O Hutzinger, LH Van Lelyveld, BCJ Zoeteman, pp. 483–486. New York: Pergamon, 1978.

Binder RL, Stegeman JJ: Induction of aryl hydrocarbon hydroxylase activity in embryos of an estuarine fish. Biochem Pharmacol 29:949–951, 1980.

Bjorseth A, Knutzen J, Skei J: Determination of polycyclic aromatic hydrocarbons in sediments and mussels from Saudafjord, W. Norway, by glass capillary gas chromatography, Sci Total Environ 13:71–86, 1979a.

Bjorseth A, Lunde G, Lindskog A: Long-range transport of polycyclic aromatic hydrocarbons. Atmos Environ 13:45–53, 1979b.

Black JJ, Holmes M, Dymerski PP, Zapisek WF: Fish tumor pathology and aromatic hydrocarbon pollution in a Great Lakes estuary. In: Hydrocarbons and Halogenated Hydrocarbons

in the Aquatic Environment, edited by BK Afghan, D Mackay, pp. 559–566. New York: Plenum, 1980.

Blumer M: Polycyclic aromatic compounds in nature, Sci Am 234(1):34–45, 1976.

Boehm PD, Quinn JG: The effect of dissolved organic matter in sea water on the uptake of mixed individual hydrocarbons and no. 2 fuel oil by a marine filter-feeding bivalve (*Mercenaria mercenaria*). Estuarine Coastal Mar Sci 4:93–105, 1976.

Boney AD: Aromatic hydrocarbons and the growth of marine algae. Mar Pollut Bull 5:185–186, 1974.

Boney AD, Corner EDS: On the effects of some carcinogenic hydrocarbons on the growth of sporelings of marine red algae. J Mar Biol Assoc UK 43:579–585, 1962.

Borneff J, Kunte H: Carcinogenic substances in water and soil. Part XVII: Concerning the origin and estimation of the polycyclic aromatic hydrocarbons in water. Arch Hyg (Berlin) 149:226–243, 1965 (German).

Borneff J, Selenka F, Kunte H, Maximos A: Experimental studies on the formation of polycyclic aromatic hydrocarbons in plants. Environ Res)2:22–29, 1968.

Bourne EW, Jones RW: Effects of 7,12-dimethylbenz[a]anthracene (DMBA) in fish cells *in vitro.* Trans Am Microsc Soc 92:140–142, 1973.

Bresch H, Spielhoff R, Mohr U, Barkemeyer H: Use of sea urchin egg for quick screen testing of the biological activities of substances. I. Influence of fractions of a tobacco smoke condensate on early development. Proc Soc Exp Biol Med 141:747–752, 1972.

Calder JA, Lader JH: Effect of dissolved aromatic hydrocarbons on the growth of marine bacteria in batch culture. Appl Environ Microbiol 32:95–101, 1976.

Caldwell RS, Caldarone EM, Mallon MH: Effects of a seawater-soluble fraction of Cook Inlet crude oil and its major aromatic components on larval stages of the dungeness crab, *Cancer magister* Dana. In: Fate and Effects of Petroleum Hydrocarbons in Marine Ecosystems and Organisms, edited by DA Wolfe, pp. 210–220. New York: Pergamon, 1977.

Ceas MP: Effects of 3,4-benzopyrene on sea urchin egg development. Acta Embryol Exp 3:267–272, 1974.

Cerniglia CE, Hebert RL, Szaniszlo PJ, Gibson DT: Fungal transfrormation of naphthalene. Arch Microbiol 117:135–143, 1978.

Cerniglia CE, Dodge RH, Gibson DT: Studies on the fungal oxidation of polycyclic aromatic hydrocarbons. Bot Mar 23:121–124, 1980.

Chambers JE: Induction of microsomal mixed function oxidase system components in striped mullet by short-term exposure to crude oil. Toxicol Lett 4:227–230, 1979.

Collier TC, Thomas LC, Malins DC: Influence of environmental temperature on disposition of dietary naphthalene in coho salmon (Oncorhynchus kisutch): Isolation and identification of individual metabolites. Comp Biochem Physiol 61C:23–28, 1978.

Corner EDS, Harris RP, Kilvington CC, O'Hara SCM: Petroleum compounds in the marine food web: Short-term experiments on the fate of naphthalene in Calanus. J Mar Biol Assoc UK 56:121–123, 1976a.

Corner EDS, Harris RP, Whittle KJ, Mackie PR: Hydrocarbons in marine zooplankton and fish. In: Effects of Pollutants on Aquatic Organisms, edited by APM Lockwood, pp. 71–106. Cambridge, England: Cambridge Univ. Press, 1976b.

Corner EDS, Kilvington CC, O'Hara SCM: Qualitative studies on the metabolism of naphthalene in Maia squinado (Herbst). J Mar Biol Assoc UK 53:819–832, 1973.

Couch JA, Courtney LA, Winstead JT, Foss SS: The American oyster (Crassostrea virginica) as an indicator of carcinogens in the aquatic environment. In: Animals as Monitors of Environmental Pollutants, pp. 65–84. Washington, D.C.: National Academy of Sciences, 1979.

De Angelis E, Giordano GG: Sea urchin egg development under the action of benzo[a]pyrene and 7,12-dimethylbenz[a]anthracene. Cancer Res 32:1275–1280, 1974.

Delaune RD, Hambrick GA, III, Patrick WH, Jr: Degradation of hydrocarbons in oxidized and reduced sediments. Mar Pollut Bull 11:103–106, 1980.

De Lustig ES, Matos EL: Teratogenic effects induced in tail of Bufo arenarum tadpoles following treatment with carcinogens. Experientia 27:555–556, 1971.

DePierre JW, Ernster L: The metabolism of polycyclic hydrocarbons and its relationship to cancer. Biochim Biophys Acta 473:149–186, 1978.

DiMichele L, Taylor MH: Histopathological and physiological responses of Fundulus heteroclitus L. to naphthalene exposure. J Fish Res Board Can 35:1060–1066, 1978.

Dobroski CJ, Jr, Epifanio CE: Accumulation of benzo[a]pyrene in a larval bivalve via trophic transfer. Can J Fish Aquat Sci 37:2318–2322, 1980.

Doherty JJ, Khan MAQ: Hepatic microsomal mixed-function oxidase in the frog, Xenopus laevis. Comp Biochem Physiol 68C:221–228, 1981.

Donahue WH, Wang RT, Welch M, Nicol JAC: Effects of water-soluble components of petroleum oils and aromatic hydrocarbons on barnacle larvae. Environ Pollut 13:187–202, 1977.

Dunn BP, Fee J: Polycyclic aromatic hydrocarbon carcinogens in commercial seafoods. J Fish Res Board Can 36:1469–1476, 1979.

Dunn BP, Stich HF: The use of mussels in estimating benzo[a]pyrene contamination of the marine environment. Proc Soc Exp Biol Med 150:49–51, 1975.

Dunn BP, Stich HF: Monitoring procedures for chemical carcinogens in coastal waters. J Fish Res Board Can 33:2040–2046, 1976.

Dunn BP, Young DR: Baseline levels of benzo[a]pyrene in southern California mussels. Mar Pollut Bull 7:231–234, 1976.

Eganhouse RP, Calder JA: The solubility of medium molecular weight aromatic hydrocarbons and the effects of hydrocarbon co-solutes and salinity. Geochim Cosmochim Acta 40:555–561, 1976.

Ermer M: Studies with carcinogens in short-lived fish species. Zool Anz 184:175–193, 1970 (German).

Ferris JP, Fasco MJ, Stylianopoulou FL, Jerina DM, Daly JW, Jeffrey AM: Monooxygenase activity in Cunninghamella bainierii. Evidence for a fungal system similar to liver microsomes. Arch Biochem Biophys 156:97–103, 1973.

Ferris JP, MacDonald LH, Patrie MA, Martin MA: Aryl hydrocarbon hydroxylase activity in the fungus *Cunninghamella bainierri.* Evidence of the presence of cytochrome P-450. Arch Biochem Biophys 175:443–452, 1976.

Flower AR: World oil production. Sci Am 238(1): 42–49, 1978.

Fucik KW, Neff JM: Effects of temperature and salinity on naphthalene uptake in the temperate clam *Rangia cuneata* and the boreal clam *Protothaca staminea*. In: Fate and Effects of Petroleum Hydrocarbons in Marine Ecosystems and Organisms, edited by DA Wolfe, pp. 305–312. New York: Pergamon, 1977.

Gehrs CW: Enironmental implications of coal-conversion technologies: Organic contaminants. In: Energy and Environmental Stress in Aquatic Systems, edited by JH Thorp, JW Gibbons, pp. 157–175. CONF-771114, Springfield, Va.: National Technical Information Center, 1978.

Gerarde HW, Gerarde DF: The ubiquitous hydrocarbons. Assoc Food Drug Offic US 25–26:1–47, 1962.

Gerhart EH, Carlson RM: Hepatic mixed-function oxidase activity in rainbow trout exposed to several polycyclic aromatic compounds. Environ Res 17:284–295, 1978.

Gibson DT: Biodegradation of aromatic petroleum hydrocarbons. In: Fate and Effects of Petroleum Hydrocarbons in Marine Ecosystems and Organisms, edited by DA Wolfe, pp. 36–46. New York: Pergamon, 1977.

Goldacre RJ: The effects of detergents and oils on the cell membrane. In: The Biological Effects of Oil Pollution on Littoral Communities, edited by JD Carthy, DR Arthur, pp. 131–139. London: Field Studies Council, 1968.

Graf W, Diel H: Concerning the naturally caused normal level of carcinogenic polycyclic aromatics and its cause. Arch Hyg 150:49–59, 1966 (German).

Graf W, Nowak W: Promotion of growth in lower and higher plants by carcinogenic polycyclic aromatics. Arch Hyg 150:513–528, 1966 (German).

Green FA, Jr, Neff JM: Toxicity, accumulation and release of three polychlorinated naphthalenes (Halowax 1000, 1013, and 1099) in postlarval and adult grass shrimp, *Palaemonetes pugio*. Bull Environ Contam Toxicol 17:399–407, 1977.

Griest WH: Multicomponent polycyclic aromatic hydrocarbon analysis of inland water and sediment. In: Hydrocarbons and Halogenated Hydrocarbons in the Aquatic Environment, edited by BK Afghan, D Mackay, pp. 173–183. New York: Plenum, 1980.

Grimmer G, Bohnke H, Borwitzky H: Profile-analysis of polycyclic aromatic hydrocarbons in sewage sludge by gas chromatography. Fresenius Z Anal Chem 289:91–95, 1978.

Grimmer G, Duval D: Endogenous formation of polycyclic hydrocarbons in higher plants. 8. Carcinogenic hydrocarbons in the environment of humans. Z Naturforsch 25b:1171–1175, 1970 (German).

Gruger EH, Jr, Wekell MM, Numoto PT, Craddock DR: Induction of hepatic aryl hydrocarbon hydroxylase in salmon exposed to petroleum dissolved in seawater and to petroleum and polychlorinated biphenyls, separate and together, in food. Bull Environ Contam Toxicol 17:512–520, 1977a.

Gruger EH, Jr, Wekell MM, Robisch PA: Effects of chlorinated biphenyls and petroleum hydrocarbons on the activity of hepatic aryl hydrocarbon hydroxylase of coho salmon (*Oncorhynchus kisutch*) and chinook salmon (*O. tshawytscha*). In: Fate and Effects of Petroleum Hydrocarbons in Marine Ecosystems and Organisms, edited by DA Wolfe, pp. 323–331. New York: Pergamon, 1977b.

Guerin MR, Elper JL, Griest WH, Clark BR, Rao TK: Polycyclic aromatic hydrocarbons from fossil fuel conversion processes. In: Carcinogenesis. A Comprehensive Survey, vol. 3, Polynuclear Aromatic Hydrocarbons. Second International Symposium on Analysis, Chemistry, and Biology, edited by PW Jones, RI Freudenthal, pp. 21–34. New York: Raven, 1978.

Hamelink JL, Spacie A: Fish and chemicals: The process of accumulation. Annu Rev Pharmacol Toxicol 17:167–177, 1977.

Hansen N, Jensen VB, Appelquist H, Morch E: The uptake and release of petroleum hydrocarbons by the marine mussel *Mytilus edulis*. Prog Water Technol 10:351–359, 1978.

Harris RP, Berdugo V, Corner EDS, Kilvington CC, O'Hara SCM: Factors affecting the retention of a petroleum hydrocarbon by marine planktonic copepods. In: Fate and Effects of Petroleum Hydrocarbons in Marine Ecosystems and Organisms, edited by DA Wolfe, pp. 286–304. New York: Pergamon, 1977.

Harrison RM, Perry R, Wellings RA: Polynuclear aromatic hydrocarbons in raw, potable and waste waters. Water Res 9:331–346, 1975.

Harrison RM, Perry R, Wellings RA: Effect of water chlorination upon levels of some polynuclear aromatic hydrocarbons in water. Environ Sci Technol 10:1151–1156, 1976a.

Harrison RM, Perry R, Wellings RA: Chemical kinetics of chlorination of some polynuclear aromatic hydrocarbons under conditions of water treatment processes. Environ Sci Technol 10:1156–1160, 1976b.

Hase A, Hites RA: On the origin of polycyclic aromatic hydrocarbons in recent sediments: Biosynthesis by anaerobic bacteria. Geochim Cosmochim Acta 40:1141–1143, 1976.

Hase A, Hites RA: On the origin of polycyclic aromatic hydrocarbons in the aqueous environment. In: Identification of Organic Pollutants in Water, edited by LH Keith, pp. 205–214. Ann Arbor, Mich.: Ann Arbor Science, 1977.

Hass BS, Applegate HG: The effects of unsubstituted polycyclic aromatic hydrocarbons on the growth of *Escherichia coli.* Chem Biol Interact 10:265–268, 1975.

Hawkes JW, Gruger EH, Jr, Olson OP: Effects of petroleum hydrocarbons and chlorinated biphenyls on the morphology of the intestine of chinook salmon *Oncorhynchus tshawytscha).* Environ Res 23:149–161, 1980.

Hayatsu R, Scott RG, Moore LP, Studier MH: Aromatic units in coal. Nature (Lond) 257:378–380, 1975.

Heidelberger C: Studies on the mechanisms of carcinogenesis by polycyclic aromatic hydrocarbons and their derivatives. In: Carcinogenesis—A Comprehensive Survey, vol. 1, Polynuclear Aromatic Hydrocarbons, edited by R Freudenthal, PW Jones, pp. 1–8. New York: Raven, 1976.

Herbes SE: Partitioning of polycyclic aromatic hydrocarbons between dissolved and particulate phases in natural waters. Water Res 11:493–496, 1977.

Herbes SE, Risi GF: Metabolic alteration and ex-

cretion of anthracene by *Daphnia pulex.* Bull Environ Contam Toxicol 19:147–155, 1978.

Herbes SE, Schwall LR: Microbial transformation of polycyclic aromatic hydrocarbons in pristine and petroleum-contaminated sediments. Appl Environ Microbiol 35:306–316, 1978.

Hites RA: Sources of polycyclic aromatic hydrocarbons in the aquatic environment. In: Sources, Effects and Sinks of Hydrocarbons in the Aquatic Environment, pp. 325–332. Washington, D.C.: American Institute of Biological Sciences, 1976.

Hites RA, Laflamme RE, Windsor JG, Jr: Polycyclic aromatic hydrocarbons in marine/aquatic sediments: Their ubiquity. In: Petroleum in the Marine Environment, edited by L Petrakis, FT Weiss, pp. 289–311. Washington, D.C.: American Chemical Society, 1980.

Hodgins HO, McCain BB, Hawkes JW: Marine fish and invertebrate diseases, host disease resistance, and pathological effects of petroleum. In: Effects of Petroleum on Arctic and Subarctic Marine Environments and Organisms, edited by DC Malins, vol. 2, pp. 95–174. New York: Academic, 1977.

Huberman E, Sachs L, Yang SK, Gelboin HV: Identification of mutagenic metabolites of benzo[a]pyrene in mammalian cells. Proc Natl Acad Sci USA 73:607–612, 1976.

Hutchinson TC, Hellebust JA, Tam D, Mackay D, Mascarenkas RA, Shiu WY: The correlation of the toxicity to algae of hydrocarbons and halogenated hydrocarbons with their physical-chemical properties. In: Hydrocarbons and Halogenated Hydrocarbons in the Aquatic Environment, edited by BK Afghan, D Mackay, pp. 577–586. New York: Plenum, 1980.

International Agency for Research on Cancer: Monograph on the Evaluation of Carcinogenic Risk of the Chemical to Man: Certain Polycyclic Aromatic Hydrocarbons and Heterocyclic Compounds, vol. 3. Geneva, Switzerland: World Health Organization, 1973.

James MO, Bend JR: Polycyclic aromatic hydrocarbon induction and cytochrome P-450-dependent fixed-function oxidases in marine fish. Toxicol Appl Pharmacol 54:117–133, 1980.

James MO, Bowen ER, Dansette PM, Bend JR:

Epoxide hydrase and glutathione *S*-transferase activities with selected alkene and arene oxides in several marine species. Chem Biol Interact 25:321–344, 1979.

Jerina DM, Daly JW: Arene oxides: A new aspect of drug metabolism. Science 185:573–578, 1974.

Jerina DM, Daly JW, Jeffrey AM, Gibson DT: Cis-1,2-dihydroxy-1,2-dihydronaphthalene: A bacterial metabolite from naphthalene. Arch Biochem Biophys 142:394–396, 1971.

Jerina DM, Yagi H, Lehr RE, Thakker DR, Schafer-Ridder M, Karle JM, Levin W, Wood AW, Chang RL, Conney AH: The bay-region theory of carcinogenesis by polycyclic aromatic hydrocarbons. In: Polycyclic Hydrocarbons and Cancer, vol. 1, Environment, Chemistry, and Metabolism, edited by HV Gelboin, POP Ts'o, pp. 173–188. New York: Academic, 1978.

Jones RW, Huffman MN: Fish embryos as bioassay material in testing chemicals for effects on cell division and differentiation. Trans Am Microsc Soc 76:177–183, 1957.

Khan MAQ, Stanton RH, Reddy G: Detoxication of foreign compounds by invertebrates. In: Survival in Toxic Environments, edited by MAQ Khan, JP Bederka, Jr, pp. 177–201. New York: Academic, 1974.

Kreiger RI, Lee PW: Properties of the aldrin epoxidase system in the gut and fat body of a caddisfly larva. J Econ Entomol 66:1–6, 1973.

Kurelec B, Britvic S, Rijavec M, Muller WEG, Zahn RK: Benzo[a]pyrene monooxygenase induction in marine fish—molecular response to oil pollution. Mar Biol 44:211–216, 1977.

Kurelec B, Matijasevic Z, Rijavec M, Alacevic M, Britvic S, Muller WEG, Zahn RK: Induction of benzo[a]pyrene monooxygenase in fish and the *Salmonella* test as a tool for detecting mutagenic/carcinogenic xenobiotics in the aquatic environment. Bull Environ Contam Toxicol 21:799–807, 1979.

Kusk KO: Effects of crude oils and aromatic hydrocarbons on the photosynthesis of three species of *Acrosiphonia* grown in the laboratory. Bot Mar 23:587–593, 1980.

Lake JL, Hershner C: Petroleum sulfur-containing compounds and aromatic hydrocarbons in the

marine mollusks *Modiolus demissus* and *Crassostrea virginica*. In: Proceedings of the 1977 Oil Spill Conference (Prevention, Control, Cleanup), pp. 627–632. Washington, D.C.: American Petroleum Institute, 1977.

Larson RA, Blankenship DW, Hunt LL: Toxic hydroperoxidases: Photochemical formation from petroleum constituents. In: Sources, Effects and Sinks of Hydrocarbons in the Aquatic Environment, pp. 298–308. Washington, D.C.: American Institute of Biological Sciences, 1976.

Larson RA, Hunt LL, Blankenship DW: Formation of toxic products from a #2 fuel oil by photooxidation. Environ Sci Technol 11:492–496, 1977.

Laughlin RB, Jr, Neff JM: Interactive effects of salinity, temperature and polycyclic aromatic hydrocarbons on the survival and development rate of larvae of the mud crab *Rhithropanopeus harrisii*. Mar Biol 53:281–291, 1979.

Laughlin RB, Jr, Neff JM: Influence of temperature, salinity, and phenanthrene (a petroleum derived polycyclic aromatic hydrocarbon) on the respiration of larval mud crabs, *Rhithropanopeus harrisii*. Estuarine Coastal Mar Sci 10:655–669, 1980.

Lech JJ, Bend JR: Relationship between biotransformation and the toxicity and fate of xenobiotic chemicals in fish. Environ Health Perspect 34:115–131, 1980.

Lee RF: Fate of petroleum hydrocarbons in marine zooplankton. In: Proceedings of the 1975 Conference on Prevention and Control of Oil Pollution, pp. 549–554. Washington, D.C.: American Petroleum Institute, 1975.

Lee RF: Mixed function oxygenases (MFO) in marine invertebrates. Mar Biol Lett 2:87–105, 1981.

Lee RF, Gardner WS, Anderson JW, Blaylock JW, Barwell-Clarke J: Fate of polycyclic aromatic hydrocarbons in controlled ecosystem enclosures. Environ Sci Technol 12:832–838, 1978.

Lee RF, Lehsau D, Madden M: Polycyclic aromatic hydrocarbons in oysters (*Crassostrea virginica*) from Georgia coastal waters: Analysis by high pressure liquid chromatography. In:

Proceedings of the 1981 Oil Spill Conference, pp. 341–346. Washington, D.C.: American Petroleum Institute, 1981.

Lee RF, Ryan C, Neuhauser ML: Fate of petroleum hydrocarbons taken up from food and water by the blue crab *Callinectes sapidus*. Mar Biol 37:363–370, 1976.

Lee RF, Sauerheber R, Benson AA: Petroleum hydrocarbons: Uptake and discharge by the marine mussel *Mytilus edulis*. Science 177:344–346, 1972a.

Lee RF, Sauerheber R, Dobbs GH: Uptake, metabolism and discharge of polycyclic aromatic hydrocarbons by marine fish. Mar Biol 17:201–208, 1972b.

Lee RF, Singer SC, Tenore KR, Gardner WS, Philpot RM: Detoxification system in polychaete worms: Importance in the degradation of sediment hydrocarbons. In: Marine Pollution: Functional Responses, edited by WB Vernberg, FP Thurberg, A Calabrese, FJ Vernberg, pp. 23–38. New York: Academic, 1979.

Lee WY, Nicol JAC: Individual and combined toxicity of some petroleum hydrocarbons to the marine amphipod, *Elasmopus pectenicrus*. Mar Biol 48:215–222, 1978.

Lehr RE, Jerina DM: Metabolic activations of polycyclic hydrocarbons. Structure-activity relationships. Arch Toxicol 39:1–6, 1977.

Lehr RE, Kumar S, Levin W, Wood AW, Chang RL, Buening MK, Conney AH, Whalen DL, Thakker DR, Yagi H, Jerina DM: Benzo[e]-pyrene dihydrodiols and diol epoxides: Chemistry, mutagenicity and tumorigenicity. In: Polynuclear Aromatic Hydrocarbons: Chemistry and Biological Effects, edited by A Bjorseth, AJ Dennis, pp. 675–688. Columbus, Ohio: Battelle Press, 1980.

Leo A, Hansch C, Elkins DE: Partition coefficients and their uses. Chem Rev 71:525–616, 1971.

Levitan WM, Taylor MH: Physiology of salinity-dependent naphthalene toxicity in *Fundulus heteroclitus*. J Fish Res Board Can 36:615–620, 1979.

Lindstrom-Seppa P, Koivusaari U, Hanninen O: Metabolism of xenobiotics by vendace (*Coregonus albula*). Comp Biochem Physiol 68C: 121–126, 1981.

Lunde G, Bjorseth A: Polycyclic aromatic hydrocarbons in long-range transported aerosols. Nature (Lond) 268:518–519, 1977.

Lyes MC: Bioavailability of a hydrocarbon from water and sediment to the marine worm *Arenicola marina*. Mar Biol 268:518–519, 1979.

MacKenzie MJ, Hunter JV: Sources and fates of aromatic compounds in urban stormwater runoff. Environ Sci Technol 13:179–183, 1979.

Mackie PR, Hardy R, Whittle KJ, Bruce C, McGill AS: The tissue hydrocarbon burden of mussels from various sites around the Scottish coast. In: Polynuclear Aromatic Hydrocarbons: Chemistry and Biological Effects, edited by A Bjorseth, AJ Dennis, pp. 379–394. Columbus, Ohio: Battelle Press, 1980.

Mallet L (ed): Pollution of the living world by polycyclic aromatic hydrocarbons of the benzo-3,4-pyrene type. Paris: Maloine, 1972.

May WE: The solubility behavior of polycyclic aromatic hydrocarbons in aqueous systems. In: Petroleum in the Marine Environment, edited by L Petrakis, FT Weiss, pp. 143–192. Washington, D.C.: American Chemical Society, 1980.

May WE, Wasik SP, Freeman DH: Determination of the aqueous solubility of polynuclear aromatic hydrocarbons by a coupled column liquid chromatographic technique. Anal Chem 50: 175–179, 1978.

Meineke I, Klamberg H: On the degradation of polycyclic aromatic hydrocarbons. I. Reaction products of ozonolysis of polycyclic aromatic hydrocarbons in aqueous systems. Fresenius Z Anal Chem 293:201–204, 1978 (German).

Meyers PA, Quinn JG: Association of hydrocarbons and mineral particles in saline solutions. Nature (Lond) 244:23–24, 1973.

Mix MC, Schaffer RL: Benzo[a]pyrene concentrations in mussels (*Mytilus edulis*) from Yaquina Bay, Oregon, during June 1976–May 1978. Bull Environ Contam Toxicol 23:677–684, 1979.

Mix MC, Riley RT, King KI, Trenholm SR, Schaffer RL: Chemical carcinogens in the marine environment. Benzo[a]pyrene in economically-important bivalve mollusks from Oregon estuaries. In: Fate and Effects of Petroleum Hydrocarbons in Marine Ecosystems and Organisms, edited by DA Wolfe, pp. 421–431. New York: Pergamon, 1977.

Moles A: Sensitivity of parasitized coho salmon fry to crude oil, toluene, and naphthalene. Trans Am Fish Soc 109:109–293, 1980.

Moore MN, Livingstone DR, Donkin P, Bayne BL, Widdows J, Lowe DM: Mixed function oxygenases and xenobiotic detoxication/toxication systems in bivalve molluscs. Helgol Wiss Meeresunters 33:278–291, 1980.

Moore MN, Lowe DM, Fieth PEM: Lysosomal responses to experimentally injected anthracene in the digestive cells of *Mytilus edulis*. Mar Biol 48:297–302, 1978.

National Academy of Sciences: Particulate Polycyclic Organic Matter. Washington, D.C.: National Academy Press, 1972.

National Academy of Sciences: Petroleum in the Marine Environment. Washington, D.C.: National Academy Press, 1975.

Neely WB, Branson DR, Blau GE: Partition coefficient to measure bioconcentration potential of organic chemicals in fish. Environ Sci Technol 8:1113–1115, 1974.

Neff JM: Polycyclic Aromatic Hydrocarbons in the Aquatic Environment. Sources, Fates, and Biological Effects. London: Applied Science, 1979.

Neff JM, Anderson JW: Responses of Marine Animals to Petroleum and Specific Petroleum Hydrocarbons. London: Applied Science, 1981.

Neff JM, Anderson JW, Cox BA, Laughlin RB, Jr, Rossi SS, Tatem HE: Effects of petroleum on survival, respiration and growth of marine animals. In: Sources, Effects and Sinks of Hydrocarbons in the Aquatic Environment, pp. 515–539. Washington, D.C.: American Institute of Biological Sciences, 1976a.

Neff JM, Cox BA, Dixit D, Anderson JW: Accumulation and release of petroleum-derived aromatic hydrocarbons by four species of marine animals. Mar Biol 38:279–289, 1976b.

Neukomn S: The newt test for studying certain categories of carcinogenic substances. In: Experimental Model Systems in Toxicology and Their Significance to Man. Proc Eur Soc Study Drug Toxicity Int Conf 15:228–235, 1974.

Nicholls TP, Perry R, Lester JN: The influence of heat treatment on the metallic and polycyclic aromatic hydrocarbon content of sewage sludge. Sci Total Environ 12:137–150, 1979.

Orr WL, Grady JR: Perylene in basin sediments off southern California. Geochim Cosmochim Acta 31:1201–1209, 1967.

Ott FS, Harris RP, O'Hara SCM: Acute and sublethal toxicity of naphthalene and three methylated derivatives to the estuarine copepod *Eurytemora affinis*. Mar Environ Res 1:49–58, 1978.

Palmork KH, Solbakken JE: Accumulation and metabolism of phenanthrene in Norway lobster (*Nephrops norvegicus*). Proc Int Counc Explor Sea CM 1979/E, 53: 1979.

Palmork KH, Solbakken JE, Neppelberg T: Accumulation and metabolism of phenanthrene by saithe (*Pollachius virens*). Proc Int Counc Explor Sea CM 1978/E 42: 1978.

Pancirov RJ, Brown RA: Analytical methods for polynuclear aromatic hydrocarbons in crude oils, heating oils, and marine tissues. In: Proceedings of the 1975 Conference on Prevention and Control of Oil Pollution, pp. 103–115. Washington, D.C.: American Petroleum Institute, 1975.

Patterson AM, Capell LT, Walker DF: The Ring Index: A List of Ring Systems Used in Organic Chemistry, 2d ed. Washington, D.C.: American Chemical Society, 1960.

Payer HD, Soeder CJ, Kunte H, Karuwanna P, Nonhoff R, Graf W: Accumulation of polycyclic aromatic hydrocarbons in cultivated microalgae. Naturwissenschaften 62:536–538, 1975.

Payne JF: Field evaluations of benzopyrene hydroxylase induction as a monitor for marine petroleum pollution. Science 191:945–946, 1976.

Payne JF: Mixed function oxidases in marine organisms in relation to petroleum hydrocarbon metabolism and detection. Mar Pollut Bull 8:112–114, 1977.

Payne JF, Martins I, Rahimtula A: Crankcase oils: Are they a major mutagenic burden in the aquatic environment. Science 200:329–330, 1978.

Payne JF, May N: Further studies on the effect of petroleum hydrocarbons on mixed-function oxidases in marine organisms. In: Pesticide and Xenobiotic Metabolism in Aquatic Organisms, edited by MAQ Khan, JJ Lech, JJ Menn, pp.

339–347. Washington, D.C.: American Chemical Society, 1979.

Pearson WII, Olla BL: Detection of naphthalene by the blue crab, *Callinectes sapidus*. Estuaries 2:64–65, 1979.

Pearson WH, Olla BL: Threshold for detection of naphthalene and other behavioral responses by the blue crab, *Callinectes sapidus*. Estuaries 3: 224–229, 1980.

Pedersen MG, Hershberger WK, Zachariah PK, Juchau MR: Hepatic biotransformation of environmental xenobiotics in six strains of rainbow trout (*Salmo gairdneri*). J Fish Res Board Can 33:666–675, 1976.

Pelkonen O, Boobis AR, Nebert DW: Genetic differences in the binding of reactive carcinogenic metabolites to DNA. In: Carcinogenesis, vol. 3, Polynuclear Aromatic Hydrocarbons: Chemistry, Metabolism and Carcinogenesis, edited by RI Freudenthal, PW Jones, pp. 383–400. New York: Raven, 1978.

Platt HM, Mackie PR: Analysis of aliphatic and aromatic hydrocarbons in Antarctic marine sediment layers. Nature (Lond) 280:576–578, 1979.

Pohl RJ, Bend JR, Guarino AM, Fouts JR: Hepatic microsomal mixed function oxidase activity of several marine species from coastal Maine. Drug Metab Dispos 2:545–555, 1974.

Pupp C, Lao RC, Murray JJ, Pottie RF: Equilibrium vapour concentrations of some polycyclic aromatic hydrocarbons, arsenic trioxide (As_4O_6) and selenium dioxide and the collection efficiencies of these air pollutants. Atmos Environ 8:915–925, 1974.

Radding SB, Mill T, Gould CW, Liu DH, Johnson HL, Bomberger DC, Fojo CV: The environmental fate of selected polynuclear aromatic hydrocarbons. EPA-560/5-75-009, 1976.

Roesijadi G, Anderson JW, Blaylock JW: Uptake of hydrocarbons from marine sediments contaminated with Prudhoe Bay crude oil: Influence of feeding type of test species on availability of polycyclic aromatic hydrocarbons. J Fish Res Board Can 35:608–614, 1978.

Rose FL: Tissue lesions of tiger salamanders (*Ambystoma tigrinum*): Relationship to sewage effluents. In: Aquatic Pollutants and Biologic Effects with Emphasis on Neoplasia, edited by HF Kraybill, CJ Dawe, JC Harshbarger, RG Tardiff, Ann NY Acad Sci 298:270–279, 1977.

Rossi SS: Bioavailability of petroleum hydrocarbons from water, sediments and detritus to the marine annelid, *Neanthes arenaceodentata*. In: Proceedings of the 1977 Oil Spill Conference (Prevention, Behavior, Control, Cleanup). pp. 621–626. Washington, D.C.: American Petroleum Institute, 1977.

Rossi SS, Anderson JW: Accumulation and release of fuel oil-derived diaromatic hydrocarbons by the polychaete *Neanthes arenaceodentata*. Mar Biol 39:51–55, 1977.

Rossi SS, Neff JM: Toxicity of polynuclear aromatic hydrocarbons to the marine polychaete, *Neanthes arenaceodentata*. Mar Pollut Bull 9: 220–223, 1978.

Roubal WT: Spin-labeling of living tissue—a method for investigating pollutant-host interaction. In: Pollution and Physiology of Marine Organisms, edited by FJ Vernberg, WB Vernberg, pp. 367–380. New York: Academic, 1974.

Roubal WT, Collier TK: Spin-labeling techniques for studying mode of action of petroleum hydrocarbons on marine organisms. Fish Bull 73: 299–305, 1975.

Sanborn IIR, Malins DC: Toxicity and metabolism of naphthalene: A study with marine larval invertebrates. Proc Soc Exp Biol Med 154:151–155, 1977.

Sanborn HR, Malins DC: The disposition of aromatic hydrocarbons in adult spot shrimp (*Pandalus platyceros*) and the formation of metabolites of naphthalene in adult and larval spot shrimp. Xenobiotica 10:193–200, 1980.

Schmeltz I, Hoffman D: Formation of polynuclear aromatic hydrocarbons from combustion of organic matter. In: Carcinogenesis—A Comprehensive Survey, vol. 1, Polynuclear Aromatic Hydrocarbons. Chemistry, Metabolism, and Carcinogenesis, edited by R Freudenthal, PW Jones, pp. 225–240. New York: Raven, 1976.

Schoor WP, Couch J: Correlation of mixed-function oxidase activity with ultrastructural changes in the liver of a marine fish. Cancer Biochem Biophys 4:95–103, 1979.

Schwarz FP, Wasik SP: Fluorescence measurement of benzene, naphthalene, anthracene, pyrene, fluoranthene, and benzo[a]pyrene in water. Anal Chem 48:425–428, 1976.

Seilern-Aspang F, Kratochwil K: Induction and differentiation of an epithelial tumor in the newt (*Triturus cristatus*). J Embryol Exp Morphol 10:337–356, 1962.

Seilern-Aspang F, Kratochwil K: Spontaneous healing of an infiltrating and metastasizing epithelial tumor of *Triturus cristatus*. Arch Geschwulstforsch 21:292–300, 1963.

Shaw DG, McIntosh DJ, Smith ER: Arene and alkane hydrocarbons in nearshore Beaufort Sea sediments. Estuarine Coastal Mar Sci 9:435–449, 1979.

Sims P, Grover LL, Swaisland A, Pal K, Hewer A: Metabolic activation of benzo[a]pyrene proceeds by a diol-epoxide. Nature (Lond) 252:326–328, 1974.

Singer SC, Lee RF: Mixed function oxygenase activity in blue crab, *Callinectes sapidus:* Tissue distribution and correlation with changes during molting and development. Biol Bull Woods Hole, Mass. 153:377–386, 1977.

Singer SC, March PE, Gonsoulin JF, Lee RF: Mixed function oxygenase activity in the blue crab, *Callinectes sapidus:* Characterization of enzyme activity from stomach tissue. Comp Biochem Physiol 65C:129–134, 1980.

Solbakken JE, Palmork KH: Distribution of radioactivity in the Chondrichthyes *Squalus acanthus* and the Osteichthyes *Salmo gairdneri* following intragastric administration of (9-^{14}C)-phenanthrene. Bull Environ Contam Toxicol 25:902–908, 1980.

Solbakken JE, Palmork KH, Neppelberg T, Scheline RR: Urinary and biliary metabolites of phenanthrene in the coalfish (*Pollachius virens*). Acta Pharmacol Toxicol 46:127–132, 1980.

Soto C, Hellebust JA, Hutchinson TC: Effect of naphthalene and aqueous crude oil extracts on the green flagellate *Chlamydomonas angulosa*. II. Photosynthesis and the uptake and release of naphthalene. Can J Bot 53:118–126, 1975.

Southworth GR, Beauchamp JJ, Schmieder PK: Bioaccumulation potential of polycyclic aromatic hydrocarbons in *Daphnia pulex*. Water Res 12:973–977, 1978.

Speers GC, Whitehead EV: Crude petroleum. In: Organic Geochemistry: Methods and Results,

edited by G Eglinton, MRJ Murphy, pp. 638–675. Berlin: Springer Verlag, 1969.

Statham CN, Melancon MJ, Jr, Lech JJ: Bioconcentration of xenobiotics in trout bile: A proposed monitoring aid for some waterborne chemicals. Science 193:680–681, 1976.

Stegeman JJ: Fate and effects of oil in marine animals. Oceanus 20:59–66, 1977.

Stegeman JJ: Influence of environmental contamination on cytochrome P-450 mixed-function oxygenases in fish: Implications for recovery in the Wild Harbor marsh. J Fish Res Board Can 35:668–674, 1978.

Stegeman JJ: Temperature influence on basal activity and induction of mixed function oxygenase activity in *Fundulus heteroclitus*. J Fish Res Board Can 36:1400–1405, 1979.

Stegeman JJ: Mixed-function oxygenase studies in monitoring for effects of organic pollution. Rapp. PV Reun Cons Int Explor Mer 179:33–38, 1980.

Stegeman JJ, Binder RL: High benzo[a]pyrene hydroxylase activity in the marine fish *Stenotomus versicolor*. Biochem Pharmacol 28:1686–1688, 1979.

Stegeman JJ, Chevion M: Sex differences in cytochrome P-450 and mixed-function oxygenase activity in gonadally mature trout. Biochem Pharmacol 29:553–558, 1980.

Stegeman JJ, Kaplan HB: Mixed-function oxygenase activity and benzo[a]pyrene metabolism in the barnacle *Balanus eburneus* (Crustacea: Cirripedia). Comp Biochem Physiol 68C:55–62, 1981.

Stich HF, Dunn BP: The carcinogenic load of the environment: Benzo[a]pyrene in sediments of Arctic waters. Arctic 33:807–814, 1980.

Suess MJ: The environmental load and cycle of polycyclic aromatic hydrocarbons. Sci Total Environ 6:239–250, 1976.

Thomas JF, Mukai M, Tebbens BD: Fate of airborne benzo[a]pyrene. Environ Sci Technol 2:33–39, 1968.

Thomson RH: Naturally Occurring Quinones, 2nd ed. London: Butterworth, 1981.

Vandermeulen JH, Penrose WR: Absence of aryl hydrocarbon hydroxylase (AHH) in three marine bivalves. J Fish Res Board Can 35:643–647, 1978.

Van Overbeek J, Blondeau R: Mode of action of phytotoxic oils. Weeds 3:55–65, 1954.

Varanasi U, Gmur DJ: Metabolic activation and covalent binding of benzo[a]pyrene to deoxyribonucleic acid catalyzed by liver enzymes of marine fish. Biochem Pharmacol 29:753–761, 1980.

Varanasi U, Gmur DJ, Treseler PA: Influence of time and mode of exposure on biotransformation of naphthalene by juvenile starry flounder (*Platichthys stellatus*) and rock sole (*Lepidopsetta bilineata*). Arch Environ Contam Toxicol 8:673–692, 1979.

Varanasi U, Malins DC: Metabolism of petroleum hydrocarbons: Accumulation and biotransformation in marine organisms. In: Effects of Petroleum on Arctic and Subarctic Marine Environments and Organisms, vol. 2, Biological Effects, edited by DC Malins, pp. 175–270. New York: Academic, 1977.

Varanasi U, Uhler M, Stranahan SU: Uptake and release of naphthalene and its metabolites in skin and epidermal mucus of salmonids. Toxicol Appl Pharmacol 44:277–289, 1978.

Wakeham SG: Synchronous fluorescence spectroscopy and its application to indigenous and petroleum-derived hydrocarbons in lacustrine sediments. Environ Sci Technol 11:272–276, 1977.

Wallcave L, Garcia H, Feldman R, Lijinsky W, Shubik P: Skin tumorigenesis in mice by petroleum asphalts and coal-tar pitches of known polynuclear aromatic hydrocarbon content. Toxicol Appl Pharmacol 18:41–52, 1971.

Walters JM, Cain RB, Higgins IJ: Cell-free benzo[a]pyrene hydroxylase activity in marine zooplankton. J Mar Biol Assoc UK 59:553–563, 1979.

Walton DG, Penrose WR, Green JM: The petroleum-inducible mixed-function oxidase of cunner (*Tautogolabrus adspersus* Walbaum 1792): Some characteristics relevant to hydrocarbon monitoring. J Fish Res Board Can 35:1547–1552, 1978.

Ward DM, Atlas RM, Boehm PD, Calder JA: Biodegradation and chemical evolution of oil from the *Amoco* spill. Ambio 9:227–283, 1980.

Whittle KJ, Murray J, Mackie PR, Hardy R, Farmer J: Fate of hydrocarbons in fish. In:

Petroleum Hydrocarbons in the Marine Environment, edited by AD McIntyre, KJ Whittle, Cons Int Explor Mer 171:139–142, 1977.

Willis DE, Zinck ME, Darrow DC, Addison RF: Induction of mixed function oxidase enzymes in fish by halogenated and aromatic hydrocarbons. In: Hydrocarbons and Halogenated Hydrocarbons in the Aquatic Environment, edited by BK Afghan, D Mackay, pp. 531–536. New York: Plenum, 1980.

Wiser WH: Some chemical aspects of coal liquification. Cited by JT Enminger, Coal: Origin, classification and physical and chemical properties. In: Environmental Health and Control Aspects of Coal Conversion: An Information Overview, edited by HM Braunstein, ED Copenhaver, HA Pfuderer. ORNL/EIS-94. Oak Ridge, Tenn.: Oak Ridge National Laboratory, 1973.

Woo CS, Dsilva AP, Fassel VA, Oestreich GJ: Polynuclear aromatic hydrocarbons in coal—identification by their X-ray excited optical luminescence. Environ Sci Technol 12:173–174, 1978.

Yang SK, Deutsch J, Gelboin HV: Benzo[a]pyrene metabolism: Activation and detoxification. In: Polycyclic Hydrocarbons and Cancer, vol. 1, Environment, Chemistry, and Metabolism, edited by HV Gelboin, POP Ts'o, pp. 205–232. New York: Academic, 1978.

Yang SK, McCourt DW, Leutz JC, Gelboin HV: Benzo[a]pyrene diol epoxides: Mechanism of enzymatic formation and optically active intermediates. Science 196:1199–1201, 1977.

Yevich PP, Barszcz CA: Neoplasia in soft-shell clams (*Mya arenaria*) collected from oil-impacted sites. Ann NY Acad Sci 298:409–426, 1977.

Young GP: Effects of naphthalene and phenanthrene on the grass shrimp *Palaemonetes pugio* (Holthuis). M.A. thesis, Texas A&M Univ., College Station, Texas, 1977.

Youngblood WW, Blumer M: Polycyclic aromatic hydrocarbons in the environment: Homologous series in soils and recent marine sediments. Geochim Cosmochim Acta 39:1303–1314, 1975.

Zedeck MS: Polycyclic aromatic hydrocarbons: A review. J Environ Pathol Toxicol 3:537–567, 1980.

Zepp RG, Schlotzhauer PF: Photoreactivity of

selected aromatic hydrocarbons in water. In: Polynuclear Aromatic Hydrocarbons. Third International Symposium on Chemistry and Biology—Carcinogenesis and Mutagenesis, edited by PW Jones, P Leber, pp. 141–158. Ann Arbor, Mich.: Ann Arbor Science, 1979.

Zitko V: Aromatic hydrocarbons in aquatic fauna. Bull Environ Contam Toxicol 14:621–631, 1975.

SUPPLEMENTAL READING

Andelman JB, Snodgrass JE: Incidence and significance of polynuclear aromatic hydrocarbons in the water environment. CRC Crit Rev Environ Control 4(1):59–83, 1972.

Blumer M: Polycyclic aromatic compounds in nature. Sci Am 234(1):34–45, 1976.

Hodgins HO, McCain BB, Hawkes JW: Marine fish and invertebrate diseases, host disease resistance, and pathological effects of petroleum. In: Effects of Petroleum on Arctic and Subarctic Marine Environments and Organisms, vol. 2, edited by DC Malins, pp. 95–174. New York: Academic, 1977.

Lee RF: Mixed function oxygenases (MFO) in marine invertebrates. Mar Biol Let 2:87–105, 1981.

National Academy of Sciences: Petroleum in the Marine Environment. Washington, D.C.: National Academy Press, 1975.

Neff JM: Polycyclic Aromatic Hydrocarbons in the Aquatic Environment. Sources, Fates and Biological Effects. London: Applied Science, 1979.

Stegeman JJ: Polynuclear aromatic hydrocarbons and their metabolism in the marine environment. In: Polycyclic Hydrocarbons and Cancer, vol. 3, edited by HV Gelboin, POP Ts'o, pp. 1–60. New York: Academic, 1981.

Suess MJ: The environmental load and cycle of polycyclic aromatic hydrocarbons. Sci Total Environ 6:239–250, 1976.

Zedeck MS: Polycyclic aromatic hydrocarbons: A review. J Environ Pathol Toxicol 3:537–567, 1980.

Chapter 15

Ammonia, Nitrite, and Nitrate

R. C. Russo

INTRODUCTION

Ammonia (NH_3) is one of the most important pollutants in the aquatic environment because of its relatively highly toxic nature and its ubiquity in surface water systems. It is discharged in large quantities in industrial, municipal, and agricultural waste waters. Nitrite (NO_2^-) is not considered such a severe environmental problem because, although it is extremely toxic to aquatic life, it does not usually occur in natural surface water systems at concentrations considered deleterious to aquatic organisms. Nitrate (NO_3^-) is a less serious environmental problem; it can be found in relatively high concentrations in surface waters, but is relatively nontoxic to aquatic organisms.

These three compounds are interrelated through the process of nitrification, the biological oxidation of ammonia to nitrate. In this process nitrite is produced as an intermediate product. Under aerobic conditions ammonia is readily oxidized to nitrite by *Nitrosomonas* bacteria. Nitrite is, in turn, oxidized to nitrate by *Nitrobacter* bacteria:

$$2NH_3 + 3O_2 \xrightarrow{\textit{Nitrosomonas}} 2NO_2^- + 2H^+ + 2H_2O$$

and

$$2NO_2^- + O_2 \xrightarrow{\textit{Nitrobacter}} 2NO_3^-$$

In relatively stable, oxygenated natural water systems the oxidation of nitrite to nitrate is rapid, but the conversion of ammonia to nitrite is the rate-limiting step in the total process.

These chemical species can exist in two different forms:

1 Ionized: the dissociated, charged form of the chemical species. For example, the ammonium ion, NH_4^+, is the ionized form of ammonia.

2 Un-ionized: the undissociated, uncharged form. The ammonia molecule, NH_3, is the un-ionized form of ammonia.

AMMONIA

Ammonia can enter natural water systems from several sources, including industrial wastes, sewage effluents, alternative fuel conversion processes, and agricultural discharges. It is a natural biological degradation product of nitrogenous organic matter.

In order to understand the toxicity of ammonia in aqueous media, it is important to understand its chemical equilibrium in water. In aqueous solutions ammonia assumes two chemical forms, illustrated by the equation

$$NH_3 + nH_2O \rightleftharpoons NH_3 \cdot nH_2O \rightleftharpoons NH_4^+ + OH^-$$

$$+ (n-1)H_2O$$

These species are the un-ionized form (NH_3), hydrogen-bonded to at least three ($n \geqslant 3$) water molecules (Butler, 1964), and the ionized form (NH_4^+). Total ammonia is the sum of NH_3 and NH_4^+, and it is total ammonia that is measured analytically in aqueous solution.

The relative concentrations of ionized and un-ionized ammonia in a given ammonia solution are principally a function of the pH, temperature, and ionic strength of the aqueous solution. As pH increases, the equilibrium is shifted toward the un-ionized species, and the concentration of NH_3 increases while that of NH_4^+ decreases. For example, a pH increase from 7.0 to 8.0 in the temperature range 0 to 30°C results in a nearly tenfold increase in the concentration of NH_3 (Emerson et al., 1975; Thurston et al., 1979). Temperature in-

crease also favors the NH_3 species but to a lesser extent; a temperature increase of 5° between 0 and 30°C at pH 7.0 results in an NH_3 concentration increase of 40–50% (Emerson et al., 1975). An ionic strength increase (increase in total salt content) at low concentrations favors the NH_4^+ species. In natural waters with low to moderate amounts of dissolved solids (200–1000 mg/l), this effect will slightly lower the concentration of NH_3. The magnitude of this effect will vary with the composition of the water (Thurston et al., 1979).

When the concentration of total ammonia and the pH and temperature are measured in a solution, the relative concentrations of NH_3 and NH_4^+ can be calculated from the formulas of Emerson et al. (1975). A table is available (Thurston et al., 1979) that provides the percentage of NH_3 in solutions of total ammonia over the pH range 5–12 and temperature range 0–40°C in increments of 0.01 pH unit and 0.2°C.

Toxicity

Ammonia is clearly toxic to fish and has many effects. Fish mortality caused by ammonia may be due to different effects in different cases, and it is likely that ammonia has a different mode of action at high than at low concentrations. A great deal of information on the toxicity of ammonia to fish and other aquatic organisms is available in the literature; however, much of this does not include sufficient information on the pH and temperature of the test water.

Acute exposure of fish to a high concentration of ammonia causes an increase in gill ventilation, hyperexcitability, convulsions, and then death. These effects are most likely the result of a direct effect of ammonia on the central nervous system. Effects of chronic exposure of fish to lower concentrations of ammonia include deleterious histological changes, a decrease in reproductive capacity (numbers of eggs produced, egg viability, delay in spawning), a decrease in growth and morphological development, and an increase in susceptibility to disease. Chronic exposure may cause progressive deterioration of several physiological functions, any one of which may be the ultimate cause of death.

Acute Toxicity

Table 1 gives some typical examples of the acute toxicity of un-ionized ammonia to several families of aquatic organisms including invertebrates and vertebrates. There is some evidence that salmonid fish species are more susceptible to ammonia than are nonsalmonid species, at least on an acute toxicity basis. For a test duration of 96 h, LC50 values reported for two salmonid species fall in the range 0.08–1.1 mg/l NH_3; LC50 values for nonsalmonid species fall in the range 0.5–4.6. Although, in general, nonsalmonids are less sensitive to NH_3 than salmonids, the lower values for nonsalmonids are only slightly higher than the lowest value for salmonids, suggesting that sensitivity differences between these groups are not large.

Results of acute sublethal exposures of aquatic organisms to ammonia have also been reported. The effect of ammonia on clams was investigated by Anderson et al. (1978), who found that lethal concentrations of 0.036–0.011 mg/l NH_3 caused a reduction in ciliary beating rate of fingernail clam (*Musculium transversum*) gills. Freshwater mussels were exposed for 165 h to 0.32 mg/l NH_3 and a range of tolerance to ammonia was found; the more tolerant species generally had their shells tightly shut, whereas the least tolerant species continued siphoning or had their mantles exposed (Horne and McIntosh, 1979).

There can be susceptibility differences among species and among specific life stages of a particular species. Moreover, a number of factors can affect the toxicity of un-ionized ammonia to aquatic organisms. These include pH, dissolved oxygen concentration, temperature, calcium concentration, salinity, previous acclimation to ammonia, fluctuation or intermittency of exposures, and presence of other toxicants.

pH Effects

Chipman (1934), Wuhrmann et al. (1947), and Wuhrmann and Woker (1948) observed that the

Table 1 Representative Acute Toxicity Values for Un-ionized Ammonia

Species	48- or 96-h LC50 (mg/l NH_3)	Reference
Cladoceran (*Daphnia pulicaria*)	1.2	DeGraeve et al. (1980)
Crayfish (*Orconectes nais*)	3.2–3.8	Hazel et al. (1979); Evans (1979)
Riffle beetle (*Stenelmis sexlineata*)	8.0	Hazel et al. (1979)
Pink salmon (*Oncorhynchus gorbuscha*)	0.08–0.1	Rice and Bailey (1980)
Rainbow trout (*Salmo gairdneri*)	0.2–1.1	Calamari et al. (1977); Broderius and Smith (1979); DeGraeve et al. (1980); Thurston et al. (1981a,b)
Bluegill (*Lepomis macrochirus*)	0.49–4.6	Emery and Welch (1969); Roseboom and Richey (1977)
Red shiner (*Notropis lutrensis*)	2.8	Hazel et al. (1979)
Channel catfish (*Ictalurus punctatus*)	1.8–3.8	Colt and Tchobanoglous (1976); Roseboom and Richey (1977)
Largemouth bass (*Micropterus salmoides*)	0.9–1.4	Roseboom and Richey (1977)

toxicity of total ammonia solutions was greater at higher pH values; because increasing pH increases the concentration of NH_3, they concluded that NH_3 was the toxic form of ammonia to aquatic organisms. They considered NH_4^+ to be nontoxic or appreciably less toxic. This conclusion was based on the ease of NH_3 diffusion across gill membranes, which are much less permeable to NH_4^+ (Wuhrmann et al., 1947; Wuhrmann and Woker, 1948; Fromm and Gillette, 1968; Hillaby and Randall, 1979). There is evidence, however, that NH_4^+ is excreted across the gills in exchange for Na^+ (Maetz and Garcia-Romeu, 1964; Girard and Payan, 1980). A number of researchers observed that the toxicity of NH_4^+ and/or the effect of pH on the toxicity of NH_3 is greater than reported earlier. This has been shown with both invertebrates (prawn larvae and *Daphnia*) and fish (rainbow trout, fathead minnows, coho salmon, and channel catfish) (Tabata, 1962; Robinson-Wilson and Seim, 1975; Armstrong et al., 1978; Hillaby and Randall, 1979; Tomasso et al., 1980; Thurston et al., 1981a). Figure 1 shows results of tests with rainbow trout (*Salmo gairdneri*) (Thurston et al., 1981a), demonstrating increased toxicity of total ammonia with increasing pH (due to an increased concentration of NH_3), and a correlation between pH and acute toxicity of NH_3 over the pH range 6.5–9. Water quality criteria for ammonia (U.S. EPA, 1977; European Inland Fisheries Advisory Commission, 1970) are expressed in terms of NH_3. The U.S. Environmental Protection Agency's forthcoming water quality criteria document for ammonia in fresh water based on acute toxicity test data is expected to be an equation for NH_3 versus pH, reflecting the increased toxicity of NH_3 at lower pH values.

Dissolved Oxygen

The interaction between ammonia and dissolved oxygen is an important factor in ammonia toxicity to aquatic life. Discharge of ammonia is frequently associated with a reduction of oxygen levels in the receiving water. This is brought about by several causes, including the oxygen demand of the am-

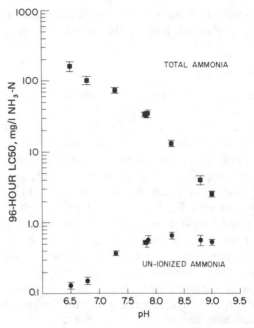

Figure 1 Acute toxicity of ammonia to rainbow trout: 96-h LC50 versus pH. Error bars are 95% confidence intervals. *[Reprinted with permission from Thurston et al. (1981a); copyright 1981, American Chemical Society.]*

monia as it is converted by natural microbial oxidation to nitrite and nitrate, the chemical and biological oxygen demand of other chemicals that may be, and frequently are, discharged along with ammonia, and the reduction in oxygen-carrying capacity of the receiving water caused by a high-temperature discharge. If the receiving water is rich in nutrients and highly productive, as is frequently the case downstream from a sewage treatment plant, diurnal and seasonal fluctuations in dissolved oxygen caused by plant growth can also occur.

Several researchers, working with a variety of fish species, have reported that the toxicity of ammonia increases when dissolved oxygen concentrations decrease (Wuhrmann, 1952; Wuhrmann and Woker, 1953; Downing and Merkens, 1955; Merkens and Downing, 1957; Alabaster et al., 1979; Thurston et al., 1981b). Figure 2 illustrates the effect of dissolved oxygen on the acute toxicity of ammonia to rainbow trout (Thurston et al., 1981b). Rainbow trout appear to be more sensitive to the combined effect of dissolved oxygen reduction and ammonia than are the nonsalmonid species tested.

Temperature

Limited information is available on the effects of temperature on ammonia toxicity to fish. Temperature affects the aqueous ammonia equilibrium, with higher temperatures resulting in a greater fraction of total ammonia present as NH_3.

Several studies were performed to investigate the effect of temperature on the toxicity of NH_3 itself, independent of the effect of temperature on NH_3 concentration. Although data have been reported that indicate little or no effect of temperature on the toxicity of NH_3 to certain fish species, it is reasonable to expect that at marginal temperatures a species will not be able to function optimally to resist the toxic effects of ammonia. From the few studies addressing this question, it appears that the acute toxicity of ammonia to channel catfish (*Ictalurus punctatus*) decreases with an increase in temperature over a range (20–30°C) tolerated by the fish (Colt and Tchobanoglous, 1976). Bluegill (*Lepomis macrochirus*), channel catfish, and largemouth bass (*Micropterus*

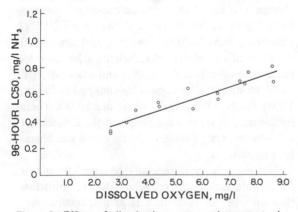

Figure 2 Effect of dissolved oxygen on the acute toxicity of ammonia to rainbow trout: 96-h LC50 versus dissolved oxygen. *[Reprinted with permission from Thurston et al. (1981b).]*

salmoides) were reported by Roseboom and Richey (1977) to be less susceptible to ammonia at 28–30°C than at 22°C. Survival time of minnows (*Phoxinus*) was reported to be shortened by an increase in temperature from 2–27°C (Wuhrmann and Woker, 1953). The European Inland Fisheries Advisory Commission (1970) pointed out that the toxic effect of NH_3 may be greater below 5°C than above 5°C. It is important that the relationship between temperature and NH_3 toxicity be studied further, particularly at low temperatures.

Other Effects

From studies with channel catfish, Tomasso et al. (1980) reported that elevated calcium concentrations in the water decrease ammonia toxicity. An increase in water salinity reduced the toxicity of ammonia to Atlantic salmon (*Salmo salar*) smolts (Alabaster et al., 1979). These observations may be related to the favorable osmotic condition resulting from the addition of salts to the fish's medium.

Fluctuating Concentrations and Acclimation

Aquatic life in streams receiving ammonia-containing effluents are subjected to daily fluctuations in ammonia concentration, as opposed to steady or constant concentrations. Also, when accidental spills of ammonia occur, aquatic organisms are subjected to slugs of ammonia for short periods of time. It is therefore important to consider the toxic effects of fluctuating or intermittent ammonia exposure on aquatic life. Brown et al. (1969) tested rainbow trout in static bioassays in which the fish were moved from tanks with a lower ammonia concentration to tanks with ammonia concentrations three times higher. They reported that the median period of survival was the same as that for constant exposure if fish were transferred on an hourly basis, but was less if the fish were transferred at 2-h intervals. Thurston et al. (1981c), in tests with rainbow and cutthroat (*Salmo clarki*) trout, found that fish were better able to withstand a fixed concentration of ammonia over 96 h than fluctuating concentrations having mean values comparable to that of the fixed concentration. Thurston and co-workers also reported that fish were able to withstand short-term excursions slightly above acutely toxic ammonia concentrations without any apparent long-term adverse effects, provided the high levels were followed by periods during which the ammonia concentration was lower. Evidence of increased tolerance due to acclimation was also shown by this work. For example, fish subjected for 96-h periods to cyclic pulses of ammonia at concentrations below acutely toxic ones were better able to withstand subsequent exposure to acutely lethal pulses than were fish not previously acclimated.

Acclimation of fish to sublethal concentrations of ammonia resulting in increased resistance to subsequent exposure to acutely toxic concentrations has also been reported by Vámos (1963), Mălăcea (1968), Schulze-Wiehenbrauck (1976), and Redner and Stickney (1979).

Mixtures of Ammonia and Other Chemicals

Effects of other chemicals in water solution on the toxicity of ammonia have not been well studied. There is some evidence (Herbert and Vandyke, 1964) that a combination of ammonia and copper is more toxic than either toxicant individually. Studies of solutions containing both ammonia and zinc (Ministry of Technology, UK, 1962) indicated that the toxicity of the two chemicals in combination was greater than that of each chemical separately. Ammonia and nitrate in combination were reported (Rubin and Elmaraghy, 1977) to have additive toxicity, except when ammonia-to-nitrate ratios were very low. Wuhrmann and Woker (1948) and Broderius and Smith (1979) studied combinations of ammonia and hydrogen cyanide (HCN) and reported synergistic effects of the two toxicants. Information on NH_3 in combination with organic chemicals is limited to studies with phenol (Herbert, 1962). The toxicity of ammonia and phenol combined was reported to approxi-

mate the toxicity of either ammonia or phenol when tested separately. Brown et al. (1969) tested a mixture of three pollutants—ammonia, zinc, and phenol—and observed that the toxicity of the mixture was greater than the sum of the individual toxicity of each of these three pollutants. It is apparent from these studies that the toxicity of ammonia is affected by the presence of other pollutants and that the toxicity of ammonia in combination with several other toxic chemicals can be synergistic.

Chronic Toxicity

Much less information is available from long-term toxicity tests with ammonia and aquatic organisms, and very few data are available from partial chronic or chronic studies. Data from long-term tests indicate that ammonia has deleterious effects at fairly low concentrations. Tests lasting from 1 wk to 3 mo at sublethal concentrations have been reported for both salmonid and nonsalmonid fish species (Department of the Environment, UK, 1972; Robinette, 1976; Schulze-Wiehenbrauck, 1976; Burkhalter and Kaya, 1977; Thurston et al., 1978; Rice and Bailey, 1980). At exposure concentrations as low as 0.002–0.15 mg/l NH_3, fish showed reduced food uptake and assimilation, accompanied by growth inhibition. Histological changes attributed to ammonia exposure have also been reported. In the range 0.04–0.4 mg/l NH_3, reported effects including swelling and diminished numbers of red blood cells, inflammation and degeneration of gills and kidneys, and lowered resistance to disease (Reichenbach-Klinke, 1967; Flis, 1968; Smart, 1976; Thurston et al., 1978). These histological changes were observed for a variety of fish species, tested under a variety of water chemistry conditions.

Not enough data are available from chronic or subchronic studies to provide definitive information on whether such factors as pH, acclimation, dissolved oxygen, and salt concentration, which have demonstrated effects on acute toxicity, also affect chronic toxicity.

NITRITE

Nitrite is usually present only in trace amounts in most natural freshwater systems, because it is rapidly oxidized to nitrate. In sewage treatment plants using the nitrification process to convert ammonia to nitrate, the process may be impeded, causing discharge of nitrite at elevated concentrations into receiving waters. Increased nitrite concentrations may also occur in water reuse systems in fish culture facilities employing the nitrification process to reduce ammonia concentrations. The conversion process is affected by several factors, including pH, temperature, dissolved oxygen, number of nitrifying bacteria, and presence of inhibiting compounds. Depending on the effectiveness of the conversion process, the amount of nitrite discharged may raise the concentration of nitrite in the receiving water to levels toxic to aquatic organisms.

It has been demonstrated (Anthonisen et al., 1976) that the nitrification process can be inhibited by the presence of nitrous acid (HNO_2) and NH_3. Total ammonia in a waste water treatment system consists of NH_4^+ and NH_3. If the pH of the solution increases, either naturally or by addition of a base, the concentration of un-ionized ammonia will increase. Un-ionized ammonia inhibits nitrobacters at concentrations (0.1–1.0 mg/l NH_3) appreciably lower than those (10–150 mg/l) that inhibit nitrosomonads. This situation impedes the conversion of nitrite to nitrate, causing nitrite to accumulate. When the pH decreases, as ammonium and nitrite are oxidized, an increase in HNO_2 concentration occurs. Nitrous acid inhibits both nitrobacters and nitrosomonads at concentrations between 0.22 and 2.8 mg/l. This inhibition can also result in an increase in nitrite.

Several organic compounds likely to be found in significant concentrations in industrial wastes were shown to inhibit the nitrification process. Hockenbury and Grady (1977) found that dodecyclamine, aniline, and n-methylaniline at concentrations less than 1 mg/l caused 50% inhibition of ammonia oxidation by *Nitrosomonas;* p-nitro-benzaldehyde, *p*-nitroaniline, and *n*-methylaniline at 100 mg/l inhibited nitrite oxidation by *Nitrobacter*. Loss of nitrification flora, resulting from use of antibiotics, has also been mentioned (Patrick et al., 1979) as a potential cause of large amounts of nitrite accumulating in natural waters.

Nitrite may thus be present under some circumstances in natural waters at concentrations high enough to be deleterious to freshwater aquatic life. Some field data are available on environmental concentrations of nitrite. Klingler (1957) reported nitrite concentrations $\geqslant$30 mg/l NO_2-N (nitrite nitrogen) in waters receiving effluents from metal, dye, and celluloid industries. McCoy (1972) measured concentrations up to 73 mg/l NO_2-N in Wisconsin lakes and streams. A concentration of 0.1 mg/l NO_2-N was also found in a reasonably clean cold-water trout stream in Montana (Russo and Thurston, 1974).

In aqueous nitrite solution the following equilibrium is established:

$$NO_2^- + H^+ \rightleftharpoons HNO_2$$

This equilibrium is affected by pH, and thus the relative concentrations of ionized nitrite (NO_2^-) and un-ionized nitrous acid (HNO_2) are pH-dependent. Total nitrite is the sum of these ($NO_2^- + HNO_2$), and concentrations of the HNO_2 species can be calculated from the equation

$$\log[HNO_2] = \log[NO_2^-] + pK_a - pH$$

where [NO_2^-] is the analytically measured nitrite concentration (mol/l), pH is the measured pH, and pK_a is the equilibrium constant (Russo et al., 1981). This constant, pK_a, has not been accurately measured as a function of temperature, but values at different temperatures were compiled (Sillén and Martell, 1964). At 10°C, a best estimate of pK_a is 3.39 (Russo et al., 1981). The concentration of HNO_2 is 4–5 orders of magnitude less than the concentration of NO_2^- in the pH range 7.5–8.5; in going from pH 7.5 to 8.5, the NO_2^- concentration remains essentially constant, whereas the HNO_2 concentration decreases tenfold.

Toxicity

Nitrite impairs the ability of fish blood to transport oxygen. Oxygen is transported in fish blood by the respiratory blood pigment hemoglobin. The iron in hemoglobin is present in the ferrous, Fe(II), state. Hemoglobin combines loosely with oxygen to form the easily dissociated compound oxyhemoglobin, in which iron is still in the Fe(II) state. Transport of oxygen by blood is dependent on the ease with which hemoglobin unites with oxygen and with which oxyhemoglobin gives up oxygen. If the iron in hemoglobin is oxidized to the ferric, Fe(III), state, methemoglobin is formed. Methemoglobin is not capable of combining reversibly with oxygen, and thus sufficiently high concentrations can cause hypoxia and death. Nitrite oxidizes hemoglobin to methemoglobin (Bodansky, 1951; Jaffé, 1964; Kiese, 1974), increasing the amount of methemoglobin present and impairing oxygen transport by the blood.

The total hemoglobin present as methemoglobin in rainbow trout (*Salmo gairdneri*) under normal conditions (not under stress from environmental nitrite) generally falls in the range 1–4% (Shterman, 1970; Cameron, 1971; Smith and Russo, 1975; Brown and McLeay, 1975), although a value as high as 17% has been reported (Cameron, 1971). Increased environmental nitrite concentrations, even as low as 0.015 mg/l NO_2-N, produce increased methemoglobin levels in fish blood (Smith and Williams, 1974; Smith and Russo, 1975; Brown and McLeay, 1975; Crawford and Allen, 1977; Perrone and Meade, 1977; Bortz, 1977). Brown and McLeay (1975) also observed a decrease in total hemoglobin at NO_2-N concentrations above 0.1 mg/l. The presence of high levels of methemoglobin in fish blood is visually apparent in that the blood becomes brown-colored (methemoglobinemia). Different concentrations of methemoglobin have been reported as causing mortality in fish. Species differences and differences in overall physical condition may influence the tolerance of fish to different methemoglobin levels.

Some work has been done on treatment of methemoglobinemia. Ascorbic acid administered intravenously reduced methemoglobin in rainbow trout blood (Cameron, 1971). Methylene blue administered either by injection (Bortz, 1977) or by addition to test water (Wedemeyer and Yasutake, 1978) also reduced methemoglobin levels. Removal of fish to nitrite-free water resulted in a reduction of methemoglobin level, although to a smaller extent than was found with methylene blue treatment (Wedemeyer and Yasutake, 1978). Methylene blue reduced methemoglobin levels rapidly, within a few hours. The effect was apparently temporary, as methemoglobin levels gradually rose again (Bortz, 1977).

Methemoglobinemia represents one mechanism by which nitrite is toxic to fish, although probably not the only mode of toxic action. Smith and Williams (1974) observed mortality of some rainbow trout with blood methemoglobin levels lower than those of other rainbow trout that survived, and this led them to suggest that the fish died from a toxic reaction to nitrite itself rather than from methemoglobinemia. Crawford and Allen (1977) observed that in seawater with added nitrite, chinook salmon (*Oncorhynchus tshawytscha*) had high methemoglobin levels (74%) but very low mortality (10%); in fresh water with added nitrite, lower methemoglobin levels (44%) were found in salmon, but 70% mortality occurred. They further observed that fish that died in fresh water often had red gill lamellae, rather than the brown color typically caused by methemoglobinemia. This indicates that the toxicity of nitrite in fresh water may be attributable to some other mechanism or something in addition to methemoglobinemia. More research is needed to investigate this mechanism.

Nitrite has been implicated in the formation of *N*-nitroso compounds (Archer et al., 1971; Wolff and Wasserman, 1972; Mirvish, 1975), and nitrosamines have been shown to be carcinogenic in zebrafish (*Brachydanio rerio*), rainbow trout, and guppy (*Poecilia reticulata*) (Stanton, 1965; Ashley and Halver, 1968; Sato et al., 1973). Nitrite was also reported to induce cancer in rats directly, rather than through formation of nitrosamines (Newberne, 1979).

The amount of published information on nitrite toxicity to fishes is limited, and much of the available data is from tests of short duration (≤48 h). Representative results from acute toxicity tests for a variety of aquatic organisms are presented in Table 2. These data indicate that, except for the sculpin, there is an order of magnitude (0.1–13 mg/l) difference among LC50 values for freshwater fish from several different families. The sculpin was apparently less sensitive to nitrite than the other species. This range of species sensitivity is probably attributable both to differences in water chemistry for the different tests and to differences in susceptibility among species. Salmonids (trout and salmon) appear to be the most susceptible fish species, and nonsalmonids are somewhat more tolerant. McCoy (1972) tested 13 fish species, presumably using the same dilution water in all cases, and observed a wide variation in susceptibility. At 5 mg/l NO_2-N, mortality occurred in less than 3 h in logperch (*Percina caprodes*) and in 3–5 h in brook stickleback (*Culaea inconstans*). In contrast, 100% of carp (*Cyprinus carpio*) survived 40 mg/l for 48 h, and white sucker (*Catostomus commersoni*) survived 100 mg/l for 48 h (McCoy, 1972). Although there was some indication from limited data that younger rainbow trout and coho salmon (*Oncorhynchus kisutch*) were somewhat less susceptible to nitrite than older fish of the same species (Russo et al., 1974; Smith and Williams, 1974; Perrone and Meade, 1977), more recent findings (Russo, 1980) with rainbow trout over a larger size range (2–387 g), under similar water chemistry conditions, showed no relationship between fish size and susceptibility to nitrite.

Effects of Water Chemistry on Toxicity of Nitrite

In addition to species susceptibility to nitrite, researchers have examined the effect of water chemistry conditions on nitrite toxicity. The principal factors studied were pH, chloride, and calcium; the effects of several other anions were also addressed to a limited extent.

pH Effects

The aqueous nitrite equilibrium is pH-dependent, as mentioned above, and the effect of pH on nitrite toxicity was examined by Wedemeyer and Yasutake (1978) and Russo et al. (1981). It was

Table 2 Representative Acute Toxicity Values for Nitrite

Species	48- or 96-h LC50 (mg/l NO_2-N)	Reference
Rainbow trout (*Salmo gairdneri*)	0.1–0.4	Russo et al. (1974); Brown and McLeay (1975); Russo (1980)
Cutthroat trout (*Salmo clarki*)	0.5–0.6	Thurston et al. (1978)
Chinook salmon (*Oncorhynchus tshawytscha*)	0.9	Westin (1974)
Mosquitofish (*Gambusia affinis*)	1.6	Wallen et al. (1957)
Fathead minnow (*Pimephales promelas*)	2.3–3.0	Russo and Thurston (1977)
Channel catfish (*Ictalurus punctatus*)	7.5–13	Konikoff (1975); Colt and Tchobanoglous (1976)
Mottled sculpin (*Cottus bairdi*)	>67	Russo and Thurston (1977)

shown by Russo et al. (1981) that over the pH range 6.4–9.0 the toxicity of total nitrite decreases as pH increases. If the concentrations of the un-ionized and ionized species comprising total nitrite are calculated separately, this might be expressed in another way: as pH increases, toxicity in terms of NO_2-N decreases and toxicity in terms of HNO_2-N increases (Fig. 3). However, neither of these species alone is entirely responsible for the toxicity of nitrite; if it were, its plot (Fig. 3, a and b) would be a horizontal line. It has been concluded that in the pH range 6.4–9.0 both species contribute significantly to the total toxicity and the toxicity of HNO_2 must be higher per unit weight than that of the ion.

Chloride and Other Ions

Nitrite toxicity decreases with increasing chloride ion (Cl^-) concentration, and the relationship between them is linear. For rainbow trout, the 96-h LC50 increased from 0.46 mg/l NO_2-N in the presence of 1 mg/l Cl^- to 12.4 mg/l NO_2-N at 41 mg/l Cl^- (Russo and Thurston, 1977) (see Fig. 4). Similar results were reported for coho salmon (Perrone and Meade, 1977), steelhead trout (*Salmo gairdneri*) (Wedemeyer and Yasutake, 1978), and channel catfish (*Ictalurus punctatus*) (Tomasso et al., 1979). Other anions have been found to inhibit nitrite toxicity to different degrees; these include bromide (Br^-), sulfate (SO_4^{2-}), phosphate (PO_4^{3-}), and nitrate (NO_3^-) (Russo et al., 1981). Crawford and Allen (1977) studied the effect of Calcium (Ca^{2+}) and seawater on nitrite toxicity to chinook salmon (*Oncorhynchus tshawytscha*). The acute toxicity of nitrite in seawater was markedly less than that in fresh water, logically so in view of the chloride effect discussed above. They also found that increasing the calcium concentration in both fresh water and seawater decreased the toxicity of nitrite.

Long-Term Effects

Thurston et al. (1978) conducted 36-d exposures of cutthroat trout (*Salmo clarki*) fry and found LC50 values at 36 d to be only slightly lower than 96-h values. Wedemeyer and Yasutake (1978) exposed steelhead trout to low NO_2-N concentrations (0.015–0.060 mg/l) over a 6-mo period and found no serious deleterious effects. Growth and the ability of the fish to adapt to seawater were not impaired. Varying degrees of gill hyperplasia and lamellar separation were observed early in the test, but the fish seemed to recover and after 28 wk these abnormalities were no longer observed.

It is apparent that the aquatic toxicity of nitrite is highly dependent on the chemical composition of the water. More research is needed on nitrite toxicity to examine other water chemistry effects, to study chronic toxicity more definitively, to obtain toxicity data for additional species (especially species other than fish), and to define the mechanism(s) of nitrite toxicity.

NITRATE

The nitrate ion, NO_3^-, is formed by complete oxidation of ammonia through the nitrification process. High concentrations of nitrate can be found in natural surface waters—for example, 10–60 mg/l NO_3-N (McCoy, 1972)—and in fish culture waters—for example, 70 mg/l NO_3-N (Knepp and Arkin, 1973). Nitrate does not form an un-ionized species in aqueous solution (i.e., HNO_3 is completely dissociated to H^+ and NO_3^-).

Toxicity

Nitrate is considerably less toxic to aquatic organisms than are ammonia and nitrite. It is considered essentially nontoxic, and consequently there are few reports of studies of its toxicity. Indeed, nitrate compounds are often the chemicals of choice for assessing the toxicities of metals and other cations, because it is assumed that NO_3^- will not contribute additional toxicity to the system. A compilation of acute toxicity data is presented in Table 3. From the limited data available, nitrate appears to be relatively innocuous as an aquatic toxicant. Trama (1954) found that bluegill (*Lepomis macrochirus*) were most susceptible to potas-

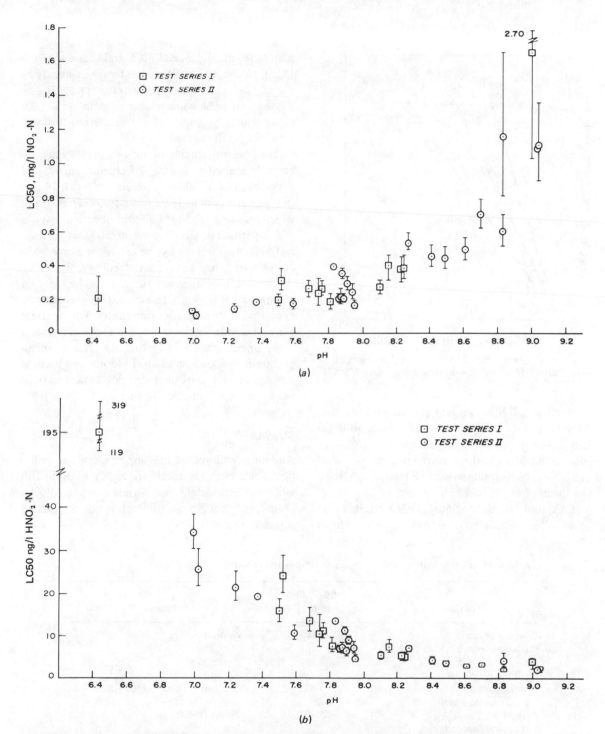

Figure 3 (a) Acute toxicity to rainbow trout of nitrite over the pH range 6.4–9.0: LC50 as NO_2–N versus pH. Error bars are 95% confidence intervals. (b) Acute toxicity to rainbow trout of nitrite over the pH range 6.4–9.0: LC50 as HNO_2–N versus pH. Error bars are 95% confidence intervals. *[Reprinted with permission from Russo et al. (1981).]*

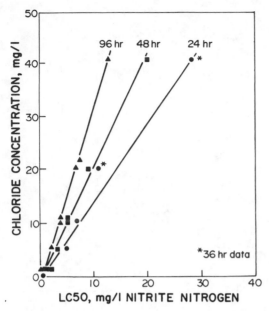

Figure 4 Effect of chloride on nitrite toxicity to rainbow trout (*Salmo gairdneri*). *[Reprinted from Russo (1980).]*

sium nitrate, KNO_3; sodium and calcium nitrates, $NaNO_3$ and $Ca(NO_3)_2$, were less toxic. Bluegill had 100% survival when exposed for 96 h to sodium nitrate solutions containing up to 1650 mg/l NO_3–N. Guppies were the most sensitive of the species tested (Table 3).

Colt and Tchobanoglous (1976) studied the toxicity of nitrate to channel catfish (*Ictalurus*

punctatus) at 22, 26, and 30°C and found the 96-h ·LC50 to be independent of temperature. They stated that the toxicity of nitrate appears to be related to the fish being unable to maintain normal osmoregulatory ability when transferred to water with a high salt content.

Longer-term studies of nitrate toxicity are apparently limited to a study of channel catfish and largemouth bass (*Micropterus salmoides*) held in a fish culture system (Knepp and Arkin, 1973) in which gradual nitrate buildup occurred over a 164-d period. A nitrate concentration of 96 mg/l NO_3–N was tolerated by the catfish and bass without affecting their growth and feeding activity.

Nitrates may increase the net productivity of aquatic systems. To a certain extent this may be beneficial to the aquatic community. When nitrate concentrations become excessive, however, and other essential nutrient factors are present, eutrophication and associated algal blooms can become a problem even though the nitrate concentrations per se may not be toxic to fish.

SUMMARY

Ammonia and nitrite are important water pollutants, and both chemicals are highly toxic to fish and aquatic invertebrates. Nitrate is a related compound, but it is not significantly toxic to fish and invertebrates.

Table 3 Representative Acute Toxicity Values for Nitrate

Species	96-h LC50 (mg/l NO_3–N)	Reference
Chinook salmon (*Oncorhynchus tshawytscha*)	1310	Westin (1974)
Rainbow trout (*Salmo gairdneri*)	1360	Westin (1974)
Channel catfish (*Ictalurus punctatus*)	1400	Colt and Tchobanoglous (1976)
Bluegill (*Lepomis macrochirus*)	420–2000	Trama (1954)
Guppy (*Poecilia reticulata*)	180–200	Rubin and Elmaraghy (1977)

Acute toxicity of ammonia to aquatic organisms is affected by water pH, dissolved oxygen, temperature, fluctuating concentrations, previous acclimation to ammonia, calcium, salinity, and the presence of other chemicals. Whether these factors also affect chronic toxicity has not yet been investigated.

Acute toxicity of nitrite is affected by water pH, chloride, and calcium. More research is needed on the effects on toxicity of other water chemistry variables and on long-term effects of nitrite exposure.

LITERATURE CITED

Alabaster JS, Shurben DG, Knowles G: The effect of dissolved oxygen and salinity on the toxicity of ammonia to smolts of salmon, *Salmo salar* L. J Fish Biol 15:705–712, 1979.

Anderson KB, Sparks RE, Paparo AA: Rapid assessment of water quality, using the fingernail clam, *Musculium transversum*. WRC Res Rep 133. Urbana, Ill.: Water Resources Center, Univ. of Illinois, 1978.

Anthonisen AC, Loehr RC, Prakasam TBS, Srinath EG: Inhibition of nitrification by ammonia and nitrous acid. J Water Pollut Control Fed 48:835–852, 1976.

Archer MC, Clark SD, Thilly JE, Tannenbaum SR: Environmental nitroso compounds: Reaction of nitrite with creatine and creatinine. Science 174:1341–1343, 1971.

Armstrong DA, Chippendale D, Knight AW, Colt JE: Interaction of ionized and un-ionized ammonia on short-term survival and growth of prawn larvae, *Macrobrachium rosenbergii*. Biol Bull Woods Hole Mass 154:15–31, 1978.

Ashley LM, Halver JE: Dimethylnitrosamine-induced hepatic cell carcinoma in rainbow trout. J Natl Cancer Inst 41:531–552, 1968.

Bodansky O: Methemoglobinemia and methemoglobin-producing compounds. Pharmacol Rev 3:144–196, 1951.

Bortz BM: The administration of tetramethylthionine chloride as a treatment for nitrite-induced methemoglobinemia in rainbow trout (*Salmo gairdneri*). M.S. thesis, American Univ., Washington, D.C., 1977.

Broderius SJ, Smith LL, Jr: Lethal and sublethal effects of binary mixtures of cyanide and hexavalent chromium, zinc, or ammonia to the fathead minnow (*Pimephales promelas*) and rainbow trout (*Salmo gairdneri*). J Fish Res Board Can 36:164–172, 1979.

Brown DA, McLeay DJ: Effect of nitrite on methemoglobin and total hemoglobin of juvenile rainbow trout. Prog Fish Cult 37:36–38, 1975.

Brown VM, Jordan DHM, Tiller BA: The acute toxicity to rainbow trout of fluctuating concentrations and mixtures of ammonia, phenol, and zinc. J Fish Biol 1:1–9, 1969.

Burkhalter DE, Kaya CM: Effects of prolonged exposure to ammonia on fertilized eggs and sac fry of rainbow trout (*Salmo gairdneri*). Trans Am Fish Soc 106:470–475, 1977.

Butler JN: Ionic Equilibrium. Reading, Mass.: Addison-Wesley, 1964.

Calamari D, Marchetti R, Vailati G: Effetti di trattamenti prolungati con ammoniaca su stadi di sviluppo del *Salmo gairdneri*. (Effects of prolonged treatments with ammonia on stages of development of *Salmo gairdneri*.) Nuovi Ann Ig Microbiol 28:333–345, 1977 (English translation).

Cameron JN: Methemoglobin in erythrocytes of rainbow trout. Comp Biochem Physiol 40A:743–749, 1971.

Chipman WA, Jr: The role of pH in determining the toxicity of ammonium compounds. Ph.D. thesis, Univ. of Missouri, Columbia, 1934.

Colt J, Tchobanoglous G: Evaluation of the short-term toxicity of nitrogenous compounds to channel catfish, *Ictalurus punctatus*. Aquaculture 8:209–224, 1976.

Crawford RE, Allen GH: Seawater inhibition of nitrite toxicity to chinook salmon. Trans Am Fish Soc 106:105–109, 1977.

DeGraeve GM, Overcast RL, Bergman HL: Toxicity of underground coal gasification condenser water and selected constituents to aquatic biota. Arch Environ Contam Toxicol 9:543–555, 1980.

Department of the Environment, UK: Effects of pollution on fish. In: Water Pollution Research

1971, p. 37. London: H.M. Stationery Office, 1972.

Downing KM, Merkens JC: The influence of dissolved-oxygen concentration on the toxicity of un-ionized ammonia to rainbow trout (*Salmo gairdneri* Richardson). Ann Appl Biol 43:243–246, 1955.

Emerson K, Russo RC, Lund RE, Thurston RV: Aqueous ammonia equilibrium calculations: Effect of pH and temperature. J Fish Res Board Can 32:2379–2383, 1975.

Emery RM, Welch EB: The toxicity of alkaline solutions of ammonia to juvenile bluegill sunfish (*Lepomis macrochirus* Raf.). Chattanooga, Tenn.: Water Quality Branch, Division of Health and Safety, Tennessee Valley Authority, 1969.

European Inland Fisheries Advisory Commission: Water quality criteria for European freshwater fish. Report on ammonia and inland fisheries. EIFAC Tech Pap 11, 1970; also in Water Res 7: 1011–1022, 1973.

Evans JW: The construction and use of a continuous-flow bioassay apparatus to determine a preliminary un-ionized ammonia 96-hour LC50 for the crayfish, *Orconectes nais*. M.S. thesis, Univ. of Kansas, Lawrence, Kans., 1979.

Flis J: Anatomicohistopathological changes induced in carp (*Cyprinus carpio* L.) by ammonia water. Part II. Effects of subtoxic concentrations. Acta Hydrobiol 10:225–238, 1968.

Fromm PO, Gillette JR: Effect of ambient ammonia on blood ammonia and nitrogen excretion of rainbow trout (*Salmo gairdneri*). Comp Biochem Physiol 26:887–896, 1968.

Girard JP, Payan P: Ion exchanges through respiratory and chloride cells in fresh water- and seawater-adapted teleosteans. Am J Physiol 238: R260–R268, 1980.

Hazel RH, Burkhead CE, Huggins DG: The Development of Water Quality Criteria for Ammonia and Total Residual Chlorine for the Protection of Aquatic Life in Two Johnson County, Kansas Streams. Washington, D.C.: Office of Water Research and Technology, Dept. of Interior, 1979.

Herbert DWM: The toxicity to rainbow trout of spent still liquors from the distillation of coal. Ann Appl Biol 50:755–777, 1962.

Herbert DWM, Vandyke JM: The toxicity to fish of mixtures of poisons. II. Copper-ammonia and zinc-phenol mixtures. Ann Appl Biol 53: 415–421, 1964.

Hillaby BA, Randall DJ: Acute ammonia toxicity and ammonia excretion in rainbow trout (*Salmo gairdneri*). J Fish Res Board Can 36: 621–629, 1979.

Hockenbury MR, Grady CPL, Jr: Inhibition of nitrification—effects of selected organic compounds. J Water Pollut Control Fed 49:768–777, 1977.

Jaffé ER: Metabolic processes involved in the formation and reduction of methemoglobin in human erythrocytes. In: The Red Blood Cell, edited by C Bishop, DM Surgenor, pp. 397–422. New York: Academic, 1964.

Kiese M: Methemoglobinemia: A comprehensive treatise. Cleveland, Ohio: CRC, 1974.

Klingler K: Natriumnitrit, ein langsamwirkendes Fischgift. (Sodium nitrite, a slow-acting fish poison.) Schweiz Z Hydrol 19:565–578, 1957 (English translation).

Knepp GL, Arkin GF: Ammonia toxicity levels and nitrate tolerance of channel catfish. Prog Fish Cult 35:221–224, 1973.

Konikoff M: Toxicity of nitrite to channel catfish. Prog Fish Cult 37:96–98, 1975.

Maetz J, Garcia-Romeu F: The mechanism of sodium and chloride uptake by the gills of a fresh-water fish, *Carassius auratus*. II. Evidence for NH_4^+/Na^+ and HCO_3^-/Cl^- exchanges. J Gen Physiol 47:1209–1227, 1964.

Mălăcea I: Untersuchungen über die Gewöhnung der Fische an hohe Konzentrationen toxischer Substanzen. (Studies on the acclimation of fish to high concentrations of toxic substances.) Arch Hydrobiol 65:74–95, 1968 (English translation).

McCoy EF: Role of bacteria in the nitrogen cycle in lakes. Water Pollut Control Res Ser 16010 EHR 03/72. Washington, D.C.: Office of Research and Monitoring, U.S. EPA, 1972.

Merkens JC, Downing KM: The effect of tension of dissolved oxygen on the toxicity of un-ionized ammonia to several species of fish. Ann Appl Biol 45:521–527, 1957.

Ministry of Technology, UK: Effects of pollution on fish. Toxicity of mixtures of zinc sulphate and ammonium chloride. In: Water Pollution Research 1961, pp. 90–93. London: H.M. Stationery Office, 1962.

Mirvish SS: N-Nitroso compounds, nitrite, and nitrate: Possible implications for the causation of human cancer. In: Proceedings of a Conference on Nitrogen as a Water Pollutant, vol. 1, Analysis, Sources, Public Health, August 18–20, 1975, Copenhagen. London: International Association on Water Pollution Research, 1975.

Newberne PM: Nitrite promotes lymphoma incidence in rats. Science 204:1079–1081, 1979.

Patrick R, Colt JE, Crawford RE, Manny BA, Russo RC, Thurston RV, Wedemeyer GA: Nitrates, nitrites. In: A Review of the EPA Red Book: Quality Criteria for Water, edited by RV Thurston, RC Russo, CM Fetterolf, Jr, TA Edsall, YM Barber, Jr. pp. 158–162. Bethesda, Md.: Water Quality Section, American Fisheries Society, 1979.

Perrone SJ, Meade TL: Protective effect of chloride on nitrite toxicity to coho salmon (*Oncorhynchus kisutch*). J Fish Res Board Can 34:486–492, 1977.

Redner BD, Stickney RR: Acclimation to ammonia by *Tilapia aurea*. Trans Am Fish Soc 108:383–388, 1979.

Reichenbach-Klinke HH: Untersuchungen über die Einwirkung des Ammoniakgehalts auf den Fischorganismus. (Investigations on the influence of the ammonia content on the fish organism.) Arch Fischereiwiss 17:122–132, 1967 (English translation).

Rice SD, Bailey JE: Survival, size, and emergence of pink salmon, *Oncorhynchus gorbuscha*, alevins after short- and long-term exposures to ammonia. Fish Bull 78:641–648, 1980.

Robinette HR: Effect of selected sublethal levels of ammonia on the growth of channel catfish (*Ictalurus punctatus*). Prog Fish Cult 38:26–29, 1976.

Robinson-Wilson EF, Seim WK: The lethal and sublethal effects of a zirconium process effluent on juvenile salmonids. Water Resour Bull 11:975–986, 1975.

Roseboom DP, Richey DL: Acute toxicity of residual chlorine and ammonia to some native Illinois fishes. Ill State Water Surv Rep Invest 85, 1977.

Rubin AJ, Elmaraghy GA: Studies on the toxicity of ammonia, nitrate and their mixtures to guppy fry. Water Res 11:927–935, 1977.

Russo RC: Recent advances in the study of nitrite toxicity to fishes. In: Proceedings of the Third USA–USSR Symposium on the Effects of Pollutants upon Aquatic Ecosystems, July 2–6, 1979, Borok, Jaroslavl Oblast, USSR, edited by WR Swain, VR Shannon, pp. 226–240. EPA Ecol Res Ser EPA 600/9-80-034. Duluth, Minn.: U.S. EPA, 1980.

Russo RC, Thurston RV: Water analysis of the East Gallatin River (Gallatin County), Montana 1973. Tech Rep 74-2. Bozeman, Mont.: Fisheries Bioassay Laboratory, Montana State Univ, 1974.

Russo RC, Thurston RV: The acute toxicity of nitrite to fishes. In: Recent Advances in Fish Toxicology, edited by RA Tubb, pp. 18–131. EPA Ecol Res Ser EPA-600/3-77-085. Corvallis, Ore.: U.S. EPA, 1977.

Russo RC, Smith CE, Thurston RV: Acute toxicity of nitrite to rainbow trout (*Salmo gairdneri*). J Fish Res Board Can 31:1653–1655, 1974.

Russo RC, Thurston RV, Emerson K: Acute toxicity of nitrite to rainbow trout (*Salmo gairdneri*): Effects of pH, nitrite species, and anion species. Can J Fish Aquat Sci 38:387–393, 1981.

Sato S, Matsushima T, Tanaka N, Sugimura T, Takashima F: Hepatic tumors in the guppy (*Lebistes reticulatus*) induced by aflatoxin B, dimethylnitrosamine, and 2-acetylaminofluorene. J Natl Cancer Inst 50:767–778, 1973.

Schulze-Wiehenbrauck H: Effects of sublethal ammonia concentrations on metabolism in juvenile rainbow trout (*Salmo gairdneri* Richardson). Ber Dtsch Wiss Komm Meeresforsch 24:234–250, 1976.

Shterman L Ya: Methemoglobin in fish blood. J Ichthyol 10:709–712, 1970.

Sillén LG, Martell AE: Stability Constants of Metal-Ion Complexes. London: Chemical Society, 1964.

Smart G: The effect of ammonia exposure on gill structure of the rainbow trout (*Salmo gairdneri*). J Fish Biol 8:471–475, 1976.

Smith CE, Russo RC: Nitrite-induced methemoglobinemia in rainbow trout. Prog Fish Cult 37: 150–152, 1975.

Smith CE, Williams WG: Experimental nitrite toxicity in rainbow trout and chinook salmon. Trans Am Fish Soc 103:389–390, 1974.

Stanton MF: Diethylnitrosamine-induced hepatic degeneration and neoplasia in the aquarium fish, *Brachydanio rerio*. J Natl Cancer Inst 34: 117–130, 1965.

Tabata K: Suisan dobutsu ni oyobosu amonia no dokusei to pH, tansan to no kankei. (Toxicity of ammonia to aquatic animals with reference to the effect of pH and carbon dioxide.) Tokai-ku Suisan Kenkyusho Kenkyu Hokoku 34:67–74, 1962 (English translation).

Thurston RV, Russo RC, Smith CE: Acute toxicity of ammonia and nitrite to cutthroat trout fry. Trans Am Fish Soc 107:361–368, 1978.

Thurston RV, Russo RC, Emerson K: Aqueous ammonia equilibrium—tabulation of percent un-ionized ammonia. EPA Ecol Res Ser EPA-600/3-79-091. Duluth, Minn.: U.S. EPA, 1979.

Thurston RV, Russo RC, Vinogradov GA: Ammonia toxicity to fishes: Effect of pH on the toxicity of the un-ionized ammonia species. Environ Sci Technol 15:837–840, 1981a.

Thurston RV, Phillips GR, Russo RC, Hinkins SM: Increased toxicity of ammonia to rainbow trout (*Salmo gairdneri*) resulting from reduced concentrations of dissolved oxygen. Can J Fish Aquat Sci 38:983–988, 1981b.

Thurston RV, Chakoumakos C, Russo RC: Effect of fluctuating exposures on the acute toxicity of ammonia to rainbow trout (*Salmo gairdneri*) and cutthroat trout (*S. clarki*). Water Res 15: 911–917, 1981c.

Tomasso JR, Goudie CA, Simco BA, Davis KB: Effects of environmental pH and calcium on ammonia toxicity in channel catfish. Trans Am Fish Soc 109:229–234, 1980.

Tomasso JR, Simco BA, Davis KB: Chloride inhibition of nitrite-induced methemoglobinemia in channel catfish (*Ictalurus punctatus*). J Fish Res Board Can 36:1141–1144, 1979.

Trama FB: The acute toxicity of some common salts of sodium, potassium and calcium to the common bluegill (*Lepomis macrochirus* Raf-inesque). Proc Acad Nat Sci Philadelphia 106: 185–205, 1954.

U.S. Environmental Protection Agency: Ammonia. In: Quality Criteria for Water, pp. 10–13. Washington, D.C.: Office of Water and Hazardous Materials, U.S. EPA, 1977.

Vámos R: Ammonia poisoning in carp. Acta Biol Szeged 9(1–4):291–297, 1963.

Wallen IE, Greer WC, Lasater R: Toxicity to *Gambusia affinis* of certain pure chemicals in turbid waters. Sewage Ind Wastes 29:695–711, 1957.

Wedemeyer GA, Yasutake WT: Prevention and treatment of nitrite toxicity in juvenile steelhead trout (*Salmo gairdneri*). J Fish Res Board Can 35:822–827, 1978.

Westin DT: Nitrate and nitrite toxicity to salmonoid fishes. Prog Fish Cult 36:86–89, 1974.

Wolff IA, Wasserman AE: Nitrates, nitrites, and nitrosamines. Science 177:15–19, 1972.

Wuhrmann K: Sur quelques principes de la toxicologie du poisson. (Concerning some principles of the toxicology of fish.) Bull Cent Belge Etude Doc Eaux 15:49–60, 1952 (English translation).

Wuhrmann K, Woker H: Beiträge zur Toxikologie der Fische. II. Experimentelle Untersuchungen über die Ammoniak- und Bläusaurevergiftung. (Contributions to the toxicology of fishes. II. Experimental investigations on ammonia and hydrocyanic acid poisoning.) Schweiz Z Hydrol 11:210–244, 1948 (English translation).

Wuhrmann K, Woker H: Beiträge zur Toxikologie der Fische. VIII. Über die Giftwirkungen von Ammoniak- und Zyanidlösungen mit verschiedener Sauerstoffspannung und Temperatur auf Fische. (Contributions to the toxicology of fishes. VIII. On the toxic effects of ammonia and cyanide solutions on fish at different oxygen tensions and temperatures.) Schweiz Z Hydrol 15:235–260, 1953 (English translation).

Wuhrmann K, Zehender F, Woker H: Über die fischereibiologische Bedeutung des Ammonium- und Ammoniakgehaltes fliessender Gewässer. (Biological significance for fisheries of ammonium ion and ammonia content of flowing bodies of water.) Vierteljahrsschr Naturforsch Ges Zurich 92:198–204, 1947 (English translation).

SUPPLEMENTAL READING

Alabaster JS, Lloyd R: Ammonia. In: Water Quality Criteria for Freshwater Fish, pp. 85–102. London: Butterworth, 1980.

National Research Council: Ammonia. Subcommittee on Ammonia, Committee on Medical and Biological Effects of Environmental Pollutants, National Research Council. Baltimore, Md.: University Park, 1979.

Patrick R, Colt JE, Crawford RE, Manny BA, Russo RC, Thurston RV, Wedemeyer GA: Nitrates, nitrites. In: A Review of the EPA Red Book: Quality Criteria for Water, edited by RV Thurston, RC Russo, CM Fetterolf, Jr, TA Edsall, YM Barber, Jr, pp. 158–162. Bethesda, Md.: Water Quality Section, American Fisheries Society, 1979.

Russo RC: Recent advances in the study of nitrite toxicity to fishes. In: Proceedings of the Third USA–USSR Symposium on the Effects of Pollutants upon Aquatic Ecosystems, July 2–6, 1979, Borok, Jaroslavl Oblast, USSR, edited by WR Swain, VR Shannon, pp. 226–240. EPA Ecol Res Ser EPA-600/9-80-034. Duluth, Minn.: U.S. EPA, 1980.

Russo RC, Thurston RV: The acute toxicity of nitrite to fishes. In: Recent Advances in Fish Toxicology, edited by RA Tubb, pp. 118–131. EPA Ecol Res Ser EPA-600/3-77-085. Corvallis, Ore.: U.S. EPA, 1977.

U.S. Environmental Protection Agency: Ammonia. In: Quality Criteria for Water, pp. 10–13. Washington, D.C.: Office of Water and Hazardous Materials, U.S. EPA, 1977.

Willingham WT, Colt JE, Fava JA, Hillaby BA, Ho CL, Katz M, Russo RC, Swanson DL, Thurston RV: Ammonia. In: A Review of the EPA Red Book: Quality Criteria for Water, edited by RV Thurston, RC Russo, CM Fetterolf, Jr, TA Edsall, YM Barber, Jr, pp. 6–18. Bethesda, Md.: Water Quality Section, American Fisheries Society, 1979.

Chemical
Distribution/Fate

Chapter 16
Analytical Chemistry

T. R. Gilbert and J. P. Kakareka

INTRODUCTION

Reliable measurements of toxicant concentrations are vital to the interpretation of toxicological data. In studies of bioaccumulation or biotransformation of toxicants, analytical chemistry supplies the principal measure of chemical exposure. This chapter provides summaries of the techniques commonly used to measure toxicant concentrations in aqueous test media and in the tissues of aquatic test organisms. Total analysis schemes including sampling strategies, sample pretreatment and concentration, methods of quantification, data interpretation, and quality assurance are discussed.

In formulating an analytical protocol one must consider the nature of the samples, the concentra-

The authors would like to acknowledge Ms. Beth Penney and Ms. Lisa Urry for their comments during the preparation of this manuscript.

tions of the pollutant of interest, the capabilities of the available methods of quantification, and the measures of data verification to be used. It must be emphasized that each protocol should be carefully considered and decided upon before any samples are taken. The protocol must then be faithfully followed at each step of every analysis.

Field monitoring programs will not be discussed in detail in this chapter. In common with laboratory toxicity tests, such surveys include procedures for the preparation of sample containers, sample documentation, and sample preservation. However, field surveys usually require more sophisticated sampling regimes than are needed to support toxicity tests. A protocol for field sampling includes selection of sampling sites and sampling frequencies, which are functions of such time-dependent variables as toxicant discharge rates and the movement of the water mass being

475

sampled. Site selection must take into account local dispersion patterns and any vertical stratification of the water column. When possible, "field blanks," that is, samples containing less than detectable levels of the toxicant(s) of interest, should also be taken (MacDougall et al., 1980).

All samples taken for chemical analysis must be stored and handled in a manner that minimizes changes in toxicant concentration. Greater care is required with field samples because toxicant concentrations are usually much lower than in laboratory samples. Both types of samples must be divided and preserved, and the two portions prepared for analysis independently when both organic and inorganic toxicants are to be measured.

In selecting a quantification method, priority should be given to those that require minimal sample manipulation. In this way sample contamination or loss of the toxicant is reduced. The method should have high specificity (freedom from interference) and high sensitivity. Whatever the method, the analyst must be thoroughly familiar with its capabilities and limitations and must institute a program of data verification to control or compensate for experimental errors. One component of such a program is routine system calibration through the processing of complete procedural blanks and spiked blanks. To verify the accuracy of the methodology, samples of known composition should be analyzed periodically. Finally, the reporting of analytical results should include expressions of uncertainty that reflect all sources of error and not just the variability observed when the final measurement is repeated with the same sample. In the following sections the features of analytical protocols described above will be discussed in detail in relation to the measurement of toxic trace metals and organic toxicants.

TERMINOLOGY

Procedural blank or *method blank.* An appropriate volume of analyte-free water that has been processed in exactly the same way as a sample.

Limit of detection. Lowest concentration of the analyte that can be reliably detected. In practice, this is the concentration that produces an instrumental signal (S_L) which equals the sum of the background (or method blank) signal (S_b) plus three times the variability in the background (or method blank) measurement (σ_B)

$$S_L = S_b + 3\sigma_B$$

Accuracy. Nearness of an analytical result to the true or accepted value.

Precision. Nearness of two or more measurements that have been performed in the same manner.

Systematic errors or *determinate errors.* Errors related to improper adjustment of apparatus, improper method design, or mistakes by the analyst. Such errors degrade accuracy by systematically skewing the analytical results.

Random errors or *indeterminate errors.* Errors inherent in all measurements, reflecting the uncertainties associated with each sample treatment and with the final measurement. The analyst's goal is to reduce these errors to acceptable levels by proper method design, good analytical technique, and use of a sufficiently large number of measurements.

DETERMINATION OF TRACE METALS

Sample Preparation

Toxicity Test Media

In most toxicity tests the toxicant is introduced into the test medium in dissolved form. To measure dissolved chemical species, an aliquot of medium (usually taken daily when monitoring static or flow-through toxicity tests) is filtered through membrane with a pore size of 0.4 μm. The first 50–100 ml of filtrate is used to rinse the filter flask and is discarded. The desired volume of filtrate is then collected, acidified with redistilled nitric acid to pH <1.5, and transferred to a Teflon or polyethylene bottle. To reduce sample contamination, the filtration apparatus should contain no metallic components. Plastic or glass parts should be cleaned by one of the methods described below for cleaning storage containers. Use of neoprene rubber O-rings should be avoided if zinc is to be measured (Robertson, 1968a).

Acidified water samples may be stored in either polyethylene or Teflon containers. Financial considerations argue for routine use of the former material. The literature contains many procedures for cleaning new or used polyethylene containers so that elements will not be leached into water samples. Most approaches include cleaning with detergent, rinsing with tap water and deionized water, and then soaking in hydrochloric and/or nitric acid prior to a final rinse with deionized water. In an evaluation of 13 methods for cleaning polyethylene bottles, Laxen and Harrison (1981) found that a 48-h soak in 10% (v/v) HNO_3 adequately cleaned both new and used bottles of leachable lead, cadmium, copper, and zinc. However, Moody and Lindstrom (1977) reported that 50% (v/v) HCl was more effective than 50% (v/v) HNO_3 in leaching lead from conventional polyethylene (CPE) and linear polyethylene (LPE) containers. They recommended a sequential cleaning process that included a 1-wk soak in 50% (v/v) HCl and a 1-wk soak in 50% (v/v) HNO_3 followed by several weeks of soaking in the highest purity water available.

The cleaning procedure best suited for routine analyses in support of toxicological studies depends on toxicant concentrations in the test media. If storage-related contamination in the range 10–50 ng/l is acceptable, then the relatively short cleaning procedure of Laxen and Harrison (1981) should be adequate. If more rigorous avoidance of contamination is required, one should review the methods developed by Settle and Patterson (1980).

Storage of freshwater or seawater samples without pH adjustment or another mode of sample preservation may result in loss of trace elements due to adsorption on container surfaces (Robertson, 1968b; Subramanian et al., 1978). If samples have been stored at their natural pH, addition of the chelator ethylenediaminetetraacetic acid (EDTA) has been shown to be more effective than acidification in desorbing metals from polyethylene containers (Hoyle and Atkinson, 1979).

It should be noted that adsorption of toxicant can also occur in the toxicity test tanks (Barker and Smith, 1979). Since acidification of the test media is out of the question, the tanks should be conditioned by soaking in media spiked with the toxicant. This can be accomplished most easily in flow-through tests by allowing the test medium to cycle through the system for several days prior to initiation of the test. Equilibrium of toxicant concentrations in exposure aquaria can be confirmed analytically. Concentrations slightly in excess of those to be used in the toxicity test may be necessary during conditioning to saturate all adsorption sites.

Because some elements elicit toxic responses at very low concentrations, toxicity test media may contain levels of elements too low to be measured reliably. Therefore, the toxicant must first be concentrated from the samples collected. Appropriate methods may be as straightforward as evaporation or freeze-drying, but often involve extraction into a second phase. Two of the most commonly used methods, solvent extraction and resin chelation, are described below.

The American Society for Testing and Materials (ASTM) (1980) and the U.S. Environmental Protection Agency (U.S. EPA) (1979b) methods for water analysis include procedures for extracting cadmium, copper, silver, nickel, lead, and zinc, using the chelator pyrrolidinecarbodithioic acid (PCDA) or its ammonium salt. This reagent may also be used to extract vanadium and hexavalent chromium (Stolzberg, 1975). The acid form of the reagent is prepared by mixing pyrrolidine and carbon disulfide in chloroform (ASTM, 1980). Alternatively, the commercially available ammonium salt may be dissolved in deionized water. The aqueous solution is washed with methyl isobutyl ketone to remove metal contamination. A portion of the aqueous solution is mixed with the sample, and the metal-PCDA complexes are extracted with more methyl isobutyl ketone. The latter approach produces unacceptably high blank values for lead and cadmium (Stolzberg, 1975) and requires daily preparation of fresh reagent. PCDA solutions in chloroform are less susceptible to contamination and are stable for several months with refrigeration.

One disadvantage of solvent extraction is that the preconcentration factor is limited to about 10:1 to 30:1. At larger volume ratios of sample to solvent, recovery of the solvent (and analyte) becomes difficult. When greater concentration factors are required, chelating resins may be used. The iminiodiacetate resin Chelex-100 is commonly used for analyses of natural waters. The calcium form of the resin offers better pH control than the sodium and ammonium forms (Figura and McDuffie, 1977). However, Kingston et al. (1978) separated sodium, calcium, and magnesium from several transition metals including cadmium, nickel, lead, and zinc with the ammonium form of the resin after water samples were first buffered to pH 5.0–5.5 with nitric acid, ammonia, and ammonium acetate. Davey and Soper (1975) also used the ammonium form of the resin to concentrate the above metals from 4-l samples of seawater into 10-ml final volumes.

More recently, Colella et al. (1980a) described the synthesis of a poly(acrylamidoxime) resin for chelating metals from aqueous solution. This resin does not have the affinity for alkali and alkaline earth elements that Chelex-100 does. Therefore, elution of poly(acrylamidoxime) with strong acid produces a final sample with fewer matrix salts. The resin has been used to concentrate copper, cadmium, lead, and zinc from seawater and pond water samples (Colella et al., 1980b).

Tissue Samples

Analysis of tissues for bioaccumulated trace elements requires care in sample handling if serious contamination is to be avoided. In biological studies tissue samples are often excised with stainless steel scalpel blades. If blending of tissues is

required, it is usually done in a blender with a stainless steel rotor. Both of these instruments can impart massive doses of nickel and chromium contamination. If these metals are to be measured, glass blades may be used to remove tissues and a Teflon rod can be used to grind and blend freeze-dried samples.

The literature contains many methods for the destruction of organic matter in the analysis of tissue samples. These methods may be divided into two categories: wet digestion and dry ashing. Ashing of solid samples at 500–550°C provides complete destruction of organic matter. In the measurement of many elements this is the method of choice. However, for mercury, arsenic, and selenium, which form volatile compounds in organic matrices, significant losses may occur during dry ashing. Most approaches to tissue dissolution for multiple element analyses involve wet digestion.

The most commonly used reagent for wet digestion is redistilled nitric acid. Tissue-acid mixtures can be heated to reflux temperatures (121°C) without loss of volatile elements. While hot nitric acid alone does not destroy all organic material, that which remains has usually been degraded to water-soluble species. Such a sample can be analyzed directly provided the presence of nitrogen oxides and covalent organic compounds of the element does not interfere with analysis. If the formation of hydride derivatives or elemental mercury is required, then the methods for further sample treatment described in the section on atomic absorption are necessary.

Methods for more complete tissue digestion are not always necessary and may cause loss of some trace elements. For example, addition of sulfuric acid to nitric acid digestates followed by evaporation until fumes of SO_3 are produced will result in loss of mercury. Perchloric acid may be used following nitric acid treatment, but may result in loss of chromium as CrO_2Cl_2 (Sinex et al., 1980). A method that has proved satisfactory in our laboratory consists of overnight digestion of tissue samples in nitric acid at room temperature, followed by slow heating for 1 h and then evaporation of the acid until a moist residue remains. A second volume of acid is added and the heating cycle is repeated. The remaining residue is solubilized in nitric acid and taken to volume with a solution of sea salt and deionized water (the sea salt is added as a buffer because of the enhancement effects described below for measurements by direct-current plasma emission spectrometry).

Methods of Quantification

It is beyond the scope of this chapter to describe all the instrumental methods that could be used to measure toxic elements in toxicity test media and digested tissue samples. Instead, three techniques have been selected because they are widely used and form the basis for standard methods published by the U.S. EPA (1979a,b) and the ASTM (1980). These three are atomic absorption spectrophotometry, plasma emission spectrometry, and anodic stripping voltammetry. Other techniques, such as spark source mass spectrometry (SSMS), offer much greater sensitivity. Some methods provide high sensitivity without requiring extensive sample preparation; an example is neutron activation analysis. Methods employing isotopic internal standards, such as isotope dilution/SSMS, are free from uncertainties connected with analyte recovery during sample preparation. These alternative techniques are also capable of simultaneously measuring several of the elements considered to be priority pollutants. Unfortunately, these and other methods require analytical and/or reactor facilities that are beyond the means of most toxicology laboratories. For this reason they are not included in the following discussion.

Atomic Absorption Spectrophotometry

Since its inception in the 1950s, atomic absorption spectrophotometry (AAS) has become the most commonly used technique for measuring trace elements in aqueous samples. Its popularity is based on several factors: low cost, ease and speed of operation, relative freedom from interference, and good degree of sensitivity (Table 1). Modern instruments offer automated sampling and data

Table 1 Comparison of Detection Limits for Atomic Absorption and Plasma Emission Spectrometry

	Limit of detection (μg/l)		
	Atomic absorption[a]		
Element	Flame	Electrothermal atomization	Plasma emission[b]
Antimony	200	3	30
Arsenic		1	10
Beryllium	5	0.2	0.05
Cadmium	5	0.1	0.9
Chromium	50	1	1
Copper	20	1	0.4
Lead	100	1	20
Mercury		0.2	25
Nickel	40	1	2
Selenium	2	2	70
Silver	10	0.2	7
Thallium	100	1	7
Zinc	5	0.05	0.2

[a]From U.S. EPA (1979b).
[b]From Floyd et al. (1980); values for silver and mercury are from Winge et al. (1979).

acquisition and enhanced sensitivity through electrothermal atomization.

The components of a modern atomic absorption spectrophotometer are shown in Fig. 1. Liquid sample is aspirated into a nebulizer, the resulting aerosol mixes with the combustion gases and is sprayed into the flame. Energy from the flame desolvates the sample and atomizes the analyte. A beam of light from a narrow-line

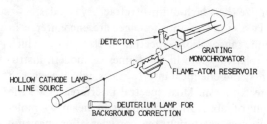

Figure 1 Optical diagram of a single-beam atomic absorption spectrometer. *[Courtesy of Instrumentation Laboratory, Inc.]*

source, such as a hollow cathode lamp (HCL) or an electrodeless discharge lamp (EDL), is aimed through the flame and into a grating monochromator, which has been aligned to the analytical wavelength of the line source. Analyte atoms in the path of the beam absorb some of the light; the resulting loss in signal provides a measure of the concentration of analyte atoms in the flame and in the liquid sample.

STOP

For some elements absorption is a linear function of concentration over fairly wide concentration intervals, and the spectrophotometer can be calibrated with only a few standard solutions. To achieve linear response, the width of the absorption line in the flame must not change with concentration and must always be greater than the width of the emission line from the HCL or EDL source. In addition, the degree of vaporization of the analyte cannot change with varying concentration. In many cases these criteria are not met, resulting in a nonlinear response. A series of up to five standard solutions with concentrations bracketing those of the samples must then be used for calibration. The resulting curve is approximated by a second- or higher-order calibration equation, using the curve correction routines available with most modern instruments.

The choice of flame conditions depends on the volatility of the compounds the element is likely to form in the flame. Measurements of chromium, for example, usually require a fuel-rich air-acetylene flame to inhibit the formation of chromium oxides. For elements such as beryllium and vanadium, the higher temperatures of a nitrous oxide-acetylene flame are needed to atomize their high-boiling (refractory) oxides.

Two types of interferences are encountered in atomic absorption: spectral interferences, which are relatively rare in the flames of modern instruments, and chemical interferences, which are much more common. Most spectral interferences are the result of absorption of the light beam by molecules and scattering by particles. For measurements at wavelengths below 420 nm a deuterium arc lamp may be used to simultaneously compensate for interfering species producing up to 1.5 absorption units. The beam of continuum radiation from the deuterium arc is also absorbed by the analyte and attenuated by interfering species, but the band pass of a typical atomic absorption spectrometer is so wide that the loss in signal from the arc is due almost entirely to background absorption and scatter. At longer wavelengths background correction may be achieved by measuring the intensity of a nonabsorbing emission line in spectral proximity to the analytical line.

A chemical interference may be defined as a matrix-dependent change in the number of ground-state analyte atoms in the flame produced by a given concentration of analyte in solution. For example, if the atom is partially ionized in the flame, the presence of other easily ionized elements may increase the density of ground-state analyte atoms. The net reaction may be written:

$$M^{\circ} \text{ concomitant} + M^{+} \text{ analyte}$$

$$\rightarrow M^{+} \text{ concomitant}$$

$$+ M^{\circ} \text{ analyte}$$

The effect of the reaction is an enhancement in the measure of the analyte. Fortunately, the flames used in atomic absorption are not hot enough to significantly ionize most elements, and this effect is usually limited to measurements of alkali and alkaline earth elements.

Suppression of signal can result from reaction of the analyte with a matrix component to form a compound that is less easily vaporized in the atom reservoir. The classic example of this effect is decreased calcium absorption due to concomitant phosphorus and the formation of calcium phosphate. To compensate for these chemical interferences, the sample matrix may be duplicated in the preparation of standard additions, either through the method of standard addition or by preparing a synthetic sample matrix. The latter approach is generally less desirable; even when the composition of the matrix is completely known, the reagent grade chemicals used to simulate it may be contaminated with intolerably high levels of the toxicant. Ultrahigh-purity chemicals may be available, but they are usually quite expensive.

Matrix modifications may be made to reduce chemical interferences. For example, the phosphate interference with calcium can be ameliorated by adding excess lanthanum. This results in the formation of lanthanum phosphate rather than calcium phosphate in the flame. The ASTM (1980) procedure for the measurement of chromium in water includes the addition of ammonium chloride to eliminate interferences from iron and other elements.

To achieve greater sensitivity in atomic absorption, electrothermal atom reservoirs were developed. Use of these devices is commonly referred to as flameless atomic absorption spectrophotometry (FAAS). Measurements by FAAS require small sample volumes, usually between 5 and 50 μl. Samples are injected with a micropipette into a pyrolytically coated graphite tube. The tube is then heated in an inert atmosphere by passing an electrical current through it. The heating process occurs in several stages to produce desolvation and ashing of the sample, atomization of the analyte, and finally high-temperature cleaning of the tube. The cleaning step is not always necessary, particularly if temperatures in excess of 3000°C are needed to vaporize the analyte. Some losses of the more volatile elements, such as cadmium and arsenic, may occur during the ashing step. To avoid this problem, the sample matrix may be modified to reduce the volatility of the analyte. Concomitant nickel, for example, raises the temperatures at which arsenic and selenium are vaporized.

The rapid heating that produces high sensitivities can also result in so much molecular absorption and light scattering that conventional background correction is inadequate. To reduce these effects ammonium nitrate has been added to brackish water and seawater samples. During the ashing step most of the sodium chloride in these samples is volatilized as ammonium chloride and sodium nitrate. According to Montgomery and Peterson (1980), the use of ammonium nitrate degrades the pyrolytic coating of graphite tubes, resulting in decreased sensitivity. However, new coatings may be applied by the analyst.

A second approach to increasing sensitivity involves generation of volatile derivatives of trace elements. The elements may then be purged from 5 to 100 ml of sample into the atom reservoir in only a few seconds. The most commonly produced derivatives are the hydrides of arsenic, antimony, and selenium, and elemental mercury. Methods for preparing these species have been published (ASTM, 1980; U.S. EPA, 1979a,b).

The principal sources of interferences in these methods are concomitants that consume sodium borohydride or stannous chloride, the reducing agents commonly used. Among the potential interfering species are the oxides of nitrogen remaining in nitric acid digestates of tissue samples. To eliminate these oxides, sulfuric acid is added and the digestate is evaporated until fumes of SO_3 are evolved. Care must be taken to maintain an excess of nitric acid until all organic matter is destroyed (ASTM, 1980). The volatility of mercury compounds precludes taking this approach, so digestion with nitric acid, permanganate, and persulfate is usually carried out at temperatures below boiling. Residual levels of the oxidizing agents are reduced with a salt of hydroxylamine just before divalent mercury is reduced to the elemental form with stannous chloride.

Arsenic, antimony, and selenium can exist in natural waters in more than one oxidation state. The highest of these—As(V), Sb(V), and Se(VI)—react more slowly with borohydride than do the lower states—As(III), Sb(III), and Se(IV). To reduce each element to its more reactive state, samples are treated with potassium iodide prior to generation of the hydrides.

Plasma Emission Spectrometry

Operationally, plasma emission spectrometry (PES) resembles combustion flame techniques such as atomic absorption in that a liquid sample is pumped or aspirated into a nebulizer and the resulting aerosol is swept into a high-temperature atom reservoir. In PES the aerosol is atomized and the analytes are excited and/or ionized by an argon plasma. These plasmas are partially ionized regions of gas in which electrons are heated either by a radio-frequency magnetic field, as in the inductively coupled plasma (ICP) shown in Fig. 2, or by the flow of direct current between two or more electrodes, as in direct current plasmas (DCPs). In both sources high-temperature electrons sustain the plasmas through collisional ionization of argon atoms. The result is more electrons, more collisions, and so on until an equilibrium of ionization and ion recombination is established.

Sample aerosols are heated to 6000 K in both ICPs (Abercrombie and Cruz, 1979) and DCPs (Gilbert and Stacey, 1979), or to temperatures about 3000° above those produced by combustion flames and electrothermal atomizers. At plasma temperatures, nearly complete dissociation of refractory substances occurs and fewer chemical interferences are observed than with atomic absorption. One interference encountered with DCPs is enhancement of analyte emission when salts of other, easily ionized elements are present. This

effect can influence analyses of marine toxicity test media (Nygaard, 1979).

Another advantage of PES is the capacity for simultaneous, or rapid sequential, multielement detection. Commercial spectrometers (Fig. 3) capable of measuring up to 48 elements simultaneously are available. The high temperatures of plasmas result in enhanced sensitivities for elements that form refractory compounds in combustion flames. For instance, the limit of detection for barium by direct nebulization is 0.1 mg/l by atomic absorption (EPA, 1979) but is 0.0005 mg/l by PES (Floyd et al., 1980). Comparison of the limits of detection for flame and electrothermal atomic absorption and plasma emission (see Table 1) indicates that PES is generally more sensitive than flame atomic absorption and, for some elements, matches the exceptional signal-to-noise properties of electrothermal atomic absorption. The methods used to enhance sensitivity in FAAs, such as hydride generation, may also be used in PES.

However, emission techniques have generally been more susceptible to spectral interferences than atomic absorption. A major type of interference is stray light—that is, a matrix-induced shift in background emission intensity. This occurs when radiation of wavelengths other than that for which the spectrometer is aligned reaches the detector. Such interferences may be reduced, but not necessarily eliminated, by the use of precisely ruled spectrometer gratings and by double dispersion of the emission spectrum. The latter approach was taken by Instrumentation Laboratory in the design of the Plasma 100 spectrometer and is an inherent feature of the echelle grating spectrometers produced by SpectraMetrics and Leeman Laboratories. Stray light can also be reduced by installing optical baffles in the spectrometer or filters over entrance or exit slits. If stray light effects cannot be adequately reduced at the wavelength of one emission line of the analyte, another line less influenced by matrix emission may be selected.

Spectral interferences may also be caused by

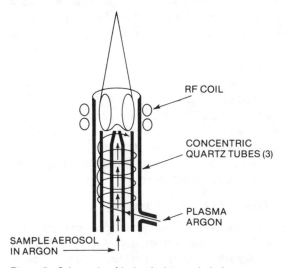

RF COIL

CONCENTRIC QUARTZ TUBES (3)

PLASMA ARGON

SAMPLE AEROSOL IN ARGON

Figure 2 Schematic of inductively coupled plasma.

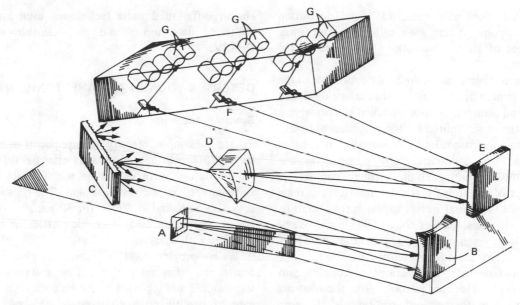

Figure 3 Optical schematic of an echelle grating spectrometer for plasma emission spectrometry: A, entrance slit; B, collimating mirror; C, echelle grating; D, prism-lens; E, folding mirror; F, focal plane; G, photomultiplier tube. *[Courtesy of Leeman Laboratories, Inc.]*

overlap of the analyte line by matrix-derived band emission, line emission, or continuum radiation. Of these, shifts in the intensity of continuum radiation are most likely to affect measurements with high-resolution spectrometers. Continuum radiation in plasmas is produced by radiative recombination of electrons with argon ions and with ionized matrix elements. Shifts in continuum radiation produced by the sample matrix can be evaluated by scanning the wavelength region of the analytical line. Most commercial plasma emission spectrometers have a wavelength modulation device to generate these scans. Wavelength modulation can also provide dynamic correction for shifts in background emission due to stray light or to changes in continuum radiation intensity. Therefore, most of the spectral interferences encountered in the analysis of water or digested tissue samples by PES are effectively eliminated.

Anodic Stripping Voltammetry

Voltammetric methods for measuring trace elements in environmental waters have been popular in some laboratories for decades. However, they did not become widely used until the introduction of a commercial polarograph capable of performing normal pulse and differential pulse polarography and anodic stripping voltammetry—the Princeton Applied Research model 174. Since then, a method based on differential pulse anodic stripping voltammetry (DPASV) has been developed and evaluated by ASTM Committee D-19 on water. It is now approved by ASTM for the measurement of cadmium and lead in water (ASTM, 1980).

Quantification by anodic stripping voltammetry begins by transferring an aliquot of aqueous sample to an electrolysis cell and deoxygenating it with O_2-free nitrogen. The metal ions are deposited into a stationary mercury electrode held at a relatively negative potential, for example, -0.8 to -1.2 V versus the standard calomel electrode. After several minutes of deposition, the potential of the electrode is scanned positively and the deposited metals are stripped back into the solution. The resulting current-potential curve is recorded. For calibration, additional deposition and stripping cycles are performed after small volumes of standard solutions are added to the sample.

The technique is theoretically applicable to the measurement of any element that can be deposited into and stripped from a mercury electrode in a potential range limited by the reduction of hydrogen ion and the oxidation of mercury. In addition to lead and cadmium, these elements include antimony, bismuth, indium, thallium, copper, and zinc. ASV methods for the determination of these elements in natural waters appear in the literature. Other elements, such as cobalt and nickel, may be deposited, but are stripped at potentials more positive than that at which mercury is oxidized.

Simultaneous determinations of copper, zinc, cadmium, and lead are possible, given the adequate separation of their stripping potentials. However, reduced copper and zinc form an intermetallic compound in the mercury electrode, which reduces the current of the zinc stripping peak while it increases and distorts the copper stripping peak (Bradford, 1972). To reduce this interference the analyst may use a sequential rather than a simultaneous approach. In the sequential method, a deposition potential is selected at which copper but not zinc is deposited. After copper has been determined, gallium is added to the sample and copper, zinc, and gallium are all codeposited at a more negative potential. Copper in the mercury preferentially forms an intermetallic compound with gallium, allowing the zinc to be stripped without interference (Abdullah et al., 1976).

While ASV is not applicable to the determination of many toxic elements, it offers the analyst several advantages when one of the electrochemically detectable metals is to be measured. Instrumentation is quite inexpensive, and the technique requires little sample pretreatment and is extremely sensitive. Using a 5-min deposition interval and a linear voltage sweep, Poldoski and Glass (1978) reported limits of detection for copper and lead of 0.03 $\mu g/l$ and for cadmium of 0.005 $\mu g/l$. Because of the better signal-to-noise ratios inher-

ent in differential pulse techniques, even lower limits of detection should be attainable with DPASV.

DETERMINATION OF ORGANIC TOXICANTS

Sample Preparation

To ensure sample integrity, all equipment in contact with the sample should be glass or Teflon. All laboratory ware should be washed with the solvents used in sample treatment. The glassware may also be baked at 400°C for 30 min. No plasticware should be used; leachable plasticizers may interfere with analyses.

Water samples must be stored in glass containers and refrigerated at 4°C. Chemical preservatives should not be used indiscriminately. In the case of specific polar compounds, however, pH may be adjusted to a range suitable for maximum sample preservation and analyte extraction efficiency. Water samples should be analyzed as soon as possible, and all samples must be analyzed within 7 d of collection (Federal Register, 1979). Whole test organisms or tissue samples should be frozen immediately to retain sample integrity.

Toxicity Test Media

In aquatic toxicological testing, concentrations of toxicant in the test systems generally are in the range of parts per billion (ppb) to low parts per million (ppm). Such low values usually necessitate concentration prior to quantification.

Liquid-liquid extraction is the most common method of concentrating organic compounds from aqueous samples. First, the pH of the sample is adjusted to promote maximum efficiency of extraction of the analyte from the aqueous matrix. For example, if a phenolic (acidic) compound is to be extracted, the pH is adjusted to ~2.0. Next, a suitable solvent for extraction is chosen. Organic compounds that are common in aquatic toxicological testing can be classified by degree of polarity. Substituted phenolics, acidic/basic pesticide derivatives, carboxylic acids, and aliphatic/aroma-

(evaporation)

steam concentration

tic amines are polar organic compounds. Plasticizers; organochlorine, -nitrogen, -phosphorus, and -sulfur pesticides; polynuclear aromatic hydrocarbons; and chlorinated hydrocarbons are toxicologically significant classes of nonpolar organic chemicals. The polarity of the toxicant to be analyzed will influence the choice of solvent polarity. The sample matrix and the detection method must also be considered when selecting the solvent. Proper judgment of the analyst is essential in choosing the solvent and in altering standard procedures when improvements in technique are presented in the literature.

A large selection of polar and nonpolar solvents is available (ASTM, 1980). Methylene chloride (dichloromethane) is a polar, low-boiling-point solvent frequently used for extraction. If the method of quantification employs a detector sensitive to chlorinated compounds, this solvent is a poor choice and hexane may be preferable. Moreover because hexane is nonpolar, it is less soluble in water than dichloromethane.

After selection of an appropriate extraction solvent, the aqueous sample is extracted in a separatory funnel at a ratio of water to sample between 20:1 and 40:1 (v/v). The solvent phase is drawn off and collected. The aqueous phase is extracted at least twice with similar volumes of solvent to improve recovery of the analyte. The extracts are combined and dried over anhydrous sodium sulfate. The extract can then be measured or subjected to further chemical preparation.

Nonconventional extraction procedures can be performed provided the same extraction efficiency is attained. An example is the extraction of a 40-ml portion of aqueous test solution in a Teflon-lined capped test tube. The analyte is concentrated in 5.0 ml hexane through vigorous shaking. This method may be preferred because of its procedural ease and simplicity.

Concentration of the solvent extract by evaporation is often necessary. Solvents (usually of boiling point $<80°C$) are evaporated on a steam bath. Sample extracts are concentrated over steam in a standard solvent concentration apparatus, a Kuderna-Danish (K–D) flask equipped with a concentrator tube. For example, 100 ml sample extract would be reduced to a 5-ml concentrate that retains all of the analyte. After steam concentration the volume can be further reduced to less than 1 ml by passing dry nitrogen over the sample concentrate.

An alternative extraction method recommended for analysis is the purge-and-trap extraction of volatile compounds from aqueous solutions (Bellar and Lichtenberg, 1979). Briefly, an inert gas is bubbled through a water sample contained in a specially designed purging chamber. Volatile components are transferred to the vapor phase and adsorbed onto a short sorbent trap. The trap is heated and back-flushed with gas to desorb the analyte into a gas chromatographic system.

Tissue Samples

Extraction of organic toxicants from tissue samples involves homogenization of the sample with a suitable extraction solvent. Homogenization, or blending, requires a high-speed grinding device to break up the tissue structure, providing maximum contact with the extracting solvent. As in aqueous sample extraction, solvent choice will vary with the analyte of interest and the sample matrix. For example, liver tissue containing an organometallic pesticide may require a very polar solvent to extract the parent compound and possible degradation products. Acidified methylene chloride, however, may coextract excessive biogenous lipid material with the analyte. Therefore, an alternative method of extraction would be chosen.

Another method of preparing tissue for analysis is digestion of the sample in hot 4 N NaOH followed by solvent extraction (Warner, 1976). Both the homogenization/extraction procedure and the digestion process result in large amounts of biogenous lipid material in the extracting solvent, requiring sample cleanup prior to quantitative analysis.

In aqueous samples as well as tissues, interfering substances may be coextracted with the analyte from the sample. These compounds can cause qualitative and quantitative analytical errors.

Therefore, a cleanup procedure is recommended before complex sample analyses.

One approach to extract cleanup is separation of constituent compounds by adsorption chromatography. A glass chromatographic column is packed with a solid adsorbent. Florisil and silica gel are two preferred adsorbents. The adsorbent-packed column is prewashed with the eluting solvent. The sample extract (1–2 ml in volume) is transferred onto the column. The column is next eluted with a nonpolar solvent, usually hexane, at a flow rate of 1–2 ml/min. If the analyte does not elute with nonpolar solvent, the polarity of the eluting solvent can be increased until an effective separation from interfering biogenous compounds is attained. One example of this technique is the elution of polychlorinated biphenyls (PCBs) from a Florisil column with 6% diethyl ether in petroleum ether (U.S. Department of Health, Education, and Welfare, 1968). Increasing the solvent polarity (15% diethyl ether in petroleum ether) elutes the more polar organochlorinated pesticides (e.g., aldrin, endrin, and dieldrin) from the column; biogenous extracted material is retained on the adsorbent.

Silica gel-packed columns can be used for more elaborate separations of chemical classes. By increasing the polarity of the eluting solvent, fractionation of analyte from other extractable compounds can be easily accomplished.

Additional column chromatography cleanup procedures are available in the literature (McMahon and Burke, 1978; Snook et al., 1975; Picer and Anel, 1978). Adsorbent supports and differing elution schemes are the parameters distinguishing these methods. Thus, formation of the analytical protocol requires that the analyst select the appropriate adsorbent, decide whether the adsorbent is to be activated or deactivated, and select the elution scheme for separating the compounds of interest. Proper selection of the correct conditions for sample cleanup will result in an easier, more dependable qualitative and quantitative analysis.

Quantitative Analysis

The principal methods for qualitative or quantitative analysis of organic toxicants are gas chromatography and liquid chromatography. The choice between gas chromatography and liquid chromatography for quantification of the analyte depends on the sample matrix, physical and chemical properties of the analyte, and sensitivity required. A polar aromatic chemical in an aqueous test medium at levels greater than 1 ppm could be measured by liquid chromatography without extraction. Gas chromatographic determination of the same compound would require extraction, concentration, and derivatization to a volatile compound; the former technique is obviously preferable. On the other hand, a nonpolar chlorinated pesticide in a tissue sample at parts per billion or lower levels would preferably be quantified by gas chromatography. The low concentration of the analyte necessitates an extraction and concentration step, and the analysis is improved by the greater sensitivity of the gas chromatographic detector. The variety of combinations of toxicants, sample matrix, and concentrations employed in aquatic toxicity testing calls for a large and flexible set of protocols for analysis of organic toxicants. In order to obtain reliable results, the analyst must choose the best set of procedures.

Gas Chromatography

Gas chromatography was established as an instrumental analytical technique before the development of liquid chromatography. Hence there is more information available on its capabilities, which results in a general preference for its use. A diagram of a gas chromatographic system is presented in Fig. 4.

The sample extract (1–5 μl) is introduced into the chromatographic column by injection from an accurately calibrated syringe. If the purge-and-trap method has been used, the sample is introduced by heating the trap and flushing it with carrier gas. In the column, the carrier gas flows over a stationary

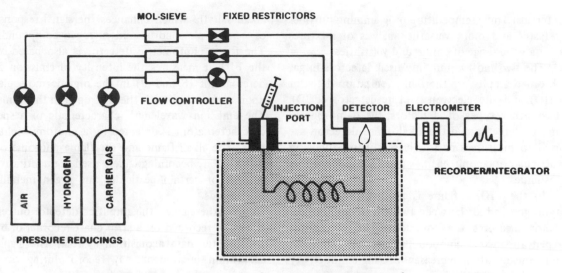

Figure 4   Diagram of a gas chromatographic system. *[Courtesy of Hewlett-Packard.]*

liquid phase on a solid support. The stationary phase retains each component of the sample mixture to a degree dependent on its distribution coefficient—an empirical value affected by volatility, polarity, and functionality. The sample components partition into and out of the liquid phase at a rate determined by these characteristics and are carried through the length of the column. Each component of the sample mixture is then eluted from the column by the carrier gas, after a characteristic retention time, and measured. The identity of each component is deduced on the basis of its relative retention time in comparison with standards of known retention times under the given instrument conditions.

The capacity of the column packing for effective separations and the sensitivity of the detector to specific compounds have established the utility of gas chromatography as an analytical technique. Basic reference books list the types of column stationary phases and solid supports that can provide effective separations of various nonpolar and polar compounds (McNair and Bonelli, 1969; Lynn, 1975). In addition, manufacturers of chromatographic supplies (e.g., Supelco, Analabs,

and Alltech) provide information about particular separations on selected column packings. These packings will not be discussed in detail here because of the abundance of supports and stationary phases available. Generally, greater difficulty is encountered in separating polar classes of chemicals. Fewer column packings are available for these separations. Therefore, it is recommended that derivatives of organic acids and bases that are more volatile than the parent compound be prepared. More versatile, easily analyzed derivatives of phenols, alcohols, and organic acids are obtained by alkylation (substitution of an alkyl group for an active hydrogen) and silylation (substitution of an $-SiR_3$ group for an active hydrogen). Similarly, acylation [substitution of a $-C(O)R$ group for an active hydrogen] provides suitable derivatives of the more basic compounds (e.g., amines). On specific instruments, programmed variation of the column oven temperature is available. In many cases separations can be improved through the use of temperature programming. For example, a linear increase of column temperature during a chromatographic analysis can effectively separate members of any homologous series at constant intervals. Thus, temperature programming provides a faster and more versatile analysis of mixtures over a wide range of compound volatilities.

The two most commonly used detectors in gas chromatography are the flame ionization detector (FID) and the electron capture detector (ECD). Two other types of detectors, the flame photometric detector and the alkali flame detector, are used to measure a narrow class of compounds, in particular organonitrogen, -sulfur, and -phosphorus pesticides.

In the FID, a flame is produced by burning hydrogen and air between two electrodes. The detector measures the conductivity of the flame. When an organic compound enters the flame the ion concentration increases, causing conductivity to increase, and the increased current flow is measured. The FID is sensitive to compounds with easily dissociated bonds (e.g., C–H, C–C) and without effective electron-capturing substituents, which decrease the ion concentration disproportionately. Therefore, when measuring aliphatic or aromatic hydrocarbons, the FID is the preferred detector.

In the ECD a radioactive source, usually ^{3}H or ^{63}Ni, ionizes the carrier gas. This produces a steady current, which can be monitored. As electron-absorbing or -capturing molecules are eluted from the column and reach the detector, the current decreases. This detector is extremely sensitive to halogen-substituted compounds and also to compounds containing phosphorus, silicon, and nitro-, carbonyl-, and organometallic functional groups. Pesticides containing chlorine (e.g., DDT, dieldrin, and endrin) are particularly well suited to ECD detection.

Through derivitization of polar compounds, it is possible to introduce halogens or silicon into a compound for increased response. For example, polar acids can be silylated, producing a more easily separated and quantitated silyl ester; amines can be treated with fluorinated acid anhydrides to produce a more easily chromatographed amide derivative.

The alkali flame detector is an FID with an alkali salt tip which enhances the signal response of certain phosphorus and nitrogen compounds. The flame photometric detector is also based on the FID; it measures the intensity of emission of heteroatoms (S and P) in the organic molecules upon combustion with the hydrogen in the flame. The emission wavelength characteristic of a specific heteroatom is detected by a photomultiplier tube. The alkali flame and the flame photometric detectors are becoming widely used in quantitative analysis of certain pesticides and organometallic compounds.

In all these cases, the amplified detector output is usually recorded on a strip chart recorder or by a computer data acquisition system. The signal acquisition instrument may record eluting compounds on the basis of peak height or peak area (or both). A calibration curve is prepared by plotting response versus concentration of analyte at three concentrations. The concentration of the analyte in the test sample is then calculated from this calibration curve.

Liquid Chromatography

High-performance liquid chromatography (HPLC) is becoming very useful for quantification of organics in aqueous samples. Direct injection of aqueous media with minimal sample preparation provides an inexpensive, reliable, and fast method of quantification with minimal loss of analyte. A diagram of a liquid chromatographic system is shown in Fig. 5.

Whereas mobile and stationary phases are fixed and temperature may vary in gas chromatography, in HPLC the stationary phase (column packing) is fixed, but the mobile phase can be changed during analysis (e.g., to gradually increase solvent polarity). Temperature can also be controlled (usually near room temperature) to avoid degradation of organic compounds or column packing.

A 25- to 100-μl volume of sample extract or aqueous test medium is injected into a sample loop and washed onto the column by the mobile phase, which is frequently a solvent such as hexane or methanol, at high pressure (140 kg/cm^2). The

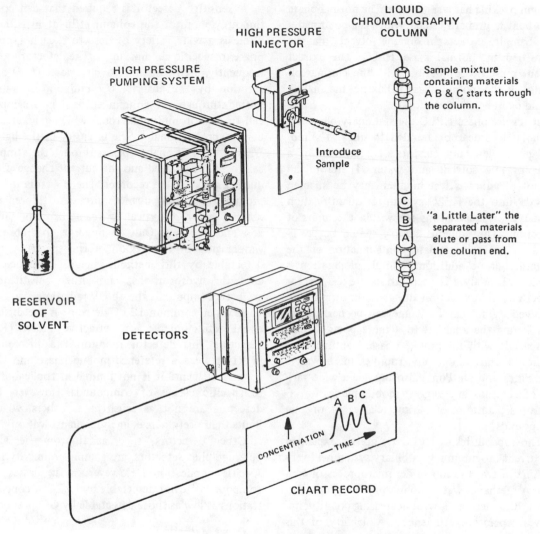

Figure 5   Diagram of a liquid chromatographic system. *[Courtesy of Waters Associates, Inc.]*

chromatographic column packing is either normal- or reversed-phase.

In normal-phase chromatography, a nonpolar mobile phase is used to elute the sample from a polar stationary phase; nonpolar compounds are eluted first. For example, in a mixture of aliphatic and aromatic hydrocarbons, hexane will elute the saturated compounds first, then the aromatic fraction. In reversed-phase chromatography a polar mobile phase is paired with a nonpolar support; polar compounds are eluted first. Benzidine, an acid degradation product of hydrazobenzene, is more polar and is eluted before the parent compound by a mobile phase consisting of 80% methanol and 20% water. A variety of reference books discuss adsorption and partition phenomena and properties of column supports and elution solvents (Snyder and Kirkland, 1974; Perry et al., 1976).

In both forms of liquid chromatography, the

column packing has a silica base. The normal-phase adsorbent is primarily silica, which is a polar material. Sample extracts in organic solvents may be quantified by normal-phase HPLC. The extract solvent must be compatible with the eluting solvent(s). If the mobile phase is hexane, the analyte should be in hexane solution.

In reverse-phase HPLC the stationary phase is a nonpolar hydrocarbon bonded to silica. The mobile phase generally consists of a mixture of a polar organic solvent and water. Therefore, an aliquot of aqueous test medium may be injected directly into the HPLC system for quantification if analyte concentrations are within the limits of detection. The aqueous sample should be prefiltered to avoid particulate contamination on the column, but no additional sample preparation is required. If analyte concentrations are too low for detection, an extraction and concentration step followed by solvent exchange can be performed, transferring the analytes to a more polar solvent compatible with the mobile phase. Manufacturers of liquid chromatography supplies (e.g., Waters Associates and Du Pont) also provide a wide variety of columns and suggest mobile phases for effective separations of various classes of organic compounds.

The capabilities of HPLC are greatly expanded by solvent programming. A binary system will vary the mix of two solvents under microprocessor control. A methanol-water mobile phase varying from 30 to 70% methanol, with decreasing polarity, improves separation efficiency. Availability of this feature in addition to a growing variety of column packings with different properties has helped to increase the popularity of HPLC as a method of quantification.

Another factor contributing to the increased use of HPLC is that polar compounds may be effectively separated without derivatization. However, a derivative may be used to enhance sample detection (e.g., an aromatic derivative of a compound that does not absorb ultraviolet radiation may be produced to allow the use of an ultraviolet-absorption detector).

A sensitive detector is required that can continuously monitor the column effluent in HPLC. There is a wide variety of detectors, each appropriate to specific circumstances. The detector most frequently used responds to ultraviolet (UV) absorption by the analyte. UV radiation is transmitted through the column effluent in a sample cell to a photomultiplier tube, which generates a current proportional to the intensity of the light. When a band of analyte passes through the sample cell, light is absorbed and the current change produces a peak on the recorder. The UV radiation is produced by a broadband source and filtered to obtain useful analytical wavelengths, especially 254 and 280 nm. Only compounds that absorb wavelengths in this region of the spectrum are detectable by this method. Phenols, polynuclear aromatic hydrocarbons, and other substituted aromatic compounds absorb UV radiation.

Another common HPLC detector is the differential refractometer, or refractive index (RI) detector. This detector monitors the difference in RI between a reference mobile phase and the column effluent. It is not limited in applicability to specific classes of compounds. However, RI detectors are not as sensitive as others, which limits their usefulness in analyte quantification.

Other detectors, such as fluorometric and polarographic detectors, are gaining popularity for specific applications. However, most classes of compounds are not detectable by HPLC at concentrations as low as those detectable by GC methods.

Other Methods

Gas chromatography and liquid chromatography are the most common methods of quantification in aquatic toxicology testing. However, they are separation techniques that provide qualitative identification by comparison to known standards. Alternative methods exist that can provide additional information. Gas chromatography-mass spectrometry (GC–MS) provides identification of unknown compounds. In GC–MS separation is provided by a gas chromatograph, which is interfaced with a mass spectrometer, a highly sophisticated detector that gives positive identification of the sample components.

In the quantification of organometallic compounds, the analyst can choose an organic or inorganic methodology. For example, a triphenyltin compound in aqueous test media may be analyzed by HPLC with a UV detector because of the aromatic portion of the compound, or a volatile derivative of the compound may be produced and quantified by gas chromatography. Finally, an inorganic methodology utilizing atomic absorption spectroscopy for quantitative analysis of the metal component may be used. Once again, it is left to the analyst to select the most appropriate method of quantitative analysis.

QUALITY ASSURANCE

Quality assurance (QA) programs are set up to check the accuracy and precision of analytical results and to maintain an acceptable level of analytical reliability. When a method is first developed or an existing method is applied in a new way, the first function of a QA program is method validation. If the new method does provide acceptable levels of precision and accuracy, it may be applied routinely. Then a quality control (QC) program is initiated to maintain the reliability of the measurement process.

The purity of the reagents used should match the needs of the analysis. This may require the purchase of special purity reagents or the purification of standard reagent chemicals. For example, reagent grade nitric acid may be used to clean laboratory ware for trace element measurements, but redistilled or higher-purity acid must often be used in sample pretreatment.

Some of the ways in which results are checked were alluded to above. One of the most important methods is periodic analysis of standard reference materials (SRMs). Replicate analyses of SRMs provide measures of precision and accuracy. When either of these performance checks gives results that fall below acceptable standards, the analyst must identify the source of error and reduce random error or eliminate systematic error.

QC measures are routinely applied to reduce the occurrence of error. These measures include processing of complete procedural blanks and spiked blanks with each set of samples. In this way, an unexpected increase in the level of sample contamination during pretreatment or decrease in analyte recovery can be detected and the measurement can be corrected accordingly. Spiked blanks or standard solutions prepared in the final sample matrix can be used for detector calibration. To reduce the occurrence of determinate error, the calibration of all apparatus, including balances and pipettes, should be checked and adjusted according to manufacturers' suggested schedules.

Such QC measures are part of the overall analytical protocol. They must be proposed, validated, documented, and faithfully carried out if measurements are to be precise and accurate.

SUMMARY

Before toxicity testing begins, analytical protocols for monitoring toxicant concentrations must be thoroughly evaluated and established. Samples should be taken and prepared in ways designed to minimize contamination or loss of analyte through adsorption, precipitation, or volatilization.

Toxic trace metals can be determined in liquid samples at or even below the level of micrograms per liter. Graphite furnace atomic absorption spectrophotometry may be used to measure most toxic trace metals at such low levels. However, the high salt content of marine or digested tissue samples may produce one or more severe matrix effects with graphite furnace atomization. To reduce these effects, matrix modification may be employed.

Cadmium and lead can also be measured by differential pulse anodic stripping voltammetry. This technique is well suited for analyses of marine samples since the matrix elements provide a natural electrolyte that does not react electrochemically at the sensing electrode. However, the technique is limited to elements that can be reduced and reoxidized in a potential range limited by reduction of the hydrogen ion and oxidation of the mercury-sensing electrode.

If simultaneous multielement detection is more important than high sensitivity, plasma emission spectrometry may be the technique of choice. The high temperatures of plasma sources provide greater freedom from chemical interferences than in flame or graphite furnace atomic absorption, but spectral interferences, including stray light effects and changes in continuum background emission intensity, require routine use of dynamic background correction for trace analyses. Analytical sensitivity can be improved by such preconcentration techniques as solvent extraction or ion exchange chromatography.

Similarly, trace organic toxicants can be determined in various samples in the range of parts per billion to parts per million. These low values usually necessitate extraction and concentration before quantification. The concentration step must provide maximum efficiency of extraction of the analyte from the sample matrix. In many complex sample analyses, the extraction-concentration step causes interfering substances to be coextracted with the analyte, thus requiring cleanup by adsorption chromatography. Proper selection of the correct conditions for sample cleanup will result in an easier, more dependable, qualitative and quantitative analysis.

The principal methods for qualitative and quantitative analyses of organic toxicants are gas chromatography and liquid chromatography. The choice between these methods for quantification of the analyte depends on the sample matrix, physical and chemical properties of the analyte, and sensitivity required.

Gas chromatography requires extraction, concentration, and, if necessary, derivatization of the analyte to a volatile compound. Generally, gas chromatography with one of a wide variety of specific detectors provides greater sensitivity than

liquid chromatography for substances present at the level of parts per billion or less.

Liquid chromatography is becoming increasingly popular in qualitative and quantitative analyses. Although less sensitive, it offers the capability of analyzing polar compounds without derivatization.

LITERATURE CITED

Abdullah MI, Reusch Berg B, Klimek R: The determination of zinc, cadmium, lead and copper in a single sea-water sample by differential pulse anodic stripping voltammetry. Anal Chim Acta 84:307–317, 1976.

Abercrombie FN, Cruz RB: Determination of trace inorganic toxic substances by inductively-coupled plasma-atomic emission spectroscopy. In: Monitoring Trace Substances, edited by D Schuetzle, pp. 113–135. Washington, D.C.: American Chemical Society, 1979.

American Society for Testing and Materials: 1980 Annual Book of ASTM Standards: Part 31, Water. Philadelphia, Pa.: ASTM, 1980.

Barker AJ, Smith K: Toxicity testing: Interlaboratory comparison with marine animals. Final Report, EPA Contract 68-03-2724, New England Aquarium, Boston, Ma., 1979.

Bellar T, Lichtenberg J: Semi-automated headspace analysis of drinking waters and industrial waters for purgeable volatile organic compounds. In: Measurement of Organic Pollutants in Water and Wastewater, edited by CE Van Itall, Denver, Colo.: American Society for Testing and Materials, 1979.

Bradford WL: A study on the chemical behavior of zinc in Chesapeake Bay water using anodic stripping voltammetry. Chesapeake Bay Institute, The Johns Hopkins University, Tech. Rep. 76, Ref. 72-7.

Colella MB, Siggia S, Barnes RM: Synthesis and characterization of a poly(acrylamidoxime) metal chelating resin. Anal Chem 52:967–972, 1980a.

Colella MB, Siggia S, Barnes RM: Poly(acrylamidoxime) resin for determination of trace metals in natural waters. Anal Chem 52:2347–2350, 1980b.

Davey EW, Soper AE: Apparatus for the sampling and concentration of trace metals from seawater. In: Analytical Methods in Oceanography, edited by TRP Gibb, Jr, pp. 16–21. Washington, D.C.: American Chemical Society, 1975.

Figura P, McDuffie B: Characterization of the calcium form of Chelex-100 for trace metal studies. Anal Chem 49:1950–1953, 1977.

Floyd MA, Fassel VA, Winge RK, Katzenberger JM, D'Silva AP: Inductively coupled plasma-atomic emission spectroscopy: A computer controlled, scanning monochromator system for the rapid sequential determination of the elements. Anal Chem 52:431–438, 1980.

Gilbert TR, Stacey GM: The effect of centimolar levels of barium on the measurement of trace elements by dc plasma emission spectrometry. In: Applications of Plasma Emission Spectrochemistry, edited by RM Barnes, pp. 79–89. Philadelphia, Pa.: Heyden, 1979.

Hoyle WC, Atkinson A: Retardation of surface adsorption of trace metals by competitive complexation. Appl Spectrosc 33:37–40, 1979.

Kingston HM, Barnes IL, Brady TJ, Rains TC, Champ MA: Separation of eight transition elements from alkali and alkaline earth elements in estuarine and sea water with chelating resin and their determination by graphite furnace atomic absorption spectrometry. Anal Chem 50:2064–2070, 1978.

Laxen DPH, Harrison RM: Cleaning methods for polyethylene containers prior to the determination of trace metals in freshwater samples. Anal Chem 53:345–350, 1981.

Lynn T: Guide to Stationary Phase for Gas Chromatography. North Haven, Conn.: Analabs, 1975.

MacDougall D, Amore FJ, Cox GV, Crosby DG, Estes FL, Freeman DH, Gibbs WE, Gordon GE, Keith LH, Lal J, Langner RR, McClelland NI, Phillips WF, Pojasek RB, Sievers RE: Guidelines for data acquisition and data quality evaluation in environmental chemistry. Anal Chem 52:2242–2249, 1980.

McMahon B, Burke JA: Analytical behavior data for chemicals determined using AOAC multiresidue methodology for pesticide residues in foods. J Assoc Off Anal Chem 61:640–652, 1978.

McNair H, Bonelli E: Basic Gas Chromatography. Palo Alto, Calif.: Varian Aerograph, 1969.

Montgomery JR, Peterson GN: Effects of ammonium nitrate on sensitivity for determinations of copper, iron and manganese in seawater by atomic absorption spectrometry with pyrolytically coated graphite tubes. Anal Chim Acta 117:397–401, 1980.

Moody JR, Lindstrom RM: Selection and cleaning of plastic containers for storage of trace element samples. Anal Chem 49:2264–2267, 1977.

Nygaard DD: Plasma emission determination of trace heavy metals in saltwater matrices. Anal Chem 51:881–884, 1979.

Perry S, Amos R, Brewer P: Practical Liquid Chromatography. New York: Plenum, 1976.

Picer M, Anel M: Separation of polychlorinated biphenyls from DDT and its analogues on a miniature silica gel column. J Chromatogr 150:119–127, 1978.

Poldoski JE, Glass GE: Anodic stripping voltammetry at a mercury film electrode: Baseline concentrations of cadmium, lead and copper in selected natural waters. Anal Chim Acta 101:79–88, 1978.

Robertson DE: Role of contamination in trace element analysis of sea water. Anal Chem 40:1067–1072, 1968a.

Robertson DE: The adsorption of trace elements in seawater on various container surfaces. Anal Chim Acta 42:533–536, 1968b.

Settle DM, Patterson CC: Lead in albacore: Guide to lead pollution in Americans. Science 207:1167–1176, 1976.

Sinex SA, Contillo AY, Helz GR: Accuracy of acid extraction methods for trace metals in sediments. Anal Chem 52:2342–2346, 1980.

Snook M, Chamberlain W, Severson R, Chortyk O: Chromatographic concentration of polynuclear aromatic hydrocarbons of tobacco smoke. Anal Chem 47:1155–1157, 1975.

Snyder L, Kirkland J: Introduction to Modern Liquid Chromatography. New York: Wiley, 1974.

Stolzberg RJ: Ammonium pyrrolidinecarbodithioate-methyl isobutyl ketone extraction system for some trace metals in seawater. In: Analytical Problems in Oceanography, edited by TRP Gibb, Jr, pp. 30–43. Washington, D.C.: American Chemical Society, 1975.

Subramanian KS, Chakrabarti CL, Sueiras JE, Maines IS: Preservation of some trace metals in samples of natural water. Anal Chem 50:444–448, 1978.

U.S. Department of Health, Education, and Welfare: Pesticide Analytical Manual, vol. 1. Washington, D.C.: Food and Drug Administration, 1968.

U.S. Environmental Protection Agency: Guidelines establishing test procedures for the analysis of pollutants; proposed regulations. Fed Regist 44:69464–69575, 1979a.

U.S. Environmental Protection Agency: Methods for Chemical Analysis of Water and Wastes. EPA-600/2-79-020. Cincinnati, Ohio: U.S. EPA, 1979b.

Warner JS: Determination of aliphatic and aromatic hydrocarbons in marine organisms. Anal Chem 48:578–583, 1976.

Winge RK, Peterson VJ, Fassel VA: Inductively coupled plasma-atomic emission spectroscopy: Prominent lines. Appl Spectrosc 33:206–219, 1979.

SUPPLEMENTAL READING

American Society for Testing and Materials: Annual Book of ASTM Standards, Part 3: Water. Philadelphia: American Society for Testing and Materials, 1980.

APHA, AWWA, and WPCF: Standard Methods for the Examination of Water and Wastewater, 14th ed., Washington, D.C.: American Public Health Association, American Water Works Association, and Water Pollution Control Federation, 1975.

U.S. Environmental Protection Agency: Guidelines establishing test procedures for the analysis of pollutants; proposed regulations, Fed Regist 44:69464–69575, 1979.

U.S. Environmental Protection Agency: Handbook for Analytical Quality Control in Water and Wastewater Laboratories. EPA-600/4-79-019. Cincinnati, Ohio: Environmental Monitoring and Support Laboratory, Office of Research and Development, 1979.

U.S. Environmental Protection Agency: Methods for Chemical Analysis of Water and Wastes. EPA-600/4-79-020. Cincinnati, Ohio: Environmental Monitoring and Support Laboratory, Office of Research and Development, 1979.

Chapter 17

Bioaccumulation

A. Spacie and J. L. Hamelink

INTRODUCTION

Bioaccumulation of pollutants first gained public attention in the 1960s with the discovery of DDT, DDD, and methyl mercury residues in fish and wildlife. Mortalities and reproductive failures in fish and fish-eating birds were linked to unusually high concentrations of DDT or its metabolites in the fat of these animals. Since the top-level carnivores, especially birds, had higher residue concentrations of these chemicals than the food they consumed, it was logical to postulate that accumulation occurred primarily by transfer through the food chain. This idea was supported indirectly by the observation that DDT residues increased in a stepwise fashion from one trophic level to the next (Woodwell et al., 1967). The net efficiency of energy transfer between trophic levels is only about 10%. If the transfer efficiency for a chemical contaminant from food to consumer were greater, say 50–100%, and if there were no significant losses from the organism, then residues would continue to accumulate throughout the life of the consumer. The higher the trophic level, the greater would be the body burden of residues. Although the actual mechanism for such a process was not clear, the concept of "biomagnification" or "transfer up the food chain" became popular.

Later, when laboratory and microcosm experiments failed to show the same degree of magnification, debates arose over the relative importance of food and water in the accumulation process. This was the situation until quite recently, when detailed dynamic models were used to distinguish the various routes of uptake. It is now clear that the degree of accumulation in aquatic organisms depends on the type of food chain, on the availability and persistence of the contaminant in water, and especially on the physical-chemical properties of the contaminant.

water soluble → degradable
& polar

Persistent contaminants such as DDT and the highly chlorinated PCBs share several characteristics, including poor biodegradability, low water solubility, and high lipid solubility. When such nonpolar chemicals are allowed to partition or distribute between aqueous and organic solvents, nearly all of the molecules diffuse into the organic phase. For example, about 562,000 times more DDT will accumulate in octanol than in water in the same system. Nonpolar chemicals also partition into the fat of aquatic animals exposed to them in water. The degree of bioaccumulation is generally correlated with the partition coefficient (P) measured in an octanol-water mixture. Chemicals with very large partition coefficients are more likely to be bioaccumulated than those with low P values.

Nevertheless, the distribution of a chemical in aquatic organisms is not quite as simple to model or measure as it is in organic solvents. Since animals move about, feed, grow, and actively transport and transform chemicals within their tissues, it is more difficult to describe the factors that affect chemical uptake and distribution. Mass balance or kinetic models are required to describe the various steps in accumulation, distribution, and elimination of residues. Models similar to those used by pharmacologists to describe the time course of drugs in the human body are transferable to aquatic systems. They are especially useful for describing residue dynamics over time and for distinguishing the routes of uptake from food and water.

This chapter introduces the use of kinetic models in describing bioaccumulation. It emphasizes the application of models and physical-chemical correlations to the design of appropriate test methods for measuring bioaccumulation potential.

TERMINOLOGY

Uptake. Transfer of a chemical into or onto an aquatic organism. The uptake phase of an accumu-

lation test is the period during which test organisms are exposed to the chemical.

Depuration. Elimination of a chemical from an organism by desorption, diffusion, excretion, egestion, biotransformation, or another route. The depuration phase of a test is the period during which previously exposed organisms are held in uncontaminated water.

Half-life or half-time. Time required for an organism held in clean water to eliminate 50% of the total body burden or tissue concentration of a chemical.

Bioavailable. Term used for the fraction of the total chemical in the surrounding environment which is available for uptake by organisms. The environment may include water, sediment, suspended particles, and food items.

Partitioning. Distribution of a chemical between two immiscible solvents. The partition coefficient (P or K_{ow}) is the ratio of the chemical concentrations in the two solvents at equilibrium. Partition coefficients are commonly measured between n-octanol and water.

Steady state or dynamic equilibrium. The state at which the competing rates of uptake and elimination of a chemical within an organism or tissue are equal. An apparent steady state is reached when the concentration of a chemical in tissue remains essentially constant during a continuous exposure. Bioconcentration factors are usually measured at steady state.

Compartment. Quantity of chemical that displays uniform rates of uptake and elimination in a biological system and whose kinetics can be distinguished from those of other compartments (Moriarty, 1975).

THE PROCESS OF ACCUMULATION

Bioaccumulation can occur only if the rate of uptake of a chemical by an organism exceeds its rate of elimination. It is important to consider all the possible routes of chemical uptake so that appropriate models and test methods can be designed. Although many of the biochemical processes involved in xenobiotic transport are poorly understood, the general patterns of uptake from water, sediment, and food are clear enough to be modeled in a reasonably realistic way. This section describes the major features of the uptake process.

Uptake from Water

Direct uptake of chemicals from water has been shown for many aquatic organisms including algae, annelids, arthropods, mollusks, and fish. Considering the tremendous size range and structural diversity of aquatic organisms, a variety of uptake sites and mechanisms would be expected. Nevertheless, the discussion can be simplified by concentrating on the three most significant transport processes: diffusion, special transport, and adsorption.

Diffusion

Most xenobiotics are taken into the body by passive diffusion through semipermeable membranes such as the gill, lining of the mouth, or gastrointestinal tract. Fish gills are especially vulnerable to foreign chemicals because their design maximizes diffusion. Gill membranes are thin (2-4 μm) and typically represent 2-10 times the surface area of the body. In contrast, the fish skin, crustacean carapace, and insect cuticle are relatively impermeable because of their dense, nonliving layers composed of hydrophobic and hydrophilic regions. Factors governing the transport of toxicants through insect cuticles have been studied intensively but are still not well understood (Matsumura, 1975).

Passive diffusion can occur across any barrier that is permeable to the chemical and across which a concentration gradient (ΔC) exists. It is a physical process that requires no energy expenditure by the organism. The lipid bilayer of simple biological membranes permits rapid diffusion of nonpolar (lipophilic) organic molecules, but little diffusion of water, ions, or polar molecules. Weak acids and bases cross the membrane primarily in their unionized form. Proteinaceous pores in the membrane, however, allow passage of water, small ions such as chloride, and small molecules up to a mo-

lecular weight (MW) of approximately 100. The permeability of these membrane pores can vary with salinity and with the physiological state of the organism.

According to Fick's law, the rate of diffusion is proportional to

$$\frac{\Delta C \times \text{area} \times \text{temperature}}{\text{distance}} \tag{1}$$

Isolated membranes would be quickly saturated and the rate of diffusion would decline if the chemical were allowed to accumulate locally. The countercurrent blood flow pattern at the gill, which transports substances away from the site of diffusion, is especially effective in maintaining a large concentration gradient. The rate of passive uptake at the gill tissue (dC/dt) is directly proportional to the difference between the chemical concentration in water (C_w) and that in blood (C_b). Since the initial value of C_b for a xenobiotic substance is usually zero at the beginning of an exposure,

$$\frac{dC}{dt} = k_u C_w \tag{2}$$

initially. Here the rate coefficient k_u incorporates all the physical factors that affect the rate of diffusion. Not only surface area and membrane thickness, but also characteristics such as the respiration rate and the size and lipid solubility of the chemical molecule, are involved. Assuming that the chemical concentration in water is held constant, the initial rate of diffusion into the organism is also constant. Later we will see that Eq. (2) forms the basis for a simple bioconcentration model.

Experiments with isolated perfused trout gills showed diffusion of the insecticide dieldrin from water to blood (Fromm and Hunter, 1969). The transport into blood apparently requires the presence of plasma proteins to help bind the dieldrin. Passive diffusion of cadmium was also shown with isolated gills of the mussel *Mytilus edulis* (Carpene and George, 1981). The uptake was linear over time and directly proportional to the external cadmium concentration.

In vivo uptake at the gill has been observed for DDT in salmonids (Premdas and Anderson, 1963; Holden, 1962), methyl mercury and mercuric chloride in rainbow trout (Olson et al., 1973), surfactants in carp (Kikuchi et al., 1980), copper in sunfish (Anderson and Spear, 1980), and fish anesthetics (Hunn and Allen, 1974). In general, measured uptake rates are greater for living than for dead animals because of the role of the blood circulation in transport.

Arthropods can apparently absorb some chemicals through the general body surface. Derr and Zabik (1974) found passive diffusion of DDE through the cuticle of midge larvae. Uptake was related to the surface area and was similar for both living and dead animals. DDT also accumulates through the integument of dragonfly nymphs (Wilkes and Weiss, 1971) and *Daphnia* (Crosby and Tucker, 1971), where uptake is proportional to exposure concentration. Dead *Daphnia* accumulate about half as much DDT in 24 h as live *Daphnia*.

The molting process can affect body burdens, at least for metals. Jennings and Rainbow (1979) found that the gills of the crab *Carcinus maenas* absorbed cadmium, but 59–80% of the total body burden was sorbed to the exoskeleton. Zinc may also be taken up by the gills of *C. maenas* (Bryan, 1976), but 61% is lost at each molt (Renfro et al., 1975). About half of the cadmium concentration in shrimp *Lysmata seticaudata* was also lost at each molt (Fowler and Benayoun, 1974). PCBs were taken up across the general integument of *Gammarus oceanicus*, but in this case no effect of molting was noted (Wildish and Zitko, 1971).

Special Transport

Special transport of chemicals into the body includes both active and facilitated transport. Active transport can occur against a concentration gradient, while facilitated transport cannot. In both processes the chemical forms a reversible complex with a macromolecular carrier in the membrane. Thus the kinetics of special transport can be

saturated at high chemical concentrations. Competitive inhibition of the uptake of a chemical in the presence of chemically similar substances is also possible. There are numerous examples of metals interacting to affect uptake. For example, cadmium tends to reduce the uptake of zinc and copper. Cobalt and manganese can compete for uptake via the iron transport system (Klaassen, 1980).

Since active transport requires energy to move the chemical against a gradient, it is a true concentrating mechanism. Metabolic blocking agents can be used experimentally to prevent active transport. In contrast, facilitated transport requires no cellular energy input and cannot concentrate chemicals against a gradient (Klaassen, 1980). The two special transport processes are intended to regulate biologically important materials such as essential metals, sugars, and amino acids. Metals can be accumulated by both active and passive transport processes and it is not clear which is more common.

Regardless of mechanism, metal uptake in aquatic organisms is usually directly proportional to the metal concentration in water (C_w), at least initially. Bryan (1976) showed linear rates of uptake for mercury, copper, silver, manganese, zinc, cadmium, and arsenic in the marine worm *Nereis diversicolor*. Direct proportionality between uptake and C_w for lead was also found with aquatic insects (Spehar et al., 1978). In the same study, cadmium residues in insects after 28 d were proportional to exposure concentration at low C_w but approached a constant concentration at the upper end of the range tested. This suggests saturation of binding sites on or in the insects. Cadmium uptake in perfused trout gills also decreased at high exposure concentrations (Part and Svanberg, 1981).

Low salinity can increase the rate of uptake of cadmium by marine organisms that actively accumulate salt as salinity declines (O'Hara, 1973; Jackim et al., 1977). Low salinity also enhances the uptake of cesium in aquatic organisms because of reduced competition from the similar ion, potassium (Thomann, 1981). Thus it may be difficult to generalize about bioaccumulation of metals in aquatic organisms because of the importance of water chemistry and the active role played by organisms in regulating normal body constituents.

Adsorption

Adsorption is the binding of a chemical to a surface by covalent, electrostatic, or molecular forces. Since it is a surface phenomenon, it is important mainly as the initial step in the accumulation process. Substances that bind to the integument of an animal contribute to the total body burden and may affect vulnerable functions of the epithelium, but they do not generally contribute to the toxic effect level within the body.

Adsorption is especially important for microorganisms because of their extremely high surface-to-volume ratio. Sodergren (1968) found initial rapid adsorption of DDT onto *Chlorella* cells followed by absorption across the cell membrane. Similarly, zinc was adsorbed on diatoms and immediately transported by diffusion into the cytoplasm (Davies, 1973). Diffusion rather than adsorption controlled the overall rate of zinc uptake. Adsorption mechanisms have been cited for bacteria with certain PCBs and toxaphene (Paris et al., 1977, 1978) and for algae with TCDD (Isensee and Jones, 1975) and DDT (Hamelink et al., 1971; Cox, 1970). Because adsorption is a physical process, it should be equally effective in living and dead organisms. Paris et al. (1978) found very little difference in the degree of accumulation of PCB between bacteria, nonliving seston, and sediment. Sodergren (1968) reported similar rates of DDT uptake for living and dead algal cells.

A common method of expressing adsorption to a substrate is the Freundlich isotherm:

$$\frac{X}{M} = kC_w^{1/n} \quad \text{or} \quad \log\frac{X}{M} = \log k + \frac{\log C_w}{n}$$

$$(3)$$

where X/M is the mass of chemical sorbed per gram of sorbent at equilibrium, k is the Freundlich

adsorption constant, C_w is the equilibrium solution concentration of the chemical, and $1/n$ represents the slope of the isotherm. The slope may be found by plotting $\log (X/M)$ against $\log C_w$ for various concentrations. The higher the intercept ($\log k$), the greater the degree of adsorption, and the larger the slope, the greater the efficiency of adsorption.

It is important to note that this relationship assumes a constant ratio of sorbent to water. Higher sorbent concentrations tend to produce proportionately less adsorption. If the constant k is thought of as a type of concentration factor, then that factor may vary with the quantity of sorbent in the system tested. A good example of this mass effect is the uptake of 2,4,5,2',5'-pentachlorobiphenyl by marine phytoplankton, which follows a Freundlich-type relationship (Harding and Phillips, 1978). The quantity of PCB adsorbed (X/M) decreases linearly with increasing density of the algal suspension when plotted logarithmically (Fig. 1). Ellgehausen et al. (1980) also found a Freundlich relationship for the uptake of p,p'-DDT by algae,

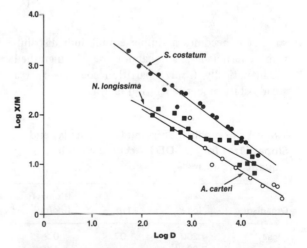

Figure 1 Relationships between algal density as log *D* (micrograms of cell carbon per liter) and equilibrium concentration of 2,4,5,2',5'-pentachlorobiphenyl (PCB) in phytoplankton as log *X/M* (micrograms of PCB per gram of cell carbon). Suspensions of *Skeletonema costatum*, *Nitzschia longissima*, and *Amphidinium carteri* were incubated at 12°C with an initial PCB concentration of 0.31 µg/l. *[From Harding and Phillips (1978).]*

Daphnia, and fish (Table 1). The algae appeared to have a greater binding capacity (k) than the other organisms because they were tested at a lower biomass concentration (0.2 mg/ml). When expressed on the basis of equivalent weight (1 mg/ml), all three taxa showed approximately the same degree of accumulation. Thus the relative proportions of chemical, water, and biomass can affect the outcome of bioaccumulation experiments. Field studies may also show this mass effect. For example, lower DDT concentrations in marine phytoplankton were associated with higher densities of the phytoplankton standing crop (Cox, 1970).

The slope of the isotherm ($1/n$) is often close to 1.0 under equilibrium conditions (Table 1). Harding and Phillips (1978) found slopes ranging from 0.8 to 2.5 for various algal species, with most values near 1.0. A value of 1.0 indicates a direct proportionality between the concentration of a chemical in or on the organism (C) and its concentration in water (C_w):

$$C = \frac{X}{M} = kC_w \qquad (4)$$

so that k becomes a simple equilibrium distribution coefficient that cannot be distinguished mathematically from a partition coefficient or a steady-state bioconcentration factor:

Table 1   Freundlich Sorption Constants (k) and Slopes ($1/n$) for p,p'-DDT Accumulation in Aquatic Organisms[a]

Organism	log k	$1/n$	Biomass (mg/ml)
Algae	4.200	1.07	0.2
Algae	3.322[b]	—	1.0
Daphnia	3.350	1.09	1.0
Catfish	3.539	1.21	1.0

[a]Adapted from Ellgehausen et al. (1980).
[b]Calculated from an experimentally determined regression relating DDT residue in algae to algal biomass.

$$\text{Partition coefficient} = \frac{\text{concentration in solvent 1}}{\text{concentration in solvent 2}} \qquad (5)$$

Bioconcentration factor

$$= \frac{\text{concentration in organism}}{\text{concentration in water}} \qquad (6)$$

Thus adsorption isotherms with slopes near unity do not necessarily represent simple physical adsorption, but rather may describe a more general distribution or partitioning phenomenon. Although PCB uptake by marine plankton can be described by a Freundlich relationship, the accumulation is certainly not limited to surface adsorption (Pavlou and Dexter, 1979).

Bioavailability in Water

Transport into biological membranes requires that the xenobiotic in the surrounding water be available in a dissolved form. Environmental factors that reduce the amount of chemical in true solution (C_w) will also reduce the rate of uptake [Eq. (2)]. Among the most important processes that reduce bioavailability are adsorption to suspended solids, adsorption to sediments, adsorption to humic acids and other macromolecules, formation of colloidal suspensions, chelation, complexation, and ionization.

Lipophilic chemicals with a strong tendency to be bioconcentrated are also likely to partition into the organic fraction of sediment or suspended solids (Baughman and Lassiter, 1978; Kenaga and Goring, 1980; Hamelink, 1980; Kenaga, 1980). The concentration factor (K) for a chemical adsorbed to sediments or soil (C_a) at equilibrium can be defined as

$$K = \frac{C_a}{C_w}$$

or, normalized for the organic content of the soil,

$$K_{oc} = \frac{K}{\text{fraction of organic content}}$$

The adsorption-desorption process for lipophilic organics is rapid (equilibrium in minutes or a few hours) and usually reversible (Baughman and Lassiter, 1978). Kenaga and Goring (1980) measured the concentration factors (K_{oc}) for a number of pollutants, mostly pesticides, as a function of water solubility (S, ppm) or octanol-water partition coefficient (P):

$$\log K_{oc} = 3.64 - 0.55 \log S \qquad (7)$$

$$\log K_{oc} = 1.377 + 0.544 \log P \qquad (8)$$

Thus association with soil or sediments is greatest for chemicals with low water solubility and high P values. Bioconcentration factors (BCFs) were also expressed as functions of S or P, giving correlations such as

$$\log \text{BCF} = 2.791 - 0.564 \log S \qquad (9)$$

The slopes of Eqs. (7) and (9) are remarkably similar, illustrating the tendency of aquatic organisms to "compete" with sediments for the same dissolved chemicals.

Sorption of organics and cations increases as the particle size of the soil becomes smaller (Baughman and Lassiter, 1978). For example, the concentration factor (K_{oc}) for methoxychlor increases from 22,000 for sand to 93,000 for fine silt. Thus the nature of the sediments may profoundly influence the availability of a chemical in the environment. For example, Lynch (1979) found that amphipods exposed to hexachlorobiphenyl in the sediments of a stream microcosm accumulated substrate-desorbed residues directly from water. Bioaccumulation was greatest in amphipods exposed to sediments with the least organic content and the largest particle sizes. Suspended particulates and adsorbents such as humic acids should have a similar effect of reducing uptake of lipophilic chemicals in the environment by reducing C_w. For example, the presence of humic acids reduces the rate of uptake of benzo[a]pyrene from water by sunfish but does not

affect the uptake of anthracene, which is less lipophilic (Spacie et al., 1983). Lower total DDT residues were measured in fish taken from hypereutrophic lakes than from the same species taken from nearby oligotrophic lakes (Vanderford and Hamelink, 1977). Differences in plankton standing crop and organic content of the water and sediments may explain this result.

The importance of complexation in reducing the uptake and toxicity of trace metal ions is well documented (Sprague, 1968; Sunda et al., 1979; Zitko et al., 1973; Pagenkopf et al., 1974). Greater accumulation of metals usually occurs in soft water and at lower pH values, as reported for cadmium (Kinkade and Erdman, 1975), lead (Merlini and Pozzi, 1977), and mercury (Tsai et al., 1975). Part and Svanberg (1981) found that an organic complexing agent EDNTA (Na_2-(ethylenedinitrilo)tetraacetate) reduced the rate of cadmium diffusion through perfused trout gills. While it is generally correct to assume that the free metal ion is the available form, some metal-ligand complexes may be sufficiently lipophilic to accumulate as well. For example, uptake of cadmium by *Daphnia* was increased by the formation of a nonpolar complex with diethyldithiocarbamate (Poldoski, 1979).

Uptake from Food

Chemicals that are taken in at the gill or outer membranes should also be readily absorbed in the gastrointestinal tract. The same models of uptake by diffusion and special transport function in the gut. In addition, certain macromolecules such as carrageenans (MW ~ 40,000) and polystyrene particles (2200 Å) can apparently be absorbed in the intestine by a process similar to pinocytosis (Guthrie, 1980). Lipophilic organics in food are expected to transfer efficiently because of the relatively long time of contact between food and membranes. However, efficiency of assimilation from food has been measured for very few xenobiotics in aquatic species.

Weak organic acids and bases are absorbed mainly in the un-ionized form, according to the pH of the gut environment. The acidic conditions of the stomach favor diffusion of weak acids that are protonated at pH 1–3. The intestinal pH is higher, although variable, and tends to favor absorption of neutral or weakly basic chemicals.

Absorption of metals from food is highly variable because of the variety of free and bound forms of the ions that are possible in food. Competition between related elements for active transport sites is a further variable. The type of food and method of its contamination can have a very large effect on the amount of uptake measured experimentally. Plaice, *Pleuronectes platessa,* fed zinc in gelatin or starch pellets absorbed greater amounts of zinc than those fed zinc-contaminated *Nereis* worms (Pentreath, 1973). Sunfish, *Lepomis gibbosus,* also accumulated more zinc from an artificial diet than from a natural diet of snails contaminated with the same levels (Merlini et al., 1976). Apparently, the organically bound fraction of metal in the food is relatively unavailable for uptake in the gut.

THE PROCESS OF ELIMINATION

Both the toxicity and the bioaccumulation potential of a foreign compound are greatly affected by the rate of elimination from the organism. If an unaltered chemical can be eliminated rapidly, residues will not accumulate and tissue damage is less likely. In vertebrates, elimination can proceed by several routes, including transport across the integument or respiratory surfaces, secretion in gallbladder bile, and excretion from the kidney in urine. Biotransformation to more polar metabolites is also an important means of eliminating foreign chemicals (see Chapter 18). The metabolites may have rates and routes of elimination different from those of the parent material. Two other elimination processes are important in certain situations. Arthropods may lose residues in exuviae through the process of molting (Renfro et al., 1975; van Weers, 1975). Furthermore, fish and invertebrates eliminate lipid-soluble chemicals through egg deposition (Derr and Zabik, 1974; Guiney et al., 1979). Surprisingly few attempts

have been made to distinguish between the various routes of elimination in aquatic organisms, perhaps because of experimental difficulties. At least a few chemicals are known to proceed by each of the principal routes in certain species. But considering the importance of elimination processes in both toxicity and bioaccumulation, it is clear that more work needs to be done in this area.

Gill

Passive elimination of lipid-soluble chemicals can occur across the skin and gills by the same partitioning process involved in uptake. The physical characteristics of the gill make it the principal organ for elimination of this type. Gill elimination appears to be most important for nonpolar compounds that are not biotransformed rapidly. Their rates of elimination are generally a function of the partition coefficient (Maren et al., 1968). In the case of weak electrolytes, gill elimination depends on the relative proportions of protonated and unprotonated forms, as well as the difference between blood and external pH (Lo and Hayton, 1981). The nonionized form of the weak base tricane methanesulfonate (MS-222) ($pK_a = 3.5$) diffuses rapidly across the gills of the dogfish shark (*Squalus acanthias*) (Maren et al., 1968), rainbow trout (*Salmo gairdneri*), and channel catfish (*Ictalurus punctatus*) (Hunn and Allen, 1974). Quinaldine ($pK_a = 5.4$) is another base that is eliminated at the gill (Hunn and Allen, 1974; Allen and Hunn, 1977). Studies of elimination of phenol, DDT, and di-2-ethylhexylphthalate (DEHP) from dogfish shark suggest significant elimination through gill or other body surfaces (Guarino and Arnold, 1979). Approximately half of the pentachlorophenol residue in goldfish (*Carassius auratus*) is eliminated through the gill, and the remainder is eliminated equally in bile and urine (Kobayashi, 1979). Both free and conjugated forms may be excreted.

Liver and Gallbladder

Polar chemicals and metabolites of nonpolar substances are usually excreted more effectively by the liver or the kidney. Metabolites formed in the vertebrate liver are transported to the gallbladder, where they are discharged with bile into the small intestine. Although some metabolites in bile are eventually eliminated with the feces, a significant portion may be reabsorbed in the intestine and returned to the blood. This short-circuiting of the biliary excretion process, termed enterohepatic cycling, complicates the study of elimination routes.

Statham et al. (1976) recommended analysis of fish bile as an aid to water quality monitoring because a wide variety of pollutants tend to accumulate in bile. Metals such as mercury, lead, and arsenic are actively transported to the gallbladder. Furthermore, the liver is capable of conjugating many organic chemicals that are bound to plasma proteins and are thus unavailable for excretion by other routes. These conjugates are secreted into the bile. Benzo[a]pyrene is a nonpolar organic that is effectively biotransformed and eliminated in bile. Chemicals of moderate to high molecular weight (>400) tend to be eliminated in bile, whereas those of lower weight are often excreted more readily in urine. Despite this general pattern, there are significant differences among species in their ability to biotransform and eliminate foreign chemicals. Aquatic invertebrates seem especially variable in transformation abilities, and the role of the hepatopancreas in elimination is still not clear.

Kidney

The kidney eliminates chemicals in the course of urine formation, either by glomerular filtration or by diffusion or secretory processes in the kidney tubules. Most xenobiotics (MW <60,000) dissolved in the blood are small enough to be removed by glomerular filtration. However, binding of chemicals to plasma proteins reduces elimination by this route, because plasma proteins are retained by the glomeruli. Thus the urinary excretion of many lipid-soluble organics and metals is impeded by their affinity for proteins. Furthermore, nonpolar chemicals in the glomerular filtrate may be reabsorbed by passive diffusion across tubular membranes. Weak organic acids and bases are excreted or reabsorbed, depending on urinary pH. Renal tubules are also capable of actively secreting certain organic acids and bases into the urine. Protein binding does not prevent this type of active transport. However, competition between similar chemicals for the same transport sites may affect the overall rate of elimination (Klaassen, 1980).

The importance of physical-chemical properties is shown by a study comparing the distribution and excretion of DDT and its polar metabolite DDA (Pritchard et al., 1977). After administration of equal doses to the winter flounder (*Pseudopleuronectes americanus*), DDA was excreted into the urine 250 times as quickly as DDT. The difference could not be explained by plasma binding, which was similar for both chemicals (97%). *In vitro* studies with isolated renal tubules showed that DDA was actively accumulated by the renal organic acid transport system. Some of the accumulation could be blocked by metabolic inhibitors. The more lipid-soluble DDT was not actively transported and was probably reabsorbed from tubular fluids.

It is important to distinguish between the primary routes of elimination in aquatic organisms because the routes can be affected differently by temperature, water chemistry, tissue damage, preexposure to toxicants, or the presence of competing chemicals. Such complications are common for exposed populations in the field. Changes in elimination pathways can affect the success of laboratory tests as well as the ability of models to predict the degree of bioaccumulation found in nature.

COMPARTMENT MODELS

A compartment model is a mathematical description of the quantity of a chemical within a uniform system, as determined by competing rates of chemical input and output. Compartment models are commonly used in pharmacokinetic studies and the properties of such models are discussed elsewhere (Levy and Gibaldi, 1975; Moriarty, 1975; Roland, 1977; Tuey, 1980).

This section outlines the compartment models

that are most frequently used in bioaccumulation studies. Throughout this discussion the reader should note the data requirements and assumptions incorporated in each model, since these will apply directly to the design of bioaccumulation experiments. Compartment models are not descriptions of biological processes, but rather descriptions of the data set collected by the experimenter. They can be used successfully as predictive tools provided they are used in situations that do not violate the original constraints on the data. Many environmental and physiological factors, including those discussed in the previous sections, can modify the results predicted by such models.

One-Compartment Bioconcentration Model

The simplest technique for modeling residue dynamics is to treat each organism as a single compartment (Fig. 2). Uptake of the chemical from water is the only input considered, and it is assumed to be directly proportional to the exposure concentration (C_w). All residues in the organisms are assumed to belong to a common pool, where they are equally available for depuration. The rate of depuration, regardless of mechanism, is assumed to be first-order, that is, directly proportional to the concentration in the organism (C). The volume of the compartment must be constant (no growth). In this case the rate of change in residues over time is given by

$$\frac{dC}{dt} = \text{uptake} - \text{loss} = k_u C_w - k_d C \qquad (10)$$

where C_w = concentration of chemical in water (μg/ml)

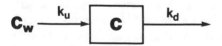

Figure 2 Representation of a one-compartment model for accumulation of a chemical concentration (C) in a whole organism exposed to a constant concentration in water (C_w).

C = concentration of chemical in animal (μg/g)
t = time (h)
k_u = uptake rate constant (ml/g·h or, assuming a tissue density of 1 g/ml, h^{-1}).
k_d = first-order rate constant for depuration (h^{-1}).

During initial uptake, when C is very small, the increase in residues over time should be linear and proportional to C_w. As C becomes larger, the uptake rate (dC/dt) declines and eventually reaches zero. Steady state occurs when the rate of uptake balances the rate of loss, so that

$$\frac{dC}{dt} = 0 = k_u C_w - k_d C_{ss}$$

Therefore, after a sufficient duration of exposure,

$$C_{ss} = \frac{k_u}{k_d} C_w \qquad (11)$$

where C_{ss} is the residue concentration in the body at steady state. The steady-state bioconcentration factor can then be conveniently defined as

$$\text{BCF} = \frac{C_{ss}}{C_w} = \frac{k_u}{k_d} \qquad (12)$$

To integrate Eq. (10), it is necessary to assume that the coefficients k_u and k_d as well as the concentration in water remain constant. The integrated form is

$$C = \frac{k_u}{k_d} C_w [1 - \exp(-k_d t)] \qquad (13)$$

where $\exp(-k_d t)$ represents the base of natural logarithms (e) raised to the power $-k_d t$. Equivalent forms combining Eqs. (12) and (13) are

$$C = C_{ss} [1 - \exp(-k_d t)] \qquad (14)$$

$$C = \text{BCF} \, C_w [1 - \exp(k_d t)] \qquad (15)$$

Equations (13)-(15) describe a curvilinear increase in C, with an asymptotic approach to a "plateau" at later times (Fig. 3).

The time required to approach steady state is determined solely by the depuration rate constant (k_d). For example, 90% of steady state will be reached when $C = 0.9 C_{ss}$. Substituting this into Eq. (14), the time required may be found from

$$t_{90} = -\frac{\ln 0.1}{k_d} = \frac{2.303}{k_d} \tag{16}$$

Figure 3 illustrates the relationship between k_d, the shape of the uptake curve, and the time to steady state. A useful graph for estimating time to steady state is given in Fig. 4. If an apparent steady state is reached during a continuous exposure experiment, the value of k_d may be estimated by finding the time (t_{50}) required to reach 50% of C_{ss}:

$$k_d = -\frac{\ln 0.5}{t_{50}} = \frac{0.693}{t_{50}}$$

provided there are sufficient observations during uptake to fit a smooth curve with confidence. Unfortunately, uptake curves resembling Fig. 3 may be produced by mechanisms other than simple exchange processes, and such cases do not fit the one-compartment model.

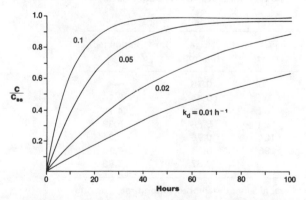

Figure 3 Influence of k_d on time required to approach a steady-state concentration of chemical (C_{ss}) in a one-compartment model.

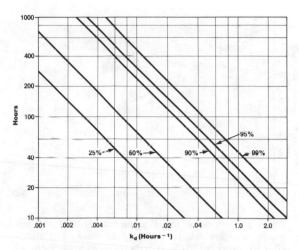

Figure 4 Relationship between depuration rate constant (k_d) and time required to reach a given percentage of steady state within an organism.

Graphical Method

For this reason it is usually better to verify k_d directly by transferring exposed animals to uncontaminated water. The organisms do not need to be at steady state when this depuration phase is initiated. A plot of the decline in C, on a logarithmic scale, against depuration time can be used to calculate k_d from the slope of the straight line:

$$\ln C = \ln C_0 - k_d t \tag{17}$$

where C_0 is the residue concentration at the start of the depuration phase (Fig. 5). If logarithms to the base 10 are plotted instead of natural logarithms, the slope must be multiplied by 2.303 to determine k_d. A depuration half-life ($t_{1/2}$) can be found from

$$t_{1/2} = \frac{\ln 0.5}{k_d} = \frac{0.693}{k_d} \tag{18}$$

This direct method has several advantages. First, a line can be fitted to the data points by using a simple linear least-squares regression that provides confidence limits for the slope. Second, if the depuration phase does not fit a straight line with a

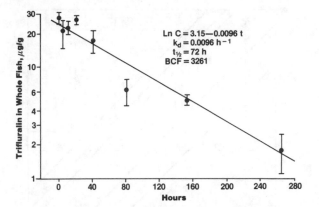

Figure 5 Depuration of trifluralin from fathead minnows (*Pimephales promelas*) transferred to clean water after a 40-h exposure to 20 µg/l trifluralin. Bars represent ±1 standard error. *[From Spacie (1975).]*

measurable slope, the simple one-compartment model is in question and other models should be sought (see the following section).

Once k_d is determined, the uptake coefficient k_u can be calculated manually by measuring the tangent to the uptake curve ($\Delta C/\Delta t$) at several points (Blanchard et al., 1977). Each tangent is an approximation of dC/dt that can be used to calculate a value of k_u from Eq. (10), as shown in Table 2. The k_u estimates for each sample time are

then averaged. Small variations in C_w during the experiment can be accommodated by this method of calculating k_u.

Nonlinear Method

It is also possible to find both k_u and k_d directly from the uptake phase of the test without using a separate depuration experiment. In this approach the quantity C/C_w is followed over time:

$$\frac{C}{C_w} = \text{BCF}\,[1 - \exp(-k_d t)] \qquad (19)$$

The two parameters k_d and BCF must be evaluated by a nonlinear least-squares regression procedure such as those available in the Biomedical Computer Programs (Dixon and Brown, 1979), SPSS (Nie et al., 1975), or similar programs written specifically for kinetic models (Metzler et al., 1974; Blau and Agin, 1978). Such iterative programs require the input of reasonably good initial estimates for k_d and BCF (or k_u). An initial estimate of k_d can be obtained graphically from the depuration curve. Alternatively, it can be calculated by choosing two separate data points C_1,t_1 and C_2,t_2 on the uptake curve. The parameter k_d that appears in

Table 2 Sample Calculation of k_u Based on Hypothetical Data for Uptake Phase of an Experiment[a]

Exposure time (h)	Tangent ($\Delta C/\Delta t$)	k_d (h⁻¹)	C (mg/g)	C_w (mg/ml)	Estimated k_u[b]
0	—	—	0	0.76	—
12	2.8	0.015	52	0.44	8.14
24	2.0	0.015	82	0.78	4.14
48	1.7	0.015	124	0.66	5.39
72	1.6	0.015	164	0.76	5.34
96	1.0	0.015	195	0.64	6.13
Means				0.67	5.83

[a]The tangent to the uptake curve was determined graphically at each observation time. The rate constant k_d was found previously from the depuration phase.
[b]Estimated $k_u = (\Delta C/\Delta t + k_d C)/C_w$; BCF $= k_u/k_d = 5.83/0.015 = 388$; $C_{ss} = \text{BCF} \times C_w = 260$ µg/g. Time to 90% of steady state $= 2.303/k_d = 154$ h.

$$\frac{C_1}{C_2} = \frac{1 - \exp(-k_d t_1)}{1 - \exp(-k_d t_2)} \qquad (20)$$

can be determined numerically by trial and error on a hand calculator. A rough estimate for k_d is substituted into the right-hand side of Eq. (20) and the expression calculated. The process is repeated with better estimates of k_d until the expression approaches C_1/C_2. For example, a k_d estimate of 0.0175 h^{-1} was obtained with the 24- and 96-h data in Table 2. Once k_d is determined, an initial estimate for k_u or BCF can be made by using the method of Table 2.

One drawback of nonlinear estimation procedures is that they do not provide a unique solution of the equation representing the model. There is always a chance that the iterative program will converge on an unrealistic answer, particularly if the initial parameter estimates are poor. Thus the researcher should check that the original model is justified and that the numerical results make sense biologically.

Growth

Chemicals such as DDT and PCB with large partition coefficients approach steady state slowly. Results of long-term bioconcentration tests designed for these materials must be corrected for the growth of the test animals, since growth has the effect of diluting the accumulated residues. Growth can be incorporated as a loss term in the simple model:

$$\frac{dC}{dt} = k_u C_w - k_d C - gC \qquad (21)$$

In this relationship, growth (dW/dt) is assumed to be an exponential function:

$$\frac{dW}{dt} = W_0 \exp(gt) \qquad (22)$$

where W_0 is the weight at the start of the growth period or test and g (d^{-1}) is the growth rate constant (other growth functions could be substituted for the exponential one). For convenience, the two loss coefficients in Eq. (21) may be combined as

$$k' = k_d + g \qquad (23)$$

so that the simple compartment model with growth can be integrated to yield

$$C = \frac{k_u}{k'} C_w [1 - \exp(-k't)] \qquad (24)$$

Since growth contributes to the overall decline of residue concentration, rapid growth of test organisms may cause a reduction in the time required to approach an apparent steady state and also reduce the depuration half-life.

Examples of the application of one-compartment models to the study of bioconcentration are given by Harding and Vass (1979); Kimerle et al. (1981); McLeese et al. (1979); Spacie and Hamelink (1979); and Wong et al. (1981).

Two-Compartment Bioconcentration Model

Tissue residues do not always behave as if they belong to a common pool. Often a portion of the chemical is eliminated rapidly while the remainder takes considerably longer to depart. Metals may bind strongly to proteins or other cell components (Miettinen, 1974); organics in poorly perfused adipose tissue may require longer to be eliminated than those circulating in the blood. Biphasic or biexponential kinetics are recognized by a noticeable change in slope of the depuration curve, representing loss from "fast" and "slow" compartments (Fig. 6). The transport process can be visualized as a two-compartment design such as Fig. 7, where uptake and elimination by the body occur only through the fast or central compartment. Residues in the slower peripheral compartment accumulate as a function of the concentration in compartment 1. It is important to realize that a compartment does not necessarily represent an anatomic unit

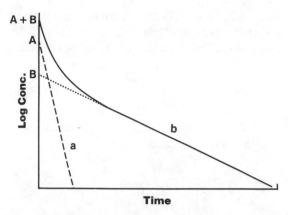

Figure 6 Illustration of a depuration curve showing bi-phasic kinetics. The slopes of the "fast" and "slow" phases are a and b, respectively.

(although it is convenient to think in terms of blood, fat, etc.). It represents a quantity of chemical with identifiable kinetics.

The total residue concentration in the animal at any time during depuration (Fig. 6) is described by Eq. (25):

$$C = A \exp(-at) + B \exp(-bt) \qquad (25)$$

where A and B are the intercepts of the lines with slopes a and b, respectively, plotted logarithmically. The quantity $A + B$ is equivalent to C_0, the initial body concentration of chemical at the start

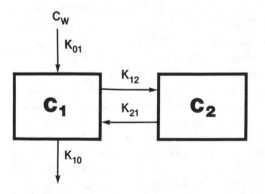

Figure 7 Representation of a two-compartment model for accumulation of residues in an organism exposed to a chemical in water. It is assumed that uptake from water and elimination can occur only through compartment 1.

of depuration. The two lines can be resolved from the experimental points by first using a linear regression on the later portion of the slow phase. Once B and b are found, the remaining line can be found by subtracting the calculated values of C at each observation time from the experimental points during the early period. A plot of the differences will yield a straight line with slope a and intercept A. The graphically determined values are related to the rate constants for the model shown in Fig. 6 according to the following equations:

$$k_{21} = \frac{Ab + Ba}{A + B} \qquad (26)$$

$$k_{10} = \frac{ab}{k_{21}} \qquad (27)$$

$$k_{12} = a + B - k_{21} - k_{10} \qquad (28)$$

The uptake rate constant k_{01} must be measured independently by using the initial portion of the uptake curve. If it is known, the BCF can be calculated as

$$\text{BCF} = \frac{k_{01}}{ab} (a + b - k_{10}) \qquad (29)$$

or

$$\text{BCF} = \frac{k_{01}}{ab} (k_{12} + k_{21}) \qquad (30)$$

In the special case where the peripheral compartment clears rapidly ($k_{21} \gg k_{12}$), the model reduces to a one-compartment type.

One practical drawback of the two-compartment model is the requirement for many data points during the later phases of depuration. The added time and expense of providing these later samples, though, are often justified by the added realism of the model. The work of Könemann and van Leeuwen (1980) on the bioconcentration of chlorobenzenes is a good illustration of the use of the two-compartment model. Nagel and Urich

(1980) describe the use of a slightly different type of two-compartment analysis to study the accumulation of substituted phenols in goldfish.

Verifying Kinetics

The compartment models presented in this section assume constant rate coefficients (k_u and k_d) over the range of experimental conditions. This assumption should be tested by measuring k_u and k_d at several exposure levels and, perhaps, temperatures. One method of verifying a constant rate of uptake is to rearrange Eq. (13) as

$$C = k_u C_w \left[\frac{1 - \exp(-k_d t)}{k_d} \right] \tag{31}$$

A plot of the function in brackets against C during the experiment should yield a linear relationship if k_u and C_w are both constant. An example of this approach for the uptake of methyl mercury at several temperatures is shown in Fig. 8.

First-order elimination kinetics should be verified by plotting the logarithm of C/C_0, the fraction of the initial tissue concentration for the depuration phase, against time at several levels of exposure. The depuration lines for the various exposure concentrations should all coincide and

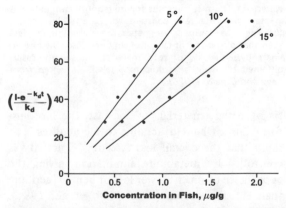

Figure 8 Demonstration of zero-order kinetics during the uptake of methyl mercuric chloride in whole rainbow trout (*Salmo gairdneri*) at three temperatures. The estimated k_d is 0.00099 h⁻¹. *[From Hartung (1976), using data of Reinert et al. (1974).]*

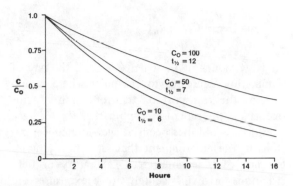

Figure 9 Hypothetical depuration of residues at several initial residue concentrations in the organism (C_0). The long half-life at the highest initial concentration suggests Michaelis-Menten or saturation kinetics during elimination.

should have the same slope and half-life if depuration is first-order.

Elimination often involves special transport or a series of enzyme-mediated biotransformation steps. Unlike simple diffusion, these processes can become saturated at high residue concentrations. As a result, elimination at high doses may be slower than elimination at lower doses (Fig. 9). In such cases the depuration half-life appears to increase at the upper concentrations. For example, Mayer (1976) found somewhat slower elimination of DEHP from fathead minnows at the highest exposure concentration tested.

Under such circumstances, elimination can often be described by Michaelis-Menten kinetics:

$$-\frac{dC}{dt} = \frac{V_m C}{K_m + C} \tag{32}$$

where V_m = maximum or "saturated" rate of elimination

K_m = concentration of contaminant that can be eliminated at half the maximum rate

First-order elimination can be viewed as a special case of Eq. (32) for which $C \ll K_m$, so that elimination is directly proportional to C:

$$\frac{dC}{dt} = -\frac{V_m}{K_m}C = -k_u C \qquad (33)$$

At large values of C, when $C \gg K_m$, the rate of elimination decreases to the point where saturation of the transport or transformation systems occurs and the rate of loss approaches V_m (Fig. 9).

Most xenobiotics occur at such low concentrations in the environment that saturation kinetics are not often encountered. Laboratory or field situations involving acutely toxic exposures are more likely to require a Michaelis-Menten type of model.

Rates of Metabolite Elimination

Bioaccumulation tests are commonly performed with chemicals labeled with radioactive carbon (^{14}C) or another radioisotope (e.g., ^{3}H, ^{36}Cl, ^{35}S) because it is easy to analyze for these atoms. If the labeled material is biotransformed to a labeled metabolite during the experiment, results based on total isotope activity may lead to an incorrect estimate of k_d for the parent compound. Metabolites carrying the ^{14}C label may be eliminated at rates (k_m) that are greater or less than that of the parent (k_d). Figure 10 shows elimination patterns for two extreme cases. When $k_m \gg k_d$, the overall elimination process will be controlled by loss of parent material. Only a small proportion of the ^{14}C body burden will consist of metabolite and the slope of the depuration line will yield an appropriate value of k_d (Fig. 10a). However, if $k_m \ll k_d$, metabolite residues will persist longer than parent residues and a plot of total ^{14}C activity will produce a slope that underestimates k_d for the parent material (Fig. 10b). The latter case can be resolved only by direct analysis of either the parent compound or total activity plus metabolite.

The elimination of the phthalate DEHP and the hydrocarbon benz[a]acridine from fathead minnow (*Pimephales promelas*) illustrates the two situations. Mayer (1976) found that the half-life for DEHP elimination was approximately the same whether it was based on total ^{14}C activity or analy-

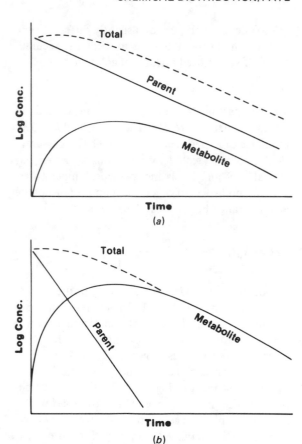

Figure 10 Elimination of a parent chemical and its metabolite from an organism following transfer to clean water. (a) The rate constant for metabolite elimination is greater than the rate constant for parent elimination. (b) The rate constant for metabolite elimination is less than that of the parent chemical. In both cases the dashed line shows quantity of total material, such as the result obtained by using a radioisotope label. [Adapted from Levy and Gibaldi (1975).]

sis of parent material. In contrast, the biotransformation of benz[a]acridine to metabolites is so rapid that the overall loss rate of ^{14}C activity is controlled by metabolite elimination, giving the appearance of much slower loss of benz[a]acridine than actually occurs (Southworth et al., 1981). Chemicals such as benz[a]acridine can give variable results in bioconcentration tests, depending on the rate of biotransformation in the test organisms.

Bioaccumulation Model

A term for the assimilation of contaminant from food can be incorporated into the simple one-compartment model with growth [Eqs. (21)–(23)] according to the analysis of Thomann (1981):

$$\frac{dC}{dt} = k_u C_w + \alpha R C_f - k'C \qquad (34)$$

where α = assimilation efficiency of contaminant from food (micrograms absorbed divided by micrograms ingested)

R = weight-specific ration for feeding rate (grams ingested per gram of body weight per day)

C_f = concentration of contaminant in food ($\mu g/g$)

A similar expression can be written for the rate of accumulation of the total body burden:

$$\frac{dX}{dt} = k_u C_w W + \alpha R C_f W - k_d X \qquad (35)$$

where X is the total weight of residue (μg) in the body and W is body weight. The integrated forms of the two expressions are

$$C = \frac{k_u C_w + \alpha R C_f}{k'} [1 - \exp(-k't)]$$
$$+ C_0 \exp(-k't) \qquad (36)$$

$$X = \frac{(k_u C_w + \alpha R C_f)W_0}{k'} [\exp(gt) - \exp(-k_d t)]$$
$$+ X_0 \exp(-k_d t) \qquad (37)$$

where X_0, W_0, and C_0 represent the total residue, body weight, and residue concentration, respectively, at the beginning of the experiment or observation period.

Equations (36) and (37) are helpful for evaluating the relative contributions of food, water, and growth to the overall bioaccumulation of a chemi-cal. At long exposure times, as $t \to \infty$, the term $\exp(-k_d t)$ of Eq. (37) approaches zero. Thus the total body burden (X) can continue to increase as long as growth [$\exp(gt)$] continues. A steady state of X cannot be reached unless growth is zero. Even with growth, however, the residue concentration (C) can reach a steady state as $t \to \infty$:

$$C_{ss} = \frac{k_u C_w + \alpha R C_f}{k'} \qquad (38)$$

Referring to the bioconcentration factor defined in Eq. (12),

$$\text{BCF} = N_w = \frac{k_u}{k'} \qquad (39)$$

where N_w represents the bioconcentration factor for uptake from water only. An analogous bioaccumulation factor (N) for total uptake from food and water can be derived from Eqs. (38) and (39):

$$N = \frac{C_{ss}}{C_w} = \frac{k_u}{k'} + \frac{\alpha R}{k'}\frac{C_f}{C_w} \qquad (40)$$

or

$$N = N_w + \frac{\alpha R}{k'}\frac{C_f}{C_w} \qquad (41)$$

Equation (41) shows that bioaccumulation will exceed bioconcentration (according to this model) whenever the food term ($\alpha R C_f$) is nonzero. In practice, though, the contribution from food will be insignificant if the loss term (k') is large—that is, whenever the chemical has a short half-life of depuration. For substances with long half-lives, k' will be very small, causing the expression for food intake ($\alpha R/k'$) to increase in importance.

This model assumes that the food and water sources of a chemical are additive. Macek et al. (1979) concluded, on the basis of experimental evidence, that additivity is a good assumption for most residues. Nevertheless, there may be special situations where chemicals from the two sources compete or interfere with each other's uptake.

The model also assumes that elimination rates of food- and water-derived residues are first-order and identical. Experiments on the bioaccumulation of metals (Giesy et al., 1980; Vighi, 1981) suggest that metals derived from food may be eliminated more slowly than those derived from water.

In actual field situations, the uptake, assimilation, and elimination rates are also affected by the metabolic rate of the animal, which may vary (Roberts et al., 1979). Thus, water temperature influences respiration and caloric intake, which in turn control contaminant uptake, growth, and lipid content of trout (Spigarelli et al., 1983). Elimination rates may also slow as an animal grows and accumulates fat, so that it may be necessary to normalize chemical concentrations and rate constants according to size or lipid content (Bruggeman et al., 1981).

Food Chain Transfer

The bioaccumulation model can be expanded to represent the transfer of a chemical through an aquatic food chain with trophic levels such as (1) phytoplankton, (2) zooplankton, (3) small fish, and (4) large fish. The concentration of chemical at each trophic level (i) is determined by the bioconcentration factor for that level (N_{iw}) plus the chemical contributed by feeding on the next lower level $(i-1)$. In general,

$$C_i = \frac{k_{ui}}{k_i'} C_w + \frac{\alpha_{i,i-1} R_{i,i-1}}{k_i'} C_{i-1} \tag{42}$$

The bioaccumulation factor for level i can also be derived:

$$N_i = \frac{C_i}{C_w} = N_{iw} + \frac{\alpha_{i,i-1} R_{i,i-1}}{k_i'} \frac{C_{i-1}}{C_w}$$

or

$$N_i = N_{iw} + \frac{\alpha_{i,i-1} R_{i,i-1}}{k_i'} N_{i-1,w} \tag{43}$$

where $N_{i-1,w}$ = bioconcentration factor for trophic level $i-1$

N_{iw} = bioconcentration factor for trophic level i

The notation can be simplified by substituting

$$f_i = \frac{\alpha_{i,i-1} R_{i,i-1}}{k_i'} \tag{44}$$

into Eq. (43) to give the general expression

$$N_i = N_{iw} + f_i N_{i-1} \tag{45}$$

Expressions for the overall accumulation at each trophic level, derived by Thomann (1981), show the cumulative effect of food sources to successive trophic levels:

Level 1: $N_{1w} = \dfrac{k_{u1}}{k_1'}$ (no feeding)   (46)

Level 2: $N_2 = N_{2w} + f_2 N_{1w}$ (47)

Level 3: $N_3 = N_{3w} + f_3 N_{2w} + f_3 f_2 N_{1w}$ (48)

Level 4: $N_4 = N_{4w} + f_4 N_{3w} + f_4 f_3 N_{2w}$

$$+ f_4 f_3 f_2 N_{1w} \tag{49}$$

Thus the bioaccumulation at any trophic level can be calculated from a knowledge of the bioconcentration factors (N_{iw}) at each level and the food chain transfer numbers (f_i) for the consumers. Values of f_i greater than 1.0 increase the food contribution at successive trophic levels, causing biomagnification. The longer the food chain, the greater the magnification can be. However, if $f_i < 1$, the contribution of phytoplankton residues to the upper trophic levels becomes insignificant.

A numerical example can be used to illustrate the biomagnification effect. Thomann (1981) employed rate constants from the literature to calculate PCB residues in a four-step food chain (Table 3). The rate constants k_u, k_d, and α were not measured directly. Nevertheless, the resulting bioaccumulation factors agreed within an order of magnitude with residues measured in the field. Trophic levels 2, 3, and 4 showed stepwise magnification of residue concentrations caused by the important contributions from food. In contrast, calculations for plutonium (^{239}Pu) showed that transfer through food did not contribute significantly to the bioaccumulation of plutonium in upper trophic levels.

One cautionary note should be mentioned in discussing food chain transfer. The model is highly sensitive to the relative values of α and k'. A small error in estimating either coefficient will affect the outcome significantly, especially at the higher trophic levels. Rates of depuration and assimilation from food have been measured for few organic pollutants in fewer species. The larger predaceous fish are especially inconvenient for laboratory testing. Thus calculations such as those in Table 3 should be viewed as a helpful guide in analyzing food chain transfer, not as proof of a particular mechanism.

Macek et al. (1979) reviewed data on bioaccumulation in simple experimental food chains and concluded that most chemicals are not biomagnified. Most organic compounds have depuration rate constants of 0.1 d^{-1} or more, with half-lives of hours or a few days (Zitko, 1979). Even assuming efficient assimilation from food (e.g., $\alpha = 0.8$ or 0.9), the rate of loss from the body will exceed the rate of intake from food, giving $f_i \ll 1$. Organochlorines such as DDT and PCB are unusual because of their large bioconcentration factors and half-lives of 1 wk or more in fish. Hence, slow-growing, long-lived species have the potential to accumulate such residues from their food at a rate exceeding that of depuration. Bruggeman et al. (1981) evaluated the relative importance of bioaccumulation from food and water, concluding that food chain biomagnification is likely only for organics with octanol-water partition coefficients of approximately 10^5 or greater.

PREDICTING BIOCONCENTRATION FACTORS

Correlations between the partition coefficients (P) of toxicants such as alcohol and ether and their

Table 3 Sample Calculation of Food Chain Transfer from Parameters for PCB Estimated by Thomann (1981)[a]

Parameter	Trophic level			
	1	2	3	4
k_d, 1/d	—	0.01	0.004	0.001
g, 1/d	—	0.0092	0.0048	0.0018
R, g/g·d	—	0.105	0.017	0.009
α	—	0.9	0.9	0.9
N_w	$10^{5.5}$	$10^{5.29}$	$10^{4.59}$	$10^{4.9}$
N	$10^{5.5}$	$10^{6.24}$	$10^{6.49}$	$10^{6.95}$
Magnification (N/N_w)	—	8.9X	79X	112X

[a]Sample calculation for level 3: $N_3 = N_{3w} + f_3 N_{2w} + f_3 f_2 N_{1w}$; $N_3 = 10^{4.59} + (1.74)10^{5.29} + (1.74)(4.92)10^{5.5}$; $N_3 = 10^{6.49}$; where $f_3 = \alpha_3 R_3/(k_d + g) = (0.9)(0.017)/(0.004 + 0.0048) = 1.74$.

effective concentrations in organisms have been recognized for many years. Partitioning is also the dominant process governing bioconcentration of trace organics in algae, fish and invertebrates (Hamelink et al., 1971; Neely et al., 1974; Pavlou and Dexter, 1977; Southworth et al., 1978; Voice et al., 1983). Veith et al. (1979a) reported a good correlation between the bioconcentration factor and the partition coefficient for a group of 84 organics in fish:

$$\log BCF = 0.76 \log P - 0.23 \quad r = 0.907 \quad (50)$$

This relationship is illustrated in Fig. 11. More recently, Mackay (1982) reexamined the available data on bioconcentraton and concluded that BCF is approximately 5% of the octanol-water partition coefficient. Such relationships are useful because the expected BCF of a new chemical can be estimated before laboratory tests are designed. Detailed methods for using partition coefficients to predict bioconcentration potentials are given by Bysshe (1982). The partition coefficients used in these estimates must be either measured directly (Chiou et al., 1977; Veith and Morris, 1978) or calculated from structural constants. In general, the calculated values are more reliable because of practical difficulties in measuring equilibrium concentrations of the chemical in the partitioning

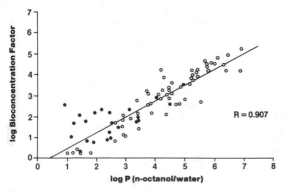

Figure 11 Correlation between bioconcentration factor and n-octanol-water partition coefficient (*P*) for a variety of organic chemicals in whole fish. *[From Veith et al. (1979a).]*

phases. Methods for calculating *P* values are described by Leo et al. (1971), Lyman (1982), and Rekker (1977). Compilations of *P* values are also available (Leo et al., 1971; Veith et al., 1979b; Kenaga and Goring, 1980).

Partition coefficients can be estimated indirectly from a knowledge of water solubility, since the two properties are directly related. Regression equations such as the one published by Chiou et al. (1977) can be used to calculate *P*:

$$\log P = 5.00 - 0.670 \log S \qquad (51)$$

where *S* is the water solubility (μmol/l). Solubilities of a number of organics are tabulated by Kenaga and Goring (1980), Kenaga (1980), Chiou et al. (1977), and Martin and Worthington (1977).

Equation (50) is most appropriate for relatively inert compounds that do not undergo rapid biotransformation in the body. Degradable chemicals usually have a lower BCF because elimination is enhanced. For example, Southworth et al. (1980) found a lower than predicted BCF for azaarenes in fish because of rapid biotransformation and elimination.

The rate constants k_u and k_d can also be predicted for certain organics. Neely (1979) analyzed uptake rates in fish as a function of log *P* and respiration rate. A direct correlation between k_u and log *P* for organochlorines and several other chemicals is also available (Fig. 12). Based on the relationship provided by these few substances, it appears that k_u is relatively constant over a wide range of partition coefficients. By comparison, the depuration rate constant (k_d) is highly dependent on log *P* (Fig. 13). A regression such as the one shown in Fig. 13 is especially useful for designing bioconcentration tests because the predicted k_d can be used to estimate the time required to approach steady state [Eq. (16)] and to reach the depuration half-life [Eq. (18)]. The length of the uptake and depuration phases of the test, sampling intervals, and number of organisms required can be judged from the predicted rate constants.

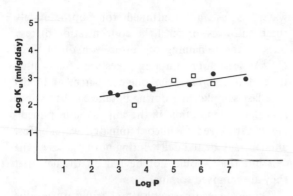

Figure 12 Correlation between uptake rate constant (k_u) and n-octanol-water partition coefficient (P) for several organic chemicals in fish. Data are for (●) rainbow trout (Neely et al., 1974) and (□) guppies (Könemann and van Leeuwen, 1980) converted to the basis of whole fish weight. *[From Spacie and Hamelink (1982).]*

TEST METHODS

Plateau Method for Bioconcentration

The most direct way to measure bioconcentration is to expose a group of test organisms to a constant concentration of a chemical in water until accumulation reaches an apparent steady state. The test usually consists of an uptake phase followed by a depuration phase. During uptake, randomized groups of test organisms are exposed to one or more chemical concentrations in a system

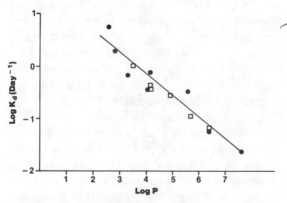

Figure 13 Correlation between depuration rate constant (k_d) and n-octanol-water partition coefficient (P) for several organic chemicals in fish. Symbols as in Fig. 12. *[From Spacie and Hamelink (1982).]*

with continuous or intermittent flow, as described for the acute toxicity tests (see Chapters 1 and 2). Basic procedures for handling and exposing the organisms are also similar to those used in toxicity tests (see Chapters 2, 3, and 4). The flow of water provided should be sufficient that the organisms do not significantly deplete either the test chemical or the oxygen in their surroundings. The test water should be analyzed before and during the uptake phase to verify the exposure concentration. A control group consisting of untreated animals should be maintained throughout the experiment to provide uncontaminated samples for analysis and to demonstrate the acceptability of the living conditions.

In situations where a flow-through aquarium system is impractical, a static exposure is sometimes adequate for measuring the accumulation of stable materials. Recommendations for conducting static bioconcentration tests with bivalves are discussed by Ernst (1977, 1979). Since the concentration of test chemical in a static system usually declines exponentially during the test, the actual analytical data for chemical concentrations over time must be fitted to an exponential equation. The bioconcentration results must then be interpreted according to the changing value of C_w. Static exposures are not recommended for long-term tests or for materials that degrade rapidly in water.

Choice of exposure levels in a bioconcentration test depends on several practical constraints. First, the chemical must be tested at a concentration high enough to permit residue analyses in both water and tissue. Nevertheless, the concentration should not be so high that it exceeds the solubility limit of the chemical in water. Concentrations that are toxic to the organisms during the test period should also be avoided, since organisms that are stressed or damaged by the material may exhibit unusual rates of accumulation. Finally, whenever possible, the test concentration should be reasonably close to those anticipated or observed in the environment, so that the bioconcentration results provide some degree of realism.

The bioconcentration test can best be designed if a preliminary estimate of k_d is available. If k_d is unknown, a pretest may be performed by exposing a small number of organisms to the chemical for several hours under static or flow-through conditions. All organisms are then transferred to uncontaminated water, where they are sampled periodically for analysis. A preliminary estimate of k_d may be found from Eq. (17).

The length of the uptake phase of the plateau test is determined by the time required to reach an apparent steady state. In practice, it is the time (t_{95}) to reach approximately 95% of C_{ss}, where $t_{95} = 3.0/k_d$. Organisms are usually sampled at least five times during the uptake phase, with the fifth sample near t_{95}. In addition, samples at two or more times after t_{95} should be taken to establish the plateau or steady-state concentration (Fig. 14). In general, if t_{95} is 12 d or less, the additional samples may be taken at 1-d intervals; if t_{95} is greater than 12 d, the interval can be two or more days. Steady state is demonstrated when replicate samples at three or more sampling intervals do not differ significantly, according to an analysis of variance test.

The depuration phase of the test, following transfer of exposed organisms to uncontaminated water, is usually continued for approximately three half-lives, or until the concentration of residues in the remaining organisms is about 10% of C_{ss}. At least four sampling times are usually used to establish k_d for the one-compartment model (the last sample time during uptake can be used as $t = 0$ for depuration if the animals are immediately transferred to uncontaminated water). Test animals may be fed daily during both phases of the test but they should not be fed on the day that they are removed for analysis.

Duplicate water samples and triplicate residue analyses of the organisms are typically taken at each sampling time. Each residue analysis can represent an individual, if the organisms are sufficiently large, or it can consist of a group of pooled organisms. The animals should be removed from the tanks, rinsed, killed, weighed, and preserved by an acceptable method. Residues are ordinarily reported on a whole-body, wet-weight basis. However, for special studies, residues in separate tissues (e.g., muscle, fat, blood, and fillet) or concentrations expressed on the basis of dry weight or lipid weight may be desirable. If other bases are used, a conversion factor for whole body, wet weight should be reported.

Results of the plateau test are easily calculated, since the BCF is the mean of the residue concentrations during steady state, C_{ss}, divided by the mean C_w for the uptake phase. The standard deviation should be calculated as well. The k_d for a one-compartment model is found from a regression of $\ln C$ versus time during depuration [Eq. (17)]. Multiple-compartment models may also be applied if the data warrant such treatment. An estimate of k_u can be calculated from BCF $\times k_d$.

The plateau test has the advantage of measuring a steady-state BCF directly. It requires no assumptions about the type of compartment model or rates of metabolism. On the other hand, it is an expensive test, lasting up to 1 mo or more for chemicals with high bioconcentration potentials. The information gained in a long exposure may not justify the time and expense. Long tests may also require a correction for growth of the organisms.

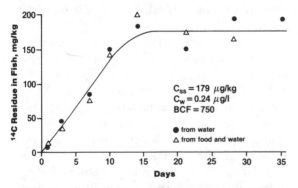

Figure 14 Accumulation of ^{14}C-labeled leptophos in bluegill sunfish (*Lepomis macrochirus*) during continuous exposure through water or food plus water. The steady-state residue concentration (C_{ss}) and bioconcentration factor are for the aqueous exposure. *[Drawn from data of Macek et al. (1979); copyright ASTM, Philadelphia, Pa. Adapted with permission.]*

Accelerated Bioconcentration Test

Branson et al. (1975) described a shorter method for measuring BCF based on the one-compartment model. The uptake phase is terminated after 4 d whether or not steady state has been reached. The depuration phase is performed as for the plateau test. After calculation of k_d, the value of k_u is calculated as illustrated in Table 2 or by a nonlinear least-squares regression. The projected BCF is k_u/k_d.

The accelerated method is more economical than the plateau test and is especially good for biologically stable materials with large BCF values. It can also be used as a range-finding test for more elaborate studies. Its limitations are those of the one-compartment model, which fails to account for "fast" and "slow" tissues, changes in biotransformation rate, irreversible binding, saturation kinetics, or other nonideal processes.

Uptake from Water and Sediment

Tests can be designed to measure the bioavailability of contaminants incorporated in sediments. It is often possible to use a simple static system containing sediments or soil equilibrated with water. Organisms are added in quantities that do not seriously deplete the total supply of test chemical or the available dissolved oxygen. The organisms can either be given direct access to the sediments or separated from the sediments by screening (Halter and Johnson, 1977).

Aquarium-scale tests typically employ about 1 kg soil for 10–15 kg water. In contrast, lakes usually have sediment-to-water proportions closer to 1:100 or 1:1000. For chemicals with a moderate to high bioconcentration potential (log P = 4–6), a 1:10 soil-water system in an aquarium leaves very little of the total chemical in solution (Table 4). The resulting low values of C_w may cause analytical problems and slow uptake by the test organisms. To avoid such problems, the equilibrium water concentration (C_w) may be estimated before designing the test, according to:

Table 4 Effect of Partition Coefficient and Soil: Water Ratio on the Proportion of Test Chemical Remaining in Water[a]

log P	K[b]	Percent of chemical in water for soil/water ratio		
		1:10	1:100	1:1000
1	4.2	70	95	99
2	14.6	40	86	98
4	179	5	36	84
6	2190	0.5	4	31

[a]Each system contains enough fish to accumulate 1% of total chemical added.
[b]Calculated from Eq. (8) with 5% organic matter.

$$C_w = \frac{X_T}{G_w + G_s K} \tag{52}$$

where X_T = total grams of chemical added to the system

G_w = weight of water (g)

G_s = weight of sediment or soil (g)

K = distribution coefficient for that soil, calculated from log P or water solubility [Eqs. (7) and (8)]

The desirable biomass loading in a static uptake experiment is also influenced by log P and the soil-water ratio (Table 5). If the values of log P and ex-

Table 5 Effect of Partition Coefficient and Soil: Water Ratio on Biomass of Fish Used in Model Ecosystems[a]

log P	BCF[b]	Grams of fish per kilogram of water for soil:water ratio		
		1:10	1:100	1:1000
1	3.4	4.1	3.06	2.95
2	19.5	1.3	0.59	0.52
4	646	0.3	0.04	0.018
6	21,380	0.1	0.01	0.0015

[a]The fish accumulate 1% of the total chemical added to each test, as for Table 4.
[b]Calculated from Eq. (50).

pected BCF are high, fewer animals can be added to the system without seriously depleting the dissolved chemical. For example, Table 5 shows the weight of fish (G_f) that will accumulate 1% of the total chemical in a static system, according to:

$$G_f = \frac{0.01}{\text{BCF}} (G_w + G_s K) \qquad (53)$$

At a log P of 6 (similar to that of DDT) and a soil-water ratio of 1:10, a loading of only 0.1 g of organisms per kilogram of water will accumulate approximately twice as much chemical as the amount dissolved in water. This limitation presents a serious problem in the physical design of tests to show accumulation rates over time. Isensee and Jones (1975) found a wide range of "bioaccumulation factors," depending on the soil-water ratio of static tests.

Soil-water tests can be done in flow-through systems to maintain concentrations of unstable materials or to simulate conditions in rivers or estuaries. Unless the influent test water contains a level of contaminant equal to C_w at equilibrium with the sediments, the system may continually release contaminant from the sediment. Thus the concentration in both water and sediment may change over time, making it difficult to calculate the rate constants for bioconcentration.

Aquarium-scale microcosms containing soil, water, plants, and animals of several trophic levels have been widely used to screen environmental chemicals (Metcalf et al., 1971; Isensee and Jones, 1975; Metcalf, 1977a,b). Generally they are not recommended for measuring bioaccumulation potential in aquatic animals because of their very high ratios of soil to water and of biomass to water. Larger organisms such as fish often do not reach a steady-state body burden because they are exposed to a continually changing C_w following the single or multiple applications of chemical. Such aquarium-scale microcosms are not steady-state and are difficult to replicate, it is usually more informative to use a simpler, larger system where the soil-water and biomass-water ratios can

be controlled and rate constants for uptake and depuration can be measured (Ribeyre et al., 1979).

Large-scale microcosms or field enclosures designed to simulate specific portions of lake, stream, or oceanic habitats have more representative proportions of water, sediment, and biomass. Some are able to reproduce physical characteristics (such as thermal stratification, light extinction, and eddy diffusion) that are impossible to mimic in aquaria (see, for example, Hamelink and Waybrant, 1976). Large systems may be used to measure the bioconcentration and fate of a chemical, provided precautions are taken to prevent release of hazardous materials into the surrounding environment. Advantages and disadvantages of working with microcosms for chemical testing have been reviewed by Giesy (1980) and others (National Research Council, 1981). While large-scale microcosms offer a high degree of realism for chemical fate testing and for measuring responses of aquatic communities. they are often too cumbersome and costly to be used simply for bioconcentration testing.

Regardless of the physical design of the system, soil-water bioaccumulation tests should be based on a careful analysis of the dissolved contaminant concentration. The analyst must distinguish between dissolved material and material that is bound to sediments and suspended particulates. The substrate should also be characterized according to percent organic matter and particle size.

Bioaccumulation Tests

Bioaccumulation or food chain transfer tests should be undertaken only for chemicals showing a high degree of bioconcentration or for especially hazardous and persistent environmental contaminants. The relative contributions of food and water to overall bioaccumulation for a particular species can be measured by a plateau test with three groups of test organisms. Two of the groups, fed uncontaminated food, serve as the control group and the treatment group for aqueous exposure. The third group is exposed to both contaminated water and food. The water concentration (C_w) should be the same for both treated groups. The food usually consists of living organisms such as algae or microcrustaceans that have been exposed to the same C_w and are at steady state. They may be exposed in an individual chamber of the same flow-through system or, if they equilibrate rapidly, they may be exposed separately in a static system. The contaminated food can be fed alive or frozen. However, the feeding rates and type of food should be identical for all three treatment groups. The food organisms should be characterized in terms of percentages of lipid and protein. The terms R and C_f in Eq. (41) are measured directly, while the term α is found by comparing the steady-state body burdens in the "water-only" and "food-plus-water" treatments [Eq. (38)].

It is important to perform the depuration phases for both the water-only and food-plus-water groups, because the depuration rate constants may not be the same for both sources. For example, Vighi (1981) found an overall half-life of 27 d for lead in *Poecilia* fish. The lead acquired from water was eliminated with a half-life of only 9 d, while the food-derived lead required 40 d.

Experimental designs for feeding studies have been described by Johnson (1975), Petrocelli (1975), Bryan (1976), Jarvinen et al. (1977), Jarvinen and Tyo (1978), Canton et al., (1978), Macek et al. (1979), Giesy et al. (1980), and Skaar et al. (1981).

Food Chain Transfer

The bioaccumulation test may be expanded to a simple three-step food chain by using the same three treatment groups for the highest trophic level. The organisms are typically exposed in a flow-through system of tanks connected in series, with the lowest trophic level receiving the test water first. A good example of such a design is given by Vighi (1981). Other designs are described by Canton et al. (1975), Reinert (1972), Chadwick and Brocksen (1969), Ribeyre et al. (1979), and Klumpp (1980).

Feeding rates (R_i) and contaminant concentra-

tions (C_{i-1}) at each level must be monitored throughout the test. Since the top-level organisms usually require the longest time to reach steady state, it may be a good idea to equilibrate the first two levels with the chemical first. The third-level organisms can then be brought to steady state more rapidly, saving time and the number of samples used for analysis.

If the parameters R, k_d, g, C_{i-1}, and α_i have been determined over the course of the experiment at each level, the food chain transfer numbers (f_i) can be determined for each trophic level [Eq. (44)].

CONCLUSIONS

A small number of the trace contaminants in aquatic ecosystems pose an environmental hazard because of their great toxicity or persistence. Nevertheless, it is now possible to measure bioaccumulation potential and, in many cases, to predict potential residue problems before they develop. New organic chemicals can be evaluated according to their partition coefficients and rates of biodegradation. Those with moderate to high partition coefficients can be tested for bioconcentration and, if necessary, bioaccumulation potential. Depuration rate constants can also be used to predict loss of residues from contaminated organisms following pollution abatement.

The type of kinetic model and testing scheme chosen for measuring bioaccumulation depends largely on the level of detail required. One-compartment models, log P correlations, and short-term tests are adequate for prescreening the great majority of chemicals. Those that "look suspicious" in preliminary tests can be scrutinized more carefully in bioaccumulation or food chain transfer tests. The internal dynamics of residues within the body can also be studied for especially hazardous materials. Whatever the level of detail, the primary goal in designing a bioaccumulation test should be to produce data that can be interpreted and evaluated in terms of a clearly defined conceptual model.

LITERATURE CITED

Allen JL, Hunn JB: Renal excretion in channel catfish following injection of quinaldine sulphate or 3-trifluoromethyl-4-nitrophenol. J Fish Biol 10:473–479, 1977.

Anderson PD, Spear PA: Copper pharmacokinetics in fish gills. I. Kinetics in pumpkinseed sunfish, *Lepomis gibbosus,* of different body sizes. Water Res 14:1101–1105, 1980.

Baughman GL, Lassiter RR: Prediction of environmental pollutant concentration. In: Estimating the Hazard of Chemical Substances to Aquatic Life, edited by J Cairns, Jr, KL Dickson, AW Maki, ASTM STP 657, pp. 35–54. Philadelphia, Pa.: ASTM, 1978.

Blanchard FA, Takahashi IT, Alexander HC, Bartlett EA: Uptake, clearance, and bioconcentration of ^{14}C-*sec*-butyl-4-chlorodiphenyl oxide in rainbow trout. In: Aquatic Toxicology and Hazard Evaluation, edited by FL Mayer, JL Hamelink, pp. 162–177. ASTM STP 634. Philadelphia, Pa.: ASTM, 1977.

Blau GE, Agin GL: A User's Manual for BIOFAC: A Computer Program for Characterizing the Rates of Uptake and Clearance of Chemicals in Aquatic Organisms. Midland, Mich.: Dow Chemical, 1978.

Branson DR, Blau GE, Alexander HC, Neely WB: Bioconcentration of 2,2',4,4'-tetrachlorobiphenyl in rainbow trout as measured by an accelerated test. Trans Am Fish Soc 104:785–792, 1975.

Bruggeman WA, Martron LBJM, Kooiman D, Hutzinger, O: Accumulation and elimination kinetics of di-, tri- and tetra chlorobiphenyls by goldfish after dietary and aqueous exposure. Chemosphere 10:811–832, 1981.

Bryan GW: Some aspects of heavy metal tolerance in aquatic organism. In: Effects of Pollutants on Aquatic Organisms, edited by APM Lockwood, pp. 7–34. London: Cambridge, 1976.

Bysshe SE: Bioconcentration factor in aquatic organisms. In: Handbook of Chemical Property Estimation Methods, edited by WJ Lyman, WF Reehl, DH Rosenblatt, pp. 5-1–5-30, New York: McGraw-Hill, 1982.

Canton JH, Greve PA, Slooff W, van Esch GJ: Toxicity, accumulation and elimination studies of γ-hexachlorocyclohexane (γ-HCH) with freshwater organisms of different trophic levels. Water Res 9:1163–1169, 1975.

Canton JH, Wegman RCC, Vulto TJA, Verhoef CH, van Esch GJ: Toxicity, accumulation, and elimination studies of γ-hexachlorocyclohexane (γ-HCH) with saltwater organisms of different trophic levels. Water Res 12:687–690, 1978.

Carpene E, George SG: Absorption of cadmium by gills of *Mytilus edulis* (L.). Mol Physiol 1:23–34, 1981.

Chadwick GG, Brocksen RW: Accumulation of dieldrin by fish and selected fish-food organisms. J Wildl Manage 33(3):693–700, 1969.

Chiou CT, Freed VH, Schmedding DW, Kohnert RL: Partition coefficient and bioaccumulation of selected organic chemicals. Environ Sci Technol 11:475–478, 1977.

Cox JL: DDT residues in marine phytoplankton: Increase from 1955 to 1969. Science 170:71–73, 1970.

Crosby DG, Tucker RK: Accumulation of DDT by *Daphnia magna.* Environ Sci Technol 5:714–716, 1971.

Davies AG: In: Radioactive Contamination of the Marine Environment, pp. 403–420. Vienna: International Atomic Energy Agency, 1973.

Derr SK, Zabik MJ: Bioactive compounds in the aquatic environment: Studies on the mode of uptake of DDE by the aquatic midge, *Chironomus tentans* (Diptera: Chironomidae). Arch Environ Contam Toxicol 2(2):152–164, 1974.

Dixon WJ, Brown MB (eds.): BMDP Biomedical computer programs, P-series. Berkeley: Univ. of California Press, 1979.

Ellgehausen H, Guth JA, Essner HO: Factors determining the bioaccumulation potential of pesticides in the individual compartments of aquatic food chains. Ecotoxicol Environ Saf 4:134–157, 1980.

Ernst W: Determination of the bioconcentration potential of marine organisms—a steady state approach. I. Bioconcentration data for seven chlorinated pesticides in mussels (*Mytilus edulis*) and their relation to solubility data. Chemosphere 6:731–740, 1977.

Ernst W: Factors affecting the evaluation of chemicals in laboratory experiments using marine organisms. Ecotoxicol Environ Saf 3: 90–98, 1979.

Fowler SW, Benayoun G: Experimental studies on cadmium flux through marine biota. In: Comparative Studies of Food and Environmental Contamination, pp. 159–178. Vienna: International Atomic Energy Agency, 1974.

Fromm PO, Hunter RC: Uptake of dieldrin by isolated perfused gills of rainbow trout. J Fish Res Board Can 26:1939–1942, 1969.

Giesy JP, Jr (ed.): Microcosms in Ecological Research. DOE CONF-781101. Springfield, Va.: National Technical Information Service, 1980.

Giesy JP, Jr, Bowling JW, Kania HJ: Cadmium and zinc accumulation and elimination by freshwater crayfish. Arch Environ Contam Toxicol 9:685–699, 1980.

Guarino AM, Arnold ST: Xenobiotic transport mechanisms and pharmacokinetics in the dogfish shark. In: Pesticide and Xenobiotic Metabolism in Aquatic Organisms, edited by MAQ Khan, JJ Lech, JJ Menn, ACS Symp Ser 99: 131–143, 1979.

Guiney PD, Melancon MJ, Jr, Lech JJ, Peterson RE: Effects of egg and sperm maturation and spawning on the distribution and elimination of a polychlorinated biphenyl in rainbow trout (Salmo gairdneri). Toxicol Appl Pharmacol 47: 261–272, 1979.

Guthrie FE: Absorption and distribution. In: Introduction to Biochemical Toxicology, edited by E Hodgson, FE Guthrie, pp. 10–39. New York: Elsevier, 1980.

Halter MT, Johnson HE: A model system to study the desorption and biological availability of PCB in hydrosoils. In: Aquatic Toxicology and Hazard Evaluation, edited by FL Mayer, JL Hamelink, pp. 178–195. ASTM STP 634. Philadelphia, Pa.: ASTM, 1977.

Hamelink JL: Bioavailability of chemicals in aquatic environments. In: Biotransformation and Fate of Chemicals in the Aquatic Environment, edited by AW Maki, KL Dickson, J Cairns, Jr, pp. 56–62. Washington, D.C.: American Society of Microbiology, 1980.

Hamelink JL, Waybrant RC: DDE and lindane in a large-scale model lentic ecosystem. Trans Am Fish Soc 105:124–134, 1976.

Hamelink JL, Waybrant RC, Ball RC: A proposal: Exchange equilibria control the degree chlorinated hydrocarbons are biologically magnified in lentic environments. Trans Am Fish Soc 100: 207–214, 1971.

Harding GCH, Vass WP: Uptake from seawater and clearance of p,p'-DDT by marine planktonic crustacea. J Fish Res Board Can 36:247–254, 1979.

Harding LW, Jr, Phillips JH, Jr: Polychlorinated biphenyl (PCB) uptake by marine phytoplankton. Mar Biol 49:103–111, 1978.

Hartung R: Pharmacokinetic approaches to the evaluation of methylmercury in fish. In: Toxicity to Biota of Metal Forms in Natural Water, edited by RW Andrew, PV Hodson, DE Konasewich, pp. 233–248. Windsor, Ontario: International Joint Commission, 1976.

Holden AV: A study of the absorption of ^{14}C-labeled DDT from water by fish. Ann Appl Biol 50:467–477, 1962.

Hunn JB, Allen JL: Movement of drugs across the gills of fishes. Annu Rev Pharmacol 14:47–55, 1974.

Isensee AR, Jones GE: Distribution of 2,3,7,8-tetrachlorodibenzo-p-dioxin (TCDD) in aquatic model ecosystem. Environ Sci Technol 9:668–672, 1975.

Jackim E, Morrison G, Steele R: Effects of environmental factors on radiocadmium uptake by four species of marine bivalves. Mar Biol 40: 303–308, 1977.

Jarvinen AW, Hoffman MJ, Thorslund TW: Long-term toxic effects of DDT food and water exposure on fathead minnows (Pimephales promelas). J Fish Res Board Can 34:2089–2103, 1977.

Jarvinen AW, Tyo RM: Toxicity to fathead minnows of endrin in food and water. Arch Environ Contam Toxicol 7:409–421, 1978.

Jennings JR, Rainbow PS: Studies on the uptake of cadmium by the crab Carcinus maenas in the laboratory. I. Accumulation from seawater and food source. Mar Biol 50:131–139, 1979.

Johnson BT: Aquatic food chain models for estimating bioaccumulation and biodegradation of xenobiotics. Columbia, Mo.: U.S. Dept. of Interior, Fish and Wildlife Service, Fish-Pesticide Research Laboratory, 1975.

Kenaga EE: Predicted bioconcentration factors

and soil sorption coefficients of pesticides and other chemicals. Ecotoxicol Environ Saf 4:26–38, 1980.

Kenaga EE, Goring CAI: Relationship between water solubility, soil sorption, octanol-water partitioning, and concentration of chemicals in biota. In: Aquatic Toxicology, edited by JG Eaton, PR Parrish, AC Hendricks, pp. 78–115. ASTM STP 707. Philadelphia, Pa.: ASTM, 1980.

Kikuchi M, Wakabayashi M, Kojima H, Yoshida T: Bioaccumulation profiles of ^{35}S-labeled sodium alkylpoly(oxyethylene) sulfates in carp (*Cyprinus carpio*). Water Res 14:1541–1548, 1980.

Kimerle RA, Macek KJ, Sleight BH, III, Burrows ME: Bioconcentration of linear alkylbenzene sulfonate (LAS) in bluegill (*Lepomis macrochirus*). Water Res 15:251–256, 1981.

Kinkade ML, Erdman HE: The influence of hardness components (Ca^{2+} and Mg^{2+}) in water on the uptake and concentration of cadmium in a simulated freshwater ecosystem. Environ Res 10(2):308–313, 1975.

Klaassen CD: Absorption, distribution, and excretion of toxicants. In: Toxicology: The Basic Science of Poisons, 2nd ed, edited by J Doull, CD Klaassen, MO Amdur, pp. 28–55. New York: Macmillan, 1980.

Klumpp DW: Accumulation of arsenic from water and food by *Littorina littoralis* and *Nucella lapillus*. Mar Biol 58:265–274, 1980.

Kobayashi K: Metabolism of pentachlorophenol in fish. In: Pesticide and Xenobiotic Metabolism in Aquatic Organisms, edited by MAQ Khan, JJ Lech, JJ Menn, ACS Symp Ser 99:131–143, 1979.

Könemann H, van Leeuwen K: Toxicokinetics in fish: Accumulation and elimination of six chlorobenzenes by guppies. Chemosphere 9:3–19, 1980.

Leo A, Hansch C, Elkins D: Partition coefficients and their uses. Chem Rev 71:525, 1971.

Levy G, Gibaldi M: Pharmacokinetics. In: Concepts in Biochemical Pharmacology: Handbook of Experimental Pharmacology, edited by JR Gillette, JR Mitchell, pp. 1–34. Berlin: Springer Verlag, 1975.

Lo IH, Hayton WL: Effects of pH on the accumulation of sulfonamides by fish. J Pharmacokinet Biopharmacol 9:443–459, 1981.

Lyman WJ: Octanol/water partition coefficient. In: Handbook of Chemical Property Estimation Methods, edited by WJ Lyman, WF Reehl, DH Rosenblatt, pp. 1-1–1-54. New York: McGraw-Hill, 1982.

Lynch TR: Residue dynamics and availability of 2,4,5,2′,4′,5′-hexachlorobiphenyl in aquatic model ecosystems. Ph.D. thesis, Michigan State Univ., Ann Arbor, Mich., 1979.

Macek KJ, Petrocelli SR, Sleight BH, III: Considerations in assessing the potential for, and significance of, biomagnification of chemical residues in aquatic food chains. In: Aquatic Toxicology, edited by LL Marking, RA Kimerle, pp. 251–268. ASTM STP 667. Philadelphia, Pa.: ASTM, 1979.

MacKay, D: Correlation of bioconcentration factors. Environ Sci Technol 16:274–278, 1982.

Maren TH, Embry R, Broder LE: The excretion of drugs across the gill of the dogfish, *Squalus acanthias*. Comp Biochem Physiol 26:853–864, 1968.

Martin H, Worthing CR: Pesticide Manual, 5th ed. Worcestershire, England: British Crop Protection Council, 1977.

Matsumura F: Toxicology of Insecticides. New York: Plenum, 1975.

Mayer FL: Residue dynamics of di-2-ethylhexylphthalate in fathead minnows (*Pimephales promelas*). J Fish Res Board Can 33:2610–2613, 1976.

McLeese DW, Zitko V, Sergeant DB: Uptake and excretion of fenitrothion by clams and mussels. Bull Environ Contam Toxicol 22:800–806, 1979.

Merlini M, Pozzi G: Lead and freshwater fishes. Part 1. Lead accumulation and water pH. Environ Pollut 12:168–172, 1977.

Merlini M, Pozzi G, Brazzelli A, Berg A: The transfer of ^{65}Zn from natural and synthetic foods to a freshwater fish. In: Radioecology and Energy Resources. Ecol Soc Am Spec Publ 1:226–229, 1976.

Metcalf RL: Model ecosystem approach to insecticide degradation: A critique. Annu Rev Entomol 22:241–261, 1977a.

Metcalf RL: Model ecosystem studies of bioconcentration and biodegradation of pesticides. In: Pesticides in Aquatic Environments, edited by

MAQ Khan, pp. 127–144. New York: Plenum, 1977b.

Metcalf RL, Sangha GK, Kapoor IP: Ecosystem for the evaluation of pesticide biodegradability and ecological magnification. Environ Sci Technol 5:709–713, 1971.

Metzler CM, Elfring GL, McEwen AJ: A package of computer programs for pharmacokinetic modeling. Biometrics 30:562–563, 1974.

Miettinen JK: The accumulation and excretion of heavy metals in organisms. In: Ecological Toxicology Research, edited by AD McIntyre, CF Mills, pp. 215–229. New York: Plenum, 1974.

Nagel R, Urich K: Kinetic studies on the elimination of different substituted phenols by goldfish (*Carassius auratus*). Bull Environ Contam Toxicol 24:374–378, 1980.

National Research Council: Testing for Effects of Chemicals on Ecosystems. Washington, D.C.: National Academy Press, 1981.

Neely WB: Estimating rate constants for the uptake and clearance of chemicals by fish. Environ Sci Technol 13:1506–1510, 1979.

Neely WB, Branson DR, Blau GE: Partition coefficient to measure bioconcentration potential of organic chemicals in fish. Environ Sci Technol 8:1113–1115, 1974.

Nie NII, Hull CH, Jenkins JG, Steinbrenner K, Bent DH: SPSS statistical package for the social sciences, 2nd ed., New York: McGraw-Hill, 1975.

O'Hara J: Cadmium uptake by fiddler crabs exposed to temperature and salinity stress. J Fish Res Board Can 30(6):846–848, 1973.

Olson KR, Bergman HL, Fromm PO: Uptake of methyl mercuric chloride and mercuric chloride by trout: A study of uptake pathways into the whole animal and uptake by erythrocytes in vitro. J Fish Res Board Can 30:1293–1299, 1973.

Pagenkopf GK, Russo RC, Thurston RV: Effect of complexation on toxicity of copper to fishes. J Fish Res Board Can 31:462–465, 1974.

Paris DF, Lewis DL, Barnett JT: Bioconcentration of toxaphene by microorganisms. Bull Environ Contam Toxicol 17:564–572, 1977.

Paris DF, Steen WC, Baughman GL: Rate of physico-chemical properties of Aroclors 1016 and 1242 in determining their fate and transport in aquatic environments. Chemosphere 7:319–325, 1978.

Part P, Svanberg O: Uptake of cadmium in perfused rainbow trout (*Salmo gairdneri*) gills. Can J Fish Aquat Sci 38:917–924, 1981.

Pavlou SP, Dexter RN: Distribution of polychlorinated biphenyls (PCB) in estuarine ecosystems. Testing the concept of equilibrium partitioning in the marine environment. Environ Sci Technol 13:65–70, 1979.

Pentreath RJ: The accumulation and retention of ^{65}Zn and ^{54}Mn by the plaice, *Pleuronectes platessa* L. J Exp Mar Biol Ecol 12:1–18, 1973.

Petrocelli SR: Biomagnification of dieldrin residues by food-chain transfer from clams to blue crabs under controlled conditions. Bull Environ Contam Toxicol 13:108–116, 1975.

Poldoski JE: Cadmium bioaccumulation assays. Their relationship to various ionic equilibria in Lake Superior water. Environ Sci Technol 13:701–706, 1979.

Premdas FH, Anderson JM: The uptake and detoxification of C^{14}-labeled DDT in Atlantic salmon, *Salmo salar*. J Fish Res Board Can 20:827, 1963.

Pritchard JB, Karnaky KJ, Jr, Guarino AM, Kinter WB: Renal handling of the polar DDT metabolite DDA (2,2-bis[*p*-chlorophenyl] acetic acid) by marine fish. Am J Physiol 233:F126–F132, 1977.

Reinert RE: Accumulation of dieldrin in an alga (*Scenedesmus obliquus*), *Daphnia magna*, and the guppy (*Poecilia reticulata*). J Fish Res Board Can 29:1413–1418, 1972.

Reinert RE, Stone LJ, Willford WA: Effect of temperature on accumulation of methylmercuric chloride and *p,p'*-DDT by rainbow trout (*Salmo gairdneri*). J Fish Res Board Can 31:1649–1652, 1974.

Rekker RF: The Hydrophobic Fragmental Constant. Amsterdam: Elsevier, 1977.

Renfro WC, Fowler SW, Heyraud M, La Rosa J: Relative importance of food and water in long-term zinc^{65} accumulation by marine biota. J Fish Res Board Can 32:1339–1345, 1975.

Ribeyre F, Boudou A, Delarche A: Interest of the experimental trophic chains as ecotoxicological models for the study of the ecosystem contaminations. Ecotoxicol Environ Saf 3:411–427, 1979.

Roberts JR, deFreitas ASW, Gidney, MAJ: Control factors on uptake and clearance of xenobiotic chemicals by fish. In: Animals as monitors of environmental pollutants, pp. 3–14. Washington, D.C.: National Academy of Sciences, 1979.

Rowland M: Pharmacokinetics. In: Drug Metabolism—From Microbe to Man, edited by DV Parke, RL Smith, pp. 123–145. London: Taylor and Francis, 1977.

Skaar DR, Johnson BT, Jones JR, Huckins JN: Fate of Kepone and mirex in a model aquatic environment: Sediment, fish, and diet. Can J Fish Aquat Sci 38:931–938, 1981.

Sodergren A: Uptake and accumulation of C^{14}-DDT by *Chlorella* sp. (Chlorophyceae). Oikos 19:126–138, 1968.

Southworth GR, Beauchamp JJ, Schmieder PK: Bioaccumulation potential of polycyclic aromatic hydrocarbons in *Daphnia pulex*. Water Res 12:973–977, 1978.

Southworth GR, Keffer CC, Beauchamp JJ: Potential and realized bioconcentration. A comparison of observed and predicted bioconcentration of azaarenes in the fathead minnow (*Pimephales promelas*). Environ Sci Technol 14:1529–1531, 1980.

Southworth GR, Keffer CC, Beauchamp JJ: The accumulation and disposition of benz(a)acridine in the fathead minnow, *Pimephales promelas*. Arch Environ Contam Toxicol 10:561–570, 1981.

Spacie A: The bioconcentration of trifluralin from a manufacturing effluent by fish in the Wabash River. Ph.D. thesis, Purdue Univ., West Lafayette, Ind., 1975.

Spacie A, Hamelink JL: Dynamics of trifluralin accumulation in river fishes. Environ Sci Technol 13:817–822, 1979.

Spacie A, Hamelink JL: Alternative models for describing the bioconcentration of organics in fish. Environ Toxicol Chem 1:309–320, 1982.

Spacie, A, Landrum PF, Leversee GJ: Uptake, depuration, and biotransformation of anthracene and benzo(a)pyrene in bluegill sunfish. Ecotoxicol Environ Safety 7:330–341, 1983.

Spehar RL, Anderson RL, Fiandt JT: Toxicity and bioaccumulation of cadmium and lead in aquatic invertebrates. Environ Pollut 15:195–208, 1978.

Spigarelli SA, Thommes MM, Prepejchal W: Thermal and metabolic factors affecting PCB uptake by adult brown trout. Environ Sci Technol 17:88–94, 1983.

Sprague JB: Promising anti-pollutant: Chelating agent NTA protects fish from copper and zinc. Nature (London) 220:1345–1346, 1968.

Statham CN, Melancon MJ, Jr, Lech JJ: Bioconcentration of xenobiotics in trout bile: A proposed monitoring aid for some waterborne chemicals. Science 193:680–681, 1976.

Sunda WG, Engel DW, Thuotte RM: Effects of chemical speciation on toxicity of cadmium to grass shrimp *Palaemonetes pugio:* Importance of free cadmium ion. Environ Sci Technol 12:409–413, 1979.

Thomann RV: Equilibrium model of fate of microcontaminants in diverse aquatic food chains. Can J Fish Aquat Sci 38:280–296, 1981.

Tsai SC, Boush GM, Matsumura F: Importance of water pH in accumulation of inorganic mercury in fish. Bull Environ Contam Toxicol 13:188–193, 1975.

Tuey DB: Toxicokinetics. In: Introduction to Biochemical Toxicology, edited by E Hodgson, FE Guthrie, pp. 40–66. New York: Elsevier, 1980.

Vanderford MJ, Hamelink JL: Influence of environmental factors on pesticide levels in sport fish. Pestic Monit J 11:138–145, 1977.

Van Weers AW: The effect of temperature on the uptake and retention of ^{60}Co and ^{65}Zn by the common shrimp (*Crangon crangon* L.). In: Combined Effects of Radioactive, Chemical and Thermal Releases into the Environment, pp. 35–49. Vienna: International Atomic Energy Agency, 1975.

Veith GD, Morris RT: A rapid method for estimating log P for organic chemicals. Ecol Res Series EPA-600/3-78-049. Duluth, Minn.: U.S. Environmental Protection Agency, 1978.

Veith GD, Macek KJ, Petrocelli SR, Carroll J: An evaluation of using partition coefficients and water solubility to estimate bioconcentration factors for organic chemicals in fish. Fed Regist 44:15926–15981, 1979a.

Veith GD, DeFoe DL, Bergstedt BV: Measuring and estimating the bioconcentration factor of chemicals in fish. J Fish Res Board Can 36: 1040–1048, 1979b.

Vighi M: Lead uptake and release in an experimental trophic chain. Ecotoxicol Environ Saf 5: 177–193, 1981.

Voice TC, Rice CP, Weber WJ, Jr: Effect of solids concentration on the sorptive partitioning of hydrophobic pollutants in aquatic systems. Environ Sci Technol 17:513–518, 1983.

Wildish DJ, Zitko V: Uptake of polychlorinated biphenyls from seawater by *Gammarus oceanicus.* Mar Biol 9:213–218, 1971.

Wilkes FG, Weiss CM: The accumulation of DDT by the dragonfly nymph, *Tetragoneuria.* Trans Am Fish Soc 100:222–236, 1971.

Wong PTS, Chau YK, Kramar O, Bengert GA: Accumulation and depuration of tetramethyllead by rainbow trout. Water Res 15:621–625, 1981.

Woodwell GM, Wurster CF, Jr, Isaacson PA: DDT residues in an East Coast estuary: A case of biological concentration of a persistent insecticide. Science 156:821–824, 1967.

Zitko V: Relationships governing the behavior of pollutants in aquatic ecosystems and their use in risk assessment. Can Tech Rep Aquat Sci, 1979.

Zitko V, Carson WV, Carson WG: Prediction of incipient lethal levels of copper to juvenile Atlantic salmon in the presence of humic acid by cupric electrode. Bull Environ Contam Toxicol 10:265–271, 1973.

SUPPLEMENTAL READING

Clark B, Smith DA: An introduction to pharmacokinetics. Oxford: Blackwell Scientific Publications, 1981.

Hodson PV, Blunt BR, Borgmann U, Minns CK, McGaw S: Effect of fluctuating lead exposures on lead accumulation by rainbow trout (*Salmo gairdneri*). Environ Toxicol Chem 2:225–238, 1983.

Oliver BG, Niimi AJ: Bioconcentration of chlorobenzenes from water by rainbow trout: Correlations with partition coefficients and environmental residues. Environ Sci Technol 17:287–291, 1983.

Phillips GR, Russo RC: Metal bioaccumulation in fishes and aquatic invertebrates: A literature review. EPA-600/3-78-103. Duluth, Minn.: Environmental Research Laboratory, U.S. Environmental Protection Agency, 1978.

Pritchard PH: Model ecosystems. In: Environmental Risk Analysis for Chemicals, edited by RA Conway, pp. 257–353. New York: Van Nostrand Reinhold, 1982.

Chapter 18

Biotransformation

J. J. Lech and M. J. Vodicnik

INTRODUCTION

It has been known for many years that chemical compounds can alter normal physiological functions of mammals, but only in the recent past has it been recognized that contact with biological material can significantly affect the structure of a chemical compound.

Biotransformation may be defined as the biologically catalyzed conversion of one chemical into another. It should be differentiated from purely physical-chemical processes that can also effect chemical conversions, such as photolysis, and oxidations and reductions that do not involve the biological catalysts known as enzymes. The distinguishing feature of chemical conversions in a biological system is that most of the reactions are carried out under the influence of enzymes. Although the term "metabolism" has been used to describe the biological conversion of one chemical into another, the term "biotransformation" is preferable, since metabolism is more appropriately used in connection with the biochemical reactions of carbohydrates, proteins, fats, and other normal body constituents.

Although the biotransformation of drugs and xenobiotic compounds has been studied in mammals (Jakoby, 1980; LaDu et al., 1971), it is only in recent years that appreciable attention has been focused on the rates and pathways of biotransformation of xenobiotic chemicals in aquatic species (Bend and James, 1979; Chambers and Yarbrough, 1976; Khan et al., 1979; Lech and Bend, 1980). Nevertheless, it will become apparent from the information presented in this chapter that biotransformation is a significant phenomenon which is directly related to the fate and pharmacological and toxicological effects of xenobiotic chemicals in aquatic species.

TERMINOLOGY

Xenobiotic compound. A foreign compound not normally considered a constitutive component of a specified biological system.

Biotransformation. Enzyme-catalyzed conversion of one xenobiotic compound to another.

Enzyme. A biological catalyst, generally a protein plus a prosthetic group.

Microsomes. Subcellular fragments of the smooth endoplasmic reticulum of cells that are isolated by ultracentrifugation after cell disruption.

Residue. The concentration of a xenobiotic chemical measured in a species in the environment.

Toxicokinetics. Qualitative, quantitative, and temporal aspects of the behavior of a toxic xenobiotic chemical in a given organism.

Induction. The process of initiating the de novo synthesis of an enzyme.

In vivo. Within an intact animal or organism.

In vitro. Outside the intact organism; generally applied to experiments involving biochemical events occurring in tissue fragments or fractions.

Metabolite. The product of a biotransformation reaction.

Endogenous. Normally occurring in an organism.

Exogenous. From a source external to an organism.

Polar/hydrophilic. Having an affinity for aqueous systems.

Nonpolar/hydrophobic. Having an affinity for lipoidal rather than aqueous systems.

Substrate. A chemical that interacts with an enzyme and is biochemically transformed to a product.

GENERAL PRINCIPLES OF BIOTRANSFORMATION

When a specific chemical compound within an organism undergoes biotransformation to another chemical substance, several important changes in the original parent compound may also take place. These changes may occur through a series of sequential reactions in which one or more products (or metabolites) are created with chemical and/or physical properties distinct from those of the original compound. Therefore, the new compound may behave differently within the organism with respect to [1] tissue distribution, [2] bioaccumulation, [3] persistence, and [4] route and rate of excretion. In addition to affecting these parameters which dictate the fate of a chemical, biotransformation reactions may significantly alter its pharmacological and toxicological properties. There is considerable evidence that biotransformation may lead to the following alterations in pharmacological and toxicological properties of a chemical or drug:

1 Conversion of an active compound to an inactive compound.

2 Conversion of an inactive compound to an active compound.

3 Conversion of an inactive compound to another inactive compound.

4 Conversion of one active compound to another active compound.

Biotransformation reactions are also often a significant prerequisite to excretion. In general, the ease with which a compound is excreted depends on its solubility in water. Compounds in the body that are soluble in water (polar) are often more easily excreted than lipid-soluble (nonpolar) compounds. Biotransformation reactions tend to make lipid-soluble compounds more water-soluble and thus more easily excreted by intact organisms. Several reactions may do the opposite, and from the point of view of chemical persistence, the conversion of a compound to a more lipid-soluble form is not desirable. In addition, although many biotransformation reactions tend to decrease the biological activity of a compound or "detoxify" it, several reactions actually produce metabolites that are more toxic than the parent compound (Jakoby, 1980).

Biotransformation of chemicals is of importance in aquatic toxicology since these biologically catalyzed chemical conversions form the basis for the underlying mechanisms that govern persistence, bioaccumulation, residue dynamics, and toxicity of chemicals. There are wide variations among chemical classes and species in terms of biotransformation pathways and the rates at which these reactions proceed, and the toxicokinetic behavior of a chemical is an important consideration in its toxicological evaluation. If one steps back from the individual organism for a moment and views the behavior of a chemical in an entire ecosystem, it becomes obvious that biotransformations effected by aquatic organisms, including fish, insects, and microorganisms, along with physical processes such as photolysis and nonenzymatically catalyzed oxidations and reductions are all chemical reactions that dictate the overall fate of the chemical. However, biotransformation within most aquatic organisms, with the exception of bacteria, rarely, if ever, leads to complete degradation of chemicals to carbon dioxide and water. In many instances biotransformation products are excreted from organisms as relatively intact molecules that may or may not be degraded further by other components of an ecosystem.

TYPES OF ENZYME–CATALYZED BIOTRANSFORMATION REACTIONS

Biotransformation reactions involving xenobiotic compounds and drugs are often catalyzed by enzymes that occur in the soluble, mitochondrial, or microsomal fractions of the liver. These enzyme systems are also present in the intestine, lung, and kidney of many living species. In general, biotransformation reactions are catalyzed by enzymes with a relatively low degree of substrate specificity compared to reactions catalyzed by enzymes involved in the metabolism of constitutive chemicals of a specific organism. For example, the enzyme glucose-6-phosphatase recognizes glucose 6-phosphate and will remove the phosphate group only from this compound; it will

not be effective in removing the phosphate group from, say, fructose 6-phosphate. In contrast, the less specific enzymes involved in the biotransformation of xenobiotic substances tend to catalyze reactions after recognition of functional groups within a molecule, rather than recognition of the entire molecule itself. Investigators have often pondered the biological reasons for the presence of these enzymes, and it is thought that they evolved as a protective device against chemical insults encountered in the environment or that they are relatively nonspecific biological catalysts which normally biotransform certain body constituents but have relatively low substrate specificity. The fact remains that many organisms are able to biotransform a wide variety of chemicals that differ greatly in structure but have many functional groups in common.

Enzymatic biotransformation reactions can be broadly divided into two types (Williams, 1947): phase I nonsynthetic reactions, involving oxidation, reduction, and hydrolysis; and phase II synthetic reactions, involving conjugation. Oxidation, hydrolysis, and reduction can occur enzymatically and nonenzymatically. Conjugations are generally enzyme-catalyzed. Phase I reactions convert compounds to products that can undergo phase II reactions. Conjugation involves the combination of phase I products with an endogenous polar or ionic moiety. In the following sections prototype reactions are illustrated. Only general formulas are given for the chemical to emphasize the functional group conversions that take place.

Hydrolysis

Hydrolytic reactions occur in many species of fish, and the enzymes involved are diverse and have been shown to occur in several organs including liver, kidney, and plasma. The types of chemicals that undergo hydrolytic reactions include esters, epoxides, and amides, as shown in Fig. 1.

Reduction

Reduction of several chemical classes, including halogenated organic chemicals, ketones, nitro com-

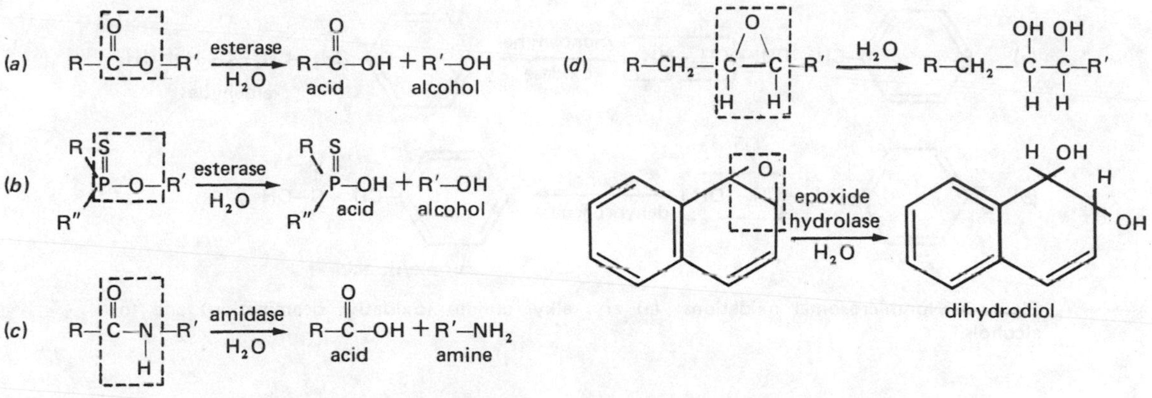

Figure 1 Chemicals that undergo hydrolysis: (a) aromatic and aliphatic esters, (b) organophosphate esters, (c) amides, and (d) aliphatic and aromatic epoxides.

pounds, and azo compounds, has been described in detail with enzymes from mammalian sources. In recent years some of these reactions have been described in fish tissues. Reduction reactions usually occur in the microsomal fraction of the liver. Examples are shown in Fig. 2.

Oxidation

Oxidation of many organic compounds with diverse functional groups has been observed in many species of fish. Some oxidations are catalyzed by nonmicrosomal enzymes in the mito-

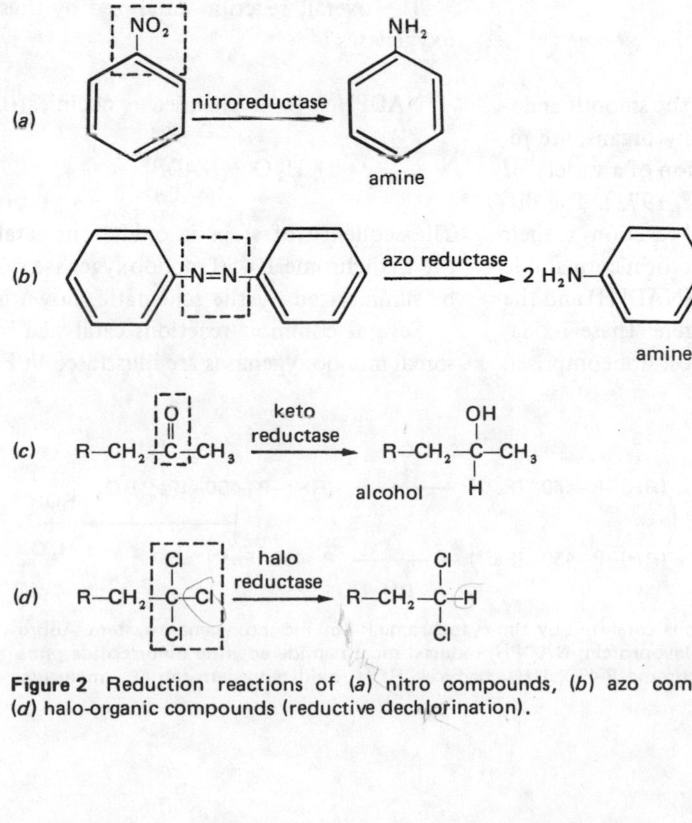

Figure 2 Reduction reactions of (a) nitro compounds, (b) azo compounds, (c) ketones, and (d) halo-organic compounds (reductive dechlorination).

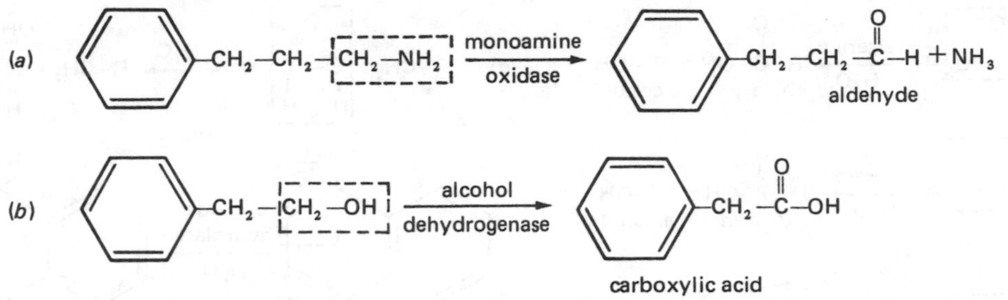

Figure 3 Nonmicrosomal oxidations: (a) aryl alkyl amines (oxidative deamination) and (b) alcohols.

chondrial and soluble fractions of tissue and others by membrane-bound microsomal monooxygenases. Usually xenobiotic oxidation rates in aquatic organisms are lower in extrahepatic organs than in hepatic tissues. Oxidations catalyzed by microsomal enzymes are important biotransformation reactions for many xenobiotic chemicals and may lead to compounds of increased toxicity, depending on the specific chemical and the reaction. Nonmicrosomal oxidations are illustrated in Fig. 3.

Microsomal Oxidations

Microsomal enzymes, located in the smooth endoplasmic reticulum of cells of many organs, are responsible for the biotransformation of a variety of drugs and chemicals (LaDu et al., 1971). The distinguishing feature of microsomal reactions is their dependence on the reducing cofactor nicotinamide adenine dinucleotide phosphate (NADPH) and the requirement for molecular oxygen. These oxidative enzymes, or monooxygenases, are comprised

of a group of hemoproteins collectively termed cytochrome P-450. The P-450 terminology is derived from the observation that these hemoproteins, in reduced form, can combine with carbon monoxide to form products that have an absorption peak at 450 nm (Gillette, 1966). The activity of these enzymes can be increased (induced) or decreased (inhibited) by specific drugs and xenobiotic chemicals (Netter, 1980; Snyder and Remmer, 1979).

The overall reaction catalyzed by these monooxygenases is

$$NADPH + O_2 + chemical \rightarrow chemical \cdot OH$$

$$+ H_2O + NADP^+$$

The sequence of steps in oxidations catalyzed by the cytochrome P-450 monooxygenase system can be summarized by the schematic shown in Fig. 4. Several common reactions catalyzed by microsomal monooxygenases are illustrated in Fig. 5.

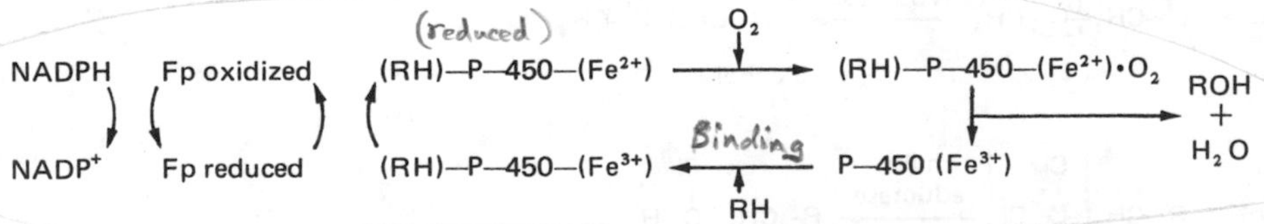

Figure 4 Steps in oxidations catalyzed by the cytochrome P-450 monooxygenase system. Abbreviations: Fp, microsomal flavoprotein; NADPH, reduced nicotinamide adenine dinucleotide phosphate; P-450 (Fe$^+$), cytochrome P-450; RH, chemical; ROH, oxidized chemical; O$_2$, molecular oxygen.

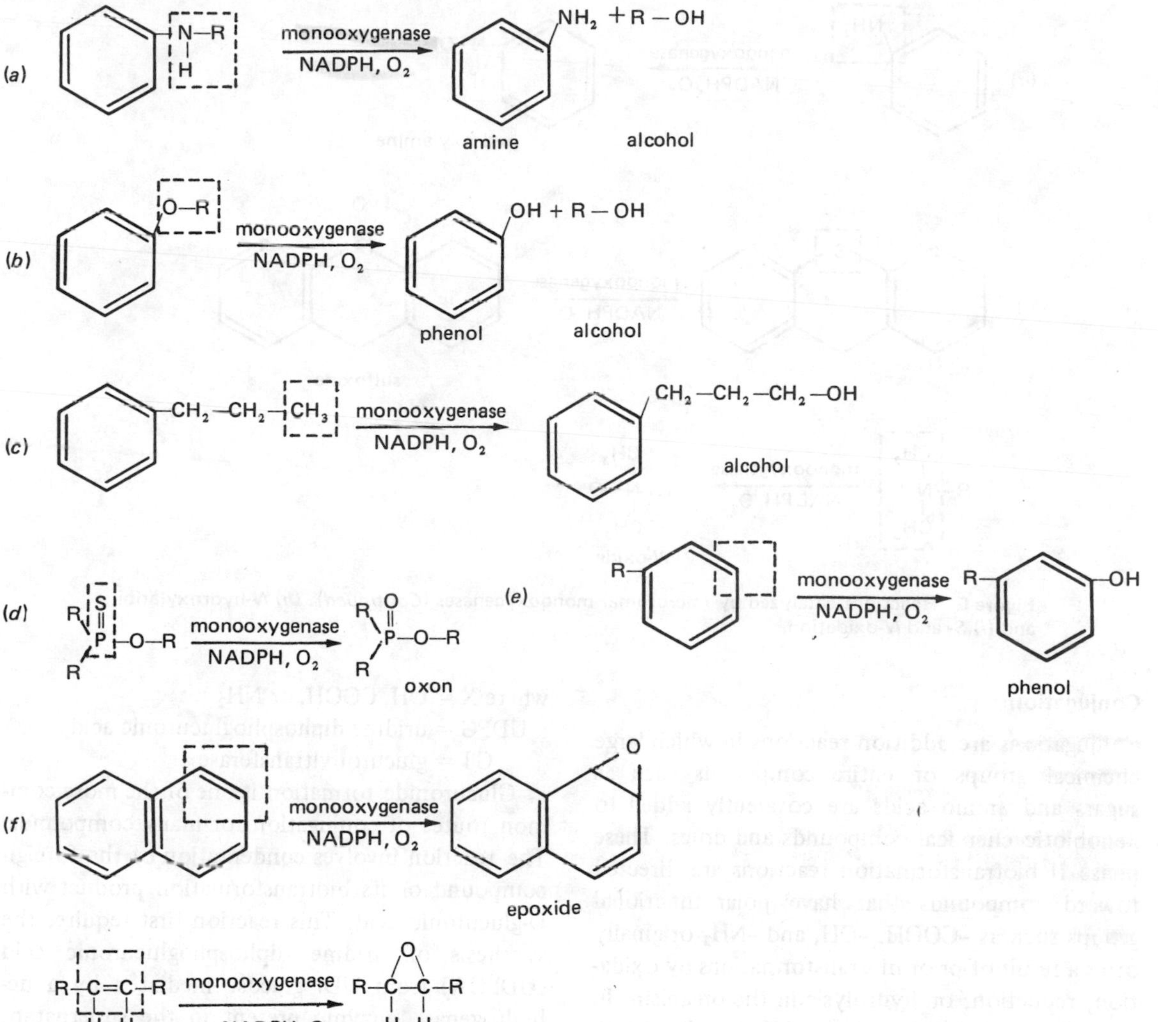

Figure 5 Reactions catalyzed by microsomal monooxygenases: (a) N-dealkylation, (b) O-dealkylation, (c) alkyl chain hydroxylation, (d) S-O exchange, (e) ring hydroxylation, (f) epoxidation, (g) deamination.

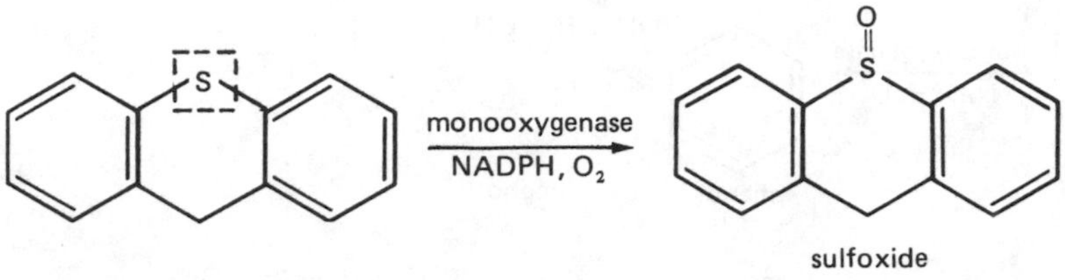

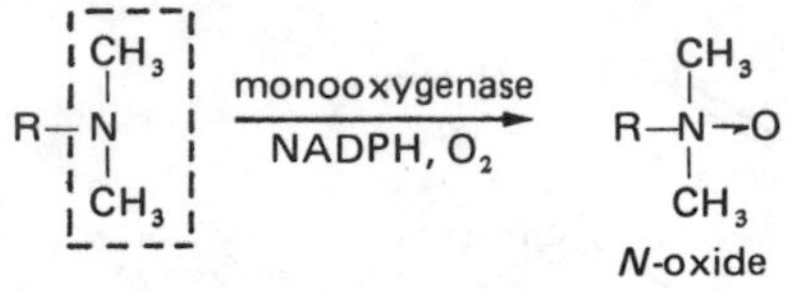

Figure 5 Reactions catalyzed by microsomal monooxygenases (*Continued*): (*h*) *N*-hydroxylation, and (*i*) *S*- and *N*-oxidation.

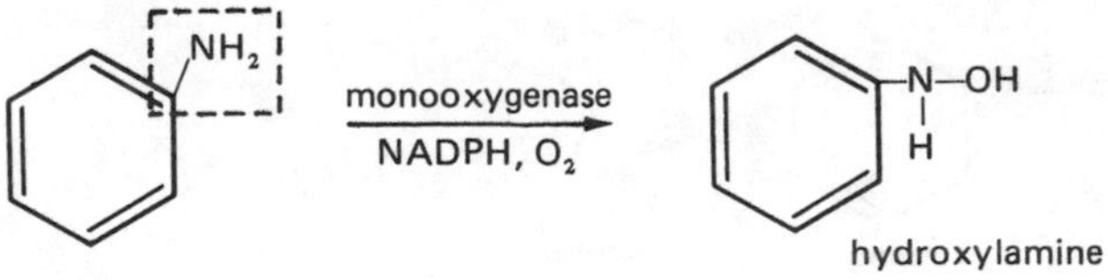

Phase II

Conjugation

Conjugations are addition reactions in which large chemical groups or entire compounds such as sugars and amino acids are covalently added to xenobiotic chemical compounds and drugs. These phase II biotransformation reactions are directed toward compounds that have polar functional groups such as –COOH, –OH, and –NH$_2$ originally or as a result of prior biotransformations by oxidation, reduction, or hydrolysis in the organism. In general, conjugation reactions tend to make chemicals more water-soluble so they are more easily excreted and often, but not always, to make them less toxicologically and pharmacologically active. The different types of conjugation reactions are explained below.

Type I

1) ### Glucuronic Acid Conjugation

The general reaction for glucuronic acid conjugation is

$$\text{UDPGA} + \text{R-X} \xrightarrow{\text{GT}} \text{R-X-GA} + \text{UDP}$$

where X = OH, COOH, or NH$_2$
  UDPG = uridine diphosphoglucuronic acid
  GT = glucuronyltransferase

Glucuronide formation is one of the more common routes of conjugation for many compounds. The reaction involves condensation of the foreign compound or its biotransformation product with D-glucuronic acid. This reaction first requires the synthesis of uridine diphosphoglucuronic acid (UDPGA) from UDP-glucose mediated by a dehydrogenase enzyme present in the supernatant fraction of the liver. The interaction of UDPGA with the acceptor compound is catalyzed by glucuronyltransferase, a microsomal enzyme that occurs mainly in liver but also in other organs. Several types of substrates (X = OH, COOH, NH$_2$), may form glucuronides in the reaction above, as illustrated in Fig. 6.

2) ### Sulfate Conjugation

The general reaction for sulfate conjugation is

$$\text{PAPS} + \text{R-XH} \xrightarrow{\text{ST}} \text{R-X-SO}_3\text{H} + \text{PAP}$$

where X = OH or NH$_2$

PAPS = 3′-phosphoadenosyl-5′-phosphosulfate

ST = sulfotransferase

PAP = 3′,5′-adenosine diphosphate

To form a sulfate derivative of a compound, sulfate is activated to phosphoadenosyl phosphosulfate (PAPS) and is added to the substrate by a reaction mediated by sulfotransferases, which are usually found in the soluble fraction of cells. Several types of substrates (X = OH or NH$_2$) may

form sulfate derivatives in this reaction, as shown in Fig. 7.

Type II

Amino Acid Conjugation

These reactions involve the addition of endogenous amino acids to aromatic or aliphatic carboxylic acids. They take place in two steps: (a) activation of the acid with acetyl coenzyme A and (b) condensation of the activated acid with the amino acid. The general reaction scheme is

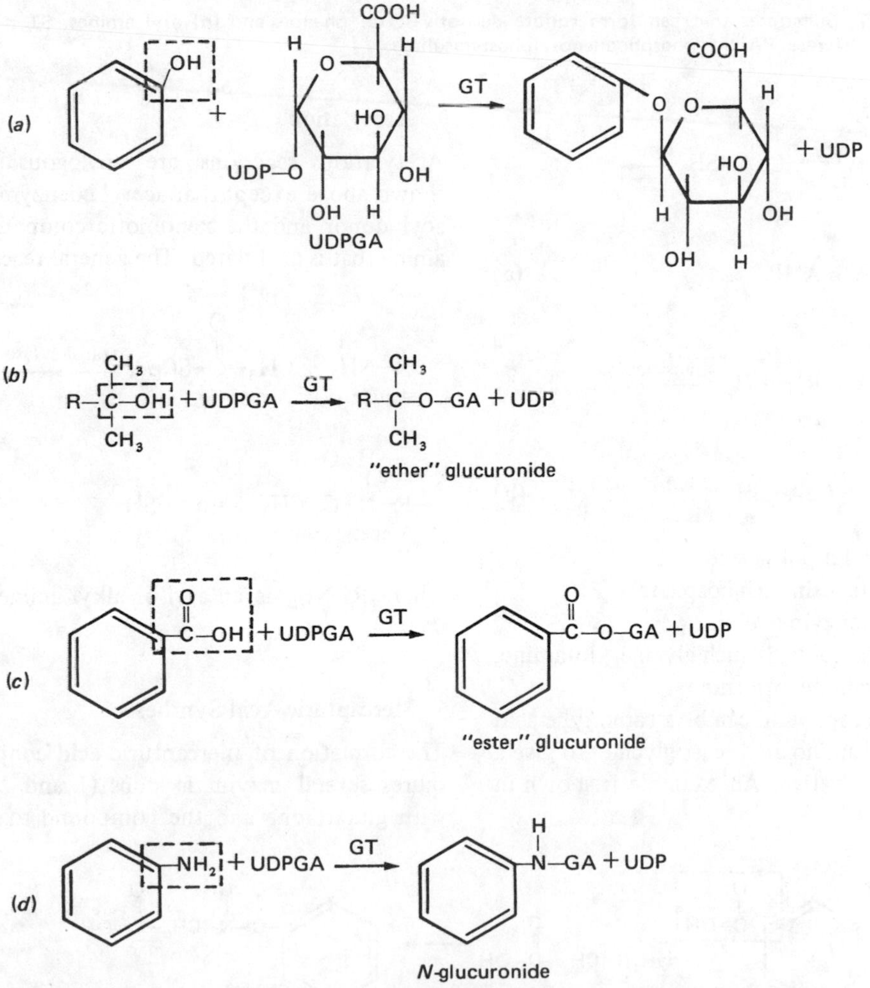

Figure 6 Substrates that can form glucuronides: (a) phenols, (b) alcohols, (c) carboxylic acids, and (d) aryl amines. GT = glucuronyl transferase, UDPGA = Uridine diphosphoglucuronic acid.

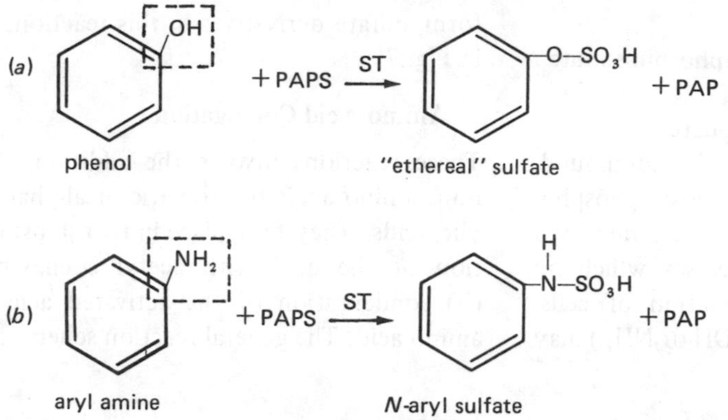

Figure 7 Substrates that can form sulfate derivatives: (*a*) phenols and (*b*) aryl amines. ST = sulfotransferase, PAPS = phosphoadenosylphosphosulfate.

$$R{-}\overset{O}{\overset{\|}{C}}{-}OH + ATP + CoA{-}SH \xrightarrow{\text{ligase}}$$

$$R{-}\overset{O}{\overset{\|}{C}}{-}S{-}CoA + AMP \qquad \text{(a)}$$

$$R{-}\overset{O}{\overset{\|}{C}}{-}S{-}CoA + R^1{-}NH_2 \xrightarrow{\text{transferase}}$$

$$R{-}\overset{O}{\overset{\|}{C}}{-}\overset{H}{\overset{|}{N}}{-}R^1 + CoA{-}SH \qquad \text{(b)}$$

where R = aryl or alkyl acid
ATP = adenosine triphosphate
CoA—SH = coenzyme A
$R^1{-}NH_2$ = amino acids such glycine, glutamine, arginine, ornithine

The foreign compound can be a carboxylic acid that acylates an amino acid (e.g., glycine) to give a hippuric acid derivative. An example is shown in Fig. 8.

Acetylation

Acetylation reactions are analogous to those shown above except that acetyl coenzyme A is the acyl donor and the xenobiotic compound is the amine that is acetylated. The general reaction is

$$\underset{\text{Amine}}{R{-}NH_2} + \underset{\text{Acetyl CoA}}{CH_3{-}\overset{O}{\overset{\|}{C}}{-}SCoA} \xrightarrow{\text{transacylase}}$$

$$\underset{N\text{-acetyl amine}}{R{-}\overset{H}{\overset{|}{N}}{-}\overset{O}{\overset{\|}{C}}{-}CH_3} + CoA{-}SH$$

where $R{-}NH_2$ is an aryl or alkyl amine (see Fig. 9).

Mercapturic Acid Synthesis

The formation of mercapturic acid conjugates requires several enzymatic steps (1 and 2) starting with glutathione and the compound to be conju-

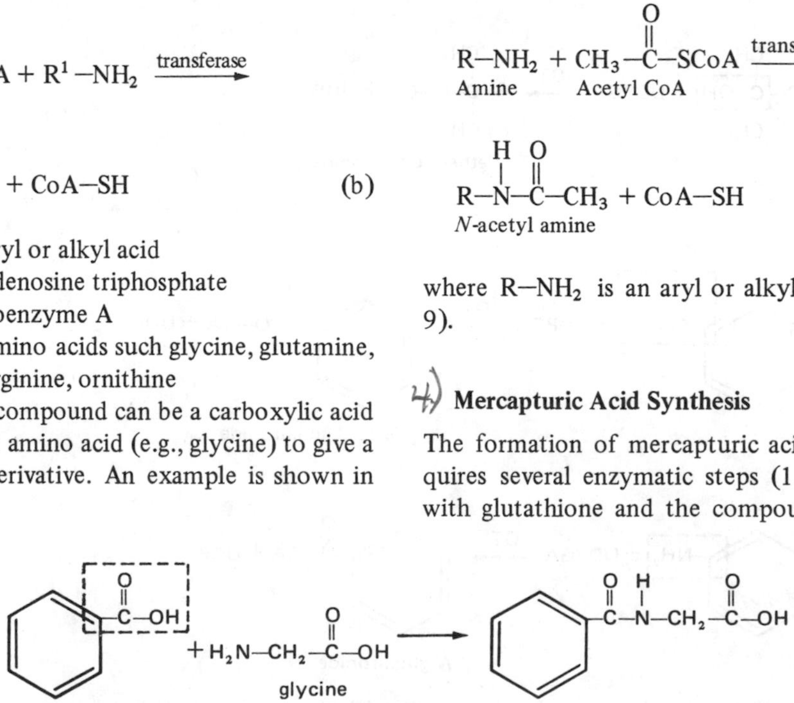

Figure 8 Example of amino acid conjugation reaction.

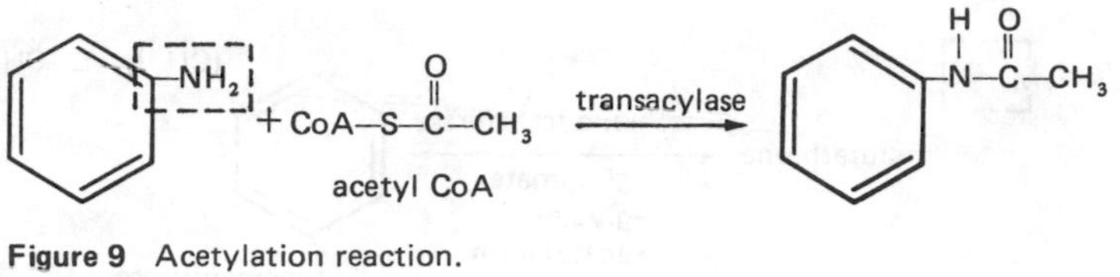

Figure 9 Acetylation reaction.

gated. In addition to making some compounds more polar, conjugation with glutathione has been thought to reduce the toxicity of certain chemicals and their metabolites. The general scheme for mercapturic acid formation is

$$RX + glutathione \xrightarrow{\text{transferase}} R\text{-}S\text{-glutathione} \tag{a}$$

$$R\text{-}S\text{-glutathione} \xrightarrow[\text{acetylase}]{\text{peptidases}} R\text{-}S\text{-mercapturate} \tag{b}$$

where RX is an aromatic ring or a halide compound (see Fig. 10).

BIOTRANSFORMATION OF CHEMICALS BY TISSUES *IN VITRO*

A method frequently used in studying enzyme-catalyzed biotransformation reactions of xenobiotic compounds is to prepare specific tissue fractions by centrifugation after disruption of the tissues by homogenization. The prepared fractions are incubated with a foreign compound and appropriate cofactors. After a specified incubation time, the reaction mixture is analyzed to isolate, identify, and quantify biotransformation products. A chromatographic technique is usually employed for qualitative and quantitative analysis of the products formed. Thin-layer chromatography, gas-liquid chromatography, and high-pressure liquid chromatography have been used in studies of this type (Tjessum and Stegeman, 1979).

In recent years, radioactive isotopes (^{3}H, ^{14}C) and stable isotopes (^{13}C), with appropriate means for detecting the isotopically labeled products (e.g., scintillation counting), have been widely used in *in vitro* biotransformation studies. The advantage of this approach is that it is possible to conveniently and reliably account for all products formed from the original compound.

Although investigation of the biotransformation of specific chemical compounds by use of *in vitro* techniques may be simple and convenient, it has several disadvantages. *In vitro* techniques provide preliminary information on the possible metabolites formed from a given compound, but the results can be misleading if projected to an intact animal. From a qualitative point of view, some biotransformation products formed *in vitro* may not be formed to an appreciable extent in the whole animal. In addition, the quantitative aspects of the rates of biotransformation in the whole animal are difficult to determine from *in vitro* studies alone. Important characteristics of the behavior of a compound in the intact animal such as compartmentalization, bioaccumulation, persistence, and half-life are difficult, if not impossible, to determine by *in vitro* techniques alone. However, *in vitro* studies are extremely valuable for the study of enzymes that catalyze biotransformation reactions. It is known that certain chemical compounds inhibit or induce biotransformation enzymes and that these enzymes can also be affected by variables such as age, sex, temperature, and/or nutritional status. Since these enzymes determine the quantitative and qualitative aspects of chemical biotransformations, it is likely that their relative activities influence the toxicity of chemical compounds as well as the compounds' behavior in an organism with respect to bioaccumulation, persistence, and excretion.

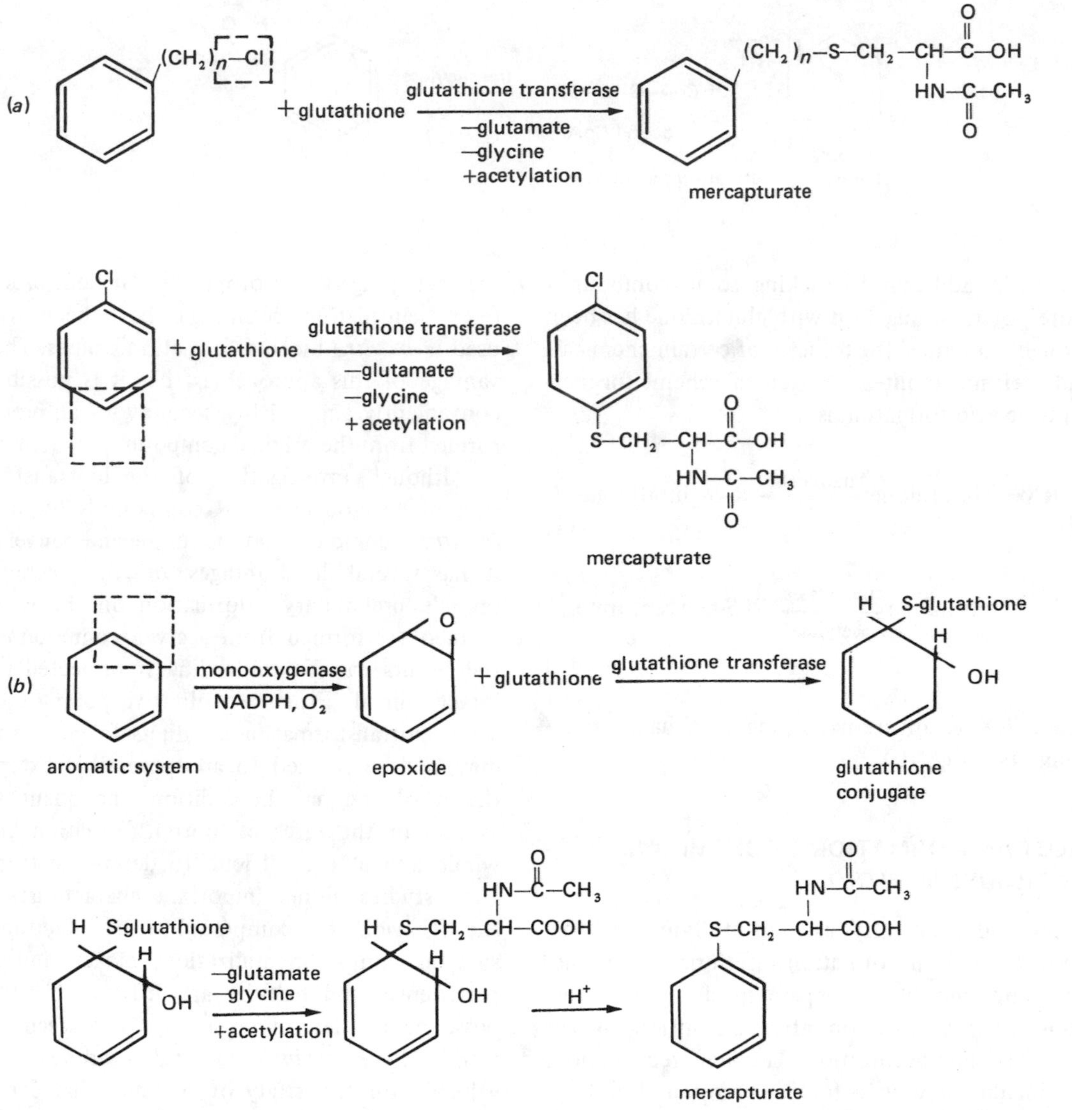

Figure 10 Formation of mercapturates with (a) halogenated organic compounds and (b) aromatic ring systems.

Prototype Monooxygenase Substrates

The activity of biotransformation enzymes has been studied with substrates that undergo specific functional group transformations which are conveniently measured analytically. A focal point for such studies in mammals and in several aquatic organisms, including fish, has been the development of prototype substrates for the measurement of cytochrome P-450–related monooxygenase activities in microsomes isolated from various tissues (Lu and Levin, 1974; Burke and Mayer, 1974). Substrates have also been developed for the assay of specific monooxygenase activities, since several forms of microsomal P-450–dependent monooxygenase enzymes may be present in tissues and these enzymes have a degree of substrate specificity (Lu and Levin, 1974; Burke and Mayer, 1974). Furthermore, since certain chemical compounds are capable of inducing different forms of cytochrome P-450–dependent monooxygenase enzymes with different substrate specificities, it is often desirable to study the types of monooxygenase activity in a particular tissue through the use of specific substrates. This concept will be discussed more completely later, but it is important to recognize that the choice of substrates is an important consideration in investigating both the levels of biotransformation enzymes in specific organs and the effect of altering these enzymes on the biotransformation pathway and toxicity of specific chemical compounds.

Several prototype substrates and the monooxygenase reaction measured by each substrate are shown in Fig. 11. The rate of an enzymatic reaction is determined by measuring the amount of product formed or quantity of substrate that has disappeared per unit time. Usually, with saturating levels of substrate, determination of the quantity of product formed is preferred. The results are usually expressed as micrograms, micromoles, or nanomoles of product formed per milligram or gram (wet weight) of liver (or amount of product formed per milligram of microsomal protein) per unit of time. In the dealkylation reactions illustrated in Fig. 11, although the immediate oxidation product may be an alcohol, an aldehyde is shown since the latter is often measured in some assay procedures (i.e., CH_3–OH versus $CH_2 = O$).

Levels of hepatic monooxygenase activities in marine species estimated by use of some of the prototype substrates are illustrated in Table 1. It should be noted that the enzyme activities vary considerably depending on the species and substrate used (Bend and James, 1979).

Table 2 shows the effects of various hepatic monooxygenase inducers on enzyme activities measured with the most commonly used prototype substrates. Substrates 1 and 2 in the table are specific for inducers of the phenobarbital class, and substrate 8 is specific for inducers that act like 3-methylcholanthrene (P-448-type inducers). On the other hand, substrates 3-7, which would show changes in enzyme activity, would lack specificity for the different types of inducers (Lech et al., 1983).

Table 3 shows the response of trout liver monooxygenase activity on prototype substrates to a variety of chemical compounds that are known to be monooxygenase inducers. Fish do not appear to be "inducible" by phenobarbital-type inducers, and this is illustrated by the lack of response to phenobarbital of enzyme activity measured with specific (EMD, BeND) and nonspecific (AHH, ECOD) prototype substrates (Lech et al., 1983; Addison et al., 1977; James and Bend, 1980).

Some industrial chemicals and pesticides, such as the Aroclors (polychlorinated biphenyls) and Firemaster (polybrominated biphenyls), induce biotransformation in mammals and fish. In mammals the induction is often referred to as "mixed type," since oxidations dependent on cytochrome P-450 and P-448 are induced as well as other pathways of xenobiotic transformation (Chambers and Yarbrough, 1979; Forlin, 1980). Freshwater and saltwater organisms are often exposed to many of these chemicals and pesticides in polluted waters. Aroclors 1242 and 1254, Firemaster BP6, and β-naphthoflavone all induce hepatic aryl hydrocarbon hydroxylase activity in fish. Ethoxycoumarin-O-deethylase and ethoxyresorufin-O-deethylase activities are also induced by Aroclors 1242 and 1254, Firemaster BP6, and β-naphthoflavone (Binder and Stegeman, 1980; Stegeman and Chevion, 1980; W. R. Penrose, personal communication).

Factors Influencing Monooxygenase Activity

The qualitative and quantitative aspects of biotransformation of specific chemical compounds have been shown to be influenced by a variety of factors, as measured by using prototype substrates *in vitro*. As would be expected from the literature on mammals, many variables affect the activity of

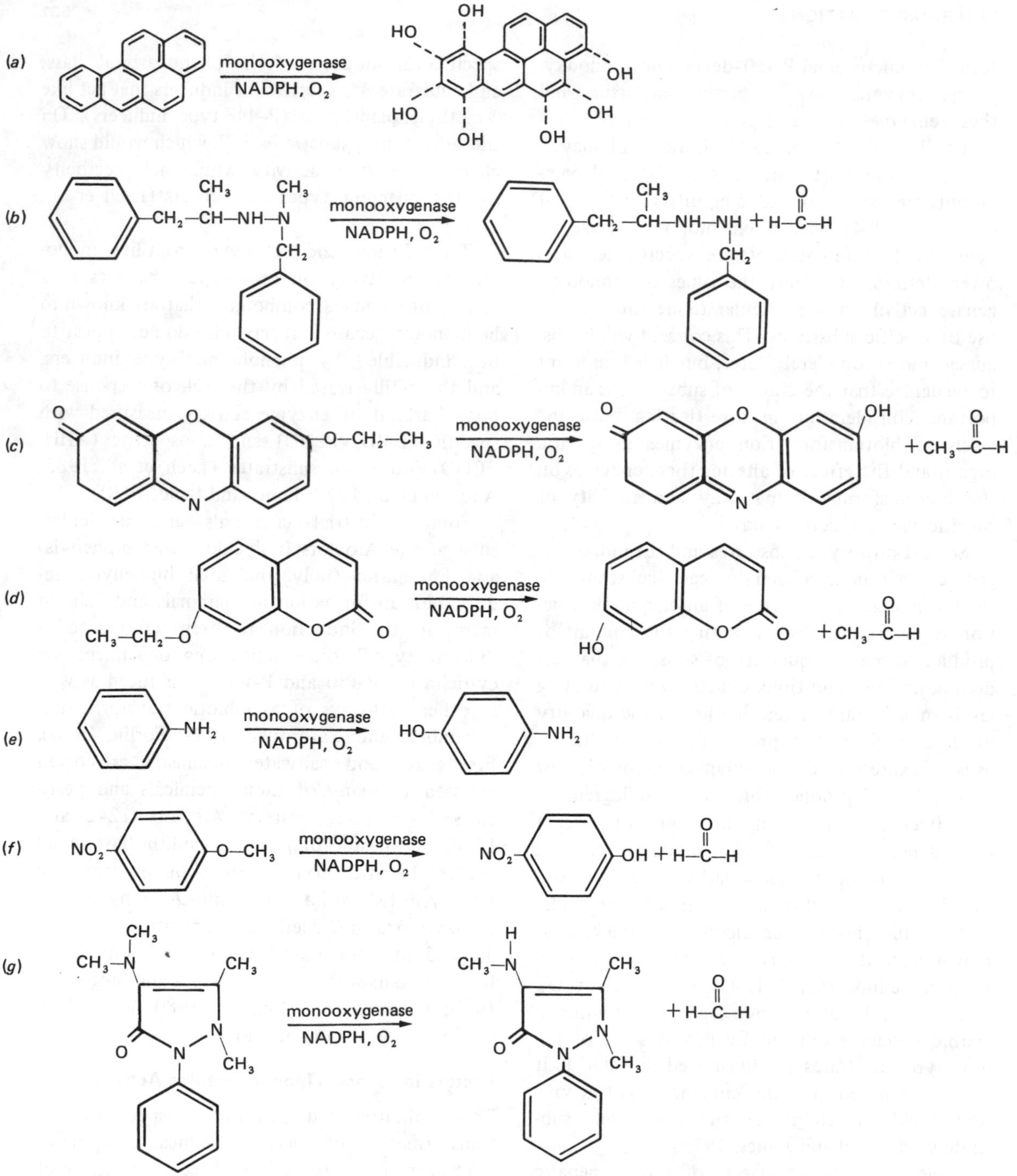

Figure 11 Monooxygenase reactions with prototype substrates: (a) benzo[a]pyrene hydroxylase (aryl hydrocarbon hydroxylase or AHH), (b) benzphetamine-N-demethylase (BeND), (c) ethoxy-coumarin-O-deethylase (ECOD), (d) ethoxyresorufin-O-deethylase (EROD), (e) aniline hydroxy-lase, (f) p-nitroanisole-O-demethylase, and (g) aminopyrine-N-demethylase.

Table 1 Hepatic Microsomal Cytochrome P-450-Dependent Monooxygenase Activity in Selected Marine Vertebrate Species with Several Substrates, Relative to the Rabbit[a]

Species	Temperature (°C)	Specific activity				
		Benzo[a]pyrene hydroxylase[b]	Benzphetamine demethylase[c]	7-Ethoxycoumarin deethylase[c]	Aldrin epoxidase[c]	Aniline hydroxylase[c]
Mangrove Snapper *Lutjanus griseus*	35	6.6	1.7	0.16	–	–
Killifish *Fundulus heteroclitus*	30	4.1	1.1	0.49	0.25	0.16
Winter flounder *Pseudopleuronectes americanus*	30	2.5	0.59	0.32	–	0.19
Black Drum *Pogonias cromis*	35	1.6	0.45	0.06	–	–
Sheepshead *Archosargus probatocephalus*	35	1.4	1.1	0.05	–	–
Atlantic stingray *Dasyatis sabina*	35	0.86	0.98	0.05	–	0.49
Large skate *Raja ocellata*	30	0.30	1.5	0.47	–	0.13
Eel *Anguilla rostrata*	30	0.21	0.44	0.89	–	0.12
Hagfish *Myxine glutinosa*	30	0.18	0.12	0.20	–	–
Bluntnose stingray *Dasyatis sayi*	35	0.17	0.23	N.D.[d] -0.01	–	0.56
Little skate *Raja erinacea*	30	0.17	1.1	0.32	–	–
Scup *Stenotomus versicolor*	30	0.13	–	–	–	–
Thorny skate *Raja radiata*	30	0.12	0.45	0.12	–	0.16
Dogfish shark *Squalus acanthias*	30	0.07	0.15	0.08	–	0.07
King of Norway *Hemitripterus americanus*	30	0.01	0.16	0.06	–	0.01
Rabbit	37	5.0	6.5	3.5	–	0.9

[a]From Bend and James (1979); copyright, Academic Press, Inc. (London) Ltd.
[b]Fluorescence units per minute per milligram of protein.
[c]Nanomoles per minute per milligram of protein.
[d]Non-detectable.

Table 2   Responses of Liver Monooxygenase Activities to Phenobarbital and 3-Methylcholanthrene[a]

Monooxygenase activity	Phenobarbital induction[b]	3-MC induction[b]
Benzphetamine-N-demethylase	+	−
Ethylmorphine-N-demethylase	+	−
Aniline hydroxylase	+	+
p-Nitroanisole-O-demethylase	+	+
Aminopyrine-N-demethylase	+	+
Arylhydrocarbon (benzo[a]pyrene) hydroxylase	+	+
Ethoxycoumarin-O-deethylase	+	+
Ethoxyresorufin-O-deethylase	−	+

[a]From Lech et al. (1983).
[b]+, increase in activity; −, no change or decrease.

biotransformation enzymes in fish tissues. Although these will be discussed briefly below, it should be recognized that very few of these variables have been investigated systematically for their influence on biotransformation rates and pathways during exposure of intact fish to selected chemicals.

Diet

Numerous studies in mammals have demonstrated that alterations in the dietary content of protein, carbohydrate, and fat can markedly influence drug and xenobiotic biotransformation, but few investigations have been carried out to examine the relationship between nutrient supply and monooxygenation reactions in aquatic organisms.

Earlier studies indicated that neither starvation nor alterations in protein or carbohydrate content of the diet affected drug-metabolizing reactions to any significant degree in the fish species studied (Dewaide, 1971). More recent evidence, however, suggests that increased dietary protein content de-

Table 3   Induction of Liver Microsomal Monooxygenase in Rainbow Trout[a]

Treatment of fish	Dose (mg/kg)	Activity (% of control)				
		EMD[b]	BeND[c]	AHH[d]	ECOD[e]	EROD[f]
Control (corn oil, 1 ml/kg)	−	100	100	100	100	100
Phenobarbital	65	81	ND[g]	104	64	65
Aroclor 1242	150	98	133	1059	808	1367
Aroclor 1254	150	105	49	1300	509	1460
FireMaster BP6	150	89	110	700	547	1564
β-Naphthoflavone	100	88	ND	4081	1178	4455

[a]Adapted from Lech et al. (1983).
[b]Ethylmorphine-N-demethylation.
[c]Benzphetamine-N-demethylation.
[d]Arylhydrocarbon (benzo[a]pyrene) hydroxylation.
[e]Ethoxycoumarin-O-deethylation.
[f]Ethoxyresorufin-O-deethylation.
[g]Not determined.

creases epoxide hydrolase, cytochrome c reductase, and aldrin epoxidase activities but elevates hepatic microsomal cytochrome P-450 content in rainbow trout. Trout fed cyclopropene fatty acids also showed depressed cytochrome c reductase and aldrin epoxidase activities with decreased cytochrome P-450 content. Furthermore, both treatment regimens resulted in alterations in the rate and route of microsomal metabolism of aflatoxin B_1, a potent hepatocarcinogen in rainbow trout (Loveland et al., 1979; Stott and Sinnhuber, 1978).

Because of the scarcity of information in this area, it is far too early to determine the role of dietary factors in normal metabolism or in the response of fish species to inducers of monooxygenase activity.

Season/Temperature/Photoperiod

Many aquatic species, notably those from temperate latitudes, are exposed to pronounced fluctuations in the environmental parameters associated with changing seasons. These environmental variations influence a variety of physiological functions. However, the correlation between seasonal changes in the environment and the rate and/or pattern of hepatic microsomal biotransformation has not been thoroughly investigated.

Early studies suggested that drug-metabolizing enzyme activities were significantly higher in the summer than in the winter in the wild roach (*L. rutilis*) (Dewaide, 1971), but this observation could not be correlated with temperature changes. Specifically, fish obtained in summer or winter and acclimated to 5°C had higher hepatic microsomal monooxygenase activity than those acclimated to 23°C. Similarly, killifish (*F. heteroclitus*) maintained in cold water had elevated monooxygenase activities compared to their warm-acclimated counterparts, but those exposed to 6.5°C did not respond to induction by benzo[*a*]-pyrene, while those maintained at 16.5°C had elevated hepatic microsomal aryl hydrocarbon hydroxylase activity and cytochrome P-450 content (Stegeman, 1979). The apparent lack of induction at low temperatures may have been

related to when the animals were killed after exposure to the inducer; investigations in the sheepshead (*A. probatocephalus*) indicated that although induction of monooxygenase activity was observed in all animals after administration of 3-methylcholanthrene, those killed in winter (14°C) responded more slowly to the inducer than those killed in summer (26°C) (James and Bend, 1980).

Contrary to what was described in the wild roach, hepatic microsomal monooxygenase activity in the mosquito fish (*G. affinis*) was reported to be greater in fall and winter than in summer (Chambers and Yarbrough, 1979), but environmental temperatures were not given. The possibility that species differences exist must also be considered.

A major difficulty in interpreting these data is in the lack of correlation of other factors that vary with season. For example, in temperate latitudes, dramatic photoperiod changes occur yearly, and the interaction between photoperiod and temperature affects a variety of physiological parameters. The photoperiod under which experimental fish are maintained is seldom reported, and whether photoperiod alone influences the hepatic microsomal monooxygenase system of these animals has not been investigated. Furthermore, the reproductive cyclicity exhibited seasonally in many fish species has been shown to be dependent on photoperiod-temperature interactions. The reproductive state of an animal may also influence monooxygenase activity (see below). Yearly changes have been observed in feeding behavior, resulting in variations in the ratio of liver weight to body weight. Thus, while monooxygenase activities per milligram of protein may vary, the animal's overall capacity for biotransformation may not be significantly affected.

Until each of these seasonally dependent variables has been examined methodically, it will not be possible to assess the effect of any one parameter on monooxygenase activity. However, in view of the fact that environmental conditioning modifies a number of metabolic, endocrine, and biochemical functions in poikilotherms, effects on biotransformation systems would certainly be anticipated.

Age

Although there do not appear to be pronounced differences in hepatic microsomal p-nitroanisole-O-demethylase and benzo[a]pyrene (BaP) hydroxylase activities or cytochrome P-450 content between 0.5-yr juvenile and 1.5-yr juvenile rainbow trout, significantly greater induction was observed in the older fish after treatment with Clophen A50 (PCBs) or 3-MC than in the younger animals (Forlin, 1980). Although these data suggest that more juvenile fish are less responsive to inducers of monooxygenase activity, it should be noted that hepatic and extrahepatic BaP hydroxylase activity could be induced in embryos of killifish exposed to PCBs (Binder and Stegeman, 1980), while basal levels in these animals were not detectable.

Sex

Sex differences have long been recognized to exist in the hepatic microsomal metabolism of many cytochrome P-450 substrates in mammals, with males having inherently higher enzymic activities than females. These differences in monooxygenase activity appear to be due, at least in part, to the action of sex steroid hormones.

Early studies in fish failed to show a sex-related difference in hepatic drug metabolism, possibly because of small sample sizes, substantial intraspecies variability, and/or the time in the reproductive cycle when the investigations were performed. More recently, it was shown that male rainbow and brook trout (S. fontinalis) have significantly higher hepatic microsomal cytochrome P-450 content and aminopyrine demethylase activity than females during the spawning season, although a sex difference was not observed in the activity of the NADPH-linked electron transport system as measured by NADPH–cytochrome c reductase activity (Stegeman and Chevion, 1980). Cytochrome P-450 content was also greater in kidney microsomes from male fish than from females. In addition, there was a pronounced dif-

ference between sexes in the response of hepatic microsomal BaP hydroxylase activity to in vitro inhibitors, suggesting a different form or forms of cytochrome P-450 in males and females. These differences were not significant in gonadally immature animals. Sex steroids appear to be involved in these phenomena, as in the mammalian system.

Preliminary data indicate that fish respond to inducers of monooxygenase activity differently depending on their reproductive condition at the time of exposure. Basal hepatic microsomal BaP hydroxylase activity and its inducibility by exposure to petroleum hydrocarbons were suppressed in male and female cunners (T. adsperus) during the prespawning and spawning seasons (W. R. Penrose, personal communication), when sex steroid levels presumably are high to promote spermatogenesis and vitellogenesis. The significance of this observation is not known, but it is of interest that various monooxygenase activities are reduced during pregnancy in mammals and that late-pregnant female rats become refractive to induction by various inducers. This decrease in monooxygenase activity may serve to ensure elevated steroid levels for the maintenance of pregnancy. While it is not possible to propose a common mechanism with respect to reproduction and monooxygenase activity in fish and mammals, the similarities noted are intriguing. Furthermore, the seasonal appearance of sex differences in prespawning and spawning fish suggests that they could be used as models for studying the regulation of sex steroid-dependent forms of cytochrome P-450.

Species and Strain

Strain and species differences have been recognized in the absorption, distribution, biotransformation, and excretion of xenobiotics among mammals, resulting in substantial differential toxicities of and susceptibilities to these chemical compounds.

Experiments in six geographically and genetically distinct strains of rainbow trout suggest that enzyme activities and kinetics differ with strain (Pedersen et al., 1976). Environment may thus influence gene expression, since basal monooxygenase activities were, in general, positively correlated with degree of pollution in areas where the individual strains were developed. The capacity for induction of these activities also appeared to be strain-dependent.

In another investigation (Chambers and Yarbrough, 1979), no significant differences were noted between insecticide-resistant and -susceptible strains of mosquito fish when hepatic microsomal cytochrome P-450 content and components of the NADPH-dependent electron transport system were compared. Whether specific enzyme activities differed, however, was not considered. Resistant fish had higher ratios of liver weight to body weight, and thus overall biotransformation capacity may have been greater than in the susceptible strain.

It must be emphasized that fish strains obtained from different locations or suppliers may differ because of the environmental or rearing conditions to which they were exposed just before the studies above. Therefore, it cannot be concluded that the observed differences are due to genetically determined factors alone. Furthermore, whether any of these animals may have had induced monooxygenase activities in the wild must be considered.

With respect to species differences in hepatic biotransformation systems, there have been no comprehensive studies of a broad range of parameters in a wide variety of aquatic species. While many species have been examined by many laboratories, overall comparisons are difficult to make because of differences in methodology (i.e., substrates chosen for study, dose regimens and routes of administration, environmental conditions, age, sex, etc.).

It does appear that basal enzyme activities, cytochrome P-450 content, and inducibility of the hepatic microsomal monooxygenase system can differ considerably among aquatic species. In a comparison of a number of marine fish species, basal cytochrome P-450 content ranged from 0.009–0.69 nmol per milligram of microsomal protein, with an average value of approximately 0.30 nmol/mg, and the inducibility of the monooxygenase system by various polycyclic aromatic hydrocarbons, as determined by aryl hydrocarbon hydroxylase activity, ranged from zero to 50-fold (Bend and James, 1979). However, species differences in substrate specificity have been demonstrated in induced fish, and it cannot be assumed from a lack of response in one assay system that these animals were incapable of responding to the inducers.

While only a few comparisons have been made, it appears that basal biotransformation rates and inducibility of the monooxygenase system among aquatic invertebrates are species-dependent as well. However, more studies of invertebrate systems are needed before conclusions can be drawn on the effects of environmental, physiological, or genetic factors on biotransformation rates and induction.

Finally, it must be reemphasized that the environmental conditions to which the experimental animals were exposed before and during these investigations and the physiological state of the animal can have profound effects on the biotransformation systems under study. Until each of these variables has been examined systematically, it is not possible to evaluate the contribution of any one parameter on constitutive monooxygenase activities or their inducibility.

BIOTRANSFORMATION OF CHEMICAL COMPOUNDS IN INTACT ORGANISMS

Little information is available on the qualitative and quantitative aspects of the biotransformation of specific chemicals in intact organisms other than that available from *in vitro* studies. It is important that intact animals be used in studies of the rates and pathways of biotransformation of chemicals, since *in vitro* studies may often yield products different from those in intact animals. For instance, an *in vitro* study may indicate that a certain chemical is converted to a specific product, but during an actual exposure, the chemical may not be taken up appreciably by the organism under study. In such a case, even if the *in vitro* study indicated that the chemical was extensively biotransformed, lack of availability of the chemical to the biotransformation enzyme systems would preclude biotransformation.

Another factor affecting uptake of a chemical is the route of administration of the compound, even in a study with intact animals. Depending on the goals of the experimental design, the chemical may be administered by water exposure, dietary intake, or interperitoneal injection. For chemicals that are absorbed into most tissues by all exposure routes, the route of administration may not be important. However, if there are differences in uptake based on route of administration, data obtained may not be valid for all other exposure routes.

In addition to exposure design, other contributing factors within the organism may influence the overall pathway and rate of biotransformation. These factors include tissue compartmentalization and lipophilicity, extent of plasma protein binding of the compound, and the rate at which certain compounds are excreted by mechanisms unrelated to biotransformation (LaDu et al., 1971). For example, fish have active excretory transport systems for organic acids, and excretion of certain organic acids by these routes into the urinary or biliary compartment may proceed at rates that can effect rapid clearance of the compounds with little transformation. This applies equally to chemicals that are rapidly excreted via the gill by simple diffusion processes. Although there is less information on the biotransformation of specific chemicals in intact organisms than in *in vitro* preparations, it is now apparent that most of the prototype reactions observed in fish *in vitro* occur with specific chemicals in intact fish (Khan et al., 1979); representative examples are shown in Table 4.

The nature of these biotransformation reactions is best illustrated in terms of specific chemicals, as shown in Figs. 12–14. From the discussion in the

Table 4 Biotransformation Reactions Demonstrated in Fish *in Vivo*[a]

Reaction	Species	Compound
Glycine, glucuronide conjugation	Flounder, goosefish	Aminobenzoic acid
Glucuronide conjugation	Rainbow trout	3-Trifluoromethyl-4-nitrophenol
	Rainbow trout	Pentachlorophenol
Taurine conjugation	Flounder	2,4-D
Sulfate conjugation	Goldfish	Pentachlorophenol
Glutathione conjugation	Carp	Molinate
Hydrolysis	Catfish, bluegills	2,4-D esters
	Rainbow trout	Diethylhexyl phthalate
	Pinfish	Malathion
Acetylation	Dogfish shark	Ethyl *m*-aminobenzoate
	Rainbow trout	Ethyl *m*-aminobenzoate
Oxidation	Mudsucker, sculpin	Naphthalene, benzo[*a*]pyrene
	Coho salmon	Naphthalene
	Rainbow trout	Methylnaphthalene
	Carp	Rotenone
	Bluegills	4-(2,4-DB)
	Mosquito fish	Aldrin, dieldrin
O-Dealkylation	Fathead minnow	*p*-Nitrophenyl ethers
	Rainbow trout	Pentachloroanisole
	Rainbow trout	Fenitrothion
N-Dealkylation	Carp	Dinitramine

[a]From Lech and Bend (1980).

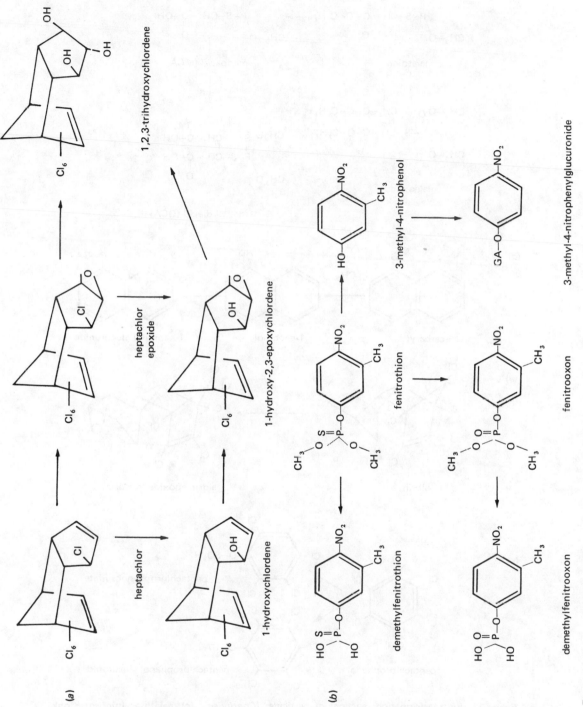

Figure 12 Biotransformation reactions of pesticides: (*a*) heptachlor (goldfish) (Khan et al., 1979), (*b*) fenitrothion (rainbow trout) (Khan et al., 1979).

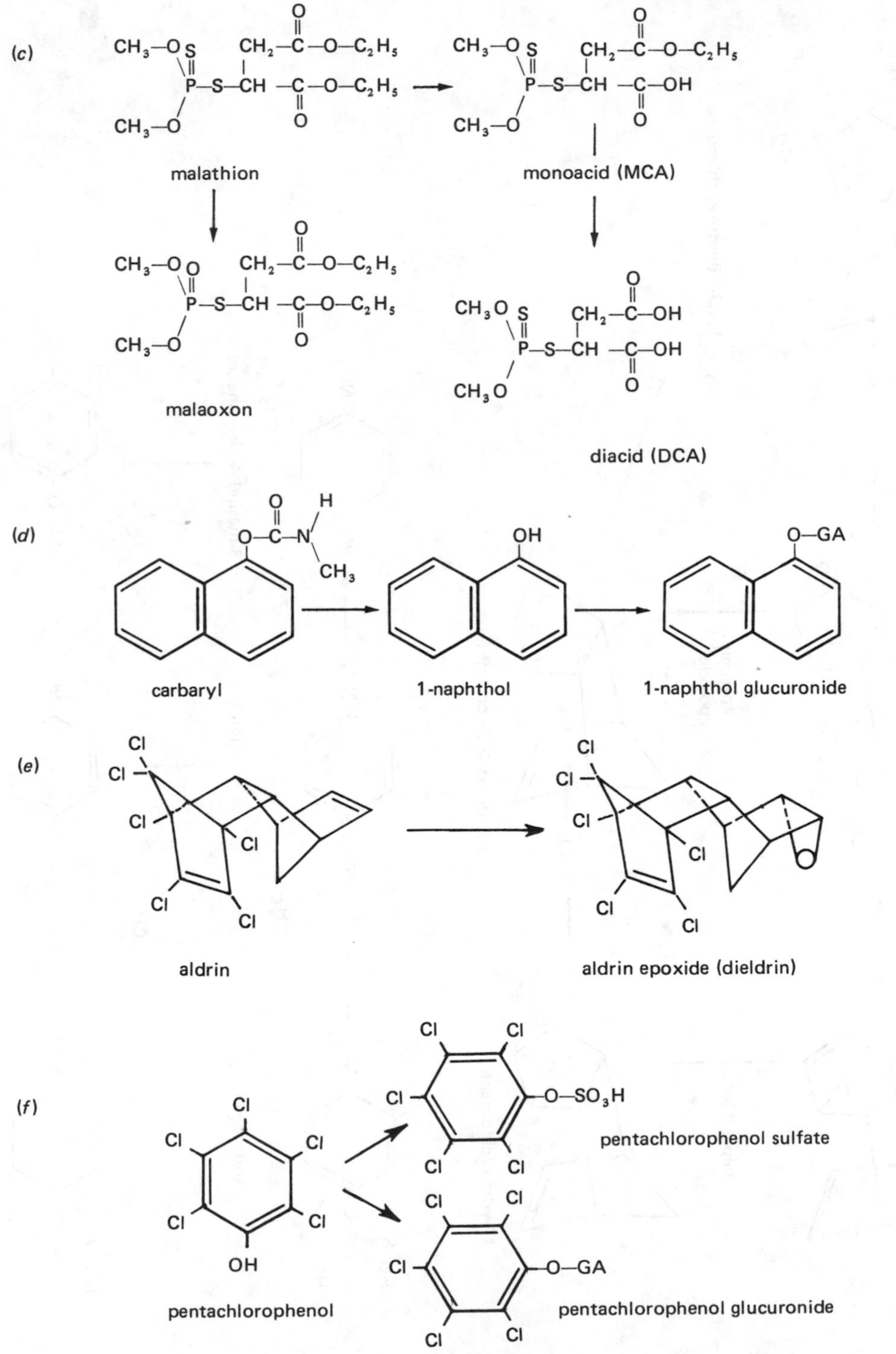

Figure 12 Biotransformation reactions of pesticides (*Continued*): (*c*) malathion (pinfish) (Cook and Moore, 1976), (*d*) carbaryl (rainbow trout) Statham and Lech, 1975), (*e*) aldrin (mosquito fish and midge) (Khan et al., 1979), and (*f*) pentachlorophenol (rainbow trout and goldfish) (Khan et al., 1979; Glickman et al., 1977).

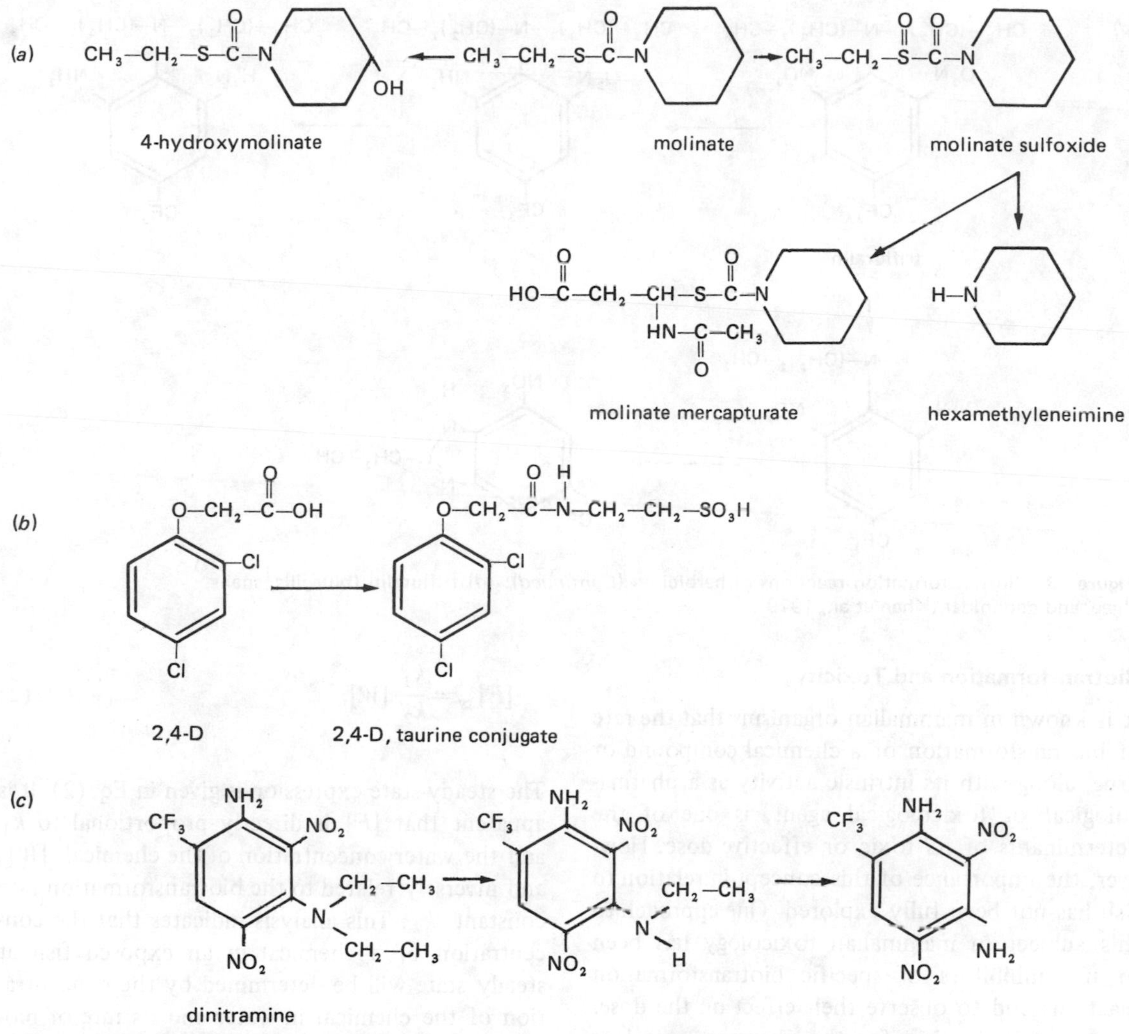

Figure 13 Biotransformation reactions of herbicides: (a) molinate (carp) (Khan et al., 1979), (b) 2,4-dinitrophenoxyacetic acid (2,4-D) (flounder) (James and Bend, 1976), (c) dinitramine (carp) (Khan et al., 1979).

section on biotransformation of chemicals *in vitro*, one should be able to identify the type of reaction and the functional groups involved.

SIGNIFICANCE OF BIOTRANSFORMATION

The enzymatic conversion of a xenobiotic chemical compound to another chemical entity within a living organism can have striking effects on its physical-chemical, pharmacokinetic, and toxicological properties. Depending on the compound, biotransformation processes may thus influence residue patterns and dynamics, bioaccumulation potential, and the intrinsic toxicity of a chemical. In the following discussion, examples from the literature will be used to illustrate how biotransformation reactions affect these parameters.

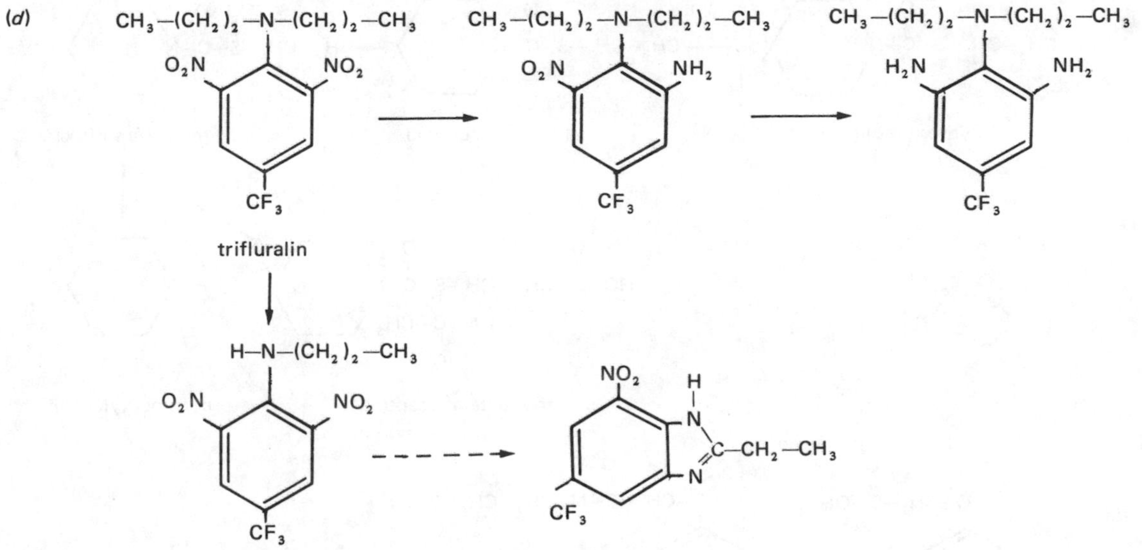

Figure 13 Biotransformation reactions of herbicides (*Continued*): (*d*) trifluralin (bluegills, snails, algae, and daphnids) (Khan et al., 1979).

Biotransformation and Toxicity

It is known in mammalian organisms that the rate of biotransformation of a chemical compound or drug, along with its intrinsic activity as a pharmacological or toxicological agent, is one of the determinants of its toxic or effective dose. However, the importance of this concept in relation to fish has not been fully explored. One approach to this subject in mammalian toxicology has been to use inhibitors of specific biotransformation reactions and to observe their effect on the dose-response relationship for the pharmacological or toxicological agent under consideration.

Equation (1) is a simplified expression for the rate of change of a chemical in an exposed fish, $[F]$. It assumes a first-order rate constant, k_1, for uptake and another, k_2, for removal by, for example, biotransformation.

$$\frac{d[F]}{dt} = k_1 [W] - k_2 [F] \tag{1}$$

$$[F] = \frac{k_1}{k_2} [W](1 - e^{-k_2 t})$$

$$[F]_{ss} = \frac{k_1}{k_2} [W] \tag{2}$$

The steady-state expression is given in Eq. (2). It is apparent that $[F]$ is directly proportional to k_1 and the water concentration of the chemical, $[W]$, and inversely related to the biotransformation rate constant, k_2. This analysis indicates that the concentration of a chemical in an exposed fish at steady state will be determined by the concentration of the chemical in water and its rate of biotransformation by the fish. One could predict, then, that perturbation of the rate of biotransformation of a chemical should affect its LC50, and the extent to which the LC50 is changed should reflect the toxicological significance of the metabolic pathway of the chemical. For illustration only, one process ($k_2 [F]$) was used for elimination; however, there are at least two processes, which will be discussed later.

Several studies with inhibitors of biotransformation have been done with fish, and the results indicate that glucuronide conjugation and sulfoxide formation in rainbow trout and mosquito fish, respectively, may be rapid enough to significantly affect the toxicity of certain chemicals (Lech, 1974; Ludke et al., 1972). Figure 15 illustrates the effect of salicylamide, an inhibitor of glucuronide formation, on the acute toxicity of 3-trifluoromethyl-4-nitrophenol (TFM, Lamprecid) in fingerling rainbow trout. Salicylamide alone at 25 mg/l had no effect on the test fish but decreased the LC50 of the phenol to approximately one-third of the control value.

One can conclude from this that glucuronide formation proceeds rapidly enough to be a significant factor in the acute toxicity of this phenol to rainbow trout. A similar phenomenon has been described in mosquito fish with the monooxygenase inhibitor, sesamex and the organophosphorus, insecticide parathion. Current evidence indicates that parathion must be activated by monooxygenases to paraoxon, which is the active cholinesterase inhibitor. It follows that the magnitude of toxicity of parathion is directly related to its rate of activation as well as inactivation. Figure 16 shows that when mosquito fish were pretreated with 2 mg/l sesamex for 24 h, the 48-h LC50 for parathion was increased from 0.11 to 1.2 mg/l. Although the LC50 curves shown in

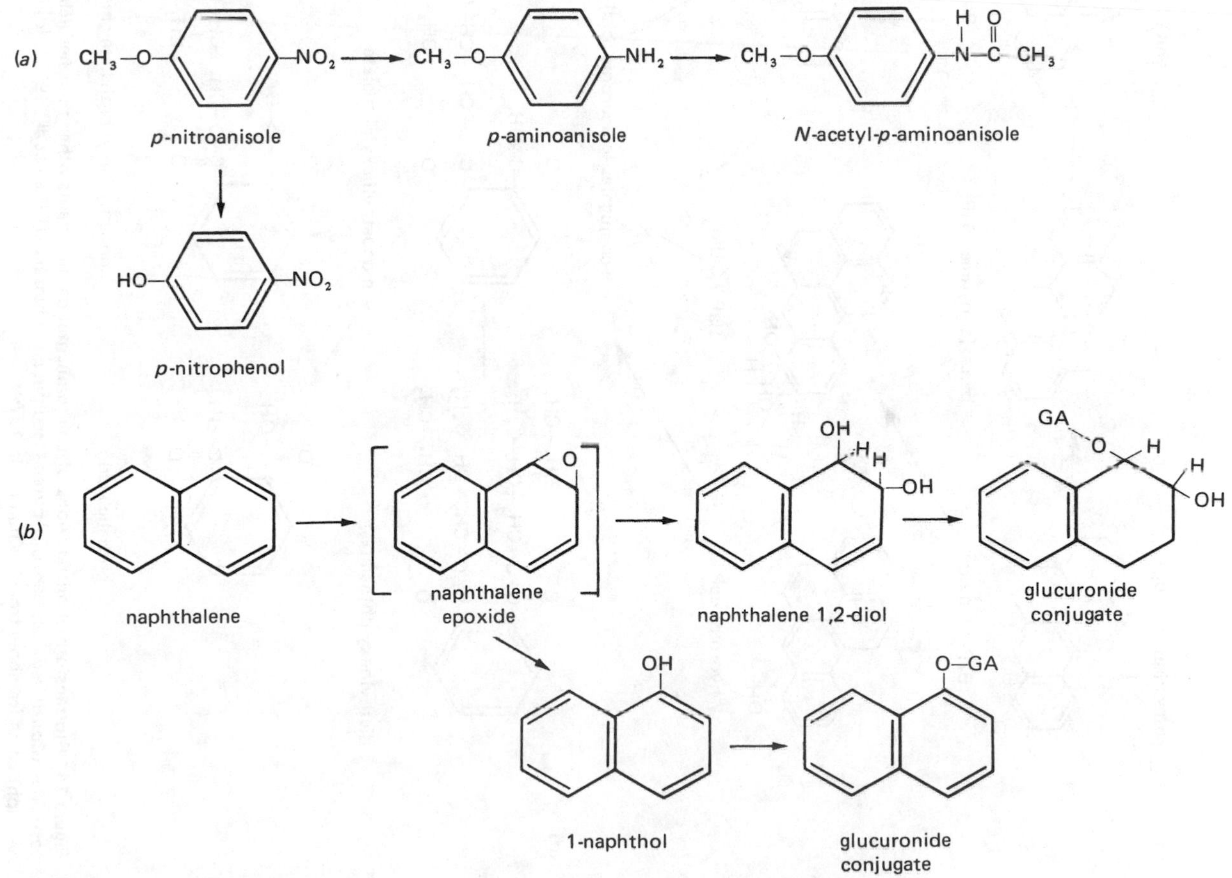

Figure 14 Biotransformation reactions of environmental contaminants other than herbicides and pesticides: (a) p-nitroanisole (sea urchin) (Khan et al., 1979), (b) naphthalene (coho salmon) (Khan et al., 1979).

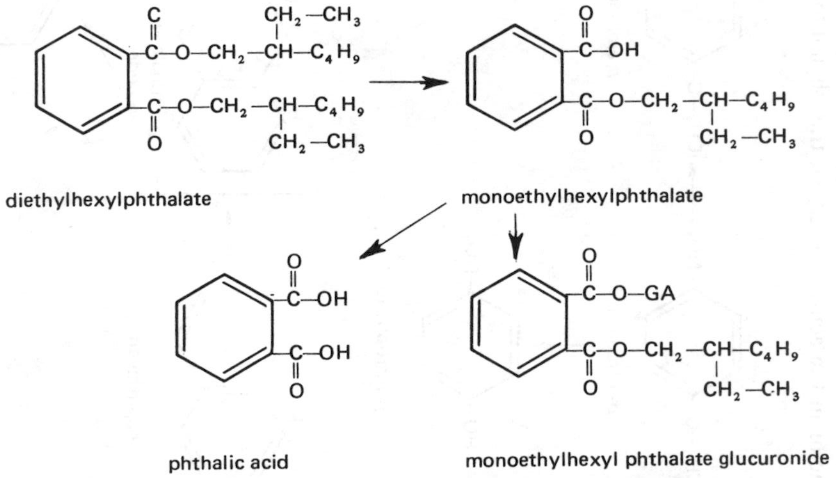

Figure 14 Biotransformation reactions of environmental contaminants other than herbicides and pesticides (*Continued*): (*c*) benzo[*a*]pyrene (sculpin and mudsucker) (Lee et al., 1972), (*d*) diethylhexylphthalate (rainbow trout) (Khan et al., 1979).

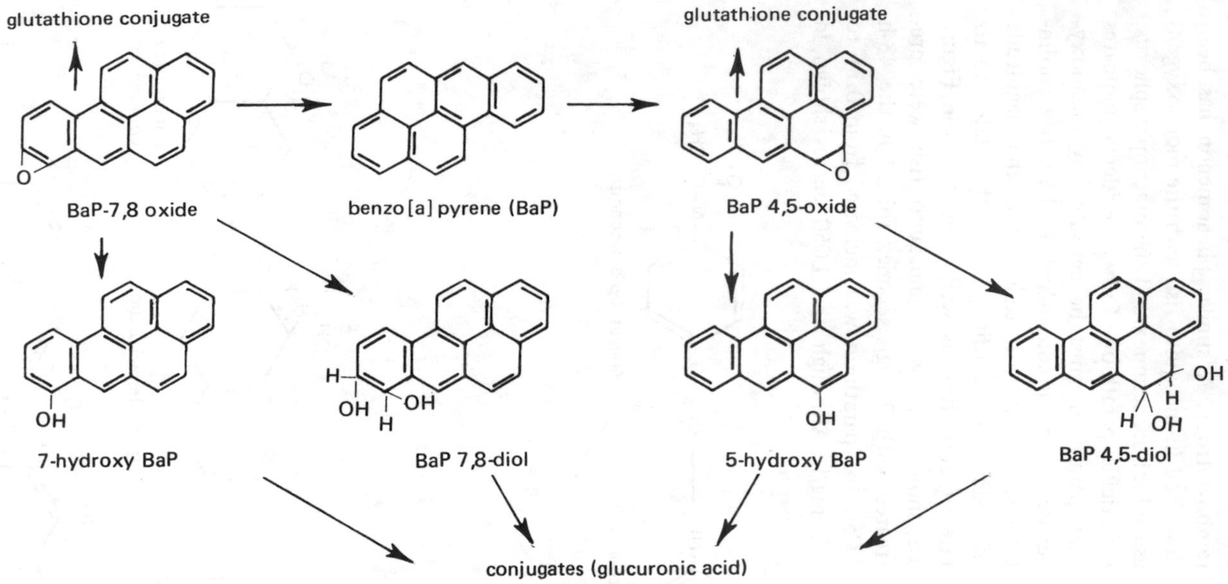

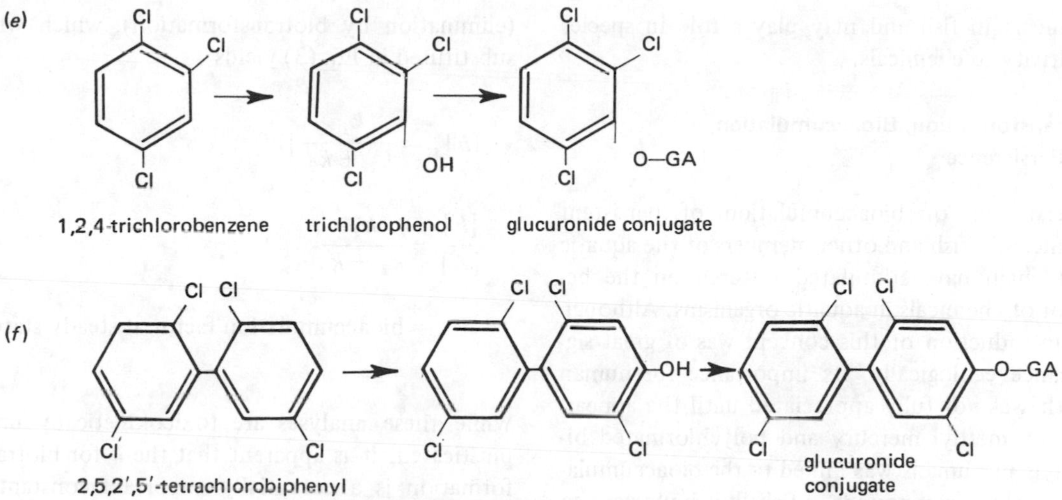

(e)

1,2,4-trichlorobenzene   trichlorophenol   glucuronide conjugate

(f)

2,5,2′,5′-tetrachlorobiphenyl

glucuronide
conjugate

Figure 14 Biotransformation reactions of environmental contaminants other than herbicides and pesticides (*Continued*): (*e*) trichlorobenzene (rainbow trout) (Melancon and Lech, 1980), and (*f*) tetrachlorobiphenyl (rainbow trout) (Melancon and Lech, 1976).

Fig. 16 are not parallel, which may indicate a further interaction of sesamex with parathion, the data show that sesamex did reduce the acute toxicity of parathion. Extracts of livers from fish pretreated with sesamex activated little or no parathion, while similar extracts from untreated fish produced enough paraoxon to inhibit 60% of brain cholinesterase activity.

In addition to the effect of biotransformation

on the acute toxicity of chemicals to fish, hepatic monooxygenase activity, which has been well characterized (Ahokas et al., 1977; Stegeman et al., 1979), has been implicated in the biotransformation of aflatoxin B_1 to an active hepatic carcinogen in rainbow trout (Schoenhard et al., 1976). Although studies of this type are rare in fish, these examples show that biotransformation may be an important determinant of the toxicity of certain

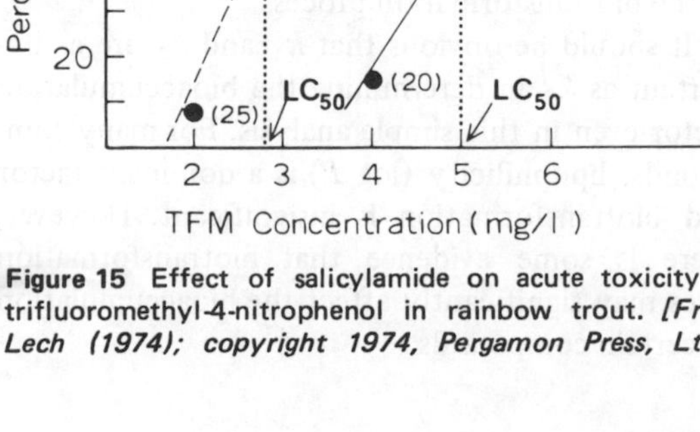

Figure 15 Effect of salicylamide on acute toxicity of trifluoromethyl-4-nitrophenol in rainbow trout. [*From Lech (1974); copyright 1974, Pergamon Press, Ltd.*]

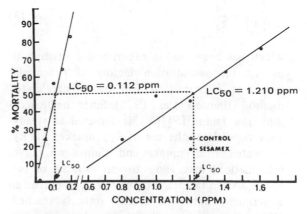

Figure 16 Effect of sesamex on acute toxicity of parathion to mosquito fish. [*From Ludke et al. (1972).*]

chemicals in fish and may play a role in species sensitivity to chemicals.

Biotransformation, Bioaccumulation, and Persistence

Observations of bioaccumulation of persistent chemicals in fish and other members of the aquatic food chain have stimulated research on the behavior of chemicals in aquatic organisms. Although the introduction of this concept was of great significance ecologically, its importance for human health was not fully appreciated until the appearance of methyl mercury and polychlorinated biphenyls in humans was linked to the bioaccumulation of these compounds in fish. It is important to recognize, however, that while bioaccumulation is important in terms of the magnification of certain chemicals within food chains, it is not the sole determinant of the hazard of chemicals to aquatic species, and therefore bioaccumulation and persistence are not necessarily synonymous with toxicity.

While bioaccumulation and persistence have often been treated as a physical-chemical problem, it is obvious from the mammalian literature that the role of biotransformation as a determinant of persistence and bioaccumulation cannot be ignored. A modification of Eq. (2) yields a form

$$\frac{[F]}{[W]} = \frac{k_1}{k_2} \tag{3}$$

which has been used in experimental attempts to predict bioconcentration factors of potentially persistent chemicals in fish by an accelerated method (Branson et al., 1975). Since the bioaccumulation factor $[F]/[W]$ is achieved at steady-state conditions, the use of k_1, (uptake) and k_2, calculated from uptake and elimination curves (elimination) may allow for an estimate of bioaccumulation factors without having to extend an experiment until the steady state is reached. Often, k_2 is composed of at least two constants: k_2 (excretion of unchanged molecule) and k_3

(elimination by biotransformation), which when substituted in Eq. (3) yields

$$[F]_{ss} = \frac{k_1}{k_2 + k_3} [W] \tag{4}$$

$$\frac{[F]}{[W]} = \frac{k_1}{k_2 + k_3}$$

= bioaccumulation factor at steady state
$$\tag{5}$$

While these analyses are toxicokinetically unsophisticated, it is apparent that the k for biotransformation is a potentially important constant in the determination of the bioaccumulation factor [Eq. (5)].

$$t_{1/2} = \frac{0.69}{k}$$

$$k = k_2 + k_3$$

$$\frac{[F]}{[W]} = \frac{k t_{1/2}}{0.69} \tag{6}$$

In addition, since the half-life ($t_{1/2}$) is equal to $0.69/k$ for a first-order elimination reaction, the relationship between the half-life of a compound and its bioaccumulation factor should become apparent [Eq. (6)]. As mentioned earlier, if this concept is valid, perturbations in the biotransformation rate should be accompanied by changes in the bioaccumulation factor, and the magnitude of the changes should reflect the relative importance of the biotransformation process.

It should be obvious that k_1 and k_2 are as important as k_3 in determining the bioaccumulation factor even in this simple analysis. For many compounds, lipophilicity (log P) is a dominant factor and biotransformation is insignificant. However, there is some evidence that biotransformation rates may significantly affect the bioaccumulation of certain compounds.

In a series of short- and long-term exposures of various organisms to BaP in a mixed aquatic ecosystem in the laboratory, it was found that BaP was rapidly metabolized by mosquito fish and slowly metabolized by snails (Lu et al., 1977). The data in Table 5 show the bioaccumulation factors for BaP by these species in an aquatic system for 3 d and an aquatic terrestrial ecosystem after 33 d.

The data indicate that the bioaccumulation factor in mosquito fish was much lower than that in snails in both systems, and the higher values in mosquito fish after 33 d in the ecosystem could be attributed to food web biomagnification. Inclusion of the monooxygenase inhibitor, piperonyl butoxide, in both systems increased the bioaccumulation factor considerably in the mosquito fish, where metabolism of BaP was most rapid, but had little effect in the snail. It is interesting that although piperonyl butoxide increased the bioaccumulation factor in the mosquito fish, presumably by inhibiting biotransformation, the bioaccumulation factor in the snail was much higher than that in the mosquito fish despite the "equalization" of the rates of metabolism of BaP by the inhibitor. Although several explanations are possible for this occurrence, the lipid solubility of the chemical and lipid content of the organism must be considered along with biotransformation in analysis of bioaccumulation.

Biotransformation and Residues

It has been established that biotransformation of xenobiotic chemicals occurs in aquatic species in vivo. The implications of this observation should be considered with regard to monitoring and residue analysis protocols. While these activities may have a common base analytically, the purposes for which they are done may be quite diverse. Data from residue analyses may be used in ecological studies to survey chemical residue levels in aquatic organisms from a particular area in order to evaluate the impact of toxicant-induced insult. They may also be used to determine the suitability of tissues of aquatic species for human or animal consumption. Most analytical methods for monitoring are designed to look for specific xenobiotic chemicals, and little attention is given to the design of the analysis to determine levels of biotransformation products. While in many cases the former approach will suffice and will indicate how much of a specific chemical is in an organism, it has limitations for chemicals that are rapidly biotransformed. It also does not consider that some biotransformation products may be more toxic than the starting chemicals. This point is illustrated with data shown in Table 6. The information in Table 6 is from a study in which pinfish (L. rhomboides) were exposed to 75 μg/l malathion in seawater for 24 h (Cook and Moore, 1976). After exposure, various organs were excised and analyzed for malathion and its possible biotransformation products. Malathion, being an ester, can be metabolized by hydrolytic pathways, and its cleavage gives rise to a carboxylic acid and an alcohol. The information in Table 6 indicates that although the fish were exposed to malathion, the analytical

Table 5   Bioaccumulation of Benzo[a]pyrene in Aquatic Systems[a]

Exposure	Aquatic system (3 d)[b]		Aquatic terrestrial ecosystem (33 d)[b]	
	Mosquito fish	Snail	Mosquito fish	Snail
Benzo[a]pyrene	<1	2177	30	4860
Benzo[a]pyrene plus piperonyl butoxide	22	3056	140	7520

[a]Data from Lu et al. (1977).
[b]Numbers indicate organism/water benzo[a]pyrene ratios at the end of the stated time periods.

Table 6 Concentrations of Malathion, Malaoxon, MCA, and DCA in Organs of Pinfish Exposed to 75 μg/l Malathion in Flowing Seawater for 24 h[a]

Organ	Malathion (μg/g)	Malaoxon (μg/g)	MCA[c] (μg/g)	DCA[d] (μg/g)
Brain	ND[b]	ND[b]	1.7	0.22
Liver	ND	ND	6.0	0.25
Gills	ND	ND	2.5	0.36
Flesh	ND	ND	3.9	0.34
Gut	ND	ND	31.4	0.7

[a]Data from Cook and Moore (1976); copyright 1976, American Chemical Society.
[b]ND, not detectable (<0.10 μg/g).
[c]Malathion monocarboxylic acid.
[d]Malathion dicarboxylic acid.

methods used did not detect malathion or its oxidation product malaoxon in various tissues of the pinfish. However, the hydrolysis products MCA and DCA, which are much more polar than the parent compound, were present in detectable amounts. If only malathion was measured in this study, the results would indicate that the fish did not contain malathion. However, the presence of malathion metabolites indicates that the fish were probably exposed to malathion. It is apparent from this example that the purpose for which a residue analysis study is done should determine whether the methods will be designed to include both the parent compound and the biotransformation products or only the parent compound.

Since a variety of biotransformation reactions have been shown to occur in aquatic species *in vivo*, it can be expected that chemical compounds will give rise to a spectrum of biotransformation products which may behave differently from the parent. Consideration should be given to biotransformation pathways in the design of residue analysis protocols, and the procolols, of course, must be matched to the overall goals of the monitoring activity.

SUMMARY

Studies over the past 10 years have indicated that, like mammals and birds, many species of fish are capable of biotransforming a variety of chemicals. The earliest studies, carried out with fish tissue fractions and model substrates *in vitro*, demonstrated phase I and phase II biotransformation reactions, although the absolute enzyme activity varied considerably among species. These studies indicated that fish can biotransform a variety of substrates, but the rates observed were generally lower than those in many mammalian species. Monooxygenase activity associated with isolated hepatic microsomes of several species of fish was found to be sensitive to inhibition by carbon monoxide and to mammalian monooxygenase modulators such as α-naphthoflavone and metyrapone.

A reasonable amount of evidence indicates that phase I reactions observed in fish *in vitro* are catalyzed by the microsomal cytochrome P-450 system, which has been extensively investigated in mammals. Although the purification and characterization of cytochrome P-450 from fish tissues have not approached the sophistication attained with mammalian systems, it appears that the substrate specificities are similar to those in mammalian systems. Benzphetamine-*N*-demethylase and ethylmorphine-*N*-demethylase activities have been observed in hepatic microsomes of fish, indicating that a system comparable to the cytochrome P-450 system of mammals exists in fish, although it appears to be refractive to induction by drugs and chemicals that produce phenobarbital-type induction in mammals. On the other hand, monooxygenase activity toward ethoxyresorufin (de-ethylation), a highly specific substrate for the polycyclic aromatic hydrocarbon–inducible (3-MC) form of cytochrome P-450 designated as cytochrome P_1-450 (P-448), was found in hepatic microsomes from several species of fish. This latter form of P-450 is inducible by 3-MC and other inducers of this class, including β-naphthoflavone,

BaP, and several coplanar PCB and PBB isomers. Phase II reactions have been demonstrated *in vitro* with tissue preparations from a variety of fish species, and it is clear that glucuronyl transferase, sulfotransferase, glutathione-*S*-transferase, and epoxide hydrolase activities are, at least qualitatively, similar to those in mammals. Although *in vitro* studies have been extremely useful in characterizing the enzymes involved in the biotransformation of chemicals in fish, an area of equal or greater importance is concerned with the functional significance of these biotransformation reactions *in vivo*. Almost every biotransformation reaction (phase I and phase II) that has been described *in vitro* in fish has been demonstrated *in vivo* during exposure of live fish to a variety of chemicals and pesticides. Metabolites arising from biotransformation reactions have been identified in fish tissues including liver, bile, and urine.

LITERATURE CITED

Addison RF, Zinck ME, Willis DE: Mixed function oxidase enzymes in trout (*Salvelinus fontinalis*) liver: Absence of induction following feeding of *p,p'*-DDT or *p,p'*-DDE. Comp Biochem Physiol C 57:39–43, 1977.

Ahokas JT, Pelkonen O, Karki NT: Characterization of benzo(a)pyrene hydroxylase of trout liver. Cancer Res 37:3737–3743, 1977.

Bend JR, James MO: Xenobiotic metabolism in marine and freshwater species. Biochem Biophys Perspect Mar Biol 4:125–188, 1979.

Binder RL, Stegeman JJ: Induction of aryl hydrocarbon hydroxylase activity in embryos of an estuarine fish. Biochem Pharmacol 29:949–951, 1980.

Branson DR, Blau GE, Alexander HC, Neeley WD: Bioconcentration of 2,2',4,4'-tetrachlorobiphenyl in rainbow trout as measured by an accelerated test. Trans Am Fish Soc 104:785–789, 1975.

Burke MD, Mayer RT: Ethoxyresorufin: Direct fluorimetric assay of a microsomal *O*-dealkylation which is preferentially inducible by 3-methylcholanthrene. Drug Metab Dispos 2:583–588, 1974.

Chambers JE, Yarbrough JD: Xenobiotic biotransformation systems in fishes. Comp Biochem Physiol C 55:77–84, 1976.

Chambers JE, Yarbrough JD: A seasonal study of microsomal mixed-function oxidase components in insecticide-resistant and susceptible mosquitofish, *Gambusia affinis*. Toxicol Appl Pharmacol 48:497–507, 1979.

Cook GH, Moore JC: Determination of malathion, malaoxon, and mono- and dicarboxylic acids of malathion in fish, oyster, and shrimp tissue. Agric Food Chem 24:631–634, 1976.

Cooper DY, Levine S, Narasimhulu S, Rosenthal O, Estabrook RW: Photochemical action spectrum of the terminal oxidase of mixed function oxidase systems. Science 147:400–402, 1965.

Dewaide JH: Metabolism of xenobiotics, Ph.D. thesis, Univ. of Nijmegen, The Netherlands, 1971.

Forlin L: Effects of Clophen A50, 3-methylcholanthrene, Pregnenolone-16α-carbonitrile, and phenobarbital on the hepatic microsomal cytochrome P-450-dependent monooxygenase system in rainbow trout, *Salmo gairdneri*, of different age and sex. Toxicol Appl Pharmacol 54:420–430, 1980.

Gillette JR: Biochemistry of drug oxidation and reduction by enzymes in hepatic endoplasmic reticulum. Adv Pharmacol 4:219–261, 1966.

Glickman AH, Statham CN, Wu A, Lech JJ: Studies on the uptake, metabolism, and disposition of pentachlorophenol and pentachloroanisole in rainbow trout. Toxicol Appl Pharmacol 41:649–658, 1977.

Jakoby WB (ed): Enzymatic Basis of Detoxication, vols. 1 and 2. New York: Academic, 1980.

James MO, Bend JR: Taurine conjugation of 2,4-dichlorophenoxyacetic acid and phenylacetic acid in two marine species. Xenobiotica 6:393–398, 1976.

James MO, Bend JR: Polycyclic aromatic hydrocarbon induction of cytochrome P-450-dependent mixed-function oxidases in marine fish. Toxicol Appl Pharmacol 54:117–133, 1980.

Khan MAQ, Lech JJ, Menn JJ (eds): Pesticide and

Xenobiotic Metabolism in Aquatic Organisms. Washington, D.C.: American Chemical Society, 1979.

LaDu BN, Mandel HG, Way EL (eds): Fundamentals of Drug Metabolism and Drug Disposition. Baltimore: Waverly, 1971.

Lech JJ: Glucuronide formation in rainbow trout, effect of salicylamide on the acute toxicity, conjugation and excretion of 3-trifluoromethyl nitrophenol. Biochem Pharmacol 23:2403–2410, 1974.

Lech JJ, Bend JR: Relationship between biotransformation and the toxicity and fate of xenobiotic chemicals in fish. Environ Health Perspect 34:115–131, 1980.

Lech JJ, Vodicnik MJ, Elcombe CR: Induction of monooxygenase activity in fish. In: Aquatic Toxicology, edited by L Weber. New York: Raven, 1982, 107–148.

Lee RF, Sauerheber R, Dobbs GH: Uptake, metabolism and discharge of polycyclic aromatic hydrocarbons by marine fish. Mar Biol 17:201–208, 1972.

Loveland PM, Nixon JE, Pawlowski NE, Eisele TA, Libbey LM, Sinnhuber RO: Aflatoxin B_1 and aflatoxicol metabolism in rainbow trout (*Salmo gairdneri*) and the effects of dietary cyclopropene. J Environ Pathol Toxicol 2:707–718, 1979.

Lu AYH, Levin W: The resolution and reconstitution of the liver microsomal hydroxylation system. Biochim Biophys Acta 344:205–240, 1974.

Lu P, Metcalf RL, Plummer N, Mandel D: The environmental fate of three carcinogens: Benzo(a)pyrene, benzidine, and vinyl chloride evaluated in laboratory model ecosystems. Arch Environ Contam Toxicol 6:129–142, 1977.

Ludke JL, Gibson JR, Lusk CI: Mixed function oxidase activity in freshwater fishes: Aldrin epoxidation and parathion activation. Toxicol Appl Pharmacol 21:89–97, 1972.

Melancon MJ, Lech JJ: Isolation and identification of a polar metabolite of tetrachlorobiphenyl from bile of rainbow trout exposed to ^{14}C-tetrachlorobiphenyl. Bull Environ Contam Toxicol 15:181–188, 1976.

Melancon MJ, Lech JJ: Uptake, metabolism and

elimination of ^{14}C-labelled 1,2,4-trichlorobenzene in rainbow trout and carp. J Toxicol Environ Health 6:645–658, 1980.

Netter KJ: Inhibition of oxidative drug metabolism in microsomes. Pharmacol Ther 10:515–535, 1980.

Pedersen MG, Hershberger WK, Zachariah PK, Juchau MR: Hepatic biotransformation of environmental xenobiotics in six strains of rainbow trout (*Salmo gairdneri*). J Fish Res Board Can 33:666–675, 1976.

Schoenhard GL, Lee DJ, Howell SE, Pawlowski NE, Libbey LM, Sinnhuber RO: Aflatoxin B_1 metabolism to aflatoxicol and derivatives lethal to *Bacillus subtilis* GSY 1057 by rainbow trout (*Salmo gairdneri*) liver. Cancer Res 36:2040–2045, 1976.

Snyder R, Remmer H: Classes of hepatic microsomal mixed function oxidase inducers. Pharmacol Ther 7:203–244, 1979.

Statham CN, Lech JJ: Biliary excretion products of 1-[1-^{14}C]naphthyl-*N*-methylcarbamate (carbaryl) in rainbow trout. Drug Metab Dispos 3:400–406, 1975.

Stegeman JJ: Temperature influence on basal activity and induction of mixed function oxygenase activity in *Fundulus heteroclitus*. J Fish Res Board Can 36:1400–1406, 1979.

Stegeman JJ, Chevion M: Sex differences in cytochrome P-450 and mixed-function oxygenase activity in gonadally mature trout. Biochem Pharmacol 29:553–558, 1980.

Stegeman JJ, Binder RL, Orren A: Hepatic and extrahepatic microsomal electron transport components and mixed-function oxygenases in the marine fish *Stenotomus versicolor*. Biochem Pharmacol 28:3431–3439, 1979.

Stott WT, Sinnhuber RO: Dietary protein levels and aflatoxin B_1 metabolism in rainbow trout (*Salmo gairdneri*). J Environ Pathol Toxicol 2:379–388, 1978.

Tjessum K, Stegeman JJ: Improvement of reverse-phase high pressure liquid chromatographic resolution of benzo(a)pyrene metabolites using organic amines: Application to metabolites produced by fish. Anal Biochem 99:129–135, 1979.

Williams RT: Detoxication Mechanisms. New York: Wiley, 1947.

SUPPLEMENTAL READING

Bend JR, James MO: Xenobiotic metabolism in marine and freshwater species. Biochem Biophys Perspect Mar Biol 4:125–188, 1979.

Chambers JE, Yarbrough JD: Xenobiotic biotransformation systems in fishes. Comp Biochem Physiol 55C:77–84, 1976.

Dewaide JH: Metabolism of xenobiotics, Ph.D. thesis, Univ. of Nijmegen, The Netherlands, 1971.

Jakoby WB (ed): Enzymatic Basis of Detoxication, vols. 1 and 2. New York: Academic, 1980.

Khan MAQ, Lech JJ, Menn JJ (eds): Pesticide and Xenobiotic Metabolism in Aquatic Organisms. Washington, D.C.: American Chemical Society, 1979.

LaDu BN, Mandel HG, Way EL (eds): Fundamentals of Drug Metabolism and Drug Disposition. Baltimore: Waverly, 1971.

Lech JJ, Bend JR: Relationship between biotransformation and the toxicity and fate of xenobiotic chemicals in fish. Environ Health Perspect 34:115–131, 1980.

Netter KJ: Inhibition of oxidative drug metabolism in microsomes. Pharmacol Ther 10:515–535, 1980.

Snyder R, Remmer H: Classes of hepatic microsomal mixed function oxidase inducers. Pharmacol Ther 7:203–244, 1979.

Williams RT: Detoxication Mechanisms. New York: Wiley, 1947.

Chapter 19

Fate Modeling

L. A. Burns and G. L. Baughman

INTRODUCTION

Toxicological investigations are prompted by a need to evaluate the environmental and public health consequences of the use and release to the environment of chemical substances. The direct effects of chemicals on individual organisms can be investigated through toxicological laboratory studies. The severity of these effects is usually a function of the magnitude of the chemical concentration to which the organism has been exposed and of the duration of the exposure (Brown, 1978). Results of toxicological studies thus must be supplemented with a knowledge of the chemical exposures experienced by organisms resident in natural systems.

When a chemical has been released into the environment for many years, exposures can be determined by direct monitoring of receiving water bodies. Safety evaluations may be required, however, for chemicals that have not been released into the environment, or that have not been used in the geographic region of concern. In these cases, exposures must be estimated or predicted from the proposed uses and potential releases of the substance, and from the physical and chemical properties of the compound and of the environments likely to receive it.

Environmental fate models can be used to assemble chemical and environmental information into an objective mathematical description of the behavior of chemical substances in aquatic ecosystems. When this information is supplemented with a knowledge of potential or actual releases of chemicals to water bodies (loadings), the resulting exposure concentrations, magnitudes of the fate processes, and persistence of the chemical can be estimated in a quantitative, systematic framework.

Much of this information, when coupled with the results of toxicological investigations, is of direct utility in evaluating the risk or hazard posed by chemical releases to the environment.

As a chemical moves through a water body, chemical and biological processes transform it into new compounds. Fate models can be used to estimate the residual concentrations of the starting materials and the concentrations of the transformation products. These concentrations can be compared to the chemical concentrations that pose a danger to aquatic organisms. The comparison is one indication of the risk due to the presence of a chemical in natural systems or in drinking-water supplies. Expected environmental concentrations (EECs) or exposure levels in receiving water bodies are thus one component of a hazard evaluation.

Toxicological and ecological effects studies are of two kinds: (1) short-term or acute experiments and (2) longer-term or chronic experiments. Acute studies are often used to determine the concentration of a chemical that results in mortality of 50% of a test population over a period of hours to days. Chronic studies examine sublethal effects on populations exposed to lower concentrations over extended periods. An EEC that is 10 times less than the acute level does not show that aquatic ecosystems will not be affected; the probability of a chronic impact increases with exposure duration. The duration of the expected exposures and the persistence of chemicals are thus of direct interest in practical toxicological investigations.

A toxicologist should also know which populations are at risk. These can to some extent be deduced from the distribution or fate of the compound, that is, by an estimate of EECs in different spatial segments of the ecosystem. A computer program can be tailored to report a separate EEC for each segment and each local population used to define the system.

The concept of the fate of a chemical in an aquatic system has an additional, equally significant, meaning. Each transport or transformation process accounts for only part of the total behavior of a chemical, and the relative importance of each process varies a great deal among systems. The relative importance can be determined by performing a total mass balance of the chemical inputs. This indicates which process is dominant in the system and thus in greatest need of accurate and precise kinetic parameters. Overall dominance by transport processes may imply contamination of downstream systems, loss of significant amounts of the chemical to the atmosphere, or pollution of ground water aquifers. In addition, the relative weights of the transformation processes indicate which transformation products deserve separate toxicological studies.

Toxicological investigations, environmental chemistry, and ecological modeling can be successfully combined in a risk analysis or a hazard assessment only when practitioners in these disciplines agree on the scientific issues involved. This chapter introduces the tools and perspectives brought to risk assessment by chemistry, mathematical modeling, and systems analysis. It provides both an overview and a detailed exposition of some of the fundamental tools of environmental chemistry and modeling. Chemical hydrolysis and acid-base equilibria are used to analyze the kinetics of transformation processes, and the application of chemical fate models in toxicological investigations is demonstrated by the example of flow-through toxicity tests of a simple mixture.

TERMINOLOGY

$[C](t)$. Chemical concentration (denoted by square brackets) of a material C, usually as molarity (M, moles per liter), or mass per unit volume (e.g., mg/l), at a specified time t.

$[C](0)$. Chemical concentration at the beginning of an interval of interest (e.g., initiation of an experiment, initial release to a water body), where $t = 0$ (compare $[C](t)$).

Chemical loading (Lo). Rate of entry, in mass per unit time, of a chemical into a water body.

Coupling variable. Measurable property of the physical world, of significance at more than one level of organization. For example, the hydrogen ion concentration (or pH) of an aqueous solution is a measurable physical-chemical property of the solution and controls the rate of hydrolytic transformation of many chemicals. In a laboratory situation, pH can be constrained to a preselected value. In a natural system, $[H^+]$ can vary by a factor of 100 (2 pH units) over diel cycles. At the ecosystem level, pH is governed by the geological structure of the drainage basis, which controls the intrinsic buffer capacity of its surface waters, and by the photosynthetic and respiratory metabolism of the biota. By understanding the role of pH in chemical kinetics, measuring pH during laboratory investigations, and describing the pH of natural systems, this parameter can be used to couple the results of laboratory investigations to events in the field—hence the term coupling variable.

E. Factor in environment controlling rate of reaction. Units depend on the process. Examples include pH and pOH (or, more precisely, $[H^+]$ and $[OH^-]$), temperature, sunlight intensity, population density and activity of microorganisms, and concentration of reactive oxidants.

First-order. See reaction order.

[H$^+$]. Molar hydrogen ion concentration, moles per liter (M).

Hydraulic residence time. Time required for a single renewal (turnover) of aqueous volume in a water body, test tank, etc. Also called detention time, renewal time, turnover time, or simply residence time. Computed as V/q, where V is volume and q is discharge (volume per unit time). The hydraulic residence time of a real water body is, to a degree, only a theoretical construct, because the use of V/q in simple mathematical transport equations assumes that the water body is very well mixed. The concept is nonetheless useful as an indicator of the approximate time available for chemical and biological reactions during the transport of a chemical through a system.

Ionization fraction. Fraction of total chemical concentration present as a particular chemical species (neutral molecules, anions, cations) of an acid or base in aqueous solution.

K_{ah}. Second-order rate constant for specific-acid (H^+) catalyzed hydrolytic reactions, with units M^{-1} t^{-1} or $/M \cdot t$ ["per mole (H^+) per time," e.g., $/M \cdot s$].

K_{bh}. Second-order rate constant for specific-base (OH^-) catalyzed hydrolytic reactions, with units M^{-1} t^{-1} or $/M \cdot t$.

K_{obs}. Observed first-order (or pseudo-first-order) rate constant of a transformation process under fixed conditions, with units of reciprocal time (t^{-1} or $/t$).

K_{nh}. Pseudo-first-order rate constant for neutral hydrolysis, with units of reciprocal time (t^{-1} or $/t$).

[OH$^-$]. Molar hydroxide ion concentration, moles per liter.

Pseudo-first-order. The condition under which, for a second-order process, the product of the second-order rate constant and one of the concentration terms is invariant (e.g., acid-catalyzed hydrolysis in a buffered system of fixed pH, $k[C][H^+] = k'[C]$) (see reaction order).

Rate constant. Kinetic parameter in an equation describing the speed at which a phenomenon occurs. For example, the rate of a first-order chemical reaction can be described by the expression $k[C]$, where $[C]$ is chemical concentration and k is the first-order rate constant. Rate constants have dimensions of reciprocal time (t^{-1}), plus additional dimensionalities dependent on the character of the reaction (see reaction order).

Reaction order. Sum of the exponents of the concentration terms in a rate equation in derivative form; $-d[C]/dt$ = rate = $k[C][B]$ is second-order and rate = $k[C]$ is first order. Chemical reactions can be classified according to their order (e.g., zero-order, first-order, second-order, third-order). The order depends on the way the reaction rate is controlled by the concentrations of the reacting chemicals. First-order reactions proceed at a rate proportional to the concentration of one reactant only. For example, the rate of the reaction $C \rightarrow P$ (where P is the product) is proportional only to the concentration of C. The rate of reaction at any time t is given by the first-order rate equation $d[C]/dt = -k[C]$, where $d[C]/dt$ is the rate at which the concentration of C is changing (with units, e.g., of M/t). In this example the kinetic constant k is a first-order rate constant. First-order rate constants have dimensions of reciprocal time; they are often reported in reciprocal seconds. In second-order reactions, the rate is proportional to the product of two concentrations or to the square of the concentration of a single reactant. For example, the rate of the reaction $C + D \rightarrow P$ is proportional to the concentrations of C and D, as given by the second-order rate equation $d[C]/dt = -k[C][D]$, where k is now a second-order rate constant. Second-order rate constants have dimensions $1/(concentration \times time)$ (e.g., $M^{-1} s^{-1}$ or $/M \cdot s$). In higher-order (or fractional-order) reactions, the rate expression may be composed of several concentration terms (e.g., three reactants in a simple third-order expression) or concentrations raised to fractional powers. Under some conditions, the rate of a reaction may be independent of concentration; these are called zero-order reactions. When the concentration of one reactant is constant (e.g., because it is present in large excess over the amount consumed in the reaction), the apparent order of the reaction is reduced—hence the term pseudo-first-order for the rate constants determined in studies of second-order processes under controlled conditions.

Residence time. The time a given amount of substance remains in a particular segment or compartment of a system. The term is widely used in geochemistry. It is computed as the quotient of the total resident mass (e.g., of a chemical) and the total flux (e.g., mass per time entering the system, or total transformation plus export flux). The concept is meaningful only in reference to a dynamic equilibrium or steady-state condition or some reasonable facsimile thereof. Residence time is a useful indicator of the time scales of concern in a particular analysis. For example, if a chemical has a short residence time, the ambient concentrations must be closely correlated with emissions entering the system. At the opposite extreme, chemicals with very long residence times are only loosely coupled to current emissions; that is, ambient concentrations are poorly correlated with current chemical loadings. (Also see hydraulic residence time.)

Second-order. See reaction order.

State variable. Dynamic (time-varying) computed quantity in a simulation model. Values of the state variables at a particular time define the state of the system at that time. By definition, chemical fate models must include a vector of concentrations of the chemicals of interest as a state variable. Addition of further state variables depends on the purposes of the model and the degree to which extension of its dynamic range is needed to accomplish them. For example, a model designed to estimate effects of chemicals on fish populations must include those populations among its state variables; that is, population sizes must be subject to treatment as an explicit, dynamic (time-varying) variable in the model.

Steady state. The ultimate dynamic equilibrium achieved by a system under fixed conditions of the system driving forces.

Turnover rate. Reciprocal of residence time, with units of reciprocal time (t^{-1}). The turnover rate represents the fractional renewal of a quantity in the system per unit time.

COUPLING VARIABLES AND HIERARCHIES OF SCALE

Scientific disciplines can be classified according to the level of organization at which their investigations are typically conducted. These levels extend from the subatomic world of particle physics, through the molecular world of chemistry and biochemistry, to the macroscopic world of regional ecosystems and earth history. The phenomena that constitute the primary subject matter of each discipline are investigated in accord with the precepts, methods, and traditions of its practitioners. At each level of organization, however, the causal mechanisms of phenomena must be sought at lower levels, and the meaning of the phenomena must be sought at higher levels of organization.

In toxicology, for example, studies of the acute toxicity of chemicals enumerate deaths in a group of animals as a function of chemical concentration. Toxicological results must then be applied in the context of natural populations. In the study of population dynamics, the deaths of individual organisms are summed to yield an entirely new property—a death rate. At the organismic level, the idea of a death rate is meaningless: each individual lives or dies; it cannot have a death rate. Furthermore, in order to infer the lethality of a chemical to natural populations, a suite of additional demographic techniques may be required, including survivorship curves, competition theory, predator-prey theory, fishery dynamics, and others. Attention to lower levels of organization (e.g., molecular chemistry and organ physiology) is also necessary. When the mechanisms of chemical lethality are neglected, the toxicological data often cannot be extrapolated with confidence to natural situations. For example, the toxicity of pentachlorophenol depends on ambient pH, which affects the relative concentrations of neutral (uncharged) pentachlorophenol and its phenolate anion (Kobayashi and Kishino, 1980). Pentachlorophenol toxicity can only be understood in terms of equilibrium chemistry.

Systems analysis combines chemistry, toxicology, and ecology in a unified approach to analysis of the consequences of release of chemicals into the environment. For this union of disciplines to be effective, three central concepts must be understood: (1) system, (2) hierarchy of organization, and (3) coupling variables. A system is defined in a dictionary (Webster's unabridged, third edition) as a "complex unity formed of many often diverse parts subject to a common plan or serving a common purpose." Systems analysis expands this definition, viewing a system as being composed of several elements, including the system objectives, components, environment, and resources.

Delineation of the system objectives is the first step in a systems analysis. This problem can be stated as an explicit question: What are the actual inputs and outputs of this system—that is, what in fact does the system do? Note that a systems analysis need not incorporate all possible behaviors of the system. In most cases, it is focused on a small number of objectives that are of immediate interest. The importance of definition of objectives as an initial step in systems analysis is that it focuses the analysis on a particular set of input and output behaviors. These behaviors define the "unity" and "common purpose" referred to in Webster's definition of a system. Thus, for example, the digestive system accepts raw foodstuffs as inputs and produces simpler compounds (and waste residuals) as outputs.

The idea of system objectives must be understood because the remaining elements of a systems analysis are defined with reference to the system objectives. The components of a system are the physically distinct entities that contribute, through their own local input-output behaviors and interactions, to the overall system objectives. For example, in the study of nutrient dynamics in aquatic systems, each phytoplankter absorbs mineral nutrients and incorporates them into cell tissue, thus contributing to overall nutrient capture by a system that also includes macrophytes, animals, and purely chemical phenomena.

The environment of a system is composed of factors affecting system objectives over which the system exercises no control. These factors are also called forcing functions or driving variables (e.g., solar irradiance, rainfall). The resources of a system also affect the input-output behaviors but are not wholly beyond system control, although that control may be effected through complex feedback mechanisms.

The importance of a systems view in chemical risk analysis derives from the dependent concepts of a hierarchical scale in levels of organization, and the idea of formal coupling variables that link results of investigations at different levels. Systems analyses are conducted, of necessity, at a single level of organization. Each component of the system, however, is itself a system (hence the term "subsystem"), and can be analyzed in terms of its local input-output behaviors and resources. For example, an organism is composed of several subsystems (e.g., digestive, circulatory, nervous), each of which can be studied in isolation from the others. In addition, every system is a subsystem of a system at some higher level of organization, as an individual is a member of a population.

Two important observations, with direct implications for toxicology, can now be stated. First, the environment of one system is often a resource at a higher level or scale of organization, and in this sense levels of organization can be ordered in a systematic way (i.e., in a causal hierarchy). Second, these environment/resource parameters are the coupling variables that allow results at one level of organization to be extrapolated and interpreted outside the domain of investigations in a single discipline.

The application of these concepts can perhaps be best appreciated through a concrete example. Aqueous-phase hydrolytic transformations and ionization of many chemicals are controlled by the pH of the solution. At molecular scales of organization, and when a chemical is present at trace levels, the pH of the solution is part of the chemical's environment; that is, pH affects the processing and state of the chemical in the system (beaker, toxicity test tank, or lake), but the chemical has no effect on pH. When the toxicities of chemical species or reaction products differ, the results of toxicity tests will vary as a function of pH. The pH of aqueous solutions couples events at molecular chemical scales of organization to toxicological events involving whole organisms.

At the level of entire ecosystems, pH is a resource factor, rather than a purely environmental variable in the sense used in formal systems analysis. In freshwater aquatic systems, pH is governed by the carbonate chemistry of the water. The metabolic processes of organisms involve the uptake and release of carbon dioxide, which can, in some circumstances (e.g., some eutrophic lakes), effect a 100-fold diel variation in the concentration of hydronium and hydroxide ions.

Suppose that a chemical toxic to phytoplankton, and rapidly degraded to innocuous forms at alkaline pH, is continuously released into such a lake. Initially, the chemical will be transformed sufficiently rapidly that little effect on the phytoplankton population will be observed. If, however, there is sufficient impact to decrease the productivity of the system, the pH of the water will decrease. As the pH decreases, the rate of breakdown of the chemical will slow, its concentration will increase, and more plankters will succumb. This will again decrease productivity and pH and again slow the chemical breakdown. This kind of phenomenon, in which an initially trivial perturbation ultimately produces collapse of the system, is called a positive feedback loop.

The point of this illustration is that successful risk analysis requires chemists, toxicologists, and ecologists to cooperate in the identification, measurement, and evaluation of the parameters linking phenomena between disciplines and across levels of organization of the natural world.

TRANSPORT AND TRANSFORMATION PROCESSES IN AQUATIC SYSTEMS

The processes governing residual aqueous-phase concentrations of organic chemicals can be divided into three classes: irreversible processes that convert the parent compound into chemical daughter or transformation products; reversible processes (e.g., ionization, sorption, complexation) that involve continuous exchanges among a number of chemical states within the system; and transport processes that move the chemical through the water body, and transfer it among relatively distinct spatial zones (e.g., benthic sediments, epilimnion, hypolimnion).

Transformation Processes

Transformation processes of importance in aquatic systems include reactions mediated by sunlight (direct and indirect photolysis), metabolic transformations (see Chapters 8 and 18), reduction reactions largely confined to anaerobic subsystems, and hydrolytic reactions with water itself and with its normal dissolved constituents (Baughman and Burns, 1980).

Direct photolysis is a process of absorption of light by the chemical molecule, followed by chemical reactions that break the molecule into smaller fragments (Zepp and Cline, 1977). During indirect or "sensitized" photolysis, in contrast, sunlight is not absorbed directly by the target chemical. Indirect photolysis can be divided into two general types of reactions. First, during what might strictly be called sensitized photolysis, sunlight is absorbed by a "sensitizer" molecule, which is often a component of the naturally occurring dissolved organic matter (e.g., humic substances). Chemical interaction between the light-excited state of the sensitizer and the target molecule then results in the formation of products by a variety of possible reaction pathways (Zepp and Baughman, 1978). In the second type of indirect photolysis, transformations arise through reactions with chemical oxidants created by the interaction of sunlight, humic materials, and dissolved oxygen. The most important oxidant species in natural waters are peroxy and hydroxyl radicals (Mill et al., 1980) and singlet oxygen (Zepp et al., 1977).

Microbial biotransformation of synthetic chemicals is an important reaction pathway in many aquatic systems (see Chapter 8). In some cases, microbial populations use synthetic organic chemicals as sources of dietary energy. When this is so, classical microbiological techniques, including Michaelis-Menten-Monod equations for growth kinetics of bacterial populations, can be used in chemical fate modeling (Slater, 1979). The results of laboratory investigations in which the synthetic compound is used as a sole source of carbon and dietary energy can be difficult to extrapolate to field situations, however. The population dynamics, viability, and metabolic status of specialized subpopulations of microbial degraders cannot currently be predicted with much confidence (Burns, 1982). In addition, in many cases synthetic compounds are degraded by multispecies microbial assemblages under natural conditions, despite the fact that no individual species capable of using the compound as a sole carbon source can be isolated (Alexander, 1981). Paris et al. (1981) described the rate of transformation of several synthetic organic chemicals by natural bacterial assemblages with a simple second-order expression, using total microbial population size as the environmental parameter in the rate equation. Algal transformations have also been detected for some compounds, but the pathways are not well understood or quantified (O'Kelley and Deason, 1976).

Although no causal mechanistic description has yet been derived, reductive dechlorination of synthetic compounds (e.g., DDT) has been observed in anaerobic sediments (Tinsley, 1979). It has not been conclusively determined whether the process is biological, or a chemical reaction proceeding under anoxic conditions created by biological activities. The ability of chemical fate models to represent this process is consequently in a comparatively immature state.

Hydrolysis of synthetic organic compounds occurs by a variety of pathways. Specific-acid and specific-base catalyzed processes, which are accelerated by hydroxide and hydrogen ions, respectively, can easily be described in terms of the pH and temperature of water bodies (Wolfe, 1980). Neutral hydrolysis (i.e., pH-independent hydrolytic reactions) can proceed by several mechanisms, including reactions in which the water molecule affects the rate-determining step, and reactions in which water is involved as a simple (non-rate-limiting) reactant. (Both can be described as a simple linear function of chemical concentration.) General acids and bases may also contribute to chemical hydrolysis in some cases; this phenomenon can be a particular problem when buffers are used to control pH in experimental systems (Perdue and Wolfe, 1983).

Hydrolytic reactions are among the best understood of chemical processes (Kirby, 1972); reactions with water thus serve as a good example of the techniques used to investigate and model transformation processes in aquatic systems. In natural waters three hydrolytic reactions predominate:

those involving hydrogen ion, hydroxide ion, and direct reactions with water (Wolfe, 1980; Tinsley, 1979). Because the concentrations of hydrogen ion $[H^+]$ and hydroxide ion $[OH^-]$ change (by definition) with the pH of the water, the speed of hydrolytic transformations is directly dependent on this property of a water body.

The actual "pseudo-first-order" hydrolytic rate constant (K_{obs} with units of reciprocal time t^{-1}) observed in a particular aqueous solution of fixed pH is the sum of contributions from each of the constituent processes. The formal relationship between K_{obs} and pH is given by

$$K_{obs} = K_{ah}[H^+] + K_{nh} + K_{bh}[OH^-] \qquad (1)$$

In this equation K_{ah} and K_{bh} are the second-order acid and alkaline (base) hydrolytic rate constants. The species $[H^+]$ and $[OH^-]$ are molar quantities, so K_{ah} and K_{bh} have units $M^{-1}\,t^{-1}$ or $/M \cdot t$. The neutral contribution (K_{nh}) is dependent only on the presence of water. Because water is the solvent or carrier material in aquatic systems, it is always present in excess, and K_{nh} can be treated as a simple (pseudo-) first-order rate constant with units t^{-1}.

Most of the chemical information needed to model hydrolytic reactions in natural waters can be encapsulated in a pH-rate profile. In this approach, a known quantity of the compound is introduced into a solution of fixed pH and the disappearance of the compound is followed over time (Fig. 1). The concentration of the chemical typically declines exponentially with increasing time (Fig. 1a), a situation that can be described by the first-order decay equation

$$[C](t) = [C](0)e^{-(K_{obs})t} \qquad (2)$$

In this equation, $[C](0)$ is the concentration of the chemical at the beginning of the experiment (the "initial condition," at $t = 0$), $[C](t)$ is the concentration at any later time t, K_{obs} is the observed (pseudo-) first-order rate constant (units t^{-1}), and e is the base of natural logarithms. When

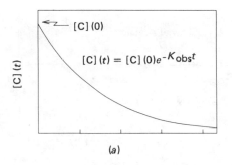

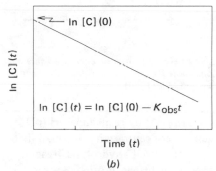

Figure 1 Characteristic pseudo-first-order (fixed pH) disappearance curves of compounds subject to hydrolytic transformation: (a) Linear plot; (b) semilogarithmic plot.

the experimental data are plotted on a semilog scale (Fig. 1b), the resulting straight line has a slope of $-K_{obs}$, as defined by

$$\ln [C](t) = \ln [C](0) - K_{obs}t \qquad (3)$$

[When base-10 logarithms of chemical concentrations are used, the slope of the line is (log e) (K_{obs}), i.e., $0.4343(K_{obs})$.] From the results of a series of such experiments at different pH, a pH-rate profile can be constructed by plotting the logarithms of the observed rate constants (K_{obs}) against the pH of the experimental solutions.

Figure 2 is the pH-rate profile of phenyl acetate; hydrolytic transformation of this compound yields acetic acid and phenol. Under acid conditions (pH < 3), specific-acid catalysis is the dominant hydrolytic mechanism. The logarithm of K_{obs} decreases with a unit slope -1.0 with increasing pH, that is, K_{obs} decreases in exact proportion

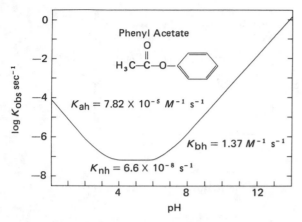

Figure 2 Hydrolysis pH-rate profile of phenyl acetate at 25°C. Profile constructed from rate constant data summarized by Mabey and Mill (1978).

with decreases in $[H^+]$. At more alkaline pH (pH > 4), the hydrogen ion concentration is so small that the specific-acid catalyzed hydrolytic reaction is too slow to be seen in the profile. Between a pH of 4 and 6, the neutral mechanism, which is independent of pH, imposes a flat plateau on the pH-rate profile. Finally, at pH > 8, specific-base catalysis imposes a +1.0 slope on the profile as K_{obs} increases in direct proportion with increases in $[OH^-]$.

The numerical value of the second-order hydrolytic rate constants [Eq. (1)] can be calculated by dividing K_{obs} by the molar concentration of the appropriate catalytic species (H^+ or OH^-), at a relevant section of the pH-rate profile. For example, at pH 10, where transformation of phenyl acetate is dominated by alkaline hydrolysis, K_{obs} is $10^{-3.86}$ or 1.37×10^{-4} s^{-1}. At pH 10, the concentration of hydroxide ion is $10^{-(14-10)}$ or 10^{-4} M, and the second-order rate constant for alkaline hydrolysis (K_{bh}) is therefore $1.37 \times 10^{-4}/10^{-4} = 1.37$ M^{-1} s^{-1}. K_{ah}, K_{bh}, and K_{nh} for phenyl acetate are indicated on Fig. 2. These numerical values can be substituted into Eq. (1), giving

$$K_{obs} = 0.82 \times 10^{-5} [H^+] + 6.6 \times 10^{-8}$$

$$+ 1.37 [OH^-] \qquad (4)$$

Many compounds are not transformed by all three of these hydrolytic pathways. In this situation, Eq. (1) can be modified either by deletion of inoperative terms or by setting the inappropriate rate constants to zero.

The pH of water bodies is a commonly measured water quality parameter. Normal, environmental pH can be as low as 2.5–3 in some peat bogs and marshlands and as high as 10.5–11 in some shallow eutrophic lakes. The relevant environmental parameters are, of course, $[H^+]$ and $[OH^-]$, rather than pH itself [Eq. (1)]. Both can be computed from a point measurement of pH, because the sum of pH and pOH is always a fixed value. It is nearly 14 at 25°C; this value is somewhat temperature-dependent, however.

Preparation of pH observations for use in environmental models is subject to some pitfalls. Although mean pH is sometimes used as a descriptive statistic, summing pH values and dividing by the number of observations is not correct, because the factor controlling the rate of hydrolytic reactions is $[H^+]$ (and/or $[OH^-]$), rather than pH per se. Instead, observed pH values must first be converted to $[H^+]$ or $[OH^-]$ before statistical treatment of the data. The negatives of the logarithms of the resulting mean concentrations are then the proper values of pH and pOH for use in computer programs or environmental models in which these parameters are input data. Proper treatment of field data is particularly important in highly productive water bodies, where pH can vary by 2 units or more over a daily cycle. A change of 2 pH units represents a 100-fold change in $[H^+]$ and $[OH^-]$ and consequently a 100-fold change in the speed of hydrolytic transformations.

Reversible Reactions

Ionization

Many synthetic organic chemicals are acids or bases that dissociate to yield charged species. The extent of dissociation is controlled by the pH of the water body. The toxicity and the chemical reactivity of the uncharged (neutral) molecule and its charged ions can be very different. For this reason, it is important to control pH during toxicity investigations and to express the results in terms of the appropriate chemical species, rather than as simplified functions of the total exposure concentration of the test compound.

Ionization equilibria of acids and bases can be computed fairly easily. Consider, for example, an acid HA (H the hydrogen atom and A the remainder of the molecule). In contact with water, this molecule will exist both as free HA and as the A$^-$ anion. Chemically, this phenomenon can be represented as

$$HA + H_2O \leftrightarrow H_3O^+ + A^- \tag{5}$$

The ionization constant or acidity constant (K_a) is a commonly measured quantity; it is defined by an equation that gives the ratio of equilibrium concentrations of the interacting chemical species:

$$K_a = \frac{[H_3O^+][A^-]}{[HA]} \tag{6}$$

Ionization constants are generally reported as the negative of their base-10 logarithms, that is, as pK_a values.

The ionization of hydrogen cyanide (HCN) in aqueous solution, as a function of pH, is shown in Fig. 3. HCN is 50% dissociated into H$^+$ and CN$^-$ at a hydrogen ion concentration equal to its acidity

constant (in other words, pH = pK_a). The pK_a of HCN is 9.1; at pH 8.1, 91% of the total is present as free HCN and 9% as CN$^-$ ions. At pH 10.1, only 9% of the compound occurs as free HCN; most of it has been converted to ionic CN$^-$.

In any aqueous solution, the total concentration [C_{tot}] of a chemical is given by the sum of the constituent species, in this instance free [HCN] and its conjugate anion [CN$^-$]:

$$[C_{tot}] = [HCN] + [CN^-] \tag{7}$$

The fraction of the total that is present in the unionized form [HCN] is given by [HCN]/[C_{tot}], and the fraction present as the anion is given by [CN$^-$]/[C_{tot}].

The distribution of HCN between its un-ionized and ionized species is controlled by the pH of the solution. This distribution can be simply but rigorously described: Letting I denote the ionization fractions (Stumm and Morgan, 1970):

$$I(0) = \frac{[HCN]}{[C_{tot}]} = \frac{[HCN]}{[HCN] + [CN^-]} \tag{8}$$

According to Eq. (6), however, [CN$^-$] = (K_a) $\times$ [HCN]/[H$^+$], so

$$I(0) = \frac{1}{1 + K_a/[H^+]} = \frac{[H^+]}{[H^+] + K_a} \tag{9}$$

The mass conservation law requires that the ionization fractions sum to 1.0. The remaining fraction $I(1) = [CN^-]/[C_{tot}]$ must therefore be equal to $1 - I(0)$; this fraction can also be expressed as

$$I(1) = \frac{K_a}{[H^+] + K_a} \tag{10}$$

This concept of ionization fractions (or, more generally, equilibrium species distribution fractions) can easily be extended to include the simultaneous occurrence of singly and doubly charged anions and cations and sediment-sorbed and bio-

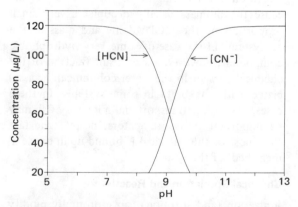

Figure 3 Equilibrium distribution of hydrogen cyanide between HCN and the CN$^-$ anion as a function of pH. Total concentration 120 μg/l.

sorbed chemical species. Notice that the ionization fractions [Eqs. (9) and (10)] are mathematically independent of the concentration of the chemical itself. This adds to the convenience of ionization fractions in relating toxicity to pH, but limits their utility to situations in which the concentration of the chemical is not so high as to affect the pH of the water. Fortunately, this is usually the case in environmentally significant situations.

Ionization fractions are useful in analyzing the specific toxicities of individual chemical species. The concept is also widely used in environmental modeling. For example, ionized species are relatively nonvolatile, and environmental models incorporate this fact through the parameter $I(0)$ (Burns et al., 1982).

Sorption

Many organic compounds bind extensively with nonliving sedimentary and detrital materials, a process generally known as sorption. Within aquatic systems, hydrophobic mechanisms drive neutral (uncharged) compounds from the water phase into association with the solid phases of the system. The extent of capture of neutral compounds by solid phases is strongly correlated with the organic carbon content of the solids (Karickhoff et al., 1979). Ionic species become associated with solids through exchanges with the naturally occurring ions, and the extent of sorption can be described fairly well as a function of pH and the exchange capacity of the solids (Brown, 1984).

Sorption equilibria can be described with the same techniques used for ionic equilibria. The chemical processes can be represented as

$$C + P \leftrightarrow CP \qquad (11)$$

in which a molecule of chemical C associates with the particulate matter in the system P to yield a sorbed complex CP. The equilibrium state of this process is often described by a partition coefficient, with units (mg/l)/(mg/kg). In this convention, the partition coefficient K_p is the ratio of chemical concentration in the aqueous phase

(mg/l), to that in the sorbed phase (milligrams of chemical per kilogram dry weight of solids), at equilibrium. The equilibrium distribution fraction can be calculated from

$$I(0) = \frac{1}{1 + K_p R} \qquad (12)$$

where R is the concentration of solids (kilograms dry weight per liter of water) in the system. [Note the similarity to Eq. (9).]

Although an equilibrium treatment of sorption phenomena is adequate for many purposes, in some cases the release of sorbed materials to the aqueous phase can be slow enough to hinder the free expression of the chemical reactivity of a compound. When the speed of release of a compound from the sorbed state is rate-limiting in this sense, environmental models may require explicit equations describing the kinetics of sorption itself (Karickhoff, 1980).

Living organisms can acquire significant body burdens of synthetic chemicals either by direct uptake from contaminated water or by consumption of contaminated food items. Small organisms with a large surface-to-volume ratio often equilibrate rapidly with their milieu, hence the term biosorption for this phenomenon (Baughman and Paris, 1981). Transfers of synthetic chemical compounds to living organisms generally do not have a major effect on the overall fate of the compound, because the biomass usually occupies a very small proportion of the total volume and mass of the ecosystem. In the case of some very hydrophobic compounds, however, a significant fraction of the chemical present in the water column can be associated with the biota in some systems. In these cases, planktonic transport and migratory fish may be important transport vectors, despite the fact that most of the chemical is bound up in the sediment beds of the system.

Chemical Speciation and Reactivity

Ionization (and sorption) can profoundly modify the lability of a chemical in a decomposition or transformation process. Figure 4 is the pH-rate profile for hydrolysis of HND, a substituted phenyl dioxane. Up to a pH of about 6, this profile resembles the usual pH-rate profiles discussed in connection with Fig. 2. Above pH 6, however, the neutral plateau turns downward and resumes a slope of −1.0, rather than showing the expected +1.0 slope of alkaline hydrolysis or a continued neutral plateau.

HND is a weak organic acid, with a pK_a of 6.63. Bender and Silver (1963) showed that HND is subject only to a specific-acid catalyzed hydrolytic reaction; alkaline and neutral hydrolytic pathways do not effect its transformation. The phenolate anion is 2300 times more reactive than the un-ionized form of HND (the second-order acid-catalyzed hydrolytic rate constants for both forms are indicated on Fig. 4). The initial descending limb (pH < 4) of the pH-rate profile reflects the effect of decreasing $[H^+]$ on the specific-acid hydrolytic decomposition of un-ionized HND. The descending limb in the region pH > 7 reflects acid catalysis of the phenolate anion transformation pathway; both descending limbs have a slope of −1.0. The central plateau in this profile reflects the ionization of neutral HND to its phenolate anion. As the fraction present in the ionic form becomes progressively more important, reaction of

this form begins to dominate the observed rate constant. The result is the relatively stable value of K_{obs} seen between pH 4 and 6 (Fig. 4; K_{obs} is ~10^{-5}).

This state of affairs can be represented by combining Eqs. (1), (9), and (10), that is, by a simultaneous treatment of hydrolysis kinetics and ionization equilibria. Combining equations gives

$$K_{obs} = I(0)K_{ah}(0)[H^+] + I(1)K_{ah}(1)[H^+] \quad (13)$$

where $K_{ah}(0)$, the second-order, specific-acid catalyzed rate constant for un-ionized HND, is 0.15 M^{-1} s^{-1} (Fig. 4) and $K_{ah}(1)$, the rate constant for the phenolate anion, is 130 M^{-1} s^{-1}. The rate of hydrolytic transformation of HND, as a function of pH is

$$\frac{d[C]}{dt} = -\{0.15I(0) + 130I(1)\}[H^+][C] \quad (14)$$

For convenience in a particular experimental investigation—for example, in a static toxicity test— Eqs. (9) and (10), the expressions for $I(0)$ and $I(1)$, could be inserted into Eq. (14) and the result simplified to yield

$$\frac{d[C]}{dt} = -\frac{0.15[H^+] + 130K_a}{K_a + [H^+]}[H^+][C] \quad (15)$$

In most cases, of course, chemicals are subject to many additional fate processes, including sorption, photolysis, oxidation/reduction, metabolic transformations, transport, and other processes. This example case of ionization and hydrolytic reactions should, however, suggest the strength and usefulness of the general analytical tools available to the toxicologist familiar with chemical kinetics and equilibrium computations.

Transport Processes

The physical transport phenomena important in aquatic systems include hydrodynamic fluid motions, the movement of solid phases carried by the

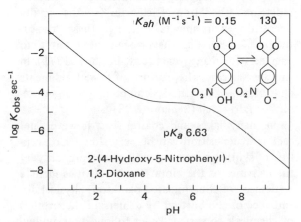

Figure 4 Hydrolysis pH-rate profile of 2-(4-hydroxy-5-nitrophenyl)-1,3-dioxane. Profile constructed from data of Bender and Silver (1963).

waters, transfers of chemicals between the water column and sediment beds, and transfers of chemicals across the air-water interface. Biological transport vectors, such as the sinking of contaminated plankton or food chain transmission of chemicals, can be important in the evaluation of toxic impacts. In addition, transport across the benthic boundary layer is strongly influenced by biological activity. Most environmental models incorporate biotic effects only indirectly, although some specialized models of selected aspects of biotic transport have been described (e.g., Aller, 1977).

The study of transport processes in aquatic systems is a major discipline in itself. In many instances, water and its associated solids can be regarded as simple carriers of dissolved and sorbed chemicals, respectively. Transport processes can be accommodated in environmental models either by directly incorporating transport equations, or by using a transport model to compute fluid and solid movements and then computing chemical transport by linking the results of the physical transport model to a model of chemical kinetics in the system. A thorough review of transport models is beyond the scope of this chapter; the interested reader should consult the works referenced below.

Hydrodynamic Transport

Hydrodynamic transport processes have been of interest to hydrologists for many years (e.g., Eagleson, 1970; Gibbs, 1977; Shen, 1979). Hydrodynamic transport has often been modeled as a combination of advective and dispersive processes. Advection, the flow of water through the system, is usually represented by the mean flow velocity of a river or hydraulic discharge from a lake or pond. Dispersive processes, which are modeled by analogy with molecular diffusion, are used to account for the macroscale effects of physical turbulence, storm surges, internal waves, and other complex processes that are not amenable to detailed, fully mechanistic mathematical descriptions. The hydrodynamic flows carry dissolved chemicals through the system, and models of the transport of chemical compounds can be produced by direct

linkage to hydrodynamic models or descriptions of hydrologic transport.

Sediment Transport

Similarly, sediment transport, particularly in fluvial (river) systems, is of direct interest in the engineering profession (e.g., Simons and Senturk, 1976; Garde and Ranga Raju, 1977). As with hydrodynamic motions, the transport of sorbed compounds can be modeled by linking chemical transport to a sediment transport model (e.g., Onishi et al., 1980). Sediment transport is very different for particles of different sizes, so this modeling strategy requires a careful evaluation of the effects of particle size on sorption. Alternatively, for some purposes a description of the sorptive properties and transport of whole sediments is sufficient (Burns et al., 1982).

Exchange across the Benthic Boundary Layer

In nonfluvial water bodies (e.g., lakes and ponds), interactions between benthic sediments and chemical contaminants often cannot be completely described by sediment transport dynamics, because direct sorption from the water column to the bed surface and biological, rather than physical, transport phenomena dominate the process. The simplest situation occurs in impounded waters behind dams, which trap large quantities of river-borne sediments. The "trap efficiencies" of the rapidly depositing environments typical of these "run-of-the-river" reservoirs have been of interest to engineers for many years (e.g., Borland, 1971). In this special case, the capture of fluvial sediments and burial of synthetic compounds can be described fairly well (Schnoor, 1981).

In many lakes and coastal seas, however, net sediment deposition can be very slow. Here, capture of synthetic compounds is driven primarily by the activities of the biota. These activities include settlement of contaminated plankton, physical disturbance of the bottom by demersal fish, sorption of chemicals to surface layers followed by subduction and mixing of contaminated layers by crustacea and worm populations, and irrigation of the sediments by benthic macrofauna (Aller, 1977). In addition, exchanges across the benthic interface can be driven by physical stirring or sediment "bursting" (Heathershaw, 1974, 1976). Transport across the benthic boundary layer has been described by an advection-dispersion equation (Berner, 1980). In this approach, the advection term is used to account for ground-water flow and compaction of the sediments, and the exchange events are described by a dispersion term.

Atmospheric Exchange Processes

Transfers of chemicals across the air-water interface can result in either net gain or loss of a chemical, although in many cases the bulk concentration in the air above a contaminated water body is low enough to be neglected (Mackay and Leinonen, 1975). The two-film or two-resistance approach originally proposed by Whitman (1923) has been applied to a number of environmental situations (Liss and Slater, 1974; Mackay and Leinonen, 1975; Mackay, 1978). In this approach (Fig. 5), transport across the air-water interface is viewed as a two-stage process, in which both the aqueous and gaseous phases of the interface can offer resistance to transport of the chemical. The rate of transfer of a chemical compound depends on turbulence in the water body and in the atmosphere, the Henry's law constant (or vapor pressure and solubility) of the chemical, and the molecular velocity of the compound in the near-surface regions.

FUNDAMENTALS OF ENVIRONMENTAL MODELING

Mathematics and mathematical modeling are nothing more than a concise language for summarizing factual information. The advantage of mathematical notation over less formal expressions is that mathematics provides a set of tools for deriving the implications of the facts in a logical, objective, and repeatable way. In addition, mathematical models incorporate facts from chemistry, physics, toxicology, and ecology into a single uni-

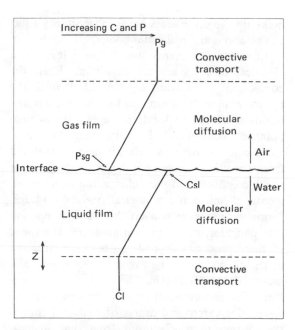

Figure 5 Two-resistance or two-film model of a gas-liquid interface. Abbreviations: C1, concentration (mol/m³) in bulk water, and Pg, partial pressure (atm) in bulk air, in both of which transport of a volatilizing substance is controlled by physical turbulence; Cs1, aqueous concentration in liquid near the interface; and Psg, partial pressure on the atmospheric side of the interface. In the interface zones events at molecular scales control movement of a volatilizing substance. *[From Liss and Slater (1974).]*

fied framework. This mathematical framework can be built into a computer program or "code" that can be tailored to forecast the probable consequences of real-world events. A unified mathematical framework allows for interactions among fate processes (e.g., photolysis and sorption) and makes possible an evaluation of the most significant events likely to occur when a synthetic chemical is released into an aquatic ecosystem. In contrast, when individual fate processes are considered in isolation, conclusions must be limited to statements of what is possible or what can conceivably happen when potentially toxic chemicals enter water bodies. A single factual observation (e.g., breakdown of a chemical observed in a laboratory experiment) has limited value until it is put in the context of the other processes and events that make up the differences between laboratory aqueous solutions and real water bodies.

Consider the events that follow release of a chemical into an aquatic ecosystem. First, the compound is immediately entrained into the hydrodynamic transport field of the system and begins to spread to locations beyond the original point of release. As the compound encounters biota and nonliving particles, it may be captured from the water column and begin to contaminate benthic systems and food chains. During its movements, chemical and biological (metabolic) transformation processes convert the parent compound into daughter transformation products. The speed of these processes depends on both the structure of the chemical and the strength of environmental factors in the ecosystem. The transport and transformation processes act together to determine the geographic extent and degree of contamination of the system that will result from the chemical loadings.

In the face of constant emissions or loadings, the receiving system evolves toward a steady-state condition. At steady state, the chemical concentrations are in a dynamic equilibrium, with the loadings balanced by the transport and transformation processes; that is, each new increment of chemical entering the system is balanced by an export loss or conversion of the parent compound to a daughter product. More generally, chemical loadings and environmental conditions can vary from day to day, and there are major differences between seasons. In this case the chemical may never reach a steady state. Instead, it may always be on a changing trajectory toward the steady-state end point defined by the current environmental conditions; the steady-state end point is itself changing through time.

Conservation of Mass and Differential Equations

When a synthetic organic chemical is first released into an aquatic ecosystem, the transport and reversible and irreversible transformation processes begin at once to act on the chemical. Transport from the point of entry into the bulk of the system takes place by advection and by turbulent dispersion. Transfers to sorbed forms and irreversible transformation processes take place simultaneously with the transport of the chemical. After a sufficient time, the chemical will be distributed throughout the system, with relatively smooth concentration gradients resulting from dilution, speciation, and transformation. The most efficient way to describe the parallel action of the processes is to combine them into a mathematical description of their total effect on the rate of change of chemical concentration in the system, through a set of coupled differential equations.

The simplest, and perhaps most important, principle used in constructing environmental models is the conservation law: matter can be neither created nor destroyed. This means that every molecule of a chemical compound that enters a defined spatial zone (e.g., a laboratory tank or beaker, the epilimnion of a lake, the earth's atmosphere) must ultimately either leave the system, be transformed into another compound, or take up residence in the system. The behavior of a chemical in an aquatic system thus can be rigorously described by using the conservation law as an accounting principle. Imagine, first, an accounting boundary drawn around some segment of the environment (Fig. 6). This imaginary boundary encloses a "control volume," or accounting unit to be used in a model. In real cases, boun-

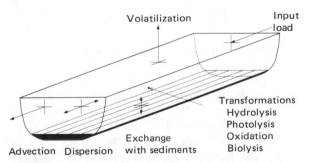

Figure 6 Segment of aquatic system used as a control volume for constructing a mass balance equation. The rate of change of chemical concentration in the segment is governed by chemical loadings, transport processes, and transformation sinks for the chemical.

daries are often chosen to correspond with actual physical discontinuities, such as riverbanks, the air-water interface, the benthic sediment–water column interface, or the depth of bioturbation of sediments. In many cases, however, the accuracy and detail of a model can be improved by including many relatively small accounting units bounded only by arbitrary lines drawn on a map or vertical profile of the water body.

Every chemical molecule entering the control volume now has three courses available: export (movement out of the control volume), transformation, or residence. Environmental modeling begins by writing a mass balance around the control volume. This mass balance expresses the changes in concentration (increases and decreases in the number of chemical molecules per unit volume of the segment) that result from loadings (inputs), exports, and transformations. The product of concentration [C] (mass/volume) and volume V is the accountable mass, so, using the usual notation of differential equations to denote a rate of change, one can write:

$$V \frac{d[C]}{dt} = \text{Lo} - \text{Ex} - VKE[C] \qquad (16)$$

that is, mass change rate = load − export − transformations, where E is the environmental factor driving the transformation of the compound (e.g., $[H^+]$), and K is the kinetic constant of the reaction pathway.

The terms in this equation must have consistent physical units for the equation to be valid. For example, when V is expressed in liters and [C] in milligrams per liter, the input loadings (Lo) and the exports (Ex) must have units of milligrams per unit time (e.g., mg/s). If we consider waterborne exports only, Ex can be set equal to $(F)[C]$, where (F) is the flow rate of water leaving the system in liters per second. The second-order transformation process $KE[C]$ must have units of milligrams per liter per second; multiplication by V converts it to the proper mass units (mg/s).

Dividing both sides of Eq. (16) by V gives a unit equation for modeling chemical concentrations in real systems:

$$\frac{d[C]}{dt} = \frac{\text{Lo}}{V} - \frac{F}{V}[C] - KE[C] \qquad (17)$$

(The reciprocal of the term F/V has units of time; when V and F apply to an entire system, V/F is often called the "hydraulic residence time" or "detention time" of the water body.)

Models of real ecosystems often consist of many unit control volumes coupled by transport equations. An export from one unit then becomes a load on another. The loadings on each control volume can thus be the sum of many terms, including "external" chemical loadings from industrial or agricultural discharges or contaminated rainfall plus "internal" loadings due to hydrodynamic motions and other transport cycles within the system that move chemicals from one control volume to another. In models that include both parent compounds and daughter transformation products, the rate of transformation of the parent to the daughter compound ($KE[C]$) is also an internal loading (Lo/V) of the daughter compound.

Export processes are often more complicated than the expression given in Eq. (17), for many chemicals can escape across the air-water interface (volatilize) or, in rapidly depositing environments, be buried for indeterminate periods in deep sediment beds. Still, the vast majority of environmental models are nothing more than elegant, complex variations on the mass balance theme expressed by Eq. (17). Furthermore, as we shall see, even this simplified equation has important implications for toxicological investigations.

Space and Time Scales

Synthetic chemicals enter the aquatic environment by many routes, including accidental spills, industrial effluents, runoff from agricultural fields, leaching from landfills and disposal sites, leaching of materials deposited on soils from the atmosphere, and sewage treatment plants. The rate, magnitude, and duration of releases by these pathways can be very different. The toxic impact of a substance and the speed of chemical transformations are functions of the magnitude of current environmental concentrations, however, rather than the precise route of entry of the material. Even so, in some circumstances variable magnitudes and durations of chemical releases, in combination with variable transport regimes, result in highly variable exposures that can only be evaluated by detailed simulation models. In other cases, concentrations and exposure durations are relatively independent of short-term variations in releases, and very long-term or steady-state analyses are required. Consequently, it is not possible to unambiguously specify a single environmental model or computer program suitable for risk analysis or hazard evaluation. Models and programs are, of necessity, designed in the context of specific problems, and systematic risk assessments usually must employ a variety of tools in order to address the whole range of concerns at issue.

Chemical spills and, to a lesser degree, early postapplication agricultural runoff, typically require an "event-oriented" model. One approach to this problem is to treat the "event" as a sudden injection of a given quantity of the chemical into the system. The time course of dilution and breakdown of the chemical can then be modeled to predict, among other things, the extent of contamination of downstream areas as a result of a chemical spill. For example, Neely et al. (1976) derived an analytical expression for transport and volatilization of soluble chemicals in flowing waters. They used the model to evaluate the consequences of a spill of chloroform in the Mississippi River. Thibodeaux (1979) summarized approaches needed to expand this analysis to account for the formation of pools of liquid chemical on the bottom of watercourses.

For many chemicals, relatively small but long-term releases are a more significant route of entry into aquatic systems than are sudden, massive accidents. Examples include runoff of field-persistent agricultural chemicals, industrial effluents from manufacturing plants, and dispersed consumer products entering aquatic systems from sewage treatment plants. In these situations, environmental evaluations must be projected over years or decades to assess the ultimate aquatic concentrations and fate of chemicals likely to result. These situations often require kinetic steady-state models, rather than the event-oriented models needed to evaluate the transient consequences of accidental spills.

Many significant fate processes occur so rapidly that their time-dependent behavior is almost never of interest in environmental situations. Ionization reactions of acids and bases typically reach equilibrium in a matter of seconds. Because the time scales of interest in toxicological investigations are seldom shorter than hours or days, ionization can usually be assumed to be in a continuous, constant equilibrium state. This is often true of sorption to nonliving sedimentary materials and of complexation reactions as well, although some exceptions to this rule have been discovered.

Models must be tailored to fit the problem-specific characteristics of the chemical and the timing and duration of chemical loadings. For example, a full evaluation of the possible risks posed by manufacture and use of a new chemical could begin from a detailed time series describing the expected releases of the compound into aquatic systems over the projected duration of its manufacture. Given an equivalently detailed time series for environmental variables, machine integration would yield a detailed picture of estimated or expected environmental concentrations (EECs) in the receiving water body over this period. The model could also be used to forecast the time required for dissipation of the chemical residuals present in the system when manufacture is terminated. This approach is very costly, however, and errors accumulate in very large-scale simulation studies.

More realistically, then, risk analysis must begin from a general evaluation of the behavior of a chemical in the environment and the associated patterns of chemical loadings. Consider, for example, a chemical that is relatively labile in the environment. Suppose also that the chemical is released only sporadically and then only for limited periods. The manufacture of some low-volume specialty chemicals is one example fitting this description. In this case, transient lethal conditions (i.e., acute effects) are the primary frame of reference. Models patterned after classical analyses of dissolved oxygen problems in streams and rivers could be used to assess the risk associated with such a chemical.

Chemicals that are very persistent in the environment, or are released at a steady rate over long periods, fall at the opposite extreme. In this case, the primary toxicological frame of reference is usually that of chronic effects. For chemicals that are extensively sorbed as well, the long-term impact on the benthos may be a major consideration in risk analysis. Models for analyzing these kinds of chemicals must include steady-state approaches; that is, the analysis must consider the long-term, ultimate residual concentrations to be expected in the environment.

Regardless of the time frame used, models that describe spatially heterogeneous systems, and the associated transport processes, lead to partial differential equations. These equations usually must be solved by numerical techniques with digital and analog computers, rather than by explicit analytic solution of the differential equations. Standard numerical techniques in one way or another divide the system, which is continuously varying in space and time, into a set of discrete elements. Spatial discrete elements are often referred to as grid points, nodes, segments, or compartments. In a compartmental or "box" model, the physical space of the system is subdivided into a series of physically homogeneous segments (compartments) connected by advective and dispersive fluxes. Each compartment is a particular volume element of the system, containing water, sediments, biota, and dissolved and sorbed chemicals. Loadings and exports can then be represented as mass fluxes across the boundaries of the volume elements; reactive properties can be regarded as point processes centered within each compartment. Similarly, continuous time is often represented by fixing the system driving functions (e.g., rainfall or sunlight intensity) for a short interval, integrating over the interval, and then "updating" the forcing functions before evaluating the next time step.

In describing an aquatic system for simulation modeling, the number and sizes of the spatial segments must be prescribed. In most simulation techniques, each physical segment is sized so that it can be assumed to be well mixed, that is, so that the speed of chemical reactions in the segment does not depend on how rapidly materials circulate in the segment. In effect, the physical segments must not be so large that internal gradients in the forcing functions have a major effect on the calculated transformation rate of the compound. Physical boundaries that can be used to demarcate system segments include the air-water interface, the thermocline, the benthic interface, and perhaps the depth of bioturbation of sediments. Some processes, however, are driven by environmental factors that occur as gradients in the system, and some processes are controlled by conditions at interfaces. For example, sunlight intensity decreases exponentially with depth in the water column, and volatilization occurs only at the air-water interface.

In well-mixed situations, gradients and processes at interfaces can easily be modeled. For example, the net rate of photochemical reaction in a well-mixed zone of a lake can be calculated by computing the average light intensity in the well-mixed zone. Similarly, volatilization models compute the flux of chemicals across the air-water interface by assuming that some depth of water below the interface zone continually renews the supply of chemical at the interface (Fig. 5). The rate of resupply of chemical does not affect the rate of volatilization, because vertical turbulence moves the chemical into the interface zone faster than it is lost to the atmosphere. In very quiescent lakes, however, relatively fine-scale vertical segmentation may be needed in order to arrive at an accurate estimate of photolysis or volatilization rates. In these cases, the speed of vertical transport processes, which move the chemical to the interface or move it along a gradient in sunlight intensity, may control the overall speed of photochemical transformation or volatilization loss of chemical from the lake. Thus, although physical boundaries help define the appropriate segmentations for use in models, slow transport processes in physically homogeneous areas of the water body may require that each zone be subdivided, for computational purposes, into many additional segments.

Regardless of the temporal and spatial horizons involved, mathematical models designed to evaluate the behavior of chemicals must include descriptions of the physical, chemical, and biological processes governing the transport and fate of chemicals in aquatic environments. These process models must be stated as a combination of the properties of the chemical and as functions of independently measurable environmental driving forces or coupling variables (e.g., pH, temperature). This approach makes it possible to study the fundamental chemistry of compounds in the laboratory and then, based on independent studies of the kinetics and intensity of driving forces in aquatic systems, the probable behavior of the compound can be evaluated for systems that have never been exposed to it.

Evaluative Models

The concept of "evaluative models" was introduced into chemical risk assessment by Baughman and Lassiter (1978). These models are intended to generate a behavioral profile of a chemical in typical environmental situations. The information produced by an evaluative model can be used in several ways. General estimates of chemical persistence can be used to select appropriate time scales for more detailed modeling studies. Evaluations of chemical fate serve to isolate the dominant fate processes and thus guide the design of detailed chemical studies. Given a general loading pattern, the order of magnitude of chemical exposures and the relative distribution of residual chemical con-

centrations in the environment can be estimated and used to guide toxicological investigations.

Mackay (1979) and Mackay and Paterson (1981) developed a series of general evaluative models to characterize the behavior of synthetic chemicals in the entire biosphere (including air, water, and solid phases). In these models the chemical concept of "fugacity" is used as an organizing principle in calculating the tendency of compounds to accumulate in different environmental sectors (e.g., atmosphere, soil, lakes, sediment, and aquatic biota). Fugacity "can be regarded as the 'escaping tendency' of a chemical from a phase. It has units of pressure, and can be related to concentration" (Mackay and Paterson, 1981).

Fugacity calculations can be performed as a level I, level II, or level III analysis. Level I provides a general indication of the sectors of the environment likely to be of concern; it is computed in terms of the thermodynamic equilibrium state to be expected if the compound is globally persistent. In a level II analysis the chemical is allowed to degrade, but interphase transport processes are assumed not to be rate-controlling; that is, transfer of the compound between phases is so fast that an equilibrium distribution of the chemical is maintained. This analysis elucidates the residence time of the chemical, giving some idea of its persistence. In level III calculations, transport processes are added to the analysis, resulting in a nonequilibrium, steady-state system that includes the possibility of kinetic hindrance of chemical breakdown of the substance due to slow transport between reactive and nonreactive zones in the environment.

One example of a level III model for aquatic systems is the "exposure analysis modeling system" (EXAMS) which was designed primarily as a screening tool for identifying and characterizing chemicals as potential aquatic pollutants (Burns et al., 1982). Inputs to the EXAMS computer program include the chemistry of the substance of concern [e.g., hydrolytic rate constants, as in Eq. (1)], characterization of an aquatic environment (e.g., pH, pOH, temperature, hydrologic inputs), and the chemical loadings entering the system. From these data, the program estimates EECs, the fate of the compound, and the persistence of the compound in that system. Persistence in this case is approximated as the time required to remove about 95–98% of the chemical mass resident in the system at steady state by the combined action of transport and transformation processes in the system.

A typical output summary from the EXAMS program is shown in Fig. 7. The program was asked to evaluate the behavior of benzo[f]quinoline in a eutrophic lake, under a total chemical loading of 100 g/d. The program divides its summary output into exposure, fate, and persistence sections; additional, more detailed outputs are available in separate tabulations.

The interpretation of this information for a hazard assessment and a guide to more detailed studies is fairly obvious. First, for this ecosystem the exposure concentration in the water column amounts to about 0.61 μg/l; this value can be compared with the results of appropriate toxicity investigations. Next, chemical reactions account

for most of the transformation activity in this system; the more detailed transformation summaries of the program could be used to identify the most significant daughter product or products. Third, most (84%) of the mass of the chemical resides in the benthic subsystem, so investigations of toxic effects on bottom-dwelling organisms might be needed for a thorough hazard evaluation. Finally, the program estimates the "self-purification" time to be about 31 mo. The chemical is thus fairly persistent (at least in this type of system), and studies of chronic effects, particularly on benthic organisms, might be warranted.

TOXICOLOGICAL APPLICATIONS OF ENVIRONMENTAL MODELING

Chemical and mathematical modeling can be used directly in toxicological investigations as well as in risk or hazard analyses. Equilibrium chemistry is useful for explaining the effects of pH on toxicological results, and for comparing chemical concentrations measured in laboratory and field situations. Chemical kinetics can be used to improve

```
     AERL-ESB MODEL OF FATE OF ORGANIC TOXICANTS IN AQUATIC ECOSYSTEMS
     CHEMICAL: BENZO[f]QUINOLINE
     ECOSYSTEM: EUTROPHIC LAKE, AERL DEVELOPMENT PHASE TEST DEFINITION
     ----------------------------------------------------------------------
     TABLE 17.   EXPOSURE ANALYSIS SUMMARY.
     ----------------------------------------------------------------------
     EXPOSURE:
       A. MAXIMUM CONC. IN WATER COLUMN: 6.13E-04 MG/L DISSOLVED, 6.29E-04 TOT
          MAX. CONC. IN BOTTOM SEDIMENT: 5.58E-04 MG/L DISSOLVED IN PORE WATER
       B. BIOSORPTION - MAX. CONCENTRATION - PLANKTON: 0.31      UG/G
                                             BENTHOS:  0.27      UG/G
       C. MAXIMUM TOT. CONC. IN SEDIMENT DEPOSITS: 0.70      MG/KG (DRY WEIGHT)
     FATE:
       A. TOTAL STEADY-STATE ACCUMULATION:   13.      KG; 15.66% IN WATER COL.,
          84.34% IN BOTTOM SEDIMENTS.
       B. TOTAL LOAD: 0.10     KG/DAY - DISPOSITION:  64.86% VIA CHEMICAL
          TRANSFORMATIONS,  28.11% BIOTRANSFORMED,   0.03% VOLATILIZED,
          7.00% EXPORTED VIA OTHER PATHWAYS.
     PERSISTENCE:
       A. AT THE END OF A  180.     DAY RECOVERY PERIOD, THE WATER COLUMN HAD
          LOST  68.38% OF ITS INITIAL TOXICANT BURDEN; THE SEDIMENTS HAD
          LOST  45.34% OF THEIR INITIAL BURDEN ( 48.95% REMOVAL OVERALL).
       B. SYSTEM SELF-PURIFICATION TIME IS ROUGHLY 31. MONTHS.
```

Figure 7 Example output summary from the EXAMS computer program. *[From Burns et al. (1982).]*

the design of toxicological experiments by ensuring that toxicological results are not distorted by extraneous chemical reactions.

Toxicological Applications of Equilibrium Chemistry

The aqueous concentration of a potentially toxic chemical is not always the same as the total mass per unit volume, because concentration can be affected by nonliving detrital and sedimentary materials or by competitive equilibria in the system. For example, the 96-h LC50 of hydrogen cyanide to juvenile fathead minnows (*Pimephales promelas*) as a function of the pH of test water is shown in Fig. 8. The LC50 of HCN drops sharply with increasing pH. Comparison of Fig. 8 with the ionic speciation of HCN (Fig. 3) suggests that the toxicities of HCN and CN⁻ are very different. A rational hazard assessment must take this difference into account.

Because pH varies from place to place and time to time, toxicity calculations must be related to the exposure concentrations of individual chemical species, rather than simply to the total environmental concentration of a compound. Cyanides (Fig. 8) are not unique in this respect. Most organic acids and bases, and metals with several valence states, are subject to chemical speciation, which can affect their toxic impact.

Chemical equilibrium calculations can refine toxicological observations in a way that facilitates extrapolation to natural ecosystems. This approach is increasingly evident in the toxicological literature. For example, Kobayashi and Kishino (1980) observed that in goldfish (*Carassius auratus*), the toxicity of pentachlorophenol, an organic acid with $pK_a = 4.8$, changes with the pH of the test water. These changes are largely due to differences in the bioconcentration of uncharged pentachlorophenol and its anionic species, a phenomenon that can be described through Eqs. (9) and (10) (Kishino and Kobayashi, 1980). In such cases, toxicological results can be extrapolated to real systems from a knowledge of pH in the toxicity test water and in natural systems.

Complexation reactions and sorption of chemicals on particulate materials, like ionizations, are often very fast and can be approximated as equilibrium processes. Sorption (and complexation) equilibria can be computed in much the same way as ionization equilibria. Consequently, reduced bioavailability of sorbed chemicals in sediment phases, for example, can be evaluated in field situations when concentrations of sorbed and dissolved chemicals and dissolved solids, and properties of the solids (e.g., organic carbon content), have been measured during laboratory toxicological investigations.

In many cases—for example, with metals that can participate in a large number of competing reactions—the equations describing the equilibrium distribution of chemical species are intricate. The principle of computation is the same in all cases, however, and computer programs that can compute speciation in a toxicity test water from its composition are now readily available [e.g., the REDEQL family of computer programs, as described by Morel and Morgan (1972) and Ingle et al. (1978, 1980)]. Magnuson et al. (1979) described a technique for identifying toxic species by factor analysis of the results of toxicity experiments, in conjunction with the computer program REDEQL2.

In very complex situations, it may be impossible to specify the toxicity of each chemical species, even when its concentration can be computed. In many cases, however, speciation is

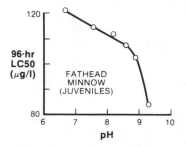

Figure 8 Hydrogen cyanide (HCN) 96-h LC50 for juvenile fathead minnows (*Pimephales promelas*) as a function of solution pH. *[From Smith et al. (1979).]*

dominated by a small subset of the possible chemical forms. Statement of toxicity in terms of the predominant species can improve the reliability and utility of aquatic toxicity data. The most important chemical parameters to specify usually include pH, carbonate alkalinity, chloride, organic carbon content, complexation capacity, and hardness.

Laboratory toxicological investigations often rely on the addition of a known quantity of test compound to a given volume of water, giving a nominal total concentration of the compound. In contrast, measured or predicted concentrations are usually used to assess potential toxicity at a field site. When, as is usually the case, speciation differs between the water in the toxicity test chamber and that at the field site, ancillary chemical analyses must be used to determine the chemical speciation in the test chamber, or ancillary variables (e.g., pH) must be measured in the test medium to allow calculation of chemical species distributions. It is important to remember that every method of chemical analysis incorporates chemical speciation either implicitly or explicitly. Unfortunately, most commonly used methods quantify the sum of neutral and ionic species (e.g., $[HA] + [A^-]$) and thus do not provide adequate information for extrapolation unless supplemented with additional data such as pH and pK_a. In these cases, the "total" concentration of potential toxicant can be the same in two different waters, but the concentration of a particular toxic species may be very different. An example is the measurement of total metal in a test tank, where the metal occurs only in dissolved forms, followed by an erroneous comparison with the "total" (suspended plus dissolved) metal in a natural water.

Toxicological Applications of Chemical Kinetics

Although fast reactions (equilibrium processes) are of first importance in improving the generality of toxicity tests, slower reactions (kinetic processes) often cannot be neglected. Flow-through toxicity test chambers are usually operated so that the water is well mixed, and the entire volume is re-

newed 4–10 times each day. With a hydraulic residence time of only 2.4 h (10 volume renewals in 24 h), it can usually be safely assumed that chemical transformations will not seriously disturb the toxicological results. This assumption should be critically evaluated in every case, however, and the tools of environmental chemistry and mathematical modeling can be used for this test. In a completely mixed, flow-through toxicity test tank, Eq. (17) becomes

$$\frac{d[C]}{dt} = \frac{F}{V}[C_i] - \frac{F}{V}[C] - KE[C] \qquad (18)$$

where the load Lo [Eq. (17)] is now the product of the inflow rate F (liters per unit time) and the concentration of chemical in the inflowing waters $[C_i]$ in milligrams per liter. If chemical transformations are unimportant, the steady-state concentration $[C]$ will be the same as the inlet concentration $[C_i]$ when the tank reaches hydrodynamic equilibrium and chemical steady state. The steady-state condition is defined by $d[C]/dt = 0$, or

$$C = \frac{[C_i]F/V}{F/V + K(E)} \qquad (19)$$

Clearly $[C] = [C_i]$ only when the system is transport-dominated, that is, when transformations have a negligible effect on concentration. This condition holds only when F/V is much less than $K(E)$; this explicit criterion can be evaluated a priori from a knowledge of the chemistry of the toxicant via Eq. (19). Of course, this approach can also be used to select appropriate experimental conditions for a toxicity test.

It is sometimes suggested that mixtures (such as commercial formulations) should be used for toxicological investigations in preference to pure chemicals. This would allow for possible toxicological interactions among the components of the mixture and would seem to eliminate the need for a factorial investigation of the toxicities of the components and their toxic interactions. The resulting data, however, are exceedingly difficult to apply to real systems if the component toxicities have not also been investigated.

Consider, for convenience, a 1:1 mixture of two compounds, Y and X. Chemical Y is a neutral organic compound subject to alkaline hydrolysis, with a second-order rate constant (K_{bh}) of $10\ M^{-1}$ s^{-1}. Compound X is an organic acid ($pK_a = 8.0$) that is subject to specific-acid hydrolysis with a rate constant (K_{ah}) of $10\ M^{-1}\ s^{-1}$. The toxicity of the anionic species $[X^-]$ is negligible, so the effective toxicity of pure X is controlled by the concentration of the uncharged species $[HX]$, that is, by the pH of the solution. The concentration of the toxic species $[HX]$ can be computed from the total concentration $[X]$ by use of Eq. (9):

$$[HX] = \frac{[H^+]}{[H^+] + K_a}\,[X] \qquad (20)$$

The chemical behavior of both components of the mixture can be described by Eq. (17). For compound Y,

$$\frac{d[Y]}{dt} = \frac{F}{V}\,[C_i] - \frac{F}{V}\,[Y] - K_{bh}[OH^-]\,[Y]$$
$$(21)$$

For compound X, assuming that its chemical reactivity is not affected by ionization,

$$\frac{d[X]}{dt} = \frac{F}{V}\,[C_i] - \frac{F}{V}\,[X] - K_{ah}[H^+]\,[X] \qquad (22)$$

In this case, F, V, and C_i are the same for both compounds. At steady state, $d[X]/dt = d[Y]/dt = 0$ by definition. By equating Eqs. (21) and (22), the steady-state ratio of total concentrations $[X]/[Y]$ can be simply stated:

$$\frac{[X]}{[Y]} = \frac{F/V + K_{bh}[OH^-]}{F/V + K_{ah}[H^+]} \qquad (23)$$

This simple result implies that the 1:1 total concentration ratio can be maintained only when the system is transport-dominated (i.e., $K_{bh}[OH^-]$ and $K_{ah}[H^+]$ are both much less than F/V, so that the transport terms, F/V, control the steady-state concentrations), or when the transformation rates happen to be the same (in this example, $K_{bh}[OH^-] = K_{ah}[H^+]$ only at pH 7.0).

Furthermore, what is of concern in a toxicological investigation of this mixture is the ratio $[HX]/[Y]$ rather than the ratio of total concentrations $[X]/[Y]$ or $([HX] + [X^-])/[Y]$ per se. Substitution of Eq. (23) gives an expression for the steady-state ratio of true toxicant concentrations as a function of detention time (V/F) and pH:

$$\frac{[HX]}{[Y]} = \frac{[H^+](F/V + K_{bh}[OH^-])}{([H^+] + K_a)(F/V + K_{ah}[H^+])} \qquad (24)$$

Figure 9 illustrates the effect of hydraulic residence time and pH on the concentration ratio $[HX]/[Y]$, computed from Eq. (24). At pH 7, hydrolytic transformation of both compounds proceeds at the same rate, and the 1:1 mixture in the inflowing waters is preserved. In this case, 91% of the total concentration of X occurs as un-

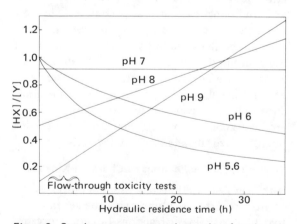

Figure 9 Steady-state concentration ratio of toxic species in a chemical mixture as a function of hydraulic residence time.

ionized HX [Eq. (20)], and [HX]/[Y] is 0.91 for all residence times.

Pure water in equilibrium with atmospheric CO_2 (315 ppm) has a pH of about 5.6; in this situation X is preferentially degraded and the concentration ratio drops sharply with increasing residence time. When the pH of the water is greater than 7, compound Y breaks down faster than compound X, and the concentration ratio increases with hydraulic residence time. The intercepts of the curves in Fig. 9 (at a residence time of zero) show the ratio of toxic chemical species, [HX]/[Y], in a transport-dominated system, that is, when the hydraulic residence time is so short that chemical concentrations are not affected by hydrolytic transformations. In this case, pH affects the ratio of toxic species only through its effect on the speciation of compound X [Eq. (20)].

Flow-through test systems are typically operated at 4–10 volume turnovers per day, corresponding to hydraulic residence times of 2.4–6 h. Figure 9 indicates that an adequately transport-dominated toxicity test could be set up for many purposes, once Eq. (20) has been used to account for ionization of compound X. A turnover rate of 4 volumes per day would be somewhat unsatisfactory, however, for a clean, unbuffered water in equilibrium with atmospheric CO_2 (pH 5.6). In this test system, the steady-state value of [HX]/[Y] is 0.65, compared to a concentration ratio in the incoming water of 0.996.

A transport-dominated toxicity test would also be difficult to achieve with an alkaline test water of pH 9.0. In the incoming waters, the ratio [HX]/[Y] is 0.91: most of compound X would be present in its (nontoxic) anionic form. A toxicity test tank operated at 10 volume turnovers per day (2.4-h residence time) would experience a steady-state [HX]/[Y] ratio of 0.17, an increase of 1.9 times. If operated at a residence time of 6 h (4 volume turnovers per day), the steady-state ratio of toxic compounds [HX]/[Y] would increase to 0.29, a factor of 3 increase over that computed by

a simple application of Eq. (20). Thus the results of toxicity tests with this mixture would depend strongly on the water formulation and flow rate used in the experiments.

Notice, moreover, that the abscissa of Fig. 9 extends to only 36 h. Lakes and ponds generally have hydraulic residence times much longer than 36 h, perhaps 30 d to several years. Taking a 30-d residence time as an environmental minimum, the concentration ratio [HX]/[Y] would then be only 0.017 in pure water (pH 5.6) and would reach 23.0 at pH 9.0. Under acidic conditions, as in a very pure water (e.g., an oligotrophic lake), the toxic effect of this mixture would be dominated by HX toxicity. In contrast, in an alkaline water (e.g., a hard-water lake), compound Y would completely dominate the final residual mixture in the system.

Clearly the toxicities of the components of a mixture must be investigated separately if the toxicity results are to be applied to natural systems. When a mixture enters the environment, it cannot be expected to maintain its original concentration ratio, for changes in pH or differential chemical reactivities produce substantial changes in the actual and relative concentrations of the components. Furthermore, partitioning to sediment phases is rarely the same for all components of a chemical mixture, and differential sorption can also have profound effects on the aqueous phase concentration ratio of a mixture introduced into a real system. The toxicity of the mixture itself may, of course, be well worth investigating. Such results, however, must be supplemented with studies on the components, proof that the toxicity test system is indeed transport-dominated, and direct investigation of the toxic interactions among the components of the mixture.

SUMMARY AND CONCLUSIONS

The results of toxicological and chemical investigations are strongly dependent on characteristics of the experimental system analyzed. An approach in which the relevant system parameters and coupling variables are carefully identified, monitored, and controlled provides a common scientific framework for environmental chemistry and toxicology. Within this framework, chemists and toxicologists can achieve a logical, realistic, and objective evaluation of the consequences of releases of synthetic chemicals into the environment. Thorough understanding of the underlying mechanisms governing toxicity and chemical processes is a requirement for success in this enterprise, because models and predictions can never be anything more than derivations of the implications of understanding. What is not understood cannot be modeled, predicted, or effectively controlled.

The tools of environmental chemistry and mathematical modeling can be applied directly to refine the sophistication and environmental applicability of laboratory toxicity investigations. Both ionic equilibria and chemical kinetics modify the exposure concentrations experienced by test organisms and natural populations. When the toxicity test tank is treated as a system in itself, however, toxicologists and ecologists gain access to a common body of tools and approaches. To the extent that aquatic toxicology or "ecotoxicology" evolves as a distinct discipline, its practitioners must develop a common view of the scientific problems involved in hazard assessment. Systems analysis, environmental chemistry, and mathematical modeling provide a convenient focus for accelerating the maturation of the discipline.

LITERATURE CITED

Alexander M: Biodegradation of chemicals of environmental concern. Science 211:132–138, 1981.

Aller RC: The influence of macrobenthos on chemical diagenesis of marine sediments. Ph.D. thesis, Yale Univ., New Haven, Conn., 1977.

Baughman GL, Burns LA: Transport and transformation of chemicals: A perspective. In: The Handbook of Environmental Chemistry, vol. 2, part A, Reactions and Processes, edited by O Hutzinger, pp. 1–17. Berlin: Springer-Verlag, 1980.

Baughman GL, Lassiter RR: Prediction of environmental pollutant concentration. In: Estimating the Hazard of Chemical Substances to Aquatic Life, edited by J Cairns, Jr, KL Dickson, AW Maki, pp. 35–54. ASTM STP 657. Philadelphia: American Society for Testing and Materials, 1978.

Baughman GL, Paris DF: Microbial bioconcentration of organic pollutants from aquatic systems. CRC Crit Rev Microbiol 8:205–228, 1981.

Bender ML, Silver MS: The hydrolysis of substituted 2-phenyl-1,3-dioxanes. J Am Chem Soc 85:3006–3010, 1963.

Berner RA: Early Diagenesis: A Theoretical Approach. Princeton, NJ: Princeton Univ Press, 1980.

Borland WM: Reservoir sedimentation. In: River Mechanics, edited by HW Shen, pp. 29-1–29-38. Fort Collins, Colorado: HW Shen, P.O. Box 606, 1971.

Brown CC: The statistical analysis of dose-effect relationships. In: Principles of Ecotoxicology (SCOPE 12), edited by GC Butler, pp. 115–148. Chichester, UK: Wiley, 1978.

Brown DS: Relationship for predicting extent of cation exchange. Submitted to J Environ Qual, 1984.

Burns LA: Identification and evaluation of fundamental transport and transformation process models. In: Proceedings of a Workshop on Modeling the Fate of Chemicals in the Aquatic Environment, Pellston, Mich., August 17–21, 1981, edited by KL Dickson, AW Maki, J Cairns, Jr., pp. 101–126. Ann Arbor, Mich.: Ann Arbor Science, 1982.

Burns LA, Cline DM, Lassiter RR: Exposure Analysis Modeling System (EXAMS): User Manual and System Documentation. Athens, Ga.: U.S. EPA Office of Research and Development, Athens Environmental Research Laboratory, 1982. EPA-600/3-82-023.

Eagleson PS: Dynamic Hydrology. New York: McGraw-Hill, 1970.

Garde RJ, Ranga Raju KG: Mechanics of Sediment Transportation and Alluvial Stream Problems. New York: Wiley, 1977.

Gibbs RJ (ed): Transport Processes in Lakes and Oceans. New York: Plenum, 1977.

Heathershaw AD: "Bursting" phenomena in the sea. Nature (Lond) 248:394–395, 1974.

Heathershaw AD: Measurements of turbulence in the Irish Sea boundary layer. In: The Benthic Boundary Layer, edited by IN McCave, pp. 11–31. New York: Plenum, 1976.

Ingle SE, Schuldt MD, Schults DW: A User's Guide for REDEQL.EPA—A Computer Program for Chemical Equilibria in Aqueous Systems. EPA-600/3-78-024; NITS PB 280 149/6BE. Corvallis, Ore.: U.S. EPA Office of Research and Development, Corvallis Environmental Research Laboratory, 1978.

Ingle SE, Keniston JA, Schults DW: REDEQL. EPAK—Aqueous Chemical Equilibrium Program. EPA-600/3-80-049. Corvallis, Ore.: U.S. EPA Office of Research and Development, Corvallis Environmental Research Laboratory, 1980.

Karickhoff SW: Sorption kinetics of hydrophobic pollutants in natural sediments. In: Contaminants and Sediments, vol. 2, edited by RA Baker, pp. 193–205. Ann Arbor, Mich.: Ann Arbor Science, 1980.

Karickhoff SW, Brown DS, Scott TA: Sorption of hydrophobic pollutants on natural sediments. Water Res 13:241–248, 1979.

Kirby AJ: Hydrolysis and formation of esters of organic acids. In: Comprehensive Chemical Kinetics, vol. 10, Ester Formation and Hydrolysis and Related Reactions, edited by CH Bamford and CFH Tipper, pp. 57–207. Amsterdam: Elsevier, 1972.

Kishino T, Kobayashi K: A study on the absorption mechanism of pentachlorophenol in goldfish relating to its distribution between solvents and water. Bull Jpn Soc Sci Fish 46:1165–1168, 1980.

Kobayashi K, Kishino T: Effect of pH on the toxicity and accumulation of pentachlorophenol in goldfish. Bull Jpn Soc Sci Fish 46:167–170, 1980.

Li Y-H: Vertical eddy diffusion coefficient in Lake Zurich. Schweiz Z Hydrol 35:1–7, 1973.

Liss PS, Slater PG: Flux of gases across the air-sea surface. Nature (Lond) 247:181–184, 1974.

Mabey W, Mill T: Critical review of hydrolysis of organic compounds in water under environmental conditions. J Phys Chem Ref Data 7:383–415, 1978.

Mackay D: Volatilization of pollutants from water. In: Aquatic Pollutants: Transformation and Biological Effects, edited by O Hutzinger, IH van Lelyveld, BCJ Zoeteman, pp. 175–185. Oxford: Pergamon, 1978.

Mackay D: Finding fugacity feasible. Environ Sci Technol 13:1218–1223, 1979.

Mackay D, Paterson S: Calculating fugacity. Environ Sci Technol 15:1006–1014, 1981.

Mackay D, Leinonen PJ: Rate of evaporation of low-solubility contaminants from water bodies to atmosphere. Environ Sci Technol 9:1178–1180, 1975.

Magnuson VR, Harriss DK, Sun MS, Taylor DK, Glass GE: Relationships of activities of metal-ligand species to aquatic toxicity. In: Chemical Modeling in Aqueous Systems—Speciation, Sorption, Solubility, and Kinetics, edited by EA Jenne, ACS Symp Ser 93, pp. 635–656. Washington, D.C.: American Chemical Society, 1979.

Mill T, Hendry DG, Richardson H: Free-radical oxidants in natural waters. Science 207:886–887, 1980.

Morel F, Morgan J: A numerical method for computing equilibria in aqueous chemical systems. Environ Sci Technol 6:58–67, 1972.

Neely WB, Blau GE, Alfrey T, Jr: Mathematical models predict concentration-time profiles resulting from chemical spill in a river. Environ Sci Technol 10:72–76, 1976.

O'Kelley JC, Deason TR: Degradation of Pesticides by Algae. EPA-600/3-76-022. Athens, Ga.: U.S. Environmental Protection Agency, 1976.

Onishi Y, Schreiber DL, Codell RB: Mathematical simulation of sediment and radionuclide transport in the Clinch River, Tennessee. In: Contaminants and Sediments, vol. 1, Fate and Transport, Case Studies, Modeling, Toxicity, edited by RA Baker, pp. 393–406. Ann Arbor, Mich.: Ann Arbor Science, 1980.

Paris DF, Steen WC, Baughman GL, Barnett JT, Jr: Second-order model to predict microbial degradation of organic compounds in natural waters. Appl Environ Microbiol 41:603–609, 1981.

Perdue EM, Wolfe NL: Prediction of buffer catalysis in field and laboratory studies of pollutant hydrolysis reactions. Environ Sci Technol 17: 635–642, 1983.

Schnoor JL: Fate and transport of dieldrin in Coralville Reservoir: Residues in fish and water following a pesticide ban. Science 211:840–842, 1981.

Shen HW (ed): Modeling of rivers. New York: Wiley, 1979.

Simons DB, Senturk F: Sediment transport technology. Fort Collins, Colo.: Water Resource Publications, 1977.

Slater JH: Microbial population and community dynamics. In: Microbial Ecology: A Conceptual Approach, edited by JM Lynch, NJ Poole, pp. 45–63. Oxford: Blackwell Scientific, 1979.

Smith LL, Jr, Broderius SJ, Oseid DM, Kimball GL, Koenst WM, Lind DT: Acute and chronic toxicity of HCN to fish and invertebrates. EPA Ecol Res Ser Rep EPA-600/3-79-009. Duluth, Minn.: U.S. EPA Environmental Research Laboratory, 1979.

Stumm W, Morgan JJ: Aquatic Chemistry, an Introduction Emphasizing Chemical Equilibria in Natural Waters. New York: Wiley-Interscience, 1970.

Thibodeaux LJ: Chemodynamics—Environmental Movement of Chemicals in Air, Water, and Soil. New York: Wiley, 1979.

Tinsley IJ: Chemical Concepts in Pollutant Behaviour. New York: Wiley, 1979.

Wetzel RG: Limnology. Philadelphia: Saunders, 1975.

Whitman WG: A preliminary experimental confirmation of the two-film theory of gas absorption. Chem Metallurg Eng 29:146–148, 1923.

Wolfe NL: Determining the role of hydrolysis in the fate of organics in natural waters. In: Dynamics, Exposure and Hazard Assessment of Toxic Chemicals, edited by R Haque, pp. 163–178. Ann Arbor, Mich.: Ann Arbor Science, 1980.

Zepp RG, Baughman GL: Prediction of photochemical transformation of pollutants in the aquatic environment. In: Aquatic Pollutants: Transformation and Biological Effects, edited by O Hutzinger, IH van Lelyveld, BCJ Zoeteman, pp. 237–263. Oxford: Pergamon, 1978.

Zepp RG, Cline DM: Rates of direct photolysis in aquatic environment. Environ Sci Technol 11: 359–366, 1977.

Zepp RG, Wolfe NL, Baughman GL, Hollis RC: Singlet oxygen in natural waters. Nature (Lond) 267:421–423, 1977.

SUPPLEMENTAL READING

Neely WB: Chemicals in the Environment—Distribution, Transport, Fate, Analysis. New York: Dekker, 1980.

Hazard Evaluation

Chapter 20

Environmental Legislation

R. B. Foster

INTRODUCTION

The evolution of the discipline of aquatic toxicology has been greatly influenced by the enactment of several pieces of major legislation related to the regulation of chemicals in the environment. Implementation of these environmental regulations accelerated efforts of the scientific community to develop and adopt standardized procedures for evaluating the effects of chemicals on aquatic life and to establish good laboratory practice and quality assurance procedures for ensuring accurate and verifiable records of the data developed. This approach was intended to provide not only comparable, replicable, and reliable data but also data that are legally defensible and which can be applied uniformly in the enforcement of regulations.

Environmental legislation dramatically increased the use of toxicity tests with aquatic organisms for regulatory purposes and led to growth in the development of standardized tests. This expanded the comparative toxicity data base, which improved our understanding of the response of organisms to chemicals and also led to a better understanding of the utility of such tests in assessing the potential hazard of chemicals. Furthermore, this legislation provided a focal point for the development of hazard evaluation procedures, which include consideration of the data on the effects of a substance on aquatic organisms and also integrate an understanding of environmental concentrations and exposure into the assessment of environmental safety. In addition to these major advances, environmental legislation motivated the development and refinement of innovative techniques for evaluating toxicity to aquatic organisms, offered a framework for international cooperation in the development of test protocols and chemical safety assessment procedures, and stimulated the development of consensus standardization.

This chapter presents a record of legislative events since the late 1960s. The record provides a means of measuring the influence of environmental legislation on developments in aquatic toxicology and of differentiating the positive, constructive changes from those that have emanated from the enforcement of environmental statutes.

BACKGROUND

In the late 1960s, growing public awareness of problems associated with environmental quality led to the enactment of two cornerstones in U.S. environmental legislation, namely the National Environmental Policy Act (NEPA) of 1969 and the Environmental Quality Improvement Act (EQIA) of 1970. By enacting NEPA, Congress first recognized the importance of creating a framework within which a national environmental improvement policy could be effectively coordinated and managed.

Today, there are more than a dozen federal statutes that directly or indirectly bear on applications of aquatic toxicology. These statutes, which employ the techniques of aquatic toxicology as both assessment and enforcement tools, regulate discharge of chemicals in industrial effluents, commercialization of new chemicals, development and application of pesticide products, disposal of hazardous wastes, and dumping of materials in the oceans and navigable fresh waters of the United States. Clearly, enactment of NEPA was the initial step which provided close scrutiny of nearly all of society's activities that could result in the contamination of aquatic environments.

Before 1970, responsibility for ensuring the protection of aquatic resources was shared among several federal agencies, including the Public Health Service, Department of Agriculture, Department of Interior, and Army Corps of Engineers. Frequently, this fragmentation of authority led to bureaucratic overlap, administrative inefficiency, and insufficient resources to address the national issue of environmental quality improve-

ment. Attempts to alleviate these problems were made by Congress in late 1970 with the creation of a central focal authority for coordinating government action on behalf of the environment. Authority for implementing environmental control legislation in a coordinated and systematic manner was given to one independent federal agency, the Environmental Protection Agency (EPA).

No other single event in the history of environmental legislation catalyzed U.S. efforts to protect public health and the environment as did the establishment of EPA. Under its direction, four major pieces of legislation directly affecting the development of aquatic toxicology were implemented. Previous enactments, such as the Federal Insecticide, Fungicide, and Rodenticide Act of 1947 (FIFRA) and the Federal Water Pollution Control Act of 1948 (FWPCA), which had been the responsibility of other agencies, were now under the control of EPA. Amendments in 1972 to both of these acts enabled the agency to initiate the coordinated effort required to control the widespread endangerment of aquatic resources in the United States. Further control was provided by the enactment, again in 1972, of the Marine Protection Research and Sanctuaries Act (MPRSA), which was intended to augment the protection of open ocean resources within the statutory limits of U.S. authority. Finally, the passage in 1976 of the Toxic Substances Control Act (TSCA) brought within the jurisdiction of EPA regulatory control over the use of commercial chemicals. Other recent enactments, such as the Resource Conservation and Recovery Act (RCRA) and Superfund legislation, although of major significance within the context of EPA's mandate to control all sources of pollution, had only a marginal effect on developments in the discipline of aquatic toxicology and hazard assessment.

FEDERAL INSECTICIDE, FUNGICIDE, AND RODENTICIDE ACT

Before the passage of FIFRA in 1947, pesticide use in the United States was regulated under the Insecticide Act of 1910, which focused on consumer protection from poor and mislabeled products, and the Food, Drug, and Cosmetic Act of 1938, which enabled the U.S. Food and Drug Administration (FDA) to establish tolerance limits for pesticide residues in agricultural commodities and processed foods. The rapid increase in pesticide usage after World War II, mainly as a result of demands for improved agricultural productivity, left a void in the ability of the federal government to control the distribution of pesticide products and led to the enactment of FIFRA. Implementing FIFRA was the responsibility of the U.S. Department of Agriculture (USDA) where interstate commerce was involved. Thus both FDA and USDA were required to approve pesticides for use. This two-party registration system came under heavy criticism in the late 1960s because there were fundamental conflicts between these agencies and they often failed to place adequate emphasis on pesticide safety in the registration process. This criticism led in 1970 to the assignment of principal regulatory activity for pesticides to EPA. Subsequently, FIFRA was amended three times (1972, 1975, and 1978) over a 6-yr period, and EPA's regulatory task was fundamentally expanded. These amendments placed specific data submission requirements on the pesticide manufacturer and directed EPA to determine whether a pesticide's use could cause "unreasonable adverse effects" on human health and the environment. The pertinent FIFRA statutes, policies, and evolving requirements are outlined in Table 1.

Unlike other environmental statutes bearing on the effects of chemicals or pollutants on aquatic life, FIFRA imposes specific data requirements on the manufacturer. Pesticide producers must supply (1) information from tests with animals to show whether the products have the potential to cause acute effects (e.g., on skin and eyes), birth defects, tumors, reproductive effects, or other harmful long-term effects, and (2) data on exposure to pesticides that might affect nontarget species, including birds and aquatic life. The 1975 and 1978 amendments defined the types of data considered necessary by EPA to judge the acceptability of a registration; they may include acute toxicity to

Table 1 Federal Insecticide, Fungicide, and Rodenticide Act

Legislative History, 61 Stat. 163

    Enacted 1947, PL92-516 (1972) as amended by PL94-51 (1975), PL94-109 (1975), PL94-140 (1975), PL95-396 (1978), PL96-539 (1980).

Goals or Policy

- No person in any state may distribute, sell, offer for sale, ship, deliver for shipment, or receive and (having so received) deliver or offer to deliver to any person any pesticide which is not registered with the Administrator.
- Procedures for registration include submission by the applicant of a statement consisting of identifying information, name, labeling, data in support of claims, complete formula, and request for classification.
- The Administrator shall publish guidelines specifying the kinds of information which will be required to support the registration of a pesticide.

Relevant Sections

    Sec. 3. Registration of pesticides

        (c) Procedures for registration

            2—Data in support of registration

        (d) Classification of pesticides

    Sec. 5. Experimental use permits

Evolving Requirements

- Development of registration standards
- Data in support of pesticide registration

Guidelines under Development Influencing Aquatic Toxicology

    Subpart E. Hazard evaluation: wildlife and aquatic organisms

    Subpart F. Good laboratory practices

    Subpart J. Hazard evaluation: nontarget plants and microorganisms

    Subpart M. Data requirements for biorational pesticides

    Subpart N. Chemistry requirements: environmental fate

freshwater, estuarine, and marine fish and invertebrates; embryo-larval and life cycle studies of fish and aquatic invertebrates; toxicity to nontarget aquatic plants and algae; aquatic organism toxicity and residue studies; and simulated or actual field testing. The registration guidelines proposed by EPA in 1978 for wildlife and aquatic organisms are contained in the Federal Register (U.S. EPA, 1978a), as are the 1980 guidelines pertaining to algae and other nontarget plants (U.S. EPA, 1980b).

Responsibility for the development and publication of these guidelines is held within EPA by the Office of Pesticides and Toxic Substances. This group is responsible for scientific review of studies submitted in support of registration and periodic revision of new test protocols and methods to meet registration and enforcement requirements. This commitment to ongoing activities enables the agency to improve the registration guidelines with technological advances in the discipline of aquatic toxicology.

Use of the concepts of hazard assessment is one area in which the regulatory agency has benefited from these advances. Before 1975, EPA did not use this integrated approach to evaluate hazards associated with pesticide use in the aquatic environment and rarely merged aquatic toxicology considerations with factors bearing on the environmental behavior, fate, and exposure characteristics of a pesticide product. The concept of hazard assessment emerged during the period 1976–1978, in part as a result of EPA's attention to test protocol development for evaluating the aquatic hazards of pesticides (American Institute of Biological Sciences, 1978) but in greater part as a consequence of developments within the industrial and academic communities in anticipation of expanding regulatory control over the production, use, and disposal of all commercial chemicals, not just pesticides (Cairns et al., 1978; Kimerle et al., 1977). These developments came about mainly as a reaction to TSCA legislation, but they were also considered suitable for evaluating pesticide safety.

FEDERAL WATER POLLUTION CONTROL ACT

Potential endangerment of the aquatic resources of the United States was recognized as early as 1899 with the passage of the Rivers and Harbors Act, which prohibited the deposition of waste materials in or on the banks of navigable waters and their tributaries. This act was followed in 1912 by the first Federal Water Pollution Control Act (FWPCA) and assignment of responsibility for its implementation to the U.S. Public Health Service.

The activities of the Public Health Service were considerably expanded when the 80th Congress passed the Water Pollution Control Act of 1948. This was the first act of a comprehensive nature in the environmental field and included the concept of joint federal and state program development and financial assistance. The 1948 act was amended in 1956, at which time further emphasis was placed on the study of pollution problems and matching federal grants to local sewage disposal plants were made available. The act was further amended in 1961, and increased emphasis was placed on the overall aspects of the federal water pollution control program. These amendments also shifted responsibility for the administration of pollution control activities from the Public Health Service to the Department of Health, Education and Welfare. In 1965 the Water Quality Act was passed, clarifying state and federal responsibilities with respect to establishing water quality standards for interstate and coastal waters.

The WPCA amendments of 1972 were the first attempt by Congress to comprehensively address the environmental pollution control needs of the country, and they fundamentally changed the required approach. The objective of the 1972 amendments was to "restore and maintain the chemical, physical and biological integrity of the Nation's waters." Vital aquatic resources were to be protected and enhanced by the attainment of two primary goals: (1) that the discharge of pollutants into navigable waters be eliminated by 1985 and (2) that water quality sufficient to provide for the protection and propagation of fish, shellfish, and wildlife be attained. Furthermore, national policy would now prohibit the discharge of toxic pollutants in toxic amounts. As is typical of enabling legislation, the 1972 amendments and the 1977 amendments (Clean Water Act or CWA) specified the goals of the legislation but not the specific methods by which these goals were to be attained. Consequently, the congressional mandate left implementation of the FWPCA up to interpretation by EPA. Table 2 is an outline of the pertinent FWPCA statutes, policies, and evolving requirements.

Initially, this interpretation focused tremendous resources on the assessment of water quality for controlling sources of pollution. This emphasis led to a proliferation of techniques and procedures for the biological monitoring of pollution sources (American Society for Testing and Materials, 1973). However, most of these procedures did not include toxicological assessments but rather focused on in-stream evaluations of the biological integrity of the receiving water community. During the period 1972-1975, regulatory limitations on industrial discharges applied mainly to pollutants typified as "conventional" and included parameters such as pH, dissolved oxygen, biochemical oxygen demand, and total suspended solids. Although recommended water quality criteria for many nonconventional pollutants were published in 1968 (National Technical Advisory Committee Green Book), 1973 (National Academy of Sciences Blue Book), and 1976 (EPA Red Book) under EPA sponsorship, these recommendations were not translated into industrial effluent limitations.

This traditional focus on water quality failed to recognize the congressional mandate to prohibit toxic discharges in "toxic amounts." This fact, coupled with increasing public concern over the presence of toxic chemicals in the environment, prompted litigation challenging the agency's implementation of Section 304 of the FWPCA concerning Water Quality Criteria as the primary approach to pollution control. Under paragraph 11 of the settlement agreement reached by this litigation (NRDC et al. *v.* Train 8 ERC 2120 D.D.C., 1976), EPA was required to publish criteria for 65 nonconventional pollutants, the so-called priority pollutants, stating the maximum allowable water concentrations consistent with the protection of aquatic life. This agreement forced EPA to abandon the traditional focus on water quality and

Table 2 Federal Water Pollution Control Act

Legislative History

Enacted June 30, 1948, Chapter 758 as amended by PL92-500 (1972), PL93-207 (1973), PL93-243 (1974), PL93-611 (1975), PL94-238 (1976), and PL95-217 Clean Water Act Amendments of 1977 and 1978 to Sections 104 and 311.

Goals or Policy

- The discharge of pollutants into navigable waters be eliminated by 1985.
- Wherever attainable, an interim goal of water quality which provides for the protection and propagation of fish, shellfish, and wildlife and provides for recreation in and on the water be achieved by July 1, 1983.
- The discharge of toxic pollutants in toxic amounts be prohibited.
- Federal financial assistance be provided to construct publicly owned waste treatment works.
- Areawide waste treatment management planning process be developed and implemented to assure adequate control of sources of pollutants in each state.
- Major research and demonstration effort be made to develop technology transfer necessary to eliminate the discharge of pollutants into navigable waters, waters of the contiguous zone, and the oceans.

Relevant Sections

    Title III—Standards and enforcement

Sec. 301. Effluent limitations for point sources

Sec. 302. Water quality related effluent limitations

Sec. 303. Water quality standards and implementation plans

Sec. 304. Quality criteria for water

Sec. 307. Toxic and pretreatment effluent standards

Sec. 311. Oil and hazardous substances liability

    Title IV—Permits and licenses

Sec. 402. National pollutant discharge elimination systems (NPDES)

Sec. 403. Ocean discharge criteria

Sec. 404. Permits for dredged or fill material

Evolving Requirements

- 1976 Natural Resources Defense Council "Settlement Agreement" (consent decree)
- 1980 Report by the Subcommittee on Oversight and Review of the Committee on Public Works and Transportation, U.S. House of Representatives, "Implementation of the Federal Water Pollution Control Act"
- 1982 Congressional amendments

adopt a more systematic approach to deriving criteria for evaluating the toxicity of water pollutants to aquatic organisms. A criterion is a qualitative or quantitative estimate of the concentration of a chemical or other constituent in water which, if not exceeded, will permit water quality sufficient to protect a specified water use. Numerical criteria can be used by EPA to develop enforceable water pollution standards under Sections 302, 303, and 307(a) (see Table 2).

Subsequently, EPA published (U.S. EPA, 1978b) uniform rules for deriving water quality criteria from scientific data on the toxic effects of a chemical constituent on aquatic organisms. Prior to the settlement agreement, EPA derived the criteria for a chemical constituent by reducing the lowest concentration known to have caused acute lethal effects in a toxicity test by a factor, usually 0.01, to protect aquatic organisms against chronic effects. The new guidelines were intended to make the rationale for the proposed numerical criteria less arbitrary and also to provide a basis for deriving criteria specifically referring to different water characteristics. Criteria were to be derived from standardized laboratory tests with individual aquatic species, including tests of acute toxicity to fish, acute toxicity to invertebrates, chronic toxicity to fish, chronic toxicity to invertebrates, toxicity to plant life, and bioconcentration.

EPA's focus on laboratory studies created an immediate need for standardized laboratory tests to determine the acute and chronic effects of the 65 pollutants identified in the settlement agreement. Development of this data base was imperative if EPA were to carry out the mandate provided in the court order. The resulting efforts clearly established the value of toxicity tests with aquatic organisms for determining water quality criteria, but also illustrated the importance of site-specific characteristics as a factor in the numerical criteria. As a result, EPA proposed procedures (U.S. EPA, January 1981) which, by employing previously published guidelines (U.S. EPA, 1978), could be used to develop site-specific water quality criteria in cases where local conditions

(e.g., water hardness) dictated that application of national criteria was too stringent and therefore an unwarranted approach. The site-specific modifications necessitate a demonstration of the potential effects of the whole effluent, rather than a chemical-by-chemical assessment as traditionally used in the National Pollutant Discharge Elimination System (NPDES) permit process. These effects are evaluated on the basis of results of acute, chronic, and bioconcentration tests conducted under site-specific conditions.

Under Section 402 of the Clean Water Act, EPA issues permits to industry allowing the discharge of waste water into the navigable waterways of the nation. These permits must be consistent with the primary pollution control mechanisms, that is, numerical effluent limitations (Section 301) and water quality criteria (Section 304) and standards (Section 303) identified in the act. During the first round of NPDES permit issuance (before 1981), EPA focused on technology-based effluent limitations, established permit conditions, and assessed compliance with these conditions by use of chemical analysis. Toxicity tests with aquatic organisms were used sporadically in the permit process at the discretion of the permit writer, but there was no uniform national policy on when to require effluent toxicity testing, what methods to use to conduct these tests, and how to use the test results in issuing permits. Although a national effluent toxicity testing (biomonitoring) policy had not been adopted, a number of EPA regions expressed interest in toxicity testing by implementing autonomous regional programs requiring toxicity testing, either as an assessment tool for establishing permit conditions or as a monitoring tool for determining compliance with these conditions. Generally, these tests consisted of static or flow-through acute tests with fish or invertebrates, but on occasion they also included exposures of longer duration for empirically evaluating the potential chronic effects of the discharge on aquatic organisms.

Recognition of the value of toxicity testing prompted several industries in the late 1970s to undertake extensive research programs designed to evaluate the toxic effects of their discharges on the aquatic environment. The programs were often comprehensive acute and chronic assessments of effluent quality and, although not directly related to NPDES permit compliance, were an indirect consequence of the regulations. Frequently, these effluent assessments used process data, chemical analyses, and toxicity tests to establish the source, duration, variability, and intensity of toxic effects in the discharge; thus they provided a better understanding of the effectiveness of waste water treatment in reducing effluent toxicity.

During the second round of NPDES permit issuance (1981–1984), EPA has proposed (U.S. EPA, 1981b) that acute aquatic toxicity tests be used on a case-by-case basis as a pollution control parameter in the development of technology- or water quality-based effluent limitations. The agency thus recognizes that while acute toxicity tests cannot be substituted for numerical chemical standards, they are extremely useful because they integrate the effects of all toxic pollutants contained in a discharge, which cannot be measured by chemical analysis. Toxicity testing is then an important means of identifying and measuring effluent toxicity and complements the present system of numerical chemical standards and limitations.

Standardized procedures for conducting effluent toxicity tests are necessary for EPA to implement its NPDES strategy. Standardized procedures have been published (U.S. EPA, 1978c, 1980d) for static and flow-through acute toxicity tests with fish and invertebrates. Adoption of these procedures provides a baseline against which the results of effluent toxicity tests can be compared and ensures the development of data in a consistent and reproducible manner. The standardized procedures are, however, limited in scope and do not address the relationship between the concentration of an effluent in the receiving water and the potential hazard to indigenous aquatic communities. These limitations are recognized by EPA and by the scientific community (Buikema et al., 1982), and efforts to better understand

these relationships through the application of more advanced procedures are recommended (Fava et al., 1982). Advanced procedures are currently under development.

MARINE PROTECTION, RESEARCH, AND SANCTUARIES ACT

Unregulated ocean disposal of municipal and industrial wastes posed a major threat to the marine resources of the United States until passage of the Marine Protection, Research, and Sanctuaries Act (MPRSA) of 1972. Commonly referred to as the Ocean Dumping Act, this legislation enabled EPA to regulate the transport of materials for ocean disposal by requiring permits based on an evaluation of the potential ecological impact of the applicant's material on the marine environment. Table 3 is an outline of the pertinent MPRSA statutes, policies, and evolving requirements.

The statute provides for the regulation of ocean disposal seaward of the 3-mile boundary of the territorial sea and is the U.S. counterpart of the International Convention on the Prevention of Marine Pollution from the Dumping of Wastes and Other Matter. Disposal within the 3-mile limit of material such as power plant effluents or discharges from oil and gas exploration and production rigs is regulated by permit under Section 402 of the Clean Water Act (National Pollutant Discharge Elimination System).

Initially, ocean dumping regulations (U.S. EPA, 1973) stated that criteria promulgated under Section 102 of MPRSA were also to function as ocean discharge guidelines, but this approach proved unworkable and EPA separated the guidelines regulating these forms of ocean pollution. The ocean discharge regulations published by EPA in 1973 were revised in 1980 (U.S. EPA, 1980a) and discharge criteria established under Section 403 of the CWA. These criteria, although not mandating the use of toxicity tests in the permit process, did recognize the importance of determining the effect of toxic pollutants discharged from stationary point sources and provided the agency with the

Table 3 Marine Protection, Research, and Sanctuaries Act

Legislative History
  Enacted October 23, 1972, PL92-532 as amended by
  PL93-254, PL93-472 (1974), PL94-62 (1975), PL94-
  326 (1976), and PL95-153 (1977)
Finding
  Unregulated dumping of material into ocean waters
  endangers human health, welfare, and amenities and
  the marine environment, ecological systems, and eco-
  nomic potentialities.
Goals or Policy
  • Regulate the dumping of all types of materials into
    ocean waters.
  • Prevent or strictly limit the dumping of any mate-
    rial which would adversely affect human health,
    welfare, or amenities, or the marine environment,
    ecological systems, or economic potentialities.
Relevant Sections
  Sec. 102. Environmental Protection Agency permits
    (a) Determination that dumping of material will
         not unreasonably degrade or endanger human
         health, welfare, or amenities, or the marine
         environment . . .
    (c) Establish criteria for evaluating effect of
         materials, excluding dredged materials, on
         fisheries, plankton, shellfish, and wildlife . . .
  Sec. 103. Corps of Engineers permits
    (a) Determination that dumping of dredged mate-
         rial will not unreasonably degrade or endanger
         human health, welfare, or amenities, or the
         marine environment . . .
    (b) Apply evaluative criteria established by EPA
         pursuant to Sec. 102 for making determina-
         tion of unreasonable degradation or endanger-
         ment.
Evolving Requirements
  • Assessment criteria and techniques for evaluating
    adverse effects on the marine environment
  • Relationship between ocean dumping criteria (this
    act) and ocean discharge criteria (1977 Clean Water
    Act)

authority and flexibility to conduct toxicity tests on a case-by-case basis.

Unlike the ocean discharge regulations, Section 102 enabled EPA to require that certain ecological evaluations be made prior to disposal of any material in the ocean. Ocean disposal regulations and criteria published by EPA in 1977 (U.S. EPA, 1977) established toxicity tests with marine organisms as the primary means of assessing the potential ecological impact of a candidate waste. Section 227.6 of these regulations also specified the framework to be used (e.g., liquid phase toxicity tests with appropriate sensitive marine organisms) and provided criteria for determining the acceptability of ocean disposal based on the results of the toxicity assessment. Although EPA was provided with widespread permit authority under MPRSA, the Army Corps of Engineers (COE) retained authority over the permit issuance and assessment of dredged material disposal into the ocean.

Section 103 of the act provided that, in collaboration with EPA, the Army Corps of Engineers require submission of certain ecological evaluations before permitting ocean disposal of dredged material. As specified by U.S. EPA (1977), this interagency collaboration led to the publication of an implementation manual (U.S. EPA/Corps of Engineers, 1977) giving national guidance for the conduct of physical, chemical, and toxicity test analyses considered applicable to the evaluation of the potential environmental impact of ocean disposal of dredged materials. These procedures consisted of detailed technical descriptions of methods for sample collection and preparation; liquid phase chemical analysis; liquid phase, suspended particulate phase, and solid phase toxicity tests; and assessment of bioaccumulation potential. In addition, recommendations were made for test organism selection, including representative plankton, crustacea, polychaetes, mollusks, and fish. Widespread use of the implementation manual in the ocean disposal permit process resulted in a number of Corps of Engineers districts adapting the procedures to meet regional needs. This additional guidance was considered necessary to inform permit applicants about procedural details such as test organism selection and chemical constituents for bioaccumulation analysis that were of particular concern in the COE district. Consequently, although a national implementation manual was published by EPA/COE, regional adaptations are currently being used (e.g., U.S. Army

Corps of Engineers, 1981) in evaluating potential environmental impacts of ocean disposal of dredged material. The preparation of these regional manuals illustrates the important role the Corps of Engineers has played in shaping the permit review process and in its commitment to the mandate of the MPRSA.

Disposal of dredged or fill material in the navigable (freshwater) environment is regulated under Section 404 of the Clean Water Act as amended in 1977, and not under the MPRSA. Furthermore, Section 404 does not mandate the use of toxicity tests in the permit process but, like other CWA regulations, accommodates assessment of the toxicological effects of dredging on a case-by-case basis. No standard procedures have been promulgated by the EPA or the Corps of Engineers, but comprehensive guidelines for the specification of disposal sites were published in 1979 (U.S. EPA, 1979c).

TOXIC SUBSTANCES CONTROL ACT

Recognition of the potential hazard associated with the widespread distribution of chemicals in commerce which were not regulated by extant legislation (e.g., chlorofluorocarbons) led to the enactment in 1976 of the landmark Toxic Substances Control Act. This act was intended to regulate commercial chemicals, other than pesticide products, that present a hazard to human health or the environment. Before this law, regulatory authority for hazardous chemicals was specified according to their particular use (e.g., drugs, pesticides, consumer products, food additives). Under TSCA, the EPA was charged with administering and implementing these regulations and is responsible for determining whether the manufacture, processing, distribution in commerce, use, or disposal of a chemical substance or mixture presents or will present an unreasonable risk of injury to human health or the environment. To assist the agency in this assessment, Congress provided that adequate data should be developed with respect to the effects of chemicals on human health and the

environment and that this development should be the responsibility of those who manufacture the chemical substances (Table 4). The sections of TSCA that have significantly affected developments in aquatic toxicology are those dealing with the testing of chemical substances (Section 4) and premanufacture notification (Section 5).

Section 4 of TSCA enables EPA to require testing of an existing or new chemical substance if it is believed that commercialization presents an unreasonable risk to human health or the environment and there are insufficient data or experience to reasonably determine the certainty of the risk.

Table 4 Toxic Substances Control Act

Legislative History
Enacted October 11, 1976, PL94-469
Goals or Policy
- Adequate data should be developed with respect to the effect of chemical substances and mixtures on health and the environment and the development of such data should be the responsibility of those who manufacture and those who process such chemical substances and mixtures.
- Adequate authority should exist to regulate chemical substances and mixtures which present an unreasonable risk of injury to health or the environment, and to take action with respect to chemical substances or mixtures which are imminent hazards.
- Authority over chemical substances and mixtures should be exercised as not to impede unduly or create unnecessary economic barriers to technological innovation while fulfilling the primary purpose of this act to assume that such innovation and commerce in such chemical substances and mixtures does not present an unreasonable risk of injury to health or the environment.

Relevant Sections
Sec. 4. Testing of chemical substances and mixtures— test rules development
Sec. 5. Manufacturing and processing notices—premanufacture notification
Sec. 8. Reporting and retention of records—significant adverse reactions and notice of substantial risk
Sec. 27. Development and evaluation of test methods

Evolving Requirements
- Interagency testing committee selections
- Test rule development activities
- Implementation of test standards

This requires the development of a rule comprehensively specifying the human health and environmental effects testing that must be performed by the manufacturer. Furthermore, the agency is responsible for developing the standards under which these test data must be developed. Under Section 5 of TSCA, manufacturers of new commercial chemicals must submit premanufacture notices to the agency describing the basic features of the new substance and its anticipated production volume, use, distribution, and human and environmental exposure. In turn, the agency must make a determination on the potential for unreasonable risk to human health or environment that may result from commercialization. If such a determination is not forthcoming, manufacture may commence within 90 d.

Although EPA has no regulatory authority requiring the submission of test data on human health or environmental effects along with a premanufacture notice, the development of guidance documents (U.S. EPA, 1979a) for use by the manufacturers spurred much activity in the area of aquatic toxicology and hazard evaluation. Activities within the scientific community had already underlined the importance of developing testing methodologies and rational integrated approaches for efficiently assessing the potential hazard to aquatic life of the use of chemical substances, and the passage of TSCA encouraged interaction between industry and EPA in the development of a uniform testing policy. Industry participation in the development of methodologies for ecological effects and chemical fate testing acknowledged the importance of environmental safety data in decisions on product commercialization and established a precedent for industry's relationship with EPA. This relationship resulted from the active role many chemical manufacturers assumed in verifying and standardizing testing methodologies that could be recommended by EPA.

Initial EPA policy guidance adopted many of the standard measurement and assessment techniques used to evaluate pesticides under the FIFRA guidelines (e.g., acute toxicity tests with fish and macroinvertebrates), but also suggested a number of methodologies of unproved reliability or value for assessing the hazard of chemicals (*Lemna* sp. inhibition and seed germination and early growth studies). It encouraged the development and validation of a variety of toxicity test procedures, but also offered the scientific community the opportunity to refine and apply the integrated aquatic hazard evaluation approach to investigating chemical safety. Standardization groups, such as the American Society for Testing and Materials (ASTM), established standard practices for evaluating the hazard of chemicals to aquatic organisms and sponsored annual symposia (beginning in 1976) on aquatic toxicology and hazard assessment. These activities provided industry and EPA with the opportunity to interact in a scientific forum, to profit from exchanges on the various hazard evaluation approaches in use (Reisa, 1978), and to help establish the credibility of this concept for assessing chemical hazards.

Consensus standards, although highly desirable within the context of regulatory enforcement, have not always been available for use by EPA. This lack of standards generally resulted from (1) the time required to develop a consensus method, (2) the unavailability of a specific method to meet the agency's need, and (3) the regulatory mandate to develop test standards in conformance with the Section 4 schedule of test rules. Consequently, EPA has prepared standards, including procedures for conducting static and flow-through acute toxicity tests, early life stage (embryo-larval) tests with fish, and bioconcentration studies, specific for the development of test data under Section 4 of TSCA. These are considered state-of-the-art procedures for evaluating chemical effects, but they include requirements that would not be consistent with existing consensus standards or be suitable for widespread, economic use in routine testing.

TSCA regulatory needs for reliable and uniform test procedures and assurances that the data are both accurate and verifiable were addressed by EPA in the development of proposed good laboratory practice (GLP) standards for the acquisition of data on physical, chemical, ecological effects, and persistence of chemical substances (U.S. EPA, 1980c). Published under the authority of Section 4, these standards were proposed to overcome problems encountered by FDA inspections in the early 1970s, including inadequate test data and unacceptable laboratory practices such as selective reporting of data, lack of adherence to specified protocols, and poor record-keeping in nonclinical laboratory studies.

The importance of adhering to standard protocols and maintaining accurate and verifiable records of aquatic toxicity tests was apparent in the late 1970s, and many testing laboratories adopted FDA standards (U.S. Department of Health, Education and Welfare and U.S. Food and Drug Administration, 1978) while awaiting the proposed TSCA regulations. Regardless of when GLP programs were instituted in these facilities, the impact of compliance was a considerable, although not necessarily unwarranted, burden. Today GLP standards are prescribed for the selection, handling, and storage of the test substance; personnel qualifications and organization of the laboratory; appropriate laboratory facilities; equipment operation and maintenance; development of and adherence to a study plan; record-keeping and reporting requirements; and audit and inspection of data. Adherence to GLP ensures an accurate and reliable account of the circumstances, conditions, and results of a study, and the benefits of adherence to GLP are shared by regulatory agencies charged with protecting human health and the environment and the industries that they regulate. Responsible testing facilities must therefore be prepared not only to address the statutory requirements of TSCA but also to apply these standards to pesticide (FIFRA), industrial effluent (FWPCA), and hazardous waste (RCRA) evaluations.

INTERNATIONAL REGULATIONS

International regulation of chemical manufacture, use, and disposal is embodied in a variety of laws specific to certain foreign nations. For example, chemical use is regulated in Japan under the Chemical Substances Control Law (1973) by the Ministries of Health, Welfare, Trade, and Industry; in the United Kingdom under the Proposed Scheme for Notification of Toxic Properties of Substances (1977) by the Health and Safety Commission and Executive; and in Canada under the Environmental Contaminants Act (1978) administered by the Ministry of Environment. These countries and the remaining 24 member nations (including the United States) of the Organization for Economic Cooperation and Development (OECD) recognized the need for a concerted international effort to protect humans and the environment from exposure to hazardous chemicals and identified the need for consistent data requirements as early as 1977 (OECD, 1981). Development of such data requirements was encouraged to promote international trade in chemicals and the mutual economic advantages that accrue from the harmonization of testing guidelines. Although implementation of chemical control laws was left to the individual nations, harmonization of chemical testing methods among the OECD members was planned to improve national controls, efficiently utilize scarce resources, and avoid unnecessary barriers to international trade. Consequently, it was agreed that data generated on a particular chemical substance in one OECD member country in accordance with OECD test guidelines and GLP principles would be accepted in other member countries.

The effort to reach agreement on test guidelines and good laboratory practices took place during 1978–1981 and resulted in the publication of a recommended premarket base set of data called the Minimum Premarket Data (MPD) set (OECD, 1981) to be used in the assessment of chemicals. The base set of tests included tests conducted to acquire data in the categories of physical and chemical properties and ecotoxicology (e.g., fish acute, algal inhibition, and daphnid reproduction tests and chemical degradation or accumulation studies), as well as long-term and short-term mammalian toxicology tests which, when integrated with information on use and exposure, would permit an initial assessment of the potential health and environmental effects of commercial chemicals.

The OECD guidelines and testing requirements were published under the laws of the European Economic Community, specifically the 6th Amendment (Table 5). Unlike its U.S. counterpart (TSCA, 1976), the 6th Amendment enabled member states to require the submission of specific test data on new and existing chemical substances. However, in forming U.S. policy on the voluntary

Table 5   European Economic Community (EEC)

Council Directive 79/831/EEC (September 18, 1979)
Amending for the sixth time directive 67/548/EEC on the approximation of the laws, regulations, and administrative provisions relating to the classification, packaging, and labeling of dangerous substances in member states.

Goals or Policy
In order to control the effects on man and the environment, it is advisable that any new substance placed on the market be subjected to a prior study by the manufacturer or importer and a notification to the competent authorities conveying mandatorily certain information; whereas it is, moreover, important to follow closely the evolution and use of new substances placed in the market, and that in order to do this it is necessary to institute a system which allows all new substances to be listed.

Relevant Sections
Article 3. Physio-chemical properties, toxicity, and ecotoxicity of substances and preparations shall be determined according to methods specified in ANNEX V(A), (B), and (C), respectively.

Evolving Requirements
* Developments in member states, e.g., Health and Safety Commission of the United Kingdom; consultative document: notification of new substances 1981, draft regulations and approved codes of practice
* Organization for Economic Cooperation and Development (OECD): Data requirement and test guidelines
* Chemicals Inspection and Testing Institute; Ministry of International Trade and Industry, Japan

development of premanufacture testing under Section 5 of TSCA, EPA recommended in 1981 that manufacturers subject to premanufacture notification (PMN) requirements utilize the base set as a starting point for designing a premanufacture testing program (U.S. EPA, 1981a). This policy included not only the chemical and biological parameters contained in the base set but also the recommended test guidelines and procedures.

Today, EPA continues to participate in the harmonization process, and more advanced test guidelines than the base set are under development by the OECD. EPA's contributions to this international standardization effort have been and will continue to be beneficial, ultimately providing the basis for mutual understanding and the commitment to protect the aquatic environment from exposure to hazardous chemicals.

SUMMARY

Interest in the use of toxicity tests with aquatic organisms as indicators of adverse environmental conditions began in the early 1940s. Use of this measurement tool over the next 25–30 yr was, however, limited to relative indications of acute toxic effects among species and among pollutants, and rarely were issues of regulatory compliance or enforcement in question. Emergence in the early 1970s of the FIFRA, FWPCA, and MPRSA legislation created an immediate demand for reliable techniques for measuring biological response and burdened a small but capable group of government, industry, and academic laboratories with the responsibility for developing and validating these methods. The need created by regulatory demand undoubtedly strained a limited set of resources, but also made available many opportunities for evaluating the impact of pollutants on aquatic life. Inevitably, it was the regulation of all forms of potential environmental contamination (TSCA, 1976) that forced aquatic toxicology and the application of toxicity tests to evaluate environmental safety to experience the quantum leap to the prominence they hold today.

Quantity is, however, not quality, and although there is little question that legislation accelerated the effort to develop and adopt standard procedures, these procedures may not always be suitable for addressing the array of questions that can arise in evaluating the hazard of a new pesticide, chemical, or industrial discharge. Continued improvement in the ability to predict the consequences of exposure to environmental contaminants is necessary if those charged with protecting the environment are to succeed. Improvements, however, require change, and change in the form of new and innovative approaches to assessing biological response can be discouraged by the regulatory bureaucracy with mechanistic demands for uniformity and standardization (Macek, 1982). Now that U.S. environmental legislation has been implemented which regulates all forms of environmental pollution, it is time to reassess this approach and strive to provide a better vehicle for long-range research and development of new testing methodologies. The evolution of aquatic toxicology and its use in the hazard evaluation process during the next 10-15 yr will be contingent on this reassessment.

LITERATURE CITED

American Institute of Biological Sciences: Criteria and rationale for decision making in aquatic hazard evaluation (third draft). In: Estimating the Hazard of Chemical Substances to Aquatic Life, edited by J Cairns, Jr, KL Dickson, AW Maki, pp. 241–273. ASTM STP 657. Philadelphia: American Society for Testing and Materials, 1978.

American Society for Testing and Materials: Biological Methods for the Assessment of Water Quality, edited by J Cairns, Jr, KL Dickson. ASTM STP 528. Philadelphia: ASTM, 1973.

Buikema AL, Jr, Niederlehner BR, Cairns J, Jr: Biological monitoring, part IV—toxicity testing. Water Res 16:239–262, 1982.

Cairns J, Jr, Dickson KL, Maki AW: Summary and conclusions. In: Estimating the Hazard of Chemical Substances to Aquatic Life, edited by J Cairns, Jr, KL Dickson, AW Maki, pp. 191–197. ASTM STP 657. Philadelphia: American Society for Testing and Materials, 1978.

Fava JA, Kapp RM, Gift JJ, Flyn CR, DelPup JA: A biological risk assessment approach to establishing water quality based effluent limits. In: Aquatic Toxicology and Hazard Assessment: Fifth Conference, edited by JG Pearson, RB Foster, WE Bishop, pp. 341–355. ASTM STP 766. Philadelphia: American Society for Testing and Materials, 1982.

Kimerle RA, GJ Levinskas, Metcalf JS, Scharf LG: An industrial approach to evaluating environmental safety of new products. In: Aquatic Toxicology and Hazard Evaluation, edited by FL Mayer, JL Hamelink, pp. 36–43. ASTM STP 634. Philadelphia: American Society for Testing and Materials, 1977.

Macek KJ: Aquatic toxicology: Anarchy or democracy? In: Aquatic Toxicology and Hazard Assessment: Fifth Conference, edited by JG Pearson, RB Foster, WE Bishop, pp. 3–8. ASTM STP 766. Philadelphia: American Society for Testing and Materials, 1982.

National Academy of Sciences, National Academy of Engineering: Water Quality Criteria 1972 (Blue Book). A Report of the Committee on Water Quality Criteria. Ecol Res Ser EPA-R3-73-033. Washington, D.C.: U.S. Environmental Protection Agency, 1973.

National Technical Advisory Committee to the Secretary of the Interior: Water Quality Criteria (Green Book). Washington, D.C.: Federal Water Pollution Control Administration, 1968.

OECD: Guidelines for Testing of Chemicals by the Organization for Economic Cooperation and Development. ISBN 92-64-12221-4. Paris: Director of Information, 1981.

Reisa JJ: Margins of safety in the assessment of aquatic hazards of chemicals—some regulatory viewpoints. In: Aquatic Toxicology and Hazard Assessment: Fourth Conference, edited by DR Branson, KL Dickson, pp. 15–27. ASTM STP 737. Philadelphia: American Society for Testing and Materials, 1978.

U.S. Army Corps of Engineers: Guidance for Performing Tests on Dredged Material to be Disposed of in Ocean Waters. Regulatory Branch

New York District in conjunction with U.S. EPA Region II, 1981.

U.S. Department of Health, Education and Welfare and U.S. Food and Drug Administration: Nonclinical laboratory studies. Good laboratory practice regulations. Fed Regist 43:59986–60025, 1978.

U.S. EPA: Subchapter H. Ocean dumping. Final regulations and criteria. Transportation for dumping and dumping of materials into ocean waters. Fed Regist 38:28610–28621, 1973.

U.S. EPA: Quality Criteria for Water (Red Book). Washington, D.C.: Office of Water and Hazardous Materials, U.S. EPA, 1976.

U.S. EPA: Ocean dumping regulations and criteria. Fed Regist 42:2468–2493, 1977.

U.S. EPA: Proposed guidelines for registering pesticides in the United States: Subpart E. Hazard evaluation: Wildlife and aquatic organisms. Fed Regist 43:29724–29741, 1978a.

U.S. EPA: Water quality criteria. Fed Regist 43:21506–21518, 1978b.

U.S. EPA: Methods for Measuring the Acute Toxicity of Effluents to Aquatic Organisms. EPA-600/4-78-012. Cincinnati, Ohio: Environmental Monitoring and Support Laboratory, 1978c.

U.S. EPA: Toxic Substances Control Act premanufacture testing of new chemical substances. Fed Regist 44:16240–16292, 1979a.

U.S. EPA: Water quality criteria. Fed Regist 44:15926–15981, 1979b.

U.S. EPA: Guidelines for specification of disposal sites for dredged or fill material. Fed Regist 44:54222–54251, 1979c.

U.S. EPA: Interim NPDES Compliance Biomonitoring Inspection Manual. MCD-62. Washington, D.C.: Office of Water Enforcement, Enforcement Division, 1979d.

U.S. EPA: Ocean discharge criteria. Fed Regist 45:9548–9555, 1980a.

U.S. EPA: Proposed guidelines for registering pesticides in the United States: Subpart J. Hazard evaluation: Nontarget plants and microorganisms. Fed Regist 45:72948–72978, 1980b.

U.S. EPA: Physical, chemical, persistence and ecological effects testing: Proposed good laboratory practice standards. Fed Regist 45:77353–77365, 1980c.

U.S. EPA: Effluent Toxicity Screening Test Using *Daphnia* and Mysid Shrimp. EPA 600/4-81-000. Cincinnati, Ohio: Office of Research and Development, Environmental Monitoring and Support Laboratory, 1980d.

U.S. EPA: New chemical substances: Premanufacture testing policy. Fed Regist 46:8986–8993, 1981a.

U.S. EPA: Use of Effluent Toxicity Testing in the Second Round of NPDES Permit Issuance. Draft Policy Guidance Document. Washington, D.C.: Industrial Permits Branch, Office of Water Enforcement, 1981b.

U.S. EPA–Corps of Engineers: Ecological Evaluation of Proposed Discharge of Dredged Material into Ocean Waters; Implementation Manual for Section 103 of PL92-532. Vicksburg, Miss.: Technical Committee on Criteria for Dredged and Fill Material, Environmental Effects Laboratory, U.S. Army Engineers Waterways Experiment Station, 1977.

Chapter 21

Field Validation

W. M. Sanders, III

INTRODUCTION

The former administrator (Gorsuch, 1981) of the U.S. Environmental Protection Agency, in testimony before a subcommittee of the Committee on Science and Technology, U.S. House of Representatives, stated, "Elected and appointed public officials are called upon almost daily to make difficult decisions on major environmental policy issues involving a great deal of scientific controversy and uncertainty. The more uncertainty there

The author gratefully acknowledges the assistance provided by the following members of the Athens Environmental Research Laboratory staff: Mr. Lee A. Mulkey for consulting on the preparation of material for the chapter; Dr. R. R. Swank, Dr. Larry Burns, Mr. Tom Barnwell, and Mr. Bob Ambrose for their technical review and comments; Mr. Bob Ryans for his editorial assistance; and Miss Brenda Strickland and Miss Pam Wright for typing and proofreading the manuscript.

is, the more difficult it is to estimate the proper balance between public safety on the one hand, and the often enormous costs of pollution control on the other. We simply cannot afford to err badly in *either* direction. Better knowledge of the scientific and technical facts almost always reduces the likelihood of such error."

Scientists and developers of new chemicals, materials, analytical methods, toxicity test procedures, protocols, and exposure and risk assessment models are anxious to evaluate the performance of their products against a variety of real world conditions to assure their scientific validity and acceptability in environmental decision-making. Thus, demands increase for a variety of "field validation" studies to be carried out in conjunction with aquatic toxicology programs.

As with any new and emerging technology, there are currently many divergent views on what constitutes an acceptable field validation program, especially when one considers the varied needs of environmental decision-makers or scientists and developers. These differences, combined with the reality that field studies can be expensive, time-consuming, frustrating, and often unrewarding, require that careful consideration be given to the field validation process prior to the commitment of time and resources. The purposes of this chapter are to (1) explore the validation process and (2) present a systematic approach for planning and executing a field validation program for an *environmental risk assessment protocol.*

ELEMENTS OF A FIELD VALIDATION PROGRAM AND TERMINOLOGY

The concept of validation is an integral part of the basic "scientific method" by which hypotheses are tested and either accepted or rejected on the basis of specific predetermined criteria. In most scientific studies, these criteria of acceptability are very strict, and the hypotheses are stated in such a way that the outcome of the scientific evaluation is a definite "yes, the hypothesis is acceptable," or "no, the hypothesis is rejected."

In applying the concept of validation to evaluate tools for environmental decision-making, users need to know whether a particular method, test, or model is applicable to the solution of a specific problem. Their criteria of acceptability are based on the conditions of the specific problem to be addressed and are as strict as possible because of the human or environmental risks and economic considerations associated with the decision. Thus, from a legal, moral, and economic position, environmental decision-makers need rigorous, problem-oriented applications of the validation process to ensure that the tools they use are scientifically valid for the problems they face.

Concurrently, scientists-developers are usually interested in providing scientific evaluations of the performance of their methods, toxicity tests, or models for application over a broad range of conditions that might occur in time and space, rather than the application to one specific problem. Here the question focuses on "how well" the product performs over a range of applications. Thus, instead of establishing a rigid set of acceptability criteria prior to initiation of the evaluation process, the scientists-developers would like to establish *confidence limits* for the performance of their product for situations representing both normal and extreme conditions of application.

Ideally, the scientists-developers would provide a large inventory of environmental decision tools, each with stated confidence limits for a wide range of field applications. Decision-makers faced with an environmental problem and armed with problem-specific acceptability criteria could examine this inventory and, matching the criteria with the confidence limits, select a scientifically valid tool to solve a problem. (Of course, most decision officials would not make the selections themselves but would rely on technical experts to carry out the detailed operations.)

In reality, there are very few decision tools that have adequate documentation of critical evaluations over a wide range of environmental conditions, decision officials who have developed valid acceptability criteria for evaluating available tools, or scientists and developers who have the necessary resources to conduct field evaluation studies over a sufficiently broad range of field conditions to ensure extrapolation of the use of their product in time and space. Thus, at present, one finds a profusion of needs, desires, expectations, demands, acceptances, competencies, and misunderstandings related to the process of field validation.

Within the scientific-technical community, the terms "verification" and "validation" are often used interchangeably, especially when dealing with mathematical models. Because both processes are important and necessary to the evaluation of decision tools, the definitions of the General Accounting Office (1979) will be followed. *Verification* is an examination to determine whether a method, test, or model operates as desired or intended. *Validation* is the process of comparing the overall result or output of a method, toxicity test, or model with data representing perceived reality, and *field validation* restricts the process to comparisons with data obtained from real-world environments. (The use of a decision tool will be valid or invalid based on problem-oriented *criteria of acceptability* selected before initiation of the comparison.) In the same context, *scientific field evaluation* is a comparison of the overall results of a method, toxicity test, or model with field data in order to determine the degree of correspondence and to establish confidence limits for the decision tool under investigation. Thus, field validation studies will include scientific evaluatons; however, scientific evaluations may not constitute validations, depending on whether acceptability criteria are preselected and used to judge the results of the comparisons.

Building on these stated definitions, five major elements must be considered in the development and execution of a field validation program. First, the method, test, or model must be verified and shown to provide theoretically consistent and desirable results. Second, a set of acceptability criteria must be developed. Third, proper field sites must be selected to serve as adequate bases for validation purposes. Fourth, the field evaluation program must provide statistically acceptable measures of the important parameters and state variables characterizing the perceived real-world conditions to serve as the basis for the validation comparison. And last, sufficient resources must be available to complete the field evaluation program in a manner consistent with the criteria of acceptability. A breakdown in any one of these key elements, including economic feasibility, will result in an "invalid" and futile field validation program.

Verification of the method or model to be validated is probably the easiest task, because many analytical methods or toxicity tests have been in use for sufficient time to have accumulated a body of information that may already have achieved scientific acceptance or that can serve as a data base for statistical evaluation. Newer methods may be subjected to statistically designed studies to determine their overall precision. Models, on the

other hand, can be verified to determine the completeness of their assumptions, the mathematical and logical constructs, the calibration data requirements, their computational efficiency, and their overall strengths and weaknesses. Such verification is necessary to determine the effectiveness of a particular model when applied to a specific problem or field condition.

Establishing the criteria of acceptability for judging validity is a key element in the whole validation process. The criteria should establish (1) the gross magnitude or range of environmental conditions over which the specific decision tool must be valid (needed in the selection of field sites) and (2) the minimum acceptable level of comparability between the overall result of applying a method, toxicity test, protocol, or model and the field-derived data base representing perceived truth or reality. Thus, the selection of the criteria must be influenced by the nature, scope, and severity of the specific problem (decision) being addressed as well as the type of method, test, or model application being validated. As an example, the range of environmental conditions to be included in a validation comparison will be much smaller for the application of an estuarine toxicity test involving a pesticide to be applied to crops only in the Mississippi Delta region than for the application of a risk assessment model involving a toxic chemical expected to receive national distribution. Likewise, the acceptability criteria (level of comparability) will be more stringent when the consequences of the decision have grave human health, environmental, and economic impacts than when the impacts are nominal.

The most difficult part of the process may be the development of a correct theoretical correspondence between the application of decision tools to be validated and the selection of appropriate field conditions to serve as the basis for comparison. For the validation of analytical measurement methods, environmental loading estimates of point source discharges, simple predictions of environmental exposures, or acute toxicological tests, the selection of appropriate field conditions will be straightforward. For other situations, the state of the art makes the task much more difficult, if not impossible. Among these difficult situations are complicated estimates of exposures where the toxic chemical interacts with environmental parameters to drastically change the system; complex microcosm effects studies; or environmental risk assessment models for subtle, chronic, or delayed impacts. Lassiter (1982) pointed out that neither coherent theories nor analytical techniques currently exist to permit the prediction or measurements of effects of toxic chemicals at the ecosystem level. Under these conditions it may be currently impossible to select appropriate ecosystem field conditions, or measurable parameters for validation purposes. If this is the case, a management decision should be made not to attempt a field validation study until the state of the art permits. The state of the art is changing rapidly in this area, however, and the selection process should not be written off without a thorough analysis.

Once the theoretical feasibility of conducting appropriate comparisons has been determined, and candidate field sites selected, available field methods to measure or characterize those relevant parameters must be evaluated on both a technical and an economic basis. From a technical standpoint, analytical methods suitable for survey work may not provide the precision or accuracy required to develop quantitatively acceptable data bases. Thus, more rigorous and often state-of-the-art methods must be utilized. Other factors that should be considered include the capability to obtain representative samples in time and space, to determine extraction and concentration efficiencies, to maintain sample integrity, and to provide quality assurance records for all analytical methods from an economic standpoint.

Field sampling is an expensive process, especially when dealing with replicate samples required for statistically acceptable results; identification and quantification of low levels of toxic chemicals requiring analytical methods such as gas chromatography–mass spectrometry (GC–MS)

[some comprehensive techniques may cost up to $1000 per sample (EPA, 1979a, 1979b; Schwab et al., 1981)]; and biological sampling including population survey studies, which are labor-intensive and often require several years to complete. For empirically based decision tools, it may also be important to consider natural seasonal and annual variations in environmental factors caused by changes in temperature and the hydrologic cycle, because a statistically acceptable field data base may require sampling over several years (Toebes and Ouryvaev, 1970). C. N. Smith (1978), calculating the field sampling costs for five U.S. EPA multiyear agricultural pesticide runoff studies (for model calibration), found that the total average cost per parameter per solution per year ranged from $2,000 to $19,000. The total average field sampling cost for the pesticides alone ranged from $11,000 to $20,500 per pesticide per solution per year. Thus, it is essential to develop realistic cost estimates, not only for the analytical methods but also for the entire field validation program including labor, equipment, support services, and logistics.

The last element in the development of a field validation program is a benefit-cost analysis to ensure that the value of the analytical method, toxicity test, or model for a particular environmental decision is worth the expenditure of time and resources required to meet the acceptability criteria established for the field validation study. When the human or environmental risks and/or the socioeconomic costs of failure to control or clean up an environmental problem greatly exceed the cost of the study, field validations may be recommended. More important, if sufficient time or resources are not available to develop minimally acceptable field data bases for the validation comparisons, management decisions must be made to accept and use the methods, assays, or models on their current merits and not to waste valuable resources on ineffective field validation programs. It should be recognized, however, that reliance on techniques that have not been validated may lead to costly adverse environmental effects on the one hand, or to the expenditure of large sums in the promulgation and enforcement of needless regulations on the other.

PLANNING AND EXECUTING A FIELD VALIDATION PROGRAM

Once it has been established that a field validation study is desirable, technically achievable, and economically feasible, the next step is to develop the simplest and most cost-effective study plan that will provide data meeting the criteria of acceptability to serve as the basis for the validation comparisons. To this end, a systems approach to planning and executing the validation program should be adopted.

The same basic concept

$$\text{Loading} \rightarrow \text{Exposure} \rightarrow \text{Effects} \qquad (1)$$

underlying aquatic "toxicity tests" [observed organism effects are related to the exposure concentration of toxicant in the test system, which in turn is related to the loading (amount) of toxicant added to the test system during a given period of time] may be extrapolated to the field and used as a framework for planning and conducting field validation studies where determinations of either exposures or effects are involved. In field situations, chemically induced human or environmental toxicological effects may be related to the multimedia loading of implicated chemicals through exposure analysis techniques, including direct ambient measurements and predictive modeling.

By including exposure as one of the three key elements in the logic, important transport and fate process information is incorporated into toxicological cause-and-effect relationships, and the concept becomes more flexible in both scale and complexity. Thus, common features can be identified in the test or model system being validated and the natural environmental system selected as the field prototype.

Another unique feature of using this concept as a systems framework for validating exposure or toxicological effects methodologies is its ready application in the development and evaluation of regulatory and control options that may be associated with solving an environmental problem. The addition of a control loop to the basic concept is illustrated in Eq. (2):

$$\text{Multimedia loadings} \rightarrow \text{Exposure} \rightarrow \underset{\text{effects}}{\overset{\text{Human or}}{\text{environmental}}} \qquad (2)$$

$$\underset{\longleftarrow \text{Control} \longrightarrow}{}$$

Thus, the same tools and field-derived data bases used in validation processes can also be used as part of the system needed to evaluate alternative control options and the social and economic costs and benefits associated with each.

For the purpose of this discussion, a protocol will be developed for planning and executing a large-scale field study to provide a data base against which the application of a complex multimedia risk assessment methodology can be validated. It is assumed that the problem, the risk assessment methodology, and the criteria of acceptability are available. Applicable portions of this protocol may be scaled down and adapted to simpler field studies required in the validation of less complex methods, toxicity tests, or exposure models.

To apply the cause-and-effect logic [Eq. (1)] to the collection of field data, chemical-specific and environment-specific data are required to quantify and characterize the loading, exposure, and effects elements. The following steps should offer a cost-effective protocol for obtaining and analyzing the needed information.

- Site selection
- Existing records survey—data inventory
- Initial screening sampling program
- Preliminary modeling and analysis
- Detailed sampling program
- Detailed modeling and analysis

Site Selection

The primary objective of site selection is to locate a geographic area that will provide suitable environmental conditions to serve as a prototype data base for comparison with the laboratory methods, tests, or model applications that must be validated. Following the simple loadings-exposure-effect logic, each major component must be identifiable and measurable in order to complete the cause-and-effect relationship within the selected area. Other factors to be considered are the following.

• The area should be sized according to data needs and should be located as close to analytical facilities as possible to minimize sampling costs.

• The area should be selected to minimize the complicating influence of external factors such as widely fluctuating environmental conditions, upstream or upwind sources, and target organisms that move in and out of the area.

• Government (city, county, state) officials, local citizens, landowners, and industrial managers in the study area should be amenable to the proposed field study and should be encouraged to participate if possible.

Existing Records Survey—Data Inventory

A survey of existing records and environmental data relative to the study site should be conducted in order to:

• Identify and characterize possible sources of pollutants such as waste treatment facilities, direct discharge sites, non-point and mobile sources, landfills, storage areas, and sludge beds.

• Quantitatively characterize the physical, chemical, and biological properties of the environment that could influence the source loadings; the transport, transformation, degradation, and distribution of the toxicants; and the normal habitat of the indigenous organisms. Such data include stream flow; storm frequency and intensity; local meteorological conditions; land use, cover, and topography; farming practices; municipal and industrial operations; water, air, and soil quality;

and types, number, and distribution of indigenous biota.

• Confirm perceived human health or environmental problems and identify new problems as the data permit. These data include results of local or regional epidemiologic studies, morbidity and mortality data, autopsy and pathology reports, farm animal and crop data, fish and wildlife reports, and water quality and air quality reports.

• Develop an initial list of target chemicals that may be present in measurable quantities in the study area. These data include identification of toxic chemicals in municipal and industrial waste discharges; ambient river, stream, lake, or estuary waters; agricultural materials applied within the area; rain, snow, and ambient air; human, farm animal, fish, and wild animal tissues; food and crop residues; and soils and sediment.

• Identify and evaluate results of any special environmental studies conducted in the area, including listing mathematical models (water quality, air quality, soil loss, non-point-source runoff, demographic, exposure, risk, etc.) that may have been calibrated for conditions in the study site.

• Assemble specific data on each chemical believed to be present in the study area. These data should include physical-chemical properties, human and environmental effects, and fate and transport process rate and equilibrium constants.

Data searches should be comprehensive. It is useful to locate and catalog pertinent information sources even though it may be unnecessary to obtain the data until it is certain that they will be used. Many excellent sources of data are often overlooked, and a little extra time and expense at this phase of the project may yield large savings during the data collection and evaluation phases. When cataloging the various types of data, an initial subjective evaluation (i.e., good, fair, or poor) should be recorded to assist in later planning and assessments.

One of the primary information needs is a complete set of area maps providing both large- and small-scale representations of the area. The U.S. Geological Survey (USGS), state highway departments, Soil Conservation Service (SCS),

National Oceanic and Atmospheric Administration (NOAA), and local planning agencies such as Area-wide 208 (Public Law 92-500, Section 208, Water Quality Program) organizations and planning commissions are excellent sources of maps.

Comprehensive waste inventories may be scarce, but U.S. EPA regional offices, state environmental protection offices, and Areawide 208 or other planning offices would have any available data files. Reports such as the 303(e) Basin Plans prepared under PL92-500 may also be useful. Individual discharge data may be obtained from local municipal sewage treatment plants, incinerators, or power plant records and from cooperating industrial plants. Non-point-source data may be more difficult to locate, although recent statewide and/or Areawide 208 plans should incorporate some estimates of non-point-source inputs. Recent hazardous waste inventories developed by individual states and the U.S. EPA under Section 3004 of the Resource Conservation and Recovery Act (RCRA) should identify the locations of landfills and other hazardous-waste disposal sites.

Information needed to characterize the aquatic, terrestrial, and atmospheric environments may be obtained from a number of sources. For example, both the USGS and the U.S. Corps of Engineers collect stream flow data regularly, and many federal, state, and local agencies, such as the U.S. EPA, the SCS, state environmental protection departments, river basin commissions, sanitary districts, and Areawide 208 organizations, may gather flow data for short-term intensive studies or on a geographically limited basis. The same organizations may also provide water quality data, as may the U.S. Fish and Wildlife Service (FWS), local drinking-water and waste water treatment plants, hydropower companies, and local or regional colleges or universities. The U.S. EPA's STORET data base contains a very large amount of water quality information on a national basis, and identifies each stream, river, lake, or estuary sampling site with longitude and latitude coordinates. Quality control is difficult to maintain on data provided by so many diverse local, state, and federal sources, and

it is recognized that some of the data collected before the mid-1970s in STORET are of questionable value. Nevertheless, the STORET system is a valuable source of information. Another source of information about aquatic systems will be the U.S. EPA Canonical Environments Data Base (Hedden et al., 1981), which, when completed, will contain basic physical, chemical, and biological characterizations of the 15 major river basins nationwide. Environmental Impact Statements, if available for the area of interest, may also be of use.

Land use, vegetation cover, and topographic information may be compiled from local planning and development agencies, county agents, the SCS, the Forest Service, and national statistical services such as the Census Bureau and the National Crop Reporting Service. Information about business and industrial activities available from area chambers of commerce may also provide valuable insights into area characteristics. Historical and current remote sensing data can be useful in establishing "before and after" scenarios. The U.S. EPA Environmental Resources Information Center (ERIC), NOAA, and the National Aeronautics and Space Administration (NASA) may be able to provide this type of data.

Certain meteorological data are available from the National Climatic Center in Asheville, N.C., and local information may be provided by local airports and TV stations. Most states maintain a state meteorological agency that can also provide historical data in summary form. Air quality information is compiled by state and local environmental protection agencies and by the U.S. EPA. In addition, detailed meteorological and air quality data may be available from special studies conducted by state or federal agencies and local or regional colleges or universities.

Information required to identify and characterize important indigenous populations of aquatic and terrestrial biota may be maintained by state and federal fish and wildlife services, state natural resource departments, forest services, state land grant colleges or universities including schools of veterinary medicine, and natural history museums (Smithsonian Institution, etc.). Likewise, many states have entomology programs that maintain records of both beneficial and problem insect populations. Water quality data may be scanned for information on bacteria, phytoplankton, zooplankton, fish, and floating and rooted aquatic plants.

Information related to human health problems may be available through local health officials, hospitals, state health departments, and the U.S. Public Health Services (PHS) Centers for Disease Control (CDC) in Atlanta, Georgia. Additional information may be provided through special studies conducted by federal agencies [the U.S. EPA, Food and Drug Administration (FDA), and National Institutes of Health (NIH)] and national health-related organizations such as the American Heart Association and the American Lung Association. In some locations industrial health units and labor unions may also be able to provide occupational health data.

One of the most important products of the records survey is an initial inventory of toxic chemicals that may be found within the study area. The format for the inventory should serve for the entire study and should be arranged so that chemicals may be added or deleted as additional information becomes available. Useful information for each chemical listed includes the common name, chemical name, structure and state, concentration, location and media, possible source or sources, identification of information source, and evaluation of data quality. The inventory should also provide space for addition of information about physical-chemical properties, fate process rates or equilibrium constants, and human and environmental toxicological effects data for each chemical.

In developing chemical inventories, investigators should consider not only the chemicals that may be produced, discharged, stored, or accumulated within an area, but also those that may be advected or transported by prevailing air movements or upstream water flows into the study area. Sources of this information include those listed above which characterize the aquatic, terrestrial, and atmospheric environments and the identification and location of waste sources. Direct monitoring data are preferable; however, a preliminary list of chemicals may be compiled from supplemental information, including U.S. EPA reports listing chemical constituents in typical industrial waste discharges (e.g., from textile and fertilizer manufacturing); master lists of chemicals found in surface waters and industrial wastes (e.g., U.S. EPA Water Drop file and Effluent Guidelines lists); information from county extension agents or Farm Bureau representatives about agricultural chemicals applied in the area; and information from garden center operators, wholesale grocery distributors, chemical suppliers, and pharmacists about chemicals used in urban areas.

Data on physical-chemical properties and transport, transformation, degradation, and distribution rates or equilibrium constants for specific chemicals may be obtained from the scientific literature, U.S. EPA reports (Mabey et al., 1981), or computerized data files being developed by the EPA. If the process rate information for a chemical cannot be located, then coefficients may be estimated from structure-activity relationships or may be determined in the laboratory by following American Society for Testing and Materials (ASTM) or U.S. EPA test protocols (Mill et al., 1982).

In analyzing the data obtained in the records survey to identify data gaps and to develop optimum sampling strategies, it is useful to transfer as much information as possible onto area maps or map overlays. These maps should be used as the basis for a field inspection trip by as many members of the investigation team as possible. It is beneficial to have at least one staff member on the survey team who is experienced in field reconnaissance techniques. Aerial reconnaissance in a helicopter or light plane is useful in visualizing the major geologic features, roads, buildings, industries, treatment plants, outfalls, landfills, farms, land use and crop patterns, and so on. Stream, river, and lakeshore lines should then be walked or viewed at close range from boats, and the perimeter and cross sections of the area should be traversed to help identify optimum sampling sites and access routes.

Initial Screening Sampling Program

Once the available information base has been evaluated and data gaps identified, a well-planned initial sampling program should be carried out in conjunction with preliminary modeling and data analysis activities. This survey and analysis will ultimately guide the entire validation program, and it is important that it be well designed in order to establish a baseline from which extrapolations can be made forward or backward in time. A systems approach to planning and executing this survey will prove to be a wise investment. This program should be designed to (1) confirm the presence of the chemicals enumerated on the preliminary list and identify others that may be present, (2) develop a preliminary multimedia mass balance for chemicals entering and leaving the study areas, (3) confirm or quantify ranges in both chemical loadings from discharges previously identified and exposure concentrations in various media, (4) establish preliminary exposure routes (5) confirm the presence or absence of critical biological species indigenous to the area, (6) measure or estimate gross toxicities of major effluents by using screening tests, (7) identify probable populations at risk, and (8) assemble information required to select appropriate loading, exposure, and risk assessment models.

To minimize analytical problems during this preliminary identification phase, sampling sites should be selected where pollutant loading or ambient exposures are expected to be at or near maximum levels. Such sites may include locations downstream from industrial complexes and outfalls; urban and agricultural drains, landfills, and dump sites; points of collection or concentration such as sludge banks or areas of organic sediment deposition; turbidity maxima in estuarine rivers; soils from chemical storage areas; insects, plants, or animals known to accumulate certain types of chemicals; fly ash from coal burning facilities and incinerators; and residues from wet and dry fall collectors such as rain gauges, plate precipitation collectors, and ambient air samplers.

Because a primary objective of this initial sampling is to determine what toxic or hazardous chemicals may be present in significant concentrations, state-of-the-art techniques for characterizing and quantifying the broadest spectrum of organic and inorganic chemicals in each sample should be employed. Although the costs per sample will be relatively high, the costs per chemical remain low. Such procedures will focus on the most important cause-effect relationships. The need for broad-spectrum analyses, however, should not preclude the use of specific analytical procedures for particular target chemicals. Combinations of the best broad-spectrum techniques [e.g., the U.S. EPA Master Analytical Scheme (Garrison et al., 1979, 1981), and Huggett's (1981) capillary column gas chromatography and high-pressure liquid chromatography (HPLC) for organics and spark source mass spectrometry (SS–MS), plasma emission spectrometry, and activation analyses for metals and other inorganics] will provide characterization, quantitative analysis, and identification for only about 40% of the chemicals that could be distributed within areas affected by current industry. This 40%, however, represents a large proportion of the chemicals known to have toxic impact. Because many of these analytical techniques are state of the art and still being improved, generalized procedure manuals are not available and analysts will have to refer to the scientific literature, consultants, or contract laboratories for assistance.

The U.S. EPA Master Analytical Scheme provides protocols for sample collection, handling, extraction and separation, cleanup, and analysis by various gas chromatography–mass spectrometry (GC–MS) procedures, including automated spectral matching for more than 40,000 volatile organic chemicals. The system is being improved, especially in the areas of sample handling and extraction. Current levels of detection range from 10 $\mu g/l$ for organics in sediment and sewage to 0.1

μg/l in drinking water. As with any system involving extraction of chemicals from complex media, interlaboratory testing indicates that the lower the concentration and the more complex the sample, the poorer the precision and accuracy of the procedure.

The capillary column gas chromatographic system developed by Huggett to characterize organic chemicals in Chesapeake Bay sediments has a similar range with confirmed detection limits of 1–5 μg/kg for materials such as polynuclear aromatics.

Detection systems for nonvolatile organics rely on liquid chromatographs coupled with various detectors including low-resolution mass spectrometers. The sensitivity of the liquid chromatography–mass spectrometry (LC–MS) system is far from ideal, and the detection level is currently at least 100 times less than that of GC–MS instruments. Another problem is lack of spectra for specific nonvolatile organics in the data banks for automated matching and identification. Work is continuing in this area, and broad-based LC systems are improving.

Of the three techniques recommended for characterizing inorganic chemicals in a screening study, SS–MS can identify the greatest number of elements per sample (up to 80) with a sensitivity of 10–100 μg/l. The major drawback of this technique is the cost of the instrumentation and the limited number of samples that can be analyzed per work shift. Current systems can handle only 5–10 samples per day. Plasma emission spectrometry is a much more economical procedure with high productivity; however, only about 40 elements can be readily measured. The sensitivity is about the same as that of SS–MS and, in either case, samples are restricted to elements that can be solubilized to increase their homogeneity.

Neutron activation analysis (Moore and Propheter, 1977) falls somewhere between the spark source and plasma emission procedures. The instrumentation requires use of a nuclear reactor; however, university and commercial reactor facilities are available for contract work. The number of samples that can be processed is much higher than

in SS–MS, and the number of elements that can be analyzed is between 50 and 55, depending on interferences from some elements. An advantage of the activation procedures is their ability to analyze nonhomogeneous materials such as non-mixed sediments, which reduces the need for laborious sample preparation. Some field screening programs have used plasma emission systems with a few samples split and run through activation analysis for confirmation.

Unfortunately, none of the procedures that provides broad elemental coverage can detect or quantify the chemical species of the elements as they exist in the original matrix. This is unfortunate because the toxicity of a heavy metal varies widely according to speciation. For this phase of the program, however, information on the concentration of total metals present in the sample will be sufficient for planning the detailed sampling program.

Good reference manuals (U.S. EPA, 1973) are available to help plan and execute the initial sampling to identify and quantify aquatic and terrestrial organisms indigenous to the study area. Complete taxonomic characterization should not be required; however, if the design of the study requires detailed individual identifications, then time and resources will probably be saved by obtaining the services of expert consultants on the taxonomy of the species of concern. Universities and museums of natural history are good sources of assistance. The identification and quantification of key organisms or group relationships may serve as measures of community variability. If time and resources permit, toxicological and necroptic examinations may be made on a small subset of the organisms collected to identify possible sublethal chemical impacts.

Chemical exposure concentration data and biological samples should be collected concurrently to help establish any cause-effect relationships that may be quantifiable. If none is evident, selected toxicity tests may be performed on the effluents from the major discharges within the study site. Positive toxicity results obtained during the screening study provide valuable information on sources requiring in-depth investigations during the full-scale study. Protocols for conducting the screening toxicity tests may be found in test guidelines published by U.S. EPA in the Federal Register in response to either the Federal Insecticide, Fungicide, and Rodenticide Act or the Toxic Substances Control Act of 1976. Protocols may also be found in the scientific literature, including ASTM publications and U.S. EPA research reports.

Preliminary Modeling and Analysis

Preliminary chemical loading, exposure, and risk modeling should be conducted in parallel with the records survey and initial sampling program to (1) serve as a guide for data collection; (2) provide a systems framework for assessing the data; (3) provide preliminary sensitivity analyses of the major environmental parameters, chemical loadings, chemical properties, chemical mass balances, exposure routes, exposure concentrations, and exposure-effects coupling; (4) identify possible localized toxic hot spots; (5) rank and select significant chemicals to be investigated in the full field study; and (6) provide initial insights into environmental loadings—observed or perceived human and environmental effects.

Depending on the overall purpose of the field validation project, either a single-medium or a multimedia risk analysis model should be selected for use in screening and sensitivity analysis. Because state-of-the-art multimedia risk analysis models are currently being assembled and tested, it may be necessary to select an appropriate exposure model and then manually link the relevant effects data. Unfortunately, the more scientifically precise the simulation of real-world conditions is, the more calibration data are required and the higher the setup and operating costs. Thus, model selection and application in screening and sensitivity analysis becomes extremely important for this phase of the project, and when properly executed this step can result in significant savings in time, facilities, and labor in the field.

Ambrose (1981), in his paper on selecting models to meet management needs, describes the three main phases in model selection as analysis of the problem, evaluation of available models, and selection of appropriate models. In analysis of the problem he suggests that the problem be defined in simple terms, the informational needs listed, and the data and cost constraints analyzed. To evaluate available models he suggests that models that address the subject areas be listed, and that the list be screened and models ranked according to the informational needs of the problem. Next, the scientific capabilities, operational characteristics, and operational costs for each of the top-ranked models should be assessed. Finally, if more than one model has to be used, the compatibility among models should be evaluated. With this information, the most cost-effective modeling packages can be selected which balance the best scientific structural concepts with minimum data requirements and operation difficulties. The same process can be used to select the model sets for both the initial screening study and the detailed modeling task required in the latter parts of the validation program.

When evaluating the appropriate sets of models for screening analysis an investigator should look for the simplest package that contains transport, transformation, and degradation process reactions; operates in a steady-state mode for ease of use; and provides reasonable time steps to ensure adequate integration of chemical loadings, exposure, and biological effects. Models designed to provide monthly average data will be of little use in predicting exposures for compounds having a half-life of 10 d. Conversely, models that provide time steps on the order of minutes to hours will be very costly to run when only daily or weekly averages are required.

After appropriate model sets have been selected for the preliminary modeling task, the first two objectives (using the model to guide data collection and providing a framework for assessing the data) can best be accomplished in terms of providing a screening and sensitivity analysis tool. This process evaluates the relative importance of the various environmental loading factors, exposure and effects processes, rate coefficients, equilibrium constants, and physical-chemical properties of the suspected toxic chemicals within the context of the specific environment of the field validation site.

Once set up, the screening models can be roughly calibrated with the data obtained from the records survey or from estimated values based on literature reports. Although it is important to use realistic parameter values, the temptation to provide detailed and costly calibration should be avoided because this task requires only ballpark estimates.

The sensitivity analysis process for parameter screening simply involves running the model while changing each input parameter (e.g., loading rates, locations, stream or river flows, residence times, wind speed and directions, dispersion rates, temperatures, light intensities, pH values, numbers of organisms, fate process rates or equilibrium constants, sediment concentrations, solubilities, Henry's law constants, molecular diameters) either by orders of magnitude or within ranges of expected maximum or minimum values for the given field site, and observing the impact of each change on the model output. Thus, the most sensitive and therefore significant input parameters for the field site and toxic chemical combination can be identified and the detailed sampling program planned or adjusted to obtain consistent ambient data. Consistency here may require statistically ordered numbers of samples in both time and space as well as the degree of precision, level of sensitivity, and sample quality control.

Sensitivity analyses run in this manner for each toxic chemical on the preliminary priority list will provide a ranking of possible point source discharges, exposure pathways, media distribution, and environmental exposure concentrations. These preliminary findings are invaluable in developing the full-scale field sampling plan and selecting the proper modeling packages for the final data analysis.

One multimedia modeling package that may be included in the initial model selection process is the Air Land Water Analysis System (ALWAS). This model is comprised of (1) an atmospheric transport, degradation, dispersion, and deposition module, (2) a land surface runoff module (modified EPA non-point-source model) that partitions toxic organic chemicals onto sediment and predicts sediment transport into receiving waters, and (3) a fresh surface water exposure model [modified dynamic EPA Exposure Analysis Modeling System (EXAMS)] that simulates equilibrium partitioning of natural and ionic forms between dissolved, sediment-sorbed, or biosorbed phases and volatilization, hydrolysis, biolysis, photolysis, and oxidation as first-order processes. Hedden et al. (1982) recently combined ALWAS with a water treatment process model to provide a multimedia model for predicting human exposure to pollutants in drinking water.

Field Sampling Program

Because the primary purpose of the field validation program is to compare a given set of results, extrapolations, or predictions with data representing perceived real-world conditions, the objective of the field sampling program is to collect the most comprehensive, accurate, and precise data sets required to complete the validation process within the limits of variability selected at the beginning of the study. In reality, each of the previous tasks was designed to ensure that the planning and execution of this task would provide a scientifically valid data set for a minimum of expended resources. It should also be reiterated that one's perception of real-world conditions is limited by one's ability to identify and measure relevant characteristics and that if the data collected in this exercise are inapplicable or inaccurate, the validation process itself will become invalid and a great deal of time and resources will have been wasted.

It is recommended that this ultimate sampling program be planned and executed in conjunction with the final modeling and analysis activity to further reduce sampling costs. Again, in a systems context, properly selected exposure or risk models may serve as explicit quantitative statements of the extrapolation or prediction being validated, and the model framework will serve as an excellent planning and analysis tool.

Building on the results of the initial sampling and analysis activities, the planning and execution of the sampling program should include the following steps:

- Final selection of target chemicals
- Statistical design of the sampling plan
- Development of a logistic support plan
- Redevelopment and analysis of benefit-cost data
- Execution of the data collection programs

The first step involves a thorough analysis of the results of the initial sensitivity analysis runs for each of the top-ranked target chemicals. Lists should be made of the physical-chemical properties, fate process coefficients, and species-specific effects data that require additional laboratory measurements or verifications. Cost estimates for these studies should be obtained and included in the economic analysis. If the final ranking of the target toxic chemicals cannot be completed without these data, the necessary laboratory studies should be conducted and the data factored into the final selection of chemicals to be included in the sampling plan.

Likewise, the significant environmental parameters identified by the sensitivity analyses should be listed for each chemical evaluated and the *projected* multimedia source locations and loads, exposure routes, mass balances, exposure concentrations, and identified human and environmental effects should be collated and used as a basis for developing a composite list of chemicals and parameters to be measured. With this list, sampling, extraction, and analysis procedures may be selected and the spatial and temporal sampling plan developed.

Humenik et al. (1980), investigating the feasibility of using probability sampling to measure water quality parameters (e.g., velocity, tempera-ture, suspended solids, dissolved oxygen, total organic carbon, total phosphorus, total nitrogen) related to non-point-source discharges in the Chowan River basin, found that flow and advective transport were highly variable in time and space. They found that the precision of measurements increased as the sample size (number of samples) increased and, as predicted by statistical theory, the increase in precision was proportional only to the square root of the increase in sample size. This means that in order to increase the level of precision one unit, the number of samples taken must increase by the square of the original number. Thus, the cost of gaining added precision increases dramatically. They also found that the statistically valid number of samples required to reach the same relative end point (e.g., 1 standard deviation) varied with each parameter tested. Thus a consulting statistician who is familiar with field sampling procedures and a quality assurance expert should be engaged to help develop the final sampling and analysis plan so that the accuracy and precision of the data collected will meet or surpass the criteria of acceptability selected for the overall validation process.

Once the sampling and analysis plan has been completed, an accompanying logistic support plan must be developed covering the scheduling, operation, and maintenance of the field crews and equipment, laboratory personnel and instrumentation, transportation, data handling and processing, and so on. For large field sampling programs it is difficult to find laboratory facilities to process all of the samples in a reasonable time, so that sample storage becomes a problem and long delays may be experienced before all the data are available for processing. Some adjustments may have to be made in the sampling plan and the delays must be factored into the project planning and budgeting. Again, it is wise to seek the assistance of an experienced field program manager when developing the logistics plan and the final budget.

Unfortunately, economics govern the design and execution of most field programs, and sampling and logistic support activities are often reduced to the point where the precision and accuracy of the resulting data are so poor that the validation process itself becomes technically invalid. For this reason it is imperative that a final benefit-cost analysis be conducted for the entire validation process as soon as the cost estimates for the field sampling and logistic support plans have been completed. If the costs of collecting and analyzing the data exceed the projected benefits of applying the validated method, test, extrapolation, or model, the project should be terminated. If the expected benefits exceed the costs, every effort should be made to secure the appropriate resources, using the scientific and economic justifications developed thus far. If, as often happens, only part of the projected laboratory, equipment, or economic resource needs can be obtained, a very difficult management decision must be made: scale down the project to fit the budget and sacrifice scientific credibility, or terminate the project until adequate resources become available. Again, the scientific decision is clear: *do not attempt an invalid study*.

Detailed Modeling and Analysis

As stated earlier, the selection and application of exposure and risk assessment models should be conducted in conjunction with the field sampling program to (1) serve as a quantitative statement of the hypothesis being validated; (2) provide a guide for planning and executing the field sampling program so that only essential data will be collected, and (3) provide a framework for assessing and presenting the data for comparative purposes. Execution of this phase of the program should include:

- Model selection
- Preliminary calibration and sensitivity analysis
- Final calibration and execution
- Comparison of results for validation
- Report preparation and recommendations

The model selection criteria proposed by Ambrose (1981) and the general discussion presented earlier concerning the selection of preliminary screening models are also applicable to the selection of the detailed model or model sets. Of course, by this point in the overall validation process, the problem has been well defined. Thorough analysis of the results from the preliminary sampling and screening modeling tasks will have identified the significant toxic chemicals; provided estimates of the range of environmental loading for each chemical of interest, identified probable exposure pathways, quantified ranges in exposure concentrations in various environmental media, and identified possible human and environmental effects and cause-and-effect relationships. Also, evaluation of available exposure and risk models for the preliminary modeling step will have been completed. Thus, the remaining work in the model selection task is to match the available model characteristics with the environmental loading, exposure, and effects information listed above. Again, based on the state of the art in multimedia exposure and risk modeling, individual model routines may have to be coupled to meet the specific needs of the validation process. Of course, if the purpose of the field study is to validate an exposure or risk model as described in this chapter, then the model selection step will not be required.

Compared to the preliminary screening models, models selected for this phase of the study will be more complex in simulating the dynamics of environmental loadings, transport, exposure, and effects (e.g., rather than steady state, continuous time-varying simulations will mimic actual environmental variables such as rainfall and runoff, municipal discharges, and industrial process variation). These models will also be more complicated in both the number of environmental fate processes simulated and the order of the process rate expressions (second-order versus first-order kinetics).

Once the model or model sets have been selected, the next step is to calibrate the models, using the environmental data developed in the preliminary sampling and modeling steps, and to conduct sensitivity analysis runs to guide the selection of locations, frequencies, and parameters for the field sampling program. This is a very important task and, if properly executed, can result in substantial savings in time and resources by focusing the sampling efforts on critical points in time and space. It should also increase the opportunity to run additional replicate samples at the critical points.

Data from the sampling program can be used to recalibrate the models and to evaluate the sampling plan and make midcourse corrections as required.

The steps involved in identifying and gathering the various kinds of data produced by large field validation studies have been discussed. Now the task becomes one of assembling and processing the huge masses of information in forms amenable to comparison with results or predictions derived from the methodology being validated. A number of manual procedures are available for handling field data, but because of the large volumes it is recommended that one of several automated data management systems (storage, retrieval, and processing) be used. It is also highly recommended that the data management system be selected and implemented early in the development of the field study so that information may be entered directly as it is collected. For example, the U.S. EPA Chesapeake Bay Program (Talbot et al., 1980) developed a data management system around the STORET computerized data base system and a minicomputer used for local processing, data entry, archival storage, and high-speed transfer from one system to the other. The joint U.S.-Egyptian project on "Evaluation of the Environmental Impacts of the Aswan High Dam" (Younis et al., 1979) utilized only a minicomputer for the entire data management process. (This project is processing more than 35,000 individual computer printout sheets of data accumulated in a 5-yr study.) Both of these systems include computer software subroutines that provide statistical and graphic data processing and display. Also included in the Chesapeake Bay Program is a subsystem designed to accept, archive, and report textual information (descriptive or other than tabular data). This subroutine, EPALIT, enables the entire data base to be searched (using standard English) and selected information retrieved within seconds.

Other stand-alone computer software packages available for use in processing field data include BMPD (Dixon and Brown, 1979); SPSS (Statistical Package for the Social Sciences, 1975), and SAS and SAS/ETS (SAS Institute, 1979). These packages provide the capability to aggregate, analyze, and display data including plots and histograms, frequency tables, tests and one-way analysis of variance, linear and nonlinear regressions, analysis of variance and covariance, nonparametric analyses, cluster analysis, multivariate analysis, survival analysis, and so on. Some of the newer water quality and exposure models, Hydrologic Simulation Program-Fortran (HSP–F) and WASP, have built-in data processing subroutines that will accept both calibration and evaluation data.

Once the field data have been processed, various comparisons may be made, depending on the nature of the data (e.g., time- and space-varying) and the criteria of acceptability established for the validation process (e.g., standard deviations, percentages, frequencies, and probabilities). After appropriate comparisons have been made, the results are measured against the criteria of acceptability, and the application of the method, toxicity test, or model to the particular problem is judged to be valid or invalid.

The validative process does not stop at this point. Final reports have to be written, and the raw data and processed data should be archived so that others may benefit from their use at some later time. This is especially true if some control or regulatory activity may be recommended and implemented with follow-up studies conducted to evaluate the effectiveness of the decision process. Experience with two large field programs (Chesapeake Bay Program and U.S.-Egyptian Project) has shown that the final report writing is difficult to complete for a number of reasons, including overcommitted resources during data gathering, loss of key investigators near the end of the project, loss of interest, and lack of commitment from sponsoring organizations after the result is obtained.

SUMMARY

There is a present and continuing need to develop and utilize field-validated methods, tests, protocols, and models when making decisions that have significant health, social, economic, or environmental consequences. Because of the diverse backgrounds and interests of the scientists-developers and the array of different problems facing environmental decision-makers, there is confusion about the basic validation process and general disagreements about the definition of common terms.

In this chapter a distinction is made between a scientific evaluation of a method, test, or model with field data where the objective is to determine the degree of correspondence, goodness of fit, or confidence limits, and a field validation study where the results of using a method, test, or model to solve a particular problem are compared to data collected in the field (representing perceived reality) and judged to be valid or invalid on the basis of preselected criteria of acceptability. These criteria of acceptability should be set by decision officials and the strength of the criteria should correspond to the consequences of the decision.

Locating adequate field sites to provide the theoretical correspondence between the significant elements in the method, test, or model being applied and similar parameters, variables, processes, and so on that can be measured in the field becomes a major task. A basis for identifying corresponding elements, however, can be found in the concept that observed human and environmental effects can be related to environmental loading of implicated toxic or hazardous chemicals through environmental fate (transport, transformation, and distribution) calculation or estimations. In setting up the sampling program, it is necessary to collect sufficient kinds of data to assure that observed effects are truly related to projected sources and not caused by natural phenomena or interfering materials or processes. If statistically acceptable field measurements cannot be made, then the validation process itself becomes invalid.

Field sampling and analysis programs are time and resource intensive; large programs can overwhelm laboratory facilities so that without good logistical planning, long delays may be experienced in obtaining analytical results. It is recommended that a systems approach be applied to planning and executing the entire field program and, if available, exposure or risk models should be utilized in a screening or sensitivity analysis mode in developing cost-effective sampling plans. Automated data analysis systems should be used in receiving, storing, analyzing, and comparing the collected data.

Because of the high costs (manpower, facilities, equipment, and dollars) associated with field sampling programs, benefit-cost analyses should be conducted as part of the planning exercise and only those studies that show benefits in excess of costs should be undertaken. If adequate resources are not available, the field validation studies should not be attempted.

In the last two decades, many scientific field evaluation projects have been conducted in which analytical methods, tests, protocols, and models were applied and evaluated to determine their degree of correspondence with real world data. On the other hand, only a few true field validation studies, in which a problem is defined and criteria of acceptability established prior to the initiation of a field data collection program, have been performed because resources have generally not been available for these large, expensive projects.

LITERATURE CITED

Ambrose RB: Models for Analyzing Eutrophication in Chesapeake Bay Watersheds: A Selection Methodology. Annapolis, Md.: Chesapeake Bay Program, U.S. Environmental Protection Agency, 1981.

Dixon WJ, Brown MB (eds): Biomedical Computer Program P-Series. Berkeley, Calif.: Univ. of California Press, 1979.

Garrison AW, Pope JD, Jr, Alford AL, Doll CK: An automated analytical scheme, and a registry system for organics in water. In: Trace Organic Analysis: A New Frontier in Analytical Chemistry, pp. 65–78. NBS Spec Publ 519. Gaithersburg, Md.: National Bureau of Standards, 1979.

Garrison AW, Pellizzari ED, Ryan JF: The master analytical scheme: An overview of interim procedures. In: Advances in the Identification and Analysis of Organic Pollutants in Water, edited by LH Keith, vol. 1, chap. 2, pp. 17–30. Ann Arbor, Mich.: Ann Arbor Science, 1981.

Gorsuch AM: Statement of Anne M. Gorsuch, Administrator, U.S. Environmental Protection Agency, before the Subcommittee on Natural Resources, Agriculture Research and Environment of the Committee on Science and Technology, U.S. House of Representatives, October 22, 1981.

Hedden KF, Mulkey LA, Tucker WA: Application of multimedia exposure assessment to drinking water. Environmental Monitoring and Assessment. 2(1 & 2):57–69, 1982.

Hedden KF, Skaggs RL, Brown SM: Development of a canonical environmental data base for rivers, lakes and reservoirs. In: Paper presented, 6th Aquatic Toxicology Symposium, St. Louis, Mo., October 13–16, 1981.

Huggett RD: Investigations of Organic Pollutants in the Chesapeake Bay. Preliminary Final Report, Cooperative Agreement R80612. Annapolis, Md.: Chesapeake Bay Program, U.S. Environmental Protection Agency, March, 1981.

Humenick FD, Hayne DW, Overcash MR, Gilliam JW, Witherspoon AM, Galler WS, Howells DH: Probability Sampling to Measure Pollution from Rural Land Runoff, North Carolina State University, Raleigh, NC. EPA-600/3-80-035. Prepared for the U.S. Environmental Protection Agency, Athens, Ga., 1980.

Lassiter RR: Testing Models of the Fate of Chemicals in the Aquatic Environments. In: Proceedings of a Workshop on Modeling the Fate of Chemicals in the Aquatic Environment, Pelston, Mich., August 16–21, 1981, edited by A Maki, K Dickson, J Cairns, pp. 287–301. Ann Arbor, Mich.: Ann Arbor Science, 1982.

Mabey WR, Smith JH, Podoll RT, Johnson HL, Mill T, Chow TW, Gates J, Partridge IW, Vandenbury D: Aquatic Fate Process Data for Organic Priority Pollutants, EPA Final Draft Report. Washington, D.C.: Office of Water Regulations and Standards, U.S. Environmental Protection Agency, 1981.

Mill T, Mabey WR, Bomberger PI, Chow TW, Hendry DG, Smith JH: Laboratory Protocols for Evaluating the Fate or Organic Chemicals in Air and Water. SRI International, Menlo Park, Calif. EPA-600/3-82-022. Prepared for U.S. Environmental Protection Agency, Athens, Ga., 1982.

Moore RV, Propheter OW: Nondestructive Multielement Instrumental Neutron Activation Analysis. EPA-600/4-77-011. Athens, Ga.: U.S. Environmental Protection Agency, 1977.

SAS Institute: SAS User's Guide. Raleigh, N.C., 1979.

Schwab GM, Coop PG, Rider E, Spokes GN, Tordini A, Pierpaoli AR, Posner R: Feasibility Study for a National Comprehensive Water Quality Monitoring Program. Project 68-03-2909, Draft Final Report. Athens, Ga.: U.S. Environmental Protection Agency, 1981.

Smith CN: Summary of the Athens Environmental Research Laboratory's Agricultural Runoff Field Studies. Unpublished report, Technology Development and Applications Branch, Environmental Research Laboratory, U.S. Environmental Protection Agency, Athens, Ga., 1978.

Smith JH: Environmental Pathways of Selected Chemicals in Freshwater Systems: Part II, Laboratory Studies, SRI International, Menlo Park, Calif. EPA-600/7-780-74. Prepared for the U.S. Environmental Protection Agency, Athens, Ga., 1978.

SPSS: Statistical Package for the Social Sciences, 2d ed. New York: McGraw-Hill, 1975.

Talbot R, Oglesby J: Chesapeake Bay Program data management. Presented at the 1980 Trimester Peer Review Panel Meeting, Ocean City, Md., October 12–17, 1980.

Toebes C, Ouryvaev V (eds): Representative and Experimental Basins—An International Guide for Research and Practices. New York: Unipub, 1970.

U.S. Environmental Protection Agency: Biological

Field and Laboratory Methods for Measuring the Quality of Surface Waters and Effluents. EPA-670/4-73-001. Washington, D.C.: U.S. EPA, 1973.

U.S. Environmental Protection Agency: Guidelines Establishing Test Protocols. 40 CFR 136. Fed Regist 44:69532–69552, 1979a.

U.S. Environmental Protection Agency: National Pollutant Discharge Elimination System; Revision of Existing Regulations. 40 CFR 122. Fed Regist 44:34408–34416, 1979b.

U.S. General Accounting Office: Guidelines for Model Evaluation. PAD-79-17. Washington, D.C., January 1979.

Younis MI, Mancy KH: Water Quality Data Bank— River Nile Project. Cairo, Egypt: Egyptian Academy of Scientific Research and Technology, 1979.

Chapter 22
Chemical Safety Evaluation

A. W. Maki and W. E. Bishop

INTRODUCTION

In recent years much attention has been directed toward assessment of the hazards associated with the manufacture, distribution, use, and disposal of chemicals. Many countries are evolving legislation to regulate the introduction of new chemicals and to provide for the review of existing chemical compounds. It has been estimated that there are more than 4,000,000 distinct chemical entities, that approximately 63,000 of these are in common use, and that several hundred new chemicals annually have the potential for environmental release (Maugh, 1978; Maki et al., 1979). The need to formalize procedures for assessing chemical hazards and deciding whether a particular chemical presents a reasonable or unreasonable risk to human health or the environment is apparent. References to many of the plans advanced in recent years for assessing chemical safety are given in the bibliographies at the end of this chapter. Rather than review these published plans in detail, the purpose of this chapter is to identify and discuss the principles involved in assessing the hazard of chemical substances to aquatic life and to describe the conceptual framework underlying specific safety assessment procedures.

In dealing with this subject it is important to have a thorough understanding of the terminology involved. For this discussion the terms *hazard* and *risk* may be used interchangeably. Both are synonyms of the word danger, and each implies an element of chance that an adverse effect will occur under a particular set of conditions. *Hazard assessment* of a chemical has been defined as prediction of the magnitude and duration of chemical concentrations in various segments of the environment resulting from use of the compound compared with the concentrations of the chemical in food, water, or air which are known to be harmful to representative species, populations, and ecosystems (Kenaga, 1980). Such a definition clearly indicates the kind of information that is essential for assessing the hazards of a chemical to aquatic life (Fig. 1).

Toxicity is defined as the potential of the chemical to induce unwanted or deleterious effects in biological systems. Toxicity is an inherent, unalterable property of the chemical and is a function of the exposure concentration, or dose, and the nature of the biological system that is exposed. Toxicity and hazard are not synonymous terms. It is unfortunate that the redundant terms "toxic substance" and "toxic chemical" enjoy such widespread use, for scientists recognize that all chemicals have the potential to be toxic to some biological system under appropriate exposure conditions. It is, of course, essential to learn about the inherent toxicity patterns associated with a chemical in order to complete the risk assessment.

It is equally important to learn about the nature and degree of exposures that might result from the manufacture, use, or disposal of the chemical. This requires a thorough understanding of the *environmental fate* of the chemical. The fate of a chemical in the aquatic environment may be thought of as the concentrations resulting from all point source and non-point source inputs, as modified by the chemical, physical, and biological transport and transformation processes that are active in the environment.

Safety may be defined as a value judgment of

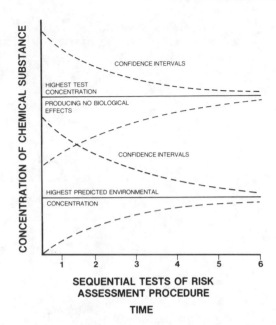

Figure 2 Diagrammatic representation of the risk assessment process, showing the increasingly narrower confidence limits for predicted environmental concentration and estimates of no adverse biological effects concentration. *[From Cairns et al. (1978)]*

the acceptability of risk. A chemical is regarded as "safe" if its associated risks are judged to be acceptable. Such a definition implies that two different activities are required for determining safety. First, a risk assessment is necessary to evaluate potential harm to aquatic organisms. Second, a value judgment regarding the acceptability of that risk must be made.

THE RISK ASSESSMENT PROCESS

In any risk assessment process, basically two lines of scientific investigation seek to relate observed biological effects to predicted exposure concentrations (Fig. 2). Theoretically, there exists a concentration of a particular chemical substance that can be determined to have no adverse effects on survival, growth, or reproduction of representative aquatic life. This concentration is typically referred to as the no observed effect concentration (NOEC) and is determined from laboratory toxic-

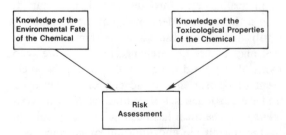

Figure 1 Information needs for the risk assessment process.

ity testing of fish, macroinvertebrate, or plant species. Similarly, there exists a highest predicted environmental concentration (PEC) that will result from the normal anticipated use of the chemical during manufacture, transport, and consumer use. It is thus basic to the risk assessment procedure to accurately measure or estimate these two concentrations so that a comparison of the difference between the known biological effects and the environmental concentrations can be made.

Figure 2 represents these two concentrations by parallel lines and demonstrates that increasingly accurate and statistically reliable estimates of these concentrations will result from a sequential series of tests. In the early phases of the risk assessment process, biological effects and environmental concentrations are estimated; however, the wide and overlapping confidence intervals indicate that additional data are needed to determine whether the two concentrations are statistically significantly different. As the risk assessment proceeds, increasingly accurate estimates of fate and effects can be made, to the point where it becomes possible to state with a high degree of confidence that environmental concentrations and biological effect concentrations are indeed different. It then becomes a matter of judgment to determine just how far into the assessment process the investigator should proceed to further narrow the confidence intervals around fate and effect concentrations.

SAFETY ASSESSMENT PROGRAMS

Many factors and their appropriate combination must be considered to carry out an effective yet efficient safety assessment program. A generalized safety assessment program may be presented as a flow chart consisting of a number of distinct phases (Fig. 3). Each phase is designed to accomplish certain scientific purposes, and all the phases are interrelated. In each phase there are provisions for acquiring and organizing information and for making certain kinds of decisions. Flexibility is provided so that the key issues for any particular chemical are addressed. Experimentation flows

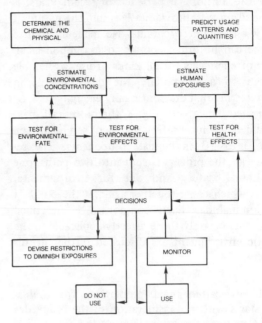

FLOW CHART FOR SAFETY ASSESSMENT

Figure 3 Flow chart for the generalized safety assessment process. [From Beck et al. (1981)]

from relatively simple screening tests to increasingly complicated confirmatory studies. The amount and kind of information needed in each phase are largely independent of those needed in other phases, even though the phases are closely integrated. After consideration of the physical and chemical characteristics of the material and potential routes of exposure, important questions are identified and tests are selected to answer those questions. As more information is developed, a point is reached at which a decision can be made regarding the safety of the substance. The decision may be that the substance presents too high a risk, or that there is an acceptable risk, or that more work needs to be carried out. Scientific judgment is used in deciding which tests to do and when sufficient testing has been conducted. The collection of decisions is then integrated into an overall decision concerning the acceptability of the material in terms of human and environmental health.

The generalized outline provided here, derived from the authors' experience of recent years, is intended only to provide insight into the nature of safety assessment programs. No made-in-advance outline can be broad enough to accommodate all kinds of chemicals for all kinds of uses or flexible enough to accommodate the developments in safety testing that are continually emerging.

In accordance with Fig. 3, the process of making and reviewing a safety judgment can be broken down into 10 individual components. The sequence of the process is split into two paths, one for human safety and one for environmental safety, which come together again at the point of decision-making. Each component is described briefly below; only those directly applicable to the aquatic environment are discussed further in this chapter.

1 Physical/chemical properties: The evaluation starts with a consideration of the properties of the material, ascertained from the literature if possible and determined in the laboratory if necessary. Estimates may suffice in the early stages, but more precise determinations will generally be needed later. This is the time for initial development of the analytical methodology that will be needed.

2 Usage patterns: How and in what quantities the material will be used must be considered, since usage patterns (and such related matters as manufacturing, shipping, and disposal) determine the routes and amounts of human and environmental exposure.

3 Environmental concentrations: From anticipated usage patterns and physical-chemical properties, the concentrations in various environmental compartments are predicted. These estimates can be helpful in projecting human exposures, but their chief value is in suggesting how extensively the materials should be tested for environmental fate. Then, from the results of the environmental fate tests, more refined predictions of environmental concentrations can be made. These estimates are necessary both for predicting human exposures and for interpreting the results of the tests that will be done to evaluate environmental effects.

4 Environmental fate: Tests for environmental fate reveal what happens to the material after it is released into the environment. This kind of information is necessary for making the refined estimates of environmental concentration referred to above, and this is one of the factors influencing the estimate of human exposure.

5 Human exposure: Estimates of human exposure can be made from information about manufacturing, transport, and usage patterns and the estimates of environmental concentration. A number of estimates are needed to cover such diverse situations as exposure of factory workers, intentional and accidental exposures of consumers, and incidental exposures of humans from drinking water or air. Exposure may be by the oral, respiratory, ocular, or dermal route. These estimates of exposure are of value in determining which health effects tests should be carried out and are essential in evaluating the results of those tests.

6 Health effects: Tests for health effects are concerned with the possible effects of the material on human health, but most of the tests are carried out with laboratory animals. From information about the kinds of effects produced in these animals and the dosages of material necessary to produce them, it is possible to determine the dosages of material that would be safe for humans.

7 Environmental effects: Tests for environmental effects indicate whether the concentrations expected may cause harm to the environment, particularly to the living creatures in it; the kinds of injury that may occur; and the species most likely to be affected. These tests include acute and chronic tests with marine and freshwater fish, macroinvertebrates, and algae.

8 Decision-making: The first step in decision-making is to compare the dosages of a material that are predicted to cause harm to humans or the environment with the dosages that will result from using the material. From this comparison it is possible to assess the risk of causing harmful effects. Finally, a decision is made about whether the risks are acceptable. It is not necessary to do all possible tests before making this decision. Sound scientific judgment may be used at many points in the process to decide that no further testing is necessary.

9 Monitoring: If the decision is to use the material, field monitoring may be needed to deter-

mine whether the resulting environmental concentrations correspond to those predicted on the basis of laboratory testing. Medical follow-up of consumer comments and surveillance of employee health can also be useful ways to check on the correctness of the decision to proceed.

10 Restrictions on use: If any of the risks associated with using the material as originally planned are judged unacceptable, it may be possible to devise restrictions on the use of the material that would diminish the anticipated exposure and thereby lower the risk. The restrictions might range from use of warning labels to construction of containment dikes around storage tanks. Once such restrictions have been devised, it will be necessary to review parts of the decision-making process to see whether the risks are now acceptable.

SAFETY ASSESSMENTS FOR THE AQUATIC ENVIRONMENT

Material Characteristics

The first step in evaluating any compound is to assemble and evaluate all available information. Sources of information include (1) published literature as obtained through Chemical Abstracts, Biological Abstracts, Toxline, Medline, etc.; (2) information supplied by vendors; (3) information supplied by investigators who have worked with the compound; and (4) predictions that can be based on the material's physical and chemical similarity to more familiar materials (i.e., structure-activity relationships). The information can be assembled under the following headings.

Identity

The material is identified by the following information.

Definitive chemical name, common names, Chemical Abstracts registry number, or other designations.

Molecular formula, structural formula, and molecular weight, if the material is a distinct chemical species.

Origin, preparation, or isolation. This information is especially relevant for materials that cannot be defined chemically, such as crude reaction products, naturally occurring materials, or polymers.

Composition of the material, including the nature and concentration of its minor components. If there is more than one supplier, possible differences in composition should be considered.

Analytical methods available to confirm the identity of the material and to determine the degree of purity. Limits of sensitivity for the various methods should be ascertained.

Physical Properties

The properties of interest usually include physical form, color, odor, density, melting and boiling points, vapor pressure, solubility in water and organic solvents, octanol-water partition coefficient, and sorption characteristics on pertinent surfaces. Not all of these properties will need to be examined for all materials. Many of them may be ascertained from existing information; others can be estimated from the chemical structure or determined approximately with little experimental effort. These approximations may be adequate for planning the program, but may need to be refined by more precise measurements later.

Chemical Properties

Depending on the nature of the material, the chemical properties to be considered may include some or all of the following: acidity or basicity; ionization or dissociation properties; ion-exchange characteristics; complexation properties; susceptibility to hydrolysis, oxidation, thermal degradation, and photolysis, together with consideration of the products of these reactions. Not all of these properties are pertinent for all materials. Many may be ascertained from published information; others may be estimated from the chemical structure of the material or may be approximated with minimum experimental effort. These estimates and approximations may be adequate for planning the program, but may need to be supplemented by more precise determinations as the decision-making phases of the program are approached.

Biological Characteristics

These may include information about mammalian toxicity, absorbability from the gut or through the skin or lungs, microbial toxicity, biodegradability, aquatic toxicity, microbiological contamination, and the likelihood of forming biologically significant metabolites or degradation products. Some of this information may be available from the literature or from vendors; some may be inferred from what is known about familiar materials that are chemically similar to the material of interest; some will be unknown, and its acquisition is a major goal of the risk evaluation program.

Review

All the available information should be reviewed to predict what kinds of problems, if any, the material may ultimately present. Of particular interest is whether it resembles materials that are known to be safe or that have problems associated with them. Particular attention should be given to the adequacy of existing analytical methods with complex matrices such as body fluids and waste and surface waters and to whether more sophisticated methods or isotopically labeled material will be required in the testing program.

Manufacture, Use, and Disposal

The ways in which a material is manufactured and used profoundly influence human and environmental exposure to it and must be considered in choosing and interpreting the tests that comprise a safety testing program. Therefore, the objective of this part of the assessment is to assemble as much information as possible about how a material will be handled in order to predict as accurately as possible how much of it will enter the environment.

It is not possible to specify in advance just what information about usage should be brought together for all materials. Accordingly, the following questions should be considered suggestive. The answers will ultimately define the priority and scope of the environmental testing program.

Manufacture

Where will the material be manufactured?
What quantities will be manufactured?
What opportunities exist for loss or escape of the material during manufacture?
What measures will be taken to control such exposure?
Does the manufacture of the material induce production or handling of other substances—intermediates or raw materials—that require safety assessment?

Shipping

How will the material be shipped?
What quantities will be shipped?
How large will the containers be?
What opportunities exist for environmental exposure during shipping?
What is the likelihood of accidental spillage?
What measures will be taken to control such exposures?

Storage

Where will the material be stored?
Under what conditions will it be stored?
What quantities will be stored?
How large will the containers be?
What opportunities exist for environmental exposure during storage?
What is the likelihood of accidental spillage?
What measures will be taken to control such exposures?

Usage

For what purpose will the material be used?
Which of its properties make it suitable for that use?
Will it replace another material now used for that purpose?
Is the material so similar to another material already in use that their effects may be additive?
Might other companies use or offer the same material for a similar purpose? For a different purpose? If so, what quantities are likely to be involved?
Is the material to be used under conditions that prevent or restrict its escape into the environment?

Is the material so altered during usage as to lose its chemical identity? If so, what is it changed into? Do the transformation products need to be evaluated for safety?

Misuse

In what ways might the material be accidentally or deliberately misused?

What environmental exposures might result from misuse?

How can the possibility of misuse be minimized?

Disposal

By what routes will the material be disposed of after use?

What quantities will be disposed of by each route?

Will disposal be localized or general?

What is the likelihood of accidental spillage during disposal?

What environmental concentrations will result from disposal?

Will disposal involve chemical transformation of the materials? If so, to what products? Do these products need to be evaluated for safety?

Prediction of Environmental Concentrations

The concentration of a chemical in the environment is one of the factors influencing human exposure and the major factor influencing the exposure of plants and animals. Since the risk evaluation ultimately depends on comparison of exposure concentrations with those causing a measurable biological response, it is necessary that a safety testing program predict the environmental concentrations that a chemical is likely to attain when it is used. These estimates become part of the criteria for deciding which environmental fate and effects tests are appropriate.

Most of the authors' experience in predicting environmental concentrations has involved chemicals that are broadly distributed and used in consumer products which are disposed of in waste water. The following simplified example is based on this experience; the approach would certainly need to be modified for chemicals that are distributed differently or used for other purposes.

Influent Waste Water

The concentration of a chemical in raw or influent waste water (C_{Iw}) can be estimated from

$$C_{Iw} = \frac{M \times F}{P \times W}$$

where C_{Iw} = concentration of the chemical in influent waste water (mg/l)

M = quantity of product marketed (mg/d)

F = fraction of chemical in the product

P = population of market area (number people)

W = per capita flow rate of waste water (l/d)

For example, if a chemical is 10% of a consumer product, broadly distributed across the United States, with a market volume of 25×10^6 kg/yr, and 507 l/d per capita is the median value of W for municipal treatment plants, then the concentration of the chemical in influent waste water is projected to be:

$$C_{Iw} = [(25 \times 10^6 \text{ kg/yr})(10^6 \text{ mg/kg})(0.10)] /$$

$$[(365 \text{ d/yr})(210 \times 10^6 \text{ persons})$$

$$\times(507 \text{ l/d per capita})] = 0.064 \text{ mg/l}$$

Different values of W and the other variables in this equation can be used if they are more appropriate for a specific situation. For example, a value of 200 l/d per capita is appropriate for domestic (as opposed to municipal) waste water flow.

Effluent Waste Water

The first estimate of the chemical concentration in effluent waste water (C_{Ew}) can be made by assuming that none of the chemical is removed during sewage treatment; thus

$$C_{Iw} = C_{Ew}$$

As information from environmental fate tests becomes available, more refined estimates of C_{Ew} may be developed which will account for the fraction of the material that is removed during the treatment process (Holman, 1981).

Surface Water

An estimate of a chemical's concentration in surface water is needed early in the safety testing program to guide decisions concerning the scope of testing for environmental fate and effects. Effluents from waste water treatment plants are discharged predominantly (~84%) to surface water, with the balance going to ocean outfalls, ground water recharge, and land disposal (Metcalf and Eddy, 1979). The predictions discussed here pertain only to surface waters, specifically to rivers. An estimate of the concentration of a chemical in surface waters can be obtained from

$$C_{SW} = \frac{C_{EW}}{\text{SDF}} \qquad (1)$$

where C_{SW} = concentration of the chemical in surface water below the outfall of a waste water treatment plant

SDF = stream dilution factor, which equals the stream flow rate at the plant site divided by the effluent discharge flow rate

Using SDF = 10, 100, and 1000 in Eq. (1) gives an estimate of C_{SW} that is exceeded in 9, 46, and 90% of U.S. river basins, respectively, under real-world conditions (Holman, 1979). Use of SDF = 10 has therefore been suggested as conservative for U.S. dilution ratios (Beck et al., 1981).

Based on the data from the example above, where C_{Iw} was predicted to be 0.064 mg/l, and the assumption that there is no removal by sewage treatment, the concentration of the chemical in surface water is projected to be:

$$C_{Sw} = \frac{0.064 \text{ mg/l}}{10} = 0.006 \text{ mg/l}$$

The surface water concentration projected from the equations above is a conservative estimate since no attempt was made to account for removal of the chemical by subsequent in-stream degradation processes. These estimates can be refined further when degradation information becomes available. Moreover, field studies and monitoring programs can provide data to check the accuracy of the predicted concentrations and to provide the most refined values for concentration in surface waters.

Drinking Water

As a first approximation, the concentration of a chemical in drinking water may be taken as the best estimate of its concentration in surface waters that are the source of the drinking water. It is appropriate to use 100 rather than 10 as the SDF, because drinking water is taken from protected sources with a minimum input of waste water. This estimate may be refined if information about removal by drinking water treatment processes is developed or if information from field and monitoring studies is available.

Additional Predictive Techniques

The discussion above gives only one example of methods available for predicting environmental concentrations. Many other chemical fate assessment procedures have been developed (Baughman and Lassiter, 1978; Branson, 1978; Stern, 1980). Most of these procedures involve the use of physical or mathematical modeling techniques; they are reviewed in detail in Chapter 19.

Testing for Environmental Fate

A number of experimental methods are available for determining the fate of a chemical after it enters the aquatic environment. Important questions to be addressed include the chemical's transport (i.e., mobility) and persistence (i.e., removal or biodegradation). Results of environmental fate tests are used to develop refined estimates of environmental concentrations. Detailed methodologies for environmental fate tests are available (Gilbert and Lee, 1980; Stern and Walker, 1978), and a few of the more useful tests are briefly described below.

Screening Tests

The *CO₂ evolution test* indicates whether a material can be converted to carbon dioxide by microbial action and may indicate whether it inhibits microbial activity.

The *octanol-water partition coefficient* is an indicator of the potential for bioconcentration of a chemical in living organisms. A high coefficient suggests that the material may be concentrated in lipid; if it is not metabolized and excreted it may become more concentrated at higher trophic levels.

Tests for *microbial inhibition* indicate the likelihood that a material will interfere with the action of microorganisms that degrade organic materials.

The *semicontinuous activated sludge* (SCAS) test measures the extent to which a chemical is removed in a simulation of the most commonly used secondary waste water treatment process.

The *settling test* determines how much of a material may be removed from waste water by settling. It is an appropriate test for any material that will appear in influent waste water as a solid or associated with solids. The results may be useful in refining the estimate of surface water concentration and may direct attention toward sludge as an environmental compartment of interest.

Certain chemical and physical properties of the material may need to be investigated in greater detail. The chemical properties include the potential of the material to undergo hydrolysis, oxidation, reduction, photolysis, complex formation, ion exchange, chlorination, ozonation, and ionization or dissociation. The physical properties include volatility and vapor pressure, adsorptive behavior, and solubility in water. Not all of these will need to be studied for all materials. The properties that should be investigated are those that can be expected to influence the form of the material and its movement through, accumulation in, or disappearance from the environment.

Investigations of chemical and physical properties should be conducted under protocols designed to show whether a property is likely to influence the environmental concentration of the material. Results of the tests are used to refine the estimate of anticipated environmental concentration and to draw attention to the environmental compartments in which the material is likely to appear.

Confirmatory Tests

In order to gain more certain knowledge of the environmental fate of some chemicals, it may be appropriate to carry out more complex types of tests. Such a program may involve aspects of the following:

Determining the kinetics of primary and ultimate degradation in fresh, estuarine, or saline water.

Measuring the rate constants for hydrolysis, photolysis, or other removal mechanisms that the screening tests have indicated are likely to be significant.

Determining the adsorption isotherm for the material onto solids or influent sewage, the solids in biological treatment, and representative sediments.

Measuring the equilibrium constants for chelation or ion exchange with trace metals.

If the screening information suggests reactivity, determining the potential for chlorination and/or ozonation.

Treatability studies with laboratory or pilot-scale models of biological treatment processes (activated sludge and trickling filter) are conducted to predict the fate and effects of the chemical in the full-scale processes. Items to be determined may include primary degradation and removal of the chemical, mass balance for the chemical, and effects of the chemical on the efficiency of the treatment process. The capacity of the chemical to inhibit biological processes, particularly activated sludge and anaerobic digestion, may be evaluated. Studies to determine the effects of the chemical on sludge handling properties should also be considered.

The results of all the confirmatory tests are used to make a more refined estimate of the anticipated concentration of the compound in surface waters and to estimate its probable concentration in activated sludge, digester solids, soil, and sediments.

Investigative Tests

Programs designed to answer specific questions may be appropriate. These programs cannot be specified in a general outline, since each must be designed in response to a specific need. The programs may include further laboratory studies, field tests, modeling, and monitoring. Criteria for undertaking such investigative studies include:

The material is likely to be concentrated in sediment.
Significant interaction of the compound with trace metals is likely.
The chemical is likely to form biologically active metabolites or degradation products.
The chemical is predicted to occur in drinking water at biologically significant concentrations.

Information from the investigative programs is used to make the most refined estimates possible of the concentrations at which a material will appear in various environmental compartments. This information will lead to a more accurate estimate of likely environmental exposures and may become an essential element in the final decision-making process.

Testing for Environmental Effects

Although there are many materials for which toxicity testing will not be needed, such as those with adequate literature data or suitable structure-activity correlations or those that never reach the aquatic environment, a safety assessment of most materials that can reach surface waters will normally require some minimum aquatic toxicity data. This is particularly true when the available

information suggests that the chemical may be highly toxic or poorly removed by waste water treatment, or that it is bioaccumulated or complexes metals.

Aquatic toxicity test methods have been discussed in detail in earlier chapters of this book and need not be reviewed here. It is important, however, to discuss the judgments and criteria needed to guide the selection of tests and aid in the evaluation of the results obtained.

To work properly and efficiently, the safety assessment program must contain specific decision criteria or pass-fail options which will provide direction in decisions concerning the future use of, scope, and priority of additional data required in the overall evaluation (Beck et al., 1981; Maki, 1980). Without decision criteria imposed throughout the assessment, the entire process degenerates to a simple listing of tests and required data with no real direction or indication of when it has been satisfactorily completed.

The first step in an environmental effects assessment is determining the acute toxicity of the chemical to one or more species of fish. The ratio of the LC50 to the estimated surface water concentration (C_{Sw}) is used to indicate the need for additional acute toxicity testing. Some possible decisions include:

$LC50/C_{Sw} > 100$: no further tests unless there is information indicating that specific tests should be run.
$LC50/C_{Sw} = 1$: material too toxic to be used except with restriction.
$LC50/C_{Sw} > 1 < 100$: further tests should be done on appropriate organisms to more closely estimate this ratio.

The need for longer-term partial or full chronic testing is assessed by comparing the acute toxicity data with the C_{Sw} and combining the results with persistence data from biodegradability tests and the measured partition coefficient. Some criteria for deciding on the need for chronic tests are shown in Table 1.

Table 1 Criteria for Chronic Testing

$\frac{LC50}{C_{Sw}}$	Octanol-water partition coefficient	Percent theoretical CO_2 evolved	Conclusion indicated
<20	>5000	<50	A[a]
<20	>5000	>50	B[b]
<20	<5000	<50	B
<20	<5000	>50	C[c]
20–100	>5000	<50	B
20–100	>5000	>50	C
20–100	<5000	<50	B
20–100	<5000	>50	D[d]
>100	>5000	<50	C
>100	>5000	>50	C
>100	<5000	<50	C
>100	<5000	>50	D

[a]A: the material should not be used without restrictions unless the concerns can be resolved by further testing.
[b]B: full chronic toxicity testing is appropriate.
[c]C: partial chronic toxicity testing is appropriate.
[d]D: no further aquatic toxicity testing is needed.

If partial chronic tests are indicated, a species is selected that has been shown by acute tests to be susceptible and that has been shown by fate studies as likely to be exposed. The NOEC is determined and decisions are based on the criteria shown in Table 2.

A special partial chronic procedure, the oyster shell deposition test, should be considered for any material that is strongly associated with solids at the C_{Sw}, provided EC50/C_{Sw} < 20, or for any material that has a partition coefficient > 10,000 and a CO_2 < 50%. Any observation of interference with oyster shell deposition at the C_{Sw} indicates a need for caution.

Full chronic tests can be conducted with fish or invertebrate species. For a chemical associated with solids, the benthic midge (e.g., *Chironomus* sp.) should be considered. Results from full chronic studies may be evaluated as shown in Table 3. If the bioconcentration factor is determined, decisions can be made as shown in Table 4.

Usually the tests outlined above are a sufficient basis for a responsible judgment concerning en-

Table 2 Criteria for Partial Chronic Testing

$\frac{NOEC}{C_{Sw}}$	Octanol-water partition coefficient	Conclusion indicated
<1	_[d]	A[a]
1–5	>1000	B[b]
1–5	<1000	C[c]
>5	>1000	B
>5	<1000	C

[a]A: the material should not be used without restrictions unless the concerns can be resolved by further testing.
[b]B: full chronic toxicity testing is appropriate.
[c]C: no further aquatic toxicity testing is needed.
[d]If NOEC/C_{Sw} < 1, a substantial potential for hazard to aquatic species exists regardless of the partition coefficient for the chemical.

Table 3 Criteria for Evaluating Results from Full Chronic Studies

$\frac{NOEC}{C_{Sw}}$	Octanol-water partition coefficient	Conclusion indicated
<1	–	A[a]
<10	>1000	B[b]
>5	<1000	C[c]

[a]A: the material should not be used without restrictions.
[b]B: testing to determine the bioconcentration factor (BCF) should be considered.
[c]C: no further aquatic toxicity testing is needed.

Table 4 Conclusions Based on Bioconcentration Factor

BCF	Conclusion indicated
>1000	A[a]
500–1000	B[b]
<500	C[c]

[a]A: the material should not be used without restrictions.
[b]B: a careful reexamination of environmental fate and concentration data (including degradation) and of toxicity data is indicated, and an investigative program may be needed to resolve the concerns.
[c]C: no further aquatic toxicity testing is needed.

vironmental safety, but field studies, monitoring programs, and other specific investigative studies (e.g., behavioral, physiological, biochemical, histopathologic) may be needed in response to perceived needs for further assurances of safety or to clarify uncertainties in any part of the effects assessment program.

Monitoring, Surveillance, and Follow-up

The decision to use a material is based on the integration of many estimates, predictions, and extrapolations. Environmental concentrations are estimated from consumption forecasts and laboratory simulations. Toxicities are often determined in animals at relatively high doses and extrapolated to humans at much lower doses. The uncertainties inherent in these estimates and extrapolations entail risks which we try to minimize by imposing "safety factors."

The ultimate test of a chemical's safety is the outcome of its use in the natural environment. What concentrations actually occur in water? Is the material biodegraded or decomposed? Is it being used by other companies or for other purposes so that our estimates of environmental exposure are inaccurate? These questions can be addressed through environmental monitoring programs, medical follow-up of consumers' comments, and surveillance of employees' health.

This is not meant to suggest that follow-up programs are justified for all chemicals, but that the question of a material's safety is never settled or closed. We must always be sensitive to the emergence of new toxicological, epidemiologic, or environmental concentration information and to the necessity for seeking new information when there is reason to question the adequacy of existing information.

Review and Decision-making

Many decisions have already been made throughout the process outlined above. Certain test results may have indicated that a material should not be used; other test data may have indicated that concern for certain possible effects is relieved; or the

need for further testing may have been identified. It is not necessary to do all the tests listed in a particular section before reaching decisions or conclusions; there should be provisions at many points in the overall outline for determining the priority and scope of testing required for necessary use-related decisions.

Thus, repeatedly throughout the program, but finally in an overall sense at the end, it is necessary to answer the question, "Is this material safe for its intended use?" The question is answered by judging whether the risks are acceptable in view of the societal benefits associated with its use.

Restrictions

If any of the risks associated with a material appear to be unacceptable so that the material is judged unsuitable for use, it may be possible to make the risks smaller. This cannot be done by diminishing the toxicity of the material, but it can be done in some cases by diminishing the anticipated exposure to it. Among the measures that may be useful are:

Use lower concentrations of the chemical in the product.
Apply warning labels.
Handle in smaller containers.
Change the physical form of the product.
Introduce more stringent industrial hygiene measures.
Devise means to confine or neutralize spills.

Other methods might be devised that are appropriate for specific chemicals or specific circumstances. Once a restriction has been imposed, the entire decision-making process can be repeated to see whether the risk has been diminished enough to be judged acceptable.

APPLICATION OF THE GUIDELINES TO EXAMPLE CHEMICALS

To illustrate the principles developed in this outline, two materials have been selected for a retrospective review. These are sodium aluminosilicate (type A zeolite) and linear alkyl benzenesulfonate (LAS).

These materials are laundry detergent ingredients; LAS is an anionic surfactant and type A zeolite is a builder used to form complexes and reduce water hardness and to minimize effects on the detergent process. Much is known about each of these chemicals in addition to what is suggested by this outline. Although extensive human and environmental safety programs were carried out for these materials, the programs of safety assessment used when they were being developed did not follow the systematic pattern presented below. However, they illustrate how the decision-making process would work if they were presented as new chemicals at present.

These materials, as used in detergents, have similar potentials for coming in contact with humans, and they enter the environment by the same route. However, there are significant differences in their physical, chemical, and biological properties, and these differences are key factors to consider in designing individual testing programs.

Type A Zeolite

Chemical formula:

$$(AlO_2)_{12} (SiO_2)_{12} \cdot 27 H_2 O$$

+ sodium to maintain neutrality

Purity: >95%

Type A zeolite is an inorganic material in the aluminosilicate family which has characteristic cubic crystalline structure of aluminum, silicon, and oxygen atoms. It is an odorless, essentially nonhygroscopic, free-flowing, fine, crystalline white powder. The only notable impurities are small amounts of hydroxysodalite (<5%), a common by-product of zeolite synthesis, and traces of uncrystallized aluminosilicate gel (Breck et al., 1956). Its purity, as measured by X-ray techniques, is greater than 95%. The elemental ratio

Na:Al:Si is 1:1:1. The median particle size, as developed for detergents, is 3–4 μm. It is closely related to other zeolites that are accepted and used as food additives and to aluminosilicate clays. It has no characteristics or structure suggestive of carcinogenic or mutagenic properties, but the fact that it contains a form of silicate raised questions about its potential for lung damage. An analytical method had to be developed.

LAS

Chemical formula: Mean alkyl chain length: 11.8. Mean molecular weight: 345.

The alkyl chains of commercially available LAS mixtures are generally 10–14 carbons long and the phenyl group occurs at various positions on the alkyl chains. LAS was selected as a replacement for tetrapropylene-derived alkyl benzenesulfonate (ABS) because it was more rapidly and completely biodegraded in laboratory model waste water units. The molecule has no characteristics that would indicate mutagenic or carcinogenic effects. An analytical method had to be developed.

Environmental Fate Studies

Predictions of environmental concentrations for Zeolite A and LAS are based on expected concentrations in influent waste water, removability by waste water treatment as determined in laboratory studies, and dilution of the effluent upon discharge (Table 5). Predicted concentrations for influent waste water were calculated from equations given earlier.

These materials may be incorporated into detergents at levels up to 15–20%. With laundry detergent usage at 4000 million pounds per year in the

Table 5   Predicted Environmental Concentrations of Detergent Materials

	Concentration (mg/l)	
Sample	Type A zeolite	LAS
Influent waste water (C_{IW})	6.6	10.9
Removal by primary treatment (settling test), %	50	40–50
Removal by secondary treatment, first estimate (SCAS test), %	98	91
Effluent waste water (C_{EW})	0.92	1.0
Receiving water $(C_{SW\text{-}1})^a$	0.092	0.1

[a]The $C_{SW\text{-}1}$ concentration is a conservative estimate for surface waters immediately below waste water outfall with minimum dilution; $C_{SW\text{-}1}$ is a figure higher than the anticipated average concentration that will exist in most natural waters.

United States, they might therefore be consumed at a rate of 600 million pounds per year.

For type A zeolite, laboratory studies of activated sludge indicated 80–90% removal across the aeration tank and final clarifier (Hopping, 1978). Laboratory treatability studies with activated sludge units indicated 90% removal of LAS and continuing degradation during river water die-away tests designed to simulate receiving water conditions (Weaver and Coughlin, 1964).

A need for supplemental tests was indicated by the guidelines, and testing was completed for both materials to identify the biotic and abiotic interactions they would undergo in waste water and receiving water systems (Table 6). The criteria specified indicate the need for investigative studies designed to address specific issues identified during earlier screening tests. Since these are relatively high-volume chemicals, their influent waste water concentrations exceed 1.0 mg/l, indicating a need

Table 6   Summary of the Environmental Fate Testing Programs that the Guidelines Would Suggest for the Two Test Materials

Test	Type A zeolite	LAS
Screening tests		
CO_2 evolution	NA (inorganic)	>95% (theoretical CO_2)
Octanol-water partition coefficient	NA (insoluble in octanol)	125
Microbial inhibition	NA (insoluble, unreactive)	NA (CO_2 evolution tests demonstrate no inhibition)
Semicontinuous activated sludge	80–90% removal	>91% removal efficiency
Settling test	40–60% removal	NA (water-soluble)
Confirmatory tests		
Adsorption isotherms	NA	Some affinity for organics and inorganics; effective in removal from water
Hydrolysis rate	Half-life ~ 55 d	NA (theoretical CO_2 ~ 90%)
Metal complexation	Readily complexes metals	NA
Ozonation	NA	NA (theoretical CO_2 ~ 90%)
Chlorination	NA	NA (theoretical CO_2 ~ 90%)
Photolysis	NA	NA (theoretical CO_2 ~ 90%)
Biodegradation rates	NA (inorganic)	NA (theoretical CO_2 ~ 90%)
Continuous activated sludge	90% removal efficiency	>90% removal efficiency
Biological inhibition of waste water treatment process		NA (CO_2 tests demonstrate no inhibition)
Sludge properties	No effects on ability to settle	NA (water-soluble)

[a]NA: guidelines indicate test is not needed or not applicable.

for additional examination. Tests were conducted to examine the impact of type A zeolite and LAS on biotic and abiotic aspects of waste water treatment.

Environmental Effects Studies

In this section of the guidelines, the no observed effect concentrations developed from toxicity tests with aquatic species are compared with increasingly refined estimates of the environmental concentrations of the test compounds expected to result from their consumer distribution, use, and disposal.

Aquatic toxicity testing gave the data shown in Table 7.

First conclusion: For both materials the screening tests indicated that no further aquatic toxicity testing is needed. However, the estimate of influent waste water concentration and consideration of the high-volume use and potential exposures indicated that several confirmatory tests should be conducted. In addition, further aquatic toxicity

tests were conducted to verify the first estimates. Refined estimates of surface water concentrations were also made, based on results from field studies at sewage treatment plants.

Second conclusion: No further aquatic toxicity testing is indicated for these materials. In a present-day hazard evaluation program for a new chemical or one whose use is being expanded, sufficient data would be available at this point to guide usage decisions for most chemicals except those with a tendency to bioaccumulation. However, to further illustrate the application of the guidelines to these chemicals, the results of chronic studies were incorporated into the third series of criteria.

Third conclusion: These compounds, at the maximum anticipated usage, are judged to cause no harm to aquatic life. Special field studies also determined that neither material had an adverse effect on sewage treatment processes or on metal transport in surface waters. Similarly, studies in home septic and aerobic systems indicated no adverse effects.

Table 7 Summary of Environmental Fate and Effects Data for Two Case Study Materials

	Zeolite A	LAS
96-h LC50 in bluegill (mg/l)	>680	3.5
First guideline		
First estimate of C_{SW}	0.092	0.1
EC50/C_{SW}	7390	35
Partition coefficient (assumed)	<1	<1
Percent theoretical CO_2	NA	90
Second guideline		
Refined estimates:		
Removal by secondary treatment	80%	85%
C_{EW} (mg/l)	1.8	1.1
C_{SW}-2, $\frac{1}{10}$ of C_{EW} (mg/l)	0.18	0.11
Partial chronic NOEC (mg/l)	>87	0.9
NOEC/C_{SW}	>480	8.2
Partition coefficient (assumed)	<1	<1
Third guideline		
Chronic NOEC (mg/l)	>100 (midge)	0.7
	129 (*Daphnia magna*)	
NOEC/C_{SW}	>550	6.3
Partition coefficient (assumed)	<1	<1

CONCLUSIONS

A conceptual framework has been developed for assessing the hazard of chemical substances to aquatic life. A risk assessment is based on the relationship between the environmental exposure concentration of the material and the concentration showing some adverse biological effect. Any sound program or guideline for environmental safety testing must have a strong element of flexibility with respect to testing priority and test selection. Specific questions associated with each material should be identified during early comprehensive screening tests, which subsequently lead to individualized testing and experiments designed to weigh risks against intended use.

Satisfactory approaches and methods are available for predicting the environmental fate of chemicals, and test methods exist for determining adverse biological effects. However, there is a need for further refinements in both of these critical components of risk assessment. Although risk assessment procedures are in the developmental stages, it is evident that the respective approaches have reasonable philosophical foundations and are functional. They need, however, to be tested with data on chemical substances for which longer-term use has defined the safety for aquatic life. After such testing it is highly probable that refinements will be needed in the procedures. In addition, the criteria used in the procedures to make decisions on the need for additional testing must be scrutinized to establish their scientific credibility. Such scrutiny can only come after repeated applications of these assessment procedures to a wide variety of test substances that have the potential to reach surface waters.

It is unreasonable to expect that any testing program for comprehensive safety assessment could be conceived with sufficient foresight to anticipate each issue of testing that could arise during the evaluation. An extreme but impractical alternative is to specify all tests for all chemicals. The authors believe that the more reasonable and scientifically valid approach outlined in this chapter, coupled with flexibility in test selection, presents the best option for efficient decision-making.

LITERATURE CITED

Baughman GL, Lassiter RR: Prediction of environmental pollutant concentration. In: Estimating the Hazard of Chemical Substances to Aquatic Life, edited by J Cairns, KL Dickson, AW Maki, pp. 35–54. ASTM STP 657. Philadelphia: American Society for Testing and Materials, 1978.

Beck LW, Maki AW, Artman NR, Wilson ER: Outline and criteria for evaluating the safety of new chemicals. Regulat Toxicol Pharmacol 1(1):19–58, 1981.

Branson DR: Predicting the fate of chemicals in the aquatic environment from laboratory data. In: Estimating the Hazard of Chemical Substances to Aquatic Life, edited by J Cairns, KL Dickson, AW Maki, pp. 55–70. ASTM STP 657. Philadelphia: American Society for Testing and Materials, 1978.

Breck DW, Eversole WG, Milton RM, Reed TB, Thomas TL: Crystalline zeolites. I. The properties of a new synthetic zeolite, type A. J Am Chem Soc 78:5963–5971, 1956.

Cairns J, Dickson KL, Maki AW: Summary and conclusions. In: Estimating the Hazard of Chemical Substances to Aquatic Life, edited by J Cairns, KL Dickson, AW Maki, pp. 191–197. ASTM STP 657. Philadelphia: American Society for Testing and Materials, 1978.

Gilbert PA, Lee CM: Biodegradation tests: Use and value. In: Biotransformation and Fate of Chemicals in the Aquatic Environment, edited by AW Maki, KL Dickson, J Cairns, pp. 34–45. Washington, D.C.: American Society for Microbiology, 1980.

Holman WF: Estimating the Environmental Concentration of Consumer Product Components. In: Aquatic Toxicology and Hazard Assessment, edited by DR Branson, KL Dickson, pp. 159–182. ASTM STP 737. Philadelphia: American Society for Testing and Materials, 1981.

Hopping, WD: Activated sludge treatability of type-A zeolite. J Water Pollut Control Fed 50: 433–441, 1978.

Kenaga EE: Challenges to Tradition—Environmental Toxicology in the 1980's. Speech delivered to the 30th Semiannual Meeting of the Chemical Manufacturers Association, Houston, October 27–28, 1980.

Maki AW: Design and conduct of hazard evaluation programs for the aquatic environment. In: Water Chlorination Environmental Impact and Health Effects, edited by RL Jolley, WA Brungs, RB Cumming, VA Jacobs, vol. 3, pp. 979–959. Ann Arbor, Mich.: Ann Arbor Science, 1980.

Maki AW, Dickson KL, Cairns J: Introduction. In: Analyzing the Hazard Evaluation Process, edited by AW Maki, KL Dickson, J Cairns, pp. 1–6. Washington, D.C.: American Fisheries Society, 1979.

Maugh TH: Chemicals: How many are there? Science 199:162, 1978.

Metcalf and Eddy, Inc.: Wastewater Engineering: Treatment, Disposal and Reuse. New York: McGraw-Hill, 1979.

Stern AM: A proposed approach to chemical fate assessments. Ecotoxicol Environ Saf 4:404–414, 1980.

Stern AM, Walker CR: Hazard assessment of toxic substances: Environmental fate testing of organic chemicals and ecological effects testing. In: Estimating the Hazard of Chemical Substances to Aquatic Life, edited by J Cairns, KL Dickson, AW Maki, pp. 81–131. ASTM STP 657. Philadelphia: American Society for Testing and Materials, 1978.

Weaver PJ, Coughlin FJ: Measurement of biodegradability. J Am Oil Chem Soc 41:738–741, 1964.

SUPPLEMENTAL READING

Butler GC (ed): Principles of Ecotoxicology. New York: Wiley, 1978.

Cairns J, Dickson KL, Maki AW (eds): Estimating the Hazard of Chemical Substances to Aquatic Life. ASTM STP 657. Philadelphia: American Society for Testing and Materials, 1978.

Dickson KL, Maki AW, Cairns J (eds): Analyzing the Hazard Evaluation Process. Washington, D.C.: American Fisheries Society, 1979.

Hague R: Dynamics, Exposure and Hazard Assessment of Toxic Chemicals. Ann Arbor, Mich.: Ann Arbor Science, 1980.

Kates RW: Risk Assessment of Environmental Hazard. New York: Wiley, 1978.

Maki AW, Dickson KL, Cairns J (eds): Biotransformation and Fate of Chemicals in the Aquatic Environment. Washington, D.C.: American Society for Microbiology, 1980.

Chapter 23

Effluent Evaluation

K. J. Macek

INTRODUCTION

The Federal Water Pollution Control Act amendments of 1972 (Public Law 92-500) established in Section 101(a) that "it is the national *goal* that wherever attainable, an interim goal of water quality which provides for the protection and propagation of fish, shellfish, and wildlife, and provides for recreation in and on the waters be achieved." The axiomatic translation of this national goal has become "fishable, swimmable waters." Section 101(a) also states that "it is a national *policy* that the discharge of toxic pollutants in toxic amounts be prohibited." The act further required in Section 304(a) that the administrator of the U.S. Environmental Protection Agency (U.S. EPA) publish national criteria for water quality. Such criteria specify concentrations of water constituents which, if not exceeded, are expected to result in

aquatic ecosystems suitable for various specified uses of water. According to the U.S. EPA (1976) these criteria are not intended to offer the same degree of safety for survival and propagation at all times to all organisms within a given ecosystem. However, they are intended not only to protect essential and significant life in water as well as the direct uses of water, but also to protect life that is dependent on life in water for its existence or that may consume, intentionally or unintentionally, any edible portions of such life.

In retrospect, one of the most significant omissions from the act may be that Section 502, General Definitions, does not enumerate the differences intended between the terms "national goal" and "national policy." The distinction intended by Congress was that a "goal" is an objective that serves as a focal point for long-range planning and for research and development in water pollution control technology, while a "policy" is an actual method that is spelled out within the terms of the act to allow progress toward achievement of the stated goals (Feliciano and Ellicott, 1981). Conversely, one of the most significant inclusions in the act are the words "in toxic amounts." Congress could easily have stated that "it is a national policy that the discharge of toxic substances be prohibited." Implicit in the actual wording is the recognition that toxicity is not a question of the mere presence or absence of a toxic pollutant, but rather a function of the concentration of toxic pollutant to which organisms are exposed and the duration of exposure. The concentration of pollutant to which organisms are exposed is determined after mixing in the water that receives the waste water discharge, and its determination requires consideration of an appropriate mixing zone. A mixing zone is an area or location of a receiving water where waste water discharges and receiving water mix. It is contiguous to a point source (identifiable waste water discharge) where exceptions to water quality objectives and conditions otherwise applicable to the receiving water may be granted. Mixing zones are designated by the responsible regulatory agency in the area, and the primary purpose of designating mixing zones is to limit areas of degradation while not requiring excessive waste water treatment.

The utility of toxicity tests with aquatic organisms in implementing the national policy mandated by the act is obvious. One can hardly conceive of an alternative methodology to define "toxic amounts." Unfortunately, the emphasis in drafting and implementing the act to achieve the goal of fishable, swimmable waters was based on a policy that ignored, and largely continues to ignore, the utility of toxicity tests to define toxic amounts. Feliciano and Ellicott (1981) reported that during the drafting of the act, the staff of the House of Representatives was supportive of the traditional concept that regulation should be related to a defined water quality impact. That is, the use of the water in question (e.g., for drinking, agriculture, or recreation) should be defined and scientifically characterized, and a pollution abatement program should be tailored to that definition. The Senate staff, however, had adopted a concept that embodied a radical new approach to pollution abatement—namely that rather than being the goal of a program, water quality should become the measure of success of an abatement program based on relatively uniform application of pollution control technology. What emerged from Congress was legislation that primarily based treatment requirements on the current and future performance capabilities of waste water treatment technology and was only secondarily concerned with the traditional water quality considerations.

The primary thrust of the implementation strategy mandated (PL 92-500, Section 301) the installment of technology-based targets on two levels. First, a minimum of secondary waste treatment for municipal wastes and an interim level of treatment known as best practical control technology (BPT) for industry was required by 1977; more stringent targets of best available technology (BAT) economically achievable was mandated for implementation by 1983. The emphasis of BAT was to control the discharge of toxic pollutants, yet toxicity to aquatic organisms was never a significant criterion for evaluating alternative technologies. Furthermore, the implementation strategy provided that additional limitations (based on water quality) could be superimposed on the technology-based limitations where necessary to attain the national goal of fishable, swimmable waters, as authorized in Section 302 of the act. This was to be accomplished primarily by translating national water quality criteria into toxic pollutant standards. A standard differs from a criterion in that a standard connotes a legal entity (limit) for a particular effluent or receiving water. A standard may use a water quality criterion as a basis for regulation and enforcement, but it may differ from a criterion because of prevailing local conditions, the intended use of a waterway, or the degree of safety desired for a particular ecosystem.

THE PAST DECADE

With this perspective, it is easy to understand the recent evolution of the science of aquatic toxicology in general and, more specifically, the role of toxicity tests with aquatic organisms in implementing the Federal Water Pollution Control Act. Since 1972, the emphasis on water quality criteria has resulted in virtually all toxicity testing efforts being directed toward the development of aquatic toxicity test methods, resulting in exponential growth of the chemical specific acute and chronic toxicity data base. It seems to be generally agreed that there will be an increasing need for this type of chemical specific toxicity data. Conversely, the emphasis on technology-based effluent limitations on specific pollutants has resulted in the virtual absence of any comprehensive, organized, scientific investigations into the sources, nature, extent, and control of effluent toxicity. Lack of this type of information, in a regulatory environment where the basic thrust is toward more and better treatment technology, will eventually lead to the development of treatment for treatment's sake. Just such a scenario was foreshadowed in 1977, when conflicting evidence on progress to date in pollution control was presented during Congressional hearings on the implementation of the act (U.S. House of Representatives, 1978).

On one side of the debate, the EPA administrator stated that "we must still seek preventive measures on large numbers of chemicals where a certain percentage eventually will prove to be dangerous and will cause damage far beyond the point that responsible public policy should allow. For most of the toxic pollutants, the only safe and environmentally responsible solution is eventual elimination of the discharge." Clearly, this shotgun approach, which ignores concentration and duration of exposure in dealing with the concept of toxicity, is no longer economically viable or environmentally required. On the other side of the debate, a commissioner of the National Commission on Water Quality stated that "the achievement of the 1977 (treatment) requirements by

industry . . . will enable most of the nation's waterways to meet the fishable, swimmable goal of the Act" (U.S. House of Representatives, 1978).

The truth of the matter obviously lies somewhere between the extremes described above, but unfortunately it was impossible to say precisely where. Although by 1977 industry had already spent billions of dollars in treatment technology to control effluent discharges, neither industry nor government had any quantitative measure of the effectiveness of such treatment technologies in controlling the discharge of toxic pollutants in toxic amounts. How can one possibly measure progress in controlling the toxicity of effluent discharges without measuring the toxicity of effluent discharges? During the 1977 Congressional hearings (U.S. House of Representatives, 1978), one of the agency's leading scientists stated, "We are not yet giving adequate attention to the use of biological responses as a measure of effluent acceptability and completeness of treatment. The use of aquatic toxicity tests . . . will not solve all of our problems but the use of such tests in conjunction with the many analytical tests already available, will add a new dimension to our understanding and assessment of the biological significance of the treated wastes which are discharged to our nation's waters." He touched on the true status of progress in controlling toxicity when he reported, "We have been pleased to find that effluents receiving treatment, adequate to meet the 1977 guidelines and utilizing generalized measures of treatment adequacy such as biological oxygen demand [sic] (BOD) and suspended solids, have little acute toxicity (to aquatic organisms) . . . we cannot generalize from these few samples and conclude that presently required treatment will solve our problems. We urgently need more information of this type [i.e., toxicity to aquatic organisms] to assess the acceptability of treatment now being installed." He summarized by stating that "It is significant to point out that when one is concerned about toxicity, there really must be a measurement on an organism to determine if toxicity is, indeed, present." Since toxicity is a biological phenomenon, it seems evident that a biological response is the most appropriate measure.

In retrospect, it seems unconscionable that this nation could undertake an effort of such magnitude to prohibit the discharge of toxic pollutants in toxic amounts without a comprehensive effort to realistically measure the results of that effort. Yet, despite recognition of this problem within the agency in 1977, there has been no organized comprehensive scientific effort to generate this important information. During further Congressional hearings on the implementation of the act, almost a decade after the act was enacted, this author again advocated the utility of toxicity tests with aquatic organisms to help balance the need for adequate control of toxic effluent discharges against the need to avoid costly treatment for treatment's sake (U.S. House of Representatives, 1981):

> It is evident that there are many instances where industrial discharges are not currently toxic and additional treatment, i.e., BAT, would serve no useful purpose. On the other hand, I would think it entirely possible that applying BAT to a discharge which is currently toxic does not guarantee a reduction of toxicity to acceptable levels. *However, if we never measure toxicity, we will never know where BAT is required, where it is superfluous, and where it is inadequate* [emphasis added].

After 10 years, it is clear that, until Congress or the U.S. EPA recognizes the utility of such data and allows industry to use toxicity testing to evaluate and establish where adequate treatment already exists, where further effluent treatment is needed, and the degree of additional treatment necessary, this nation will blindly implement treatment for treatment's sake. Furthermore, the potential of toxicity testing with aquatic organisms to assist in the logical implementation of the act and the attainment of its goal of fishable, swimmable waters will never be realized.

THE NEXT DECADE

It seems useful to consider several aspects of the role of toxicity tests with aquatic organisms in regulating the discharge of industrial wastes into aquatic ecosystems. Specifically, the role of aquatic toxicity data will be considered with respect to three basic regulatory issues:

1 How can one estimate, on a case-by-case basis for individual industrial dischargers, a reasonable target level of toxicity control required to preclude the discharge of toxic pollutants in toxic amounts, while at the same time avoiding costly treatment for treatment's sake?

2 How can an individual industrial discharger adequately demonstrate that adequate toxicity control exists, that a particular discharge does not pose a threat of acute or chronic toxicity to the aquatic environment, and that the goals of the act are, in fact, being attained?

3 How can toxicity testing with aquatic organisms, or other surrogate techniques, be used to monitor the continuing performance of effective in-plant toxicity control systems?

The Required Degree of Toxicity Control

The required degree of toxicity control is that amount of control which will preclude the discharge of toxic pollutants "in toxic amounts." One can only determine the amount that is toxic in terms of the effects of the discharge on the quality of the receiving water. A requirement that the toxicity of an effluent be reduced is appropriate only when failure to reduce toxicity can be anticipated to have an adverse impact on water quality. The degree of reduction required need only be sufficient to reduce the toxicity of the discharge to a level that can be reasonably expected not to have any such adverse impact.

It is important to distinguish in the regulatory program between *measurable* toxicity of a discharge and toxicity that is significant to the receiving water. A regulatory philosophy that has as its goal reducing the end-of-pipe toxicity of industrial discharges to levels below those measurable by acute toxicity testing techniques clearly is advancing toward a national goal of "fishable, swimmable pipes," not "fishable, swimmable waters." Implementation of such a regulatory philosophy will mandate treatment for treatment's sake in an effort to reach such a goal. It is essential that there be a clear understanding of how one identifies the level of toxicity control that will ensure the preservation of fishable, swimmable waters, the stated goal of the act, while avoiding costly treatment for treatment's sake.

The initial requirement in evaluating the potential impact of an industrial discharge on a receiving water is to derive a conservative estimate of the concentration of the waste in the receiving water after mixing. Where acute toxic effects are of concern, one should consider the concentration of the waste at the interface of the designated mixing zone and the remainder of the receiving water body. Since a vast majority of industrial discharges do not currently pose a threat of acute toxicity to receiving waters (U.S. House of Representatives, 1978, 1981), regulatory emphasis should be on the potential chronic effects of the waste on the receiving water ecosystem. That is, it should be concerned with the concentration of the waste water in the receiving water after complete mixing with the entire receiving water body.

Such in-stream waste concentrations (IWCs) have been estimated by using the maximum daily flow for the discharge (V_w) and the mean daily flow of the receiving water during the 7-d 10-yr low flow (7Q10). However, the estimates so derived would seem to be unduly conservative. An evaluation of flow duration data for several major U.S. rivers (Table 1) indicates that mean daily flows in receiving waters exceed the 7Q10 values 99% of the time, generally exceed them by 100% as much as 90% of the time, and may exceed them by almost an order of magnitude more than 50% of the time. Such data suggest that the variation in receiving water flow be taken into account in deriving estimates of the IWC and in setting target levels for control of the toxicity of the discharge to protect receiving water quality. One might reasonably ask whether the same degree of control is

Table 1   Mean Daily Flows Occurring in Major U.S. Rivers for the 7-d Low Flow (7Q10) Period during 1971–1980, and Mean Daily Flow that Was Exceeded 99, 98, 95, 90, and 50% of the Time during 1971–1980[a,b]

River (location)	7Q10	Volume of flow exceeded for the indicated incidence				
		V99%	V98%	V95%	V90%	V50%
Susquehanna (Marietta, Pa.)	5,500	5,720	6,500	7,700	11,000	30,000
Tennessee (Savannah, Tenn.)	15,000	18,000	20,000	24,000	29,000	51,000
Mississippi (Memphis, Tenn.)	141,000	150,000	180,000	210,000	230,000	450,000
James (Richmond, Va.)	638	680	800	1,000	1,500	5,500
Kanawa (Charleston, W. Va.)	2,490	2,900	3,200	3,900	4,700	12,000
Delaware (Trenton, N.J.)	2,690	2,800	3,100	3,500	3,900	10,000
Hudson (Green Island, N.Y.)	2,900	3,300	3,900	4,400	5,300	13,000

[a]Data reported from U.S. Geological Survey, Reston, Va. (personal communication).
[b]Values are cubic feet per second.

required during the 50% of the time when the mean daily flows exceed 7Q10 values by a factor of 5–10 in volume. If, for regulatory purposes, a single numerical estimate of receiving water flow is convenient, the volume that is exceeded 90% (V90) or 95% (V95) of the time would be a reasonable, yet conservative, estimate of stream flow when one is concerned with chronic toxicity. It would also be reasonable for industry to calculate and report to the agency waste concentrations in the stream both at the mixing zone interface and after complete mixing for various sets of receiving water conditions. By using such data, the U.S. EPA could routinely consider (1) the acute and chronic toxicity of the waste water, (2) the IWC of the discharge at various times, (3) the estimated threshold concentration required for the protection of sensitive aquatic forms, and (4) the period of occurrence of these sensitive forms in the receiving water, in evaluating the degree of control required for a particular discharge.

For example, consider a hypothetical situation in which a discharge is entering a receiving water system being regulated to allow for the maintenance of a salmonid fishery. The in-stream waste concentration after mixing is estimated to be 10% (by volume) during 7Q10, less than 6.5% more than 95% of the time, less than 2.5% more than 50% of the time, and less than 1% during periods of higher flows (e.g., spring runoff). Acute toxicity studies with fingerling salmonids and principal food organisms (invertebrates) for the salmonids indicate 100% survival in 100% effluent. An embryo-larval toxicity test with trout (a salmonid) indicates that the MATC for the discharge is > 6% < 12% effluent. Traditionally, regulators would evaluate such data and conclude that more treatment is required because the estimated safe level for trout may be exceeded in the receiving water under certain extreme conditions. Realistically, does this situation really pose a threat to the salmonid population when one considers that the most sensitive life stage of the salmonid fishery probably is resident in the system during the periods of maximum flow (spring),

when the IWC (1%) may be an order of magnitude less than the chemically toxic threshold for salmonids (> 6% < 12%).

The ultimate scientific determination of whether a waste water has any adverse ecological impact on a receiving water community would be to find out whether there are any significant adverse effects on community structure and function in the stream. However, such determinations are not easily made, require prolonged (several years) intensive efforts, are extremely expensive, and frequently yield data that are inadequate to establish precise cause-and-effect relationships. An alternative approach to identifying chronically toxic threshold waste concentrations would be for industry to conduct on-site, real-time toxicity testing with several representative aquatic organisms in order to estimate the chronically toxic IWC threshold for a particular waste water. Such tests can be performed in a reasonable time (several months) but require intensive commitments of labor and equipment. Although these tests are less costly than intensive stream surveys, they still require significant expenditures. Finally, chronically toxic threshold waste concentrations could be estimated by measuring the acute toxicity of the waste water and applying an application (i.e., safety) factor to derive a chronically safe threshold concentration. The latter approach has been advocated in the regulation and control of water pollution and is a valid one (National Technical Advisory Committee, 1978; National Academy of Sciences, 1974). The problem with the approach is that selecting an appropriate application factor, in lieu of chronic toxicity data, is an arbitrary process, and it is debatable whether 0.1, 0.05, 0.01, 0.001, or some other value is an appropriate application factor.

As the science of aquatic toxicology grows, and as more and more chronic toxicity data become available, it becomes more and more apparent to aquatic toxicologists that very few chemicals are chronically toxic at 0.001 of the acutely toxic values (Macek and Sleight, 1977). In fact, for most chemicals studied, concentrations of 0.01 or less of the acutely toxic values are not chronically toxic to aquatic organisms (U.S. EPA, 1976). Although the data base for complex waste waters is limited, there is little, if any, evidence that such treated discharges are chronically toxic to aquatic organisms at concentrations equal to or less than 0.05 of the acutely toxic values. The bulk of the limited data on the chronic toxicity of treated waste waters from a variety of different industries suggests that 0.1 of the acutely toxic value is a reasonably good estimate of chronically toxic threshold concentrations.

By using a reasonable estimate of the IWC after complete mixing, and assuming an appropriate conservative application factor for estimating chronically toxic thresholds, it is possible, before any actual toxicity testing, to grossly estimate the maximum acute toxicity concentration (i.e., minimum LC50 value) not to be exceeded in a treated waste water discharge. Based on general toxicity information, a "target level" can be estimated for the minimum degree of toxicity control required. For example, consider that several industries (A, B, and C) have discharges of various indicated volumes to the indicated receiving waters (see Table 2).

Where there is no evidence to the contrary, assume that the IWC that exists only 2% of the time is just below the chronically toxic threshold concentration. Also, assume that 0.05 is a reasonable conservative application factor for relating the acute and chronic toxicities of industrial waste water to aquatic organisms. The IWC divided by the application factor (IWC/0.05) would equal the maximum acute toxicity threshold (minimum

LC50 value) to which acute toxicity of the discharge should at least be controlled (i.e., the "target" level of control) in order to begin to preclude the discharge of toxic pollutants in toxic amounts.

Considering the examples in Table 2, if periodic acute toxicity testing of plant B's waste with a representative aquatic organism (e.g., fathead minnow) indicated that the acute toxicity (LC50 value) of the waste was consistently on the order of 30–45%, there would clearly be a reasonable margin of safety between the level of actual toxicity control (LC50 of 30–45%) and the estimated minimum required degree of toxicity control (LC50 >1.5%). In such instances an NPDES permit could be issued requiring reporting of periodic toxicity test results to ensure that the apparent margin of safety is maintained or that the target level for toxicity control is not approached or exceeded. Alternatively, suppose periodic acute toxicity testing of plant C's effluent with a representative aquatic organism indicates that the acute toxicity (LC50 value) of the waste water is occasionally as low as 7.0–8.5%. Considering the assumptions involved in estimating the target level of control, a reasonable margin of safety may not exist for protection of the aquatic life indigenous to the receiving water. In such an instance the permitting agency could give the permittee the option of providing additional control to increase the margin of safety or providing site-specific chronic toxicity data to more precisely define the specific margin of safety by providing the "appropriate application factor" specific for the discharge and receiving water in question. When such an applica-

Table 2 Hypothetical Relationships for Various Industrial Discharges and Receiving Streams

Industry	River	Volume of discharge (ft³/s)	V98 of receiving water (ft³/s)	In-stream waste concentration (%)	Target level of toxicity control (LC50, % effluent)
A	James	22	>800	<2.75	55
B	Kanawa	2.4	>3200	<0.07	1.5
C	Susquehanna	19.5	>6500	<0.30	6

tion factor has been derived, it can be substituted for the general factor of 0.05 and used to estimate whether any adverse impact on the receiving water can be expected to occur with the current level of treatment. If such an impact is indicated, the specific application factor can be used to determine the required degree of additional toxicity control by more precisely establishing the target level of toxicity control for the discharge.

Undoubtedly, situations will occur in which, even after chronic toxicity data are available, there will be concern about whether there is an ample margin of safety between the toxicity of the discharge and the chronically toxic threshold concentration in the stream. In some of these situations an option to require more toxicity control may exist; in others maximum toxicity control may already be in place. In cases where there is reasonable uncertainty about whether more toxicity control should be required, or whether existing control is sufficient, the regulatory agency could ask the industry to perform the more costly and time-consuming in-stream surveys to sufficiently assess stream quality and the impact of the discharge on the receiving water.

Demonstrating the Adequacy of Toxicity Control Systems

It is evident from the examples above that there will be a number of situations in the regulatory process where it is evident to both the regulatory agency and the discharger that toxicity is being well controlled, that further control is not necessary, and that monitoring to ensure that the status quo is maintained is the only prudent action to be required of the discharger. Conversely, there will also be situations where it will be evident that additional toxicity control is required to protect the biological integrity of the receiving water. In such cases efforts will be focused on determining the required degree of additional control. However, a significant number of situations will not fit in either of these categories, and uncertainty due to lack of adequate appropriate data will plague the regulatory process. In such cases, development

of appropriate toxicity data by the discharger to reasonably demonstrate the adequacy of current treatment technology, or to quantitate the additional toxicity control required, is in the best interest of all parties.

As a result of its recent hearings on PL92-500, the House Subcommittee on Oversight and Review has recommended that the law be amended to allow for waiver from BAT if the "discharger can demonstrate on the basis of biological testing that his effluent will not pose a threat of acute or chronic toxicity to the aquatic environment" (U.S. House of Representatives, 1981). Should such an amendment be enacted, there will be considerable interest in both industry and the regulatory agency as to how such a demonstration should be conducted.

In effect, what is required is the formulation, based on an adequate amount of aquatic toxicity data, of a water quality criterion for the discharge. Such a criterion would be specific to both the receiving water and the discharge. The U.S. EPA (1980b) published a description of what it considers a minimum aquatic toxicity data base for a specific chemical for deriving water quality criteria for the protection of freshwater aquatic life. The agency subsequently published a similar document describing the minimum data base for deriving a "site-specific" water quality criterion for the protection of freshwater aquatic life for a particular chemical pollutant (U.S. EPA, 1980a). By combining these approaches and applying them to a waste water discharge as opposed to a specific chemical, a site-specific water quality criterion for the discharge can be derived on the basis of both biological and chemical considerations. Biological considerations include such factors as sensitivity of resident species of aquatic organisms, protection of sensitive life stages of resident species, and maintenance of acceptable community structure and function. Chemical considerations include effects of water chemistry variables on the toxicity and persistence of the discharge and variability in the quality of the discharge. Discharge-specific criteria could be derived in two parts: a criterion describing the waste concentration never to be exceeded at the interface of the mixing zone, and a criterion describing the maximum 24-h average waste concentration after complete mixing in the receiving water.

Industry could provide the regulatory agency with the minimum data base required to describe the acute and chronic toxicity of the waste water discharge to aquatic organisms. It could also provide information on the capacity and effectiveness of its toxicity control (treatment) system, including data on the variability in acute toxicity of the waste water resulting from normal day-to-day operation of the plant and its waste water treatment system. With these data and available EPA-formulated procedures, a two-part site-specific water quality criterion for a particular discharge could be derived, and it could be compared with IWCs under various conditions to evaluate whether the receiving water organisms are adequately protected by the current or proposed level of toxicity control. Such a demonstration based on toxicity testing with aquatic organisms would alleviate uncertainty in the regulatory process where adequate protection of water quality is not evident, or would provide information to allow industry to qualify for a waiver from BAT by demonstrating that the discharge will not pose a threat of acute or chronic toxicity to the aquatic environment.

For example, the following approach for the derivation of a site-specific waste criterion is based on methodology described for the derivation of national water quality criteria (U.S. EPA, 1980b) and guidance for modifying those procedures for the derivation of site-specific water quality criteria (U.S. EPA, 1980a) for specific chemicals. All toxicity tests would be conducted with receiving water as the diluent. The objective is at least to generate the minimum data base required to derive a maximum IWC criterion for the discharge of concern.

Acute toxicity tests could be performed with freshwater organisms from a minimum of eight families to evaluate variability in species sensitivity to acute exposure to the discharge. Ideally, these would include one salmonid, a representative of

one other fish family, one planktonic crustacean, one benthic crustacean, one benthic insect, and one detrivorous benthic species. If salmonids are not resident in the receiving water, a centrarchid could be substituted. If a species from either or both crustacean groups is not resident at the site, a resident arthropod species could be substituted. The unadjusted maximum waste concentration criterion to be met at the interface of the mixing zone and the receiving water proper is derived by calculating the geometric mean of all acute toxicity values.

However, since most industrial waste water discharges are subject to normal day-to-day variation in acute toxicity, the unadjusted maximum waste concentration derived above should be adjusted to take into account the amplitude of this variability in toxicity. Standard statistical expressions of the central tendencies of distributed toxicity values such as arithmetic mean, geometric mean, harmonic mean, median, and mode are not appropriate for describing in a single quantitative term the acute toxicity of the waste water. Regulatory concern should be not for the central tendency in the toxicity distribution, but for the most toxic portion of the toxicity distribution. This is not to suggest that one should focus on the most toxic value (LC50), but rather on the most toxic portion of the distribution. For example, one might consider the quartile of the most toxic LC50 values as representing the portion of the toxicity distribution of regulatory concern. Some expression of central tendency for that particular portion of the distribution might be a reasonable numerical estimate of the toxicity aspect of the waste water of regulatory concern. To quantify that estimate, one could perform 24-h acute toxicity tests with an aquatic organism on waste water samples taken at a minimum of 20 regular intervals (e.g., every 12 h, every 24 h, or weekly), numerically order the toxicity values (LC50 values), and calculate the geometric mean LC50 for the first quartile of the data. The effect of the inherent variability in the acute toxicity of the effluent would be taken into account by multiplying the unadjusted maximum waste concentration by the ratio of the geometric mean LC50 for the first quartile of the data set to the geometric mean LC50 for the entire data set to derive an adjusted maximum waste concentration.

It should be noted that this adjusted maximum waste concentration (percent), based solely on acute toxicity considerations, is not the "target" toxicity control value in the pipe; instead it is the maximum concentration of the waste in the stream at the interface of the mixing zone with the receiving water. The adjusted 24-h average waste concentration of the waste in the stream after complete mixing should take into account the potential chronic effects of the waste discharge and could be derived in the following manner.

Acute and chronic toxicity tests (e.g., multigeneration daphnid study, fish embryo-larval study) with three species (at least one fish and at least one invertebrate) would be conducted. The acute/chronic ratio (ACR) for each species and then the geometric mean of all acute/chronic ratios could be calculated. This geometric mean represents the waste-specific ACR and approximates the reciprocal of the waste-specific application factor. The 24-h average water quality criterion for the discharge is equal to the adjusted maximum waste concentration divided by the mean ACR.

Example

The following acute toxicity data for the waste and resident stream organisms are developed for industry C in the Susquehanna River:

Species	LC50 or EC50 (% effluent)
Bluegill	15
Fathead minnow	21
Catfish	24
Crayfish	38
Midge	11
Algae	30
Daphnia	10
Seed shrimp	9

The unadjusted maximum waste concentration is the geometric mean of these data and is equal to 17.4%.

The following acute toxicity data (24-h LC50 values, percent) are developed for daphnids and waste water samples taken daily for 32 consecutive days.

10	9	36	28
12	8	14	39
20	8	14	11
60	17	22	10
49	9	58	10
38	8	47	19
20	7	35	18
41	15	19	20

The geometric mean of all the data above is 18.6%, and the geometric mean of the lowest quartile of the data above is 8.6%. The ratio of these geometric means (lowest quartile to all data) is 0.46. Thus the adjusted maximum IWC not to be exceeded at the interface of the mixing zone and the receiving water proper is 8.0% (0.46 × 17.4%). This value (8%) is not to be confused with the target level for toxicity control in the pipe.

Suppose the following chronic toxicity data are developed:

Species	Acute: LC50 (%)	Chronic: MATC (%)	ACR[a]
Fathead minnow	21	5	4.25
Daphnia	10	2.4	4.16
Midge	11	1.6	6.87

[a]Note that the ACR as derived by the referenced EPA procedures is the reciprocal of the classically described application factor, which is generally derived by calculating the ratio of chronic and acute values.

The final ACR is the geometric mean of the individual ACRs, or 5.0. The waste-specific 24-h average water quality criterion is equal to the adjusted maximum waste concentration divided by the mean ACR (8.0%/5.0), or 1.6%, which is the concentration of waste not to be exceeded *in the stream* after complete mixing. It is evident, from the results of toxicity testing with aquatic organisms, that a reasonable margin of safety exists between the actual IWC, which exists more than 98% of the time in the receiving water (i.e., <0.30%), and the chronically toxic threshold concentration (i.e., 1.5%) of the waste from industry C.

In this particular case the empirically derived target level for in-the-pipe toxicity control (LC50) for industry C to preclude chronic toxicity in the stream is equal to the IWC (Vw/V98) multiplied by the mean waste-specific application factor, and is equal to an LC50 of 1.5% (0.30% × 5.0). A reasonable margin of safety is seen to exist between the required (target) degree and the actual degree of toxicity control. This is largely because, in this example, there is relatively little difference between waste concentrations producing acute toxicity and the chronically safe waste concentration in the stream.

A waste-specific water quality criterion, derived as shown above, represents a conservative estimate of the concentration of waste water that would not be expected to have significant adverse chronic effects on the biota of the water. It is based on direct measurement of toxicity and does not ignore toxicity measurements. It provides a solid basis for identifying the degree of toxicity control required to prohibit the discharge of toxic pollutants in toxic amounts. Furthermore, it includes a reasonable safety margin by virtue of the fact that (1) the actual acute toxicity of the effluent will, by definition, be lower than the mean value of the first quartile of the acute values approximately 87% of the time, (2) the daily volume of the discharge may frequently be less than the maximum daily discharge, (3) the volume of flow in the river will generally exceed the conservative estimate of river flow (V98) 98% of the time and may exceed it by as much as an order of magnitude 50% of the time, and (4) there are natural physical, chemical, and biological processes in the environment (e.g., absorption, complexing, degradation) which generally serve to mitigate the toxicity of a waste water, as measured by toxicity tests, after it enters the receiving water.

Monitoring the Performance of Toxicity Control Systems

Having established an appropriate target level for control of the toxicity of a waste water, as measured by acute toxicity tests, and having installed a waste water treatment system that has been shown to provide the required degree of toxicity control, there remains the requirement of monitoring the waste water discharge. The purpose of such monitoring is twofold: (1) to demonstrate that the toxicity characteristics of the influent into the waste water treatment system have not changed enough to exceed (i.e., overload) the design capacity of the waste water treatment system to control the toxicity of the discharge to the required level, and (2) to ensure that the waste water treatment system is operating as effectively as designed (i.e., that no system "failure" occurs). Both these requirements can be fulfilled by periodically monitoring, directly or indirectly, the toxicity characteristics of the waste water discharge from the treatment system.

An effective monitoring tool should be rapid, relatively cost-effective, and able to produce information on three critical variables related to the characteristics of the waste water. These variables are the frequency, intensity, and duration of significantly elevated toxicity. Nemetz and Drechsler (1978) made a comprehensive analysis of sampling design in effluent monitoring. They concluded that "composite sampling, even at frequent intervals . . . performs the ironic function of apparently measuring elevated pollutant [toxicity] releases without detecting them." As a result, composite sampling fails to fulfill either of the essential functions of an effective monitoring system, namely (1) to give an accurate representation of the effluent profile, or (2) to detect most or all pollutant releases with potential serious environmental consequences. Nemetz and Drechsler recommended that consideration be given to the cessation of composite sampling in effluent monitoring programs and their replacement by frequent grab sampling and sequential analysis. How frequent is the question. They found that with a paper mill where they were measuring a parameter having an N of 120,000 and a relative standard deviation of 50% (similar to toxicity test data), the duration of 95% of the "spills" was less than 4 h. This suggests that if one took instantaneous grab samples every day, one would still not detect 99 out of every 100 spills.

In light of this information, although aquatic toxicity testing is undoubtedly the most accurate and direct means of measuring effluent toxicity, toxicity tests will not routinely be the monitoring tool of choice because they are not rapid (requiring 24–48 h to complete), are not cost-effective (requiring expenditures of hundreds of dollars per data bit), and could not be routinely used often enough to provide the necessary information on the frequency and duration of elevated toxicity discharges. It is thus necessary to identify some other biological, chemical, or physical characteristic of the waste water which can be rapidly and economically measured and which is quantifiably related in some manner to the toxicity of the waste water to aquatic organisms.

After identifying such a surrogate parameter (or suite of parameters) and adequately establishing the quantitative relationship between that parameter and effluent toxicity, one can use the surrogate parameter with sufficient frequency to ensure reasonable monitoring of the toxicity of the waste water. Toxicity tests with an appropriate aquatic organism should also be periodically conducted to demonstrate the continuing utility of the surrogate monitoring technique. The frequency of such toxicity testing would be a function of (1) the precision of the quantitative relationship between waste water toxicity as measured by toxicity testing and the response of the surrogate technique, and (2) the margin of safety between the "actual" toxicity of the treatment waste water as measured by toxicity testing and the "target" level of toxicity control.

Suppose, for example, there was a very precise quantitative relationship between waste water toxicity and the surrogate technique, and there was routinely an order of magnitude difference between the LC50 values of the waste water and the target level for toxicity control (LC50). Then a requirement for quarterly toxicity tests might provide reasonable assurance that the toxicity of the waste water is being adequately controlled. On the other hand, if the relationship between waste water toxicity and the surrogate technique is somewhat imprecise, or the actual level of toxicity control differs from the target level by a factor of only 2–3, then more frequent toxicity testing (e.g., monthly or weekly) may be more appropriate. In extreme cases, where there is little margin for error, daily toxicity testing with a simple rapid toxicity test (e.g., 12- or 24-h daphnid or fish test) may be appropriate. As more information becomes available on the capacity, efficacy, and reliability of the waste water treatment system to control toxicity to below target levels, the requirement for toxicity testing could be reduced.

Because of the inherent variability in waste water toxicity and the lack of precision associated with toxicity testing (e.g., ±25–40%), the ability of toxicity tests to determine, for regulatory purposes, compliance with specific toxicity "limits" in an NPDES permit is questionable. However, such data do provide valuable information on waste water toxicity. When data from the required periodic toxicity testing, or the more frequently employed surrogate technique, indicate that waste water toxicity may be approaching or exceeding target control levels, the industry should investigate and accurately define the nature of the waste water toxicity. If sufficient data (i.e., more than a single or a few observations) indicate that there has been a significant change in waste water toxicity, it should be determined whether this is related to in-process changes resulting in a significant increase in toxicity in the input to the treatment system (i.e., "overload") or to failure of the waste water treatment system to operate properly. Once the source of the increased toxicity has been identified, appropriate corrective action can be taken to adequately control waste water toxicity.

CONCLUSIONS

Although the Federal Water Pollution Control Act as amended in 1972 emphasized the need to prohibit the discharge of toxic pollutants in toxic amounts, implementation of that legislation by EPA has disregarded the need to measure in meaningful terms (i.e., toxicity) the nation's progress toward that goal. Nearly a decade after the legislation was passed, neither EPA nor industry has any comprehensive quantitative measurement of whether that goal has been attained, or how much more treatment is required to attain it.

In retrospect, with the emphasis on technology-based limitations it is understandable that toxicity testing of waste water discharges with aquatic organisms has not become a barometer of progress in pollution control. However, it is clear that the time has come to evaluate and quantitate progress in controlling the toxicity of industrial waste water discharges, and this can only be accomplished by measuring their toxicity to aquatic organisms.

Toxicity testing of waste water discharges of aquatic organisms can be used to:

1 Identify the acceptable limit (target level) for toxicity control by establishing maximum safe concentrations in the receiving water.

2 Demonstrate that current treatment technology is adequate to control toxicity to within acceptable limits or to quantify the degree of additional treatment, if any, required to control effluent toxicity to within acceptable limits.

3 Establish the validity of surrogate parameters for monitoring effluent toxicity on a continuing basis.

Unless there emerges a clear and significant role for toxicity tests with aquatic organisms in this nation's effort to control effluent toxicity, regulatory progress will continue down the path of treatment for treatment's sake. Without a valid mechanism for determining when we have reached the stated goal of the act, fishable, swimmable waters, our regulatory efforts will continue to pursue the regulatory grail of fishable, swimmable pipes.

LITERATURE CITED

Feliciano DV, Ellicott A: WPCF round table discussion—Congressional staffers take a retrospective look at PL92-500. Environ Sci Technol 53(8):1264–1270, 1981.

Macek KJ, Sleight BH, III: Utility of toxicity tests with embryos and fry of fish in evaluating hazards associated with the chronic toxicity of chemicals to fishes. In: Aquatic Toxicology and Hazard Evaluation, edited by FL Mayer and JL Hamelink, pp. 137–146. ASTM STP 634. Philadelphia: ASTM, 1977.

National Academy of Sciences, National Academy of Engineering: Water Quality Criteria. U.S. EPA Ecol Res Ser EPA-R3-73-033. Washington, D.C.: U.S. Environmental Protection Agency, 1972.

National Technical Advisory Committee to the Secretary of Interior: Water Quality Criteria. Washington, D.C.: Federal Water Pollution Control Administration, 1968.

Nemetz P, Drechsler ND: The role of effluent monitoring in environmental control. Water Air Soil Pollut 10:477–497, 1978.

U.S. Environmental Protection Agency: Quality Criteria for Water. Washington, D.C.: Government Printing Office, 1976.

U.S. Environmental Protection Agency: Derivation of Site-Specific Water Quality Criteria for the Protection of Aquatic Life and Its Uses. Duluth, Minn.: Environmental Research Laboratory, 1980a.

U.S. Environmental Protection Agency: Guidelines for Deriving Water Quality Criteria for the Protection of Aquatic Life and Its Uses. Internal Publication, 1980b. Revision of version published in Fed Register 44:15970, 1979.

U.S. House of Representatives: Implementation of the Federal Water Pollution Control Act. Hearings of the Subcommittee on Investigation and Review, Committee on Public Works and Transportation, 95th Congress. Washington, D.C.: Government Printing Office, 1978.

U.S. House of Representatives: Implementation of the Federal Water Pollution Control Act. Hearings of the Subcommittee on Oversight and Review, Committee on Public Works and Transportation, 96th Congress. Washington, D.C.: Government Printing Office, 1981.

SUPPLEMENTAL READING

Cairns J, Dickson KL, Maki AW (eds): Estimating the Hazard of Chemical Substances to Aquatic Life. ASTM STP 657. Philadelphia: ASTM, 1978.

Dickson KL, Maki AW, Cairns J: (eds): Analyzing the Hazard Evaluation Process. Washington, D.C.: Water Quality Section, American Fisheries Society, 1979.

Duthie JR: The importance of sequential assessment in test programs for estimating hazard to aquatic life. In: Aquatic Toxicology and Hazard Evaluation, edited by FL Mayer and JL Hamelink, pp. 17–35. ASTM STP 634. Philadelphia: ASTM, 1977.

Pearson JG, Glennon JP, Barkley JJ, Highfill JW: An approach to toxicological evaluation of a complex industrial wastewater. In: Aquatic Toxicology, edited by LL Marking and RA Kimerle, pp. 284–301. ASTM STP 667. Philadelphia: ASTM, 1979.

Glossary

Acclimation (1) Steady state compensatory adjustments by an organism to the alteration of environmental conditions. Adjustments can be behavioral or physiological/biochemical. (2) An adaptation of aquatic organisms to some selected experimental conditions, including adverse stimuli. (3) Acclimation also refers to the time period prior to the initiation of a toxicity test in which aquatic organisms are maintained in untreated, toxicant-free dilution water with physical and chemical characteristics (e.g., temperature, pH, hardness) similar to those to be used during the toxicity test.

Acute Having a sudden onset, lasting a short time. Of a stimulus, severe enough to induce a response rapidly. Can be used to define either the exposure or the response to an exposure (effect). The duration of an acute aquatic toxicity test is generally 4 d or less and mortality is the response measured.

Additive toxicity The toxicity of a mixture of chemicals which is approximately equivalent to that expected from a simple summation of the known toxicities of the individual chemicals present in the mixture (i.e., algebraic summation of effects).

Alkalinity The acid-neutralizing (i.e., proton-accepting) capacity of water; the quality and quantity of constituents in water which result in a shift in the pH toward the alkaline side of neutrality.

Antagonism A phenomenon in which the toxicity of a mixture of chemicals is less than that which would be expected from a simple summation of the toxicities of the individual chemicals present in the mixture (i.e., algebraic subtraction of effects).

Application factor (AF) A numerical, unitless value, calculated as the threshold chronically toxic concentration of a chemical divided by its acutely toxic concentration. An AF is generally calculated by dividing the limits [no observed effect concentration (NOEC) and lowest observed effect concentration (LOEC)] on the maximum acceptable toxicant concentration (MATC) by the time-independent LC50, if available, or the 96-h LC50 (or 48-h EC50 or 48-h LC50 for daphnids) from a flow-through acute toxicity test. The AF is usually reported as a range and is multiplied by the median lethal concentration of a chemical as determined in a short-term (acute) toxicity test to estimate an expected no-effect concentration under chronic exposure.

Asymptotic threshold concentration The concentration of a chemical at which some percentage of a population of test organisms is in a state of approximate homeostasis for some prolonged period of time (not necessarily absolute). It may be demonstrated as the concentration at which the toxicity curve is approximately asymptotic (parallel) to the time axis. The asymptotic LC50 is the concentration at which acute mortality has essentially ceased and will not change substantially with exposure time. That is, there is no evidence of significantly increasing effects resulting from increasing duration of exposure.

Bioaccumulation General term describing a process by which chemicals are taken up by aquatic organisms from water directly or through consumption of food containing the chemicals.

Bioassay Test used to evaluate the relative potency of a chemical by comparing its effect on a living organism with the effect of a standard preparation on the same type of organism. Bioassays are frequently used in the pharmaceutical industry to evaluate the potency of vitamins and drugs. "Bioassay" and "aquatic toxicity test" are not synonymous—see "toxicity tests."

Bioconcentration A process by which there is a net accumulation of a chemical directly from water into aquatic organisms resulting from simultaneous uptake (e.g., by gill or epithelial tissue) and elimination.

Bioconcentration factor (BCF) A unitless value describing the degree to which a chemical can be concentrated in the tissues of an organism in the aquatic environment. At apparent equilib-

rium during the uptake phase of a bioconcentration test, the BCF is the concentration of a chemical in one or more tissues of the aquatic organisms divided by the average exposure concentration in the test.

Biomagnification Result of the processes of bioconcentration and bioaccumulation by which tissue concentrations of bioaccumulated chemicals increase as the chemical passes up through two or more trophic levels. The term implies an efficient transfer of chemical from food to consumer, so that residue concentrations increase systematically from one trophic level to the next.

Biomonitoring Use of living organisms as "sensors" in water quality surveillance to detect changes in an effluent or water and to indicate whether aquatic life may be endangered.

Chronic Involving a stimulus that is lingering or continues for a long time; often signifies periods from several weeks to years, depending on the reproductive life cycle of the aquatic species. Can be used to define either the exposure or the response to an exposure (effect). Chronic exposure typically induces a biological response of relatively slow progress and long continuance. The chronic aquatic toxicity test is used to study the effects of continuous, long-term exposure of a chemical or other potentially toxic material on aquatic organisms.

Concentration The quantifiable amount of chemical in the surrounding water, food, or sediment.

Concentration-response curve A curve describing the relationship between exposure concentration and percentage response of the test population.

Control A treatment in a toxicity test that duplicates all the conditions of the exposure treatments but contains no test material. The control is used to determine the absence of toxicity of basic test conditions (e.g., health of test organisms, quality of dilution water).

Criteria (water quality) An estimate of the concentration of a chemical or other constituent in water which if not exceeded, will protect an organism, an organism community, or a prescribed water use or quality with an adequate degree of safety.

Cumulative Brought about, or increased in

strength, by successive additions at different times or in different ways.

Delayed effects Effects or responses that occur some time after exposure. Carcinogenic effects of chemicals typically have a long latency period; the occurrence of a tumor may take years after the initial exposure.

Depuration A process that results in elimination of a material from an aquatic organism.

Dilution water (diluent) Water used to dilute the test material in an aquatic toxicity test in order to prepare either different concentrations of a test chemical or different percentages of an effluent for the various test treatments. The water (negative) control in a test is prepared with dilution water only.

Dose The quantifiable amount of a material introduced into the animal by injection or ingestion.

Dose-response curve Similar to concentration-response curve except that the dose (i.e., the quantity) of the chemical administered (e.g., by injection) to the organisms is known. The curve is plotted as dose versus response.

Effluent A complex waste material (e.g., liquid industrial discharge or sewage) which may be discharged into the environment.

Estimated (or expected) environmental concentration (EEC) The concentration of a material estimated as being likely to occur in environmental waters to which aquatic organisms are exposed as a result of planned manufacture, use, and disposal.

Exposure The contact reaction between a chemical or physical agent and a biological system.

Fate Disposition of a material in various environmental compartments (e.g., soil or sediment, water, air, biota) as a result of transport, transformation, and degradation.

Flow-through system An exposure system for aquatic toxicity tests in which the test material solutions and control water flow into and out of test chambers on a once-through basis either intermittently or continuously.

Half-life Time required to reduce by one-half the concentration of a material in a medium (e.g., soil or water) or organism (e.g., fish tissue) by transport, degradation, transformation, or depuration.

Hardness The concentration of all metallic cations, except those of the alkali metals, present in water. In general, hardness is a measure of the concentration of calcium and magnesium ions in water and is frequently expressed as mg/l calcium carbonate equivalent.

Hazard Likelihood that a chemical will cause an injury or adverse effect under the conditions of its production, use, or disposal.

Hazard evaluation Identification and assessment of the potential adverse effects that could result from manufacture, use, and disposal of a material in a specified quantity and manner.

Incipient LC50 The concentration of a chemical which is lethal to 50% of the test organisms as a result of exposure for periods sufficiently long that acute lethal action has essentially ceased. The asymptote (part of the toxicity curve parallel to the time axis) of the toxicity curve indicates the value of the incipient LC50, approximately.

Joint action Two or more chemicals exerting their effects simultaneously.

Lethal Causing death by direct action. Death of aquatic organisms is the cessation of all visible signs of biological activity.

Lethal time See survival time.

Life cycle study A chronic (or full chronic) study in which all the significant life stages of an organism are exposed to a test material. Generally, a life cycle test involves an entire reproductive cycle of the organism.

Loading Ratio of the animal biomass to the volume of test solution in an exposure chamber.

Lordosis An anteroposterior curvature of the spine, generally in the lumbar region. Also called hollow back or saddle back.

Lowest observed effect concentration (LOEC) The lowest concentration of a material used in a toxicity test that has a statistically significant adverse effect on the exposed population of test organisms as compared with the controls. When derived from a life cycle or partial life cycle test, it is numerically the same as the upper limit of the MATC.

Maximum acceptable toxicant concentration (MATC) The hypothetical toxic threshold concentration lying in a range bounded at the lower end by the highest tested concentration having no observed effect (NOEC) and at the higher end by the lowest tested concentration having a significant toxic effect (LOEC) in a life cycle (full chronic) or partial life cycle (partial chronic) test. This may be represented as NOEC < MATC < LOEC. Calculation of a MATC requires quantitative life cycle toxicity data on the effects of a material on survival, growth, and reproduction.

Median effective concentration (EC50) The concentration of material in water to which test organisms are exposed that is estimated to be effective in producing some sublethal response in 50% of the test organisms. The EC50 is usually expressed as a time-dependent value (e.g., 24-h or 96-h EC50). The sublethal response elicited from the test organisms as a result of exposure to the test material must be clearly defined. For example, test organisms may be immobilized, lose equilibrium, or undergo physiological or behavioral changes.

Median effective dose (ED50) The dose of material estimated to be effective in producing some sublethal response in 50% of the test organisms. It is appropriately used with test animals such as rats, mice, and dogs, but it is rarely applicable to aquatic organisms because it indicates the quantity of a material introduced directly into the body by injection or ingestion rather than the concentration of the material in water in which aquatic organisms are exposed during toxicity tests.

Median lethal concentration (LC50) The concentration of material in water to which test organisms are exposed that is estimated to be lethal to 50% of the test organisms. The LC50 is usually expressed as a time-dependent value (e.g., 24-h or 96-h LC50; the concentration estimated to be lethal to 50% of the test organisms after 24 or 96 h of exposure). The LC50 may be derived by *observation* (i.e., 50% of the test organisms may be observed to be dead in one test material concentration), by *interpolation* (i.e., mortality of more than 50% of the test organisms occurred at one test concentration and mortality of fewer than 50% of the test organisms died at a lower test concentration, and the LC50 is estimated by interpolation between these two data points), or by *calculation* (i.e.,

the LC50 is statistically derived by analysis of mortality data from all test concentrations).

Median lethal dose (LD50) The dose of material that is estimated to be lethal to 50% of the test organisms. It is appropriately used with test animals such as rats, mice, and dogs, but it is rarely applicable to aquatic organisms because it indicates the quantity of a material introduced directly into the body by injection or ingestion rather than the concentration of the material in water in which aquatic organisms are exposed during toxicity tests.

Median tolerance limit (TLm or TL50) The concentration of material in water at which 50% of the test organisms survive after a specified time of exposure. The TL50 (equivalent to the TLm) is usually expressed as a time-dependent value (e.g., 24-h or 96-h TL50; the estimated concentration at which 50% of the test organisms survive after 24 or 96 h of exposure). Unlike lethal concentration and lethal dose, the term tolerance limit is applicable in designating a level of any measurable lethal condition (e.g., extremes in pH, temperature, dissolved oxygen). TLm and TL50 have been replaced by median lethal concentration (LC50) and median effective concentration (EC50).

Monitoring test A test designed to be applied on a routine basis, with some degree of control, to ensure that the quality of water or effluent has not exceeded some prescribed criteria range. In a biomonitoring test, aquatic organisms are used as "sensors" to detect changes in the quality of water or effluent. A monitoring test implies generation of information, on a continuous or other regular basis.

No observed effect concentration (NOEC) The highest concentration of a material in a toxicity test that has no statistically significant adverse effect on the exposed population of test organisms as compared with the controls. When derived from a life cycle or partial life cycle test, it is numerically the same as the lower limit of the MATC.

Octanol-water partition coefficient (K_{ow}) The ratio of a chemical's solubility in n-octanol and water at equilibrium; also expressed as P. The logarithm of P or K_{ow} (i.e., log P or log K_{ow}) is used as an indication of a chemical's propensity for bioconcentration by aquatic organisms.

Parts per billion (ppb) One unit of chemical (usually expressed as mass) per 1,000,000,000 (10^9) units of the medium (e.g., water) or organism (e.g., tissue) in which it is contained. For water, the ratio commonly used is micrograms of chemical per liter of water, 1 μg/l = 1 ppb; for tissues, 1 μg/kg = 1 ng/g = 1 ppb.

Parts per million (ppm) One unit of chemical (usually expressed as mass) per 1,000,000 (10^6) units of the medium (e.g., water) or organism (e.g., tissues) in which it is contained. For water, the ratio commonly used is milligrams of chemical per liter of water, 1 mg/l = 1 ppm; for tissues, 1 mg/kg = 1 μg/g = 1 ppm.

Parts per thousand (ppt) One unit of chemical (usually expressed as mass) per 1000 (10^3) units of the medium (e.g., water) or organism (e.g., tissues) in which it is contained. For water, the ratio commonly used is grams of chemical per liter of water, 1 g/l = 1 ppt; for tissues, 1 g/kg = 1 ppt. This ratio is also used to express the salinity of seawater, where the grams of chloride per liter of water is denoted by the symbol ppt. Full-strength seawater is approximately 35 ppt.

Parts per trillion (pptr) One unit of chemical (usually expressed as mass) per 1,000,000,000,000 (10^{12}) units of the medium (e.g., water) or organism (e.g., tissues) in which it is contained. The ratio commonly used is nanograms of chemical per liter of water, 1 ng/l = 1 pptr; for tissues, 1 ng/kg = 1 pptr.

Percentage (%) One unit of material (usually a liquid) per 100 units of dilution water. In tests with industrial wastes (effluents), test concentrations are normally prepared on a volume-to-volume basis and expressed as percent of material.

Pesticide A substance used to kill undesirable and unwanted fungi, plants, insects, or other organisms. This generic term is used to describe fungicides, algicides, herbicides, insecticides, rodenticides, and other substances.

Preliminary test See screening test.

Quality assurance (QA) A program organized and designed to provide accurate and precise results. Included are selection of proper technical methods, tests, or laboratory procedures; sample collection and preservation; selection of limits; evaluation of data; quality control; and qualifications and training of personnel.

Quality control (QC) Specific actions required to provide information for the quality assurance program. Included are standardizations, calibration, replicates, and control and check samples suitable for statistical estimates of confidence of the data.

Range-finding test See screening test.

Resistance time The period of time for which an aquatic organism can live beyond the incipient lethal level.

Ring-test (or Round-robin test) (1) A conjoint test conducted under strictly standardized and uniformly applied conditions to assess the precision and accuracy with which different laboratories can determine the toxicity of a chemical or effluent. (2) A test designed to measure statistically the reproducibility of a test method, or to compare the results obtained from the use of different test methods.

Risk A statistical concept defined as the expected frequency or probability of undesirable effects resulting from a specified exposure to known or potential environmental concentrations of a material. A material is considered safe if the risks associated with its exposure are judged to be acceptable. Estimates of risk may be expressed in absolute or relative terms. Absolute risk is the excess risk due to exposure. Relative risk is the ratio of the risk in the exposed population to the risk in the unexposed population.

Round-robin test See Ring-test.

Safe concentration (SC) Concentration of material to which prolonged exposure will cause no adverse effect.

Safety The practical certainty that adverse effects or injury will not result from exposure to a material when used in the quantity and the manner proposed for its use. "Practical certainty" must be defined—for example, in terms of a numerically specified low risk. Another view is that "safety" is a value judgment of the acceptability of risk.

Scoliosis Lateral curvature of the spine.

Screening test (Preliminary test or Range-finding test) (1) A test conducted to estimate the concentrations to be used for a definitive test. (2) A short-term test used early in a testing program to evaluate the potential of a chemical (or other material) to produce some selected adverse effect (e.g., mortality).

Solvent or carrier An agent (other than water) in which the test chemical is mixed to make it miscible with dilution water before distribution to test chambers. Solvents or carriers are used in tests where the concentrations of the test chemical are extremely low and a very small amount of test material must be added to the test chambers.

Standard (water quality) The limiting concentration of a chemical (or degree of intensity of some other adverse condition, e.g., pH) which is permitted in an effluent or waterway. Standards are established for regulatory purposes and are determined from a judgment of the criteria involved. The standard is dependent on the use (e.g., potable, agricultural) of the water to be protected.

Static system An exposure system for aquatic toxicity tests in which the test chambers contain still solutions of the test material or control water.

Statistically significant effects Effects (responses) in the exposed population that are different from those in the controls at a statistical probability level of $P \leqslant 0.05$. Biological end points that are important for the survival, growth, behavior, and perpetuation of a species are selected as criteria for effect. The end points differ depending on the type of toxicity test conducted and the species used. The statistical approach also changes with the type of toxicity test conducted.

Sublethal Below the concentration that directly causes death. Exposure to sublethal concentrations of a material may produce less obvious effects on behavior, biochemical and/or physiological function, and histology of organisms.

Survival time The time interval between initial exposure of an aquatic organism to a harmful chemical and death.

Synergism A phenomenon in which the toxicity of a mixture of chemicals is greater than that which would be expected from a simple summation of the toxicities of the individual chemicals present in the mixture.

Test material A chemical, formulation, effluent, sludge, or other agent or substance that is under investigation in an aquatic toxicity test.

Test solution (or test treatment) Medium containing the material to be tested to which the test organisms are exposed. Different test solutions contain different concentrations of the test material.

Threshold concentration A concentration above which some effect (or response) will be produced and below which it will not.

Time-independent (TI) test An acute toxicity test with no predetermined temporal end point. This type of test, sometimes referred to as a "threshold" or "incipient" lethality test, is allowed to continue until acute toxicity (mortality or a defined sublethal effect) has ceased or nearly ceased and the toxicity curve (plot of effect versus time of exposure) indicates a threshold or incipient concentration. With most test materials, this point is reached within 7–10 d, but it may not be reached within 21 d. Practical or economic reasons may dictate that the test be stopped at this point and a test be designed for longer duration.

Toxic unit The strength of a chemical (measured in some unit) expressed as a fraction or proportion of its lethal threshold concentration (measured in the same unit). The strength may be calculated as follows:

toxic unit

$$= \frac{\text{actual concentration of chemical in solution}}{\text{lethal threshold concentration}}$$

If this number is greater than 1.0, more than half of a group of aquatic organisms will be killed by the chemical. If it is less than 1.0, half the organisms will not be killed. 1.0 toxic unit = the incipient LC50.

Toxicant An agent or material capable of producing an adverse response (effect) in a biological system, seriously injuring structure or function or producing death.

Toxicity The inherent potential or capacity of a

material to cause adverse effects in a living organism.

Toxicity curve The curve obtained by plotting the median survival times of a population of test organisms against concentration on a logarithmic scale.

Toxicity test The means by which the toxicity of a chemical or other test material is determined. A toxicity test is used to measure the degree of response produced by exposure to a specific level of stimulus (or concentration of chemical).

Ultimate median tolerance limit The concentration of a chemical at which acute toxicity ceases. Also called incipient lethal level, lethal threshold concentration, and asymptotic LC50.

Uptake A process by which materials are transferred into and onto an aquatic organism.

Xenobiotic A foreign chemical or material not produced in nature and not normally considered a constitutive component of a specified biological system. This term is usually applied to manufactured chemicals.

Index